Perioperative Standards and Recommended Practices

2012 Edition

Association of periOperative Registered Nurses

Manager, Standards and Recommended Practices
Ramona Conner, MSN, RN, CNOR

Clinical Editors
Joan Blanchard, MSS, BSN, RN, CNOR, CIC
Byron Burlingame, MS, BSN, RN, CNOR
Bonnie Denholm, MS, BSN, RN, CNOR
Sharon Giarrizzo-Wilson, MS, RN-BC, CNOR
Mary Ogg, MSN, RN, CNOR
Sharon A. Van Wicklin, MSN, RN, CNOR, CRNFA, PLNC

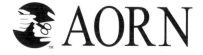

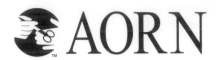

2170 South Parker Road
Suite 400
Denver, CO 80231-5711
(800) 755-2676
(303) 755-6300

Perioperative Standards and Recommended Practices
2012 Edition

Copyright © 2012 AORN, Inc.

Director of Publishing: Lynn King, MPS
Editor/Team Lead: Kimberly Retzlaff
Associate Editor: Jennifer Brusco
Associate Editor: Helen Starbuck Pashley
Graphic Design Manager: Joelle Stevens
Graphic Designer: Kurt Jones

ISBN 978-1-888460-70-4   Printed in USA

Table of Contents

**Indicates items appearing in print for the first time in 2012 and new/revised items published electronically during 2011.

2012 Perioperative Standards and Recommended Practices

iii

Table of Contents

*** Indicates items appearing in print for the first time in 2012 and new/revised items published electronically during 2011.*

AORN is committed to promoting excellence in perioperative nursing practice, advancing the profession, and supporting the professional perioperative registered nurse (RN). AORN promotes safe care for patients undergoing operative and other invasive procedures by providing practice support to the perioperative RN. Perioperative RNs function in a variety of roles that may include, but are not limited to, staff nurse, registered nurse first assistant, advanced practice RN, manager, administrator, educator, informatics nurse specialist, and researcher. This publication contains the AORN-approved standards, recommended practices, guidelines, and guidance statements.

These descriptive and comprehensive documents reflect the perioperative RN's scope of professional responsibility and provide essential information for the delivery of safe perioperative patient care and a safe work environment. AORN's standards, recommended practices, guidelines, and guidance statements guide the practice of perioperative nursing practice while allowing for flexibility and adaptability in all settings where surgical and other invasive procedures are performed.

NEW IN THIS EDITION

Two new recommended practices are included in this 2012 edition:
- ♦ Recommended Practices for Prevention of Deep Vein Thrombosis and
- ♦ Recommended Practices for Medication Safety.

Additionally, one recommended practices document was revised for this edition:
- ♦ Recommended Practices for Perioperative Health Care Information Management.

The "AORN guidance statement: 'Do-not-use' abbreviations, acronyms, dosage designations, and symbols," "AORN guidance statement: Safe medication practices in perioperative settings across the life span," and "AORN guideline for prevention of venous stasis" have been retired and do not appear in this edition.

SECTION I: STANDARDS OF PERIOPERATIVE NURSING PRACTICE

The AORN standards of perioperative nursing practice define the scope, responsibilities, and dimensions of professional perioperative nursing practice. The standards guide individual practitioners in performing safe and effective care

and are reflected in value-based behaviors and priorities of the profession.

The standards serve as the foundation for AORN's recommended practices, competency statements, and core curriculum, as well as the Perioperative Nursing Data Set (PNDS). The standards are consistent with *Nursing: Scope and Standards of Practice, Nursing's Social Policy Statement,* 2nd edition, and *Nursing Administration: Scope and Standards of Practice,* 3rd edition, published by the American Nurses Association (ANA). The "Standards of perioperative nursing" focus on the process of providing nursing care and performing professional role activities; they also provide a mechanism to delineate the responsibilities of the RN engaged in practice in the perioperative setting. The structure and content of the Standards reflect current professional perioperative nursing practice and align with the ANA Standards.

SECTION II: RECOMMENDED PRACTICES FOR PERIOPERATIVE NURSING

AORN's recommended practices for perioperative nursing represent what is believed to be optimal and achievable perioperative nursing practice, based on the highest level of evidence available. The recommended practices are intended to describe excellent perioperative nursing practices, promote patient and health care worker safety, and guide policy and procedure development in surgical and invasive procedure settings. The AORN recommended practices are authored by perioperative nurse specialists in the AORN Nursing Department and selected members of AORN in collaboration with liaisons from the American Association of Nurse Anesthetists, the American College of Surgeons, the American Society of Anesthesiologists, the Association for Professionals in Infection Control and Epidemiology, the Centers for Disease Control and Prevention, and the International Association of Healthcare Central Service Materiel Management.

SECTION III: AORN GUIDELINES AND GUIDANCE STATEMENTS

This section includes the AORN guidelines and guidance statements. Guidelines address a specific medical diagnosis or clinical condition and are based on empirical data. Guidelines assist practitioners in clinical decision making and are used to assess and ensure the quality of care and guide clinical practice. Guidelines are statements that assist practitioners in making evidence-based health care decisions in specific circumstances. Guidelines are based on a body of evidence, are necessity driven, and define a minimum set of services and actions appropriate for certain clinical conditions.

Guidance statements provide suggested strategies to assist practitioners in developing organization-specific processes related to clinical and administrative issues.

SECTION IV: ADDITIONAL RESOURCES

Additional resources include a policy and procedure template with sample policies and procedures for fire safety and correct site surgery. These policy examples reflect the recommendations found in the related recommended practices.

Other resources include a listing of AORN Position Statements, the "AACD glossary of times used for scheduling and monitoring of diagnostic and therapeutic procedures," the revised "AORN standards for RN first assistant education programs" (2011), and an updated index of important terms and concepts.

AORN and Perioperative Nursing

The Association of periOperative Registered Nurses (AORN) is the national association committed to improving patient safety in the surgical setting. AORN is the premier resource for perioperative nurses, advancing the profession and the professional with valuable guidance as well as networking and resource-sharing opportunities. AORN promotes safe patient care and is recognized as an authority for safe operating room practices and a definitive source for information and guiding principles that support day-to-day perioperative nursing practice.

AORN Vision and Mission

Vision statement
AORN will be the indispensable resource for evidence-based practice and education that establishes the standards of excellence in the delivery of perioperative nursing care.

Mission statement
AORN's mission is to promote safety and optimal outcomes for patients undergoing operative and other invasive procedures by providing practice support and professional development opportunities to perioperative nurses. AORN will collaborate with professional and regulatory organizations, industry leaders, and other health care partners who support the mission.

Core Values

AORN's core values reflect what is important to the association:
- Communication—open, honest, respectful
- Quality—reliable, timely, accountable
- Innovation—creative, risk taking, leading edge
- Collaboration—teamwork, inclusion, diversity

Standards of Perioperative Nursing

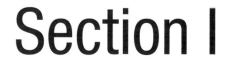

Section I

AORN Perioperative Standards and Recommended Practices, 2012 Edition

Introduction

AORN is dedicated to enhancing the professionalism of perioperative registered nurses (RNs), promoting standards of perioperative nursing practice to better serve the needs of society, and providing a forum for interaction and exchange of ideas related to perioperative health care. Standards are authoritative statements that describe the responsibilities for which RNs are accountable and that reflect the values and priorities of the profession. The history of the Standards of Perioperative Nursing is detailed in **Exhibit A**.

As recipients of care, patients are entitled to privacy, confidentiality, personal dignity, and quality health services. The delivery of patient-focused care is guided by ethical, legal, and moral principles. These inherent principles serve as a foundation for perioperative nursing practice and are paramount in achieving optimal patient outcomes.

The standards of perioperative nursing focus on the process of providing nursing care and performing professional role activities. These standards apply to all nurses in the perioperative setting and were developed by AORN using the American Nurses Association's (ANA) scope and standards of practice for nursing and nursing administration as the foundation.[1,2]

It is the perioperative RN's responsibility to meet these standards, assuming that adequate environmental working conditions and necessary resources are available to support and facilitate the nurse's attainment of these standards. It is the responsibility of health care employers to provide an appropriate environment for nursing practice. It is important to recognize the link between working conditions and the nurse's ability to deliver care.

Several related themes underlie the standards of perioperative nursing. Nursing care must be individualized to meet a patient's unique needs and situation. This care should be provided in the context of disease or injury prevention, health promotion, health restoration, health maintenance, or palliative care. The cultural, racial, and ethnic diversity of the patient always must be taken into account while providing nursing care.

The perioperative RN must respect the patient's goals and preferences in developing and implementing a plan of care. One of nursing's primary responsibilities is patient education; therefore, nurses should provide patients with appropriate information to make informed decisions regarding their care and treatment. It is recognized, however, that some state regulations or institutional policies or procedures may prohibit full disclosure of information to patients.

The perioperative RN's partnership with the patient and other health care providers is recognized in the standards. It is assumed that the nurse will work with other health care providers in a coordinated manner throughout the process of caring for patients undergoing operative or other invasive procedures. The involvement of the patient and designated support person(s) is paramount. The appropriate degree of participation that is expected of the patient, designated support person(s), and other health care providers is determined by the clinical environment and the patient's unique situation.

It is beyond the scope of documents such as these to account for all possible scenarios that the perioperative RN may encounter in practice. The nurse will need to exercise judgment based on education and experience to determine what is appropriate, pertinent, or realistic. Further direction also may be available from documents such as recommended practices, guidelines for care, agency standards, policies, procedures, protocols, and current research findings.

The standards of perioperative nursing provide a mechanism to delineate the responsibilities of RNs engaged in practice in the perioperative setting. These standards serve as the basis for quality monitoring and evaluation systems, databases; regulatory systems; the development and evaluation of nursing service delivery systems and organizational structures; certification activities; job descriptions and performance appraisals; agency policies, procedures, and protocols; and educational offerings. The standards of perioperative nursing are generic and apply to all RNs engaged in perioperative practice, regardless of clinical setting, practice setting, or educational preparation.

A. Perioperative Patient Focused Model

A.1. Conceptual Framework

The Perioperative Patient Focused Model (**Figure 1**) is the conceptual framework for perioperative nursing practice and the Perioperative Nursing

Figure 1

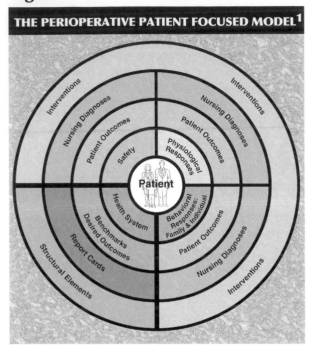

THE PERIOPERATIVE PATIENT FOCUSED MODEL[1]

1. Petersen C, ed. Perioperative Nursing Data Set. *2nd ed rev.* Denver, CO: AORN, Inc; 2007: 16, inside front cover.

Data Set (PNDS).[3] At the core of the Model, the patient and his or her designated support person(s) provide the focus of perioperative nursing care. Concentric circles expand beyond the patient and designated support person(s) representing the perioperative nursing domains and elements. The Model illustrates the relationship between the patient, designated support person(s), and care provided by the perioperative RN.

A.2. Patient Centered

The patient is at the center of the Model, which clearly represents the true focus of perioperative patient care. Regardless of practice setting, geographic location, or nature of the patient population, there is nothing more important to the perioperative RN than the patient.

A.3. Four Domains

The Model is divided into four quadrants, three representing patient-centered domains:
- patient safety,
- patient physiologic responses to operative and other invasive procedures, and
- patient and designated support person(s) behavioral responses to operative and other invasive procedures.

The fourth quadrant represents the health system in which the perioperative care is delivered. The health system domain designates administrative concerns and structure elements essential to successful perioperative outcomes.

A.4. Outcome Focused

The Model focuses on patient outcomes. This is important, because nursing theories and models should embrace and represent all elements of the nursing process. AORN's Model represents the outcomes focus of perioperative RNs by placing outcomes immediately adjacent to the patient care domains. Perioperative RNs have a unique knowledge base that supports high-quality patient outcomes. An individualized patient assessment guides the identification of nursing diagnoses and selection of nursing interventions for each patient.

B. Goal for Perioperative Nursing Practice

The goal of perioperative nursing practice is to assist patients and their designated support person(s) with achieving a level of wellness equal to or greater than that which they had before their operative or other invasive procedures.

C. Scope of Perioperative Nursing Practice

C.1. Definition of Perioperative RN

C.1.1. Perioperative RNs use the nursing process to develop individualized plans of care and to coordinate and deliver care to patients undergoing operative or other invasive procedures. Perioperative RNs identify patient needs, set goals with patients, and implement nursing interventions and activities to achieve optimal patient outcomes.

C.1.2. Perioperative RNs address the physiological, psychological, socio-cultural, and spiritual responses of patients.

C.1.3. Perioperative RNs use standards, knowledge, judgment, and skills based on scientific principles.

C.1.4. Perioperative RNs are ethical, responsible, and accountable for quality patient care.

C.1.5. Perioperative RNs use evidence as the foundation for practice.

C.1.6. Perioperative RNs assume responsibility for lifelong learning.

C.2. Definition of Perioperative Nursing Practice

C.2.1. Perioperative nursing practice is consistent with ANA's definition of nursing, which states,

> Nursing is the protection, promotion, and optimization of health and abilities, prevention of illness and injury, alleviation of suffering through the diagnosis and treatment of human response, and advocacy in the care of individuals, families, communities, and populations.[4(p6)]

C.2.2. Perioperative nursing practice is based on holistic caring relationships that facilitate health and healing within the range of human experiences.

C.2.3. Perioperative nursing practice is enhanced by interdisciplinary collaboration and appropriate resource utilization.

C.2.4. Perioperative RNs use AORN recommended practices as a foundation for practice and specialized educational preparation.

C.3. Span of Perioperative Nursing Practice

C.3.1. Perioperative RNs provide care across the surgical continuum, beginning when patients are first informed that they need an operative or invasive procedure and ending when they return to their usual roles and responsibilities.

C.3.2. Perioperative RNs focus on patients and their designated support person(s).

C.4. Settings of Perioperative Nursing Practice

Perioperative RNs provide care in a variety of clinical settings. These settings include traditional ORs, ambulatory surgery centers, physicians' offices, cardiac catheterization suites, endoscopy suites, radiology departments, and all other areas where operative and other invasive procedures may be performed.

Perioperative RNs influence community, regulatory, and legislative activities through employment or voluntary participation at the local, state, national, or international level.

C.5. Role Functions

Perioperative RNs function in a variety of roles that are dynamic and continually evolving through increased education and experience to meet the changing needs of society. These may include, but are not limited to, staff RN, RN first assistant, advanced practice RN, manager, administrator, educator, informatics nurse specialist, and researcher.

Perioperative RNs act in the public interest when providing the unique service society has entrusted to them. Accountability is accomplished through self-regulation, professional regulation, and legal regulation. Perioperative RNs positively influence health care services and delivery by promoting a safe environment.

D. Standards of Perioperative Nursing

D.1. Standard 1: Assessment

The perioperative RN collects patient health data that are relevant to the operative or invasive procedure.

Measurement

D.1.1. Perioperative RN:

D.1.1.1. Determines data collection priorities based on the patient's condition or needs, and the relationship to the proposed intervention.

D.1.1.2. Collects pertinent data using systematic, comprehensive, and evidence-based techniques.

D.1.1.3. Conducts a systematic and ongoing process for data collection.

D.1.1.4. Involves the patient, designated support person(s), and health care providers in the data-collection process.

D.1.1.5. Reviews the results of diagnostic studies relevant to the patient's current status and planned operative or invasive procedure.

D.1.1.6. Documents relevant data in a retrievable format.

Additional measurement

D.1.2. Advanced practice RN:

D.1.2.1. Uses advanced assessment techniques, independently or collaboratively, to gather appropriate data pertinent to patients and populations.

D.1.2.2. Recognizes complex physiologic responses.

D.1.2.3. Initiates diagnostic studies relevant to the patient's current status and planned operative or invasive procedure.

D.1.2.4. Interprets results of diagnostic studies relevant to the patient's current status and planned operative or invasive procedure.

D.1.2.5. Synthesizes assessment data to identify trends and improve perioperative outcomes.

D.1.2.6. Assigns American Society of Anesthesiologists (ASA) physical status classification.

D.2. Standard 2: Diagnosis

The perioperative RN analyzes the assessment data to determine nursing diagnoses.

Measurement

D.2.1. Perioperative RN:

D.2.1.1. Identifies nursing diagnoses that are consistent with the assessment data.

D.2.1.2. Sets priorities using nursing diagnoses based on assessment data.

D.2.1.3. Validates nursing diagnoses with the patient, designated support person(s), and health care providers when possible.

D.2.1.4. Documents nursing diagnoses using standardized nursing language in a retrievable format.

Additional measurement

D.2.2. Advanced practice RN:

D.2.2.1. Synthesizes assessment data using advanced knowledge and clinical judgment to formulate differential diagnoses for risk reduction and clinical problems.

D.2.2.2. Sets priorities using differential diagnoses.

D.3. Standard 3: Outcome Identification

The perioperative RN identifies expected outcomes that are unique to the patient.

Measurement

D.3.1. Perioperative RN:

D.3.1.1. Uses ethical principles to determine expected outcomes that are mutually formulated with the patient, designated support person(s), and health care providers when appropriate.

D.3.1.2. Develops culturally and age-appropriate expected outcomes based on the patient's present and potential physical capabilities and behavioral patterns.

D.3.1.3. Defines expected outcomes that are attainable with considerations to the human and material resources available to the patient.

D.3.1.4. Identifies measurable criteria to determine outcome attainment.

D.3.1.5. Sets priorities including a time estimate for attaining expected outcomes.

D.3.1.6. Modifies expected outcomes based on patient status.

D.3.1.7. Communicates expected and attained outcomes to health care providers to provide direction for continuity of care.

D.3.1.8. Documents outcomes in a retrievable format.

Additional measurement

D.3.2. Advanced practice RN:

D.3.2.1. Develops peer education that emphasizes identification and use of culturally appropriate patient outcome measures.

D.3.2.2. Acts as a resource to determine an outcome-driven plan for individual patients and patient populations.

D.3.2.3. Synthesizes evidence to determine optimal outcomes for individual patients and patient populations.

D.4. Standard 4: Planning

The perioperative RN develops an individualized plan of care to attain expected outcomes.

Measurement

D.4.1. Perioperative RN:

D.4.1.1. Uses nursing diagnoses to identify nursing interventions.

D.4.1.2. Uses current trends and scientific evidence in the planning process.

D.4.1.3. Designs a plan of care that includes strategies for health promotion and restoration.

D.4.1.4. Collaborates with the patient and designated support person(s), as appropriate, while planning care.

D.4.1.5. Creates a plan of care that supports continuity among providers.

D.4.1.6. Specifies a logical sequence of interventions to attain expected outcomes.

D.4.1.7. Identifies human and material resources necessary to implement the plan of care.

D.4.1.8. Communicates the plan of care to the patient, designated support person(s), and health care providers.

D.4.1.9. Documents plan of care using standardized language in a retrievable format.

Additional measurement

D.4.2. Advanced practice RN:

D.4.2.1. Synthesizes research findings and applies expert clinical knowledge to expand the plan of care for individuals and patient populations.

D.4.2.2. Develops priorities for care reflecting the signs, symptoms, and behavioral responses within the realm of care for the advanced practice nurse.

D.5. Standard 5: Implementation

The perioperative RN implements the identified plan of care.

Measurement

D.5.1. Perioperative RN:

D.5.1.1. Determines that the nursing interventions are consistent with the plan of care.

D.5.1.2. Verifies that nursing interventions reflect the rights and desires of the patient and designated support person(s).

D.5.1.3. Implements nursing interventions safely and efficiently.

D.5.1.4. Implements the ongoing plan of care in collaboration with the patient, designated support person(s), and health care providers based on the patient's responses.

D.5.1.5. Anticipates and responds to situational changes.

D.5.1.6. Modifies the plan of care based on the patient's responses.

D.5.1.7. Incorporates new knowledge and strategies to initiate change in nursing care practices if desired outcomes are not achieved.

D.5.1.8. Documents interventions using standardized language in a retrievable format to promote continuity of care.

Additional measurement

D.5.2. Advanced practice RN:

D.5.2.1. Integrates advanced knowledge and skills to implement the plan of care.

D.5.2.2. Performs ongoing physical examinations, selecting, ordering, and interpreting diagnostic tests.

D.5.2.3. Provides advanced interpretation of conditions and gives rationale for the procedure.

D.5.2.4. Performs interventions that apply advanced nursing therapies and include medication management and clinical procedures.

D.5.a. Standard 5a: Coordination of Care

The perioperative RN coordinates patient care continually throughout the patient's perioperative experience.

Measurement

D.5.a.1. Perioperative RN:

D.5.a.1.1. Delegates tasks and functions according to applicable laws, regulations, and standards, taking into consideration the competency of the assignee.

D.5.a.1.2. Assists the patient and designated support person(s) with identifying alternative options for care.

Additional measurement

D.5.a.2. Advanced practice RN:

D.5.a.2.1. Uses advanced knowledge to initiate new treatments or change existing treatment based on changing trends or scientific evidence.

D.5.a.2.2. Makes referrals to other health care professionals and community agencies.

D.5.a.2.3. Initiates interdisciplinary team meetings or other communication to improve the health of individual patients and patient populations.

D.5.b. Standard 5b: Health Teaching—Health Promotion

The perioperative RN promotes holistic wellness and a safe environment.

Measurement

D.5.b.1. Perioperative RN:

D.5.b.1.1. Teaches modifications for activities of daily living.

D.5.b.1.2. Provides information to patients to reduce high-risk behaviors.

D.5.b.1.3. Advocates for healthy lifestyle choices.

D.5.b.1.4. Uses teaching strategies that are appropriate to the situation and the patient's developmental level, cognitive ability, learning needs, readiness, language preference, culture, and beliefs.

D.5.b.1.5. Alters teaching strategies based on feedback.

D.5.b.1.6. Reports information to the appropriate source regarding local, state, and national health issues that affect safety according to policy, guidelines, or regulations.

Additional measurement

D.5.b.2. Advanced practice RN:

D.5.b.2.1. Uses advanced theoretical knowledge to organize and deliver educational programs for patients, designated support person(s), health care professionals, and the community.

D.5.b.2.2. Initiates referrals promoting health or risk reduction.

D.5.b.2.3. Analyzes and disseminates information regarding local, state, and national health issues that affect safety.

D.5.c. Standard 5c: Consultation

The perioperative RN seeks specialized dialogue appropriate to the patient.

Measurement

D.5.c.1. Perioperative RN:

D.5.c.1.1. Facilitates communication between health care professionals to enhance patient outcomes.

Additional measurement

D.5.c.2. Advanced practice RN:

D.5.c.2.1. Provides independent consultation services based on expertise using advanced knowledge within the scope of practice.

D.5.c.2.2. Collaborates and coordinates with medical, nursing, and other disciplines to plan and implement monitoring of physiologic responses for individuals or patient populations.

D.5.c.2.3. Consults with the appropriate health care providers to determine a need for new treatments or a change in existing treatments.

D.5.c.2.4. Initiates new treatment based on consultation.

D.5.d. Standard 5d: Prescriptive Authority

The advanced practice RN prescribes medications, treatments, and therapies in compliance with state and federal laws and regulations.

Measurement

D.5.d.1. Prescriptive authority does not apply to the perioperative RN.

Additional measurement

D.5.d.2. Advanced practice RN:

D.5.d.2.1. Uses prescriptive authority within the scope of practice.

D.5.d.2.2. Uses scientific evidence to order, prescribe, or initiate diagnostic, therapeutic, or pharmacologic interventions based on patient status.

D.5.d.2.3. Monitors the patient for therapeutic and potential adverse effects in response to diagnostic or pharmacologic interventions.

D.5.d.2.4. Modifies diagnostic, therapeutic, or pharmacologic interventions based on the patient's status and responses.

D.5.d.2.5. Educates patients and designated support person(s) about intended and potential adverse effects of proposed prescribed therapies.

D.5.d.2.6. Informs patients and designated support person(s) about potential costs, alternative treatment options, and procedures as appropriate.

D.6. Standard 6: Evaluation

The perioperative RN evaluates the patient's progress toward attaining outcomes.

Measurement Criteria

D.6.1. Perioperative RN:

D.6.1.1. Conducts a systematic and ongoing evaluation measuring the effectiveness of the interventions in relation to achieving identified outcomes.

D.6.1.2. Monitors the patient's progress toward achieving outcomes in the timeframe identified in the plan.

D.6.1.3. Documents the patient's progress toward achieving outcomes accurately and consistently using standardized language in a retrievable format.

D.6.1.4. Revises diagnoses, outcomes, and the plan of care, based on ongoing assessment and evaluation.

D.6.1.5. Documents revisions in diagnoses, outcomes, and the plan of care using standardized language in a retrievable format.

D.6.1.6. Involves the patient, designated support person(s), and health care providers in the evaluation process whenever possible.

D.6.1.7. Disseminates evaluation results as appropriate to the patient and others according to state and federal laws and regulations.

D.6.1.8. Recommends policy, procedure, protocol, process, or structural changes, as appropriate, based on evaluation data.

Additional measurement

D.6.2. Advanced practice RN:

D.6.2.1. Evaluates responses to interventions systematically and revises differential diagnoses as needed in relation to the patient's progress toward attaining outcomes.

D.6.2.2. Uses advanced knowledge of learning and change theories, human behavior, stress and coping mechanisms, crisis management, growth, and development to evaluate patient responses to care.

D.6.2.3. Modifies the patient's plan of care, recommending additional diagnostic testing and treatments if necessary to attain outcomes.

D.6.2.4. Synthesizes knowledge of diagnostic tests, therapeutic regimens, and the patient's responses as they relate to progress toward attaining expected outcomes.

D.6.2.5. Uses advanced knowledge to synthesize evaluation data that have a potential effect on current and future health care practices for individual patients and patient populations.

Standards of Perioperative Professional Practice

D.7. Standard 7: Quality of Practice

The perioperative RN systematically evaluates the quality and appropriateness of nursing practice.

Measurement

D.7.1. Perioperative RN:

D.7.1.1. Demonstrates the quality of perioperative nursing care by documenting use of the nursing process using standardized language in a retrievable format.

D.7.1.2. Participates in ongoing quality improvement activities as appropriate to the individual's position, education, and practice environment. Such activities may include, but are not limited to, the following:

– Identifying aspects of the perioperative nursing practice that are important for quality monitoring.

– Assigning responsibility for quality monitoring and evaluation activities.

– Identifying dimensions of performance related to perioperative nursing practice.

– Developing quality indicators for each identified dimension of performance.

– Establishing benchmarks to evaluate the quality indicators.

– Collecting data related to the dimensions of performance and quality indicators.

– Evaluating perioperative nursing practice and care based on the cumulative data collected.

– Identifying strategies to improve perioperative nursing care or services based on quality indicators as necessary.

– Taking action to improve perioperative nursing care or services.

– Assessing the effectiveness of the action(s) taken.

– Communicating the data collected organization-wide to other agencies, regulatory bodies, or data repositories while maintaining confidentiality.

D.7.1.3. Initiates changes in perioperative nursing practice through knowledge gained and shared via the quality and performance improvement process.

D.7.1.4. Improves perioperative nursing practice, services, and care through the quality improvement process.

D.7.1.5. Monitors perioperative nursing practice and compares it to national guidelines, standards, or existing research.

D.7.1.6. Uses internal and external data to create innovative quality indicators.

Additional measurement

D.7.2. Advanced practice RN:

D.7.2.1. Applies advanced theoretical knowledge, research findings, and assessment data to design and implement ongoing quality monitoring activities to evaluate perioperative nursing practice.

D.7.2.2. Works with multidisciplinary groups to design or implement advanced practices and alternative solutions to patient care issues based on quality monitoring data.

D.7.2.3. Synthesizes data from clinical investigations and scientific research to improve the safety, efficiency, and effectiveness of perioperative patient care.

D.7.2.4. Publishes or presents results of quality monitoring and evaluation activities to influence and improve perioperative nursing practice.

D.7.2.5. Maintains certification in advanced nursing practice.

D.8. Standard 8: Education

The perioperative RN acquires and maintains specialized knowledge and skills in nursing practice.

Measurement

D.8.1. Perioperative RN:

D.8.1.1. Completes an individualized orientation based on identified learning needs.

D.8.1.2. Demonstrates skill proficiency relevant to perioperative nursing practice.

D.8.1.3. Seeks experiences to maintain skills and competency necessary to practice perioperative nursing.

D.8.1.4. Participates in ongoing educational activities relevant to professional issues and trends in perioperative nursing.

D.8.1.5. Maintains records and documents to support competence in perioperative nursing.

D.8.1.6. Strives to achieve certification in perioperative nursing.

Additional measurement

D.8.2. Advanced practice RN:

D.8.2.1. Incorporates current research, national guidelines, standards, and evidence-based practices to develop advanced clinical knowledge and augment performance in perioperative nursing.

D.8.2.2. Develops, coordinates, implements, and evaluates educational programs for individual patients, designated support person(s), patient populations, and local, regional, or state communities based on identified needs.

D.8.2.3. Maintains educational requirements necessary for advanced certification and licensure to practice.

D.9. Standard 9: Professional Practice Evaluation

The perioperative RN evaluates his or her practice in context with current professional practice standards, rules, and regulations.

Measurement

D.9.1. Perioperative RN:

D.9.1.1. Provides care consistent with the institution's policies and procedures.

D.9.1.2. Practices nursing in accordance with the state board of nursing statutes, as well as the standards and guidelines of accrediting and regulatory bodies.

D.9.1.3. Maintains current knowledge of and adheres to ANA standards, practice guidelines, and position statements.

D.9.1.4. Maintains current knowledge of and adheres to AORN standards, recommended practices, guidelines, and position statements.

D.9.1.5. Maintains current knowledge of and adheres to standards, recommended practices, guidelines, and position statements from other nursing organizations as relevant to practice.

D.9.1.6. Participates in an ongoing evaluation process to ensure practice is current, legal, ethical, culturally competent, and age-appropriate.

D.9.1.7. Seeks evaluative input from peers, colleagues, patients, and patients' designated support person(s) regarding nursing practice.

D.9.1.8. Participates in peer review to evaluate nursing practice of fellow RN colleagues.

D.9.1.9. Identifies goals and develops an action plan for professional development as part of an ongoing evaluation process.

D.9.1.10. Interprets and facilitates staff member and agency compliance with current local, state, and federal regulations and standards.

D.9.1.11. Participates in legislative and policy-making activities that influence health services and nursing practice.
D.9.1.12. Respects diversity in all interactions.

Additional measurement

D.9.2. Advanced practice RN:
D.9.2.1. Devises innovative, evidence-based evaluation strategies to ensure that care is being delivered in a legal, ethical, culturally competent and age-appropriate manner.
D.9.2.2. Applies advanced theoretical knowledge, research findings, and assessment data to design, implement, and evaluate perioperative nursing practice.
D.9.2.3. Works with multidisciplinary groups to design or implement advanced practices and alternative solutions to patient care issues based on quality monitoring data.
D.9.2.4. Synthesizes data from clinical investigations and scientific research to improve the safety, efficiency, and effectiveness of perioperative patient care.
D.9.2.5. Publishes or presents results of quality monitoring and evaluation activities to influence and improve perioperative nursing practice.

D.10. Standard 10: Collegiality
The perioperative RN interacts with and contributes to the professional growth of peers, colleagues, and others.

Measurement

D.10.1. Perioperative RN:
D.10.1.1. Shares knowledge and skills through a variety of methods including, but not limited to,
– providing inservice education, programs, seminars, and workshops;
– precepting;
– mentoring;
– role modeling;
– participating in peer evaluation;
– publishing; and
– participating in professional associations.
D.10.1.2. Contributes to a supportive and healthy work environment by using appropriate verbal and nonverbal communication techniques.
D.10.1.3. Builds trust by being approachable, honest, and accountable.
D.10.1.4. Acts as a role model for professional behavior.
D.10.1.5. Supports colleagues' professional development.
D.10.1.6. Interacts with team members and others in a respectful and courteous manner.
D.10.1.7. Uses conflict resolution skills to manage difficult behavior, promote positive working relationships, and advocate for patient safety.

Additional measurement

D.10.2. Advanced practice RN:
D.10.2.1. Shares knowledge and skills as a role model and mentor.
D.10.2.2. Uses advanced knowledge to assist staff members with applying the nursing process to complex patient situations in the perioperative setting.
D.10.2.3. Develops evidence-based guidelines to influence policy, change practice, and support professional development of colleagues.
D.10.2.4. Acts as a preceptor for advanced practice nurses.

D.11. Standard 11: Collaboration
The perioperative RN collaborates with the patient and designated support person(s) when practicing professional nursing.

Measurement

D.11.1. Perioperative RN:
D.11.1.1. Communicates pertinent information relating to patient care to internal and external stakeholders as appropriate.
D.11.1.2. Demonstrates accountability and flexibility when interacting with others.
D.11.1.3. Includes the patient and designated support person(s) and health care team members, as appropriate, in decision making when providing perioperative nursing care.
D.11.1.4. Provides continuity of care when implementing referrals.
D.11.1.5. Supervises allied health care providers and support personnel with appropriate authority.

D.11.1.6. Delegates tasks and functions according to applicable law, regulation, and standards, taking into consideration the competency of the assignee.

Additional measurement

D.11.2. Advanced practice RN:
D.11.2.1. Participates with the interdisciplinary team to promote the use of nationally accepted clinical practice guidelines and standards in advanced nursing practice.
D.11.2.2. Serves as a resource for perioperative staff members, surgeons, ancillary departments, and community groups requiring advanced nursing expertise.
D.11.2.3. Fosters a collaborative environment and recognizes the value of each provider's contribution to comprehensive health care.
D.11.2.4. Acts in partnership with appropriate health care providers to initiate new treatments or change existing treatments to promote positive outcomes.

D.12. Standard 12: Ethics
The perioperative RN uses ethical principles to determine decisions and actions.

Measurement

D.12.1. Perioperative RN:
D.12.1.1. Practices nursing according to the ANA *Code of Ethics for Nurses with Interpretive Statements* (**Exhibit B**).
D.12.1.2. Acts as a patient advocate.
D.12.1.3. Encourages patient self-advocacy.
D.12.1.4. Maintains patient confidentiality within legal and regulatory guidelines.
D.12.1.5. Delivers care in a nonjudgmental and nondiscriminatory manner that is sensitive to cultural, racial, and ethnic diversity.
D.12.1.6. Delivers care in a way that preserves and protects patient autonomy, dignity, and human rights.
D.12.1.7. Upholds the professional and therapeutic boundaries of the nurse-patient relationship.
D.12.1.8. Formulates ethical decisions by using available resources.
D.12.1.9. Reports illegal, incompetent, or impaired practices.

D.12.1.10. Recognizes own physical and psychological limitations to provide safe, competent patient care.
D.12.1.11. Participates on ethics committees as appropriate.

Additional measurement

D.12.2. Advanced practice RN:
D.12.2.1. Develops treatment plans while instructing the patient and designated support person(s) about the risks, benefits, and possible outcomes of the plan.
D.12.2.2. Contributes to the development of consistent policies and services that are comparable in all settings and that are within the legal and ethical scope of advanced practice.
D.12.2.3. Provides independent or collaborative care that is nondiscriminatory and nonprejudicial regardless of the setting.
D.12.2.4. Initiates treatments in a nonjudgmental and nondiscriminatory manner that is sensitive to the patient's cultural, racial, socioeconomic, and ethnic diversity.
D.12.2.5. Considers ethical implications of scientific advances, cost, and clinical effectiveness, as well as patient and designated support person(s)' acceptance or satisfaction.

D.13. Standard 13: Research
The perioperative RN incorporates research findings into practice.

Measurement

D.13.1. Perioperative RN:
D.13.1.1. Uses the best available research evidence to guide practice.
D.13.1.2. Initiates change using scientific evidence to develop policies and procedures or influence perioperative nursing practice.
D.13.1.3. Supports nursing practice changes based on research evidence.
D.13.1.4. Seeks new knowledge that is evidence-based through print, web-based, and other sources.
D.13.1.5. Participates in research activities by involvement in one or more of the following:
– identifying clinical problems pertinent to perioperative nursing practice;
– participating in data collection;

– reading, analyzing, critiquing, and interpreting research findings to determine applicability to practice;

– sharing research activities and findings with others;

– participating on a research committee;

– participating in a research study; or

– joining a journal club.

Additional measurement

D.13.2. Advanced practice RN:

D.13.2.1. Collects and aggregates data to analyze care decisions, patient responses, and health outcomes for potential research projects.

D.13.2.2. Synthesizes current and emerging research findings that contribute to positive patient outcomes and incorporates them into advanced practice decisions.

D.13.2.3. Performs a literature review and critically appraises findings to advocate for analysis or review of system-wide clinical practices.

D.13.2.4. Conducts research to contribute to nursing knowledge and evidence-based practice.

D.13.2.5. Disseminates research findings through writing, publishing, and presenting to influence general and advanced nursing practice.

D.13.2.6. Pursues funding for perioperative nursing research.

D.14. Standard 14: Resource Utilization

The perioperative RN considers factors related to safety, effectiveness, efficiency, and the environment, as well as the cost in planning, delivering, and evaluating patient care.

Measurement

D.14.1. Perioperative RN:

D.14.1.1. Assigns tasks or delegates care based on knowledge and skills of perioperative team members to meet the needs of the patient and keep him or her free from harm.

D.14.1.2. Assists the patient and designated support person(s) with identifying human and material resources that are available to address perioperative patient needs.

D.14.1.3. Advocates for technical advances in clinical care to increase efficiency or improve outcomes.

D.14.1.4. Promotes the use of electronic information systems to provide perioperative patient care efficiently and safely.

D.14.1.5. Advocates for reusing, recycling, and renewing supplies whenever appropriate in the perioperative setting.

D.14.1.6. Conserves supplies to minimize waste and decrease costs without compromising safety or negatively affecting outcomes.

Additional measurement

D.14.2. Advanced practice RN:

D.14.2.1. Uses advanced knowledge to provide consultation services to the organization to achieve high-quality, cost-effective outcomes for populations of patients across settings.

D.14.2.2. Promotes system-wide communication to reduce costs by avoiding unnecessary duplication of diagnostic tests.

D.14.2.3. Collects and evaluates data regarding the effectiveness of care, cost-benefit relationship of the care being provided, and patient satisfaction.

D.14.2.4. Maintains knowledge of the organization's methods of financing the delivery of care.

D.14.2.5. Implements a cost-benefit evaluation of new technology and participates in product review committees.

D.14.2.6. Considers health care access, fiscal responsibility, efficacy, and quality when providing advanced nursing care.

D.15. Standard 15: Leadership

The perioperative RN provides leadership in the profession and professional practice setting.

Measurement

D.15.1. Perioperative RN:

D.15.1.1. Supervises peers, colleagues, allied health personnel, and support staff members as assigned and appropriate.

D.15.1.2. Delegates tasks and responsibilities according to law, regulation, and accrediting agency standards.

D.15.1.3. Holds self and team members accountable to the patient, the organization, and other internal and external stakeholders.

D.15.1.4. Creates and maintains a healthy work environment.

D.15.1.5. Embraces lifelong learning for self and others.

D.15.1.6. Advocates for a culture of safety for patients and staff members in the workplace.

D.15.1.7. Actively has input into organizational operations. Activities include, but are not limited to, the following:
- influencing policy-making to improve patient care;
- advocating for issues that affect perioperative care;
- participating in quality improvement activities;
- participating on committees;
- being a role model when new policies, procedures, or processes are implemented;
- supporting change while considering short- and long-term organizational goals;
- operationalizing the mission, vision, and values of the organization; and
- encouraging peers and colleagues to be active.

D.15.1.8. Participates in ongoing quality improvement workplace activities as appropriate to the individual's position, education, and practice environment.

D.15.1.9. Enhances perioperative nursing through involvement with professional organizations. Activities include, but are not limited to, the following:
- taking an active role in the association;
- encouraging peers and colleagues to be active;
- sharing information received through associations with team members; and
- presenting pertinent information to individuals and groups of lay and professional audiences.

D.15.1.10. Participates in legislative and policy-making activities that influence perioperative care.

Additional measurement

D.15.2. Advanced practice RN:

D.15.2.1. Uses advanced knowledge to act at the organizational level and beyond to promote change by identifying and influencing variables affecting health care practices and outcomes.

D.15.2.2. Promotes interdisciplinary cooperation and collaboration to implement outcome-based patient care programs to meet the needs of individual patients, designated support person(s), or patient populations or local, regional, or state communities.

D.15.2.3. Uses advanced team building, negotiation, and conflict resolution skills to promote teamwork to build partnerships within and across health care systems.

D.15.2.4. Initiates legislative and policy-making activities that influence perioperative care.

D.15.2.5. Collaborates to prevent and reduce the incidence of surgical site infections, health care-associated infections, and other adverse events related to surgical patients.

D.15.2.6. Facilitates staff member access to and compliance with current local, state, and federal regulations; professional standards; and accreditation guidelines.

D.15.2.7. Advances the profession through writing, publishing, and presenting pertinent information to individuals and groups of lay and professional audiences.

E. Standards of Perioperative Administrative Practice

E.1. Standard 1: Assessment

The perioperative RN administrator collects comprehensive data necessary to support perioperative and organizational services.

Measurement

E.1.1. Uses evidence-based processes to collect pertinent data in a systematic and ongoing manner to support perioperative services.

E.1.2. Sets priorities for data collection activities based on the needs of the department, the organization, and perioperative patients.

E.1.3. Involves internal and external stakeholders, as appropriate, in systematic data collection.

E.1.4. Develops mechanisms to resolve missing or insufficient data, information, and knowledge resources.

E.1.5. Develops, maintains, and evaluates retrievable data management systems to support perioperative services.

E.2.　Standard 2: Identifies Issues or Trends

The perioperative RN administrator analyzes data to develop ideas and support decisions relevant to the delivery of perioperative nursing care.

Measurement

E.2.1. Synthesizes available data to identify issues, patterns, trends, and variances involving perioperative nursing services.

E.2.2. Collaborates with internal and external stakeholders when analyzing data as appropriate.

E.2.3. Validates the issues and trends with internal and external stakeholders as appropriate.

E.2.4. Reports issues or trends to internal and external stakeholders as appropriate.

E.2.5. Documents issues and trends in a retrievable format to facilitate outcome identification and planning.

E.3.　Standard 3: Outcomes Identification

The perioperative RN administrator identifies expected outcomes for perioperative services.

Measurement

E.3.1. Develops outcomes for perioperative nursing service using assessment findings and analysis.

E.3.2. Develops and maintains policies and procedures that support the outcomes.

E.3.3. Identifies evidenced-based outcomes using standardized perioperative nursing language.

E.3.4. Supports perioperative RNs and other health care personnel to achieve quality patient care outcomes.

E.3.5. Promotes acquisition of appropriate technologies to provide patient and worker safety.

E.3.6. Identifies a physically, emotionally, and psychologically safe work environment as a priority.

E.3.7. Identifies a time frame in which to achieve the outcomes.

E.3.8. Modifies outcomes based on issues, trends, and research.

E.4.　Standard 4: Planning

The perioperative RN administrator develops the process and strategic plan to attain expected outcomes for perioperative services.

Measurement

E.4.1. Considers organizational and departmental structure, as well as lines of authority, when planning to meet the outcomes.

E.4.2. Develops a strategic plan that is consistent with the mission, vision, and values of the organization.

E.4.3. Establishes a timeline for processes and strategies to carry out the plan.

E.4.4. Uses current laws, regulations, and standards to guide the planning process.

E.4.5. Bases the plan on current research and other evidence.

E.4.6. Assigns duties and responsibilities to carry out the plan with job descriptions, scope of practice, and regulatory and accrediting agencies.

E.4.7. Considers the physical, psychosocial, and economic effect of the plan.

E.4.8. Modifies the strategic plan based on issues and trends in the department.

E.4.9. Documents the strategic plan in a retrievable format.

E.5.　Standard 5: Implementation

The perioperative RN administrator implements a strategic plan within the organizational and departmental structure.

Measurement

E.5.1. Implements the strategic plan by following the defined timeline with special consideration to the perioperative patient and workplace safety.

E.5.2. Provides those implementing the plan with sufficient time and material, as well as intellectual, human, and financial resources.

E.5.3. Uses health care organization and community resources to support implementation.

E.5.4. Coordinates and documents implementation of the plan, including modifications.

E.5.5. Communicates with internal and external stakeholders regarding implementation and modifications.

E.5.6. Encourages the development of organizational systems and processes that support implementation.

E.5.a. Standard 5a: Coordination

The perioperative RN administrator coordinates implementation of the plan, using appropriate human and capital resources.

Measurement

E.5.a.1. Organizes implementation with consideration for budgetary, health care organization, and community resources.

E.5.a.2. Promotes efficient integration of services to implement the plan.

E.5.a.3. Leads the coordination of efforts related to perioperative care and associated services when implementing the plan.

E.5.b. Standard 5b: Health Teaching and Health Promotion

The perioperative RN administrator employs strategies to promote workplace safety and health.

Measurement

E.5.b.1. Uses regulatory and evidence-based professional guidelines to implement workplace safety practices.

E.5.b.2. Promotes workplace safety by applying wellness techniques.

E.5.b.3. Commits to practicing self-care and promoting wellness with others.

E.5.c. Standard 5c: Consultation

The perioperative RN administrator provides consultation to communicate the identified plan.

Measurement

E.5.c.1. Acts as a resource to internal and external stakeholders regarding perioperative nursing care, perioperative patient outcomes, and perioperative services.

E.5.c.2. Uses assessment data, theoretical frameworks, current research, and evidence related to perioperative nursing care when providing consultation.

E.5.c.3. Provides consultation based on experience and knowledge of perioperative standards of care, recommended practices, laws, and regulations.

E.6. Standard 6: Evaluation

The perioperative RN administrator evaluates the effectiveness of the plan toward achieving desired outcomes.

Measurement

E.6.1. Measures progress toward strategic planning goals at regular intervals to determine their validity.

E.6.2. Reviews the plan for compliance with legal, regulatory, and credentialing requirements and guidelines.

E.6.3. Includes internal and external stakeholders when evaluating progress toward or achievement of outcomes.

E.6.4. Takes action based on the results of the evaluation to modify processes or structures.

E.6.5. Reports evaluation results to internal and external stakeholders.

E.6.6. Documents results of progress toward attaining outcomes.

E.7. Standard 7: Quality of Practice

The perioperative RN administrator guides improvement of care delivery using key indicators.

Measurement

E.7.1. Coordinates efforts and assigns personnel to systematically collect and record data in a retrievable format related to quality indicators.

E.7.2. Tracks data to develop performance improvement initiatives that support the delivery of high-quality patient care.

E.7.3. Develops written plans to monitor organizational or departmental outcomes at regular intervals.

E.7.4. Uses data to initiate organizational or departmental changes to provide high-quality patient care.

E.7.5. Identifies pertinent evidence to establish appropriate benchmarks.

E.7.6. Compares benchmark data to challenge current practice and organizational or departmental outcomes.

E.7.7. Incorporates research and current evidence to enhance quality and improve delivery of care.

E.7.8. Analyzes data to identify trends, variances, and patterns that affect perioperative nursing services.

E.7.9. Uses analysis to develop and enact new policies and procedures to improve perioperative nursing services.

E.7.10. Validates privileges, credentials, or certifications to schedule procedures appropriately.

E.7.11. Reports quality outcomes to internal and external stakeholders in compliance with state and federal requirements.

E.8. Standard 8: Education

The perioperative RN administrator has advanced educational preparation and management experience to direct perioperative services.

Measurement

E.8.1. Achieves advanced education in nursing or a related field.

E.8.2. Demonstrates management and leadership skills.

E.8.3. Validates experience in perioperative nursing.

E.8.4. Participates in ongoing educational activities related to leadership, management, and perioperative nursing.

E.8.5. Upholds local, state, federal, legislative, and regulatory activities affecting perioperative nursing services.

E.8.6. Recognizes professional standards, recommended practices, and guidelines pertinent to perioperative nursing services.

E.8.7. Maintains professional records to document ongoing competence.

E.9. Standard 9: Professional Practice Evaluation

The perioperative RN administrator follows regulatory, accrediting, and professional guidelines and regulations to evaluate professional practice of self and members of the department.

Measurement

E.9.1. Engages in self-evaluation of perioperative practice on a regular basis, identifying areas of strength as well as opportunities for professional development.

E.9.2. Validates competence of self and others at regular intervals.

E.9.3. Participates in a systematic peer review of self and others.

E.9.4. Provides a rationale for practice beliefs, decisions, and actions as part of the informal and formal evaluation processes.

E.9.5. Respects diversity in all interactions.

E.9.6. Ensures ongoing departmental compliance with local, state, national, and professional legislative and regulations.

E.9.7. Conducts formal performance reviews at regular intervals based on patient and departmental outcomes.

E.9.8. Solicits informal and formal feedback regarding departmental performance from appropriate internal and external stakeholders.

E.10. Standard 10: Collegiality

The perioperative RN administrator promotes the professional development of others.

Measurement

E.10.1. Serves as a professional role model and mentor to motivate, develop, recruit, and retain perioperative RNs and colleagues.

E.10.2. Establishes a learning environment that is open and respectful to others.

E.10.3. Shares expertise to advance the mission, vision, and values of the organization and promote positive perioperative outcomes.

E.10.4. Provides opportunities and support for continuing education, professional development, and formal education.

E.10.5. Promotes specialty certification.

E.10.6. Promotes active membership and participation in professional organizations.

E.10.7. Encourages staff member participation on multidisciplinary teams that improve perioperative nursing practice.

E.10.8. Enhances own professional perioperative nursing practice and role performance through interactions with peers and colleagues.

E.11. Standard 11: Collaboration

The perioperative RN administrator collaborates with internal and external stakeholders to improve perioperative services.

Measurement

E.11.1. Participates on system-wide committees as a perioperative resource to influence organizational decisions, policies, and procedures.

E.11.2. Oversees departmental activities, providing expert input regarding perioperative and organizational interests.

E.11.3. Interacts with health care providers to promote positive perioperative outcomes.

E.11.4. Partners with internal and external stakeholders to influence health care policy decisions affecting perioperative services and outcomes.

E.11.5. Documents collaborative efforts toward improving perioperative services, including planning, implementation, and effectiveness.

E.12. Standard 12: Ethics

The perioperative RN administrator ensures that ethical processes are used to deliver perioperative services.

Measurement

E.12.1. Establishes an environment where perioperative team members engage in competent, ethical, and legal practices.

E.12.2. Ensures the protection of human rights for all individuals in the perioperative setting.

E.12.3. Maintains privacy and confidentiality of individuals and health information within the perioperative setting.

E.12.4. Fosters a nondiscriminatory climate within the perioperative setting.

E.12.5. Maintains sensitivity to diversity within the perioperative setting.

E.12.6. Uses resources within the organization to address ethical issues.

E.13. Standard 13: Research

The perioperative RN administrator supports and integrates current research and other available evidence into perioperative services.

Measurement

E.13.1. Evaluates and updates practice decisions based on available evidence and current research findings.

E.13.2. Creates a supportive environment with sufficient resources for nurses to investigate research findings and initiate evidence-based best practices.

E.13.3. Promotes dissemination of knowledge gained from evidence-based activities via presentations, publications, and consultation.

E.13.4. Ensures that departmental research priorities align with the mission, vision, values, and strategic plan of the organization.

E.13.5. Aligns departmental research priorities with those set by professional nursing organizations, regulatory agencies, and accrediting bodies.

E.13.6. Incorporates evidence-based practice to improve perioperative patient outcomes.

E.13.7. Incorporates evidence-based practice to improve and support a positive work environment.

E.13.8. Supports research activities that contribute to perioperative nursing knowledge.

E.14. Standard 14: Resource Utilization

The perioperative RN administrator uses human and material resources to deliver safe, high-quality, and cost-effective perioperative services.

Measurement

E.14.1. Considers safety and effectiveness when analyzing the cost-benefit ratios that affect perioperative services.

E.14.2. Allocates resources to promote quality patient outcomes.

E.14.3. Allocates fiscal resources to support the perioperative services strategic plan.

E.14.4. Advocates for human and material resources by using patient acuity and nursing workload guidelines to deliver safe patient care.

E.14.5. Advocates for human and material resources to support a safe work environment.

E.14.6. Identifies strategies for cost-effective and efficient practices without compromising perioperative patient safety or outcomes.

E.14.7. Promotes creative thinking among staff members, peers, and colleagues to develop new and innovative devices, practices, and strategies to advance and improve perioperative nursing services.

E.14.8. Advocates for environmental consciousness when using and managing resources in the perioperative setting.

E.14.9. Provides documentation for internal and external stakeholders to demonstrate costs, risks, and benefits that support decisions for perioperative practices.

E.15. Standard 15: Leadership

The perioperative RN administrator provides leadership within the organization and the profession.

Measurement

E.15.1. Maintains membership in relevant professional organizations related to leadership and perioperative nursing.

E.15.2. Strives to achieve relevant professional specialty certification(s).

E.15.3. Acts as a leader on administrative teams participating in decision making that affects perioperative services.

E.15.4. Participates in activities to influence legislative or regulatory decisions that affect perioperative services and perioperative nursing practice.

E.15.5. Leads committees, task forces, councils, and teams to make decisions that positively influence perioperative services, perioperative nursing practice, or perioperative patient outcomes.

E.15.6. Supervises perioperative personnel and supports their roles in promoting positive patient outcomes.

E.15.7. Promotes life-long learning among personnel involved with perioperative services.

E.15.8. Inspires loyalty, teamwork, respect, and professionalism among personnel involved with perioperative services.

E.15.9. Promotes an environment that fosters independent and creative critical thinking.

E.15.10. Acts as a leader and change agent, supporting evidence-based practices in the perioperative setting.

E.15.11. Advances knowledge of perioperative services and perioperative nursing by communicating pertinent information through publishing and presenting for professional and lay audiences.

E.16. Standard 16: Advocacy

The perioperative RN administrator advocates for individuals and groups related to perioperative health and safety.

Measurement

E.16.1. Advocates for one perioperative RN circulator per patient in the intraoperative phase of care.

E.16.2. Supports perioperative patients' health care rights by involving individuals in their own care.

E.16.3. Endorses regulatory measures that provide for safe patient care and workplace safety.

E.16.4. Incorporates safe perioperative care into the design, implementation, and evaluation of policies, programs, services, and systems.

E.16.5. Allocates resources to support advocacy activities related to perioperative services and the nursing profession.

E.16.6. Supports the perioperative patient's right to access personal health data and information related to privacy, security, and confidentiality.

E.16.7. Promotes a philosophy of advocacy in the perioperative environment.

REFERENCES

1. *Nursing: Scope and Standards of Practice.* Washington, DC: American Nurses Association; 2004.
2. *Scope and Standards for Nurse Administrators.* Washington, DC: American Nurses Association; 2009.
3. Petersen C, ed. *Perioperative Nursing Data Set.* 2nd ed rev. Denver, CO. AORN, Inc; 2007.
4. *Nursing's Social Policy Statement.* 2nd ed. Washington, DC: American Nurses Association; 2003.

PUBLICATION HISTORY

Standards of Perioperative Nursing Practice

Compiled from previous editions for publication in *Perioperative Standards and Recommended Practices* (Denver, CO: AORN, Inc; 2009).

Revised October 2009 for online publication in *Perioperative Standards and Recommended Practices.*

AORN gratefully acknowledges the work of the 2007–2008, 2008–2009, and 2009–2010 Nursing Practice Committees

2007–2008, 2009–2010 CHAIR,
2008–2009 ADVISOR
Antonia Hughes, RN, BSN, MA, CNOR
Perioperative Education Specialist
Baltimore Washington Medical Center
Glen Burnie, Maryland

2008–2009 CHAIR, 2007–2010 MEMBER
Sharon L. Chappy, RN, PhD, CNOR
Associate Professor
University of Wisconsin Oshkosh
Oshkosh, Wisconsin

MEMBERS
Beth A. Beilein, RN, BSN, MSM, CNOR
(2009–2010)
Director of Clinical Operations
Naples Day Surgery, South
Naples, Florida

James (Jay) Bowers, RN, BSN, CNOR (2007–2008)
Clinical Nurse Preceptor
West Virginia University Hospitals
Morgantown, West Virginia

Judith L. Clayton, RN, CNOR (2007–2009)
Perioperative Clinical Educator
Gwinnett Medical Center
Duluth, Georgia

Nikki A. Collier, RN, CNOR, CRNFA (2008–2010)
RN First Assistant
St Joseph Hospital
Eureka, California

Joy Crouse, RN, MS, CNOR (2007–2008)
Clinical Supervisor
St Josephs Hospital and Medical Center
Phoenix, Arizona

Jim D'Alfonso, RN, MSN, CNOR (2007–2009)
Associate Vice President
Scottsdale Healthcare Shea
Mesa, Arizona

Vicki Dreger, RN, MSN, CNOR (2007–2009)
Staff Nurse
Advocate Christ Medical Center
Oak Lawn, Illinois

Elizabeth Gasson, RN, MSN, CNOR (2009–2010)
Clinical Director
River Oaks Hospital
Jackson, Mississippi

Denise M. Jackson, RN, MSN, CNS, CRNFA
(2009–2010)
RN First Assistant
Shannon Medical Center
San Angelo, Texas

Ellice M. Mellinger, RN, MS, CNOR (2008–2010)
Clinical Educator
University Medical Center
Tucson, Arizona

Barbara A. Ricker, RN, MSN, CNOR (2007–2009)
RN Clinical Development Professional
Banner Health
Phoenix, Arizona

Linda P. Voyles, RN, BSN, CNOR (2009–2010)
Perioperative Educator
Banner Estrella
Phoenix, Arizona

Dawn M. Yost, RDH, RN, BSN, CNOR (2008–2010)
Manager of Nursing Operations and Sterile
Processing
West Virginia University Hospitals
Morgantown, West Virginia

2009–2010 BOARD LIAISON
Peter Graves, RN, BSN, CNOR
Consultant
Corinth, Texas

2007–2009 BOARD LIAISON
Jane Kusler-Jensen, RN, BSN, MBA, CNOR
Director of Perioperative Services
Ozaukee and River Woods Campuses,
Columbia-St Mary's
Milwaukee, Wisconsin

2007–2010 STAFF CONSULTANT
Bonnie G. Denholm, RN, BSN, MS, CNOR
Perioperative Nursing Specialist
AORN Center for Nursing Practice
Denver, Colorado

2007–2010 ADMINISTRATIVE SUPPORT
Bonnie Kibbe

EXHIBIT A: Historical Perspectives on the AORN Standards, Competency Statements, and Certification

AORN's first "Standards of nursing practice: OR" were developed with the American Nurses Association (ANA) Division of Medical Surgical Practice and printed in 1975. In addition to these standards, AORN began publishing recommended practices in the technical aspects of perioperative nursing in March 1975. Subsequently, AORN developed a variety of programs and activities to assist perioperative registered nurses (RNs) to become aware of and use the standards to evaluate their professional practice and the recommended practices to initiate best practices in their settings.

The standards were revised after data were collected from practicing perioperative RNs to determine the applicability and usefulness of the standards. The resulting revision, titled "Standards of perioperative nursing practice," was published in 1981. These standards were augmented by "Standards of administrative nursing practice: OR" in 1982, the "Patient outcome standards for perioperative nursing" in 1985, and the "Quality and Performance Improvement Standards for Perioperative Nursing" in 2004. In 2009, the standards collection was consolidated into one document with four exhibits that included historical perspectives, perioperative patient outcomes, perioperative explications for the ANA *Code of Ethics for Nurses*, and the quality and performance improvement standards.

The Nursing Practice Committee reviewed and updated the standards collection for 2010. Advanced practice RN measurements were added and the administrative standards were revised to align with the current ANA administrative standards. The outcome statements and the quality and performance improvement standards were removed from the exhibit section of the standards collection to facilitate flexibility in updating and distributing those documents. The content changes were posted on the AORN web site for public review and comment for 30 days. The AORN Board of Directors approved the revisions in October 2009.

The standards serve as the foundation for the AORN professional competency statements, which were first published by AORN in 1986. These statements are revised periodically to provide a means for perioperative nurses to validate and measure the quality of their practice. AORN developed competency statements for the perioperative advanced practice nurse, the perioperative care coordinator, and the RN first assistant in 1994, 1999, and 2002, respectively, to define other professional roles of the perioperative nurse. All four sets of competencies were published in a collection titled *Competencies for Perioperative Practice* in 2008. Together with the *Perioperative Nursing Data Set*, recognized by ANA in 1999 and published by AORN in 2000, these resources provide a comprehensive framework for creating job descriptions, performance appraisals, competency checklists, and credentialing documents that affirm and support the contribution of the perioperative RN in providing safe, effective patient care.

Certification in perioperative nursing (CNOR®) demonstrates the perioperative RN's individual commitment to excellence in practice in the clinical setting as well as AORN's ongoing commitment to fostering excellence in the clinical setting. The first perioperative RN certification program was approved by the AORN House of Delegates in 1978 to "enhance quality patient care" and to "demonstrate accountability to the general public for nursing practice." From this vote, a Certification Council was appointed by the AORN Board of Directors to oversee the development, direction, implementation, and evaluation of the entire certification process. The Council was incorporated in January 1980. Evolution in its organizational mission and structure resulted in name changes in 1985 and 1997. In 2005, the organization became the Competency & Credentialing Institute (CCI). Today, it offers credentialing, nursing competency assessment, education, and consulting on nursing competency issues.

AORN continues to encourage the achievement and maintenance of additional certifications applicable to various arenas of perioperative practice, such as first assisting (CRNFA®), administration, nursing informatics, and other subspeciality areas. Resolutions and statements adopted by the House of Delegates consistently reiterate the primacy of the Association's concern for quality and safety in patient care. Striving for excellence in practice, perioperative nurses actively participate in shaping the practice environment and identifying clinical and organizational indicators for quality patient care, patient and workplace safety, and performance improvement.

Editor's note: *CNOR and CRNFA are registered trademarks of the Competency and Credentialing Institute, Denver, CO.*

EXHIBIT B: Perioperative Explications for the
ANA Code of Ethics for Nurses

Editor's note: *The following is reprinted with permission from American Nurses Association,* Code of Ethics for Nurses with Interpretive Statements, © 2001 *American Nurses Publishing, American Nurses Foundation/American Nurses Association, Washington, DC.*

ANA Code of Ethics for Nurses With Interpretive Statements

Preface

Ethics is an integral part of the foundation of nursing. Nursing has a distinguished history of concern for the welfare of the sick, injured, and vulnerable and for social justice. This concern is embodied in the provision of nursing care to individuals and the community. Nursing encompasses the prevention of illness, the alleviation of suffering, and the protection, promotion, and restoration of health in the care of individuals, families, groups, and communities. Nurses act to change those aspects of social structures that detract from health and well-being. Individuals who become nurses are expected not only to adhere to the ideals and moral norms of the profession but also to embrace them as a part of what it means to be a nurse. The ethical tradition of nursing is self-reflective, enduring, and distinctive. A code of ethics makes explicit the primary goals, values, and obligations of the profession.

The *Code of Ethics for Nurses* serves the following purposes:

♦ It is a succinct statement of the ethical obligations and duties of every individual who enters the nursing profession.

♦ It is the profession's nonnegotiable ethical standard.

♦ It is an expression of nursing's own understanding of its commitment to society.

There are numerous approaches for addressing ethics; these include adopting or subscribing to ethical theories, including humanist, feminist, and social ethics, adhering to ethical principles, and cultivating virtues. The *Code of Ethics for Nurses* reflects all of these approaches. The words "ethical" and "moral" are used throughout the *Code of Ethics*. "Ethical" is used to refer to reasons for decisions about how one ought to act, using the above mentioned approaches. In general, the word "moral" overlaps with "ethical" but is more aligned with personal belief and cultural values. Statements that describe activities and attributes

Preamble

The American Nurses Association (ANA) *Code of Ethics for Nurses with Interpretive Statements* expresses the moral commitment to uphold the goals, values, and distinct ethical obligations of all nurses. As nursing is practiced in a changing social context, the *Code of Ethics for Nurses* becomes a dynamic document. AORN's Ethics Task Force detailed the specific perioperative nursing explications that correspond to the nine provisions from the ANA *Code of Ethics for Nurses with Interpretive Statements* (ANA, 2001). The primary goals and values of a profession are made explicit in a code of ethics.

Together, the ANA code and the explications for perioperative nursing provide the framework within which perioperative nurses can make ethical decisions. The code establishes the profession's nonnegotiable ethical standard. This document demonstrates accountability and responsibility to the public, to

---

About This Document

The ANA *Code of Ethics for Nurses with Interpretive Statements,* updated in 2001, is composed of nine provisions, with each provision further subdivided under provision headings. In the following document, the nine ANA provisions are listed in the **left-hand column** and identified by large numerals; the provision headings are identified by numerical subheads (eg, 1.1, 1.2, 1.3, etc). AORN's *Explications* are printed in the **right-hand column** following the same format. Each "Perioperative explication" is illustrated by "Perioperative examples" that pertain to a particular ANA provision heading. The *Explications* read from the top of the right-hand column on one page to the bottom, to the top of the right-hand column on the next page to the bottom, and so on.

The ANA *Code of Ethics for Nurses with Interpretive Statements* can be viewed in its entirety, at no charge, at *http://nursingworld.org/ethics/code/protected_nwcoe813.htm.* You can purchase a copy online at *http://nursingworld.org/MainMenu Categories/ThePracticeofProfessionalNursing/Ethics Standards/CodeofEthics.aspx.*

Code of Ethics for Nurses with Interpretive Statements *reprinted with permission from American Nurses Association,* © 2001 Nursesbooks.org, Silver Spring, MD.

---

of nurses in this *Code of Ethics* are to be understood as normative or prescriptive statements expressing expectations of ethical behavior.

The *Code of Ethics for Nurses* uses the term *patient* to refer to recipients of nursing care. The derivation of this word refers to "one who suffers," reflecting a universal aspect of human existence. Nonetheless, it is recognized that nurses also provide services to those seeking health as well as those responding to illness, to students and to staff, in health care facilities as well as in communities. Similarly, the term *practice* refers to the actions of the nurse in whatever role the nurse fulfills, including direct patient care provider, educator, administrator, researcher, policy developer, or other. Thus, the values and obligations expressed in this *Code of Ethics* apply to nurses in all roles and settings.

The *Code of Ethics for Nurses* is a dynamic document. As nursing and its social context change, changes to the *Code of Ethics* are also necessary. The *Code of Ethics* consists of two components: the provisions and the accompanying interpretive statements. There are nine provisions. The first three describe the most fundamental values and commitments of the nurse, the next three address boundaries of duty and loyalty, and the last three address aspects of duties beyond individual patient encounters. For each provision, there are interpretive statements that provide greater specificity for practice and are responsive to the contemporary context of nursing. Consequently, the interpretive statements are subject to more frequent revision than are the provisions. Additional ethical guidance and detail can be found in ANA or constituent member association position statements that address clinical, research, administrative, educational, or public policy issues.

The *Code of Ethics for Nurses with Interpretive Statements* provides a framework for nurses to use in ethical analysis and decision-making. The *Code of Ethics* establishes the ethical standard for the profession. It is not negotiable in any setting, nor is it subject to revision or amendment except by formal process of the House of Delegates of the ANA. The *Code of Ethics for Nurses* is a reflection of the proud ethical heritage of nursing, a guide for nurses now and in the future.

other members of the health care team, and to the profession. This document helps perioperative nurses relate the ANA *Code of Ethics* to their own areas of practice and provides examples of behaviors that reflect the ethical obligations of perioperative nurses.

Introduction

Ethical decisions for the perioperative nurse are often difficult but necessary during the care of the surgical patient. Additionally, perioperative nurses need to be able to recognize ethical dilemmas and take action. Perioperative nurses are responsible for nursing decisions that are not only clinically and technically sound but also morally appropriate and suitable for the specific problems of the particular patient being treated. The technical or medical aspects of the decision answer the question, "What can be done for this patient?" The moral component involves the patient's wishes and answers the question, "What should be done for this patient?"

The strength of the ethical perspective is its resolute nature. It promotes an action guide for nurses to follow in the realm of patient care. Ethics, as a branch of philosophy, incorporates multiple approaches to take when dealing with or applying actions to real life situations. Thus, each perioperative nurse may experience a situation differently, as well as addressing the situation and identifying the ethical conflict issues, his or her feelings, behaviors, actions, analysis, and resolution of the situation differently.

Health care delivery provided via a team format, such as the surgical team, does not necessarily create ethical conflicts, but it may highlight the conflicts if the values of the team members emphasize different priorities. Additionally, new roles of health care team members may carry expectations about how members should interact with each other and how standards of care should be met.

The perioperative nurse, by virtue of the nurse-patient relationship, has an obligation to provide safe, professional, and ethical patient care. It is important that nurses know how to manage ethical decisions appropriately so that patients' beliefs can be honored without compromising the nurse's own moral conscience. Ethical practice is thus a critical aspect of nursing care, and the development of ethical competency is paramount for present and future nursing practice.

EXHIBIT B: Perioperative Explications

1: The nurse, in all professional relationships, practices with compassion and respect for the inherent dignity, worth, and uniqueness of every individual, unrestricted by considerations of social or economic status, personal attributes, or the nature of health problems.

1.1 Respect for human dignity

A fundamental principle that underlies all nursing practice is respect for the inherent worth, dignity, and human rights of every individual. Nurses take into account the needs and values of all persons in all professional relationships.

1.2 Relationships to patients

The need for health care is universal, transcending all individual differences. The nurse establishes relationships and delivers nursing services with respect for human needs and values, and without prejudice. An individual's lifestyle, value system, and religious beliefs should be considered in planning health care with and for each patient. Such consideration does not suggest that the nurse necessarily agrees with or condones certain individual choices, but that the nurse respects the patient as a person.

Perioperative Explications

The perioperative nurse is morally obligated to respect the dignity and worth of each individual patient. Perioperative nursing care is provided to each patient undergoing a surgical or other invasive procedure in a manner that preserves and protects patient autonomy, dignity, and human rights.[1] Each nurse has an obligation to be knowledgeable about the moral and legal rights of all patients and to protect and support those rights. As health care does not occur in a vacuum, the perioperative nurse must take into account both the individual rights and the interdependence of individuals in decision-making.

Perioperative examples

- ♦ Respects patient's decision for surgery.
- ♦ Respects patient's wishes (eg, advance directives, end-of-life choices).
- ♦ Implements institutional advance directive policy in the practice setting.
- ♦ Restrains patient only when patient poses a direct or potential danger to self or others.

Perioperative Explications

It is the responsibility of the perioperative nurse to provide care for each patient without prejudicial behavior. The care should be planned with consideration for the patient's values, religious beliefs, lifestyle choices, and age. The perioperative nurse respects the worth and dignity of the patient regardless of the diagnosis, disease process, procedure, or projected outcome. When the perioperative nurse is ethically opposed to interventions or procedures in a particular case, the nurse is justified in refusing to participate if the refusal is made known in advance and in time for other appropriate arrangements to be made for the patient's nursing care. When the patient's life is in jeopardy, the perioperative nurse is obliged to provide for the patient's safety, to avoid abandonment, and to withdraw only when assured that alternative sources of nursing care are available to the patient.

Code of Ethics for Nurses with Interpretive Statements *reprinted with permission from American Nurses Association, © 2001 Nursesbooks.org, Silver Spring, MD.*

Perioperative examples
- ♦ Applies standards of nursing practice consistently to all patients with sensitivity to disability and economic, educational, cultural, religious, racial, age, and sexual differences.[2]
- ♦ Provides nursing care respecting the worth and dignity regardless of diagnosis, disease process, procedure, or projected outcome.[3]
- ♦ Respects the Patient's Bill of Rights.
- ♦ Refrains from derogatory comments about patients, families and significant others, colleagues, and other associates.
- ♦ Seeks guidance for resolving personal belief conflicts with the patient (eg, from supervisor, ethics committee, colleagues with appropriate authority).
- ♦ Uses principles of ethical analysis and moral reasoning to resolve ethical questions.[4]
- ♦ Provides spiritual comfort, arranges for appropriate substitute nursing care if personal beliefs conflict with required care, and respects the patient's decision for surgery.

Perioperative Explications

Perioperative nurses provide nursing care directed to meet the comprehensive needs of all patients, regardless of diagnosis, taking into consideration aspects of culture, language, perception of pain, significant others, values, and beliefs.[5] Nurses, as individuals, bring to their practice assumptions from their own culture, as well as about the cultures of others. In order to provide care that is culturally relevant to a diverse patient population, it is vital that nurses recognize the importance of each patient's values, beliefs, and health practices. In many instances, nurses provide care across cultures; thus, it becomes an ethical imperative for nurses to develop the skill of culturally competent caring.

To most effectively care for patients of other cultures, the nurse must be a conscientious observer, a perceptive listener, and thorough assessor. Acquiring information about the patient's culture and gaining further personal insight provides the nurse with an increased understanding of culture and values from both perspectives (the patient's and the nurse's) as they relate to providing culturally competent care.

Perioperative examples
- ♦ Provides nursing care respecting the patient's worth and dignity regardless of diagnosis, disease process, procedure, or projected outcome.[6]

1.3 The nature of health problems

The nurse respects the worth, dignity, and rights of all human beings irrespective of the nature of the health problem. The worth of the person is not affected by disease, disability, functional status, or proximity to death. This respect extends to all who require the services of the nurse for the promotion of health, the prevention of illness, the restoration of health, the alleviation of suffering, and the provision of supportive care to those who are dying.

The measures nurses take to care for the patient enable the patient to live with as much physical, emotional, social, and spiritual well-being as possible. Nursing care aims to maximize the values that the patient has treasured in life and extends supportive care to the family and significant others. Nursing care is directed toward meeting the comprehensive needs of patients and their families across the continuum of care. This is particularly vital in the care of patients and their families at the end of life to prevent and relieve the cascade of symptoms and suffering that are commonly associated with dying.

Nurses are leaders and vigilant advocates for the delivery of dignified and humane care. Nurses actively participate in assessing and assuring the responsible and appropriate use of interventions in order to minimize unwarranted or unwanted treatment and patient suffering. The acceptability and importance of carefully considered decisions regarding resuscitation status, withholding and withdrawing life-sustaining therapies, forgoing medically provided nutrition and hydration, aggressive pain and symptom management, and advance directives are increasingly evident. The nurse should provide interventions to relieve pain and other symptoms in the dying patient even when those interventions entail risks of hastening death. However, nurses may not act with the sole intent of ending a patient's life even though such action may be motivated by compassion, respect for patient autonomy, and quality of life considerations. Nurses have invaluable experience, knowledge, and insight into care at the end of life and should be actively involved in related research, education, practice, and policy development.

1.4   The right to self-determination

Respect for human dignity requires the recognition of specific patient rights, particularly, the right of self-determination. Self-determination, also known as autonomy, is the philosophical basis for informed consent in health care. Patients have the moral and legal right to determine what will be done with their own person; to be given accurate, complete, and understandable information in a manner that facilitates an informed judgment; to be assisted with weighing the benefits, burdens, and available options in their treatment, including the choice of no treatment; to accept, refuse, or terminate treatment without deceit, undue influence, duress, coercion, or penalty; and to be given necessary support throughout the decision-making and treatment process. Such support would include the opportunity to make decisions with family and significant others and the provision of advice and support from knowledgeable nurses and other health professionals. Patients should be involved in planning their own health care to the extent they are able and choose to participate.

Each nurse has an obligation to be knowledgeable about the moral and legal rights of all patients to self-determination. The nurse preserves, protects, and supports those interests by assessing the patient's comprehension of both the information presented

♦ Overcomes communication barriers to allow patients and their significant others to express preferences for care, providing interpreters when necessary.[7]

Perioperative Explications

Patients have the right to self-determination (ie, the ability to decide for oneself what course of action will be taken in various circumstances). The perioperative nurse provides care to each patient undergoing surgical intervention in a manner that preserves and protects patient autonomy, dignity, and human rights. The patient's autonomy in the decision-making process is acknowledged and supported by the perioperative nurse, who provides accurate, appropriate, and reasonable information to assist the patient in making an informed choice.[8] The perioperative nurse elicits the patient's response regarding perception of the surgical procedure and the implications of decisions. The perioperative nurse ensures that the patient has access to additional and accurate information.[9]

When individual rights must be temporarily overridden to preserve the life of the patient or of another person, the suspension of those rights must be considered a deviation to be tolerated as briefly as possible.

Perioperative examples

♦ Provides information and explains the Patient Self-Determination Act (eg, informed consent, living will, power of attorney for health care, do-not-resuscitate order, organ procurement).[10]

♦ Confirms that informed consent has been granted for planned procedure;[11] when possible, obtains surrogate's permission for emergency surgery.

and the implications of decisions. In situations in which the patient lacks the capacity to make a decision, a designated surrogate decision-maker should be consulted. The role of the surrogate is to make decisions as the patient would, based upon the patient's previously expressed wishes and known values. In the absence of a designated surrogate decision-maker, decisions should be made in the best interests of the patient, considering the patient's personal values to the extent that they are known. The nurse supports patient self-determination by participating in discussions with surrogates, providing guidance and referral to other resources as necessary, and identifying and addressing problems in the decision-making process. Support of autonomy in the broadest sense also includes recognition that people of some cultures place less weight on individualism and choose to defer to family or community values in decision-making. Respect not just for the specific decision but also for the patient's method of decision-making is consistent with the principle of autonomy.

Individuals are interdependent members of the community. The nurse recognizes that there are situations in which the right to individual self-determination may be outweighed or limited by the rights, health, and welfare of others, particularly in relation to public health considerations. Nonetheless, limitation of individual rights must always be considered a serious deviation from the standard of care, justified only when there are no less restrictive means available to preserve the rights of others and the demands of justice.

1.5 Relationships with colleagues and others

The principle of respect for persons extends to all individuals with whom the nurse interacts. The nurse maintains compassionate and caring relationships with colleagues and others with a commitment to the fair treatment of individuals, to integrity-preserving compromise, and to resolving conflict. Nurses function in many roles, including direct care provider, administrator, educator, researcher, and consultant. In each of these roles, the nurse treats colleagues, employees, assistants, and students with respect and compassion. This standard of conduct precludes any and all prejudicial actions, any form of harassment or threatening behavior, or disregard

Code of Ethics for Nurses with Interpretive Statements *reprinted with permission from American Nurses Association, © 2001 Nursesbooks.org, Silver Spring, MD.*

- ◆ Explains procedures before initiating action.
- ◆ Restrains patient only when patient poses a direct danger to self or others.
- ◆ Respects advance directives and end-of-life choices.
- ◆ Implements institutional advance directive policy in practice setting.
- ◆ Participates in perioperative teaching; answers patient's questions accurately and honestly.
- ◆ Allows choices within RN scope of practice (eg, child's preference for transport to the operating room, wagon versus cart).
- ◆ Formulates ethical decisions with assistance of available resources (eg, ethics committee, ethicists).

Perioperative Explications

Perioperative nurses must recognize the individuality not only of their patients, but also of their colleagues and others. As health care is not provided in a vacuum, nurses must be able to interact with a variety of other professionals and ancillary providers in the perioperative environment. In working with colleagues, perioperative nurses display the same nondiscriminatory and nonjudgmental behavior as they do with their patients. Treating others with professionalism and respect will enhance the performance of the health care team.

Perioperative nurses are compelled to treat colleagues and all people in a just and fair manner regardless of disability, economic status, level of education, culture, religion, race, age, and sexuality. Just as nurses have the right not to be abused or harassed in the workplace, so must they treat others for the effect of one's actions on others. The nurse values the distinctive contribution of individuals or groups, and collaborates to meet the shared goal of providing quality health services.

2: The nurse's primary commitment is to the patient, whether an individual, family, group, or community.

2.1 Primacy of the patient's interests

The nurse's primary commitment is to the recipient of nursing and health care services—the patient—whether the recipient is an individual, a family, a group, or a community. Nursing holds a fundamental commitment to the uniqueness of the individual patient; therefore, any plan of care must reflect that uniqueness. The nurse strives to provide patients with opportunities to participate in planning care, assures that patients find the plans acceptable, and supports the implementation of the plan. Addressing patient interests requires recognition of the patient's place in the family or other networks of relationship. When the patient's wishes are in conflict with others, the nurse seeks to help resolve the conflict. Where conflict persists, the nurse's commitment remains to the identified patient.

Code of Ethics for Nurses with Interpretive Statements *reprinted with permission from American Nurses Association, © 2001 Nursesbooks.org, Silver Spring, MD.*

in their workplace with respect and compassion. The nurse recognizes the contributions of each member of the health care team and works to collaborate to achieve quality patient care.

Perioperative examples
- Integrates cultural differences of coworkers.
- Recognizes and respects the value of all team members, including students and ancillary and support staff members.
- Provides education and information to coworkers, including ancillary and support staff.
- Promotes comparable levels of care in all practice settings in which invasive procedures are performed.
- Uses medical devices in a safe manner and complies with the Safe Medical Devices Act and other laws and regulations.

Perioperative Explications

The perioperative nurse supports both the interdependence and the individual rights of the patient when making decisions. The perioperative nurse collaborates in a manner that preserves and protects the patient's autonomy, dignity, and human rights. When individual rights must be temporarily overridden to preserve the life of the patient or of another person (eg, in the case of violent patients or patients with communicable diseases), the suspension of those rights must be considered a deviation to be tolerated as briefly as possible.

Perioperative examples
- Collaborates with patient regarding health care whenever possible.
- Collects patient health data.
- Analyzes assessment data and utilizes the *Perioperative Nursing Data Set* (PNDS) to formulate a nursing diagnosis and plan nursing care.
- Identifies expected outcomes unique to the patient.[12]
- Considers assessment information, including patient preferences and unique needs, when developing an individualized plan of care to attain designated patient outcomes.[13]
- Includes family/significant others in planning care.[14]
- Provides for spiritual comfort to the patient and significant others (eg, contacts religious counselor).

♦ Acts as patient advocate.
♦ Provides interpreters when necessary.
♦ Respects patient's decision to choose or refuse care or interventions.

Perioperative Explications

Conflicts may arise from financial considerations in the perioperative setting that may contribute to conflicting loyalties between the perioperative nurse and the patient. While the perioperative nurse needs to be fiscally responsible, the perioperative nurse's primary responsibility is to ensure that the patient's safety is maintained.

The perioperative nurse does not give or imply endorsement to advertising, promotion, or sale of commercial products or services in a manner that may be interpreted as reflecting the opinion or judgment of the profession as a whole.

Perioperative examples

♦ Identifies and resolves conflicts of interest effectively.
♦ Abstains from influencing purchasing decisions involving companies in which nurses have ownership to make financial gains (eg, stocks, other equity interest).
♦ The perioperative nurse does not solicit or accept gifts, gratuities, or other items of value that reasonably could be interpreted by others as influencing impartiality.

2.2 Conflict of interest for nurses

Nurses are frequently put in situations of conflict arising from competing loyalties in the workplace, including situations of conflicting expectations from patients, families, physicians, colleagues, and in many cases, health care organizations and health plans. Nurses must examine the conflicts arising between their own personal and professional values, the values and interests of others who are also responsible for patient care and health care decisions, as well as those of patients. Nurses strive to resolve such conflicts in ways that ensure patient safety, guard the patient's best interests, and preserve the professional integrity of the nurse.

Situations created by changes in health care financing and delivery systems, such as incentive systems to decrease spending, pose new possibilities of conflict between economic self-interest and professional integrity. The use of bonuses, sanctions, and incentives tied to financial targets are examples of features of health care systems that may present such conflict. Conflicts of interest may arise in any domain of nursing activity, including clinical practice, administration, education, or research. Advanced practice nurses who bill directly for services and nursing executives with budgetary responsibilities must be especially cognizant of the potential for conflicts of interest. Nurses should disclose to all relevant parties (eg, patients, employers, colleagues) any perceived or actual conflict of interest and in some situations should withdraw from further participation. Nurses in all roles must seek to ensure that employment arrangements are just and fair and do not create an unreasonable conflict between patient care and direct personal gain.

2.3 Collaboration

Collaboration is not just cooperation, but it is the concerted effort of individuals and groups to attain a shared goal. In health care, that goal is to address the health needs of the patient and the public. The

Code of Ethics for Nurses with Interpretive Statements reprinted with permission from American Nurses Association, © 2001 Nursesbooks.org, Silver Spring, MD.

Perioperative Explications

The perioperative nurse respects the interdependence of all health care providers in achieving positive outcomes for patients undergoing a surgical or other invasive procedure. As a fundamental member of the surgical team, the perioperative nurse actively participates with other health care professionals when planning and providing patient care. The perioperative nurse, nurse managers, complexity of health care delivery systems requires a multidisciplinary approach to the delivery of services that has the strong support and active participation of all the health professions. Within this context, nursing's unique contribution, scope of practice, and relationship with other health professions needs to be clearly articulated, represented, and preserved. By its very nature, collaboration requires mutual trust, recognition, and respect among the health care team, shared decision-making about patient care, and open dialogue among all parties who have an interest in and a concern for health outcomes. Nurses should work to assure that the relevant parties are involved and have a voice in decision-making about patient care issues. Nurses should see that the questions that need to be addressed are asked and that the information needed for informed decision-making is available and provided. Nurses should actively promote the collaborative multidisciplinary planning required to ensure the availability and accessibility of quality health services to all persons who have needs for health care.

Intraprofessional collaboration within nursing is fundamental to effectively addressing the health needs of patients and the public. Nurses engaged in nonclinical roles, such as administration or research, while not providing direct care, nonetheless are collaborating in the provision of care through their influence and direction of those who do. Effective nursing care is accomplished through the interdependence of nurses in differing roles—those who teach the needed skills, set standards, manage the environment of care, or expand the boundaries of knowledge used by the profession. In this sense, nurses in all roles share a responsibility for the outcomes of nursing care.

2.4   Professional boundaries

When acting within one's role as a professional, the nurse recognizes and maintains boundaries that establish appropriate limits to relationships. While the nature of nursing work has an inherently personal component, nurse-patient relationships and nurse-colleague relationships have, as their foundation, the purpose of preventing illness, alleviating suffering, and protecting, promoting, and restoring the health of patients. In this way, nurse-patient and nurse-colleague relationships differ from those that are

educators, and researchers need to participate in direct and indirect multidisciplinary planning and decision-making regarding patient care protocols and activities.

Perioperative examples

- Collaborates with the surgeon and anesthesia care provider to plan care specific to the procedure and the patient's needs.
- Collaborates and consults with nursing colleagues in the perioperative setting and practicing in other specialty areas (eg, RN first assistant [RNFA], critical care, psychiatry, pain management, pediatrics, postanesthesia care, home health).
- Demonstrates collaborative practice among subspecialties within and outside the perioperative arena.
- Collaborates with ancillary and support staff to enhance communication and work patterns that are mutually beneficial for staff and for efficient patient care.
- Collaborates with the public, industry, and health care workers regarding environmental and cost-containment issues
- Formulates ethical decisions with assistance of available resources (eg, ethics committee, counselors, and ethicists).

Perioperative Explications

Perioperative nurses promote and maintain professional relationships with patients, peers, coworkers, and all members of the surgical team. Perioperative nurses are aware of the intimate nature of nursing care, the highly stressful nature of the surgical environment, and the collegial nature of the surgical team. The perioperative nurse respects professional boundaries in the nurse-patient relationship and does not convey undue influence on patient decisions. Perioperative nurses play a critical role in providing information to patients so that decisions affecting that patient will be appropriate and effective.

The nurse should seek the assistance of peers or supervisors, without hesitation, when professional purely personal and unstructured, such as friendship. The intimate nature of nursing care, the involvement of nurses in important and sometimes highly stressful life events, and the mutual dependence of colleagues working in close concert all present the potential for blurring of limits to professional relationships. Maintaining authenticity and expressing oneself as an individual, while remaining within the bounds established by the purpose of the relationship, can be especially difficult in prolonged or long-term relationships. In all encounters, nurses are responsible for retaining their professional boundaries. When those professional boundaries are jeopardized, the nurse should seek assistance from peers or supervisors or take appropriate steps to remove her/himself from the situation.

3 : The nurse promotes, advocates for, and strives to protect the health, safety, and rights of the patient.

3.1 Privacy

The nurse safeguards the patient's right to privacy. The need for health care does not justify unwanted intrusion into the patient's life. The nurse advocates for an environment that provides for sufficient physical privacy, including auditory privacy for discussions of a personal nature and policies and practices that protect the confidentiality of information.

boundaries are unclear or in jeopardy. Perioperative nurses deliver patient care in a nondiscriminatory and nonjudgmental manner according to published, legal, agency, professional, and regulatory standards.[15]

Perioperative examples

- ◆ Plans for appropriate substitute nursing care if personal beliefs conflict with required care.
- ◆ Avoids unprofessional behavior toward patients, coworkers, and other health care professionals.
- ◆ Demonstrates respect toward colleagues and students.
- ◆ Recognizes the professional nature of the nurse-patient relationship and its inherent boundaries.

Perioperative Explications

The perioperative nurse has an obligation to protect patients from undue exposure or unwarranted invasions of privacy. Maintaining the patient's privacy is essential to preserving the trust developed in the nurse-patient relationship. Actions demeaning the dignity of the individual could destroy this relationship and jeopardize the patient's welfare. Maintaining the patient's privacy is reflected by securing mechanisms to protect the patient's physical privacy, all forms of identifiable personal information (ie, verbal, written, electronic), personal belongings, and valuables.

Perioperative examples

- ◆ Avoids needless exposure of patient's body.
- ◆ Keeps doors to OR or procedure rooms closed except during movement of patients, personnel, supplies, or equipment.[16]
- ◆ Restricts access to patient care areas to designated, authorized personnel only.
- ◆ Provides cover, warmth, and comfort during transfer from unit to surgical suite as well as during transfer to postoperative unit.
- ◆ Provides and maintains respect for deceased.
- ◆ Provides protected area for viewing deceased by family/significant others.[17]
- ◆ Provides auditory privacy for patient and staff conversations.

3.2 Confidentiality

Associated with the right to privacy, the nurse has a duty to maintain confidentiality of all patient information. The patient's well-being could be jeopardized and the fundamental trust between patient and nurse destroyed by unnecessary access to data or by the inappropriate disclosure of identifiable patient information. The rights, well-being, and safety of the individual patient should be the primary factors in arriving at any professional judgment concerning the disposition of confidential information received from or about the patient, whether oral, written or electronic. The standard of nursing practice and the nurse's responsibility to provide quality care require that relevant data be shared with those members of the health care team who have a need to know. Only information pertinent to a patient's treatment and welfare is disclosed, and only to those directly involved with the patient's care. Duties of confidentiality, however, are not absolute and may need to be modified in order to protect the patient, other innocent parties, and in circumstances of mandatory disclosure for public health reasons.

Information used for purposes of peer review, third-party payments, and other quality improvement or risk management mechanisms may be disclosed only under defined policies, mandates, or protocols. These written guidelines must assure that the rights, well-being, and safety of the patient are protected. In general, only that information directly relevant to a task or specific responsibility should be disclosed. When using electronic communications, special effort should be made to maintain data security.

Perioperative Explications

In concert with privacy is the professional responsibility to maintain the confidentiality of the patient's personal information. The perioperative nurse has a duty to safeguard the confidentiality of all patient information. Measures must be taken to protect the confidentiality of patient information, including oral, written, and electronic forms. Information pertinent to the patient's treatment and welfare is shared only with members of the health care team directly concerned with the patient's care. While relevant patient information must be shared in an expeditious manner with other members of the health care team in order to provide safe patient care, the patient must have trust and confidence in the nurse that information related to his or her care will be protected. Safeguarding private information about patients is a core belief of nursing; however, new technologies such as electronic records have added a challenge to protecting patient information.

Perioperative examples

- Maintains confidentiality of patient information within scope of practice.
- Closes patient record and logs off whenever leaving the computer unattended to protect patient information.
- Follows facility policies regarding electronic information documentation and storage.
- Is aware of and complies with local, state, and federal privacy and security regulations.
- Limits access to patient's record and information (eg, surgery schedule) to appropriate members of the health care team.
- Shares and discusses patient information only with appropriate health care providers and those directly involved in care.
- Protects all forms of confidential patient information (ie, verbal, written, electronic).
- Secures patient's records, belongings, and valuables.
- Maintains patient's record following agency policy, procedure, or protocol.
- Completes record of disposition of belongings and valuables following agency policy, procedure, or protocol.
- Completes operative records accurately and in an objective and nonjudgmental manner.
- Releases patient information only to individuals properly identified and in compliance with established policies, mandates, or protocols.

♦ Uses information for quality improvement purposes in a manner that protects patient confidentiality.[18]

♦ Follows regulations regarding disposal of printed records (eg, perioperative schedules, laboratory reports, face sheets).

3.3 Protection of participants in research

Stemming from the right to self-determination, each individual has the right to choose whether or not to participate in research. It is imperative that the patient or legally authorized surrogate receive sufficient information that is material to an informed decision, to comprehend that information, and to know how to discontinue participation in research without penalty. Necessary information to achieve an adequately informed consent includes the nature of participation, potential harms and benefits, and available alternatives to taking part in the research. Additionally, the patient should be informed of how the data will be protected. The patient has the right to refuse to participate in research or to withdraw at any time without fear of adverse consequences or reprisal.

Research should be conducted and directed only by qualified persons. Prior to implementation, all research should be approved by a qualified review board to ensure patient protection and the ethical integrity of the research. Nurses should be cognizant of the special concerns raised by research involving vulnerable groups, including children, prisoners, students, the elderly, and the poor. The nurse who participates in research in any capacity should be fully informed about both the subject's and the nurse's rights and obligations in the particular research study and in research in general. Nurses have the duty to question and, if necessary, to report and to refuse to participate in research they deem morally objectionable.

Perioperative Explications

The nurse acts to protect the rights of patients involved in clinical research.[19] These rights include the right of adequately informed consent, the right of freedom from risk of injury, the right of privacy, and the right to the preservation of dignity. The perioperative nurse respects the patient's right to decline or discontinue participation in research. The perioperative nurse should be knowledgeable about the rights of the nurse as well as the patient regarding research studies.

Perioperative nurses have an obligation to (a) ensure that research is conducted by qualified people, (b) obtain information about the intent and nature of the research, and (c) confirm that the study is approved by appropriate review bodies. The researcher should disclose the rights and obligations of the patient and the perioperative nurse. Furthermore, the researcher has an obligation to provide information about the nature of the study to the staff members providing care to the participants. Perioperative nurses should be able to question, report, or refuse to participate in research to which they are morally opposed.

Perioperative examples

♦ Confirms informed consent of patient, by physician or responsible researcher, prior to initiation of study and before use of patient information for research.

♦ Safeguards patient's rights as a research subject.

♦ Submits research proposals to the institutional review board.

♦ Follows recommended guidelines and protocols when using investigational devices or when engaging in new procedures.

♦ Follows federal guidelines for treatment of human and animal subjects.

♦ Provides for patient confidentiality during data collection.

♦ Seeks guidance from supervisor to resolve issues regarding any research project that conflict with the nurse's personal beliefs.

♦ Plans for appropriate substitute nursing care if personal beliefs conflict with the research project.

3.4 Standards and review mechanisms

Nursing is responsible and accountable for assuring that only those individuals who have demonstrated the knowledge, skill, practice experiences, commitment, and integrity essential to professional practice are allowed to enter into and continue to practice within the profession. Nurse educators have a responsibility to ensure that basic competencies are achieved and to promote a commitment to professional practice prior to entry of an individual into practice. Nurse administrators are responsible for assuring that the knowledge and skills of each nurse in the workplace are assessed prior to the assignment of responsibilities requiring preparation beyond basic academic programs.

The nurse has a responsibility to implement and maintain standards of professional nursing practice. The nurse should participate in planning, establishing, implementing, and evaluating review mechanisms designed to safeguard patients and nurses, such as peer review processes or committees, credentialing processes, quality improvement initiatives, and ethics committees. Nurse administrators must ensure that nurses have access to and inclusion on institutional ethics committees. Nurses must bring forward difficult issues related to patient care and/or institutional constraints upon ethical practice for discussion and review. The nurse acts to promote inclusion of appropriate others in all deliberations related to patient care.

Nurses should also be active participants in the development of policies and review mechanisms designed to promote patient safety, reduce the likelihood of errors, and address both environmental system factors and human factors that present increased risk to patients. In addition, when errors do occur, nurses are expected to follow institutional guidelines in reporting errors committed or observed to the appropriate supervisory personnel and for assuring responsible disclosure of errors to patients. Under no circumstances should the nurse participate in, or condone through silence, either an attempt to hide an error or a punitive response that serves only to fix blame rather than correct the conditions that led to the error.

Perioperative Explications

The perioperative nurse's primary obligation is to promote the health, welfare, and safety of the patient. The perioperative nurse is responsible for implementing and maintaining standards of perioperative nursing practice. The nurse follows policies, practice guidelines, and laws to safeguard the health and safety of the patient. The nurse participates in the establishment and evaluation of mechanisms to review practice. Competency validation is an essential component to providing safe and effective patient care. Perioperative nurses need to be aware of their own educational and clinical capabilities and seek the assistance of colleagues without hesitation when patient care needs require additional skills. The perioperative nurse uses personal, institutional, professional, and regulatory resources to assist with the resolution of incompetent, unethical, and illegal practices in the work setting.

Perioperative examples

- Uses institutional ethics committee, practice committee, and peer review.
- Supports and participates in institutional ethics committee and institutional review boards.
- Participates in educational programs that enhance patient care (eg, morbidity/mortality conferences, ethics grand rounds, patient care conferences).
- Participates in quality and performance improvement processes.
- Participates in development and revision of professional standards of practice.
- Adheres to professional standards of practice, such as AORN's "Standards of perioperative clinical practice" and "Standards of perioperative professional performance."[20]
- Participates in multidisciplinary review of patient outcomes.
- Complies with institutional policies and procedures regarding competent performance of nursing activities.
- Complies with federal and state regulations such as Occupational Safety and Health Administration regulations, the Americans with Disabilities Act, and state boards of nursing regulations.
- Complies with accrediting agencies such as the Joint Commission and state regulatory agencies.
- Confirms clinicians' practice privileges and credentials (eg, RN first assistants, physicians, physician's assistants).

3.5 Acting on questionable practice

The nurse's primary commitment is to the health, well-being, and safety of the patient across the life span and in all settings in which health care needs are addressed. As an advocate for the patient, the nurse must be alert to and take appropriate action regarding any instances of incompetent, unethical, illegal, or impaired practice by any member of the health care team or the health care system or any action on the part of others that places the rights or best interests of the patient in jeopardy. To function effectively in this role, nurses must be knowledgeable about the *Code of Ethics*, standards of practice of the profession, relevant federal, state and local laws and regulations, and the employing organization's policies and procedures.

When the nurse is aware of inappropriate or questionable practice in the provision or denial of health care, concern should be expressed to the person carrying out the questionable practice. Attention should be called to the possible detrimental affect upon the patient's well-being or best interests as well as the integrity of nursing practice. When factors in the health care delivery system or health care organization threaten the welfare of the patient, similar action should be directed to the responsible administrator. If indicated, the problem should be reported to an appropriate higher authority within the institution or agency, or to an appropriate external authority.

There should be established processes for reporting and handling incompetent, unethical, illegal, or impaired practice within the employment setting so that such reporting can go through official channels, thereby reducing the risk of reprisal against the reporting nurse. All nurses have a responsibility to assist those who identify potentially questionable practice. State nurses associations should be prepared to provide assistance and support in the development and evaluation of such processes and reporting procedures. When incompetent, unethical, illegal, or impaired practice is not corrected within the employment setting and continues to jeopardize patient well-being and safety, the problem should be reported to other appropriate authorities such as practice committees of the pertinent professional organizations, the legally constituted bodies concerned with licensing of specific categories of health

Perioperative Explications

Care providers in the perioperative environment provide health services within the scope of legitimate and ethical practice and safeguard the health and safety of their patients. The perioperative nurse is responsible for meeting legal, institutional, professional, and regulatory standards. It is the ethical obligation of the perioperative nurse to identify and appropriately report questionable practices by any member of the health care team. There should be an established process for reporting and handling incompetent, unethical, or illegal practice within the employment setting so that such reporting can go through official channels without causing fear of reprisal. The perioperative nurse should be knowledgeable about the process and be prepared to use it if necessary. Written documentation of the observed practices or behaviors must be available to the appropriate authorities.

When incompetent, unethical, or illegal practice on the part of anyone concerned with the patient's care is not corrected within the employment setting and continues to jeopardized the patient's welfare and safety, the problem should be reported to other appropriate authorities, such as practice committees of the pertinent professional organizations or the legally constituted bodies concerned with licensing of specific categories of health workers or professional practitioners. Accurate reporting and documentation undergird all action.

Perioperative examples

- ♦ Acts as a patient advocate by protecting the patient from incompetent, unethical, or illegal practices.
- ♦ Questions care that appears inappropriate or substandard.
- ♦ Expresses concern to person carrying out the questionable practice.
- ♦ Reports incompetent, unethical, or illegal practice to responsible administrative person.
- ♦ Consults with colleagues and supervisors to resolve concerns.
- ♦ Documents observations and occurrences in an objective manner according to institutional policy.
- ♦ Complies with institutional policies in resolving problems.
- ♦ Reports verbal, psychological, and physical harassment or abuse.
- ♦ Intervenes appropriately to protect patient safety.

workers and professional practitioners, or the regulatory agencies concerned with evaluating standards or practice. Some situations may warrant the concern and involvement of all such groups. Accurate reporting and factual documentation, and not merely opinion, undergird all such responsible actions. When a nurse chooses to engage in the act of responsible reporting about situations that are perceived as unethical, incompetent, illegal, or impaired, the professional organization has a responsibility to provide the nurse with support and assistance and to protect the practice of those nurses who choose to voice their concerns. Reporting unethical, illegal, incompetent, or impaired practices, even when done appropriately, may present substantial risks to the nurse; nevertheless, such risks do not eliminate the obligation to address serious threats to patient safety.

3.6 Addressing impaired practice

Nurses must be vigilant to protect the patient, the public, and the profession from potential harm when a colleague's practice, in any setting, appears to be impaired. The nurse extends compassion and caring to colleagues who are in recovery from illness or when illness interferes with job performance. In a situation where a nurse suspects another's practice may be impaired, the nurse's duty is to take action designed both to protect patients and to assure that the impaired individual receives assistance in regaining optimal function. Such action should usually begin with consulting supervisory personnel and may also include confronting the individual in a supportive manner and with the assistance of others or helping the individual to access appropriate resources. Nurses are encouraged to follow guidelines outlined by the profession and policies of the employing organization to assist colleagues whose job performance may be adversely affected by mental or physical illness or by personal circumstances. Nurses in all roles should advocate for colleagues whose job performance may be impaired to ensure that they receive appropriate assistance, treatment, and access to fair institutional and legal processes. This includes supporting the return to practice of the individual who has sought assistance and is ready to resume professional duties.

If impaired practice poses a threat or danger to self or others, regardless of whether the individual

Perioperative Explications

The perioperative nurse has an ethical responsibility to protect the patient, the public, and the profession from potential harm that could result from a colleague's impairment. It is both caring and compassionate to take action to protect the patient and ensure that the impaired person receives appropriate assistance. Nurse should follow guidelines outlined by the profession and the policies and procedures of the employing agency.

Perioperative examples

♦ Uses institutional procedural mechanisms to report substance abuse or impairment of colleagues.
♦ Consults with supervisory personnel.
♦ Confronts the individual in a supportive, caring manner.
♦ Use agency resources for helping individual to access treatment and care.
♦ Acts as patient advocate and takes action to ensure patient safety (eg, makes arrangements to remove unsafe practitioner and replace with appropriate practitioner to continue patient care).

has sought help, the nurse must take action to report the individual to persons authorized to address the problem. Nurses who advocate for others whose job performance creates a risk for harm should be protected from negative consequences. Advocacy may be a difficult process, and the nurse is advised to follow workplace policies. If workplace policies do not exist or are inappropriate—that is, they deny the nurse in question access to due legal process or demand resignation—the reporting nurse may obtain guidance from the professional association, state peer assistance programs, employee assistance program, or a similar resource.

4 : The nurse is responsible and accountable for individual nursing practice and determines the appropriate delegation of tasks consistent with the nurse's obligation to provide optimum patient care.

4.1 Acceptance of accountability and responsibility

Individual registered nurses bear primary responsibility for the nursing care that their patients receive and are individually accountable for their own practice. Nursing practice includes direct care activities, acts of delegation, and other responsibilities such as teaching, research, and administration. In each instance, the nurse retains accountability and responsibility for the quality of practice and for conformity with standards of care.

Nurses are faced with decisions in the context of the increased complexity and changing patterns in the delivery of health care. As the scope of nursing practice changes, the nurse must exercise judgment in accepting responsibilities, seeking consultation, and assigning activities to others who carry out nursing care. For example, some advanced practice nurses have the authority to issue prescription and treatment orders to be carried out by other nurses. These acts are not acts of delegation. Both the advanced practice nurse issuing the order and the nurse accepting the order are responsible for the judgments made and accountable for the actions taken.

4.2 Accountability for nursing judgment and action

Accountability means to be answerable to oneself and others for one's own actions. In order to be accountable, nurses act under a code of ethical

Code of Ethics for Nurses with Interpretive Statements *reprinted with permission from American Nurses Association,* © 2001 Nursesbooks.org, Silver Spring, MD.

Perioperative Explications

The individual professional licensee protects the public by ensuring the basic competencies of the professional nurse. Moreover, society grants the nursing profession the right to regulate its own practice. Perioperative nurses bear primary responsibility for perioperative nursing care and are individually accountable for their own practice. The nurse is responsible for nursing decisions made regarding care and is accountable for individual actions. Perioperative nursing practice may include direct patient care, delegation, teaching, research, or administration. Nurses are responsible for judgments they make regarding care and accountable for actions taken.

Perioperative examples

♦ Maintains nursing licensure and certification.
♦ Accepts responsibility and accountability for perioperative nursing practice, staffing schedules, and on-call assignments.
♦ Assumes responsibility for continued education.

Perioperative Explications

Accountability refers to being answerable to one's self, patients, peers, the profession, and society for judgments made and actions taken as a perioperative nurse. Neither physicians' orders nor the employing agency's policies relieve the perioperative nurse of accountability for those actions and judgments. Professional accountability to society is reflected in the conduct that is grounded in the moral principles of fidelity and respect for the dignity, worth, and self-determination of patients. Nurses are accountable for judgments made and actions taken in the course of nursing practice, irrespective of health care organizations' policies or providers' directives.

ANA *Code of Ethics for Nurses*, standards of practice, educational requirements for practice, certification, and a performance evaluation.

Perioperative examples

- ♦ Provides safe and competent patient care.
- ♦ Accounts for sponges, needles, instruments, and other potential foreign bodies.
- ♦ Practices according to the ANA *Code of Ethics for Nurses*; AORN's *Standards, Recommended Practices, and Guidelines*; and hospital and departmental policies and procedures.
- ♦ Practices within scope of practice.
- ♦ Evaluates own performance and solicits peer review.
- ♦ Alerts surgeon and colleagues to potential risks to patients (eg, positioning, electrical hazards, blood loss, inadvertent laceration of blood vessel).
- ♦ Questions orders that appear incorrect or inappropriate.

4.3 Responsibility for nursing judgment and action

Responsibility refers to the specific accountability or liability associated with the performance of duties of a particular role. Nurses accept or reject specific role demands based upon their education, knowledge, competence, and extent of experience. Nurses in administration, education, and research also have obligations to the recipients of nursing care. Although nurses in administration, education, and research have relationships with patients that are less direct, in assuming the responsibilities of a particular role, they share responsibility for the care provided by those whom they supervise and instruct. The nurse must not engage in practices prohibited by law or delegate activities to others that are prohibited by the practice acts of other health care providers.

Individual nurses are responsible for assessing their own competence. When the needs of the patient are beyond the qualifications and competencies of the nurse, consultation and collaboration must be sought from qualified nurses, other health professionals, or other appropriate sources. Educational resources should be sought by nurses and provided by institutions to maintain and advance the competence of nurses. Nurse educators act in

Perioperative Explications

Responsibility refers to carrying out the duties associated with perioperative nursing. Perioperative nurse obligations are reflected in AORN's *Standards, Recommended Practices, and Guidelines*. The acceptance of responsibility for care is determined by an individual's educational preparation, professional competence, and work experience. Nurses in administration, education, and research also are responsible for care through the people they supervise.

Each perioperative nurse is responsible for maintaining competence of professional knowledge and technical skills. It is the nurse's responsibility to assess when care required is beyond an individual's knowledge and to report it to the appropriate support person.

Perioperative examples

- ♦ Consults other health care providers for assistance when necessary.
- ♦ Identifies and develops a plan of corrective action related to deficits and limitations in knowledge.
- ♦ Assumes responsibility for continuous education through personal study; attendance at institutional inservice programs, staff orientation workshops, seminars, AORN chapter and other professional meetings; and reading the *AORN Journal* and other perioperative professional journals.

collaboration with their students to assess the learning needs of the student, the effectiveness of the teaching program, the identification and utilization of appropriate resources, and the support needed for the learning process.

4.4   Delegation of nursing activities

Since the nurse is accountable for the quality of nursing care given to patients, nurses are accountable for the assignment of nursing responsibilities to other nurses and the delegation of nursing care activities to other health care workers. While delegation and assignment are used here in a generic moral sense, it is understood that individual states may have a particular legal definition of these terms.

The nurse must make reasonable efforts to assess individual competence when assigning selected components of nursing care to other health care workers. This assessment involves evaluating the knowledge, skills, and experience of the individual to whom the care is assigned, the complexity of the assigned tasks, and the health status of the patient. The nurse is also responsible for monitoring the activities of these individuals and evaluating the quality of the care provided. Nurses may not delegate responsibilities such as assessment and evaluation; they may delegate tasks. The nurse must not knowingly assign or delegate to any member of the nursing team a task for which that person is not prepared or qualified. Employer policies or directives do not relieve the nurse of responsibility for making judgments about the delegation and assignment of nursing care tasks.

Nurses functioning in management or administrative roles have a particular responsibility to provide an environment that supports and facilitates appropriate assignment and delegation. This includes providing appropriate orientation to staff, assisting less experienced nurses in developing necessary skills and competencies, and establishing policies and procedures that protect both the patient and nurse from the inappropriate assignment or delegation of nursing responsibilities, activities, or tasks.

Code of Ethics for Nurses with Interpretive Statements *reprinted with permission from American Nurses Association, © 2001 Nursesbooks.org, Silver Spring, MD.*

- ♦ Remains current on new procedures affecting practice.
- ♦ Uses the AORN competency statements in perioperative practice.
- ♦ Provides unit-based orientation.
- ♦ Provides competency-based orientation.
- ♦ Practices adult learning theory.
- ♦ Demonstrates competency in use of new technologies.
- ♦ Engages in continued professional learning.

Perioperative Explications

Perioperative nurses are accountable for patient outcomes resulting from nursing care rendered to patients during the perioperative experience. Perioperative nurses are accountable for the assignment of nursing responsibilities to other nurses and for the delegation of nursing care activities to other health care workers. The nurse retains accountability for patient outcomes resulting from delegated nursing tasks. Only the perioperative registered nurse plans and directs the nursing care of every patient undergoing operative and other invasive procedures. The core activities of perioperative nursing are assessment, diagnosis, outcome identification, planning, implementation, and evaluation. The perioperative nurse may delegate certain nursing care tasks, but the nursing activities that cannot be delegated are assessment diagnosis, outcome identification, planning, and evaluation.[21]

The nurse must be aware of specific state legal definitions and guidelines regarding delegation and assignment. The perioperative nurse follows facility policies or directives in delegating functions, but these do not relieve the nurse of accountability for making judgments about the competency of personnel and the appropriateness of delegated activities. Before delegation of patient care tasks, the perioperative nurse uses professional clinical judgment to decide to whom and under what circumstances to delegate appropriate patient care activities.[22] Prior to delegation, consideration also should be given to the patient's condition, the complexity of the procedure, the predictability of the outcome, the level of preparation and competence of the person accepting the delegation, and the amount of supervision needed.[23]

The perioperative work environment supports orientation to less experienced staff. It also provides policies to prevent nurses from accepting inappropriate assignments. This is to protect both the patient and the nurse.

Nurses functioning in educator or preceptor roles may have less direct relationship with patients. However, through assignment of nursing care activities to learners they share responsibility and accountability for the care provided. It is imperative that the knowledge and skills of the learner be sufficient to provide the assigned nursing care and that appropriate supervision be provided to protect both the patient and the learner.

5 : The nurse owes the same duties to self as to others, including the responsibility to preserve integrity and safety, to maintain competence, and to continue personal and professional growth.

5.1 Moral self-respect

Moral respect accords moral worth and dignity to all human beings irrespective of their personal attributes or life situation. Such respect extends to oneself as well; the same duties that we owe to others we owe to ourselves. Self-regarding duties refer to a realm of duties that primarily concern oneself and include professional growth and maintenance of competence, preservation of wholeness of character, and personal integrity.

Code of Ethics for Nurses with Interpretive Statements *reprinted with permission from American Nurses Association,* © *2001 Nursesbooks.org, Silver Spring, MD.*

Perioperative examples

♦ Knows state regulations and definitions regarding delegation and assignment.
♦ Knows organizational guidelines regarding assignment and delegation.
♦ Delegates nursing functions to nurses.
♦ Allows assistive personnel to assist with delegated nursing tasks only when competency has been established and when allowed by state scope of practice.
♦ Bases delegation and assignments on individual competency, patient acuity, complexity of the procedure, predictability of outcomes, amount of supervision required, staffing pattern, and staff availability.[24]
♦ Follows institutional policies for modifying patient care assignments that the nurse or other health care provider does not feel competent in performing.
♦ Participates in perioperative competency-based orientation.
♦ Perioperative nurses define and supervise the training of unlicensed assistive personnel to perform the delegated nursing care tasks.

Perioperative Explications

Perioperative nurses deliver care in a manner that is respectful not only to patients but also to themselves and their colleagues. Nurses identify areas for personal and professional development and assist others in their development. Nurses participate actively in community education about surgery, invasive procedures, and perioperative nursing, and they correct misinformation and misunderstanding about perioperative patient care.

Perioperative examples

♦ Promotes a positive image of nursing in the media and the community.
♦ Promotes professional autonomy and self-regulation of practice.
♦ Uses nursing titles according to demonstrated professional achievement (eg, CNOR®, CRNΓA®).
♦ Corrects inaccurate portrayals of and misinformation about the profession.
♦ Promotes an environment that does not tolerate harassment and abuse.

5.2 Professional growth and maintenance of competence

Though it has consequences for others, maintenance of competence and ongoing professional growth involves the control of one's own conduct in a way that is primarily self-regarding. Competence affects one's self-respect, self-esteem, professional status, and the meaningfulness of work. In all nursing roles, evaluation of one's own performance, coupled with peer review, is a means by which nursing practice can be held to the highest standards. Each nurse is responsible for participating in the development of criteria for evaluation of practice for using those criteria in peer and self-assessment.

Continual professional growth, particularly in knowledge and skill, requires a commitment to lifelong learning. Such learning includes, but is not limited to, continuing education, networking with professional colleagues, self-study, professional reading, certification, and seeking advanced degrees. Nurses are required to have knowledge relevant to the current scope and standards of nursing practice, changing issues, concerns, controversies, and ethics. Where the care required is outside the competencies of the individual nurse, consultation should be sought or the patient should be referred to others for appropriate care.

- Provides an environment that optimizes the occupational health and safety of all employees.
- Promotes empowerment and team building.
- Supports the nurse's role as a patient advocate.

Perioperative Explications

The perioperative nurse is accountable to society and the profession for appropriate, effective, and efficient nursing practice. Mechanisms are established to demonstrate professional accountability and responsibility for maintaining clinical competence. Knowledge and skill related to technological advances and surgical interventions should be incorporated into the perioperative nurse's practice. The perioperative nurse maintains responsibility for his or her own continuing education.

Perioperative examples

- Incorporates AORN's competency statements in perioperative nursing education.
- Remains current on new procedures related to perioperative clinical practice.
- Participates in certification processes (eg, CNOR, CRNFA, advanced cardiac life support).
- Acquires new knowledge from continuous education through personal study; attendance at institutional inservice programs, staff orientation workshops, seminars, AORN Congress, AORN chapter and other professional meetings; and reading the *AORN Journal, Surgical Services Management*, and other perioperative and professional literature.
- Supports competency-based orientation and annual review process.
- Demonstrates competency in use of new technologies.
- Participates in self-evaluation and peer evaluation of clinical competence, decision-making skills, and professional judgment.
- Seeks consultation as necessary to provide patient care.
- Confirms clinical privileges of all caregivers.
- Promotes individual accountability for maintaining competence.
- Promotes patient safety and other forms of patient advocacy initiatives recommended by professional organizations, legislation, and regulations.

5.3   Wholeness of character

Nurses have both personal and professional identities that are neither entirely separate, nor entirely merged, but are integrated. In the process of becoming a professional, the nurse embraces the values of the profession, integrating them with personal values. Duties to self involve an authentic expression of one's own moral point of view in practice. Sound ethical decision-making requires the respectful and open exchange of views between and among all individuals with relevant interests. In a community of moral discourse, no one person's view should automatically take precedence over that of another. Thus, the nurse has a responsibility to express moral perspectives, even when they differ from those of others, and even when they might not prevail.

This wholeness of character encompasses relationships with patients. In situations where the patient requests a personal opinion from the nurse, the nurse is generally free to express an informed personal opinion as long as this preserves the voluntariness of the patient and maintains appropriate professional and moral boundaries. It is essential to be aware of the potential for undue influence attached to the nurse's professional role. Assisting patients to clarify their own values in reaching informed decisions may be helpful in avoiding unintended persuasion. In situations where nurses' responsibilities include care for those whose personal attributes, condition, lifestyle, or situation is stigmatized by the community and are personally unacceptable, the nurse still renders respectful and skilled care.

5.4   Preservation of integrity

Integrity is an aspect of wholeness of character and is primarily a self-concern of the individual nurse. An economically constrained health care environment presents the nurse with particularly troubling threats to integrity. Threats to integrity may include a request to deceive a patient, to withhold information, or to falsify records, as well as verbal abuse from patients or coworkers. Threats to integrity also may include an expectation that the nurse will act in a way that is inconsistent with the values or ethics of the profession, or more specifically a request that is in direct violation of the *Code of Ethics*. Nurses have a duty to remain consistent with both

Code of Ethics for Nurses with Interpretive Statements *reprinted with permission from American Nurses Association,* © 2001 Nursesbooks.org, Silver Spring, MD.

Perioperative Explications

The perioperative nurse must be genuine, open, and honest in interactions with patients and other health care providers. Nurses are aware of their powerful influence and offer their opinions based on scientific principles, evidence-based practices, and clinical experiences.

Perioperative examples

- ♦ Assists patients in formulating decisions affecting care as appropriate.
- ♦ Facilitates patient participation in perioperative plan of care.
- ♦ Integrates personal philosophy of nursing into practice setting.
- ♦ Helps peers to be assertive and emotionally healthy.
- ♦ Respects views of others, but clarifies misinformation.
- ♦ Applies standards of nursing practice consistently to all patients regardless of disability, economic status, culture, religion, race, age, lifestyle choices, or sexuality.
- ♦ Plans for appropriate substitute care provider if personal beliefs conflict with required care.

Perioperative Explications

The perioperative registered nurse does not compromise professional or personal integrity. Additionally, the perioperative nurse knows that the use of the title *Registered Nurse (RN)*, as granted by state licensure, carries with it the responsibility to act in the public interest. The title *RN* and all other symbols of academic degrees or other earned or honorary professional symbols of recognition may be used in all ways that are legal and appropriate

The pressure to reduce costs, especially in surgical services, reflects the current emphasis on financial well-being. Perioperative nurses can be financially prudent and at the same time discharge their clinical, educational, and administrative duties in a manner that is consistent with ethical principles.

When the perioperative nurse is ethically and morally opposed to interventions or procedures in a their personal and professional values and to accept compromise only to the degree that it remains an integrity-preserving compromise. An integrity-preserving compromise does not jeopardize the dignity or well-being of the nurse or others. Integrity-preserving compromise can be difficult to achieve, but is more likely to be accomplished in situations where there is an open forum for moral discourse and an atmosphere of mutual respect and regard.

6: The nurse participates in establishing, maintaining, and improving health care environments and conditions of employment conducive to the provision of quality health care and consistent with the values of the profession through individual and collective action.

6.1 Influence of the environment on moral virtues and values

Virtues are habits of character that predispose persons to meet their moral obligations; that is, to do what is right. Excellences are habits of character that predispose a person to do a particular job or task well. Virtues such as wisdom, honesty, and courage are habits or attributes of the morally good person. Excellences such as compassion, patience, and skill are habits of character of the morally good nurse. For the nurse, virtues and excellences are those habits

Code of Ethics for Nurses with Interpretive Statements *reprinted with permission from American Nurses Association,* © *2001 Nursesbooks.org, Silver Spring, MD.*

particular case, the nurse is justified in refusing to participate if the refusal is made known in advance and in time for other appropriate arrangements to be made for the patient's nursing care. When the patient's life is in jeopardy, the perioperative nurse is obliged to provide for the patient's safety, to avoid abandonment, and to withdraw only when assured that alternative sources of nursing care are available to the patient.

Perioperative examples

- Facilitates a working environment conducive to learning, teaching, and education.
- Makes purchasing decisions equitably and justly to provide cost-effective, quality care.
- Uses and maintains supplies and equipment according to manufacturers' instructions.
- Resterilizes and reprocesses instruments and supplies in a manner consistent with standards and regulations.
- Accepts responsibility and accountability for perioperative nursing practices.
- Is aware of limitations and accepts assignments only when competent to function safely.
- Uses nursing titles (eg, CNOR, CRNFA) according to demonstrated professional achievement.
- Participates in risk management efforts and quality process improvement.
- Plans for appropriate substitute care provider if personal beliefs conflict with required care.

Perioperative Explications

The perioperative nurse is responsible for developing a caring environment that promotes the well-being of patients. This is accomplished by doing what is right and doing it well. The nurse provides a compassionate and therapeutic environment by promoting comfort and preventing unnecessary suffering. The working environment necessary to accomplish these goals supports the growth of virtues and excellences.

Perioperative examples

- Interacts with patients in a compassionate manner.
- Demonstrates empathy, sensitivity, and patience in difficult or stressful situations.

that affirm and promote the values of human dignity, well-being, respect, health, independence, and other values central to nursing. Both virtue and excellence, as aspects of moral character, can be either nurtured by the environment in which the nurse practices or they can be diminished or thwarted. All nurses have a responsibility to create, maintain, and contribute to environments that support the growth of virtues and excellences and enable nurses to fulfill their ethical obligations.

6.2 Influence of the environment on ethical obligations

All nurses, regardless of role, have a responsibility to create, maintain, and contribute to environments of practice that support nurses in fulfilling their ethical obligations. Environments of practice include observable features, such as working conditions, and written policies and procedures setting out expectations for nurses, as well as less tangible characteristics such as informal peer norms. Organizational structures, role descriptions, health and safety initiatives, grievance mechanisms, ethics committees, compensation systems, and disciplinary procedures all contribute to environments that can either present barriers or foster ethical practice and professional fulfillment. Environments in which employees are provided fair hearing of grievances, are supported in practicing according to standards of care, and are justly treated allow for the realization of the values of the profession and are consistent with sound nursing practice.

6.3 Responsibility for the health care environment

The nurse is responsible for contributing to a moral environment that encourages respectful interactions with colleagues, support of peers, and identification of issues that need to be addressed. Nurse administrators have a particular responsibility to assure that employees are treated fairly and that nurses are involved in decisions related to their practice and working conditions. Acquiescing and accepting unsafe or inappropriate practices, even if the individual does not participate in the specific practice, is equivalent to condoning unsafe practice. Nurses should not remain employed in facilities that routinely violate patient rights or require nurses to severely and repeatedly compromise standards of practice or personal morality.

Code of Ethics for Nurses with Interpretive Statements *reprinted with permission from American Nurses Association, © 2001 Nursesbooks.org, Silver Spring, MD.*

- ◆ Uses therapeutic communication.
- ◆ Assists families with challenging issues.
- ◆ Develops relationships with patients that support mutual involvement in planning care.
- ◆ Helps to answer patients' questions related to their care.
- ◆ Listens attentively and, when appropriate, refers patient to other resources.

Perioperative Explications

Perioperative nurses create, maintain, and contribute to a work environment that supports individuals in their nursing practice. This environment is safe and has policies, procedures, guidelines, and standards for practice. The nurse is knowledgeable about the various processes and committees to support and promote a professional working environment.

Perioperative examples

- ◆ Follows process for addressing unsafe practice.
- ◆ Follows process for addressing ethical issues.
- ◆ Participates in developing policies, procedures, and standards.
- ◆ Maintains knowledge of policies and procedures.
- ◆ Promotes a positive work environment.
- ◆ Facilitates a working atmosphere conducive to education.

Perioperative Explications

The perioperative nurse treats colleagues and peers respectfully and fairly. The nurse, in all roles, participates in decisions that will affect practice and working conditions. The perioperative nurse identifies and supports conditions of employment that promote practice in accordance with AORN standards and recommended practices. This environment also meets accrediting and other regulatory standards. As a moral agent, if the work environment does not routinely support high quality patient care and safe practice, the nurse should seek employment elsewhere.

Perioperative nurses may need to address concerns about the work environment through appropriate channels. Perioperative nurses may need to participate in collective activities (eg, collective bargaining, workplace advocacy) to address concerns about patient care, work environment, or just compensation. These activities should be consistent with AORN standards and recommended practices, accrediting standards, state nurse practice acts, and the ANA *Code of Ethics for Nurses*. In this process, the interests of both nurses and patients must be kept in balance.

Perioperative examples
- Knows chain of command.
- Promotes environment that does not tolerate harassment and abuse.
- Facilitates work environment conducive to learning.
- Collaborates with all health care team members.
- Questions unfair employee practices.
- Identifies and reports unsafe patient practices.
- Participates in strategic planning and development of departmental and institutional goals.
- Promotes empowerment.
- Belongs to state nursing organization.
- Maintains membership in AORN.

7: The nurse participates in the advancement of the profession through contributions to practice, education, administration, and knowledge development.

7.1 Advancing the profession through active involvement in nursing and in health care policy
Nurses should advance their profession by contributing in some way to the leadership, activities, and the viability of their professional organizations. Nurses can also advance the profession by serving in leadership or mentorship roles or on committees within their places of employment. Nurses who are self-employed can advance the profession by serving as role models for professional integrity. Nurses can also advance the profession through participation in civic activities related to health care or through local, state, national, or international initiatives. Nurse educators have a specific responsibility to enhance students' commitment to professional and civic values. Nurse administrators have a responsibility to foster an employment environment that facilitates nurses' ethical integrity and professionalism, and nurse researchers are responsible for active contribution to the body of knowledge supporting and advancing nursing practice.

Perioperative Explications
The perioperative nurse has a personal responsibility to contribute to the advancement of the profession by participating in professional organizations. There are various activities within employment agencies and local, state, and national organizations by which one can contribute to the profession. Perioperative educators and managers are additionally responsible for providing an environment conducive to advancing the profession. Nurses can contribute to the advancement of the profession and health care policy by participating in civic activities.

Perioperative examples
- Maintains membership in AORN.
- Serves as a committee member at place of employment.
- Actively participates in AORN local and national initiatives.
- Volunteers at schools of nursing (eg, teaching, mentoring).
- Actively seeks opportunity to be involved in activities related to patient care at place of employment (eg, patient care, product selection, safety initiatives, strategic planning, risk management, infection control, and ethics committees).
- Supports perioperative preceptor programs.
- Serves as leader or mentor on committees.

- Maintains awareness of changing health care policy at the local, state, and national levels.
- Participates in defining and revising scope of practice acts.
- Consults and collaborates with individuals who shape health care policy.

7.2 Advancing the profession by developing, maintaining, and implementing professional standards in clinical, administrative, and educational practice

Standards and guidelines reflect the practice of nursing grounded in ethical commitments and a body of knowledge. Professional standards and guidelines for nurses must be developed by nurses and reflect nursing's responsibility to society. It is the responsibility of nurses to identify their own scope of practice as permitted by professional practice standards and guidelines, by state and federal laws, by relevant societal values, and by the *Code of Ethics*.

The nurse as administrator or manager must establish, maintain, and promote conditions of employment that enable nurses within that organization or community setting to practice in accord with accepted standards of nursing practice and provide a nursing and health care work environment that meets the standards and guidelines of nursing practice. Professional autonomy and self regulation in the control of conditions of practice are necessary for implementing nursing standards and guidelines and assuring quality care for those whom nursing serves.

The nurse educator is responsible for promoting and maintaining optimum standards of both nursing education and of nursing practice in any settings where planned learning activities occur. Nurse educators must also ensure that only those students who possess the knowledge, skills, and competencies that are essential to nursing graduate from their nursing programs.

7.3 Advancing the profession through knowledge development, dissemination, and application to practice

The nursing profession should engage in scholarly inquiry to identify, evaluate, refine, and expand the body of knowledge that forms the foundation of its discipline and practice. In addition, nursing knowledge is derived from the sciences and from the

Code of Ethics for Nurses with Interpretive Statements reprinted with permission from American Nurses Association, © 2001 Nursesbooks.org, Silver Spring, MD.

Perioperative Explications

Perioperative nurses are responsible for monitoring standards of practice pertinent to their role(s) and for fostering optimal standards of practice at the local, regional, state, and national levels of the health care system: "The perioperative nurse systematically evaluates the quality and appropriateness of nursing practice."[25] Perioperative educators and managers are equally responsible to provide an environment conducive to implementing and improving standards and recommended practices.

Perioperative examples

- Uses standards in nursing practice.
- Contributes to the work of AORN committees and projects to develop standards.
- Reviews and critiques practice standards (eg, responds to proposed AORN recommended practices).
- Participates in development and revision of standards of practice.
- Participates in quality and process improvement processes.
- Participates in multidisciplinary review of patient outcomes.
- Follows investigational device protocol and regulations.

Perioperative Explications

The perioperative nurse has an obligation to the patient and to society to engage in activities that promote scholarly inquiry to identify, verify, and expand the body of perioperative nursing knowledge. Perioperative nursing roles include investigation to further knowledge, participation in research, and application of theoretical and empirical knowledge. Perioperative nurses can support the research process as content experts, data collectors, research subjects, or researchers.

humanities. Ongoing scholarly activities are essential to fulfilling a profession's obligations to society. All nurses working alone or in collaboration with others can participate in the advancement of the profession through the development, evaluation, dissemination, and application of knowledge in practice. However, an organizational climate and infrastructure conducive to scholarly inquiry must be valued and implemented for this to occur.

8: The nurse collaborates with other health professionals and the public in promoting community, national, and international efforts to meet health needs.

8.1 Health needs and concerns

The nursing profession is committed to promoting the health, welfare, and safety of all people. The nurse has a responsibility to be aware not only of specific health needs of individual patients but also of broader health concerns such as world hunger, environmental pollution, lack of access to health care, violation of human rights, and inequitable distribution of nursing and health care resources. The availability and accessibility of high quality health services to all people require both interdisciplinary planning and collaborative partnerships among health professionals and others at the community, national, and international levels.

8.2 Responsibilities to the public

Nurses, individually and collectively, have a responsibility to be knowledgeable about the health status of the community and existing threats to health and safety. Through support of and participation in community organizations and groups, the nurse assists in efforts to educate the public, facilitates informed choice, identifies conditions and circumstances that contribute to illness, injury, and disease, fosters healthy lifestyles, and participates in institutional and legislative efforts to promote health

Perioperative examples
- Uses research findings to support and improve clinical practice.
- Fosters an environment of intellectual curiosity.
- Identifies problems amenable to the research process (eg, questions outmoded practices).
- Disseminates research findings to colleagues.

Perioperative Explications

Availability of health care involves not only addressing specific health needs, but also factors that affect well-being. These factors include world hunger, environmental pollution, lack of access to care, violation of human rights, and rationing of health care. The perioperative nurse recognizes the interdependence and collaboration of all health care workers to provide quality health care to everyone.

Perioperative examples
- Collaborates with members of other professional organizations at international, national, and state levels (eg, joint education offerings, joint patient safety legislative efforts).
- Communicates with elected officials about health care needs.
- Educates elected officials about health care needs.
- Donates to health care-related charities.
- Participates in international nursing societies.

Perioperative Explications

The perioperative nurse is knowledgeable about the health status of the community and factors that threaten well-being and safety. The nurse participates in educating the public about the various factors influencing health care. The perioperative nurse recognizes cultural differences of various populations and does not allow his or her own beliefs and values to influence the care provided to patients of different beliefs and values. Nursing needs to adequately represent cultural diversity to promote the welfare and safety of all patients.

and meet national health objectives. In addition, the nurse supports initiatives to address barriers to health, such as poverty, homelessness, unsafe living conditions, abuse and violence, and lack of access to health services.

The nurse also recognizes that health care is provided to culturally diverse populations in this country and in all parts of the world. In providing care, the nurse should avoid imposition of the nurse's own cultural values upon others. The nurse should affirm human dignity and show respect for the values and practices associated with different cultures and use approaches to care that reflect awareness and sensitivity.

9: The profession of nursing, as represented by associations and their members, is responsible for articulating nursing values, for maintaining the integrity of the profession and its practice, and for shaping social policy.

9.1 Assertion of values

It is the responsibility of a professional association to communicate and affirm the values of the profession to its members. It is essential that the professional organization encourages discourse that supports critical self-reflection and evaluation within the profession. The organization also communicates to the public the values that nursing considers central to social change that will enhance health.

Perioperative examples
- Volunteers to teach wellness classes.
- Educates members of community about perioperative nursing.
- Collaborates with consumer, service, and support organizations related to health care.
- Fosters collaboration with and education of the public on local, state, and national health care issues.
- Prepares for disasters and threat to community.
- Provides explanations and answers to questions in the patient's primary language.
- Incorporates patient requests regarding religious preferences into practice as much as possible.
- Integrates cultural differences into patient care.
- Incorporates requests for alternative therapies into care, as appropriate.

Perioperative Explications

AORN's mission is to support perioperative registered nurses in achieving optimal outcomes for patients undergoing operative and other invasive procedures. To further its goals, AORN is committed to excellence in support of its mission and values education, representation, and standards that are research based, current, timely, comprehensive, applicable, and achievable.[26]

Perioperative examples
- Participates in educational programs to promote life-long learning.
- Reads professional journals and newsletters.
- Incorporates AORN's *Standards, Recommended Practices, and Guidelines* into practice.
- Uses the *Perioperative Nursing Data Set* (PNDS) to link perioperative nursing care to positive patient outcomes.
- Applies "Patient Safety First" principles to perioperative patient care.
- Provides consultative and other services to support perioperative nursing and patient care.
- Engages in legislative activities to support perioperative nursing and patient care.
- Promotes interaction with regulatory agencies (eg, FDA, CMS) to advance safe, quality patient care.
- Maintains membership in AORN.

9.2 The profession carries out its collective responsibility through professional associations

The nursing profession continues to develop ways to clarify nursing's accountability to society. The contract between the profession and society is made explicit through such mechanisms as (a) the *Code of Ethics for Nurses*, (b) the standards of nursing practice, (c) the ongoing development of nursing knowledge derived from nursing theory, scholarship, and research in order to guide nursing actions, (d) educational requirements for practice, (e) certification, and (f) mechanisms for evaluating the effectiveness of professional nursing actions.

- Participates in AORN chapters, state councils, specialty assemblies, and other organizational units to support AORN and perioperative nursing.

Perioperative Explications

AORN's purpose is to unite perioperative registered nurses for the purpose of maintaining an association dedicated to the constant endeavor of promoting the highest professional standards of perioperative nursing practice for optimum patient care. AORN cooperates with other professional associations, health care facilities, universities, industries, technical societies, research organizations, and governmental agencies in matters affecting the goals and purposes of AORN.[27]

Perioperative examples

- Practices perioperative nursing incorporating AORN's *Standards, Recommended Practices, and Guidelines*.
- Participates in nursing research.
- Becomes knowledgeable about the ANA *Code of Ethics for Nurses* and the "AORN explications for perioperative nurses."
- Collaborates with other organizations (eg, American College of Surgeons, American Association of Nurse Anesthetists, American Society of Anesthesiologists) to foster optimal perioperative patient care.
- Collaborates with other nursing organizations (eg, Nursing Organizations Alliance, American Nurses Association) to enhance the nursing profession.
- Identifies partnering opportunities with educational, health care, governmental, payer, business, and professional organizations to promote mutually beneficial patient care initiatives.

9.3 Intraprofessional integrity

A professional association is responsible for expressing the values and ethics of the profession and also for encouraging the professional organization and its members to function in accord with those values and ethics. Thus, one of its fundamental responsibilities is to promote awareness of and adherence to the *Code of Ethics* and to critique the activities and ends of the professional association itself. Values and ethics influence the power structures of the

Perioperative Explications

The ANA *Code of Ethics for Nurses*, together with the "AORN explications for perioperative nursing," expresses the values and ethics of perioperative nursing. Use of the title *RN* carries with it the individual's responsibility to act in public's best interest. The title *RN* and all other academic degrees or other earned or honorary professional symbols of recognition may be used in all ways that are legal and reflect professional achievement.

Perioperative examples

- Promotes a positive image of nursing in the media and the community.

association in guiding, correcting, and directing its activities. Legitimate concerns for the self-interest of the association and the profession are balanced by a commitment to the social goods that are sought. Through critical self-reflection and self-evaluation, associations must foster change within themselves, seeking to move the professional community toward its stated ideals.

9.4 Social reform

Nurses can work individually as citizens or collectively through political action to bring about social change. It is the responsibility of a professional nursing association to speak for nurses collectively in shaping and reshaping health care within our nation, specifically in areas of health care policy and legislation that affect accessibility, quality, and the cost of health care. Here, the professional association maintains vigilance and takes action to influence legislators, reimbursement agencies, nursing organizations, and other health professions. In these activities, health is understood as being broader than delivery and reimbursement systems, but extending to health-related sociocultural issues such as violation of human rights, homelessness, hunger, violence, and the stigma of illness.

- ◆ Promotes professional autonomy and self-regulation of practice.
- ◆ Uses nursing titles (eg, CNOR, CRNFA) according to professional achievement.
- ◆ Identifies and resolves conflicts of interest effectively.
- ◆ Corrects inaccurate portrayals of and misinformation about the profession.
- ◆ Incorporates the ANA *Code of Ethics for Nurses* into daily practice.

Perioperative Explications

To promote the welfare and safety of all people, nurses need adequate representation to support effective health care delivery. Individual patients and society as whole benefit from nursing participation in decisions made about health care.

Perioperative examples
- ◆ Participates in lobbying efforts affecting health care.
- ◆ Supports political candidates that advance health care issues.
- ◆ Participates in electoral process at the local, state, and national levels.
- ◆ Participates in institutional decision-making.
- ◆ Participates in the electoral process.
- ◆ Volunteers in community health services.
- ◆ Supports political candidates, governmental programs, and legislation agenda for improving patient care.
- ◆ Educates members of the community about perioperative nursing (eg, through health fairs, Perioperative Nurse Week activities, educational programs).
- ◆ Collaborates with consumer, service, and support organizations (eg, Lions Club, Reach to Recovery, AARP).
- ◆ Collaborates with the public, industry, and health care workers regarding environmental and cost containment issues.
- ◆ Fosters collaboration with and education of the public regarding local, state, and national issues (eg, the environment, health care costs).

Conclusion

Perioperative nurses must be familiar with the ethical issues inherent to their practice. To develop familiarity with the issues, one can discuss them with peers and ethics committee members or consult other knowledgeable resources. Nurses may find it beneficial to have a file on ethics available in the department for review. Inservice programs focusing on ethical issues can be implemented for the department by utilizing members of the hospital's nursing ethics and/or medical ethics committees. Other departments and contacts, such as social services, also can be a resource, especially in the area of advance directives. Nurses can use values clarification to identify and understand their moral beliefs and attitudes.

Ethics provides guidelines of action for behavior with others. Such guidelines are both important and necessary when dealing with issues in the context of health care. To effectively deal with ethical situations in practice, nurses must be cognizant of limitations to scope of practice and never jeopardize patient care. Nurses need to realize they have a personal accountability to the care of the patient. As guidelines for practice, nurses can utilize many resources such as the ANA *Code of Ethics for Nurses* and knowledge of patient and individual rights, policies and procedures, standards of care, and community norms. Ultimately, the nurse must provide ethical care for all patients. Utilizing guidelines and recommended practices is a means to an end—safe, competent, and ethical patient care.

Code of Ethics for Nurses with Interpretive Statements *reprinted with permission from American Nurses Association, © 2001 Nursesbooks.org, Silver Spring, MD.*

REFERENCES

1. S Beyea, ed, *Perioperative Nursing Data Set*, second ed (Denver: AORN, Inc, 2002) 182.
2. *Ibid.*
3. *Ibid.*
4. S Beyea, L Nicoll, "Using ethical analysis when there is no research," *AORN Journal* 69 (June 1999) 1261-1263.
5. S Beyea, ed, *Perioperative Nursing Data Set* (Denver: AORN, Inc, 2000) 150.
6. Beyea, *Perioperative Nursing Data Set*, second ed, 182.
7. Ibid, 184.
8. "ANA code for nurses with interpretive statements—Explications for perioperative nursing," in *Standards, Recommended Practices, and Guidelines* (Denver: AORN, Inc, 2002) 54.
9. Beyea, *Perioperative Nursing Data Set*, second ed, 178.
10. *Ibid, 182.*
11. *Ibid, 183.*
12. *Ibid, 175-176.*
13. *Ibid, 178, 180.*
14. *Ibid, 179, 181.*
15. Beyea, *Perioperative Nursing Data Set*, 125.
16. "Recommended practices for traffic patterns," in Standards, Recommended Practices, and Guidelines (Denver: AORN, Inc, 2002) 350.
17. Beyea, *Perioperative Nursing Data Set*, second ed, 184
18. Beyea, *Perioperative Nursing Data Set*, second ed, 183.
19. A Orb, L Eisenhauer, D Wynaden, "Ethics in qualitative research," *Journal of Nursing Scholarship* 33 (2001) 93-96.
20. *Standards, Recommended Practices, and Guidelines* (Denver: AORN, Inc, 2002) 157-162.
21. "AORN official statement on unlicensed assistive personnel," in *Standards, Recommended Practices, and Guidelines* (Denver: AORN, Inc, 2002) 141.
22. *Ibid.*
23. *Ibid.*
24. *Ibid.*
25. "Standards of perioperative professional performance," in *Standards, Recommended Practices, and Guidelines* (Denver: AORN, Inc, 2002) 160.
26. "AORN vision, mission, philosophy, and values," in *Standards, Recommended Practices, and Guidelines* (Denver: AORN, Inc, 2002) 5.
27. "AORN national bylaws," in *Standards, Recommended Practices, and Guidelines* (Denver: AORN, Inc, 2002) 7.

PUBLICATION HISTORY

Originally published in the 1994 edition of the AORN *Standards and Recommended Practices*.

Revised; approved by the AORN Board of Directors in November 2002.

This document was previously published as Exhibit C of the "Standards of perioperative nursing" in the 2009 edition of *Perioperative Standards and Recommended Practices*.

AORN Perioperative Standards and Recommended Practices, 2012 Edition

Recommended Practices for Perioperative Nursing

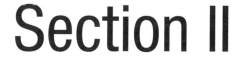

Section II

AORN Perioperative Standards and
Recommended Practices, 2012 Edition

Introduction to the AORN Recommended Practices

This section contains recommended practices for perioperative nursing practice. They are based on principles of nursing science, microbiology, research, review of the scientific literature, and the opinions of knowledgeable experts. The AORN recommended practices are authored by perioperative nurse specialists in the AORN Nursing Department and selected members of AORN in collaboration with liaisons from the American Association of Nurse Anesthetists, the American College of Surgeons, the American Society of Anesthesiologists, the Association for Professionals in Infection Control and Epidemiology, the Centers for Disease Control and Prevention, and the International Association of Healthcare Central Service Materiel Management.

These recommended practices represent the Association's official position on questions regarding optimal perioperative nursing practice. The recommended practices appearing in this edition have been approved by the AORN Recommended Practices Advisory Board. No attempt has been made to gain consensus among users, manufacturers, and consumers of any material or product. **Compliance with the AORN recommended practices is voluntary.**

AORN's recommended practices are intended as achievable and represent what is believed to be an optimal level of patient care within surgical and invasive procedure settings. These practice settings include traditional operating rooms, ambulatory surgery centers, physicians' offices, cardiac catheterization laboratories, endoscopy suites, radiology departments, and all other areas where surgery and other invasive procedures may be performed.

Each recommended practice consists of achievable recommendations based on the highest level of evidence available. The recommendations are broad statements intended to be used to guide policy and procedure development in specific work environments. Although they are considered to represent the optimal level of practice, variations in practice settings and clinical situations may limit the degree to which each recommendation can be implemented. The recommended practices are intended to describe excellent perioperative nursing practices, promote patient and health care worker safety, and guide policy and procedure development in surgical and invasive procedure settings.

Application in Practice

Application of the recommended practices in individual work settings requires close examination of existing policies and procedures. This review may indicate that revised or new policies and/or procedures are necessary. Individual commitment, professional conscience, and the setting in which perioperative nursing is practiced must guide the nurse in implementing these recommended practices. Variations in practice settings and clinical situations may determine the degree to which the recommended practice can be fulfilled.

As used within the context of the recommended practices, "may" is used to indicate that a course of action is permissible within the limits of the recommended practice; and "can" is used as a statement of possibility and capability. The use of "should" indicates that a certain course of action is recommended. "Must" is used only to describe "unavoidable" situations, including those mandated by government regulation and accreditation organization standards.

Recommended Practices and PNDS

The Perioperative Nursing Data Set (PNDS) is the structured nursing vocabulary developed by AORN and recognized by the American Nurses Association (ANA) to describe the nursing care of patients undergoing a surgical or other invasive procedure from pre-admission to discharge. As a controlled vocabulary, the PNDS enables nursing care to be documented in a standardized manner to allow for collection of reliable and valid clinical data on perioperative nurse-sensitive outcomes resulting from nursing interventions during a surgical or invasive procedure.

This standardized language consists of a collection of unique data elements reflecting the nursing process as described in the *Perioperative Standards and Recommended Practices*. The perioperative patient and his or her family members are at the core of the PNDS patient-focused conceptual model. The model depicts perioperative nursing in four domains and illustrates the relationship between the patient, his or her family members, and care provided by the professional perioperative registered nurse. Each data element in the PNDS is represented by a unique identifier. The PNDS structure consists of four domains; within each domain are associated nursing diagnoses, interventions, and outcomes.

The *Perioperative Standards and Recommended Practices* are the core of clinical knowledge from which the PNDS is derived. The PNDS forms the basis for the perioperative framework (ie, AORN SYNTEGRITY™ Standardized Perioperative Framework) that enables standardized electronic documentation. PNDS elements in the standardized framework are supported by the applicable standard or recommended practice.

An initial attempt to map the PNDS outcomes and interventions to the recommended practices is reflected in recommended practices published between 2004 and 2009, as noted in parentheses following the purpose and intervention statements. Interventions are represented by the letter "I" and a unique number; outcomes are represented by the letter "O" and a unique number. Recommended practices revised during and after 2009 no longer display the PNDS code mapping.

AORN is continuing to develop and refine the PNDS and AORN SYNTEGRITY™ Framework. Rather than continuing to map the PNDS in the recommended practices as explained above, the recommended practices are now mapped to the PNDS data elements in AORN SYNTEGRITY™ Framework.

Development, Review, and Revision Process

AORN began publishing recommended practices in March 1975. A compilation was printed in March 1978 in *AORN Standards of Practice*. The book at hand contains revisions of those previously published recommended practices as well as new ones developed since 1978.

Each recommended practice is reviewed and revised as appropriate at regular periodic intervals.

Although only a portion of the recommended practices may be updated for publication in any given year, all 32 recommended practices are under continuous scrutiny by the AORN Recommended Practices Advisory Board.

In 2006-2007, an all-digital workflow was launched to enable AORN to develop the recommended practices in an efficient, timely, and cost-effective manner and readily update them on an as-needed basis. This digital platform enables AORN to electronically publish new and revised recommended practices periodically throughout the year and make them available by electronic subscription (e-Subscription). The printed book is a snapshot in time. All updated content approved by the Recommended Practices Advisory Board as of October of the preceding year appears in the annual printed edition and on CD. These are living documents that are developed, reviewed, and revised on an ongoing basis in an effort to provide current recommendations, based on the best evidence available at the time. Differences in format and content organization may occur as the recommended practices continue to evolve over time.

Two new recommended practices have been written for this 2012 edition:

♦ Recommended Practices for Prevention of Deep Vein Thrombosis and
♦ Recommended Practices for Medication Safety.

Additionally, one recommended practices document was revised for this edition:

♦ Recommended Practices for Perioperative Health Care Information Management.

The important tasks of developing, reviewing, and updating AORN's recommended practices are ongoing. AORN continues to strive to provide recommended practices that reflect current knowledge in nursing practice, nursing and medical research, and surgical technology.

AORN Staff Support

Ramona Conner, MSN, RN, CNOR
Manager, Standards and Recommended Practices

Linda Groah, MSN, RN, CNOR, NEA-BC, FAAN
Executive Director/CEO

Janet Knox
Administrative Assistant

Melissa Kovac, MA, MLIS
Research Librarian

Kimberly Retzlaff
Editor/Team Lead

Jennifer Brusco and **Helen Starbuck Pashley**
Associate Editors

Zac Wiggy
Assistant Editor

PERIOPERATIVE NURSING SPECIALISTS
Joan Blanchard, MSS, BSN, RN, CNOR, CIC
Byron Burlingame, MS, RN, CNOR
Bonnie Denholm, MS, BSN, RN, CNOR
Sharon Giarrizzo-Wilson, MS, RN-BC, CNOR
Mary Ogg, MSN, RN, CNOR
Sharon A. Van Wicklin, MSN, RN, CNOR, CRNFA, PLNC

AORN gratefully acknowledges the work of the 2011–2012 Recommended Practices Advisory Board

COMMITTEE CHAIR
Antonia B. Hughes, MA, BSN, RN, CNOR
Perioperative Education Specialist
Baltimore Washington Medical Center
Edgewater, Maryland

COMMITTEE MEMBERS
George D. Allen, PhD, MS, RN, CNOR, CIC
Director, Infection Control
Downstate Medical Center
Clinical Assistant Professor
SUNY College of Health Related Professions
Brooklyn, New York

J. Hudson Garrett Jr., PhD, MSN, MPH, ARNP, FNP-BC, VA-BC
Senior Director, Clinical Affairs
PDI Healthcare
Atlanta, Georgia

Judith L. Goldberg, MSN, RN, CNOR, CRCST
Clinical Director Endoscopy & Sterile Processing
The William W. Backus Hospital
Norwich, Connecticut

Patricia A. Graybill-D'Ercole, MSN, RN, CNOR, CRCST, CHL
Consultant
Soyring Consulting
St Petersburg, Florida

Deborah S. Hickman Mathis, MSN, RN, CNOR, CRNFA
Director of Surgical Services
Renue Plastic Surgery
Brunswick, Georgia

Rodney W. Hicks, PhD, ARNP, RN, FAANP, FAAN
Professor
Western University of Health Science
Pomona, California

Paula J. Morton, MS, RN, CNOR
Director Perioperative Services
Sherman Health
Rockford, Illinois

Catherine M. Moses, RN, CNOR, CPHQ
QM Coordinator
Medical Arts Surgical Centers/BHSF
Miami, Florida

Rebecca M. Patton, MSN, RN, CNOR, FAAN
Atkinson Scholar in Perioperative Nursing
Case Western Reserve University
Cleveland, Ohio

Elizabeth A. Vane, MSN, RN, CNOR
Department Chair, Perioperative Nursing
Walter Reed National Military Medical Center
Bethesda, Maryland

COMMITTEE LIAISONS
American Association of Nurse Anesthetists
Leslie Ann Jeter, RN, CRNA, MSNA

American College of Surgeons
David L. Feldman, MD, MBA, CPE, FACS

American Society of Anesthesiologists
Sorin J. Brull, MD

Association for Professionals in Infection Control and Epidemiology
Marcia R. Patrick, MSN, RN, CIC

Centers for Disease Control and Prevention
Elizabeth Bolyard, MPH, RN

International Association of Healthcare Central Service Materiel Management
Paula Berrett, BS, CRCST

AORN BOARD LIAISON
Rosemarie Schroeder, BSN, RN, CNOR
Director, Surgical Services
St Josephs Hospital
Marshfield, Wisconsin

EX-OFFICIO
Anne Marie Herlehy, DNP, RN, CNOR
Administrative Director, Perioperative & Cardiovascular Services
Alexian Brothers Medical Center
Chicago, Illinois

This section contains the following AORN Recommended Practices:

**Indicates items appearing in print for the first time in 2012 and new/revised items published electronically during 2011.

The following Recommended Practices for Surgical Attire were developed by the AORN Recommended Practices Committee and have been approved by the AORN Board of Directors. They were presented as proposed recommendations for comments by members and others. They are effective November 1, 2010.

These recommended practices are intended as achievable recommendations representing what is believed to be an optimal level of practice. Policies and procedures will reflect variations in practice settings and/or clinical situations that determine the degree to which the recommended practices can be implemented.

AORN recognizes the various settings in which perioperative nurses practice. These recommended practices are intended as guidelines adaptable to various practice settings. These practice settings include traditional operating rooms (ORs), ambulatory surgery centers, physicians' offices, cardiac catheterization laboratories, endoscopy suites, radiology departments, and all other areas where surgery and other invasive procedures may be performed.

Purpose

These recommended practices provide guidelines for surgical attire including jewelry, clothing, shoes, head coverings, masks, jackets, and other accessories worn in the semirestricted and restricted areas of the surgical or invasive procedure setting. The human body and inanimate surfaces inherent to the surgical environment are major sources of microbial contamination and transmission of microbes; therefore, surgical attire and appropriate personal protective equipment (PPE) are worn to promote worker safety and a high level of cleanliness and hygiene within the perioperative environment. These recommended practices are not intended to address sterile surgical attire worn at the surgical field or all PPE.

Recommendation I

Surgical attire should be made of low-linting material, contain shed skin squames, provide comfort, and promote a professional appearance.

In a prospective interventional study of surgical attire that was motivated by an increase in endophthalmitis after cataract surgery, researchers compared several types of polyester scrub attire and cotton scrub attire. They found that surgical attire made of 100% spunbond polypropylene decreased the bacterial load in the air by 50% compared to cotton surgical attire. Researchers also found that surgical attire helps contain bacterial shedding and promotes environmental control.[1] In another study researchers found that the design of the surgical attire was not as important as the material of which it was made.[2]

I.a. Surgical attire fabrics should be tightly woven, stain resistant, and durable. Surgical attire should provide comfort in terms of design, fit, breathability, and the weight of the fabric.

Cotton fabrics with pores greater than 80 microns may allow microorganisms attached to skin squames to pass through the interstices of the material's weave.[3,4] Tightly-woven surgical attire (cotton and polyester [50/50] with 560 x 395 threads/ 10 cm) reduced the amount of bacteria shed into the air by two to five times, with the exception of methicillin-resistant *Staphylococcus epidermidis* (MRSE) from MRSE carriers.[5]

I.b. Surgical attire made of 100% cotton fleece should not be worn.

Some fabrics made of cotton fleece material collect and shed lint. Lint may harbor microbial-laden dust, skin squames, and respiratory droplets. In addition, fleece is made up of a napped surface with low density, which renders it more flammable.[6]

Cotton fiber is one of the most flammable fibers, and 100% cotton fleece without fire-retardant chemical treatment does not meet the federal flammability standard.[7,8] Cotton blended with 10% to 20% polyester may reduce the flammability,[6,7] but this is not always successful. Application of a fire-retardant chemical still may be required.[8]

Recommendation II

Clean surgical attire, including shoes, head covering, masks, jackets, and identification badges should be worn in the semirestricted and restricted areas of the surgical or invasive procedure setting.

Clean attire minimizes the introduction of microorganisms and lint from health care personnel to clean items and the environment.[9]

II.a. Facility-approved, clean, and freshly laundered or disposable surgical attire should be donned daily in a designated dressing area before entry or reentry into the semirestricted and restricted areas.

Changing from street apparel into facility-approved, clean, and freshly laundered or disposable surgical attire in a designated area decreases the possibility of cross-contamination and assists with traffic control.

II.a.1. When donning surgical attire, care should be taken to avoid contact of the clean attire with the floor or other possibly contaminated surfaces.

II.a.2. When wearing a two-piece scrub suit, the top of the scrub suit should be secured at the waist, tucked into the pants, or fit close to the body to prevent skin squames from being dispersed into the environment.

Loose scrub tops may allow skin squames to disperse into the environment from the axilla and chest. The major source of bacteria dispersed into the air comes from health care providers' skin.[10,11] When skin squames come off the body surface, they carry any microorganism that is found on the surface of the individual's skin. Every individual loses a complete layer of skin every four days (about 10^7 skin squames every day). With just the movement of walking, this may cause a loss of 10^4 squames per minute.[12,13]

II.a.3. Health care personnel should change into street clothes whenever they leave the health care facility or when traveling between buildings located on separate campuses.[9]

Surgical attire may become contaminated by direct or indirect contact with the external environment.

II.b. Jewelry including earrings, necklaces, watches, and bracelets that cannot be contained or confined within the surgical attire should not be worn.[14] Jewelry that cannot be confined within the surgical attire should be removed before entry into the semirestricted and restricted areas.

Necklaces on the skin may contaminate the front of the sterile gown if they are not confined within the surgical attire.

Wearing finger rings, nose rings, and ear piercings increases bacterial counts on skin surfaces both when the jewelry is in place and after removal. One study showed that earrings had bacterial counts more than 21 times higher beneath the earrings than on the surface of the earrings. Bacterial counts were nine times greater on the skin beneath finger and nose rings than on the rings themselves.[14]

The removal of watches and bracelets allows for more thorough hand washing. [15-17] Researchers sampled 100 wristwatch wearers in the health care environment and found that immediately after they removed their watches, 25% of the wristwatch wearers' wrists had positive cultures for *Staphylococcus aureus*.[18]

II.b.1. Rings should be removed before hand washing or using hand rubs.

Several studies have shown that wearing rings may result in colonization of health care providers' hands with gram-negative and gram-positive pathogens.[15,19,20] Finger rings have been found to increase skin surface bacterial counts. Although hand washing reduces these counts, there are more bacteria under rings than on the adjacent skin or the opposite hand. The pathogens identified in one study were coagulase-negative staphylococci, other skin flora, gram-negative cocci, Pseudomonas spp, and *Staphylococcus aureus*.[21]

Removing rings before hand washing may decrease the potential for pathogens to remain on hands after hand washing.[22] Removing rings before hand hygiene may enhance the effectiveness of the hand hygiene process.[17]

II.c. Persons entering the semirestricted or restricted areas of the surgical suite for a brief time for a specific purpose (eg, law enforcement officers, parents, biomedical engineers) should cover all head and facial hair and should don either freshly laundered surgical attire; single-use attire; or a single-use jumpsuit (eg, coveralls, bunny suit) designed to completely cover outside apparel.

Clean and freshly laundered surgical and single-use attire, or single-use jumpsuits donned before entry into the semirestricted and restricted areas may minimize the potential for contamination of the environment and cross contamination of the attire (eg, animal hair, cross contamination from other uncontrolled environments, spores in soil).

II.d. Shoes worn within the perioperative environment should be clean.[23]

Soiled shoes have been found to contribute to environmental contamination within the perioperative environment. A study of shoes worn outdoors and shoes worn only in the surgical suite showed 98% of the outdoor shoes were contaminated with coagulase-negative staphylococci, coliform, and bacillus species compared to 56% of the shoes worn only in the surgical suite. Bacteria on the perioperative floor may contribute up to 15% of colony-forming units (CFUs), which are dispersed into the air by walking. Shoes that are worn only in the perioperative area may help to reduce contamination of the perioperative environment.[23]

II.d.1. Shoes worn within the perioperative environment should have closed toes and backs, low heels, non-skid soles, and must meet Occupational Safety & Health Administration (OSHA) and the health care organization's safety requirements.[24]

Shoes that enclose the foot with backs, low heels, and non-skid soles may reduce the risk of injury from slips and falls and from dropped items. The OSHA regulations require the use of protective footwear in areas where there is a danger of foot injuries from falling or rolling objects or objects piercing the sole. The employer is responsible for determining if foot injury hazards exist and what, if any, protective footwear is required.[24,25] The OSHA regulations mandate that employers perform a workplace hazard risk assessment and ensure that employees wear protective footwear to provide protection from identified potential hazards (eg, needlesticks, scalpel cuts, splashing from blood or other possibly infectious materials).[26-28]

Shoes that have holes or perforations may not protect the feet from exposure to blood, body fluids, or other liquids that may contain potentially infectious agents. Shoes made of cloth, that are open-toed, or that have holes on the top or sides do not offer protection against spilled liquids or sharp items that may be dropped or kicked. In one study, 15 different types of shoes were tested with an apparatus that measured resistance to penetration by scalpels. The materials of the shoes included leather, suede, rubber, and canvas. Sixty percent of the shoes sustained scalpel penetration through the shoe into a simulated foot. Only six materials prevented complete penetration. These materials included sneaker suede, suede with inner mesh lining, leather with inner canvas lining, non-pliable leather, rubber with inner leather lining, and rubber.[29,30]

II.e. Identification badges should be worn by all personnel authorized to enter the perioperative setting.[31-33] Health care personnel as well as patients should be able to identify caregivers.

Identification badges assist in identifying persons authorized to be in the perioperative setting and support security measures.[32,34]

II.e.1. Identification badges should be secured on the surgical attire top, be visible, and be cleaned if they become soiled.

Badge holders such as lanyards, chains, or beads pose a risk for contamination and may be very difficult to clean. One study of identification badges and lanyards showed that the median bacterial load isolated was 10-fold greater for lanyards (3.1 CFU/cm^2) than for identification badges (0.3 CFU/cm^2). The microorganisms recovered from lanyards and identification badges were methicillin-sensitive

Staphylococcus aureus (MSSA), methicillin-resistant *Staphylococcus aureus* (MRSA), Enterococcus spp, and enterobacteriaceae.[35] As with other personal attire, such as stethoscopes, identification badges become contaminated over time.

II.f. The use of cover apparel (eg, lab coat, cover gown) may be determined at each individual practice setting based on state regulatory requirements and the culture of the health care organization.

Wearing cover apparel over surgical attire outside of the perioperative suite may be required for some health care personnel in some health care organizations for a variety of reasons, which may include professional appearance. This may be based on the belief that cover apparel decreases the risk of infection. The use of cover apparel has been found to have little or no effect on reducing contamination of surgical attire.[36]

II.f.1. Cover apparel should be laundered daily in a health-care approved or accredited laundry facility. (See Recommendation V.)

Health care personnel may carry staphylococci and enterococci on their clothing, which may include surgical attire and cover apparel.[37] Studies of cover apparel have shown that rather than protecting the clothing underneath the cover gown, cover apparel may contaminate the clothes worn under the cover apparel. Researchers have found that cover apparel is not always discarded daily after use or laundered on a frequent basis.[36,38]

In one study of cover coats worn by 100 physicians, *Staphylococcus aureus* was isolated from 25 of the cover coats. The cuffs and pockets of the coats were the most contaminated.[38]

In another study of 100 medical students, microorganisms were found on the cuffs and side pockets of the students' cover apparel. Contamination was found on their dominant hand sleeve cuffs and the backs of the cover apparel 10 cm down from the collar. These areas were contaminated with

Staphylococcus sp on all cover apparel, Acinetobacter sp on seven students' cover apparel, and diphtheroids on 12 students' cover apparel.[39]

In a study of health care practitioners' cover apparel, researchers found cover apparel in inpatient and outpatient areas, intensive care units, administration areas, and the OR were contaminated with *Staphylococcus aureus*, which included susceptible and resistant isolates. Health care personnel with colonization were more likely to have home-laundered their cover apparel. Two-thirds of the health care practitioners perceived their cover apparel to be dirty because it had not been washed in more than a week.[37]

II.g. Stethoscopes should be clean and not worn around the neck.

Inanimate objects, such as contaminated stethoscope tubing and diaphragms, may transmit pathogens such as MRSA by indirect contact (eg, by wearing the stethoscope around the neck and contaminating the skin and surgical attire).[40] Cleaning stethoscopes in combination with health care personnel washing their hands between caring for patients decreases the possibility of transmission of pathogens to patients and environmental surfaces.

Stethoscopes may be the most widely used medical device in a health care facility.[41] Although stethoscopes are not considered part of the surgical attire, health care providers often wear them around their necks as though they were part of surgical attire. Stethoscopes come in direct contact with patients' skin and could provide an opportunity for transmission of microbes from patient to patient, to health care personnel. or from health care personnel to patients. One study verified that stethoscopes could be a vector for transmission to patients.[42] Another study conducted on stethoscope diaphragms noted that, when cultured before cleaning,
- 79.8% of the cultures grew gram-positive bacilli,
- 74.8% had Staphylococcus species non-aureus,

- 2.5% of baseline cultures showed MSSA, and
- group A streptococcus was found in 1% of cultures.[43]

A study showed recontamination of stethoscopes can occur by the fifth time the stethoscope is used on different patients. The number of bacteria on a stethoscope increases with each use.[44]

Cleaning the stethoscope daily may not be adequate; cleaning stethoscopes may be required between each patient use. Several studies on contamination of stethoscope diaphragms and earpieces have been conducted and show that 66% to 100% of the diaphragms are contaminated.[41] One study noted that to avoid increasing emergent strains, routine cleaning of stethoscopes may help reduce bacterial colony counts.[45]

II.g.1. Fabric stethoscope tubing covers should not be used.

Adding fabric covers to stethoscope tubing may result in the covers acting as fomites. One study of stethoscope fabric covers isolated gram-positive aerobic bacteria, gram-negative aerobic bacteria, anaerobes, and yeast. The average length of time between stethoscope cover laundering was 3.7 months, with some fabric covers that were never laundered.[46]

II.h. Fanny packs, backpacks, and briefcases should not be taken into the semirestricted or restricted areas of the perioperative suite.

Items brought into the OR, such as fanny packs, backpacks, briefcases, and other personal items that are constructed of porous materials, may be difficult to clean or disinfect adequately and may harbor pathogens, dust, and bacteria.[47,48] Pathogens have been shown to survive on fabrics and plastics.[49,50] Dust is made up of skin particles, hair, fabric fibers, pollens, mold, fungi, insect parts, glove powder, and paper fibers, among other things. Bacteria may be transported from one location to another by carriers such as dust or liquids, and may contaminate fanny packs, backpacks, and briefcases.[48,51,52]

The type of environmental surface and its ability to support microbial growth will influence microbial carriage. Gram-positive cocci (eg, coagulase-negative staphylococci) may persist in dry settings. Settings that are moist and soiled may support gram-negative bacilli (eg, floors). Fungi favors moist, fibrous material and are also found in dust.[47]

Recommendation III

All individuals who enter the semirestricted and restricted areas should wear freshly laundered surgical attire that is laundered at a health care-accredited laundry facility or disposable surgical attire provided by the facility and intended for use within the perioperative setting.

Surgical attire helps contain bacterial shedding and promotes environmental cleanliness.[1] An individual sheds millions of skin squames daily. Five percent to 10% of skin squames carry bacteria.[53] In a study on dispersal of MRSE, carriers of MRSE were seen as possible sources of air contamination in ORs.[5]

III.a. Surgical attire should be changed daily or at the end of the shift.[54]

It has been reported that surgical attire may have bacterial colony counts that are higher when scrub clothing is removed, stored in a locker, and used again. Microbes have been shown to survive for long periods of time on fabrics such as surgical attire.[49,50,55]

III.a.1. Reusable or single-use contaminated attire should be placed in appropriately designated containers after use.[27] Worn reusable surgical attire should be left at the health care facility for laundering.

III.a.2. Surgical attire that has been penetrated by blood or other potentially infectious materials should be removed immediately or as soon as possible and replaced with freshly laundered, clean surgical attire. When extensive contamination of the body occurs, a shower or bath should be taken before donning fresh attire.[26,27]

Changing contaminated, soiled, or wet attire reduces the potential for contamination and protects personnel from prolonged exposure to potentially harmful bacteria.[26,54]

III.a.3. Wet or contaminated surgical attire should not be rinsed or sorted in the location of use.[26]

Rinsing or sorting contaminated reusable attire may expose the health care worker to blood, body fluids, or other liquids that may contain potentially infectious agents and may contaminate the patient care environment.[26]

III.a.4. Surgical attire contaminated with visible blood or body fluids must remain at the health care facility for laundering or be sent to an accredited laundry facility contracted by the health care organization.[26,48,54,56]

Controlled laundering of attire contaminated by blood or body fluids reduces the risk of transferring pathogenic microorganisms from the facility to the home or general public.[56] (See Recommendation V.)

III.b. When in the semirestricted or restricted areas, all nonscrubbed personnel should wear a freshly laundered or single-use long-sleeved warm-up jacket snapped closed with the cuffs down to the wrists.

Wearing the warm-up jacket snapped closed prevents the edges of the front of the jacket from contaminating a skin prep area or the sterile surgical field. Long-sleeved attire helps contain skin squames shed from bare arms.[1]

III.b.1. All personal clothing should be completely covered by the surgical attire. Undergarments such as T-shirts with a V-neck, which can be contained underneath the scrub top, may be worn; personal clothing that extends above the scrub top neckline or below the sleeve of the surgical attire should not be worn.

Personal clothing is not laundered by a health care accredited laundry. (See Recommendation V.)

Recommendation IV

All personnel should cover head and facial hair, including sideburns and the nape of the neck, when in the semirestricted and restricted areas.

Head coverings contain skin squames and hair shed from the scalp. It is important to prevent shed skin squames from falling onto the sterile field.[57,58] Although group A Streptococcus is isolated in less than 1% of surgical site infections (SSIs) (ie, 1 per 10,000), it is a serious cause of SSIs and can be carried on the scalp.[59] An outbreak of SSIs was attributed to group A β-hemolytic Streptococcus carried on the scalp of perioperative personnel. The report identified group A β-hemolytic Streptococcus in 20 patients with an SSI. In the outbreak investigation, 88 perioperative personnel were cultured. One was found to have erythema and scaling on the scalp and ears and under the breast. The individual was treated with medication and relocated to a non-patient work area, and the outbreak was resolved.[59]

Human hair can be a site of pathogenic bacteria such as MRSA. Routine shampooing of hair with neutral detergents does not remove MRSA or have a bactericidal effect.[60]

IV.a. A clean, low-lint surgical head cover or hood that confines all hair and covers scalp skin should be worn. The head cover or hood should be designed to minimize microbial dispersal.

Hair acts as a filter when it is uncovered and collects bacteria in proportion to its length, waviness, and oiliness. Studies have shown that *Staphylococcus aureus* and *Staphylococcus epidermidis* have a tendency to colonize hair, skin, and the nasopharynx.[60] Head coverings designed to contain hair and scalp skin will minimize microbial dispersal.[61] Skull caps may fail to contain the side hair above and in front of the ears and hair at the nape of the neck.

IV.a.1. Used single-use head coverings should be removed and discarded in a designated receptacle daily or when contaminated.

Placing contaminated head coverings in a designated receptacle assists in maintaining a clean and orderly area and decreases the possibility of cross contamination.

IV.a.2. Reusable head coverings should be laundered in a health care-accredited laundry facility after each daily use.[51] (See Recommendation V.)

Recommendation V

Surgical attire should be laundered in a health care-accredited laundry facility.

Surgical attire; street clothing; PPE; and other hospital textiles (eg, bed linens, towels, privacy curtains, washcloths) may become contaminated by bacteria and fungi during wear or use. In one study, researchers found that microbes can survive on hospital textiles for extended periods of time. These textiles included

- 100% cotton clothing;
- 60% cotton/40% polyester blends (eg, scrub suits, lab coats);
- 100% polyester clothing; and
- polyethylene plastic aprons.

Researchers inoculated these textiles with staphylococci under laboratory conditions. The textiles were allowed to remain in ambient air without any laundering for various periods of time. Results showed that the staphylococci survived one to 56 days on polyester and up to 90 days on polyethylene plastic. The larger the microbial inoculum of staphylococci on polyester and polyethylene, the longer the staphylococci survived. Even if only a few hundred staphylococci survived, they were viable for days on most textiles. The shortest time for enterococci survival on textiles was 11 days.[49,50]

Researchers in another study tested fungal survival under laboratory conditions on

- 100% cotton clothing;
- 60% cotton and 40% polyester blend (eg, scrub suits, lab coats, clothes);
- 100% polyester clothing; and
- polyethylene plastic aprons.

The microorganisms used as the inoculum were *Candida albicans, Candida tropicalis, Candida krusei, Candida parapsilosis, Aspergillus flavus, Aspergillus fumigatus, Aspergillus niger, Aspergillus terreus,* Fusarium sp, Mucor sp, and Paecilomyces sp. These pathogens were isolated in the researchers' health care facility. The data collected showed that candida, aspergillus, mucor, and fusarium, which are known to be health care-associated infectious agents, survived on fabrics and plastics for at least one day and often for weeks. The survival of these microorganisms on these textiles and plastics shows that they may serve as reservoirs or vectors for fungi.[50] Another study showed that *Staphylococcus aureus* and *Pseudomonas aeruginosa* bind to polyester and acrylic fibers.[62]

Health care-accredited laundry facilities are preferred because they follow industry standards. The Healthcare Laundry Accreditation Council (HLAC) offers voluntary accreditation for those laundry facilities that process reusable health care textiles and which incorporate OSHA and the Centers for Disease Control and Prevention (CDC) guidelines and professional association recommended practices. The HLAC standards for accreditation include, but are not limited to,

- Textile quality control procedures are defined and implemented.
- The inventory system is adequate to ensure supply.
- Soiled and contaminated textile areas are separated by a physical barrier.
- The ventilation is controlled with negative pressure in the soiled area, positive pressure from the clean textile area through the soiled textile area, six to 10 air exchanges per hour, and air vented to the outside.
- Clean textiles are stored in an area free of vermin, dust, and lint and at room temperature between 68° F to 78° F (20° C to 25.6° C).
- Storage shelves are 1 inch to 2 inches from the wall, the bottom shelf is 6 inches to 8 inches from the floor, and the top shelf is 12 inches to 18 inches below the ceiling.
- Hand washing facilities are located in all areas with soiled textiles; hand washing or antiseptic dispensers are in the clean textile area; and employees perform hand washing after glove removal and restroom use, before eating, and when hands are contaminated with blood or other potentially infectious materials.
- Working surfaces are clean and are disinfected if they become contaminated with blood or other potentially infectious materials.
- The OSHA Exposure Control Plan is in place and PPE is supplied and available.
- Personnel training is provided and documented.
- Quality control monitoring and processes are in place.
- Material Safety Data Sheets are available for each chemical used.
- Water quality is tested on a regular basis for hardness, alkalinity, iron content, and pH.
- Soiled health care textiles are handled, collected, and transported according to local, state, and federal regulations.

◆ Each wash load is monitored and applicable data for each wash are recorded, including cycle, pre-wash, wash, rinse, and final rinse times; water levels and usage; temperatures; and chemical usage.

◆ Water extraction and drying is performed using methods that preserve the integrity of the textiles and minimize bacterial growth.

◆ Cleaned textiles are packaged and stored in fluid-resistant bundles or fluid-resistant carts or hampers and are handled as little as possible.

◆ Carts used for transport or storage are kept clean and are well-maintained.

◆ Clean textiles are stored and transported separately from soiled textiles.

◆ Vehicles used to transport textiles provide separation of clean and soiled textiles, and the vehicle interiors are cleaned on a regular basis.[63]

Routine monitoring of laundry processes, including cleaning of work areas, equipment, and good hand hygiene practices are important to minimize cross-contamination of clean textiles. An accredited health care facility laundering process includes monitoring correct measurement of chemicals, sufficient water, correct temperature, mechanical action, and the duration of the washing cycle. Cleaning and disinfecting the work area includes, but is not limited to, the washers, extractors, dryers, and conveyor belts. The presence of skin bacteria on processed textiles and environmental surfaces in one study directed attention to hand hygiene of the laundry facility workers, air contamination, inadequate separation of soiled and clean work areas, and the cleaning and disinfecting of all of the equipment and work surfaces.[64] Water can be a source of bacterial transmission, which makes thorough drying of textiles vital.[65] Staphylococci, Salmonella, and Mycobacterium are fairly resistant to heat and may survive drying.[66]

Home laundering is not monitored for quality, consistency, or safety. Exposure of health care personnel and their family members to blood and other potentially infectious materials may result from improper handling and decontamination of surgical attire. Home washers may have a lower temperature (ie, < 160° F [71.1° C]) or washing parameters and temperatures may not be adjustable. Home washers may have limited capacity for chemical additives and may not have directions for using alkalis and acids.

Home laundering may not meet the specified measures necessary to achieve a reduction in antimicrobial levels in soiled surgical attire. These measures involve mechanical, thermal, and chemical components, including

◆ diluting and agitating the water to remove microorganisms and bioburden;

◆ selecting suitable chemicals, if low-temperature cycles (< 160° F [< 71.1° C]) are used;

◆ using proper chemical concentrations if low-temperature cycles are used;

◆ using water temperature > 160° F (> 71.1° C) for more than 25 minutes for hot-water cycles;

◆ using chlorine bleach, which gives added microbicidal benefit; and

◆ adding chemicals known as "sour" to the water to neutralize alkalinity in the water, soap, or detergent.

These measures cause a shift in pH from 12 to 5, inactivating some microorganisms. Low temperatures (ie, < 160° F [< 71.1° C]) may be used as long as the drying temperatures and ironing temperatures provide the additional microbicidal benefits to ensure surgical attire is clean.[51,67]

A study on bacterial contamination of home-laundered uniforms began by culturing uniforms worn at the beginning of the shift. Thirty-nine percent of the uniforms identified as "clean" had one or more microorganisms (eg, vancomycin-resistant enterococci, MRSA, *Clostridium difficile*) identified. Uniforms were tested again at the end of the shift and 54% had one or more microorganisms; some that were positive at the beginning of the shift were negative at the end of the shift. In one demonstration, bacillus spores were transferred from health care providers' aprons and cotton uniforms to a mock patient.[68]

A study of home-laundered uniforms involved taking surveillance cultures from five patients. Results showed that three of the patients were colonized with the same strain of microorganism as that cultured from the health care providers' uniforms. With uniforms contaminated with microorganisms at the beginning of a shift, the researchers suggested that inappropriate laundering practices may be the cause.[69]

Home laundering has been shown to be less effective for cleaning surgical attire than attire laundered by health care facilities or commercial laundries.[70]

A quantitative study was performed in 20 different geographical areas.[70] Eight laundering methods were studied:

- reusable clean scrubs laundered at the facility in which they were used;
- reusable worn scrubs laundered at the facility in which they were used;
- reusable clean scrubs that were home laundered;
- reusable worn scrubs that were home laundered;
- reusable clean scrubs laundered by an outside laundry facility;
- reusable worn scrubs laundered by an outside laundry facility;
- packaged, clean, single-use, non-woven scrubs; and
- packaged, worn, single-use, non-woven scrubs.

Results of the study showed that the bioburden on home-laundered surgical attire was significantly greater than surgical attire that was facility-laundered; laundered by a third party; or was single-use, disposable attire. Home-laundered clean scrubs at the beginning of the day had the same amount of organisms as worn scrubs at the end of the work day.[70]

A quantitative study was performed on cotton strips of fabric that were inoculated with 10 mL of a viral suspension to discover if enteric viruses (ie, adenovirus, rotavirus, hepatitis A virus) survived a home-laundering process. The inoculated fabric strips were washed, rinsed, and dried on a 28-minute permanent press cycle in home washers. It was found that enteric viruses remained on the fabric strips after they were washed.[71]

V.a. Laundered surgical attire should be protected during transport to the practice setting to prevent contamination.[9,65]

Proper transfer and storage of surgical attire protects surgical attire from contamination by

- preventing any physical damage to laundry,
- minimizing microbial contamination from environmental surfaces, and
- preventing any deposits from airborne sources such as dust to settle on laundry.[9,65]

V.a.1. Surgical attire should be transported in a clean vehicle and enclosed carts or containers.[9,65]

Laundry vehicles can be a source of contamination. Cleaning and disinfection on a regular basis is required.

V.b. Clean surgical attire should be stored in a clean, enclosed cart or cabinet.[9,65]

Storing clean surgical attire in a locker with personal items from outside of the hospital may contaminate the clean surgical attire. Enteric viruses have been detected in lockers where contaminated attire can act as reservoirs for viral transmission.[17,72]

V.b.1. Surgical attire may be stored in a dispensing machine. Dispensing machines should be routinely emptied and cleaned according to the manufacturer's directions.

Attire-dispensing machines may be used to increase individual accountability, promote cost containment, facilitate an adequate supply, and provide clean storage for surgical attire.[73,74]

Recommendation VI

All individuals entering the restricted areas should wear a surgical mask when open sterile supplies and equipment are present.

A surgical mask protects both the surgical team and the patient from transfer of microorganisms.[54] The surgical mask protects health care providers from droplets greater than 5 micrometers in size. Examples of diseases that produce droplets include group A Streptococcus, adenovirus, and Neisseria meningitides.[75] A single surgical mask is worn to protect the health care provider from contact with infectious material from the patient (eg, respiratory secretions, sprays of blood or body fluids) and to protect the patient from exposure to infectious agents carried in the provider's mouth or nose. Surgical masks protect surgical team members' noses and mouths from inadvertent splashes or splatters of blood and other body fluids.[26] A study involving 8,500 surgical procedures showed that 26% of exposures to blood were to the heads and necks of scrubbed personnel, and that 17% of blood exposures were to circulating personnel outside the sterile field.[76]

VI.a. The mask should cover the mouth and nose and be secured in a manner to prevent venting.

A mask that is securely tied at the back of the head and behind the neck decreases the risk of health care personnel transmitting nasopharyngeal and respiratory microorganisms to patients or the sterile field. Infectious particles can reach the wearer's nose and mouth by passing through leaks at the mask-face seal.

VI.b. A fresh, clean surgical mask should be worn for every procedure. The mask should be replaced and discarded whenever it becomes wet or soiled.

The filtering capacity of a mask is compromised when it becomes wet. In a study to determine microbial barrier efficacy of surgical masks with 95% bacterial filtration at one-, two-, three-, and four-hour intervals showed that after four hours, the masks had decreased efficacy. Avoiding unnecessary speaking and keeping in mind the patient's possible immunological status is important. This research study showed that all counts of CFUs were lower than 4X10², which could cause an SSI in patients with poor immunity or in patients with surgical wound complications (eg, ischemia, hematoma) or those undergoing surgery with an implant.[77]

VI.b.1. Masks should not be worn hanging down from the neck.

The filter portion of a surgical mask harbors bacteria collected from the nasopharyngeal airway. The contaminated mask may cross-contaminate the surgical attire top.

VI.c. Surgical masks should be discarded after each procedure. Masks should be removed carefully by handling only the mask ties. Hand hygiene should be performed after removal of masks.[17]

Removing masks by the ties prevents possible contamination of the hands. The filter portion of the mask harbors bacteria collected from the nasopharyngeal airway.

VI.d. Only one surgical mask should be worn at a time.

Masks are intended to contain and filter droplets of microorganisms expelled from the mouth and nasopharynx during talking, sneezing, and coughing.[78] Use of a double mask creates an impediment to breathing and does not increase filtration; therefore, this is not recommended.[76]

Recommendation VII

Health care personnel should receive initial and ongoing education and demonstrate competency on appropriate surgical attire.

Competency assessment verifies that health care personnel have an understanding of the articles and purpose of surgical attire. This knowledge is essential for reducing the risk of health care-associated infections.

VII.a. Health care personnel should receive education and guidance on appropriate articles of surgical attire worn in the perioperative environment at orientation and after changes are made.[26,65] Health care personnel should be informed of and be compliant with the health care organization's surgical attire policy, including laundering policies.

Ongoing education of perioperative personnel facilitates the development of knowledge, skills, and attitudes that affect patient and worker safety.

VII.a.1. Health care personnel should understand the risk of becoming colonized or infected with microorganisms from patients or the environment when surgical attire is cleaned improperly.

Recommendation VIII

Policies and procedures for surgical attire should be developed, reviewed periodically, and be readily available within the practice setting.

Policies and procedures serve as operational guidelines and establish authority, responsibility, and accountability within the organization. Policies and procedures also assist in the development of patient safety, quality assessment, and improvement activities.

VIII.a. Surgical attire polices and procedures should include, but not be limited to, requirements related to
  − facility-approved and standardized surgical attire,
  − areas where surgical attire is worn,

- infection prevention and control,
- use of PPE,
- laundering,
- transport and storage of clean attire, and
- compliance monitoring.

An understanding of surgical attire policies and procedures assists health care personnel in protecting the patient, themselves, and their family members.

VIII.b. Policies and procedures should be introduced and reviewed in the initial orientation, when new surgical attire is introduced, and during ongoing education of health care personnel.

Review of policies and procedures assists health care personnel in being knowledgeable about and compliant with the health care organization's policies and procedures.

Recommendation IX

The health care organization's quality management program should evaluate compliance with surgical attire policies and identify and respond to opportunities for improvement.

Quality management programs that enhance personal performance and monitor surgical attire practices are established to promote patient and health care personnel safety. Health care laundry processing requires specialized equipment, adequate space, qualified personnel with ongoing training, and continuous monitoring for quality assurance.[63]

IX.a.   Structure, process, and performance measures should be identified.

Structure, process, and performance measures can be used to improve surgical attire quality and monitor compliance with facility policies and procedures, national standards, and regulatory requirements.

IX.a.1.   Quality indicators for surgical attire may include, but are not limited to,
- head coverings completely cover the hair and scalp;
- warm-up jackets with wrist-length sleeves are worn and are snapped;
- identification badges are worn, visible, and clean;
- shoes are clean and protect health care personnel's feet;

- visibly soiled or wet surgical attire is removed and cleaned at an accredited health care laundry facility;
- masks, when worn, are tied securely and are discarded after each procedure; and
- cover apparel, if worn, is laundered daily at the organization or an accredited laundry facility.

IX.b.   Quality assurance monitoring of laundry processes should be ongoing.

A study of the risk of *Clostridium difficile* cross contamination in the laundry process illustrates that cross contamination occurs with the use of nonsporicidal disinfectants, but the use of sporicidal disinfectant cloths showed significantly reduced CFUs. The researcher concluded that cleaning *Clostridium difficile*-contaminated surfaces with nonsporicidal disinfectants creates a vector for cross contamination to other textiles via the laundering process. Cleaning contaminated surfaces with sporicidal disinfectant may not completely eliminate this vector, but does significantly reduce associated risk.[79]

A rare outbreak of zygomycosis in a hospital was investigated by the CDC using standard outbreak protocols. Zygomycosis is an invasive fungal infection caused by mucormycetes, which includes a Rhizopus species (ie, a group of molds that is commonly found in the environment). Infections with this microorganism are rare and usually occur in people who have underlying medical conditions. A cluster of six cases occurred from August 2008 to July 2009. Of the six cases, five patients died (ie, premature children up to age 13). All five children had risk factors for zygomycosis, which included acidosis (ie, four children) and bone marrow transplant (ie, one child). Hospital linens were the only items common to these cases. Environmental cultures taken at the hospital demonstrated Rhizopus species from 26 out of 65 swabs (40%) of clean linens and areas in contact with clean linens, and 1 out of 25 samples (4%) from items not in contact with linens. Clean linen closets were cultured, including those in the OR, where two items were found to be Rhizopus-positive. Researchers determined the hospital linens to be the most likely vehicle of transmission to patients' skin. Contamination of linens may have occurred during laundering, en route to the hospital, or during delivery to the hospital. The hospital changed commercial laundry facilities, replaced all of its linens, disinfected all linen storage closets, and used a different delivery area for its linens in an effort to prevent reoccurrence of this type of outbreak.[80]

Glossary

Restricted area: Includes the OR and procedure room, the clean core, and scrub sink areas. People in this area are required to wear full surgical attire and cover all head and facial hair, including sideburns, beards, and necklines.

Semirestricted area: Includes the peripheral support areas of the surgical suite and has storage areas for sterile and clean supplies, work areas for storage and processing instruments, and corridors leading to the restricted areas of the surgical suite.

Surgical attire: Nonsterile apparel designated for the OR practice setting that includes two-piece pantsuits, cover jackets, head coverings, shoes, masks, protective eyewear, and other protective barriers.

REFERENCES

1. Andersen BM, Solheim N. Occlusive scrub suits in operating theaters during cataract surgery: effect on airborne contamination. *Infect Control Hosp Epidemiol.* 2002;23(4):218-220.

2. Tammelin A, Hambraeus A, Stahle E. Source and route of methicillin-resistant *Staphylococcus epidermidis* transmitted to the surgical wound during cardio-thoracic surgery. Possibility of preventing wound contamination by use of special scrub suits. *J Hosp Infect.* 2001;47 (4):266-276.

3. Whyte W, Hamblen DL, Kelly IG, Hambraeus A, Laurell G. An investigation of occlusive polyester surgical clothing. *J Hosp Infect.* 1990;15(4):363-374.

4. Barrie D. How hospital linen and laundry services are provided. *J Hosp Infect.* 1994;27(3):219-235.

5. Tammelin A, Domicel P, Hambraeus A, Stahle E. Dispersal of methicillin-resistant Staphylococcus epidermidis by staff in an operating suite for thoracic and cardiovascular surgery: relation to skin carriage and clothing. *J Hosp Infect.* 2000;44(2):119-126.

6. Wu X, Yang CQ. Flame retardant finishing of cotton fleece fabric: part III—the combination of maleic acid and sodium hypophosphite. *J Fire Sci.* 2008;26(4):351-368.

7. US Department of Health and Human Services. Standard for the flammability of clothing textiles. 16 CFR §1610.

8. Yang CQ, Qiu X. Flame-retardant finishing of cotton fleece fabric: Part I. The use of a hydroxy-functional organophosphorus oligomer and dimethyloldihydroxylethyleneurea. *Fire and Materials.* 2007;31(1):67-81.

9. AAMI. *ST79: Comprehensive Guide to Steam Sterilization and Sterility Assurance in Health Care Facilities.* 2009.

10. Mitchell NJ, Evans DS, Kerr A. Reduction of skin bacteria in theatre air with comfortable, non-woven disposable clothing for operating-theatre staff. *Br Med J.* 1978;1(6114):696-698.

11. Woodhead K, Taylor EW, Bannister G, Chesworth T, Hoffman P, Humphreys H. Behaviours and rituals in the operating theatre. A report from the Hospital Infection Society Working Party on Infection Control in Operating Theatres. *J Hosp Infect.* 2002;51(4):241-255.

12. Noble WC. Dispersal of skin microorganisms. *Br J Dermatol.* 1975;93(4):477-485.

13. Noble WC, Habbema JD, van Furth R, Smith I, de Raay C. Quantitative studies on the dispersal of skin bacteria into the air. *J Med Microbiol.* 1976;9(1):53-61.

14. Bartlett GE, Pollard TC, Bowker KE, Bannister GC. Effect of jewellery on surface bacterial counts of operating theatres. *J Hosp Infect.* 2002;52(1):68-70.

15. Graves PB, Twomey CL. Surgical hand antisepsis: an evidence-based review. *Perioperative Nursing Clinics.* 2006;1(3):235-246.

16. Field EA, McGowan P, Pearce PK, Martin MV. Rings and watches: should they be removed prior to operative dental procedures? *J Dent.* 1996;24(1-2):65-69.

17. Recommended practices for hand hygiene in the perioperative setting. In: *Perioperative Standards and Recommended Practices.* Denver, CO: AORN, Inc; 2010:75-90.

18. Jeans AR, Moore J, Nicol C, Bates C, Read RC. Wristwatch use and hospital-acquired infection. *J Hosp Infect.* 2010;74(1):16-21.

19. Boyce JM, Pittet D, Healthcare Infection Control Practices Advisory Committee, HICPAC/SHEA/APIC /IDSA Hand Hygiene Task Force. Guideline for Hand Hygiene in Health-Care Settings. Recommendations of the Healthcare Infection Control Practices Advisory Committee and the HICPAC/SHEA/APIC/IDSA Hand Hygiene Task Force. Society for Healthcare Epidemiology of America/ Association for Professionals in Infection Control/Infectious Diseases Society of America. *MMWR Recomm Rep.* 2002;51(RR-16):1-45, quiz CE1-4.

20. Salisbury DM, Hutfilz P, Treen LM, Bollin GE, Gautam S. The effect of rings on microbial load of health care workers' hands. *Am J Infect Control.* 1997;25(1): 24-27.

21. Kelsall NKR, Griggs RKL, Bowker KE, Bannister GC. Should finger rings be removed prior to scrubbing for theatre? *J Hosp Infect.* 2006;62(4):450-452.

22. Trick WE, Vernon MO, Hayes RA, et al. Impact of ring wearing on hand contamination and comparison of hand hygiene agents in a hospital. *Clin Infect Dis.* 2003; 36(11):1383-1390.

23. Amirfeyz R, Tasker A, Ali S, Bowker K, Blom A. Theatre shoes—a link in the common pathway of postoperative wound infection? *Ann R Coll Surg Engl.* 2007;89(6):605-608.

24. Occupational Safety and Health Standards 1910.136: Foot protection. United States Department of Labor *http://www.osha.gov/pls/oshaweb/owadisp .show_document?p_table=STANDARDS&p_id=9786*. Accessed September 29, 2010.

25. Fairfax RE. Wearing "Crocs" brand shoes with a partially open heel and a covered toe in a pharmacy setting [letter]. July 16, 2006. *http://www.osha.gov/pls /oshaweb/owadisp.show_document?p_table=INTERPRE TATIONS&p_id=25439*. Accessed October 4, 2010.

26. Occupational exposure to bloodborne pathogens— OSHA. Final rule. *Fed Regist*. 1991;56(235):64004-64182.

27. US Health and Human Services. Bloodborne pathogens. 29 CFR §1910.1030.

28. 29 CFR 1910.132: General requirements. United States Department of Labor. *http://www.osha.gov/pls /oshaweb/owadisp.show_document?p_table=STAN DARDS&p_id=9777*. Accessed September 29, 2010.

29. Barr J, Siegel D. Dangers of dermatologic surgery: protect your feet. *Dermatol Surg*. 2004;30(12 Pt 1):1495-1497.

30. Watt AM, Patkin M, Sinnott MJ, Black RJ, Maddern GJ. Scalpel safety in the operative setting: a systematic review. *Surgery*. 2010;147(1):98-106.

31. AORN position statement on the role of the health care industry representative in the perioperative/ invasive procedure setting. *http://www.aorn.org/Prac ticeResources/AORNPositionStatements/*. Accessed September 29, 2010.

32. Recommended practices for a safe environment of care. In: *Perioperative Standards and Recommended Practices*. Denver, CO: AORN, Inc; 2010: 217-240.

33. Developing and implementing a workplace violence prevention program and policy. In: *Violence in the Workplace: Risk Factors and Prevention Strategies*. Washington, DC: National Institute for Occupational Safety and Health; 1996.

34. *Hospital Accreditation Standards*. Oakbrook Terrace, IL: The Joint Commission; 2009:47-68.

35. Kotsanas D, Scott C, Gillespie EE, Korman TM, Stuart RL. What's hanging around your neck? Pathogenic bacteria on identity badges and lanyards. *Med J Aust*. 2008;188(1):5-8.

36. Kaplan C, Mendiola R, Ndjatou V, Chapnick E, Minkoff H. The role of covering gowns in reducing rates of bacterial contamination of scrub suits. *Am J Obstet Gynecol*. 2003;188(5):1154-1155.

37. Treakle AM, Thom KA, Furuno JP, Strauss SM, Harris AD, Perencevich EN. Bacterial contamination of health care workers' white coats. *Am J Infect Control*. 2009;37(2):101-105.

38. Wong D, Nye K, Hollis P. Microbial flora on doctors' white coats. *BMJ*. 1991;303(6817):1602-1604.

39. Loh W, Ng VV, Holton J. Bacterial flora on the white coats of medical students. *J Hosp Infect*. 2000;45(1):65-68.

40. Durai R, Ng PCH, Hoque H. Methicillin-resistant *Staphylococcus aureus*: an update. *AORN J*. 2010;91(5): 599-609.

41. Wood MW, Lund RC, Stevenson KB. Bacterial contamination of stethoscopes with antimicrobial diaphragm covers. *Am J Infect Control*. 2007;35(4):263-266.

42. Bernard L, Kereveur A, Durand D, et al. Bacterial contamination of hospital physicians' stethoscopes. *Infect Control Hosp Epidemiol*. 1999;20(9):626-628.

43. Lecat P, Cropp E, McCord G, Haller NA. Ethanol-based cleanser versus isopropyl alcohol to decontaminate stethoscopes. *Am J Infect Control*. 2009;37(3): 241-243.

44. Leprat R, Minary P, Devaux V, de Waziere B, Dupond JL, Talon D. Why, when and how to clean stethoscopes. *J Hosp Infect*. 1998;39(1):80-82.

45. Sood P, Mishra B, Mandal A. Potential infection hazards of stethoscopes. *J Indian Med Assoc*. 2000;98(7): 368-370.

46. Milam MW, Hall M, Pringle T, Buchanan K. Bacterial contamination of fabric stethoscope covers: the velveteen rabbit of health care? *Infect Control Hosp Epidemiol*. 2001;22(10):653-655.

47. Recommended practices for environmental cleaning in the perioperative setting. In: *Perioperative Standards and Recommended Practices*. Denver, CO: AORN, Inc; 2010: 241-256.

48. Standards of perioperative nursing. In: *Perioperative Standards and Recommended Practices*. Denver, CO: AORN, Inc; 2010: 9-62.

49. Neely AN, Maley MP. Survival of enterococci and staphylococci on hospital fabrics and plastic. *J Clin Microbiol*. 2000;38(2):724-726.

50. Neely AN, Orloff MM. Survival of some medically important fungi on hospital fabrics and plastics. *J Clin Microbiol*. 2001;39(9):3360-3361.

51. Sehulster L, Chinn RY, CDC, HICPAC. Guidelines for environmental infection control in health-care facilities. Recommendations of CDC and the Healthcare Infection Control Practices Advisory Committee (HICPAC). *MMWR Recomm Rep*. 2003;52(RR-10):1-42.

52. Leonas KK. Effect of laundering on the barrier properties of reusable surgical gown fabrics. *Am J Infect Control*. 1998;26(5):495-501.

53. Scaltriti S, Cencetti S, Rovesti S, Marchesi I, Bargellini A, Borella P. Risk factors for particulate and microbial contamination of air in operating theatres. *J Hosp Infect*. 2007;66(4):320-326.

54. Mangram AJ, Horan TC, Pearson ML, Silver LC, Jarvis WR. Guideline for prevention of surgical site infection, 1999. Hospital Infection Control Practices Advisory Committee. *Infect Control Hosp Epidemiol*. 1999;20(4): 250-78; quiz 279-80.

55. Callaghan I. Bacterial contamination of nurses' uniforms: a study. *Nurs Stand*. 1998;13(1):37-42.

56. National Institute for Occupational Safety and Health. *Protecting Workers' Families: A Research Agenda*. DHHS(NIOSH) Pub No. 2002-113. *http://www. cdc.gov/niosh/docs/2002-113/2002-113.html*. Accessed September 29, 2010.

57. Summers MM, Lynch PF, Black T. Hair as a reservoir of staphylococci. *J Clin Path*. 1965;18(13):13-15.

58. Dineen P, Drusin L. Epidemics of postoperative wound infections associated with hair carriers. *Lancet*. 1973;2(7839):1157-1159.

59. Mastro TD, Farley TA, Elliott JA, et al. An outbreak of surgical-wound infections due to group A streptococcus carried on the scalp. *N Engl J Med*. 1990;323(14):968-972.

60. Mase K, Hasegawa T, Horii T, et al. Firm adherence of *Staphylococcus aureus* and *Staphylococcus epidermidis* to human hair and effect of detergent treatment. *Microbiol Immunol.* 2000;44(8):653-656.

61. Friberg S, Ardnor B, Lundholm R, Friberg B. The addition of a mobile ultra-clean exponential laminar airflow screen to conventional operating room ventilation reduces bacterial contamination to operating box levels. *J Hosp Infect.* 2003;55(2):92-97.

62. Takashima M, Shirai F, Sageshima M, Ikeda N, Okamoto Y, Dohi Y. Distinctive bacteria-binding property of cloth materials. *Am J Infect Control.* 2004;32(1): 27-30.

63. Healthcare Laundry Accreditation Council. Accreditation Standards for Processing Reusable Textiles for Use in Healthcare Facilities. 2006. *http://www.hlac net.org/Accredit%20Standards12.18.08.pdf.* Accessed October 6, 2010.

64. Fijan S, Sostar-Turk S, Cencic A. Implementing hygiene monitoring systems in hospital laundries in order to reduce microbial contamination of hospital textiles. *J Hosp Infect.* 2005;61(1):30-38.

65. ANSI/AAMI. ST65: Processing of reusable surgical textiles for use in health care facilities. 2008.

66. Gerba CP. Application of quantitative risk assessment for formulating hygiene policy in the domestic setting. *J Infect.* 2001;43(1):92-98.

67. Association for Linen Management. *Clinical Talking Points: Healthcare Textiles Bioburden* [educational material]. Richmond, KY: Association for Linen Management; 2009.

68. Perry C, Marshall R, Jones E. Bacterial contamination of uniforms. *J Hosp Infect.* 2001;48(3):238-241.

69. Hedin G. *Staphylococcus epidermidis*—hospital epidemiology and the detection of methicillin resistance. *Scand J Infect Dis* Suppl. 1993;90:1-59.

70. Twomey CL, Beitz H, Johnson BJ. Bacterial contamination of surgical scrubs and laundering mechanisms: infection control implications. *Infection Control Today.* 2009. *http://www.infectioncontroltoday.com /articles/bacterial-contamination-of-surgical -scrubs.html#.* Accessed September 29, 2010.

71. Gerba CP, Kennedy D. Enteric virus survival during household laundering and impact of disinfection with sodium hypochlorite. *Appl Environ Microbiol.* 2007;73(14):4425-4428.

72. Boone SA, Gerba CP. Significance of fomites in the spread of respiratory and enteric viral disease. *Appl Environ Microbiol.* 2007;73(6):1687-1696.

73. Scheuer R. Dispensing of excess scrub expenses. *Mater Manag Health Care.* 2006;15(1):24-27.

74. Akridge J. No blanket strategies in textile management. *Healthc Purchasing News.* 2007;31(12):46, 48-49.

75. 2007 Guideline for Isolation Precautions: preventing transmission of infectious agents in health care settings. Centers for Disease Control and Prevention. *http://www. cdc.gov/hicpac/2007IP/2007isolationPrecautions .html.* Accessed September 29, 2010.

76. Romney MG. Surgical face masks in the operating theatre: re-examining the evidence. *J Hosp Infect.* 2001;47(4):251-256.

77. Barbosa MH, Graziano KU. Influence of wearing time on efficacy of disposable surgical masks as microbial barrier. *Braz J Microbiol.* 2006;37(3):216-217.

78. McCluskey F. Does wearing a face mask reduce bacterial wound infection? A literature review. *Br J Theatre Nurs.* 1996;6(5):18-20, 29.

79. Carbone HL, Hellickson LA, Thomasser AL, Vu LK. Clostridium difficile cross contamination in the textile laundering process: the importance of selecting an appropriate hard surface disinfectant. Paper presented at: International Conference on Healthcare-Associated Infections; March 19, 2010; Atlanta, GA.

80. Duffy J, Harris J, Newhouse EN, et al. Zygomycosis outbreak associated with hospital linens. Paper presented at: International Conference on Healthcare-Associated Infections; March 19, 2010; Atlanta, GA.

Acknowledgements

LEAD AUTHORS

Joan Blanchard, MSS, BSN, RN, CNOR, CIC
Perioperative Nursing Specialist
AORN Center for Nursing Practice
Denver, Colorado

Melanie Braswell, DNP, MS, RN, CNS, CNOR
Full-Time Faculty School of Nursing
Purdue University
Lafayette, Indiana

CONTRIBUTING AUTHORS

George Allen, PhD, MS, RN, CNOR
Director of Infection Control
Downstate Medical Center
Brooklyn, New York

Nancy Bjerke, MPH, RN, CIC
Consultant
Association for Professionals in Infection Control
and Epidemiology, Inc (APIC)
San Antonio, Texas

Sorin Brull, MD
American Society of Anesthesiology
Professor of Anesthesiology
Mayo Clinic College of Medicine
Rochester, Minnesota

PUBLICATION HISTORY

Originally published March 1975, *AORN Journal*, as AORN "Standards for proper OR wearing apparel." Format revision March 1978, July 1982.

Revised March 1984, March 1990. Published as proposed recommended practices, August 1994.

Revised November 1998; published December 1998. *Reformatted July 2000.*

Revised November 2004; published in *Standards, Recommended Practices, and Guidelines,* 2005 edition. Reprinted February 2005, *AORN Journal.*

Revised October 2010 for online publication in *Perioperative Standards and Recommended Practices.*

AORN Perioperative Standards and Recommended Practices, 2012 Edition

Recommended Practices for Hand Hygiene in the Perioperative Setting

T he following Recommended Practices for Hand Hygiene in the Perioperative Setting were developed by the AORN Recommended Practices Committee and have been approved by the AORN Board of Directors. They were presented as proposed recommendations for comments by members and others. They are effective July 1, 2009. These recommended practices are intended as achievable recommendations representing what is believed to be an optimal level of practice. Policies and procedures will reflect variations in practice settings and/or clinical situations that determine the degree to which the recommended practices can be implemented. AORN recognizes the various settings in which perioperative nurses practice. These recommended practices are intended as guidelines adaptable to various practice settings. These practice settings include traditional operating rooms (ORs), ambulatory surgery centers, physicians' offices, cardiac catheterization laboratories, endoscopy suites, radiology departments, and all other areas where surgery and other invasive procedures may be performed.

Purpose

These recommended practices provide guidance for hand hygiene for surgical and other invasive procedures. Microorganism transfer from the hands of health care workers to patients is an important factor in health care-associated infections and has been recognized since the observations of Ignatz Semmelweis and others more than 100 years ago. Skin is a major potential source of microbial contamination in the surgical environment. Hand hygiene has been recognized as a primary method of decreasing health care-associated infections.[1] Prevention of health care-associated infections is a priority of all health care personnel. Health care-associated infections can result in untoward outcomes such as escalating cost of care, increased morbidity and mortality, longer length of stay, as well as the pain and suffering a patient may experience.[2] Hand hygiene, hand washing, and surgical hand scrubs are the most effective way to prevent and control infections and represent the least expensive means of achieving both.

The normal skin flora on the hands include transient and resident microorganisms. The transient flora are microorganisms that colonize the superficial layers of the skin. These microorganisms are acquired by health care personnel while caring for patients and from coming into contact with contaminated surfaces where patients reside. Transient bacteria are easier to remove during hand washing. Resident flora are bacteria seated in the deeper layers of skin and are more difficult to remove. The transient and resident bacteria usually maintain a constant level on individuals' hands.[3,4]

The term "hand hygiene" is used to describe all measures related to hand condition and decontamination. Decontamination of hands can be done by one or more methods:

♦ **hand washing** using
  - soap and water,
  - antiseptic and water, or
  - antiseptic hand rub if visible soil is not present, or
♦ **surgical hand scrub** using
  - water-aided brushless surgical antiseptics,
  - waterless brushless surgical antiseptics, or
  - traditional surgical hand scrub using a sponge.[3,4]

Recommendation I

All health care personnel should follow established hand hygiene practices for maintaining healthy skin and fingernail condition and regarding the wearing of jewelry in the perioperative setting.

A direct route of transmission of microorganisms occurs when person-to-person contact results in transmission of microorganisms from a person who is infectious or colonized to a susceptible host. An indirect route of transmission of microorganisms occurs when inanimate objects such as a contaminated surface, instrument, or health care personnel's hands transfer microorganisms to a susceptible host.[5,6] An example of an outbreak involved a cardiac surgeon's infected fingernail. When cultured, it grew *Pseudomonas aeruginosa*. Two patients treated by the surgeon developed a surgical site infection with the same strain of *P aeruginosa*.[7]

I.a.   Health care personnel should keep natural fingernails no more than one-quarter inch (0.64 cm) long.[3,8,9]

The subungual area of fingernails has the largest number of microorganisms on the hands. Pathogens most frequently isolated from the subungual area are coagulase-negative staphylococci, gram-negative rods (including *Pseudomonas spp*), corynebacteria, and yeasts.[10,11]

Long fingernails pose a risk of developing tears in gloves and also the possibility of injuring a patient during positioning and caring for the patient. There is also the concern that hand washing, hand rub, and surgical hand scrubbing may not be performed as well due to the health care personnel protecting their fingernails.[12,13] Short fingernails collect less debris, and debris is more easily removed when fingernails are short. Short fingernails have a decreased risk of being colonized with *P aeruginosa* compared to health care personnel with long or artificial fingernails. Long fingernails make washing and drying of hands difficult and may result in hand colonization.[9]

I.b. Chipped fingernail polish should be removed prior to entry into the restricted area of the perioperative environment.

Fingernail polish that is chipped may harbor pathogens in large numbers.[4,8,13] It has been shown that fingernail polish becomes chipped by the fourth day of wear.[13] Chipped fingernail polish should be removed to prevent possible contamination of the environment or the patient.[4,8] Glove tears occasionally occur during a surgical procedure; chipped fingernail polish could be deposited on the sterile field or in the wound.

I.c. Artificial fingernails should not be worn by health care personnel in the perioperative environment.

Any fingernail enhancement or resin bonding product is considered artificial. Fingernail extensions or tips, gels and acrylic overlays, resin wraps, or acrylic fingernails constitute types of artificial fingernails.[14] Over time, gel or acrylic fingernails can become chipped and lift from the nail plate if moisture gets under the overlay. Adding artificial fingernails to an area of fingernails that is colonized may increase the microorganisms on the native fingernails.[12] The greater the length of time artificial fingernails are worn, the greater the number of microorganisms isolated.[12] Health care personnel who wear artificial fingernails may also limit hand hygiene and surgical hand scrub practices as a result of a need to protect their manicure.[12,15] Patients at risks of infection may be at increased risk of exposure to pathogens that have been known to be colonized on artificial fingernails of health care personnel.[12,15] Studies have shown the correlation of microorganisms from health care personnel's hands to patients that result in surgical site infections. One such study showed three patients who developed a surgical site infection with *Candida albicans*; the strains isolated were identical. It was found that the surgical technician who scrubbed on all three cases had long artificial fingernails at the time of the patients' surgeries. A throat culture of the surgical technician later grew *C albicans*.[3,16]

I.d. Rings should not be worn by health care personnel in the perioperative setting.

Studies have shown that wearing rings may result in colonization of the hands with pathogens such as gram-negative and gram-positive pathogens.[2,3,4,17] With an increasing number of rings worn, the number of pathogens recovered may also increase in number.[4] In one study, isolates recovered from swabbing the area adjacent to the ring included coagulase-negative staphylococci, other skin flora, gram-negative cocci, *Pseudomonas spp* and *Staphylococcus aureus*.[18] There is a strong link between wearing rings and contamination of hands by health care personnel; removing rings will decrease the potential for pathogens remaining on hands before and after hand hygiene.[19]

I.e. Watches and bracelets should be removed prior to washing hands.[2,3,20]

One study found that persons wearing watches or bracelets wash the wrist area less. Removing watches and bracelets allows for thorough hand hygiene.[2,20]

I.f. Health care organization-approved hand lotions should be readily available and used frequently to maintain good hand skin condition following surgical hand hygiene.

Skin irritation and dermatitis from frequent hand washing can increase the risk of infection for both the health care worker and the patient.[21] Failure to follow practices that maintain intact skin may create breaks in intact epithelium, which compromises the barrier properties of the skin and presents the opportunity for microbial transmission into the tissues.[22]

I.f.1. Lotions selected for use in the perioperative setting should be evaluated and approved by an interdisciplinary group that has the designated authority to evaluate and select hand lotions.

I.f.2. Hand lotions used in the perioperative setting should
- be compatible with antiseptics and barrier products in use,
- list water as the first ingredient on the label,[23]
- contain no anionic-based materials or chemicals, and
- contain no petroleum or other ingredients with a demonstrated detrimental effect on the barrier properties of gloves in use.

Many lotions found in over-the-counter products contain an anionic-based ingredient that interferes with the residual effect of chlorhexidine gluconate and chloroxylenol. Chlorhexidine gluconate and chloroxylenol are in many hand antiseptic products used in health care organizations for their antiseptic properties.[3,23]

Petroleum may affect the barrier properties of latex gloves that may be worn by health care personnel.[24] A study on latex glove compatibility has shown petroleum to have adverse effects on the integrity of latex gloves.[25] Some gloves have been demonstrated to be compatible with some lotions.

I.g. Health care personnel with cuts, abrasions, weeping dermatitis, or fresh tattoos on exposed skin should not provide direct patient care. Health care personnel should not have patient contact until these conditions are healed and they have been cleared by an infection preventionist, employee health nurse, occupational health nurse, or other health care personnel with specialized knowledge in making a determination regarding the safety of the employee returning to work in the perioperative setting.[22,24]

Health care personnel with breaks in their skin integrity may be at risk for acquiring or transmitting infection to patients.

Recommendation II

A standardized procedure for hand washing should be followed.

The purpose of hand washing is to
- remove soil, organic material, and transient microorganisms from fingernails, hands, and forearms;
- decrease the resident microorganism count to a minimum; and
- inhibit the rapid rebound of microorganisms.[3]

Application technique, length of exposure to the product, and correct concentration of the product impact the effectiveness of hand washing.[26] Inconsistent compliance with recommended procedures may result in the transmission of pathogens to patients.

II.a. A hand wash should be performed
- upon arrival at the health care facility,
- before and after every patient contact,
- before putting gloves on and after removing gloves or other personal protective equipment,
- any time there is a possibility that there has been contact with blood or other potentially infectious materials or surfaces,
- before and after eating,
- before and after using the restroom,
- before leaving the health care facility, and
- when hands are visibly soiled.[3,27]

Hand washing remains one of the most important measures in maintaining patient and health care personnel safety. Following these hand washing practices will prevent transmission of infection and reduce health care-associated infections for the patient and health care personnel.[27]

Contamination of hands may occur
- as a result of holes or tears in gloves that are not visible;
- when gloves are removed; and
- when continuing to wear gloves following the care of a patient, which may lead to transmission of microorganisms from patient to patient.

Wearing gloves will not replace hand hygiene.[28] One study found a 15% rate of colonization from MRSA-positive patients to health care personnel's hands after removal of gloves. Another study found a 17% rate of colonization from MRSA-colonized patients to gloves of health care personnel.[29,30]

II.a.1. Hands should be washed with soap and water for at least 15 seconds.

Hand washing for 15 seconds has been shown to reduce soil, spores, and microorganism counts on the hands.[3,27,31-33]

II.a.2. Hand washing with soap and water should be performed in the following order:
(1) Remove jewelry from hands and forearms.
(2) Adjust water to a comfortable temperature.
(3) Wet hands thoroughly with water.
(4) Follow the manufacturer's directions for application of soap.
(5) Rub hands covering all surfaces including the backs of hands, fingertips, inner webs, and palms.
(6) Wash for at least 15 seconds.
(7) Rinse well to remove all soap.
(8) Dry hands thoroughly with an absorbent, non-abrasive, disposable towel.[27]
(9) Use a disposable towel to turn the water off and open the door if hands-free controls are not available.[3]

Drying hands thoroughly assists in removing soil, stratum corneum, and microorganisms that have been loosened during the process of hand washing.

Touching faucet handles provides an opportunity for cross contamination.[34] Moisture remaining on the hands can create a transfer of microorganisms remaining on the hands to surfaces in the environment.[34]

II.b. Hand washing stations should be placed in convenient locations according to local and state building codes.

Hand washing stations located close to patient care areas, medication preparation areas, and food storage and dispensing areas encourage health care personnel to wash their hands. Convenient hand washing stations result in a higher frequency of hand washing.[35]

II.b.1. Water temperature at the faucet should be controlled between 105° F to 120° F (40° C to 49° C).[35]

Dermatitis can be prevented by using tap water that is adjusted to a comfortable temperature.

II.b.2. Hand washing stations in new or remodeled facilities should have hands-free water and soap dispensing controls.[35]

Hands-free water and soap dispensing controls reduce the risk of cross-contamination.[34]

II.b.3. Paper towel dispensers should be designed to prevent recontamination when removing towels. The towel dispenser should dispense cleanly without the need to touch the towel dispenser.[36]

Paper towel dispenser design is important, as the process of drying hands is the final step in hand washing; ease of use is important in preventing recontamination of hands.[36] Towels that jam when the towel dispenser does not work properly can result in hands becoming contaminated by touching the dispenser.[36]

II.c. Hand washing may be performed using an alcohol-based antiseptic hand rub when soil is not present on hands.[3] The hand rub manufacturer's written directions for the amount of product and technique for application should be followed.[27]

Alcohol-based hand rubs are easy to use, fast acting, and provide activity against most bacteria, most viruses, and fungi.[37]

II.c.1. Care should be taken in the placement of alcohol-based hand antiseptic product dispensers in areas where surgical and other invasive procedures are performed and where oxygen and ignition sources are present.[38] Dispensers should be installed following the 2004 National Fire Protection Association (NFPA) Life Safety Code as well as state and local regulations. Alcohol-based hand hygiene product dispensers should
• be at least four feet apart;

- only hold 1.2 L in rooms, corridors, and areas open to corridors; and
- not be placed over an electrical outlet or switch.[27,39]

Hand antiseptic product dispensers containing flammable antiseptics may be a fire hazard. Following the NFPA Life Safety Code will decrease the risk of fire.[27,39]

II.c.2. Hand rubs should be performed in the following manner:
(1) Follow the manufacturer's written directions for use of product.
(2) Use the recommended amount of hand rub product.
(3) Rub hands covering all surfaces including the backs of hands, fingertips, inner webs, and palms.
(4) Rub hands until they are dry.

A sufficient amount of product is required to ensure antimicrobial effect.

Recommendation III

A surgical hand scrub should be performed by health care personnel before donning sterile gloves for surgical or other invasive procedures. Use of either an antimicrobial surgical scrub agent intended for surgical hand antisepsis or an alcohol-based antiseptic surgical hand rub with documented persistent and cumulative activity that has met US Food and Drug Administration (FDA) regulatory requirements for surgical hand antisepsis is acceptable.

The objective of a surgical hand scrub is the reduction of transient and resident flora, which also may reduce health care-associated infections.[3,26] Although the skin can never be rendered sterile, it can be made surgically clean by reducing the number of microorganisms. A surgical hand scrub will decrease transient and resident microorganisms on the hands and maintain the bacterial level below baseline.[40] The mechanical action associated with hand scrubbing removes debris and microorganisms. This can be accomplished by rubbing the skin with or without a sponge to produce friction. With the addition of a health care organization-approved antiseptic soap, which acts as a surfactant, transient and some resident microorganisms can be lifted and flushed away under running water. Surgical hand antisepsis/hand scrubs are effective only if all surfaces are exposed to the mechanical cleaning and chemical antisepsis processes.

III.a. A multiuser scrub sink should be located near the entrance to the OR. A multiuser scrub sink may serve two ORs to provide ready access to the adjacent ORs.[35]

III.b. A standardized surgical hand scrub using an alcohol-based surgical hand rub product with demonstrated persistence and cumulative activity should be performed according to the manufacturer's written directions for use. An alcohol and chlorhexidine product that is fast drying and has residual effect is preferred.[3]

III.b.1. A standardized surgical hand scrub procedure using an alcohol based surgical hand rub product should include, but may not be limited to, the following:
(1) Remove jewelry including rings, watches, and bracelets.
(2) Don a surgical mask. If others are at the scrub sink, a surgical mask should be worn in the presence of hand scrub activity.
(3) If visibly soiled, prewash hands and forearms with plain soap and water or antimicrobial agent.
(4) Clean the subungual areas of both hands under running water using a disposable nail cleaner.
(5) Rinse hands and forearms under running water.
(6) Dry hands and forearms thoroughly with a disposable paper towel.
(7) Dispense the manufacturer-recommended amount of the surgical hand rub product.
(8) Apply the product to the hands and forearms according to the manufacturer's written instructions.
(9) Repeat the product application process as directed.
(10) Rub thoroughly until completely dry.[2,27]
(11) In the OR or other invasive procedure room, don a sterile surgical gown and gloves.

III.c. A traditional, standardized, surgical hand scrub procedure should include, but may not be limited to, the following:

(1) Remove jewelry including rings, watches, and bracelets.

(2) Don a surgical mask. If others are at the scrub sink, a surgical mask should be worn in the presence of hand scrub activity.

(3) Wash hands and forearms if visibly soiled with soap and running water immediately before beginning the surgical scrub.

(4) Clean the subungual areas of both hands under running water using a disposable nail cleaner.

(5) Rinse hands and forearms under running water.

(6) Dispense the approved antimicrobial scrub agent according to the manufacturer's written directions.

(7) Apply the antimicrobial agent to wet hands and forearms using a soft, non-abrasive sponge.

(8) A three- or five-minute scrub should be timed to allow adequate product contact with skin, according to the manufacturer's written directions.

(9) Visualize each finger, hand, and arm as having four sides. Wash all four sides effectively, keeping the hand elevated. Repeat this process for opposite fingers, hand, and arm.

(10) For water conservation, turn water off when it is not directly in use, if possible.

(11) Avoid splashing surgical attire.

(12) Discard sponges, if used, in appropriate containers.

(13) Hands and arms should be rinsed under running water in one direction from fingertips to elbows as often as needed.

(14) Hold hands higher than elbows and away from surgical attire.

(15) In the OR, dry hands and arms with a sterile towel before donning a sterile surgical gown and gloves.[4]

The use of a brush for surgical hand scrubs is not necessary for adequate reduction of bacterial counts. Scrubbing with a brush is associated with an increase in skin cell shedding. The skin on hands can become damaged with the use of brushes resulting in an increase in bacterial load. Use of a sponge or soft brush rather than a hard bristle brush will reduce damage to the epidermis.[2,41] A study of the duration of surgical hand scrubs using ranges from three to five minutes showed that three-minute surgical hand scrubs are as effective as five-minute surgical hand scrubs.[42] Appropriate disposal of sponges, if used, prevents cross contamination of the surgical scrub sink area.

Hands and forearms should be held higher than the elbows and away from surgical attire to prevent contamination and allow water to run from the clean to the less clean area down the arm. A sterile gown cannot be put on over wet or damp surgical attire without resultant potential contamination of the gown by strike-through moisture.

Recommendation IV

Surgical hand hygiene products should be selected following an analysis of product effectiveness, application requirements, and user acceptance.

Acceptability of products is a key factor in health care personnel compliance with good hand hygiene practices.[21]

IV.a. Surgical hand hygiene products and hand lotions should be approved by the organization's infection prevention and control committee or designated authority with specialized knowledge in hand products.

The organization's infection prevention and control committee is made up of a multidisciplinary team that includes the infection preventionist, epidemiologist, administrative staff, perioperative member, pharmacists, as well as other department representatives. This allows for a collaborative discussion on what products would be appropriate.[3] A health care facility that does not have an infection control committee should utilize guidance from health care personnel with specialized knowledge in infection prevention and control.

IV.a.1. Written criteria should be used to evaluate surgical hand hygiene products and their application. Criteria should include, but is not limited to,
- safety,
- purpose and use,
- ease of use,
- skin comfort and reaction,
- fragrance,
- consistency,
- color,
- compatibility with other products,

- patient and health care personnel outcomes,
- efficacy,
- regulatory control, and
- cost.[21,43,44]

IV.a.2. Health care personnel's selection of products should be made with the guidance of an infection preventionist or other health care personnel with specialized knowledge in infection prevention and control.

IV.a.3. End-user evaluations should be completed to determine acceptability prior to final selection of products.

Some of the key concerns that can influence health care personnel regarding hand hygiene products include fragrance, consistency, and color.[44]

IV.a.4. Following the end-user evaluation of the products tested, written evaluations should be completed by the health care personnel and collected and reviewed by authorized personnel.[45,46]

Written questionnaires or evaluations give valuable validation on product acceptability. Written evaluations should be completed to verify acceptability.

IV.b. Surgical hand hygiene products should be selected and used according to manufacturers' written instructions.[45]

IV.b.1. Antimicrobial surgical hand hygiene products should
- significantly reduce microorganisms on intact skin,
- contain emollients and humectants to prevent skin irritation,[21]
- be broad spectrum,
- be fast acting, and
- have a persistent and cumulative effect[45] (**Table 1**).

Recommendation V

Health care personnel should receive education, training, and competency validation on surgical hand hygiene products and procedures.

Competency assessment verifies that health care personnel have an understanding of the application and purpose for surgical hand hygiene in infection prevention and control. This knowledge is essential in reducing the risk of health care-associated infections. Health care personnel also understand the potential risk of their becoming colonized or infected by microorganisms from the patient and are better able to protect themselves and the patient.

V.a. Health care personnel should receive education and guidance on hand hygiene products and their application.

Health care personnel should be knowledgeable about surgical hand hygiene products and their application. This includes the indications, contraindications, and special precautions used when handling flammable antiseptic products.[38,47]

V.a.1. Health care personnel should receive education and guidance on the identification and reporting of symptoms of irritant contact dermatitis and allergic contact dermatitis.

Skin irritation conditions may be difficult to differentiate. Skin health is related to its lipid barrier and the lipid barrier can be compromised by lipid-emulsifying detergents and lipid-dissolving alcohols.[48,49] Education to prevent skin irritation has proven to be effective. Research has shown that by providing educational theory, didactics, and evaluation of surgical hand hygiene practices, improvement in surgical hand hygiene compliance may be achieved.[50]

V.a.2. Health care personnel should participate in surgical hand hygiene product evaluation.

Participation in product evaluations assures health care personnel that they have input into choice of products. A higher level of compliance may be achieved in this manner.

V.b. Health care personnel should demonstrate proficiency in surgical hand hygiene practices and the use of surgical hand hygiene products periodically and when new products are introduced. Periodic performance monitoring also should take place.

Proficiency in surgical hand hygiene practices allows health care personnel to prevent the transmission of pathogens.

Table 1

ACTIVITY AND CONSIDERATIONS FOR HAND HYGIENE AGENTS

Antiseptic agent	Mechanism of action	Gram + bacteria	Gram – bacteria	Viruses	Rapidity of action	continued on next page
Soap and water	Cleansing activity is due to detergent property of soap and water as a solvent[1,2]	Minimal[1]	Minimal[1]		Limited	
Alcohol	Denatures proteins[1]	Excellent[1]	Excellent[1]	Good[1]	Excellent Optimal concentration 60% to 80%[2]	
Chlorhexidine	Disrupts cell membrane[1]	Excellent[1]	Good[1]	Good against enveloped viruses, less active against non-enveloped viruses[1]	Slower than alcohol[1]	
Chlorhexidine gluconate with alcohol	Disrupts cell membrane and denatures proteins[1,3]	Excellent[1]	Excellent[1]	Good	Excellent	
Chloroxylenol	Inactivates bacterial enzymes and disrupts cell walls[1]	Excellent[1]	Fair[1]	Fair[1]	Intermediate[4] Not as rapidly active as chlorhexidine or iodophors[1]	
Iodine and iodophors	Disrupts cell membrane[1]	Excellent[1]	Excellent[1]	Good[1]	Intermediate[1]	
Quaternary ammonium compounds	Believed to work by absorbing the cytoplasmic membrane, which creates leakage of the molecular weight cytoplasmic components[2]	Fair[1,2]	Good[1,2]	Fair[1]	Slow[1]	
Triclosan	Affects the cytoplasmic membrane and syntheses of RNA, fatty acids, and proteins when it enters bacterial cells[1]	Good[1]	Fair	Fair	Slow	

REFERENCES

1. Centers for Disease Control and Prevention. Guideline for hand hygiene in health-care settings. *MMWR*. October 25, 2002;51(RR-16):1-44.

2. *WHO Guidelines on Hand Hygiene in Health Care* (Advanced Draft). Geneva, Switzerland: World Health Organization; 2006. *http://www.who.int/patientsafety /information_centre/ghhad_download_link/en/*. Accessed October 19, 2009.

3. Boyce JM, Kelliher S, Vallande N. Skin irritation and dryness associated with two hand-hygiene regimens: soap-and-water hand washing versus hand antisepsis with an alcoholic hand gel. *Infect Control Hosp Epidemiol*. 2000;21(7):442-448.

4. Larson E. Guideline for use of topical antimicrobial agents. *Am J Infect Control*. 1988;16(6);253-266.

5. Sicherer SH. Risk of severe allergic reactions from the use of potassium iodide for radiation emergencies. *J Allergy Clin Immunol*. 2004;114(6);1395-1397.

6. Rotter ML. Hand washing and hand disinfection. In: Mayhall CG, ed. *Hospital Epidemiology and Infection Control*. 3rd ed. Philadelphia, PA: Lippincott Williams & Wilkins; 2004:1727-1746.

Table 1 (continued)

	Antiseptic agent	Persistent/ residual activity	Contraindications	Cautions	Soil Removal
tinued from vious page	Soap and water	None[1]		May result in an increase of bacterial counts,[1,2] can result in skin dryness and irritation with frequent use[3]	Yes
	Alcohol	None[1]		Flammable, does not penetrate organic material, very poor activity against bacterial spores[1]	No
	Chlorhexidine	Excellent[1]	Keep out of eyes and inner ears[1]	Known sensitivity to any of the ingredients; activity can be affected by natural soaps, different inorganic anions, non-ionic surfactants and hand lotions that contain anionic emulsifying agents;[3] very poor activity against bacterial spores[1]	Yes
	Chlorhexidine gluconate with alcohol	Excellent[1]	Keep out of eyes and inner ears[1]	Known sensitivity to any of the ingredients, very poor activity against bacterial spores, flammable[1]	Limited
	Chloroxylenol	Good[1]		Safe up to 5% concentration[4]	Yes
	Iodine and iodophors	Intermediate[1]	Sensitivity to providone iodine	Products prone to contamination by gram negative bacteria, shellfish allergy is not a contraindication[5]	No
	Quaternary ammonium compounds	None	Incompatible with anionic detergents[1,4]	Products prone to contamination by gram negative bacteria,[1] antimicrobial activity reduced by organic material[1]	No
	Triclosan	Good[1]		Antimicrobial activity reduced by organic material,[6] minimally effective against gram negative bacteria, product prone to contamination by gram negative bacteria[6]	Yes

V.c. Fire safety education and training should be provided to all health care personnel working in the perioperative area where alcohol and alcohol-based hand hygiene products are used. Fire safety education should include periodic fire drills.

Alcohol and alcohol/combination hand products pose a fire safety concern.

V.c.1. All members of the perioperative surgical team should participate in fire drills.[38]

Fire drills assist the surgical team in promoting a culture of fire safety.[3,38] Par-

ticipation in fire drills promotes and maintains a fire safe environment.[38]

Recommendation VI

Policies and procedures for surgical hand hygiene should be written, reviewed annually, and readily available within the practice setting.

Policies and procedures serve as a source of information for preventing health care-associated infections by delineating products to be used as well as the correct technique. Policies and procedures establish authority, responsibility, and accountability and serve as operational guidelines. Policies and procedures establish guidelines for performance improvement activities to be used when monitoring and evaluating surgical hand hygiene in the perioperative setting.

VI.a.   Policies regarding hand hygiene should be developed in collaboration with the surgical team as well as the infection preventionist and employee health nurse.

A collaborative approach to policy development and the provision of access to policies for all health care personnel will result in a better team approach to appropriate hand hygiene. The health care organization's infection prevention and control committee should be made up of a multidisciplinary team that may include the infection preventionist, epidemiologist, perioperative registered nurse, pharmacist, administrative staff, as well as nursing and other department representatives. This allows informed discussion on what products would be appropriate.[4] Smaller facilities with no infection prevention and control committee may utilize individuals with specialized knowledge in infection prevention and control.[21]

VI.a.1.   Hand hygiene policies should include, but are not limited to,
- standardized procedures for surgical hand scrub,
- removal of jewelry for hand rubs and surgical hand antisepsis,
- health care personnel education in the use of hand scrub products,
- health care organization-approved hand antiseptic products,
- identification and reporting of irritant and allergic contact dermatitis,
- maintenance and location of material safety data sheets (MSDS),
- precautions when flammable antiseptics are used,
- proper storage of flammable hand antiseptic agents,
- reporting of adverse events, and
- performance monitoring.

VI.b.   Policies and procedures should be introduced and reviewed in the initial orientation, when new products are introduced, and with ongoing education for health care personnel.

Access to policies and procedures allows health care personnel to have ongoing information. Review of policies and procedures assists health care professionals in the development of knowledge.

Recommendation VII

A quality management program should be in place to evaluate surgical hand hygiene procedures and to identify and respond to opportunities for improvement.

Quality control programs that enhance personal performance and monitor surgical hand hygiene practices are established to promote patient and health care personnel safety. It is the responsibility of professional perioperative registered nurses to ensure safe, high-quality nursing care to patients undergoing operative and invasive procedures.[43]

VII.a.   Adverse events (eg, fire, bacterial contamination of multiuse containers) related to the use of hand products should be reported to the health care organization's quality review program.

Open communication is important in determining why adverse events occur. The use of a root cause analysis will facilitate the identification of the cause of the event and assist in determining steps to be taken to prevent future adverse events.

VII.b.   Symptoms of irritant or allergic contact dermatitis should be identified and treated as soon as health care personnel report a concern.

Skin dryness, irritation, itching, cracking, and bleeding may be diagnosed as irritant contact dermatitis.[21] These symptoms should be identified and treated quickly to prevent further damage to health care personnel's hands. Allergic contact dermatitis results from an allergic reaction to ingredients in antiseptic products. Allergic contact dermatitis may be mild, localized, or severe, resulting in respiratory distress or possible anaphylaxis.[21] These symptoms should be determined quickly to prevent continued damage to health care personnel's hands and mitigate anaphylaxis reactions. A change in hand hygiene product can prevent further allergic reactions.

VII.b.1.   Cuts, abrasions, weeping dermatitis, or fresh tattoos should be documented in the employee's health record by the infection preventionist, employee health nurse, occupational health nurse, or other health care personnel with specialized knowledge in making a determination regarding the employee's returning to work in the perioperative setting.

VII.c. Barriers that may exist for surgical hand hygiene should be recognized and addressed.

Health care personnel hand washing practice studies note inadequate hand washing compliance.[51] However, another study notes that failure of health care personnel to wash their hands is not due to intentional negligence.[52] Removing barriers to hand hygiene will help improve adherence by health care personnel with these procedures. Some of the identified barriers are hand hygiene products causing irritation, sinks not conveniently located, lack of supplies, understaffing, and patient needs that take priority.[53]

VII.c.1. A study of usage patterns of surgical hand hygiene products should be done on an ongoing basis.

VII.c.2. Antiseptic products for surgical hand hygiene that minimize skin irritation should be used.

Health care personnel compliance with the recommended use of antiseptic products is improved when the product does not irritate the skin.

VII.c.3. Staffing levels of health care personnel should be evaluated as a barrier to hand washing.

Staffing levels that are inadequate may result in cross contamination when health care personnel have an increased workload. A decrease in hand washing may result. Having the right level of health care personnel available enables personnel to be compliant with hand hygiene.[54]

VII.d. Hand hygiene practices should be measured to determine compliance.

Following hand hygiene policies and procedures is an important step in infection prevention and control in protecting health care personnel and patients. Measurement involves adhering to and following the manufacturer's written product directions. Studies have been conducted but may need to be expanded.[54]

VII.d.1. Measures to evaluate surgical hand hygiene practices may include, but are not limited to,
- direct observation (considered the most effective measurement);
- measuring the amount of product used;
- monitoring by using technology plus scanning;
- electronically monitoring entrance and exits into rooms with the use of video surveillance;[55]
- electronically monitoring hand washing and surgical hand scrub dispensers;[55] and
- automated hand washing stations that read ID badges, record the length of time the process takes, and where the hand washing is performed.

Observational surveillance of surgical hand hygiene practices provides direct information on compliance by health care personnel.[3] Direct observation also can determine the areas of strengths and weaknesses in hand hygiene practices and allows for improvement in the process.[1]

A disadvantage of this method is that direct observation of hand hygiene can be labor-intensive and expensive. In addition, one study showed there was little clinical improvement because the direct observer viewed only 0.4% of the hand washing and hand scrubbing that was done.[56] The Hawthorne effect may result in health care personnel improving how they do hand hygiene while being observed.[56] Over time, however, health care personnel forget why the observer is there. The observation process, if kept simple, can monitor one type of hand hygiene at a time (eg, surgical hand scrub).[4]

Measuring the amount of hand hygiene product used requires less time and fewer productive hours to monitor but may not take into account patient-case mix.[4] Studies have shown that this method may not be as effective as direct observation and may not change hand hygiene practices.[4] Therefore, this may not be a reliable method of monitoring hand hygiene or hand antisepsis.

Electronic monitoring can be an efficient and effective method of tracking hand hygiene compliance.[55] The advantages of video surveillance is that the camera is less obvious and may prevent the Hawthorne effect. Review of the recordings can be labor-intensive,[55] however, and electronic monitoring measures may not capture all of the possible times that hand hygiene should be performed.

Automated hand washing stations that read badges and record the length of time the process takes and where hand washing is performed is a technology utilized in the food industry to measure hand hygiene practice compliance. This technology provides the ability to record and produce reports that can be evaluated for hand hygiene compliance. This method is beginning to be adopted in the health care arena. It is more expensive than other methods but may become another useful tool for monitoring hand hygiene practices within health care organizations.[57]

VII.e. The health care organization's financial plan should include sufficient funds for hand hygiene products, performance monitoring, and feedback, as well as periodic training on surgical hand hygiene and the use of surgical hand hygiene products.[4]

Health care personnel involvement in product selection and acceptance of the product can result in better hand hygiene and savings.[4] Motivating health care personnel to change and practice good hand hygiene will have no value if there are no resources to make these changes.[58]

Glossary

Alcohol-based hand rub: An alcohol-containing preparation designed for application to the hands for reducing the number of viable microorganisms on the hands.

Artificial nails: Substances or devices applied or added to the natural nails to augment or enhance the wearer's own nails. They include, but are not limited to, bonding, tips, wrapping, and tapes.

Cumulative effect: A progressive decrease over time, usually measured in days, in the number of microorganisms present after repeated applications of a product.

Hand hygiene: a generic term that applies to all measures related to hand condition and decontamination.

Persistence: Prolonged or extended antimicrobial activity, usually measured in hours, which prevents or inhibits the regrowth of microorganisms after application of the product.

Subungual: Under the nail (eg, fingernail).

Surgical hand antiseptic agent: A product that is a broad-spectrum, fast-acting, and nonirritating preparation containing an antimicrobial ingredient designed to significantly reduce the number of microorganisms on intact skin. Surgical hand antiseptic agents demonstrate both persistent and cumulative activity.

REFERENCES
1. Haas JP, Larson EL. Measurement of compliance with hand hygiene. *J Hosp Infect*. 2007;66(1):6-14.

2. Graves PB, Twomey CL. Surgical hand antisepsis: an evidence-based review. *Perioperative Nursing Clinics*. 2006;1(3):235-246.

3. Centers for Disease Control and Prevention. Guideline for hand hygiene in health-care settings. *MMWR*. October 25, 2002;51(RR-16):1-44.

4. *WHO Guidelines on Hand Hygiene in Health Care* (Advanced Draft). Geneva, Switzerland: World Health Organization; 2006. *http://www.who.int/patient safety/information_centre/ghhad_download_link/en/*. Accessed October 19, 2009.

5. Friedman C, Petersen KH. *Infection Control in Ambulatory Care*. Boston, MA: Jones and Bartlett Publishers; 2004.

6. Siegel JD, Rhinehart E, Jackson M, Chiarello L; the Healthcare Infection Control Practices Advisory Committee. *Guideline for Isolation Precautions: Preventing Transmission of Infectious Agents in Healthcare Settings 2007*. Atlanta, GA: Centers for Disease Control and Prevention; 2007. *http://www.cdc.gov/ncidod/dhqp/gl_iso lation.html*. Accessed October 19, 2009.

7. Mermel LA, McKay M, Dempsey J, Parenteau S. Pseudomonas surgical-site infections linked to a healthcare worker with onychomycosis. *Infect Control Hosp Epidemiol*. 2003;24(10):749-752.

8. Wynd CA, Samstag DE, Lapp AM. Bacterial carriage on the fingernails of OR nurses. *AORN J*. 1994; 60(5):796-805.

9. Moolenaar RL, Crutcher JM, San Joaquin VH, et al. A prolonged outbreak of *Pseudomonas aeruginosa* in a neonatal intensive care unit: did staff fingernails play a role in disease transmission? *Infect Control Hosp Epidemiol*. 2000;21(2):80-85.

10. McGinley KJ, Larson EL, Leyden JJ. Composition and density of microflora in the subungual space of the hand. *J Clin Microbiol*. 1988;26(5):950-953.

11. Hedderwick SA, McNeil SA, Lyons MJ, Kauffman CA. Pathogenic organisms associated with artificial fingernails

worn by healthcare workers. *Infect Control Hosp Epidemiol.* 2000;21(8):505-509.

12. Toles A. Artificial nails: are they putting patients at risk? A review of the research. *J Pediatr Oncol Nurs.* 2002;19(5):164-171.

13. Baumgardner CA, Maragos CS, Walz J, Larson E. Effects of nail polish on microbial growth of fingernails. Dispelling sacred cows. *AORN J.* 1993;58(1):84-88.

14. Porteous J. Artificial nails . . . very real risks. *Can Oper Room Nurs J.* 2002;20(3):16-17.

15. McNeil SA, Foster CL, Hedderwick SA, Kauffman CA. Effect of hand cleansing with antimicrobial soap or alcohol-based gel on microbial colonization of artificial fingernails worn by health care workers. *Clin Infect Dis.* 2001;32(3):367-372.

16. Parry MF, Grant B, Yukna M, et al. *Candida osteomyelitis* and diskitis after spinal surgery: an outbreak that implicates artificial nail use. *Clin Infect Dis.* 2001;32(3):352-357.

17. Salisbury DM, Hutfilz P, Treen LM, Bollin GE, Gautam S. The effect of rings on microbial load of health care workers' hands. *Am J Infect Control.* 1997;25(1):24-27.

18. Kelsall NK, Griggs RK, Bowker KE, Bannister GC. Should finger rings be removed prior to scrubbing for theatre? *J Hosp Infect.* 2006;62(4):450-452.

19. Trick WE, Vernon MO, Hayes RA, et al. Impact of ring wearing on hand contamination and comparison of hand hygiene agents in a hospital. *Clin Infect Dis.* 2003;36(11):1383-1390.

20. Field EA, McGowan P, Pearce PK, Martin MV. Rings and watches: should they be removed prior to operative dental procedures? *J Dent.* 1996;24(1-2):65-69.

21. Larson E, Girard R, PessoaSilva CL, Boyce J, Donaldson L, Pittet D. Skin reactions related to hand hygiene and selection of hand hygiene products. *Am J Infect Control.* 2006;34(10):627 635.

22. Molinari JA, Harte JA, eds. *APIC Text of Infection Control and Epidemiology. Dental services.* Washington, DC: Association for Professionals in Infection Control and Epidemiology; 2005: 51-1–51-22.

23. Marino C, Cohen M. Washington State hospital survey 2000: gloves, handwashing agents, and moisturizers. *Am J Infect Control.* 2001;29(6):422-424.

24. CPL 02-02-069–CPL 2-2.69: Enforcement procedures for the occupational exposure to bloodborne pathogens. Occupational Safety & Health Administration. *http://www.osha.gov/pls/oshaweb/owadisp.show _document?p_table=DIRECTIVES&p_id=2570.* Accessed October 19, 2009.

25. Jones RD, Jampani H, Mulberry G, Rizer RL. Moisturizing alcohol hand gels for surgical hand preparation. *AORN J.* 2000;71(3):584-587.

26. Widmer AE, Dangel M. Alcohol-based handrub: evaluation of technique and microbiological efficacy with international infection control professionals. *Infect Control Hosp Epidemiol.* 2004;25(3):207-209.

27. Hand hygiene. In: Underwood MA, ed. *APIC Text of Infection Control and Epidemiology.* Washington, DC: Association for Professionals in Infection Control and Epidemiology; 2005:19-1–19-7.

28. Kim PW, Roghmann MC, Perencevich EN, Harris AD. Rates of hand disinfection associated with glove use, patient isolation, and changes between exposure to various body sites. *Am J Infect Control.* 2003;31(2):97-103.

29. Grundmann H, Hori S, Winter B, Tami A, Austin DJ. Risk factors for the transmission of methicillin-resistant *Staphylococcus aureus* in an adult intensive care unit: fitting a model to the data. *J Infect Dis.* 2002;185(4):481-488.

30. McBryde ES, Bradley LC, Whitby M, McElwain DL. An investigation of contact transmission of methicillin-resistant *Staphylococcus aureus.* *J Hosp Infect.* 2004; 58(2):104-108.

31. Hubner NO, Kampf G, Kamp P, Kohlmann T, Kramer A. Does a preceding hand wash and drying time after surgical hand disinfection influence the efficacy of a propanol-based hand rub? *BMC Microbiol.* 2006;6:57.

32. Hubner NO, Kampf G, Loffler H, Kramer A. Effect of a 1 min hand wash on the bactericidal efficacy of consecutive surgical hand disinfection with standard alcohols and on skin hydration. *Int J Hyg Environ Health.* 2006;209(3):285-291.

33. Mangram AJ, Horan TC, Pearson ML, Silver LC, Jarvis WR. Guideline for prevention of surgical site infection, 1999. Hospital Infection Control Practices Advisory Committee. *Infect Control Hosp Epidemiol.* 1999; 20(4):250-278.

34. Griffith CJ, Malik R, Cooper RA, Looker N, Michaels B. Environmental surface cleanliness and the potential for contamination during handwashing. *Am J Infect Control.* 2003;31(2):93-96.

35. AIA Academy of Architecture for Health, Facilities Guidelines Institute. *Guidelines for Design and Construction of Health Care Facilities.* Washington, DC: American Institute of Architects; 2006.

36. Harrison WA, Griffith CJ, Ayers T, Michaels B. Bacterial transfer and cross-contamination potential associated with paper-towel dispensing. *Am J Infect Control.* 2003;31(7):387-391.

37. Hugonnet S, Pittet D. Hand hygiene-beliefs or science? *Clin Microbiol Infect.* 2000;6(7):350-356.

38. AORN guidance statement: Fire prevention in the operating room. In: *Perioperative Standards and Recommended Practices.* Denver, CO: AORN, Inc; 2009:195-203.

39. *NFPA 99 Standard for Health Care Facilities.* Quincy, MA: National Fire Protection Association; 2005.

40. Rotter ML, Kampf G, Suchomel M, Kundi M. Long-term effect of a 1.5 minute surgical hand rub with a propanol-based product on the resident hand flora. *J Hosp Infect.* 2007;66(1):84-85.

41. Gupta C, Czubatyj AM, Briski LE, Malani AK. Comparison of two alcohol-based surgical scrub solutions with an iodine-based scrub brush for presurgical antiseptic effectiveness in a community hospital. *J Hosp Infect.* 2007;65(1):65-71.

42. Hingst V, Juditzki I, Heeg P, Sonntag HG. Evaluation of the efficacy of surgical hand disinfection following a reduced application time of 3 instead of 5 min. *J Hosp Infect.* 1992;20(2):79-86.

43. Recommended practices for product selection in perioperative practice settings. In: *Perioperative Standards and Recommended Practices.* Denver, CO: AORN, Inc; 2009:387-390.

44. Larson E, Leyden JJ, McGinley KJ, Grove GL, Talbot GH. Physiologic and microbiologic changes in skin

related to frequent handwashing. *J Infect Control.* 1986;7(2):59-63.

45. Department of Health and Human Services. Tentative final monograph for healthcare antiseptic drug products: proposed rules. *Fed Regist.* 1994;59(116):31402-31452.

46. Ojajarvi J. The importance of soap selection for routine hand hygiene in hospital. *J Hyg (Lond).* 1981;86(3):275-283.

47. Recommended practices for a safe environment of care. In: *Perioperative Standards and Recommended Practices.* Denver, CO: AORN, Inc; 2009:415-437.

48. Kownatzki E. Hand hygiene and skin health. *J Hosp Infect.* 2003;55(4):239-245.

49. Boyce JM, Kelliher S, Vallande N. Skin irritation and dryness associated with two hand-hygiene regimens: soap-and-water hand washing versus hand antisepsis with an alcoholic hand gel. *Infect Control Hosp Epidemiol.* 2000;21(7):442-448.

50. Schwanitz HJ, Riehl U, Schlesinger T, Bock M, Skudlik C, Wulfhorst B. Skin care management: educational aspects. *Int Arch Occup Environ Health.* 2003;76(5):374-381.

51. Pittet D. Improving compliance with hand hygiene in hospitals. *Infect Control Hosp Epidemiol.* 2000;21(6):381-386.

52. Voss A, Widmer AF. No time for handwashing!? Handwashing versus alcoholic rub: can we afford 100% compliance? *Infect Control Hosp Epidemiol.* 1997; 18(3):205-208.

53. Pittet D. Compliance with hand disinfection and its impact on hospital-acquired infections. *J Hosp Infect.* 2001;48(Suppl A):S40-S46.

54. Kampf G. The first hand scrub: why it does not make much sense. *J Hosp Infect.* 2007;65(1):83-84.

55. Venkatesh AK, Lankford MG, Rooney DM, Blachford T, Watts CM, Noskin GA. Use of electronic alerts to enhance hand hygiene compliance and decrease transmission of vancomycin-resistant *Enterococcus* in a hematology unit. *Am J Infect Control.* 2008;36(3):199-205.

56. van de Mortel T, Murgo M. An examination of covert observation and solution audit as tools to measure the success of hand hygiene interventions. *Am J Infect Control.* 2006;34(3):95-99.

57. Paulson DS. *Independent Laboratory Studies Summary. Automated Handwashing Stations.* Bozeman, MT: BioScience Laboratories, Inc.; 2008.

58. Bandura A. Health promotion by social cognitive means. *Health Education & Behavior.* 2004;31(2):143-164.

Acknowledgements

Lead Authors
Joan Blanchard, RN, BSN, MSS, CNOR, CIC
Perioperative Nursing Specialist
AORN Center for Nursing Practice
Denver, Colorado

Renae Battié, RN, MN, CNOR
Regional Director Perioperative Services
Franciscan Health System
Tacoma, Washington

Contributing Authors
Nancy Bjerke, RN, MPH, CIC
Consultant
Association for Professionals in Infection Control and Epidemiology, Inc (APIC)
San Antonio, Texas

Elizabeth Bolyard, RN, MPH
Technical Information Specialist
Centers for Disease Control and Prevention
Atlanta, Georgia

Peter Graves, RN, BSN, CNOR
Consultant
Molnlycke Health Care US
Corinth, Texas

Ardene L. Nichols, RN, MSN, CNS, CNOR
Consultant
Association for Professionals in Infection Control and Epidemiology, Inc (APIC)
Conroe, Texas

Publication History
Originally published May 1976, *AORN Journal*, as "Recommended practices for surgical hand scrubs."

Revised March 1978, July 1982, May 1984, October 1990. Published as proposed recommended practices August 1994.

Revised November 1998; published April 1999, *AORN Journal*. Reformatted July 2000.

Revised November 2003; published in *Standards, Recommended Practices, and Guidelines*, 2004 edition. Reprinted February 2004, AORN Journal.

Revised March 2009 for online publication in *Perioperative Standards and Recommended Practices*.

Revised July 2009 for online publication in *Perioperative Standards and Recommended Practices*.

Minor editing revisions made in October 2009 for publication in *Perioperative Standards and Recommended Practices*, 2010 edition.

The following recommended practices were developed by the AORN Recommended Practices Committee and have been approved by the AORN Board of Directors. They were presented as proposed recommended practices for comments by members and others. They are effective January 1, 2006.

These recommended practices are intended as achievable recommendations representing what is believed to be an optimal level of practice. Policies and procedures will reflect variations in practice settings and/or clinical situations that determine the degree to which the recommended practices can be implemented.

AORN recognizes the numerous settings in which perioperative nurses practice. These recommended practices are intended as guidelines adaptable to various practice settings. These practice settings include traditional operating rooms, ambulatory surgery centers, physicians' offices, cardiac catheterization suites, endoscopy suites, radiology departments, and all other areas where operative and other invasive procedures may be performed.

Purpose

These recommended practices provide guidance for establishing and maintaining a sterile field. The creation and maintenance of a sterile field can directly influence patient outcomes. Adherence to aseptic practices by all individuals involved in surgical interventions aids in fulfilling the professional responsibility to protect patients from injury. Aseptic practices are implemented preoperatively, intraoperatively, and postoperatively to minimize wound contamination and reduce patient risks for surgical site infections.

Recommendation I

Scrubbed persons should function within a sterile field.

1. Before donning sterile gowns and gloves, surgical hand antisepsis should be performed according to AORN's "Recommended practices for surgical hand antisepsis/hand scrubs"[1] and the manufacturer's written instructions for the antiseptic. Surgical hand antisepsis decreases the microbial counts on the skin and will reduce the transfer of microorganisms.

2. Personnel within the sterile field should be attired according to both AORN's "Recom-

mended practices for surgical attire"[2] and "Recommended practices for standard and transmission-based precautions."[3] Personnel should wear scrub attire, caps, masks, eye protection, and sterile gowns and gloves to prevent microbial transference to the sterile field, surgical site, and patient during the surgical procedure and to reduce risk of occupational exposure to bloodborne pathogens and other potentially infectious materials.[4-7]

3. Scrubbed personnel should don sterile gowns and gloves from a sterile area away from the main instrument table to prevent contamination of the sterile field.[8-12]

4. Materials for gowns should be selected according to AORN's "Recommended practices for selection and use of surgical gowns and drapes"[13] and according to the required level of barrier protection as outlined in the Association for the Advancement of Medical Instrumentation (AAMI) guideline "Liquid barrier performance and classification of protective apparel and drapes intended for use in health care facilities."[14] Surgical gowns should be of sufficient size to adequately cover the scrubbed person. Surgical gowns should establish a barrier that minimizes the passage of microorganisms between nonsterile and sterile areas.[12,15]

5. The front of a sterile gown is considered sterile from the chest to the level of the sterile field. The sterile area of the gown front extends to the level of the sterile field because most scrubbed personnel work adjacent to a sterile bed and/or table. Gown sleeves are considered sterile from two inches above the elbow to the cuff, circumferentially.

   The neckline, shoulders, underarms, sleeve cuffs, and gown back are areas of friction and, therefore, are not considered effective microbial barriers. The gown back is considered nonsterile because it cannot be constantly monitored.

   Gowns of an adequate size to close completely in the back and a sleeve length adequate to prevent cuff exposure outside the glove should be selected.

6. Sleeve cuffs should be considered contaminated when the scrubbed person's hands pass beyond the cuff.[9,10,12]

- ◆ Cuffs of the gown should remain at or below the natural wrist area.
- ◆ Gown sleeves should not be pulled up, leaving cuffs exposed.
- ◆ Sleeves of the gown should be of sufficient length and should cover the back of the hand to avoid exposing the gown cuff when the gloves slide down.

7. Scrubbed personnel should inspect gloves for integrity after donning them. Intact gloves establish a barrier that minimizes the passage of microorganisms between nonsterile and sterile areas.[4,12,16] AORN's "Recommended practices for standard and transmission-based precautions"[3] should be followed. Policies and procedures in the practice setting should indicate when double-gloving is required to reduce the potential for hand contact with blood and body fluids.

8. Sterile gloves that become contaminated should be changed as soon as possible. The preferred method of changing gloves is assisted gloving, whereby one member of the sterile team assists another member. This technique allows a gowned and gloved team member to touch only the outside of the new glove when applying the glove to a team member's hand. If this method is not possible, the contaminated glove should be changed by the open-glove method. If it is not possible to change the glove at the moment the break in technique is noted, a new glove may be donned over the contaminated/damaged glove until it can be changed.[9,11,12]

Recommendation II

Sterile drapes should be used to establish a sterile field.

1. Surgical drapes should be selected according to AORN's "Recommended practices for selection and use of surgical gowns and drapes"[13] and the AAMI guideline "Liquid barrier performance and classification of protective apparel and drapes intended for use in health care facilities."[14] Surgical drapes should establish an aseptic barrier that minimizes the passage of microorganisms between nonsterile and sterile areas.[15,17,18]

2. To prevent transfer of microorganisms from nonsterile to sterile areas, sterile drapes should be placed on the patient, furniture, and equipment to be included in the sterile field.[19]

3. Sterile drapes should be handled as little as possible. Rapid movement of draping materials creates air currents on which dust, lint, and other particles can migrate.[20,21]

4. Draping material should be held in a compact manner, held higher than the OR bed, and placed from the surgical site to the periphery to minimize contamination of the surgical site. Some procedures may require modified draping techniques (eg, extremities).[9,10,12]

5. During draping, gloved hands should be protected by cuffing the drape material over the gloved hands to reduce the potential for contamination.[9,10,12]

6. The portion of the surgical drape that establishes the sterile field should not be moved after it is positioned. Shifting or moving the sterile drape can compromise the sterility of the field.[9,10,12]

Recommendation III

Items used within the sterile field should be sterile.

1. To ensure that only sterile items are presented to the sterile field, all items should be inspected immediately before presentation to the field for proper packaging, processing, seal, package container integrity, and inclusion of a sterilization indicator. The indicator should be inspected immediately to verify the appropriate color change for the sterilization process selected. If an expiration date is provided, the date should be checked before the package is opened and the contents are delivered to the field. Outdated items should not be used.[12,22]

   An event-related sterility system should be used. Event-related sterility is based on the concept that "sterility is not altered over time, but may be compromised by certain events or environmental conditions."[23] Shelf life refers to the time an item may remain on the shelf and still maintain its sterility. Shelf life is influenced by the type of packaging used, storage conditions (eg, open or closed shelves), humidity, temperature, transport conditions, use of dust covers, and the amount of handling the item receives.[12,22,23]

   Spaulding's criteria are used to determine the potential for transmission of infectious agents.[24] Within this classification, items contacting the vascular system, the neurological system, and/or sterile tissues pose the greatest risk of infection and are classified as critical items. Using sterile items when contacting sterile tissues minimizes the risk of infection.[12,25-28]

2. Packaging materials should meet the criteria identified in AORN's "Recommended practices for selection and use of packaging systems."[29]

3. Methods of sterilization, event-related shelf life, and handling of sterile items should be in accordance with AORN's "Recommended practices for sterilization in the perioperative practice setting."[30] Sterilization provides the highest level of assurance that surgical items are free of viable microbes. High-level disinfection reduces the risk of microbial contamination, but it does not ensure the same margin of safety that sterilization provides.[25,26,28,31,32]

Recommendation IV

All items introduced to a sterile field should be opened, dispensed, and transferred by methods that maintain item sterility and integrity.

1. All invasive surgical procedures should be performed using sterile instruments and supplies, and the surgical team should practice aseptic technique for all surgical patients.

    The mucous membranes of the mouth, urinary tract, and intestinal tract are effective bacterial barriers when intact. However, ear, nose, and throat procedures, hemorrhoidectomy, and other procedures are invasive and impair the integrity of the mucosal barrier. The normal flora found in these areas is not infectious to the individual in question, but it may be pathogenic when transferred to other tissues by contaminated surgical instruments.

    Health care-acquired surgical infections are a leading cause of patient morbidity and mortality in the United States. Rigorous adherence to the principles of asepsis is the foundation of surgical site infection prevention and should never be circumvented to save time or money. A sterile field should be prepared and maintained for every surgical patient.[4,25,26]

2. Unscrubbed individuals should open wrapped sterile supplies by opening the wrapper flap farthest away from them first, to prevent contamination from passing an unsterile arm over a sterile item. Next, they should open each of the side flaps. The nearest wrapper flap should be opened last.[9-11]

3. All wrapper edges should be secured when supplies are presented to the sterile field. Securing the loose wrapper edges prevents them from contaminating the sterile field or a sterile item.[9,10]

4. Sterile items should be presented to the scrubbed person or placed securely on the sterile field. Items tossed onto a sterile field may roll off the edge, create a hole in the sterile drape, or cause other items to be displaced, leading to contamination of the sterile field.[9,10]

   ♦ Sharps and heavy objects should be presented to the scrubbed person or opened on a separate surface. These heavy items may penetrate the sterile barrier if dropped onto the sterile field.[9,10]

   ♦ Peel pouches should be presented to the scrubbed person to prevent contamination of the contents. The edges of the package may curl and the contents may slide over the unsterile edge, contaminating the contents of the package.

   ♦ Rigid container systems should be opened on a separate surface. The external indicator should be verified for appropriate color change. Locks should be inspected for security to verify there has not been a breach of the container seal prior to use. The lid should be lifted toward the person opening the container and away from the container. The filter should be checked and changed according to the manufacturer's written instructions.

5. All items should be delivered to the surgical field in a manner that prevents nonsterile objects or people from extending over the sterile field. Skin is a source of bacteria and scurf shedding; therefore, maintaining distance from the sterile field can decrease the potential for contamination when items are passed from a nonsterile area to a sterile area.[9,10,19]

6. When solutions are dispensed, the labeled solution receptacle on the sterile field should be placed near the table's edge or held by the scrubbed person. The entire contents of the container should be poured slowly to avoid splashing. Splashing can cause strike-through and splash-back from nonsterile surfaces to the sterile field. Placing the solution receptacle near the edge of the sterile table allows the unscrubbed

person to pour fluids without contaminating the sterile field. Any remaining fluids should be discarded. The edge of a container is considered contaminated after the contents have been poured; therefore, the sterility of the contents cannot be ensured if the cap is replaced. Reuse of open containers may contaminate solutions due to drops contacting unsterile areas and then running back over container openings.[9,10]

7. Medications should be delivered to the sterile field in an aseptic manner. Stoppers should not be removed from vials for the purpose of pouring medications. Sterile transfer devices (eg, sterile vial spike, filter straw, plastic catheter) should be used to dispense medications to the sterile field. Medications should be delivered to the sterile field according to AORN's "Recommended practices for safe care through identification of hazards in the surgical environment,"[33] AORN's "Guidance statement: Safe medication practices in perioperative practice settings,"[34] the "AORN latex guideline,"[35] and the policies and procedures of the practice setting.

Recommendation V

A sterile field should be maintained and monitored constantly.

1. The sterile field should be prepared in the location in which it will be used. Moving tables stirs air currents that can contaminate the sterile field.[36]

2. Sterile supplies should be opened for only one patient at a time. Opening several cases in a room at one time increases the risk of cross-infection.

3. One patient at a time should occupy the OR. Concurrent cases performed on two patients in the same room at the same time may expose patients to a variety of hazards and increase the risk of contamination and infection. The transmission of infectious diseases can occur by airborne, contact, and droplet methods. The risk of cross contamination may be increased significantly when two sterile fields, two surgical teams, and two open surgical wounds are confined to one OR. Operating rooms in the United States are not designed to accommodate the additional personnel and equipment necessary to care for two patients simultaneously. In the United States, general ORs built to the standards of the American Institute of Architects (AIA) are 400 sq ft.[37] Some ORs may be as small as 360 sq ft. This square footage minimum is intended to accommodate the equipment and personnel necessary for one surgical field. To move around the sterile field without contaminating it, nonsterile personnel (eg, the circulating nurse) should maintain a distance of at least 12 inches from the sterile field. When two patients and two sterile fields occupy an area designed to accommodate one patient and one sterile field, contamination of the sterile field is likely.

4. Sterile fields should be prepared as close as possible to the time of use. The potential for contamination increases with time because dust and other particles present in the ambient environment settle on horizontal surfaces over time. Particulate matter can be stirred up by movement of personnel when opening the room and can settle on opened sterile supplies.[4,12,21,36,38,39] The OR environment can be breached by other vectors, such as insects, that potentially could come into contact with open sterile fields, unobserved, unless the sterile field is monitored.

   There is no specified amount of designated time that a room can remain open and not used and still be considered sterile. The sterility of an open sterile field is event-related. An open sterile field requires continuous visual observation. Direct observation increases the likelihood of detecting a breach in sterility.[12,39-41]

5. Sterile fields should not be covered. Although there are no research studies to support or discount the practice, removing a table cover may result in a part of the cover that was below the table level being drawn above the table level or air currents drawing microorganisms from a nonsterile area to the sterile field. It is important to continuously monitor all sterile areas for possible contamination.[12,21]

6. Conversations in the presence of a sterile field should be kept to a minimum to reduce the spread of droplets. Air contains microorganisms on airborne particles, such as respiratory droplets. The primary source of airborne bacteria is health care personnel.[7,12,21,31]

7. Surgical equipment (eg, cables, tubing) should be secured to the sterile field with nonperforating devices. Perforations in a barrier

provide portals of entry and exit for microorganisms, blood, and other potentially infectious body fluids.

8. Nonsterile equipment (eg, Mayo stands, microscopes, C-arms) should be covered with sterile barrier material(s) before being introduced to or brought over a sterile field. Only sterile items should touch sterile surfaces. The equipment should be covered with a barrier material on the top, bottom, and all sides. Sterile barrier material also should be applied to the portion of the Mayo stand or other equipment that will be positioned immediately adjacent to the sterile field.[11]

Recommendation VI

All personnel moving within or around a sterile field should do so in a manner that maintains the sterile field.

1. Scrubbed personnel should remain close to the sterile field.[9,10] Walking outside the sterile field's periphery or leaving the OR in sterile attire increases the potential for contamination. Using a closed container system for flash sterilization and transport of items eliminates the need for the scrubbed person to leave the sterile field to retrieve instruments from a sterilizer. Scrubbed personnel should avoid leaving the sterile field when x-rays are taken. Protective devices for reducing radiological exposure should be provided to personnel who cannot leave the room or who cannot stand approximately 6 ft away from the source of radiation.[42]

2. Scrubbed personnel should move from sterile areas to sterile areas to prevent contamination. If they must change position, they should turn back to back or face to face while maintaining safe distances from each other and the sterile field.

3. Unscrubbed personnel should face sterile fields on approach, should not walk between two sterile fields, and should be aware of the need for distance from the sterile field. By establishing patterns of movement around the sterile field and keeping sterile areas in view, accidental contamination can be reduced.

4. Scrubbed personnel should keep their arms and hands above the level of their waists at all times. Hands should remain in front of the body above waist level so the hands remain visible. Contamination may occur when arms and hands are moved below waist level. Arms should not be folded with the hands in the axilla. This area has the potential to become contaminated by perspiration, allowing for strike-through of the gown and, ultimately, contamination of the gloved hands. The gown at the axilla also is an area of friction and, therefore, is not considered an effective microbial barrier.

5. Scrubbed personnel should avoid changing levels and should be seated only when the entire surgical procedure will be performed at that level. When changing levels, exposure of the nonsterile portion of the surgical gown is likely.

6. The number and movement of individuals involved in a surgical procedure should be kept to a minimum per AORN's "Recommended practices for traffic patterns in the perioperative practice setting."[36] Bacterial shedding increases with activity. Air currents can pick up contaminated particles shed from patients, personnel, and drapes and distribute them to sterile areas.[12,21,31,43]

7. When a break in sterile technique occurs, corrective action should be taken immediately unless the patient's safety is at risk. If the patient's safety is at risk, correct the break in technique as soon as it is safe to do so.

8. When a break in sterile technique occurs and cannot be corrected immediately, the organization should determine how it should be reported and recorded, and the wound classification should be adjusted accordingly and documented on the operative record.

Recommendation VII

Policies and procedures for maintaining a sterile field should be developed, reviewed periodically, revised as necessary, and readily available in the practice setting.

1. Policies and procedures for maintaining a sterile field should be developed by each facility and should include, but not be limited to,
   - aseptic technique, including handling sterile supplies and monitoring a sterile field;
   - surgical hand antisepsis;
   - gowning and gloving with sterile gown and gloves;

- masks, head coverings, and scrub attire;
- draping;
- event-related sterility;
- traffic patterns; and
- monitoring of environmental conditions, including OR air exchange rate and pressure, temperature, and humidity.

2. These recommended practices should be used as a guideline for developing policies and procedures in the perioperative practice setting. Policies and procedures serve as operational guidelines and establish authority, responsibility, and accountability within the facility.

3. Personnel and observers should be knowledgeable about the procedures involved in developing and maintaining a sterile field. An introduction and review of policies and procedures for maintaining the sterile field should be included in orientation to the perioperative setting for personnel and observers. Continuing education should be provided when new technologies (eg, sterilization containers, barrier materials) are introduced. Ongoing education of perioperative personnel facilitates the development of knowledge, skills, and attitudes that affect surgical patient outcomes. Policies and procedures also assist in the development of quality assessment and improvement activities.

4. The Perioperative Nursing Data Set (PNDS) should be used in the development of policies and procedures and documentation of nursing interventions related to maintenance of the sterile field. The expected outcome of primary importance to this recommended practice is outcome O10, "The patient is free from signs and symptoms of infection." This outcome falls within the domain of Physiological Responses (D2). The associated nursing diagnosis is X28, "Risk for infection." The associated interventions that may lead to the desired outcome may be I21, "Assesses susceptibility for infection"; I70, "Implements aseptic technique"; and I98, "Protects from cross-contamination."[44]

Glossary

Asepsis: Process for keeping away disease-producing microorganisms.

Aseptic technique: Methods by which contamination with microorganisms is prevented.

Assisted gloving: Method by which a gowned and gloved person assists another gowned person to don sterile gloves.

Closed gloving method: Used when wearing a sterile gown to prevent exposure of bare skin during gowning and donning of sterile gloves, thereby lessening the chance of contamination.

Critical item: An item that contacts the vascular system or enters sterile tissue, posing the highest risk of transmission of infection.

Event-related sterility: Shelf life of a packaged sterile item depends on the quality of the wrapper material, the storage conditions, the conditions during transport, and the amount of handling.

Noncritical item: An item that comes in contact with intact skin but not with mucous membranes, sterile tissue, or the vascular system.

Open-gloving method: Used when changing a glove during a surgical procedure. A method of donning sterile gloves in which the everted cuff of each glove allows the gowned person to touch the inner side of the glove with ungloved fingers and the outer side of the glove with gloved fingers.

Scurf: A bran-like desquamation of the epidermis.

Semicritical item: An item that comes in contact with mucous membranes or with skin that is not intact.

Sterile: The absence of all living microorganisms.

Sterile field: Area around the site of the incision into tissue or the site of introduction of an instrument into a body orifice that has been prepared for the use of sterile supplies and equipment. This area includes all furniture covered with sterile drapes and all personnel who are in sterile attire.

Sterile technique: Methods by which contamination with microorganisms is prevented to maintain sterility throughout the surgical procedure.

Sterilization: Processes by which all pathogenic and nonpathogenic microorganisms, including spores, are killed.

Strike-through: Contamination of a sterile surface by moisture that has originated from a nonsterile surface and penetrated the protective covering of the sterile item.

Time-related sterility: Expiration dates are established to indicate the maximum duration of time within which a sterile item is considered sterile and safe to use.

REFERENCES

1. "Recommended practices for surgical hand antisepsis/hand scrubs," in *Standards, Recommended*

Practices, and Guidelines (Denver: AORN, Inc, 2005) 377-385.

2. "Recommended practices for surgical attire," in *Standards, Recommended Practices, and Guidelines* (Denver: AORN, Inc, 2005) 299-305.

3. "Recommended practices for standard and transmission-based precautions in the perioperative practice setting," in *Standards, Recommended Practices, and Guidelines* (Denver: AORN, Inc, 2005) 447-451.

4. A J Mangram et al, "Guideline for prevention of surgical site infection," *American Journal of Infection Control* 27 (April 1999) 97-134.

5. W A Rutala, D J Weber, "A review of single-use and reusable gowns and drapes in health care," *Infection Control and Hospital Epidemiology* 22 (April 2001) 248-257.

6. H Laufman, N L Belkin, K K Meyer, "A critical review of a century's progress in surgical apparel: How far have we come?" *Journal of the American College of Surgeons* 191 (November 2000) 554-568.

7. Association for Professionals in Infection Control and Epidemiology, *APIC Text of Infection Control and Epidemiology* (Washington, DC: Association for Professionals in Infection Control and Epidemiology, 2002) 27-1 to 27-4.

8. J S Heal et al, "Bacterial contamination of surgical gloves by water droplets spilt after scrubbing," *Journal of Hospital Infection* 53 (February 2003) 136-139.

9. D M Fogg, "Infection prevention and control," in *Alexander's Care of the Patient in Surgery*, 12th ed, J C Rothrock, ed (St Louis: Mosby, 2003) 97-158.

10. N F Phillips, *Berry & Kohn's Operating Room Technique*, 10th ed (St Louis: Mosby, 2004) 247-323.

11. P A Mews, "Establishing and maintaining a sterile field," in *Patient Care During Operative and Invasive Procedures*, second ed, M Phippen, M Wells, eds (Philadelphia: W B Saunders Co, 2000) 61-93.

12. B Gruendemann, S Mangum, *Infection Prevention in Surgical Settings* (Philadelphia: W B Saunders Co, 2001) 47-49, 88-97, 119-219, 250-257, 266-281, 365-371.

13. "Recommended practices for selection and use of surgical gowns and drapes," in *Standards, Recommended Practices, and Guidelines* (Denver: AORN, Inc, 2005) 371-375.

14. Association for the Advancement of Medical Instrumentation, *Liquid Barrier Performance and Classification of Protective Apparel and Drapes Intended for Use in Health Care Facilities*, ANSI/ AAMI PB70 (Arlington, Va: Association for the Advancement of Medical Instrumentation, 2003).

15. Association for the Advancement of Medical Instrumentation, *Selection of Surgical Gowns and Drapes in Health Care Facilities*, AAMI TIR no 11:1994 (Arlington, Va: Association for the Advancement of Medical Instrumentation, 2000.)

16. J Tanner, H Parkinson, "Double gloving to reduce surgical cross-infection," (Cochrane Review) in *The Cochrane Library*, issue 2 (Chichester, UK: John J Wiley & Sons, 2004). Abstract available at *http://www .cochrane.org/cochrane/revabstr/AB003087.htm* (accessed 26 Aug 2005).

17. A Lipp, "An assessment of the clinical effectiveness of surgical drapes," *Nursing Times* 99 (Dec 9, 2003) 28-31.

18. N Belkin, "Selecting surgical gowns and drapes for today's surgery," *SSM* 9 (December 2003) 41-44.

19. J Pournoor, "New scientific tools to expand the understanding of aseptic practices," *Surgical Services Management* 6 (April 2000) 28-32.

20. F Memarzadah, A P Manning "Comparison of operating room ventilation systems in the protection of the surgical site," session 4549, *ASHRAE Transactions*, proceedings of the 2002 annual meeting (Atlanta: American Society of Heating, Refrigerating, and Air-Conditioning Engineers, 2002). Abstract available at *http://resource center.ashrae.org/store/ashrae* (accessed 26 Aug 2005).

21. C Edmiston et al, "Airborne particulates in the OR environment," *AORN Journal* 69 (June 1999) 1169-1183.

22. N Japp, "Packaging: Shelf life," in *Sterilization Technology for the Health Care Facility*, second ed, M Reichert, J Young, eds (Gaithersburg, Md: Aspen Publishers, 1997) 99-103.

23. L O'Connor, "Event-related sterility assurance: An opportunity for continuous quality improvement," *The Surgical Technologist* (January 1994) 8-12.

24. E H Spaulding, "Chemical disinfection of medical and surgical materials," in *Disinfection, Sterilization, and Preservation*, C A Lawrence, S S Block, eds (Philadelphia: Lea & Febiger, 1968) 517-531.

25. W Rutala, D Weber, "Modern advances in disinfection, sterilization, and medical waste management," in *Prevention and Control of Nosocomial Infections*, fourth ed, R P Wenzel, ed (Philadelphia: Lippincott Williams & Wilkins, 2003) 542-574.

26. M C Roy, "Modern approaches to preventing surgical site infections," in *Prevention and Control of Nosocomial Infections*, fourth ed, R P Wenzel, ed (Philadelphia: Lippincott Williams & Wilkins, 2003) 369-384.

27. "Medical devices; semicritical reprocessed single-use devices; termination of exemptions from premarket notification; requirement for submission of validation data," *Federal Register* 69 (April 13, 2004) 19433-19435.

28. W Rutala, "APIC guideline for selection and use of disinfectants," *American Journal of Infection Control* 24 (August 1996) 313-342.

29. "Recommended practices for selection and use of packaging systems," in *Standards, Recommended Practices, and Guidelines* (Denver: AORN, Inc, 2005) 415-420.

30. "Recommended practices for sterilization in perioperative practice settings," in *Standards, Recommended Practices, and Guidelines* (Denver: AORN, Inc, 2005) 459-469.

31. L Sehulster, R Y Chinn, "Guidelines for environmental infection control in health care facilities," *Morbidity and Mortality Weekly Report* 52 RR-10 (June 6, 2003) 1-42.

32. "Recommended practices for high-level disinfection," in *Standards, Recommended Practices, and Guidelines* (Denver: AORN, Inc, 2005) 313-319.

33. "Recommended practices for safe care through identification of potential hazards in the surgical environment," in *Standards, Recommended Practices, and Guidelines* (Denver: AORN, Inc, 2005) 387-393.

34. "Guidance statement: Safe medication practices in perioperative practice settings," in *Standards, Recommended Practices, and Guidelines* (Denver: AORN, Inc, 2005) 196-198.

35. "AORN latex guideline" in *Standards, Recommended Practices, and Guidelines* (Denver: AORN, Inc, 2005) 117-132.

36. "Recommended practices for traffic patterns in the perioperative practice setting," in *Standards, Recommended Practices, and Guidelines* (Denver: AORN, Inc, 2005) 483-485.

37. American Institute of Architects Academy of Architecture for Health, *Guidelines for Design and Construction of Hospital and Health Care Facilities* (Washington, DC: American Institute of Architects, 2001).

38. A Tammelin et al, "Dispersal of methicillin-resistant *Staphylococcus epidermis* by staff in an operating room suite for thoracic and cardiovascular surgery: Relation to skin carriage and clothing," *Journal of Hospital Infection* 44 (February 2000) 119-126.

39. R Conner, "Washing and restringing instruments; bone debris; preparing setups; patient restraints; Group A *Streptococcus*," (Clinical Issues) *AORN Journal* 73 (April 2001) 835-838.

40. C Petersen, "Time for unused sterile setups; maintaining instrument count sheets; gowning off back tables; plants in the OR; count discrepancies," (Clinical Issues) *AORN Journal* 80 (August 2004) 321-324.

41. "Surgical site infections," in *APIC Handbook of Infection Control and Epidemiology*, third ed, J Jennings, J Wideman, eds (Washington, DC: Association for Professionals in Infection Control and Epidemiology) 312-321.

42. "Recommended practices for reducing radiological exposure in the practice setting," in *Standards, Recommended Practices, and Guidelines* (Denver: AORN, Inc, 2005) 437-442.

43. F Pryor, P Messmer, "The effect of traffic patterns in the OR on surgical site infections," *AORN Journal* 68 (October 1998) 649-660.

44. S C Beyea, ed, *Perioperative Nursing Data Set: The Perioperative Nursing Vocabulary,* second ed (Denver: AORN, Inc, 2002).

RESOURCES

American Society for Healthcare Central Service Professionals. "Eliminating sterile outdates," (self-study series) *Healthcare Purchasing News* (March 2003) 42-44.

Barrett, R; Stevens, J; Taranter, J. "A shelf-life trial: Examining the efficacy of event related sterility principles and its implications for nursing practice," *Australian Journal of Advanced Nursing* 21 (2003–2004) 8-12.

Belkin, N. "Barrier drapes and their impact on surgical site infections," *Infection Control Today* (May 2002).

Belkin, N. "Barrier materials: Their influence on surgical wound infections," *AORN Journal* 55 (June 1992) 1521-1528.

Bell, M. "Hospital uses team approach to improve processes, reduce costs," *AORN Journal* 68 (July 1998) 68-72.

Donovan, A; Turner, D W; Smith, A. "Successful, documented studies favoring indefinite shelf life," *Journal of Healthcare Materiel Management* 9 (March 1991) 34-40.

Garibaldi, R A, et al. "Comparison of nonwoven and woven gown and drape fabric to prevent intraoperative wound contamination and postoperative infection," *The American Journal of Surgery* 152 (November 1986) 505-509.

Groah, L, ed. "Limiting contamination sources in the operating room," in *Perioperative Nursing,* third ed (Stamford, Conn: Appleton & Lange, 1996) 137-162.

Gruendemann, B; Fernsebner, B. "Asepsis," in *Comprehensive Perioperative Nursing, Volume 1: Principles* (Boston: Jones and Bartlett Publishers, 1995) 180-288.

Hinchliff, S. "Innate defenses," in *Physiology for Nursing Practice,* S Hinchliff, S Montague, eds (London: Baillière Tindall, 1988) 549-578.

Mayworm, D. "Probably sterile," *Infection Control and Sterilization Technology* (March 1995) 7.

Nicolette, L. "Sterilization and disinfection," in *Perioperative Nursing,* third ed, L Groah, ed (Stamford, Conn: Appleton & Lange, 1996) 163-195.

Parker, L. "Rituals versus risks in the contemporary operating theatre environment," *British Journal of Theatre Nursing* 9 (August 1999) 341-345.

Roark, J. "Guidelines for maintaining the sterile field," *Infection Control Today* 7 (August 2003) 14-16.

Saunders, S. "Practical measures to ensure health and safety in theatres," *Nursing Times* 100 (March 16, 2004) 32-35.

Taylor, M; Campbell, C. "The multidisciplinary team in the operating department," *British Journal of Theatre Nursing* 9 (April 1999) 178-183.

Xavier, G. "Asepsis," *Nursing Standard* 13 (May 26, 1999) 49-53.

PUBLICATION HISTORY

Originally published March 1978, *AORN Journal,* as "Recommended practices for aseptic technique." Format revision July 1982. Revised March 1987, October 1991.

Revised June 1996; published November 1996, *AORN Journal.* Revised and reformatted; published February 2001, *AORN Journal.*

Revised November 2005; published in *Standards, Recommended Practices, and Guidelines,* 2006 edition. Reprinted February 2006, *AORN Journal.*

Recommended Practices for Traffic Patterns in the Perioperative Practice Setting

The following recommended practices were developed by the AORN Recommended Practices Committee and have been approved by the AORN Board of Directors. They were presented as proposed recommended practices for comments by members and others. They are effective January 1, 2006.

These recommended practices are intended as achievable recommendations representing what is believed to be an optimal level of practice. Policies and procedures will reflect variations in practice settings and/or clinical situations that determine the degree to which the recommended practices can be implemented.

AORN recognizes the numerous settings in which perioperative nurses practice. These recommended practices are intended as guidelines adaptable to various practice settings. These practice settings include traditional operating rooms, ambulatory surgery centers, physicians' offices, cardiac catheterization suites, endoscopy suites, radiology departments, emergency departments, labor and delivery units that have OR suites, and all other areas where operative and other invasive procedures may be performed.

Purpose

These recommended practices provide guidance for establishing traffic patterns in perioperative practice areas. Traffic control patterns suggest movement into and out of the surgical suite as well as movement within the suite. Clearly defined and enforced traffic control practices protect personnel, patients, supplies, and equipment from potential sources of cross contamination; safeguard the privacy of patients; and provide security.

The building design of the surgical suite often predetermines traffic patterns. Implementation of all elements of these recommended practices may not be feasible within every facility because of the physical limitations of the setting.

Recommendation I

Traffic patterns should be designed to facilitate movement of patients and personnel into, through, and out of defined areas within the surgical suite. Signs should clearly indicate the appropriate environmental controls and surgical attire required.

1. The surgical suite should be divided into three designated areas that are defined by the physical activities performed in each area. Increasing environmental controls and surgical attire as progression is made from unrestricted to restricted areas decreases the potential for cross-contamination.

   The **unrestricted** area includes a central control point that is established to monitor the entrance of patients, personnel, and materials. Street clothes are permitted in this area, and traffic is not limited. The entrance to the surgical suite should be restricted to authorized personnel based on organizational policies.

   The **semirestricted** area includes the peripheral support areas of the surgical suite. It has storage areas for clean and sterile supplies, work areas for storage and processing of instruments, scrub sink areas, and corridors leading to the restricted areas of the surgical suite. Traffic in this area is limited to authorized personnel and patients. Personnel are required to wear surgical attire and cover all head and facial hair.[1]

   The **restricted** area includes ORs, procedure rooms, and the clean core area. Surgical attire and hair coverings are required. Masks are required where open sterile supplies or scrubbed persons are located. All persons entering the restricted area should follow the AORN "Recommended practices for surgical attire."[1]

   Persons entering the semirestricted or restricted areas of the surgical suite for a brief time for a specific purpose (eg, law enforcement officers, parents, biomedical engineers) should cover all head and facial hair and may don either freshly laundered surgical attire or a single-use coverall suit (eg, jumpsuit) designed to totally cover outside apparel.

2. Movement of personnel from unrestricted areas to either semirestricted or restricted areas should be through a transition zone. A transition zone exists where one can enter the area in street clothing and exit into the semirestricted or restricted zone in surgical attire. Locker rooms serve as transition zones between the outside and inside of a surgical suite and may serve as a security point to monitor people admitted to the suite.

3. Patients entering the surgical suite should wear clean gowns, be covered with clean linens, and have their hair covered. Clean gowns, linens, and hair coverings are worn by patients to minimize particulate shedding during surgical procedures.

Patients are not required to wear masks while in the surgical suite unless they are under airborne precautions (eg, a patient with active pulmonary tuberculosis or other airborne respiratory disease).[2] While in the restricted area, the mask could hinder access to the face and airway and might increase the patient's anxiety.

Personal undergarments may be worn when they will not interfere with the surgical site. Consideration should be given for management of potential incontinence. Many health care organizations now allow specific patients to wear clean personal clothing, including socks and underwear, into the surgical suite to promote the patient's comfort and sense of dignity. The most common surgical procedures that incorporate this new patient care practice are cataract extractions and carpal tunnel releases. Access to patients below the waist usually is not necessary for these surgical procedures. In addition, sterile fields can be maintained easily without the risk of contamination from patient clothing.

Recommendation II

Operating room suites should be secure.

1. The design of perioperative areas and traffic patterns should include the following.
   ♦ Patient privacy must be provided for as required by the Health Insurance Portability and Accountability Act of 1996 (HIPAA).[3]
   ♦ Patient, personnel, and visitor safety should be ensured.
   ♦ Supplies and equipment should be protected from tampering and theft.

2. Identification badges should be worn at all times according to organizational policy.

Recommendation III

Movement of personnel should be kept to a minimum while invasive and noninvasive procedures are in progress.

1. Careful assessment of the patient and planning for patient care needs should reduce the need for excessive movement and activity during the

procedure. Air is a potential source of microorganisms that can contaminate surgical wounds. Because microbial shedding increases with activity, greater amounts of airborne contamination can be expected with increased movement of surgical team members.[4]

2. Doors to the operating or procedure rooms should be closed except during movement of patients, personnel, supplies, and equipment. The air pressure within each operating or procedure room should be greater than in the semirestricted area. The air in the OR should be maintained under positive pressure with a minimum of 15 total room air exchanges per hour.[5] When the doors are left open, the heating, ventilation, and air conditioning system is unable to maintain these critical environmental parameters. Leaving the door open can disrupt pressurization and cause turbulent airflow that could increase airborne contamination. Traffic in and out of the OR should be minimized by preplanning so that turbulence from this activity is minimized during the procedure or when sterile supplies are opened.

3. Talking and the number of people present should be minimized during procedures. An increase in airborne microorganisms can occur with an increased number of people present. Movement, talking, and uncovered skin areas can contribute to airborne contamination.[4]

Recommendation IV

The movement of clean and sterile supplies and equipment should be separated from contaminated supplies, equipment, and waste by space, time, or traffic patterns.

1. Surgical supplies prepared for surgical procedures outside the surgical suite (eg, in central processing) should be transported to the surgical suite to maintain cleanliness and sterility and to prevent physical damage. Protecting items from contamination, physical damage, and loss during transportation facilitates their safe use. Use of correct procedures for transporting items preserves the qualities of the sterile and clean environment.[6]

2. Supplies and equipment should be removed from external shipping containers and web-edged or corrugated cardboard boxes in the unrestricted area before transfer into the surgical

suite. External shipping containers and web-edged cardboard boxes may collect dust, debris, and insects during shipment and may carry contaminants into the surgical suite.[6]

3. When there is a clean core, the movement of supplies should be from the clean core through the operating or procedure room to the peripheral corridor.
   ♦ Soiled supplies, instruments, and equipment should not re-enter the clean core area. They should be contained in closed or covered carts or containers for transport to a designated decontamination area.
   ♦ The decontamination area and soiled linen and trash collection areas should be separated from personnel and patient traffic areas. Separation of clean and sterile supplies and equipment from soiled materials by space, time, and traffic patterns decreases the risk of infection.[6]

Recommendation V

During construction and renovation, specific traffic patterns should be established and maintained in accordance with applicable state regulations.

1. Specific traffic plans for construction personnel and movement of supplies, equipment, and debris should be developed and implemented following applicable guidelines for construction in health care facilities, with infection control personnel monitoring the process.[7,8] Infections have been transmitted through the dissemination of microorganisms from disruptions of environmental reservoirs (eg, drywall, ceiling tiles, flooring, casework).[9]

2. Surgical personnel should be able to move from place to place without contaminating their surgical scrubs. Clean or sterile supplies and equipment must be transported to storage areas by a route that minimizes contamination from the construction site and prevents contact with soiled or contaminated trash and linen. Since traffic patterns may not be easily altered to meet these requirements, the construction personnel may need to work during off hours. If infection control requirements still cannot be met, some areas may need to be relocated or closed temporarily.[9]

3. A multidisciplinary assessment should be completed to determine the infection control and

safety risks involved in a construction, renovation, or maintenance project. A multidisciplinary team performing the assessment should include infection control, safety, and project personnel. An infection control risk assessment (ICRA) matrix may facilitate the process. The ICRA matrix helps the team identify important preventive strategies that may include, but are not limited to,
♦ types of barriers necessary,
♦ maintenance of barrier integrity,
♦ attire for workers,
♦ special entrances and exits,
♦ negative pressure and high-efficiency particulate air filters, and
♦ other infection control prevention and surveillance measures (eg, particulate counts).[9]

Thorough planning and coordination is necessary to minimize the risk for airborne infection both during projects and after their completion.[10]

4. Compliance with barrier precautions and traffic patterns should be monitored on an ongoing basis throughout and until the completion of the construction, renovation, or repair project. Monitoring provides an opportunity to rapidly correct any barrier or traffic restriction breach.

Recommendation VI

Policies and procedures for traffic patterns for patients, personnel, supplies, and equipment should be developed, reviewed periodically, revised as necessary, and kept readily available in the practice setting.

1. These recommendations should be used as guidelines for developing written policies and procedures in the practice setting. Policies and procedures establish authority, responsibility, and accountability and serve as operational guidelines. Policies and procedures establish guidelines for performance improvement activities to be used when monitoring and evaluating traffic patterns in the surgical practice setting.

2. Information on traffic patterns and methods of handling supplies and equipment should be included in the orientation and continuing education of personnel to assist in the development of knowledge, skills, and attitudes that affect surgical patient outcomes. This education should include ancillary support or delivery personnel

whose work activities require them to be within the semirestricted or restricted areas.

3. Policies and procedures should assist in the development of patient safety and quality assessment and improvement activities.

4. The uniform perioperative nursing vocabulary should be used in the development of policies and procedures related to traffic patterns. The perioperative nursing vocabulary is a clinically relevant and empirically validated standardized language. This standardized language consists of the Perioperative Nursing Data Set (PNDS) and includes perioperative nursing diagnoses, interventions, and outcomes. The expected outcome of primary importance to these recommended practices is outcome O10, "The patient is free from signs and symptoms of infection." This outcome falls within the domain of Physiological Responses (D2). The associated nursing diagnosis is X28, "Risk for infection." The associated interventions that may lead to the desired outcome may be I121, "Initiates traffic control"; I109, "Protects from cross-contamination"; I117, "Maintains continuous surveillance"; and I111, "Minimizes the length of invasive procedure by planning care."[11]

Glossary

Corrugated cardboard box: Web-edged box used for the purpose of containing items to be shipped for use in the OR.

Jumpsuit: One-piece suit that completely covers street clothes and can be worn in the semi restricted areas of the OR. *Synonyms:* coveralls, bunnysuit.

REFERENCES

1. "Recommended practices for surgical attire," in *Standards, Recommended Practices, and Guidelines* (Denver: AORN, Inc, 2005) 299-305.

2. J S Garner, Centers for Disease Control and Prevention Hospital Infection Control Practices Advisory Committee, "Guideline for isolation precautions in hospitals," *Infection Control and Hospital Epidemiology* 17 (January 1996) 53-80.

3. "The Health Insurance Portability and Accountability Act of 1996 (HIPAA)," Centers for Medicare and Medicaid Services, *http://www.cms.hhs.gov/hipaa* (accessed 13 Dec 2005).

4. A J Mangram et al, Centers for Disease Control and Prevention Hospital Infection Control Practices Advisory Committee, "Guideline for prevention of surgical site infection, 1999," *American Journal of Infection Control* 27 (April 1999) 97-134.

5. American Institute of Architects Academy of Architecture for Health, *Guidelines for Design and Construction of Hospital and Health Care Facilities* (Washington, DC: American Institute of Architects Press, 2001).

6. Association for the Advancement of Medical Instrumentation, *Steam Sterilization and Sterility Assurance in Health Care Facilities* (Arlington, Va: Association for the Advancement of Medical Instrumentation, 2002).

7. J M Bartley, "APIC state-of-the-art report: The role of infection control during construction in health care facilities," *American Journal of Infection Control* 28 (April 2000) 156-169.

8. J Bartley, "Construction and renovation," in *APIC Text of Infection Control and Epidemiology,* rev ed, J A Pfeiffer, ed (Washington, DC: Association for Professionals in Infection Control and Epidemiology, 2002) 72-1 to 72-11.

9. S A David, J A Fernandez, L A Herwaldt, "Infection control issues in construction and renovation," in *Practical Handbook for Healthcare Epidemiologists,* second ed, E Lautenbach, K F Woeltje, eds (Thorofare, NJ: Slack, 2004) 337-360.

10. Centers for Disease Control and Prevention, *Guidelines for Environmental Infection Control in Health-Care Facilities* (Atlanta: Centers for Disease Control and Prevention, 2003).

11. S C Beyea, ed, *Perioperative Nursing Data Set: The Perioperative Nursing Vocabulary,* second ed (Denver: AORN, Inc, 2002).

RESOURCE

"Infection control risk assessment matrix of precautions for construction and renovation," US Army Health Facility Planning Agency, *http://hfpa.otsg.amedd.army.mil/refs/docs/icra_assessment_form.pdf* (accessed 9 Dec 2005).

PUBLICATION HISTORY

Originally published March 1982, *AORN Journal.* Format revision July 1982.

Revised November 1988; May 1993; November 1995. Published March 1996, *AORN Journal.*

Revised; published February 2000, *AORN Journal.* Reformatted July 2000.

Revised November 2005; published in *Standards, Recommended Practices, and Guidelines,* 2006 edition. Reprinted March 2006, *AORN Journal.*

The following Recommended Practices for Electrosurgery were developed by the AORN Recommended Practices Committee and have been approved by the AORN Board of Directors. They were presented as proposed recommendations for comments by members and others. They are effective July 1, 2009. These recommended practices are intended as achievable recommendations representing what is believed to be an optimal level of practice. Policies and procedures will reflect variations in practice settings and/or clinical situations that determine the degree to which the recommended practices can be implemented. AORN recognizes the various settings in which perioperative nurses practice. These recommended practices are intended as guidelines adaptable to various practice settings. These practice settings include traditional operating rooms (ORs), ambulatory surgery centers, physicians' offices, cardiac catheterization laboratories, endoscopy suites, radiology departments, and all other areas where surgery and other invasive procedures may be performed.

Purpose

These recommended practices provide guidance to perioperative nurses in the use and care of electrosurgical equipment, including high frequency, ultrasound, and argon beam modalities. Proper care and handling of electrosurgical equipment are essential to patient and personnel safety. Electrosurgery, using high frequency (ie, radio frequency) electrical current, is used routinely to cut, coagulate, dissect, ablate, and shrink body tissue. Ultrasonic dissectors fragment tissue by vibration. Vessel sealing devices use a combination of pressure and heat to permanently fuse vessels and tissue. These recommended practices address all of these technologies and do not endorse any specific product.

Recommendation I

Personnel selecting new and refurbished electrosurgical units (ESUs) and accessories for purchase or use should make decisions based on safety features to minimize risks to patients and personnel.

ESUs and accessories are high-risk medical devices. Minimum safety standards for ESU systems have been developed by the Association for the Advancement of Medical Instrumentation (AAMI), approved by the American National Standards Institute (ANSI), and the International Electrotechnical Commission (IEC).[1]

I.a. ESUs and accessories should be selected based on safety features that minimize patient and personnel injury.[2]

Historically, the most frequently reported patient injury has been a skin injury (eg, burn) at the dispersive electrode site.[2] The risk of this type of injury has been minimized through advances in dispersive pad design and the use of return electrode contact quality monitoring.[2,3]

I.b. ESUs and accessories should be selected to include technology that minimizes the risk of alternate site injuries.

These injuries can result from use of ground-referenced (ie, spark-gap) ESUs that allow electrical current to seek alternate pathways to complete the circuit.[1,4] The use of isolated generator ESUs has minimized this risk.[5]

I.c. ESUs and accessories should be selected to include technology that minimizes or eliminates the risk of insulation failure and capacitive coupling injuries.

During minimally invasive procedures, alternate site injuries have resulted from insulation failure and capacitive coupling.[2,4,6-9] These injuries are far more serious than skin burns and have increased in number with the increased use of minimally invasive surgery.[10] Active electrode monitoring, active electrode insulation integrity testers, active electrode indicator shafts, and visual inspection minimize these risks.[7,9,11-14]

I.d. ESUs and accessories should be designed to minimize the risk of unintentional activation.

Unintentional activation has resulted in patient and personnel injuries. Unintentional ESU activation has been reported as the cause of 56% of alternate site injuries.[2,15] Audible activation tones minimize this risk.[1,15-17]

I.e. Electrosurgical accessories should be compatible with the ESU.

Injuries have resulted when an ESU accessory intended for bipolar use was inserted into monopolar connectors and subsequently activated.[1] Appropriate matching and use of accessories specific to the ESU minimizes this risk.

I.f. Health care organizations should attempt to standardize electrosurgical equipment used within the facility.

Equipment standardization reduces the risk of error.[18]

Recommendation II

The ESU should be used in a manner that minimizes the potential for injuries.

Electrosurgical units are high-risk equipment.[1] Potential complications of electrosurgery include patient injuries, user injuries, fires, and electromagnetic interference with other medical equipment and internal electronic devices.[2] Electrosurgery safety is heightened by adhering to good practices.[18] Adverse events (eg, patient burns and fires) may be reduced by adhering to basic principles of electrosurgery safety.[15]

II.a. Instructions for ESU use, warranties, and a manual for maintenance and inspections should be obtained from the manufacturer and be readily available to users.[2,19]

Equipment manuals assist in developing operational, safety, and maintenance guidelines, as well as serve as a reference for appropriate use.[19]

II.a.1. Concise, clearly readable operating instructions specific for the device should be on or attached to each ESU.[19]

Readily available instructions reduce the risk of operator error.

II.b. The ESU should be securely mounted on a tip-resistant cart or shelf and should not be used as a shelf or table.

II.c. The ESU should be protected from liquids.[19]

Liquids entering the ESU can cause unintentional activation, device failure, or an electrical hazard.

II.c.1. Liquids should not be placed on top of the ESU.

II.c.2. Foot pedal accessories should be encased in a clean, impervious cover when there is potential for fluid spills on the floor.

II.d. Safety and warning alarms and activation indicators should be operational, audible, and visible at all times.[1,16-18,20]

Safety and warning alarms alert the operator to potential electrode failure.[5] The indicators and alarms immediately alert the perioperative team when the ESU is activated.[2,18]

II.e. The ESU should be visually inspected and the return electrode monitor tested according to manufacturer's instructions before use.[19,20]

The ESU will sound an alarm and not activate if the dispersive electrode is disconnected.[2,20]

II.f. Settings should be based on the operator's preference consistent with the intended application and the manufacturer's written instructions for patient size, active electrode type, and return electrode placement.

The ESU's power output capability is dependent on multiple variables related to the patient, generator, accessories, and the procedure.

II.f.1. The circulating nurse should confirm the power settings with the operator before activation of the ESU.

II.f.2. The ESU should be operated at the lowest effective power setting needed to achieve the desired tissue effect.[2,18,20-22]

The likelihood of arcing and capacitive coupling are increased when higher than necessary voltages are used.[22]

II.f.3. If the operator requests a continual increase in power, personnel should check the entire ESU and accessories circuit for adequate placement of the dispersive electrode and cord connections.[18,19,23]

Prolonged current at high power can cause patient injury. Common causes of ineffective coagulation and cutting are high impedance at the dispersive electrode, poor contact between the dispersive electrode and the patient, and use of an electrolytic irrigation/distention solution.[23,24]

II.f.4. The electrode tip should be visually inspected before each use and replaced if damaged.

A damaged active electrode tip may cause a buildup of eschar, creating increased resistance at the electrode tip. Cleaning a stainless steel tip with an abrasive pad or instrument may create grooves where eschar can collect.[22]

II.g. Perioperative registered nurses should be aware of potential patient safety hazards associated with specific internal implanted electronic devices (IEDs) and the appropriate patient care interventions required to protect the patient from injury.[25]

Electronic devices implanted in a patient may be affected by other IEDs or medical equipment with which a patient may come into contact in a health care facility. These devices may include cardiac pacemakers, implanted cardioverter defibrillators (ICDs), neurostimulators, implantable hearing devices, implantable infusion pumps, and osteogenic stimulators.[25]

II.h. After use, personnel should
- turn off the ESU;
- dispose of single use items;
- clean all reusable parts and accessories according to the manufacturer's directions; and
- inspect accessories and parts for damage, function, and cleanliness.

Following the manufacturer's cleaning and inspection instructions promotes safe and proper functioning of the equipment.

II.i. An ESU that is not working properly or is damaged should be removed from service immediately and reported to the designated individual responsible for equipment maintenance (eg, bioengineering services personnel).[18,19,26]

Medical device users are required to report serious injury and death related to use of a device to the Federal Drug Administration (FDA).[26]

Recommendation III

The electrical cords and plugs of the ESU should be handled in a manner that minimizes the potential for damage and subsequent patient and user injuries.

Improper handling of cords and plugs may result in breaks in the cord's insulation, fraying, and other electrical hazards.

III.a. The ESU's electrical cord should be adequate in length and flexibility to reach the electrical outlet without stress or the use of an extension cord.[19]

Tension on the electrical cord increases the risk that it will become disconnected, frayed, or move the equipment, which may result in injuries to patients and personnel.

III.a.1. The ESU should be placed near the sterile field, and the cord should reach the wall or column outlet without stress on the cord and without blocking a traffic path.[19]

Stress on the cord may cause damage to the cord, posing an electrical hazard.

III.a.2. The electrical cord should be free of kinks, knots, and bends.

Kinks, knots, and bends could damage the cord or cause leakage, current accumulation, and overheating of the cord's insulation.

III.a.3. The ESU plug, not the cord, should be held when it is removed from the outlet.

Pulling on the cord may cause cord breakage, which poses a fire hazard.

III.a.4. The ESU's cord should be kept dry.[19]

Fluids in or around the ESU connections and cord may cause an electrical hazard as a result of a short circuit.

III.b. The ESU's cord should be inspected or electrically tested for outer insulation damage.[19]

Cord failures can result in a fire or patient and personnel injuries.

III.b.1. The ESU should be removed from use if there is any evidence of breaks, nicks, or cracks in the outer insulation coating of the electrical cord.[19]

Recommendation IV

The active electrode should be used in a manner that minimizes the potential for injuries.

Incomplete circuitry, unintentional activation, and incompatibility of the active electrode to the ESU may result in patient and personnel injuries.[16,27]

IV.a. The active electrode should be visually inspected at the surgical field before use. Inspection should include but is not limited to

– identifying any apparent damage to the cord or hand piece (eg, impaired insulation),[19] and

– ensuring compatibility of the active electrode, accessories, the ESU, and the procedure.

Insulation failures allow an alternate pathway for current to leave the electrode and may result in an electrical shock or other injury.

IV.a.1. A damaged and/or incompatible active electrode, accessory, or ESU should be immediately removed from use.

IV.b. When not in use, the active electrode should be placed in a clean, dry, non-conductive safety holster.[2,15,22,28] A plastic or other non-conductive device should be used to secure the active electrode cord to the sterile drapes.[22]

Use of a non-conductive safety holster prevents the active electrode from falling off the sterile field and unintentional activation. Unintentional activation of the active electrode may cause burns of the patient, drapes, or personnel.[2,15]

IV.b.1. The protective cap of a battery-powered, hand-held cautery should be in place when the cautery is not in use.[29,30]

Application of the protective cap prevents unintended pressure on the activation button.[29,30]

IV.c. The electrode cord should be kept free of kinks and coils during use.

Kinks, knots, and bends could damage the cord, cause current leakage or accumulation, overheat the cord's insulation, or produce unanticipated changes in the surgical effect. "Hot spots" or field intensification are produced by coiling cables. Keeping the cords free of kinks and coils minimizes the risk of patient or personnel injury from conduction of stray current and capacitive current.[21]

IV.d. The active electrode should be connected directly into a designated receptacle on the ESU.

Incompatibility of the active electrode with the ESU may result in patient and personnel injuries.

IV.d.1. When needed, only adaptors approved by the manufacturers of both the ESU and the accessory should be used.

IV.e. Only the user of the active electrode should activate the device whether it is hand or foot controlled.[20,28]

Activation by the user of the active electrode prevents unintentional discharge of the device to minimize potential for patient and personnel injury.

IV.f. Active electrode tips should be used according to the manufacturer's instructions.

Failure to use the active electrode as outlined in the manufacturer's directions for use have resulted in patient injuries and surgical fires.[31-34]

IV.f.1. The active electrode tip
- should be compatible with the ESU,
- should be securely seated into the hand piece, and
- should not be altered.[34]

A loose electrode tip may cause a spark or burn tissue that comes in contact with the exposed, non-insulated section of the tip.[31,34] Bending the tip can damage the device and alter the desired function. Fires and patient injuries have resulted when insulating sheaths have been made from inappropriate material (eg, rubber catheters).[32,33]

IV.g. The active electrode tip should be cleaned away from the incision whenever there is visible eschar.[32]

Eschar buildup on the active electrode tip impedes the desired current flow, causing the entire unit to function less effectively and serving as a fuel source, which can lead to fires.[32] Debris on the electrode tip can tear tissue, cause re-bleeding, and serve as a foreign body when deposited in the wound.[22]

IV.g.1. Methods to remove debris from the active electrode tip should include but are not limited to
- a moistened sponge or instrument wipe to clean non-stick coated electrosurgical tips on the sterile field,[16,32] and
- abrasive electrode cleaning pads to remove eschar from non-coated electrodes on the sterile field.[32]

IV.g.2. The active electrode tip should not be cleaned with a scalpel blade.

Cleaning with a scalpel blade puts perioperative personnel at risk for a percutaneous injury.[35]

IV.h. If the active electrode becomes contaminated, it should be disconnected from the ESU and removed from the sterile field.

Disconnection of the contaminated active electrode minimizes the risk of unintentional activation and reduces the potential for patient and personnel injuries.[16]

IV.i. If an active monopolar electrode is being used in a fluid-filled cavity, the fluid used should be an electrically inert, near isotonic solution (eg, dextran 10, dextran 70, glycine 1.5%, sorbitol, mannitol) unless the equipment manufacturer's written directions for use instruct otherwise.[2,24]

Using an electrolyte solution instead of a nonconductive medium may render the active electrode less effective. Electrolyte solutions conduct and disperse the electrical current away from the intended site.[18,24]

IV.j. Fire safety measures should be followed when electrosurgery is in use according to local, state, and federal regulations.[36,37]

IV.j.1. Active electrodes should not be activated in the presence of flammable agents (eg, antimicrobial skin prep or hand antisepsis agents, tinctures, de-fatting agents, collodion, petroleum-based lubricants, phenol, aerosol adhesives, uncured methyl methacrylate) until the agents are dry and vapors have dissipated.[2,38-42]

Alcohol-based prep agents remain flammable until completely dry. Vapors occurring during evaporation also are flammable. Trapping of solution or vapors under incise or surgical drapes increases the risk of fire or burn injury. Alcohol-based skin prep agents are particularly hazardous because the surrounding hair or fabric can become saturated. Pooling can occur in body folds and crevices (eg, umbilicus, sternal notch). Ignition of flammable substances by active electrodes has caused fires and patient injuries. Flammable prep agents can be safely used by adhering to NFPA

standards, local fire codes, and AORN recommendations and guidance statements. Use of nonflammable prep agents will minimize this risk.[16,42-46]

IV.j.2. Caution should be used during surgery on the head and neck when using an active electrode in the presence of combustible anesthetic gases.[2,44,47]

IV.j.3. Opened suture packets containing alcohol should be removed from the sterile field as soon as possible.[16]

Ignition of flammable substances by an active electrode has caused fires and patient injuries.[16,43]

IV.k. Sponges used near the active electrode tip should be moist to prevent unintentional ignition.[32,47,48]

Fires have resulted from ignition of dry sponges near the incision site.[16,49,50]

IV.l. When battery-powered, hand-held cautery units are used, the batteries should be removed before disposal of the cautery unit.[30]

Unintentional activation of a battery-powered, hand-held cautery unit after disposal has caused fires.[29,30]

IV.m. Electrosurgery should not be used in the presence of gastrointestinal gases.

Gastrointestinal gases contain hydrogen and methane, which are highly flammable. Fires and patient injuries have occurred.[16,28,40,51,52]

IV.n. Electrosurgery should not be used in an oxygen-enriched environment.[28,32,53-55]

An oxygen-enriched environment lowers the temperature and energy at which fuels will ignite.[28,48] Fires, including airway fires, have resulted from the active electrode sparking in the presence of concentrated oxygen.[2,16,53,54]

IV.n.1. The lowest possible oxygen concentration that provides adequate patient oxygen saturation should be used.[47,48]

Mixing oxygen with nonflammable gases such as medical air reduces the risk of fire.[16,47]

IV.n.2. Surgical drapes should be arranged to minimize the buildup of oxidizers (eg, oxygen and nitrous oxide) under the drapes, to allow air circulation, and to dilute the additional oxygen.[16,47,48]

IV.n.3. The active electrode should be used as far from the oxygen source as possible.

IV.o. Personnel should be prepared to immediately extinguish flames should they occur.[16,47]

A small fire can progress to a life threatening emergency of a large fire in seconds.[16] ESUs are a potential ignition source and a common cause of surgical fires and patient injury.[28]

IV.o.1. Nonflammable material (eg, wet towel, sterile saline, water) should be available on the sterile field to extinguish the fire.[16,28]

Recommendation V

When monopolar electrosurgery is used, a dispersive electrode should be used in a manner that minimizes the potential for injuries.

Patient skin injuries at the dispersive electrode site are the most reported ESU incidents.[2] Single use dispersive electrode burns are decreasing with improved technology and the use of safety features. The reports of electrosurgical burns has decreased from 50 to 100 per month in the 1970s to one to two per month in 2007.[2]

V.a. The patient's skin condition should be assessed and documented before and after ESU use.

The most frequently reported patient injury from electrosurgery has been tissue damage (eg, burn) at the dispersive electrode site.[2] Preoperative and postoperative assessments are necessary to evaluate the patient's skin condition for possible injuries.

V.b. Return-electrode contact quality monitoring should be furnished on general purpose electrosurgery units.[18]

The technology of return-electrode contact quality monitoring inhibits the output of the ESU if the return electrode is not in contact with the patient and connected to the ESU. Return-electrode contact quality monitoring confirms that there is adequate contact between the return electrode and the patient. An audible alarm and visual indicator signals the user of a misconnection.[2,18]

V.b.1. Dual-foil return electrodes should be used.[18]

Dual-foil return electrodes are necessary for contact quality monitoring.[18] The return electrode contact quality monitoring system determines differences in impedance through patient's tissue between the two surfaces. If the impedance is too high as a result of poor contact, the alarm is triggered and the ESU stops functioning.[2]

V.c. Return-electrode continuity monitoring should be used if return-electrode contact quality monitoring is not available.

Return-electrode continuity monitoring detects breaks in the return-electrode cord or a misconnection (ie, the cord is not plugged into the ESU).[2,19]

V.c.1. If using return-electrode continuity monitoring, a single-foil electrode should be used.[2]

V.d. Dispersive electrodes should be compatible with the ESU.

Incompatibility of the electrosurgical unit and the dispersive electrode may result in patient injury.

V.e. A single-use dispersive electrode should be used once and discarded. If a single-use dispersive electrode must be repositioned, a new single-use electrode should be used.[23,56]

A reused single-use electrode may not adhere properly to the skin. Replacing the dispersive electrode provides an opportunity to examine the electrode and the patient's skin condition.

V.f. Dispersive electrodes should be an appropriate size for the patient (eg, neonate, infant, pediatric, adult) and not altered (eg, cut, folded).

Using the appropriately sized dispersive electrode reduces the concentration of current and minimizes the potential for electrosurgical injuries.

V.g. Before the application of a single-use dispersive electrode
- the manufacturer's expiration date should be verified and the dispersive electrode

should not be used if it is past the manufacturer's expiration date;[20]

- the package containing the dispersive electrode should be opened immediately before use;[19] and

- the integrity of the dispersive electrode should be checked for flaws, damage, discoloration, adhesiveness, and dryness.[18,20,23,57]

Expired, damaged, or dry single-use dispersive electrodes may fail and lead to patient injury.

V.h. The conductive and adhesive surfaces of the single-use dispersive electrode should be placed on clean, dry skin over a large, well-perfused muscle mass on the surgical side and as close as possible to the surgical site according to the manufacturer's directions for use.[19,20]

Muscle is a better conductor of electricity than adipose tissue.[23]

V.h.1. Single-use electrodes should not be placed over bony prominences, scar tissue, hair, weight-bearing surfaces, potential pressure points, or areas distal to tourniquets.[5,18,19,23,58]

Fatty tissue, tissue over bone, scar tissue, and hair can impede electrosurgical return current flow.[59] High impedance leads to heating of the tissue, arcing to the tissue under the dispersive electrode, and subsequent burns. Adequate tissue perfusion cannot be assured if the dispersive electrode is placed distal to tourniquets or over scar tissue.[23]

V.h.2. Hair should be removed following recommended practices (ie, clipping) if it interferes with single-use electrode contact with the patient's skin.[18,20,60]

Burns have resulted when electrodes have been positioned over hairy surfaces. Hair can impede electrosurgical return current flow. Hair may interfere with adequate contact between the patient and the dispersive electrode.[23,58,61]

V.h.3. The single-use electrode should not be placed over an implanted metal prosthesis.

The tissue over prostheses contains scar tissue, which impedes return of the electric current. Although there has

been no reported injury from superheating of the implant causing a tissue burn, this is a theoretical risk; therefore, it is prudent to avoid placing a dispersive electrode on the patient's skin over the site of a metal implant or prosthesis.

V.h.4. Placing the single-use dispersive electrode over a tattoo, many of which contain metallic dyes, should be avoided.

Although there have been no reported electrosurgery injuries from dispersive electrodes placed over tattoos, superheating of the tissue has occurred during magnetic resonance imaging. There is a theoretical possibility of this also happening with electrosurgery.[62-64]

V.i. Following application of the single-use dispersive electrode, uniform contact with the skin should be verified.

Injuries have been associated with inadequate adhesion of the dispersive electrode. Potential problems include tenting, gaping, and moisture, all of which interfere with adhesion to the patient's skin.[65-67]

V.i.1. Corrective measures for poor single-use dispersive electrode contact include, but are not limited to

• removing oil, lotion, moisture, or prep solution;

• removing excessive hair;

• changing sites; and

• applying a new pad.

V.i.2. Tape should not be used to hold the single-use dispersive electrode in place.

Taping the dispersive electrode may create localized pressure and increase the current concentration leading to a potential injury.[68]

V.j. The single-use dispersive electrode should be placed on the patient after final positioning.

Moving the patient after the application of the dispersive electrode may disrupt the contact to the patient's skin causing tenting, gaping, or moisture collection under the electrode. Injuries have been associated with inadequate contact of the dispersive electrode.[19,65-67]

V.j.1. If any tension is applied to the dispersive electrode cord, the perioperative registered nurse should reassess the integrity of the dispersive electrode, its contact with the patient's skin, and the connection to the ESU.

V.j.2. If the patient is repositioned, the perioperative registered nurse should verify that the dispersive electrode is in full contact with the patient's skin.

Inadequate contact of the dispersive electrode may result in a burn.[65-67]

V.k. The single-use dispersive electrode should be placed away from a warming device.[65,67]

The heat of a warming device may be cumulative with the heating of the dispersive electrode and may affect how the dispersive electrode adheres to the skin.[65,67]

V.l. Dispersive electrodes should be kept dry and protected from fluids seeping or pooling under the electrode.[23]

Liquids may prevent the electrode from adequately contacting the skin. These solutions also can cause skin injury and burns from prolonged skin exposure and concentration of electrical current.[57]

V.m. Contact between the patient and metal devices should be avoided.[69,70]

Metal devices (eg, OR beds, stirrups, positioning devices, safety strap buckles) could offer a potential alternate return path for the electrical current.[69,70]

V.m.1. Patient's metal jewelry that is between the active and dispersive electrode should be removed.

Metallic jewelry, including body piercings, presents a potential risk of burn from directed current (ie, active electrode contact); heat conducted before an electrode cools; and leakage current. Eliminating metal near the activation site minimizes this risk. Jewelry that is left in place, particularly on the hands, has the potential to cause swelling at the site during surgery or recovery.[15]

V.m.2. Patient monitoring electrodes (eg, electrocardiogram, oximetry, fetal) should be placed as far away from the surgical site as possible.[21]

Alternate pathway burns have been reported at electrocardiogram (ECG) electrode sites and temperature probe entry sites with ground-referenced electrosurgery units.[19]

V.m.3. Needle electrodes for monitoring or nonsurgical functions should be avoided.[18,21]

Stray current may flow through the small contact area of the needle electrode causing a potential alternate pathway and risk of patient burn.[18,21,71,72]

V.m.4. When use of needle monitoring electrodes is medically necessary, alternate electrosurgery technologies (eg, bipolar, laser) should be considered.[18,73]

V.n. When multiple ESUs are used simultaneously during a surgical procedure, the compatibility of equipment and proper functioning of corresponding electrode monitoring systems should be verified with the manufacturer.

V.n.1. Separate single-use dispersive electrodes should be used for each ESU.

V.n.2. The dispersive electrodes should be placed as close as possible to their respective surgical sites and the single-use dispersive electrodes should not overlap.

V.o. During high-current, long-activation-time, radio-frequency (RF) ablations and other electrosurgical procedures (eg, tumor ablation, bulk tissue resection), considerations should include, but not be limited to
- identifying surgical procedures that require the use of high-current, long-activation-time RF ablation and electrosurgical techniques;
- taking inventory of RF generators that require special or multiple dispersive electrodes;
- following the manufacturer's recommendations for use of large-size dispersive electrodes or multiple dispersive electrodes;
- ensuring proper placement and full patient contact of the dispersive electrode;
- reviewing the manufacturer's directions for use and requirements for accessories;
- using and selecting the appropriate nonconductive, near-isotonic solution (eg, sorbitol, mannitol, dextran 10 or 70,

glycine) for irrigation or distention unless contraindicated by manufacturer's directions; and

- using the lowest possible power settings and minimum activation time for obtaining the desired tissue effect.[2,24,74]

There is an increased risk of dispersive electrode site burns with high-current, long-activation-time procedures.[2,61,74-76]

V.o.1. When high current is not adequately dispersed by a single dispersive electrode and there are no specific manufacturer's directions, a second dispersive electrode with an adaptor or a return electrode with a larger conductive surface may be considered for use.[24,74]

A second dispersive electrode or a larger conductive surface increases the overall dispersive pad surface area for current to return to the generator.[74]

V.p. When removing the single-use dispersive electrode, the adjacent skin should be held in place and the dispersive electrode peeled back slowly.

Slowly removing the dispersive electrode will avoid denuding the surface of the skin. Skin injuries can result when the adhesive border pulls on the skin during electrode removal.[77]

V.q. Reusable, capacitive-coupled return electrode systems should be used according to manufacturers' written instructions for safe operation in conjunction with a compatible ESU.

V.q.1. Capacitive-coupling pads should be an appropriate size for the patient (ie, adult, pediatric).[78,79]

V.q.2. Skin preparation should not be performed unless otherwise recommended by the manufacturer's written directions.[78]

V.q.3. Adequate contact with the patient should be ensured by using minimal materials between the capacitive-coupled pad and patient.[79] The use of thick foam, gel pads, and extra linen between the patient and the capacitive-coupling pad should be avoided.

Distance and barriers (eg, positioning devices) between the patient and

electrode may increase the risk of impedance, which can result in an alternate site injury when using a capacitive-coupling pad.[78]

V.q.4. An isolated generator should be used.[78]

Use of a ground-referenced or grounded generators may cause a ground fault alarm.

V.q.5. The pad should be cleaned with the health care facility-approved and EPA-registered agent if contaminated with blood or body fluids in accordance with the manufacturer's directions. Acceptable cleaning solutions include a bleach solution diluted 1:10 and o-phenylphenol, o-benzyl-p-chlorophenol, or p-tertiary amylphenol.[78]

V.q.6. The integrity of the capacitive-coupled pad and cables should be checked for tears or breaks in the surface material before use, and

- pad cables should be replaced if damaged,
- surface damage may be repaired with the manufacturer's repair kit, and
- the pad should be replaced if superficial damage cannot be repaired.

V.q.7. When two ESUs are used, two capacitive-coupled pads or one capacitive-coupled pad with two cords should be used.

V.q.8. The pad should be replaced on its labeled expiration date.[78]

Recommendation VI

Personnel should take additional precautions when using electrosurgery during minimally invasive surgery.[18,80]

Minimally invasive surgery procedures using electrosurgery present unique patient safety risks, such as direct coupling of current, insulation failure, and capacitive coupling.

VI.a. Personnel should verify that the insufflation gas is nonflammable (ie, carbon dioxide).[81]

Carbon dioxide is noncombustible and will not ignite if the active electrosurgical electrode sparks.[81] Gases (eg, oxygen, nitrous oxide, air) are oxidizers that may support combustion. An oxidizer-enriched environment may enhance ignition and combustion.[28]

VI.b. Conductive trocar systems should be used.[7,8,11,82]

Conductive trocar cannulas provide a means for the electrosurgical current to flow safely between the cannula and the abdominal wall. This reduces high density current concentration and heating of non-target tissue.[7,8,11,82]

VI.b.1. Hybrid trocar (ie, combination plastic and metal) systems should not be used.[8,82,83]

Each trocar and cannula can act as an electrical conductor inducing an electrical current from one to the other potentially causing a capacitive coupling injury.

VI.c. Minimally invasive surgery electrodes should be examined for impaired insulation before use.[11,83-85]

Insulation failure of electrodes caused by damage during use or reprocessing provides an alternate pathway for the electrical current to leave the active electrode. Some insulation failures are not visible. This has resulted in serious patient injuries.[4,7,8,11-13,85]

VI.c.1. Methods should be used to detect insulation failure, including but not limited to
- active electrode shielding and monitoring,[11,14]
- the use of active electrode indicator shafts that have two layers of insulation of different colors,[11] and
- the use of active electrode insulation integrity testers that use high DC voltage to detect full thickness insulation breaks.[11]

Active electrode shielding continuously monitors the endoscopic instruments to minimize the risks of insulation failure or capacitive-coupling injuries.[4,7-9,12-14,83]

The inner layer of the active electrode shaft of a different color is designed to show through the outer black layer if there is an insulation break.[11]

Testing of the electrode before the procedure identifies damaged electrodes that should be taken out of service. Testing of the electrode with the sterilizable probes and cables alerts the surgeon of an insulation break. The surgical field can be explored and treated if necessary.[11,85]

VI.c.2. The lowest power setting that achieves the desired result should be selected.[83]

Lower power settings for both cut and coagulation reduce the likelihood of insulation failure and capacitive-coupling injuries. Lower power settings also minimize damage from direct coupling when the active electrode is activated while in close proximity to another metal device inserted into an adjacent trocar port.[7]

VI.d. The active electrode should not be activated until it is in close proximity to the tissue.[7,8]

Activation only when in close proximity to the tissue minimizes the risk of current arcing and contacting unintended tissue.[7,8] Activating the electrode when it is not in very close proximity to the targeted tissue increases the risk of capacitive coupling. Capacitance is reduced during closed-circuit activation.

VI.e. Patients should be instructed to immediately report any postoperative signs or symptoms of electrosurgical injury. Patient postoperative care instructions should include symptoms to look for, including but not limited to
- fever,
- inability to void,
- lower gastrointestinal bleeding,
- abdominal pain,
- abdominal distention,
- nausea,
- vomiting, and
- diarrhea.[8,86]

Symptoms of a minimally invasive electrosurgical injury can occur days after discharge from the perioperative setting and may include infection from an injured intestinal tract. Prompt reporting of electrosurgical injury symptoms ensures timely treatment and minimizes adverse outcomes.[8,84]

Recommendation VII

Bipolar active electrodes, including vessel occluding devices, should be used in a manner that minimizes the potential for injuries.

Unlike the monopolar ESU, bipolar technology incorporates an active electrode and a return electrode into a two-poled instrument, such as forceps or scissors.[6,19,53] Current flows only through the tissue contacted between two poles of the instruments; thus, the need for a dispersive electrode is eliminated.[19] This also eliminates the chance of stray or alternate pathways for current flow.[19] The bipolar ESU provides precise hemostasis or dissection at the surgical site with less potential stimulation or current spread to nearby body structures.[19]

VII.a. Molded, fixed-position pin placement bipolar cords should be used. Bipolar and monopolar plugs should be differentiated to prevent misconnections of active and return electrodes.[1,27]

Connection of a bipolar active electrode to a monopolar receptacle may activate current, causing a short circuit.

Recommendation VIII

Ultrasonic electrosurgical devices should be used in a manner that minimizes potential for injuries.

Ultrasonic devices have a generator that produces ultrasonic energy and mechanical vibrations rather than electrical energy. Ultrasonic instruments cut and coagulate by using the mechanical energy and heat that is generated to cause protein denaturation and the formation of a coagulum. A blade or probe can be used for sharp or blunt dissection, coagulation, or breaking apart of tissue without damaging adjacent tissues. Some ultrasonic dissectors incorporate an aspirator to remove tissue or fluids from the surgical field.[83,87]

VIII.a. When using an ultrasonic electrosurgical device, a dispersive electrode should not be used.

With an ultrasonic electrosurgical device, no electrical current enters the tissue; therefore, the current does not need to be returned to the generator by a dispersive electrode.[83,87]

VIII.b. Inhalation of aerosols generated by an ultrasonic electrosurgical hand piece should be minimized by implementing control measures, including but not limited to smoke evacuation systems and wall suction with an in-line ultra low penetration air (ULPA) filter.

Bio-aerosols are routinely produced by ultrasonic devices and pose a hazard to patients and perioperative professionals.

Bio-aerosols contain odorless, toxic gases; vapors; dead and live cellular debris, including blood fragments; and viruses. These airborne contaminants can pose respiratory, ocular, dermatological, and other health-related risks, including mutagenic and carcinogenic potential, to patients and OR personnel. Wall suction with an in-line ULPA filter is only appropriate for a minimal amount of aerosol (ie, aerosols generated using ultrasonic electrosurgery are within the respirable range and include blood, blood by-products, and tissue).[88]

Recommendation IX

Argon enhanced coagulation (AEC) technology poses unique risks to patient and personnel safety and should be used in a manner that minimizes the potential for injury.

Each type of AEC has specific manufacturer's written operating instructions to be followed for safe operation of the unit.

IX.a. All safety measures for monopolar electrosurgery should be used when using AEC technology.

The AEC unit uses monopolar alternating current delivered to the tissue through ionized argon gas.[89] The risks of monopolar electrosurgery are present.

IX.b. Air should be purged from the argon gas line and electrode by activating the system before use, after moderate delays between activations, and between uses.[2,89,90]

Purging the argon gas line prevents delays in coagulation, minimizing the risk of gas embolism.[89] Activating without adequately purging may present the greatest risk of embolism when operating in an open cavity.[89]

IX.c. The argon gas flow should be limited to the lowest level possible that will provide the desired clinical effect.[2,90]

Argon gas flow is most likely to be directed to tissue without simultaneous coagulation when the initiation of ionization of the argon gas is delayed due to air bubbles in the argon gas line.[89]

IX.d. The active electrode should not be placed in direct contact with tissue and should be moved away from the patient's tissue after each activation.[89,90]

There is a risk of gas emboli when the active electrode is placed in direct contact with tissue. If argon gas pressure exceeds venous pressure in the circulating system and is applied to bleeding vessels, the result is a gas emboli in open surgical procedures.[2,90,91] The flow of argon gas could enter the open vessel and enter the heart.[2]

IX.e. When using the AEC unit during minimally invasive surgical procedures, personnel should follow all safety measures identified for AEC technology.

Patient injury and death have occurred as a complication of argon enhanced technology.[90]

IX.e.1. Endoscopic CO_2 insufflators should be equipped with audible and visual over-pressurization alarms that cannot be deactivated.[2,90]

The AEC acts as a secondary source of pressurized argon gas that can cause the patient's intra-abdominal pressure to rise rapidly and exceed venous pressure, possibly creating argon-enriched gas emboli formation. This has resulted in gas emboli.[90]

IX.e.2. The active electrode and argon gas line should be purged according to the manufacturer's recommendations.[2,90]

IX.e.3. The patient's intra-abdominal cavity should be flushed with several liters of CO_2 between extended activation periods.[90]

Flushing the intra-abdominal cavity with several liters of CO_2 between extended periods of deactivation reduces the potential for argon gas emboli formation.[90]

IX.f. Personnel using the AEC technology should be knowledgeable about signs, symptoms, and treatment of venous emboli.

There is a significant risk of gas embolism when AEC is used during laparoscopic procedures from abdominal over-pressurization and displacement of CO_2 by argon gas.[90]

IX.f.1. Patient monitoring should include devices that are considered effective for early detection of gas emboli (eg, end-tidal CO_2).[2,90]

Recommendation X

Potential hazards associated with surgical smoke generated in the practice setting should be identified, and safe practices established.

Surgical smoke (ie, plume) is generated from use of heat-producing instruments such as electrosurgical devices. Airborne contaminants produced during electrosurgery have been analyzed. The electrosurgery plume contains toxic gas and vapors (eg, benzene, hydrogen cyanide, formaldehyde); bioaerosols; dead and living cell material, including blood fragments; and viruses.[92-94] Many additional hazardous chemical compounds have been noted in surgical smoke.[92,95-98]

At some level, these contaminants have been shown to have an unpleasant odor, cause problems with visibility of the surgical site, cause ocular and upper respiratory tract irritation, and demonstrate mutagenic and carcinogenic potential.[92,93,99] The possibility for bacterial and/or viral contamination of smoke plume remains controversial, but has been highlighted by different studies.[100,101]

The National Institute of Occupational Safety and Health (NIOSH) recommends that smoke evacuation systems be used to reduce potential acute and chronic health risks to personnel and patients.[92] The Occupational Safety and Health Administration (OSHA) has no separate standard related to surgical smoke. OSHA addresses such safety hazards in the General Duty Clause and Bloodborne Pathogens Standard.[97]

X.a. Surgical smoke should be removed by use of a smoke evacuation system in both open and laparoscopic procedures.

Potential health and liability risks may be reduced by the evacuation of smoke plume.[93]

X.a.1. When large amounts of plume are generated, an individual smoke evacuation unit with a ULPA filter should be used to remove surgical smoke.

X.a.2. The suction wand of the smoke evacuation system should be no greater than two inches (5.08 cm) from the source of the smoke generation.[92,93]

Close proximity of the smoke evacuation wand maximizes particulate matter and odor capture and enhances visibility at the surgical site.[99]

X.a.3. Smoke evacuation units and accessories should be used according to manufacturers' written instructions.

Detectable odor during the use of a smoke evacuation system is a signal that
- smoke is not being captured at the site where the plume is being generated,
- inefficient air movement through the suction or smoke evacuation wand is occurring, or
- the filter has exceeded its usefulness and should be replaced.[93]

X.a.4. When a minimal amount of plume is generated, a central suction system with an in-line ULPA filter may be used to evacuate the plume.[92] The in-line filter should be placed between the suction wall/ceiling connection and the suction canister.[99]

Central suction units are designed to capture liquids and should not be used without an in-line ULPA filter to remove airborne contaminants.[92] Low suction rates associated with centralized suction units limit their efficiency in evacuating plume, making them suitable only for the evacuation of small amounts of plume.[94]

X.a.5. When a centralized system dedicated for smoke evacuation is available, the smoke evacuator lines should be flushed according to the manufacturer's instructions to ensure particulate matter buildup does not occur.

Plume particulate can accumulate in the lumens of the centralized system causing decreased suction capability and potential pathogen growth.

X.b. Used smoke evacuator filters, tubing, and wands should be disposed of as potentially infectious waste following standard precautions.[93,99]

Airborne contaminants produced during electrosurgery or laser procedures have been analyzed and are shown to contain gaseous toxic compounds, bio-aerosols, and dead and living cell material. At some level, these contaminants have been shown to have an unpleasant odor, cause visual problems for physicians, cause ocular and upper respiratory tract irritation, and demonstrate mutagenic and carcinogenic potential.[99] The possibility for bacterial and/or viral contamination of smoke plume remains controversial but has been highlighted by different studies.[100,101]

X.c. Personnel should wear high-filtration surgical masks during procedures that generate surgical smoke.

High-filtration masks are specifically designed to filter particulate matter that is 0.1 micron in size and larger which may protect against residual plume in the air that has escaped smoke evacuation capture.[95] These masks should not be viewed as absolute protection from chemical or particulate contaminants found in surgical smoke and should not be used as the first line of protection against surgical smoke inhalation.[95,99]

Recommendation XI

Personnel should receive initial education and competency validation on procedures and should receive additional training when new equipment, instruments, supplies, or procedures are introduced.

Initial education on the underlying principles of electrosurgical safety provides direction for personnel in providing a safe environment. Additional, periodic educational programs provide reinforcement of principles of electrosurgery and new information on changes in technology, its application, compatibility of equipment and accessories, and potential hazards.

Electrosurgical equipment and accessories have been associated with numerous fires and patient injuries.[2,8,19,53] The National Fire Protection Association has identified ESUs as high-risk equipment, warranting training and retraining of personnel.[19]

XI.a. Personnel working with electrosurgery equipment should be knowledgeable about the principles of electrosurgery, risks to patients and personnel, measures to minimize these risks, and corrective actions to employ in the event of a fire or injury.[19]

Electrosurgical equipment and accessories have been associated with numerous fires and patient injuries.[2,8]

XI.b. Personnel should be instructed on the proper operation, care, and handling of the ESU and accessories before use.[19]

Incorrect use can result in serious injury to patients and personnel.

XI.b.1.   If multiple types of electrosurgical equipment are used within the facility, training should be provided on all of the equipment.[18]

XI.c.   Personnel should be instructed in the risks of electrosurgery during minimally invasive surgical procedures.

Direct coupling is the result of touching the laparoscopic active electrode to another anatomic structure. This can cause necrosis of underlying tissue. Insulation failure of the laparoscopic electrode can be caused by trauma during use or reprocessing. Current leaves the electrode through this alternate pathway. This can cause serious patient injury, particularly when the injury is internal. Capacitive-coupled RF currents can cause undetected burns to nearby tissue and organs outside the endoscope's viewing field. Severe patient injuries have resulted.[8]

XI.d.   Perioperative registered nurses should be knowledgeable about the types of IEDs that may be encountered in the practice setting, and the precautions that must be taken when caring for patients with these devices.[25]

Electronic devices implanted in a patient may be affected by other IEDs or medical equipment with which a patient may come into contact in a health care facility.

XI.e.   Administrative personnel should assess and document annual competency of personnel in the safe use of the ESU and accessories.

A competency assessment provides a record that personnel have basic understanding of electrosurgery, its risks, and appropriate corrective actions to take in the event of a fire or injury. This knowledge is essential to minimize the risks of misuse of the equipment and to provide a safe environment of care.

Recommendation XII

Documentation should be completed to enable the identification of trends and demonstrate compliance with regulatory and accrediting agency requirements.

Documentation of all nursing activities performed is legally and professionally important for clear communication and collaboration between health care team members and for continuity of patient care.

XII.a.   Documentation using the PNDS should include a patient assessment, a plan of care, nursing diagnoses, identification of desired outcomes, interventions, and an evaluation of the patient's response to the care provided.

Documentation provides communication among all care providers involved in planning and implementing patient care.

XII.b.   Documentation should be recorded in a manner consistent with health care organization policies and procedures and should include, but is not limited to

- electrosurgical system identification serial number;[102]
- range of settings used;
- dispersive electrode placement;
- patient's skin condition before dispersive electrode placement;
- patient's skin condition after removal of dispersive electrode;[102]
- adjunct electrosurgical devices used (eg, ultrasonic scalpel, bipolar forceps); and
- safety holster use.[18]

Recommendation XIII

Policies and procedures for electrosurgery should be developed, reviewed periodically, revised as necessary, and readily available in the practice setting.

Policies and procedures assist in the development of patient safety, quality assessment, and improvement activities. Policies and procedures establish authority, responsibility, and accountability within the facility. They also serve as operational guidelines that are used to minimize patient risk factors, standardize practice, direct staff members, and establish guidelines for continuous performance improvement activities.

XIII.a.   The health care organization's policies and procedures for electrosurgery must be in compliance with the Safe Medical Devices Act of 1990, amended in March 2000.[26]

XIII.a.1.   When patient or personnel injuries or equipment failures occur, the ESU should be removed from service and the active and dispersive electrodes retained if possible.[102]

Retaining the ESU, the active and dispersive electrodes, and packaging allows for a complete systems check to determine electrosurgical system integrity.[102]

XIII.a.2. Incidents of patient or personnel electrical injury or equipment failure should be reported as required by regulation to federal, state, and local authorities and to the equipment manufacturer.[107] Device identification, maintenance and service information, as well as adverse event information should be included in the report from the practice setting.

Documentation of details of the electrosurgical equipment and supplies allows for retrievable information for investigation into an adverse event.[102]

XIII.b. Policies and procedures for electrosurgery should include, but are not limited to the following:
  – safety features required on ESUs;
  – equipment maintenance programs;
  – required supplemental safety monitors;
  – equipment checks before initial use;
  – reporting and impounding malfunctioning equipment;
  – reporting of injuries;
  – preoperative, intraoperative, and postoperative patient assessments;
  – precautions during use;
  – ESU sanitation; and
  – documentation.

XIII.c. An introduction and review of policies and procedures for electrosurgery should be included in orientation and ongoing education of personnel to assist in the development of knowledge, skills, and attitudes that affect surgical patient outcomes.

Review of policies and procedures assists health care professionals in the development of knowledge, skills, and attitudes that affect patient outcomes.

XIII.d. A written fire prevention and management policy and procedure should be developed by a multidisciplinary group that includes all categories of perioperative personnel.[18,36]

Fire is a risk to both patients and health care workers in the perioperative setting.

XIII.d.1. The policy and procedure should describe processes to be implemented to safely manage different fire scenarios.

Recommendation XIV

A quality assurance/performance improvement process should be in place that measures patient, process, and structural (eg, system) outcome indicators.

A fundamental precept of AORN is that it is the responsibility of professional perioperative registered nurses to ensure safe, high-quality nursing care to patients undergoing surgical and invasive procedures.[103]

XIV.a. Structure, process, and clinical outcomes performance measures should be identified that can be used to improve patient care and that also monitor compliance with facility policy and procedure, national standards, and regulatory requirements.[104]

XIV.a.1. Process indicators may include, but are not limited to information about adverse patient outcomes and near misses associated with electrosurgery, which should be collected, analyzed, and used for performance improvement.[103]

XIV.b. Electrosurgical devices should be tested before initial use, inspected periodically, and receive preventive maintenance by a designated individual responsible for equipment maintenance (eg, biomedical engineering services personnel).[19]

Periodic preventative maintenance ensures continued safe operation of electrosurgical devices.[19]

XIV.c. Each ESU should be assigned an identification or serial number.

This number allows designated personnel to track function problems and document maintenance performed on individual ESUs.

XIV.d. Each health care organization should be responsible for staying abreast of evolving technology that may impact patient care and safety.

Electrosurgical technology continues to evolve, changing the way in which surgical hemostasis is achieved.

Glossary

Active electrode: The electrosurgical unit (ESU) accessory that directs current flow to the surgical site (eg, pencils, various pencil tips).

Active electrode indicator shaft: An active electrode composed of two layers of insulated material of different colors. The inner layer is a bright color, the outer layer is black. When the bright colored inner layer is evident upon visual inspection, a break in the insulation is indicated.

Active electrode insulation testing: Devices designed to test the integrity of the insulation surrounding the conductive shaft of laparoscopic electrosurgical active-electrode instruments. The devices detect full thickness breaks in the insulation layer.

Active electrode monitoring: A dynamic process of searching for insulation failures and capacitive coupling during monopolar surgery. If the monitor detects an unsafe level of stray energy, it signals the generator to deactivate.

Alternate site injury: Patient injury caused by an electrosurgical device that occurs away from the dispersive electrode site.

Argon-enhanced coagulation: Radio frequency coagulation from an electrosurgical generator that is capable of delivering monopolar current through a flow of ionized argon gas.

Bioengineering services personnel: Those individuals in an institution who are trained and qualified to check, troubleshoot, and repair medical equipment.

Bipolar electrosurgery: Electrosurgery in which current flows between two tips of a bipolar forceps that are positioned around tissue to create a surgical effect. Current passes from the active electrode of one tip of the forceps through the patient's desired tissue to the other dispersive electrode tip of the forceps—thus completing the circuit without entering another part of the patient's body.

Capacitance: Ability of an electrical circuit to transfer an electrical charge from one conductor to another, even when separated by an insulator.

Capacitive coupling: Transfer of electrical current from the active electrode through intact insulation to adjacent conductive items (eg, tissue, trocars).

Capacitively coupled return electrode: A large, nonadhesive return electrode placed close to and forming a capacitor with the patient, returning electrical current from the patient back to the electrosurgical unit (ESU).

Current: A movement of electrons analogous to the flow of a stream of water.

Direct coupling: The contact of an energized active electrode tip with another metal instrument or object within the surgical field.

Dispersive electrode: The accessory that directs electrical current flow from the patient back to the electrosurgical generator—often called the patient plate, return electrode, inactive electrode, or grounding pad.

Dual foil electrode: A dispersive return electrode that has two foil conductive surfaces on a single nonconductive adhesive pad. The two foil surfaces are connected independently through the same return electrode cord to the ESU. The dual foil design allows the return electrode quality monitor to detect impedance differences between the conductive surfaces. If a difference is detected between the two foil surfaces, the ESU will alarm and shut down. Dual foil electrodes are a necessary component of return electrode quality monitoring.

Electrosurgery: The cutting and coagulation of body tissue with a high-frequency (ie, radio frequency) current.

Electrosurgical accessories: The active electrode with tip(s), dispersive electrode, adapters, and connectors to attach these devices to the electrosurgery generator.

Electrosurgical unit: The generator that produces a high-frequency current waveform that is delivered to tissues, the foot switch with cord (if applicable), the electrical plug, cord, and connections.

Endoscopic minimally invasive: Surgical techniques that use endoscopic approaches rather than dissection.

Eschar: Charred tissue residue.

Generator: The machine that produces radio frequency waves (eg, ESU, power unit).

Ground-referenced electrosurgical unit: A system in which electrical current is sent to the patient and follows the path of least resistance back to the ground. This technology, which no longer is manufactured, produces high-frequency, high-voltage current and sometimes is referred to as a "spark gap" unit.

Insulator: A material that does not conduct electricity.

Insulation failure: Damage to the insulation of the active electrode that provides an alternate pathway for the current to leave that electrode as it completes the circuit to the dispersive electrode.

Isolated electrosurgical unit: A system in which electrical current is sent to the patient and selectively returns and is grounded through the generator.

Monopolar electrosurgery: Electrosurgery in which only the active electrode is in the surgical wound, and the electrical current is directed through the patient's body, received by the dispersive pad, and transferred back to the generator, completing the monopolar circuit.

Oxygen-enriched environment: Atmosphere containing more than 21% oxygen, frequently occurring in the oropharynx, trachea, lower respiratory tract, and near the head and neck during administration of oxygen to the patient.

Return electrode continuity monitor: A safety feature of a single foil dispersive electrode that detects an unconnected dispersive electrode or a break in the return electrode cord.

Return-electrode contact quality monitoring: A dynamic monitoring circuit measuring impedance of the dispersive return electrode. If the dispersive electrode becomes compromised, the circuit inhibits the ESU's output.

Ultra low particulate air (ULPA): Theoretically, a ULPA filter can remove from the air 99.9999% of bacteria, dust, pollen, mold, and particles with a size of 120 nanometers or larger.

Ultrasonic scalpel: A cutting/coagulation device that converts electrical energy into mechanical energy, providing a rapid ultrasonic motion.

Vessel sealing device: Bipolar technology that fuses collagen and elastin in the vessel walls and permanently obliterates the lumen of the vessel.

REFERENCES

1. Association for the Advancement of Medical Instrumentation. *ANSI/AAMI HF18:2001. Electrosurgical Devices*. Arlington, VA: Association for the Advancement of Medical Instrumentation; 2001.

2. ECRI. Electrosurgery. Healthcare Risk Control Risk Analysis. 2007;4(Surgery and Anesthesia 16).

3. Electrosurgical units. *Health Devices*. 1998;27(3): 93-111.

4. Odell RC. Pearls, pitfalls, and advancements in the delivery of electrosurgical energy during laparoscopy. *Problems in General Surgery*. 2002;19(2):5-17.

5. Jones CM, Pierre KB, Nicoud IB, Stain SC, Melvin WV 3rd. Electrosurgery. *Curr Surg*. 2006;63(6):458-463.

6. ECRI. Laparoscopic electrosurgery risks. *Operating Room Risk Management*. 1999;2(Surgery 19):1-11.

7. Guidance section: ensuring monopolar electrosurgical safety during laparoscopy. *Health Devices*. 1995;24(1):20-26.

8. Wu MP, Ou CS, Chen SL, Yen EYT, Rowbotham R. Complications and recommended practices for electrosurgery in laparoscopy. *Am J Surg*. 2000/1;179(1):67-73.

9. Vilos GA, Newton DW, Odell RC, Abu-Rafea B, Vilos AG. Characterization and mitigation of stray radiofrequency currents during monopolar resectoscopic electrosurgery. *J Minim Invasive Gynecol*. 2006;13(2):134-140.

10. Physician Insurers Association of America. *Laparoscopic Injury Study*. Rockville, Md: Physician Insurers Association of America; 2000:1-5.

11. ECRI. Safety technologies for laparoscopic monopolar electrosurgery; devices for managing burn risks. *Health Devices*. 2005;34(8):259-272.

12. Evaluation of Electroscope Electroshield System. *Health Devices*. 1995;24(1):11-19.

13. Dennis V. Implementing active electrode monitoring: a perioperative call. *Ssm*. 2001;7(2):32, 34-38.

14. Harrell GJ, Kopps DR. Minimizing patient risk during laparoscopic electrosurgery. *AORN J*. 1998;67(6): 1194-1196.

15. Electrosurgery safety issues. PA-PSRS Patient Safety Advisory. 2006;3(1):1-3.

16. ECRI. The patient is on fire! A surgical fires primer. *http://www.mdsr.ecri.org/summary/detail.aspx?doc_id =8197*. Accessed November 4, 2009.

17. Burns and fires from electrosurgical active electrodes. *Health Devices*. 1993;22(8-9):421-422.

18. Electrosurgical safety: conducting a safety audit. *Health Devices*. 2005;34(12):414-420.

19. Annex D. The safe use of high-frequency electricity in health care facilities. In: *Health Care Facilities Handbook*. 10th ed. Quincy, MA: National Fire Protection Association; 2005.

20. ECRI Institute. Electrosurgery checklist. *Operating Room Risk Management*. 2007;2(Surgery 10).

21. De Marco M, Maggi S. Evaluation of stray radiofrequency radiation emitted by electrosurgical devices. *Phys Med Biol*. 2006;51(14):3347-3358.

22. Massarweh NN, Cosgriff N, Slakey DP. Electrosurgery: history, principles, and current and future uses. *J Am Coll Surg*. 2006;202(3):520-530.

23. ESU burns from poor dispersive electrode site preparation. *Health Devices*. 1993;22(8-9):422-423.

24. Skin burns resulting from the use of electrolytic distention/irrigation media during electrosurgery with a rollerablation electrode. *Health Devices*. 1998;27(6):233-235.

25. AORN guidance statement: Care of the perioperative patient with an implanted electronic device. In: *Perioperative Standards and Recommended Practices*. Denver, CO: AORN, Inc; 2009:207-228.

26. Food and Drug Administration. Medical device reporting: Manufacturer reporting, importer reporting, user facility reporting, distributor reporting. *Fed Regist*. 2000;65:4112-4121.

27. Misconnection of bipolar electrosurgical electrodes. *Health Devices*. 1995;24(1):34-35.

28. ECRI Institute. Surgical fire safety. *Health Devices*. 2006;35(2):45-46.

29. Center for Devices and Radiological Health. Manufacturer and User Facility Device Experience (MAUDE) Database Adverse Event Report 421908. Reported October 9, 2002. *http://www.accessdata.fda .gov/scripts/cdrh/cfdocs/cfMAUDE/Detail.CFM?MDR FOI__ID=421908*. Accessed November 4, 2009.

30. Fire caused by improper disposal of electrocautery units. *Health Devices*. 1994;23(3):98.

31. Alternate-site burns from improperly seated electrosurgical pencil active electrodes. *Health Devices*. 2000;29(1):24-27.

32. Ignition of debris on active electrosurgical electrodes. *Health Devices*. 1998;27(9-10):367-370.

33. Center for Devices and Radiological Health. Manufacturer and User Facility Device Experience (MAUDE) Database Adverse Event Report 393590. Reported May 7, 2002. *http://www.accessdata.fda.gov /scripts/cdrh/cfdocs/cfMAUDE/Detail.CFM?MDRFOI __ID=393590*. Accessed November 4, 2009.

34. ECRI Institute. Hazard report. Improperly seated electrosurgical active electrodes can burn patients. *Health Devices*. 2007;36(10):337-339.

35. AORN guidance statement: sharps injury prevention in the perioperative setting. In: *Perioperative Standards and Recommended Practices*. Denver, CO: AORN, Inc; 2009:275-280.

36. Recommended practices for a safe environment of care. In: *Perioperative Standards and Recommended Practices*. Denver, CO: AORN, Inc; 2009:415-437.

37. AORN guidance statement: fire prevention in the operating room. In: *Perioperative Standards and Recommended Practices*. Denver, CO: AORN, Inc; 2009: 195-203.

38. *NFPA 99 Standard for Health Care Facilities*. Quincy, MA: National Fire Protection Association; 2002: Issue C.13.1.3.2.2:182.

39. A clinician's guide to surgical fires. How they occur, how to prevent them, how to put them out. *Health Devices*. 2003;32(1):5-24.

40. Beesley J, Taylor L. Reducing the risk of surgical fires: are you assessing the risk? *J Perioper Pract*. 2006;16(12):591-597.

41. Tentative interim amendment. In: *NFPA 99 Standard for Health Care Facilities*. Quincy, MA: National Fire Protection Association; 2005: 13.4.1.2.2-A-13.4.1.2.2.3.

42. Fire hazard created by the misuse of DuraPrep solution. *Health Devices*. 1998;27(11):400-402.

43. Center for Devices and Radiological Health. Manufacturer and User Facility Device Experience (MAUDE) Database Adverse Event Report 32071. Reported July 31, 1995. *http://www.accessdata.fda.gov /scripts/cdrh/cfdocs/cfMAUDE/Detail.CFM?MDRFOI __ID=32071*. Accessed November 4, 2009.

44. Barker SJ, Polson JS. Fire in the operating room: a case report and laboratory study. *Anesth Analg*. 2001;93(4):960-965.

45. Position statement on fire prevention. *http://www .aorn.org/PracticeResources/AORNPositionStatements /Position_FirePrevention/*. Accessed November 4, 2009.

46. *Standard for Health Care Facilities Tentative Interim Amendment: Germicides and Antiseptics*. Quincy, MA: National Fire Protection Association; 2005.

47. A Report by the American Society of Anesthesiologists Task Force on Operating Room Fires. Practice Advisory for the Prevention and Management of Operating Room Fires. *Anesthesiology*. 2008;108(5):786-801.

48. ECRI Institute. Surgical fires. *Operating Room Risk Management*. 2006;2(Safety 1):1-18.

49. Center for Devices and Radiological Health. Manufacturer and User Facility Device Experience (MAUDE) Database Adverse Event Report 441523. Reported August 23, 2002. *http://www.accessdata.fda.gov/scripts/cdrh /cfdocs/cfMAUDE/Detail.CFM?MDRFOI__ID=441523*. Accessed November 4, 2009.

50. Ortega RA. A rare cause of fire in the operating room. *Anesthesiology*. 1998;89(6):1608.

51. Soussan EB, Mathieu N, Roque I, Antonietti M. Bowel explosion with colonic perforation during argon plasma coagulation for hemorrhagic radiation-induced proctitis. *Gastrointestinal Endoscopy*. 2003/3;57(3): 412-413.

52. Smith C. Home study program. Surgical fires—learn not to burn. *AORN J*. 2004;80(1):23-27, 29-31, 33-4.

53. Smith TL, Smith JM. Electrosurgery in otolaryngology-head and neck surgery: principles, advances, and complications. *Laryngoscope*. 2001;111(5):769-780.

54. Electrosurgical airway fires still a hot topic. *Health Devices*. 1996;25(7):260-262.

55. Manufacturer and User Facility Device Experience (MAUDE) Database. Adverse event report no. 837984: Electrosurgical unit. *http://www.accessdata. fda.gov/scripts/cdrh/cfdocs/cfMAUDE/Detail.CFM?MD RFOI__ID=837984*. Accessed November 4, 2009.

56. Manufacturer and User Facility Device Experience (MAUDE) Database. Adverse event report no. 767284: Dispersive electrode. *http://www.accessdata .fda.gov/scripts/cdrh/cfdocs/cfMAUDE/Detail.CFM?MD RFOI__ID=767284*. Accessed November 4, 2009.

57. Demir E, O'Dey DM, Pallua N. Accidental burns during surgery. *J Burn Care Res*. 2006;27(6):895-900.

58. Center for Devices and Radiological Health. Manufacturer and User Facility Device Experience (MAUDE) Database Adverse Event Report 523194. Reported March 31, 2004. *http://www.accessdata .fda.gov/scripts/cdrh/cfdocs/cfMAUDE/Detail.CFM?MD RFOI__ID=523194*. Accessed November 4, 2009.

59. Manufacturer and User Facility Device Experience (MAUDE) Database Search. Adverse event report no. 115111: Dispersive electrode. *http://www.access data.fda.gov/scripts/cdrh/cfdocs/cfMAUDE/Detail.CFM ?MDRFOI__ID=115111*. Accessed November 4, 2009.

60. Recommended practices for preoperative patient skin antisepsis. In: *Perioperative Standards and Recommended Practices*. Denver, CO: AORN, Inc; 2009: 549-568.

61. Manufacturer and User Facility Device Experience (MAUDE) Database. Adverse event report no. 1021169: Grounding plate. *http://www.accessdata.fda .gov/scripts/cdrh/cfdocs/cfMAUDE/Detail.CFM?MDR FOI__ID=1021169*. Accessed November 4, 2009.

62. Ratnapalan S, Greenberg M, Armstrong D. Tattoos and MRI. *AJR Am J Roentgenol*. 2004;183(2):541.

63. Franiel T, Schmidt S, Klingebiel R. First-degree burns on MRI due to nonferrous tattoos. *AJR Am J Roentgenol*. 2006;187(5):W556.

64. Wagle WA, Smith M. Tattoo-induced skin burn during MR imaging. *Am J Roentgenol*. 2000;174(6):1795.

65. Center for Devices and Radiological Health. Manufacturer and User Facility Device Experience (MAUDE) Database Adverse Event Report 495428. Reported October 15, 2003. *http://www.accessdata .fda.gov/scripts/cdrh/cfdocs/cfMAUDE/Detail.CFM?MD RFOI__ID=495428*. Accessed November 4, 2009.

66. Center for Devices and Radiological Health. Manufacturer and User Facility Device Experience (MAUDE) Database Adverse Event Report 499965.

Reported November 25, 2003. *http://www.accessdata .fda.gov/scripts/cdrh/cfdocs/cfMAUDE/Detail.CFM?MD RFOI__ID=499965*. Accessed November 4, 2009.

67. Center for Devices and Radiological Health. Manufacturer and User Facility Device Experience (MAUDE) Database Adverse Event Report 516905. Reported February 16, 2004. *http://www.accessdata .fda.gov/scripts/cdrh/cfdocs/cfMAUDE/Detail.CFM?MD RFOI__ID=516905*. Accessed November 4, 2009.

68. Manufacturer and User Facility Device Experience (MAUDE) Database. Adverse event report no. 851317: Dispersive electrode. *http://www.accessdata .fda.gov/scripts/cdrh/cfdocs/cfMAUDE/Detail.CFM?MD RFOI__ID=851317*. Accessed November 4, 2009.

69. Center for Devices and Radiological Health. Manufacturer and User Facility Device Experience (MAUDE) Database Adverse Event Report 286226. Reported July 6, 2002. *http://www.accessdata .fda.gov/scripts/cdrh/cfdocs/cfMAUDE/Detail.CFM?MD RFOI__ID=286226*. Accessed November 4, 2009.

70. Center for Devices and Radiological Health. Manufacturer and User Facility Device Experience (MAUDE) Database Adverse Event Report 396295. Reported May 16, 2002. *http://www.accessdata .fda.gov/scripts/cdrh/cfdocs/cfMAUDE/Detail.CFM?MD RFOI__ID=396295*. Accessed November 4, 2009.

71. Russell MJ, Gaetz M. Intraoperative electrode burns. *J Clin Monit Comput*. 2004;18(1):25-32.

72. Stecker MM, Patterson T, Netherton BL. Mechanisms of electrode induced injury. Part 1: theory. *Am J Electroneurodiagnostic Technol*. 2006;46(4):315-342.

73. Patterson T, Stecker MM, Netherton BL. Mechanisms of electrode induced injury. Part 2: Clinical experience. *Am J Electroneurodiagnostic Technol*. 2007;47(2):93-113.

74. ECRI Institute. Higher currents, greater risks: preventing patient burns at the return-electrode site during high-current electrosurgical procedures. *Health Devices*. 2005;34(8):273-279.

75. Manufacturer and User Facility Device Experience (MAUDE) Database. Adverse event report no. 1069874: REM PolyHesive II electrode, ESU, dispersive. *http://www.accessdata.fda.gov/scripts/cdrh/cfdocs/cfM AUDE/Detail.CFM?MDRFOI__ID=1069874*. Accessed November 4, 2009.

76. Manufacturer and User Facility Device Experience (MAUDE) Database. Adverse event report no. 907879: Generator. *http://www.accessdata.fda.gov /scripts/cdrh/cfdocs/cfMAUDE/Detail.CFM?MDRFOI __ID=907879*. Accessed November 4, 2009.

77. Skin lesions from aggressive adhesive on Valleylab electrosurgical return electrode pads. *Health Devices*. 1995;24(4):159-160.

78. MegaDyne Mega 2000 return electrode. *Health Devices*. 2000;29(12):445-460.

79. Center for Devices and Radiological Health. Manufacturer and User Facility Device Experience (MAUDE) Database Adverse Event Report 401617. Reported June 24, 2002. *http://www.accessdata .fda.gov/scripts/cdrh/cfdocs/cfMAUDE/Detail.CFM?MD RFOI__ID=401617*. Accessed November 4, 2009.

80. Recommended practices for endoscopic minimally invasive surgery. In: *Perioperative Standards and Recommended Practices*. Denver, CO: AORN, Inc; 2009:347-359.

81. Greilich PE, Greilich NB, Froelich EG. Intra-abdominal fire during laparoscopic cholecystectomy. See comment. *Anesthesiology*. 1995;83(4):871-874.

82. Tucker RD, Voyles CR, Silvis SE. Capacitive coupled stray currents during laparoscopic and endoscopic electrosurgical procedures. *Biomed Instrum Technol*. 1992;26(4):303-311.

83. Wang K, Advincula AP. "Current thoughts" in electrosurgery. *Int J Gynaecol Obstet*. 2007;97(3):245-250.

84. Shirk GJ, Johns A, Redwine DB. Complications of laparoscopic surgery: how to avoid them and how to repair them. *J Minim Invasive Gynecol*. 2006;13(4):352-359.

85. Yazdani A, Krause H. Laparoscopic instrument insulation failure: the hidden hazard. *J Minim Invasive Gynecol*. 2007;14(2):228-232.

86. Brunner LS, Suddarth DS, Smeltzer SCO, Cheever K, eds. Management of patients with intestinal and rectal disorders. In: *Brunner & Suddarth's Textbook of Medical-Surgical Nursing*. 11th ed. Philadelphia, PA: Lippincott Williams & Wilkins; 2008:1231-1281.

87. McCarus SD. Physiologic mechanism of the ultrasonically activated scalpel. *J Am Assoc Gynecol Laparosc*. 1996;3(4):601-608.

88. Ott DE, Moss E, Martinez K. Aerosol exposure from an ultrasonically activated (Harmonic) device. *J Am Assoc Gynecol Laparosc*. 1998;5(1):29-32.

89. Matthews K. Argon beam coagulation. New directions in surgery. *AORN J*. 1992;56(5):885-889.

90. Fatal gas embolism caused by overpressurization during laparoscopic use of argon enhanced coagulation. *Health Devices*. 1994;23(6):257-259.

91. Veyckemans F, Michel I. Venous gas embolism from an Argon coagulator. *Anesthesiology*. 1996;85(2):443-444.

92. National Institute for Occupational Safety and Health. NIOSH Hazard Control/Control of Smoke From Laser/Electric Surgical Procedures-HC11. *http://www .cdc.gov/niosh/hc11.html*. Accessed November 4, 2009.

93. ECRI Institute. Smoke evacuation systems, surgical. *Healthcare Product Comparison System*. 2007.

94. Ball K. *Lasers : The Perioperative Challenge*. Denver, CO: AORN, Inc; 2004.

95. Ulmer BC. The hazards of surgical smoke. *AORN J*. 2008;87(4):721-738.

96. Hoglan M. Potential hazards from electrosurgery plume—recommendations for surgical smoke evacuation. *Can Oper Room Nurs J*. 1995;13(4):10-16.

97. US Department of Labor Occupational Safety and Health Administration. Safety and Health Topics: Laser/Electrosurgery Plume. *http://www.osha.gov/SLTC /laserelectrosurgeryplume/index.html*. Accessed November 4, 2009.

98. Alp E, Bijl D, Bleichrodt RP, Hansson B, Voss A. Surgical smoke and infection control. *J Hosp Infect*. 2006;62(1):1-5

99. American National Standards Institute. Safe use of lasers in health care facilities. Orlando, FL: Laser Institute of America; 2005.

100. Garden JM, O'Banion MK, Shelnitz LS, et al. Papillomavirus in the vapor of carbon dioxide laser-treated verrucae. *JAMA*. 1988;259(8):1199-1202.

101. Hallmo P, Naess O. Laryngeal papillomatosis with human papillomavirus DNA contracted by a laser surgeon. *Eur Arch Otorhinolaryngol.* 1991;248(7):425-427.

102. ECRI Institute. Investigating device-related skin "burns". *Operating Room Risk Management.* 2(3):1-10.

103. Quality and performance improvement standards for perioperative nursing. In: *Perioperative Standards and Recommended Practices.* Denver, CO: AORN, Inc; 2009:65-74.

104. Improving organization performance. In: *Comprehensive Accreditation Manual for Hospitals: The Official Handbook.* Oakbrook Terrace, IL: Joint Commission on Accreditation of Healthcare Organizations; 2007:PI-8–PI-9.

Acknowledgements

LEAD AUTHOR
Mary Ogg, RN, MSN, CNOR
Perioperative Nursing Specialist
AORN Center for Nursing Practice
Denver, Colorado

CONTRIBUTING AUTHOR
Cecil A. King, MS, RN, CNOR
Perioperative Clinical Educator
Cape Cod Hospital
Hyannis, Massachusetts

PUBLICATION HISTORY
Originally published March 1985, *AORN Journal.* Revised April 1991; revised July 1993.

Revised November 1997; published January 1998, *AORN Journal.* Reformatted July 2000.

Revised November 2003; published February 2004, *AORN Journal.*

Revised November 2004; published in *Standards, Recommended Practices, and Guidelines,* 2005 edition. Reprinted March 2005, *AORN Journal.*

Revised July 2009 for online publication in *Perioperative Standards and Recommended Practices.*

Minor editing revisions made in November 2009 for publication in *Perioperative Standards and Recommended Practices,* 2010 edition.

Recommended Practices for Selection and Use of Surgical Gowns and Drapes

The following recommended practices were developed by the AORN Recommended Practices Committee and have been approved by the AORN Board of Directors. They were presented as proposed recommended practices for comments by members and others. They are effective January 1, 2003.

These recommended practices are intended as achievable recommendations representing what is believed to be an optimal level of practice. Policies and procedures will reflect variations in practice settings and/or clinical situations that determine the degree to which the recommended practices can be implemented.

AORN recognizes the numerous types of settings in which perioperative nurses practice. These recommended practices are intended as guidelines adaptable to various practice settings. These practice settings include traditional operating rooms, ambulatory surgery units, physician's offices, cardiac catheterization suites, endoscopy suites, radiology departments, and all other areas where operative and other invasive procedures may be performed.

Purpose

These recommended practices provide guidelines for evaluation, selection, and use of surgical gowns and drapes. These products should provide a safe, effective means of protecting patients and health care personnel during use. Patients are at risk of contamination from both endogenous and exogenous microorganisms. Health care workers are at risk of contamination from a variety of bloodborne pathogens that can be contracted via exposure to patients' blood and body fluids. The barrier quality required of surgical gowns and drapes varies according to the planned use of the product and its anticipated exposure to blood and body fluids.

Recommendation I

Surgical gowns and drapes should be evaluated according to the AORN "Recommended practices for product selection in perioperative practice settings."[1]

1. Materials selected for construction of surgical gowns and drapes should be safe, meet identified needs, and promote patient and personnel safety.

2. Selection of gown and drape products for use in the practice setting should be based on criteria specific to the products' function and use. Surgical gowns and drapes are constructed of either single-use or reusable materials. Each of these has advantages and disadvantages. Further, in each of the two categories, design and performance characteristics vary. This variation stems from trade-offs in cost, comfort, and the amount of barrier protection provided. Both single-use and reusable gowns and drapes often are reinforced to improve their barrier quality. Reinforcements may consist of additional layers of the same material or layers of different material(s).[2]

Recommendation II

Materials used for surgical gowns and drapes should be resistant to penetration by blood and other body fluids as necessitated by their intended use.

1. Perioperative managers and purchasing agents should obtain from manufacturers data verifying that materials used in gowns and drapes are protective barriers against the transfer of microorganisms, particulates, and fluids to minimize strike-through and the potential for personnel contamination. Microorganisms can be transferred through barrier materials by wicking of fluids and/or pressure or leaning on a flooded area of the product. Mechanical action such as pressure can result in both liquid and dry penetration of microbes if the pressure exceeds the maximum level of resistance that the material provides.[3]

2. Surgical gowns should be selected for use according to the barrier quality of the item and the wearers' anticipated exposure to blood and body fluids in accordance with the Occupational Safety and Health Administration guidelines for use of personal protective equipment.[4] Short procedures during which there is little or no anticipated exposure to blood or body fluids can be completed successfully using a surgical gown with minimal barrier protection. As the complexity and length of the planned procedure increases, there may be increased potential for exposure to bloodborne pathogens, and it would be prudent to select a gown with greater barrier capability.

Recommendation III

Surgical gowns and drapes should maintain their integrity and be durable.

1. Surgical gowns and drapes should have an acceptable quality level (ie, be free of holes/ defects).

2. Surgical gowns and drapes should be resistant to tears, punctures, and abrasions. The inability to withstand tears, punctures, and abrasions may allow for passage of microorganisms, particulates, and fluids between sterile and non-sterile areas and expose patients to exogenous organisms. Health care workers may be exposed to bloodborne pathogens. Reusable materials should be inspected visually to determine their integrity before use.[5] Reusable textiles should be patched with heat-sealed patches of the same quality material as the item to which they are applied. If the item is of a single-ply material, a patch need only be applied to one side of the item. Patches must allow for penetration and removal of sterilant while maintaining the integrity of the barrier quality of the item. The percentage of exposed surface that can be patched is dependent on the sterilization method and the number of layers of patched textile.[6] Areas covered by heat-sealed patches on woven textiles should be examined carefully before the fabric is used. The patched area should maintain the original barrier properties each time the product is used. Patches of any kind should never be stitched to woven barrier materials as a method of repairing holes. Stitching creates permanent holes that reduce the barrier quality of the item.[7]

3. Surgical gowns and drapes should be low-linting. Barrier materials used for surgical gowns and drapes should be as lint-free as possible. Lint particles are disseminated into the environment where bacteria attach to them. This bacteria-carrying lint may settle in surgical sites and wounds with a resultant increase in post-operative patient complications.[8]

4. Seams of barrier materials should be evaluated to determine their capability to minimize either penetration or passage of potential contaminants. Many surgical gown seams have little or no barrier property. If wicking or pressure on a seam causes liquid transfer between sterile and unsterile surfaces, one or both sides may become contaminated.[9]

Recommendation IV

Materials used for surgical gowns and drapes should be appropriate to the method(s) of sterilization.

1. To achieve a sterile product, the sterilizing agent must contact all surfaces of the item to be sterilized. Common sterilization methodologies include
   - radiation,
   - steam, and
   - ethylene oxide.

   The primary methodologies used in health care facilities are steam and ethylene oxide. Most facilities have neither the capability of nor access to radiation as a means of sterilization.

2. Tightly woven reusable textiles will lose their protective barrier quality after repeated processing. Manufacturers' written instructions for handling, the suggested number of processings, and the useful life of barrier materials should be provided and followed. A system should be established to track the number of processings for each item. This tracking should include, but not be limited to, the number of wash cycles and sterilization processings to which the textile product is subjected. Repeated processing ultimately will diminish the protective barrier ability of reusable textiles; however, items constructed of reusable textiles should continue to meet the original barrier quality level throughout the manufacturer-recommended life cycle (ie, number of processings) for the textile. The user facility should monitor the barrier quality of reusable textiles at intervals while the product is in service. Purchasers of reusable textile gowns and/or drapes should obtain from the manufacturer instructions for testing the material to document the ongoing barrier quality of the item(s) for the entire useful life of the item(s).[10] Products that no longer meet the manufacturer-stated barrier level should be downgraded to a nonprotective category and used accordingly.

3. Unused, single-use surgical gowns and drapes should not be resterilized unless manufacturers provide specific written instructions for reprocessing or the US Food and Drug Administration (FDA) regulations are followed. Surgical gowns

and drapes intended for single use may not sterilize adequately, may be damaged during the sterilization process, or may retain toxic residues.[11] If a health care facility chooses to reprocess single-use items, including gowns and drapes, the FDA considers the facility to be the manufacturer of the item(s) and, as such, the facility is subject to the same stringent regulations as the original manufacturer of the item.[12]

Recommendation V

Surgical gowns and drapes should resist combustion.

1. Gowns and drapes selected for use should be consistent with accepted flammability standards that will provide the safest environment for patients and health care workers.[13] Specific standards for surgical materials have not been developed. All materials used in the surgical environment will burn given the right conditions.

2. Barrier materials are made of natural and/or synthetic fibers and may be flammable, needing only a combination of heat, fuel, and oxygen to ignite.[14] Care should be taken when gowns and drapes are exposed to light and heat sources, electrosurgical devices, lasers, and other power equipment. Materials ignite and burn at various rates. Even materials said to be flame-resistant might burn or melt when subjected to intense heat or an oxygen-rich environment.[15] Some materials not only ignite more easily than others but also may burn more rapidly.

Recommendation VI

Surgical gowns and drapes should be comfortable and contribute to maintaining the wearer's desired body temperature.

1. Surgical gowns and drapes should be free of toxic ingredients and allergens. Patients and/or health care workers may experience untoward reactions to toxic ingredients and/or allergens, ranging from mild discomfort to anaphylactic collapse.

2. Surgical drapes should have limited memory and be flexible enough to conform loosely to the patient's contour, allow for placement and unhampered manipulation of surgical instruments, and appropriately drape related equipment.[16] Surgical gowns should have limited memory and be flexible enough to conform loosely to the wearer's

body while at the same time protect the wearer from contamination from blood and body fluids.

3. Surgical gowns and drapes should have the ability to maintain an isothermic environment for patients and health care workers. People vary in their ability to tolerate heat and cold. Thermal comfort exists when a balance occurs between the heat the human body loses and the heat the body generates. Care must be taken to avoid hypothermia or hyperthermia in surgical patients. Normothermic or near-normothermic patients may have a more favorable postoperative course.[17]

Recommendation VII

Surgical gowns and drapes selected for use should have a favorable cost-benefit ratio.

1. Surgical gowns and drapes should not be selected on the basis of cost only. Nor should cost be the primary consideration when making a selection. In today's economic environment, however, it is imperative that after providing for patient and provider safety, fiscal factors be considered. Careful selection of the appropriate gowns and drapes for the practice setting will contribute to the fiscal soundness of the provider facility.[18] A lesser-priced product that fails consistently is not cost effective because additional volume will be required to replace the defective or poorly performing item(s).

2. Surgical gowns and drapes are considered medical devices, and failure of these devices is subject to medical device reporting requirements according to the Safe Medical Devices Act of 1990[19] (SMDA) and/or the FDA voluntary Problem Reporting Program. This voluntary program provides users with a mechanism for reporting events that do not meet the strict reporting criteria of the SMDA. Reports should be filed by telephone at (800) 638-6725. Consistent failure of a surgical gown or drape product should be reported to the manufacturer and the FDA. Any strike-through constitutes a threat of exposure to potentially harmful bloodborne pathogens.

Recommendation VIII

Policies and procedures for selecting and using surgical gowns and drapes should be developed,

reviewed regularly, revised as necessary, and readily available in the practice setting.

1. These recommended practices should be used as guidelines when developing policies and procedures. Written policies and procedures establish authority, responsibility, and accountability. They serve as operational guidelines in the practice setting. Other AORN recommended practices addressing packaging systems, sterilization, creating and maintaining a sterile field, and surgical attire also should be consulted when developing policies and procedures for the selection and use of surgical gowns and drapes.

2. Orientation and ongoing education activities for personnel should include an introduction to and/or review of policies and procedures to be applied in the practice setting. Compliance with policies and procedures helps develop and reinforce knowledge, skills, and attitudes that affect patient outcomes. Policies and procedures also may be an integral part of continuous quality assessment and improvement activities.

Glossary

Barrier material: Material that minimizes or retards the penetration of microorganisms, particulates, and fluids.

Heat-sealed patch: A patch of the same textile with an adhesive back applied to reusable textiles containing a hole or tear with high-intensity heat.

Isothermic environment: The surroundings, conditions, or influences that affect maintaining an equal temperature.

Nonwoven material: A manufactured sheet, web, or batt of directionally or randomly oriented fibers or filaments, natural or man-made, excluding paper and paper products, that are woven, knotted, tufted, or stitch bonded and have not been converted into yarns. Nonwovens are bonded to each other by friction and/or cohesion and/or adhesion. They are designed as single-use materials.

Strike-through: Penetration of microorganisms, particulates, or fluids through a barrier material.

Useful life: The anticipated life of a product, such as a woven material. Useful life is affected by the number of sterilization processing and washing cycles a product can endure and yet maintain an acceptable barrier capability.

Wicking: Absorption of a liquid by capillary action along a thread or through the material.

Woven material: Fabric constructed from yarns made of natural or synthetic fibers or filaments that are woven together to form a web in a repeated interlocking pattern.

REFERENCES

1. "Recommended practices for product selection in perioperative practice settings," in *Standards, Recommended Practices, and Guidelines* (Denver: AORN, Inc, 2004) 347-350.

2. K K Leonas, R S Jinkins, "The relationship of selected fabric characteristics and the barrier effectiveness of surgical gown fabrics," *American Journal of Infection Control* 25 (February 1997) 16-23; *Selection of Surgical Gowns and Drapes in Health Care Facilities* (Arlington, Va: Association for the Advancement of Medical Instrumentation, 2000) 4-12.

3. *Ibid.*

4. "Occupational exposure to bloodborne pathogens; Final rule," *Federal Register* 56 (Dec 6, 1991) 640004-64182; N L Belkin, "A historical review of barrier materials," *AORN Journal* 76 (October 2002) 648-653.

5. *Processing of Reusable Surgical Textiles for Use in Health Care Facilities* (Arlington, Va: Association for the Advancement of Medical Instrumentation, 2000) 23-28.

6. *Ibid,* 27-28; American Society for Healthcare Central Service Professionals of the American Hospital Association, *Training Manual for Central Service Technicians,* third ed (Chicago: American Hospital Association, 1997) 136.

7. *Ibid.*

8. *Processing of Reusable Surgical Textiles for Use in Health Care Facilities,* 24; *Selection of Surgical Gowns and Drapes in Health Care Facilities,* 16-17; C Edmiston et al, "Airborne particulates in the OR environment," *AORN Journal* 69 (June 1999) 1169-1183.

9. J Pournoor, "New scientific tools to expand the understanding of aseptic practices," *Surgical Services Management* 6 (April 2000) 28-32; J W Smith et al, "Determination of surgeon-generated gown pressures during various surgical procedures in the operating room," *American Journal of Infection Control* 23 (August 1995) 238; E A McCullough, "Methods for determining the barrier efficacy of surgical gowns," *American Journal of Infection Control* 21 (December 1993) 368; I D Learmonth, "Prevention of infection in the 1990s," *Orthopedic Clinics of North America* 24 (October 1993) 736; K W Altman et al, "Transmural surgical gown pressure measurements in the operating theater," *American Journal of Infection Control* 19 (June 1991) 147.

10. *Selection of Surgical Gowns and Drapes in Health Care Facilities,* 17, 18, 23; *Processing of Reusable Surgical Textiles for Use in Health Care Facilities,* 14, 24, 25; D Fogg, "Infection control," in *Alexander's Care of the Patient in Surgery,* 11th ed, M H Meeker, J C Rothrock, eds (St Louis: Mosby, 1999) 145.

11. *Good Hospital Practice: Steam Sterilization and Sterility Assurance* (Arlington, Va: Association for the Advancement of Medical Instrumentation, 1994) 9.

12. *Ibid;* "Reuse of single-use devices," (Clinical Issues) *AORN Journal* 73 (May 2001) 957-966; "AORN guidance statement: Reuse of single-use devices," in *Standards,*

Recommended Practices, and Guidelines (Denver: AORN, Inc, 2002) 113-119.

13. Selection of Surgical Gowns and Drapes in Health Care Facilities, 15, 16, 18; "Standard for the flammability of clothing textiles," in Code of Federal Regulations (CFR) 16: Commercial Practices, Part 1610 (Washington, DC: US Government Printing Office, 2001) 608-616; "Standard for the flammability of vinyl plastic film," in Code of Federal Regulations (CFR) 16: Commercial Practices, Part 1611 (Washington, DC: US Government Printing Office, 2001) 622-630.

14. Ibid; J R Sommers, "Flammability standards for surgical drapes and gowns: Past, present, and future," Surgical Services Management 4 (February 1998) 41-44; Fire Safety in the Perioperative Setting (Woodbury, Conn: Ciné-med, 2000) Videotape; "Surgical fires in the OR," ORRM 2 (1992).

15. Ibid; "Recommended practices for laser safety in practice settings," in Standards, Recommended Practices, and Guidelines (Denver: AORN, Inc, 2002) 277-281.

16. Selection of Surgical Gowns and Drapes in Health Care Facilities, 13, 14.

17. Ibid; A C Meling et al, "Effects of preoperative warming on the incidence of wound infection after clean surgery: A randomised controlled trial," The Lancet 358 (Sept 15, 2001) 876-880; Agency for Healthcare Research and Quality, University of California, San Francisco-Stanford Evidence-Based Practice Center, Making Health-care Safer: A Critical Analysis of Patient Safety Practices (Rockville, Md: Agency for Healthcare Research and Quality, US Department of Health and Human Services, 2001) 231-234; A Kurz, D I Sessler, R Lenhardt, "Perioperative normothermia to reduce the incidence of surgical-wound infection and shorten hospitalization," The New England Journal of Medicine 334 (May 9, 1996) 1209-1215.

18. Selection of Surgical Gowns and Drapes in Health Care Facilities, 19.

19. Safe Medical Devices Act of 1990, sec 519 (21 USC 360); "Medical device reporting," in Code of Federal Regulations (CFR) 21: Food and Drugs, Part 803 (Washington, DC: US Government Printing Office, 2002) 38-55; "Medical devices: Reports of corrections and removals," in Code of Federal Regulations (CFR) 21: Food and Drugs, Part 806 (Washington, DC: US Government Printing Office, 2002) 55-58.

PUBLICATION HISTORY

Originally published February 1988, AORN Journal. Revised March 1992.

Revised November 1995; published March 1996, AORN Journal. Reformatted July 2000.

Revised; published in Standards, Recommended Practices, and Guidelines, 2003 edition. Reprinted January 2003, AORN Journal.

AORN Perioperative Standards and Recommended Practices, 2012 Edition

Recommended Practices for
Laser Safety in Perioperative Practice Settings

The following Recommended Practices for Laser Safety in Perioperative Practice Settings were developed by the AORN Recommended Practices Committee and have been approved by the AORN Board of Directors. They were presented as proposed recommendations for comments by members and others. They are effective November 1, 2010.

These recommended practices are intended as achievable recommendations representing what is believed to be an optimal level of practice. Policies and procedures will reflect variations in practice settings and/or clinical situations that determine the degree to which the recommended practices can be implemented.

AORN recognizes the various settings in which perioperative nurses practice. These recommended practices are intended as guidelines adaptable to various practice settings. These practice settings include traditional operating rooms (ORs), ambulatory surgery centers, physicians' offices, cardiac catheterization laboratories, endoscopy suites, radiology departments, and all other areas where surgery and other invasive procedures may be performed.

Purpose

These recommended practices provide guidance to perioperative personnel in the use and care of laser equipment and to assist practitioners in providing a safe environment for patients and health care workers during use of laser technology. This document incorporates activities described in the American National Standards Institute's (ANSI's) *American National Standards for the Safe Use of Lasers in Health Care Facilities ANSI Z136.3*, which specifies standards for the use of class 3 and class 4 laser devices in the health care environment.[1] Health care facilities are encouraged to obtain *Safe Use of Lasers in Health Care Facilities ANSI Z136.3*[1] and ANSI's *American National Standard for Safe Use of Lasers ANSI Z136.1*[2] and to have them readily available in the practice environment.

Recommendation I

A laser safety program should be established for all owned, leased, or borrowed laser equipment in any location where lasers are used in the health care organization.[1,3,4]

Health care laser systems are classified by their relative hazard and the appropriate controls.[1] Class 3 and primarily class 4 lasers are used in the health care setting. Class 4 laser exposure may be hazardous to eyes and skin, and may pose a potential fire risk.[1] Class 3 lasers are potentially hazardous in the event of direct exposure or exposure to specular reflection (ie, mirror-like reflection of light).[1,4]

I.a. A formal laser safety program should include, but not be limited to,
- delegating authority and responsibility for supervising laser safety to a laser safety officer (LSO);
- establishing a multidisciplinary laser safety committee or safety committee;[3]
- establishing usage criteria and authorized procedures for all health care personnel working in laser nominal hazard zones;
- identifying laser hazards and appropriate administrative, engineering, and procedural control measures;
- educating personnel (eg, operators) regarding the assessment and control of hazards; and
- managing and reporting accidents or incidents related to laser procedures, including creating action plans to prevent recurrences.[1]

A laser safety program may minimize potential laser hazards. A multidisciplinary laser safety committee is integral to establishing and monitoring laser safety.[3]

I.a.1. The multidisciplinary laser safety committee or safety committee may include
- the chief operating officer;
- the director of patient safety;
- the patent safety coordinator;
- the director of biomedical engineering and/or clinical/biomedical engineer;[5]
- the LSO;[5]
- the deputy laser safety officer;
- the chief of surgery;
- a physician representative from each specialty group using lasers;[5]
- an anesthesia care provider;[5]
- the perioperative services director;[5]
- the perioperative educator;
- the director of medical staff education/credentialing;

- the environmental manager;[5]
- the risk manager;
- a laser safety specialist (eg, nurse, technician);[5] and/or
- the hazardous materials manager.[5]

I.a.2. The responsibilities of the laser safety committee or safety committee should include, but not be limited to,
- strategic planning (eg, technology assessment, cost analysis, product evaluation);
- credentialing;
- hazard assessment;
- laser safety program oversight;
- laser-related policy and procedure development and enforcement; and
- laser-related education.

I.a.3. The laser safety committee or safety committee members should review activities including, but not limited to,
- acquisition of laser-related technology,[5]
- design of facilities where lasers are used,
- marketing information from laser vendors,[5]
- credentialing education and competencies,
- education and training programs,[5]
- protocols,[5]
- policies and procedures,
- variance reporting,
- laser audits, and
- use of third-party laser systems.

I.a.4. The laser safety committee or safety committee should verify that any physician who operates the laser is credentialed to perform the procedure as defined by the health care organization's policy. Physician credentialing by the health care organization's medical board should include, but is not limited to,
- completing coursework in basic laser physics, laser tissue interaction, and clinical applications;[3,5]
- training in the operation and safety of the specific laser for which privileges are sought;[1,3,5] and
- completing a preceptorship (ie, training, observation, mentoring).[1]

Lasers are highly technical medical devices with potential for harm. Laser experience among physicians varies depending on the degree that residency training programs incorporate lasers into their program.[1]

I.b. An LSO should be appointed as part of a laser safety program and should be authorized by the health care organization's administrators to monitor and oversee the control of laser hazards.[1]

The LSO helps to ensure the safety of patients and personnel where lasers are used.

I.b.1. The responsibilities of the LSO should include, but not be limited to,
- verifying the manufacturer's hazard classification label of all lasers and laser systems;[1]
- performing a laser hazard evaluation before initial use;[1]
- overseeing the implementation of the health care laser system manufacturer's control measures;[1]
- developing policies and procedures for maintenance, service, and use of lasers;[1]
- verifying that protective equipment is available, used correctly, and free of defects;[1]
- ascertaining that warning signs and labels comply with the Federal Laser Product Performance Standard or international standards;[1]
- approving equipment and installation according to the manufacturer's safety recommendations;[1] and
- coordinating laser safety and education programs.[1]

I.b.2. The LSO may fulfill multiple roles (eg, laser operator, laser safety specialist [LSS]) within the health care organization depending on the scope of services provided.

I.b.3. The LSO or an appointee should assess any rented or borrowed equipment for compliance with all federal, state, local, and facility requirements.[1]

The LSO is responsible for the monitoring and oversight of laser hazards control.[1]

I.b.4. The LSO should make certain that the terms of agreements with a third-party laser equipment provider and/or operator include, but are not limited to,

- laser operator credentials that meet the health care organization's policy;
- written validation of the laser's maintenance, service, and cleaning;
- documentation of data elements regarding each laser procedure performed that meets the health care organization's policy; and
- provision of safety orientation and training of the perioperative team associated with the laser procedure.

I.c. An LSS (eg, laser resource nurse) should be designated and approved by the LSO for each area when lasers are being used in multiple sites in a health care organization.

The LSS oversees the safe laser use in each area where a laser is used. An LSS may not be needed where the laser is used only in one location and the LSO is available.

I.c.1. The responsibilities of the LSS should include, but not be limited to,

- supervising laser usage in a specific area (eg, ambulatory surgery unit, eye clinic);
- acting as a liaison between the clinical laser users and the LSO;
- troubleshooting equipment problems;[3]
- monitoring compliance with the health care organization's laser policies and procedures;
- reviewing laser-related documentation (eg, logs, laser manufacturer's directions);
- acting as a resource to staff members and laser users; and
- assessing needs for continuing education and training.

Recommendation II

All personnel should know where lasers are being used and access to these areas should be controlled.[1,4]

Identifying the laser treatment area with laser warning signs and controlling access prevents unintentional exposure to the laser beam.

II.a. A nominal hazard zone (ie, the space in which the level of direct, reflected, or scattered radiation used during normal laser operation exceeds the applicable maximum permissible exposure) should be identified.[1]

The nominal hazard zone usually is contained within the room but may extend through open doors and/or transparent windows, depending on the type of laser being used. Identification of the nominal hazard zone establishes the area where control measures are required.

II.a.1. The LSO should determine the nominal hazard zone by referencing ANSI Z136.1 and ANSI Z136.3, as well as the safety information supplied by the laser manufacturer.[1,2]

II.a.2. Personnel in the nominal hazard zone should be aware of all necessary laser safety precautions (eg, wearing appropriate eye protection) to avoid inadvertent exposure to laser hazards.[1]

II.b. Clearly marked laser signs should be placed at all entrances to laser treatment areas when lasers are in use.[3,4]

Laser signs alert health care personnel to the areas where lasers are in use.

II.b.1. Recognizable warning signs specific to the type of laser being used should be designed according to the information described in ANSI Z136.3.[1,6]

II.b.2. Warning signs should be placed conspicuously to alert bystanders to potential hazards.[1]

II.b.3. Laser warning signs should be removed when the laser procedure is completed.[4]

II.c. Doors in the nominal hazard zone should remain closed and windows, including door windows, should be covered with a barrier that blocks transmission of a beam as appropriate to the type of laser being used.[1,4,6]

Laser energy, except energy from carbon dioxide wavelength lasers, has the potential to pass through windows. Maintaining a blocking barrier stops the transmission of the laser beam.[7]

Recommendation III

Patients and health care personnel in the laser treatment area should be protected from unintentional laser beam exposure.[1]

Unintentional laser beam exposure may cause eye and skin damage.[1]

III.a. Procedures should be implemented to prevent accidental activation or misdirection of laser beams that include, but are not limited to, the following:
- access to laser keys should be restricted to authorized personnel who are skilled in laser operation;[1,3,4,7]
- lasers should be placed in standby mode when not in active use;[1,3,4,8]
- the laser foot switch should be placed in a position convenient to the operator with the activation mechanism identified; and
- the laser user should be the only one to activate the device with the foot pedal.[4,8]

Accidental activation or misdirection of the laser beam may cause eye and skin injury to the patient and health care personnel.[9] Attention to proper placement of the foot switch and use of the standby setting can reduce unintended activation of the laser beam and potential injury to the patient and health care personnel. Control of activation by the laser user prevents unintentional discharge of laser energy to minimize the potential for patient or health care personnel injury.

III.b. The laser assistant (eg, RN, laser technician) should not have competing responsibilities that would require leaving the laser unattended during active use.

Circulating responsibilities may preclude the ability to assume responsibility for laser operation. The laser assistant runs the laser console to control the laser parameters under the supervision of the laser user. The laser user operates the laser for its intended purpose within the user's scope of practice, education, and experience.[1]

III.b.1. Personnel assignments for a procedure during which a laser is used should be based on, but not limited to,
- patient assessment and acuity,
- the type of laser being used,
- the complexity and type of procedure,
- surgical site, and
- the experience and competency of the laser assistant and RN circulator.

III.c. The emergency shut off switch should be used to disable the laser in case of a component breakdown or untoward event.[1,7,10]

Immediate shut down of the laser may prevent patient and health care personnel injury as well as equipment damage.

III.d. Reflective surfaces should be minimized during laser surgery.[1]

The laser beam may refract off shiny surfaces, potentially causing skin or eye injury.[7]

III.d.1. Anodized, dull, non-reflective, or matte-finished instruments should be used near the laser site.[3,4,7]

Anodized, dull, non-reflective, or matte-finished instruments decrease the reflectivity of laser beams.[1,3,4,7]

III.d.2. Instruments that have been coated (ie, ebonized) should be inspected regularly for damage to the integrity of the coating. Instruments with damaged coating should be removed from service and repaired or replaced.[7]

Damage or scratches to the coating may allow the laser beam to refract off shiny surfaces, potentially causing skin or eye injury.[7]

III.d.3. Reflective instruments that cannot be ebonized should be covered with saline saturated materials (eg, towels, radiopaque sponges).

III.e. Exposed tissues around the surgical site should be protected with saline-saturated materials (eg, towels, sponges) when lasers with a thermal effect are being used.[1]

The solution (eg, saline) absorbs or disperses the energy of the laser beam in areas not intended for laser application.[4]

III.e.1. These materials should be remoistened periodically to prevent drying and becoming an ignition source.[7,11]

III.f. Backstops (eg, titanium rods, quartz rods) or guards should be used during CO_2 laser surgery to prevent the laser beam from striking normal tissue.[4,7]

The CO_2 laser beam continues to move through the tissue after it cuts or coagulates. A backstop or guard will prevent the laser beam from affecting non-targeted tissue.

III.f.1. Mirrors made of rhodium or stainless steel may be used as a backstop in hard-to-reach areas.

III.g. When a fiber is used to deliver laser energy through an endoscope, the end of the fiber should extend past the end of the endoscope and be in view at all times during active use.[1]

Activation of the laser fiber inside the endoscope may cause damage to the scope.

III.g.1. For rigid endoscopic delivery systems (eg, laryngoscopes, bronchoscopes, laparoscopes), care should be taken to avoid heating of the sheath wall by the laser beam.[1]

If the metallic tubular system is used improperly, the heat inside the endoscope will cause thermal damage to adjoining tissues.[1]

III.h. When using lasers with flexible endoscopic delivery systems, care should be taken to avoid laser beam exposure within the sheath.[1]

Flexible fiber-optic endoscopic sheaths may be damaged by heat. Flexible fiber-optic endoscope sheaths may be flammable.[1]

Recommendation IV

All people in the nominal hazard zone should wear appropriate eyewear selected and approved by the LSO.[1,3,4,10,12]

Scattered, diffused, and reflected laser beams, in addition to direct exposure from misdirected and damaged fibers, can cause eye injuries.[1,6]

IV.a. Selection of appropriate laser protective eyewear should be based on, but not limited to,
- the recommendations of the laser manufacturer[1] and
- the manufacturer's laser protective eyewear specifications.[1]

Laser protective eyewear protects the wearer from eye injury from direct or diffuse laser beams.[1]

IV.b. People in the nominal hazard zone must wear protective eyewear or use filters of specific wavelength and optical density for the laser in use.[1,6,12]

Eyes are vulnerable to injury from the laser beam. The part of the eye that is at risk depends on the wavelength of the laser used.[4] Color vision and/or night vision could be impaired or lost if the laser beam focuses on the retina.[6] Protective glasses are manufactured to specifications that will prevent damage to the eye by stopping the laser energy from penetrating the lens of the eye.[7] Lens filters protect the laser user from laser exposure.[1]

IV.b.1. Eyewear must be labeled with the appropriate optical density and wavelength for the laser in use.[1,4,12]

Optical density is the ability of laser protective eyewear to absorb a specific laser wavelength. The portion of the eye (eg, lens, cornea, retina) that may be injured by exposure to the laser beam depends on the laser's wavelength.[4]

IV.b.2. Correct laser wavelength and optical density eye protection should be available at the entrance to a room where a laser is in use.[1,6]

IV.b.3. Laser shutters or filters with the appropriate optical density should be used on microscopes to protect the laser user from laser exposure.[1]

Shutters and laser filters protect the laser user from laser exposure.[1]

IV.b.4. Laser filters with the appropriate optical density should be used on microscope accessory oculars. If filters are unavailable, personnel using accessory microscope view ports should wear protective eyewear.[1]

Filters protect viewers using microscope accessory oculars from laser exposure.[1]

IV.b.5. Health care personnel in the nominal hazard zone should wear protective eyewear even when a microscope eye lens filter is in use unless the LSO has determined that protective eyewear is not needed in the nominal hazard zone.[1,6,7]

IV.b.6. A lens filter of the appropriate laser wavelength may be used over the top of an endoscope viewing port.[1,4]

IV.b.7. Protective eyewear should be carefully handled and stored to prevent scratches and damage.[4,7]

IV.b.8. Protective eyewear should be inspected for damage and scratches before use. Damaged eyewear should be removed from use and reported to the LSO or LSS.[1,7]

IV.c. Patients' eyes and eyelids should be protected from the laser beam.[1,3]

The laser beam may cause injury to the patient's eyes if they are unprotected. The part of the eye at risk depends on the wavelength of the laser being used.[4]

IV.c.1. Patients who remain awake during laser procedures should wear goggles or glasses designated for the type of laser being used.[3,4,7]

IV.c.2. Patients undergoing general anesthesia should be provided with appropriate protection, such as wet eye pads, laser-specific eye shields, or as approved by the LSO.[1,3,4]

IV.c.3. Patients undergoing laser treatments on or around the eyelids should have their eyes protected by metal corneal eye shields that are approved by the US Food and Drug Administration (FDA).[1,4,6,7]

IV.d. Medical surveillance (eg, baseline eye exam, post-procedure exposure exam) should be considered for health care personnel where class 3B and class 4 lasers are used, if requested by the employing health care organization.[1,4,7,13]

A baseline eye examination provides historical information in the event of a laser injury.[1,4]

IV.d.1. The baseline exam should be performed before working with lasers, as directed by the health care organization policy and procedure.[1,14]

IV.d.2. A medical eye exam should be performed at the time of a suspected or abnormal exposure to laser radiation.[1,13,14]

Recommendation V

Potential hazards associated with surgical smoke generated in the laser practice setting should be identified and safe practices established.

Surgical smoke (ie, plume) is generated from use of lasers.[1,15] Analysis of the airborne contaminants produced during laser surgery has shown that laser plume contains toxic gas and vapors (eg, benzene, hydrogen cyanide, formaldehyde); bioaerosols; dead and living cell material, including blood fragments; and viruses.[1,16-18]

Many additional hazardous chemical compounds have been noted in surgical smoke.[17-22] At some level, these contaminants have been shown to have an unpleasant odor, cause problems with visibility of the surgical site, cause ocular and upper respiratory tract irritation, and demonstrate mutagenic and carcinogenic potential.[1,17]

Bacterial and/or viral contamination of plume has been highlighted by different studies.[18,23,24] The National Institute of Occupational Safety and Health (NIOSH) recommends that smoke evacuation systems be used to reduce potential acute and chronic health risks to health care personnel and patients.[17] The Occupational Safety and Health Administration (OSHA) has no separate standard related to surgical smoke plume, but does address related safety hazards in the General Duty Clause and Bloodborne Pathogens Standard.[25,26]

V.a. Surgical smoke should be removed by use of a smoke evacuation system in both open and minimally invasive procedures to prevent occupational exposure to laser-generated airborne contaminants.[1]

Local exhaust ventilation (LEV) is the primary means to protect health care personnel from occupational exposure to laser-generated airborne contaminants.[1] Potential health and liability risks may be reduced by the evacuation of surgical smoke.[16]

V.a.1. When surgical smoke is generated, an individual smoke evacuation unit with a 0.1 micron filter (eg, ultra-low particulate air [ULPA] or high efficiency particulate air [HEPA]) should be used to remove surgical smoke.[1,17]

During laser surgery, the cells are heated to a high temperature causing the cell membrane to rupture, releasing particles into the air. Lasers create particles approximately 0.3 microns in size.[18]

V.a.2. The capture device (eg, wand, non-flammable suction tip) of the smoke evacuation system should be positioned as close as possible, but no greater than two inches (5.08 cm) from the source of the smoke.[16,17]

Close proximity of the smoke evacuation wand maximizes particulate matter and odor capture and enhances visibility at the surgical site.[1,4]

V.a.3. Smoke evacuation units and accessories should be used according to manufacturers' written instructions.

V.a.4. When a central (wall) suction system is used to evacuate smoke, a 0.1 micron in-line filter (eg, ULPA filter) should be used.[4,17] The in-line filter should be placed between the suction connection and the suction canister.[1]

Central (ie, wall) suction units are designed to capture liquids and are used with an in-line 0.1 micron filter to remove airborne contaminants.[17] Low suction rates associated with centralized suction units limit their efficiency in evacuating plume, making them suitable only for the evacuation of small amounts of plume.[16]

V.a.5. When a centralized suction system dedicated for smoke evacuation is available, the smoke evacuator lines should be flushed according to the manufacturer's instructions to prevent particulate matter build up or contamination of the suction line.

V.b. Used smoke evacuator filters, tubing, and wands should be considered potentially infectious waste. These used devices should be handled using standard precautions and disposed of as biohazardous waste.[1,4,16,17]

Airborne contaminants produced during laser procedures have been analyzed and are shown to contain gaseous toxic compounds, bioaerosols, and dead and living cell material. At some level, these contaminants have been shown to have an unpleasant odor, cause visual problems for health care personnel, cause ocular and upper respiratory tract irritation, and demonstrate mutagenic and carcinogenic potential.[1] Bacterial and/or viral contamination of smoke plume also has been identified.[23,24]

V.c. Personnel should wear respiratory protection (ie, fit-tested surgical N95 filtering face piece respirator or high-filtration surgical mask) during procedures that generate surgical smoke as secondary protection against residual plume that has escaped capture by local exhaust ventilation.[4]

Local exhaust ventilation is the first line of protection from surgical smoke.[1,27]

Analysis of the airborne contaminants produced during laser surgery has shown that laser plume contains toxic gas and vapors (eg, benzene, hydrogen cyanide, formaldehyde); bioaerosols; dead and living cell material, including blood fragments; and viruses.[1,16-18]

Many additional hazardous chemical compounds have been noted in surgical smoke.[17-22]

V.c.1. High-filtration face masks should not be used as the first line of protection against surgical smoke inhalation or as protection from chemical or particulate contaminants found in surgical smoke plume.[1,27]

A surgical mask is intended to prevent the release of potential contaminants from the user into their immediate environment. It also is used to protect the wearer from large droplets, sprays, and splashes of body fluids.[28] High-filtration face masks are specifically designed to filter particulate matter that is 0.1 micron in size and larger. Virus particles range from about 0.01 to 0.3 micrometers.[19] Surgical and high filtration masks do not seal the face and may allow dangerous contaminants to enter the health care worker's breathing zone.[28]

A recent laboratory study of five surgical masks with bacterial filtration efficiency of 95% to 99% found that 80% to 100% of subjects failed an OSHA-accepted qualitative fit test using Bitrex (ie, a bitter tasting aerosol) and quantitative fit factors ranged from 4 to 8 (12% to 25% leakage) using a TSI Portacount.[29] In contrast, the least protective type of respirator (ie, negative pressure half mask) must have a fit factor (outside particle concentration divided by inside concentration) of at least 100 (1% leakage). A high-filtration mask provides less protection than a fit-tested N95 filtering face piece respirator.[30]

Research is pending to test the efficacy of high-filtration masks and the air quality and quantity of airborne contaminants resulting from varying energy devices (eg, laser, electrosurgery, ultrasonic).

V.c.2. Respiratory protection that is at least as protective as a fit-tested surgical N95 filtering face piece respirator should be considered for use in conjunction with LEV in disease transmissible cases (eg, human papillomavirus)[23,24,31] and during high-risk or aerosol transmissible disease procedures (eg, tuberculosis, varicella, rubeola).[32]

A fit-tested surgical N95 filtering face piece respirator is a personal protective device that is worn on the face, covers at least the nose and mouth, and is used to reduce the wearer's risk of inhaling hazardous airborne particles including infectious agents.[28] The NIOSH respirator approval regulation defines the term *N95* to refer to a filter class that removes at least 95% of airborne particles during "worse case" testing using a "most-penetrating" sized particle during NIOSH testing.[28] Filters meeting the criteria are given a 95 rating. Many filtering face piece respirators have an N95 class filter and those meeting this filtration performance are often referred to simply as N95 respirators.[28]

Recommendation VI

All people in the laser treatment area should be protected from electrical hazards associated with laser use.

Lasers may use high voltage electrical current.[7] Electrocutions and accidental shock of personnel have been reported.[3]

VI.a. The LSO should approve laser systems and equipment after they are evaluated for electrical hazards and before they are placed in service.

The LSO is responsible for administration and oversight of laser hazards.[1]

VI.b. The manufacturer's directions for laser installation, operation, and maintenance should be followed.

Some laser systems require special utilities (eg three-phase, 208 VAC, 50 ampere service).[3]

VI.b.1. The manufacturer's recommendations for electrical plugs and outlets should be followed.[3,4]

VI.c. The electrical cord and plugs of the laser should be handled in a manner that minimizes the potential for damage and subsequent patient and health care personnel injuries.

Improper handling of cords and plugs may result in breaks in the cord's insulation, fraying, and other electrical hazards.

VI.c.1. The electrical cord should be free of kinks, knots, and bends.

Kinks, knots, and bends damage the cord and cause current leakage, current accumulation, and overheating of the cord's insulation.

VI.c.2. The laser plug, not the cord, should be held when it is removed from the outlet.

Pulling on the cord may cause cord breakage, which poses a fire hazard.

VI.c.3. The laser cord and plug should be kept dry.[3]

Fluids in or around the laser connection and cord may cause an electrical hazard as a result of a short circuit.

VI.c.4. The laser's cord should be inspected before use or electrically tested for outer insulation damage.[3]

Cord failures can result in electrical shock, sparking, or a fire, which could injure the patient or health care personnel.

VI.d. Liquids should not be placed on laser units.[4,7]

Lasers are high-voltage equipment that should be protected against short circuiting associated with spillage or splatter.[4,7]

VI.e. Laser service and preventive maintenance in accordance with the manufacturer's guidelines should be performed on a regular basis by trained personnel who have knowledge of laser systems.[3]

Periodic preventive maintenance helps to support continued safe operation of laser devices.[1]

VI.e.1. The laser safety officer should review maintenance documents before allowing any laser to be reentered into service.

Recommendation VII

All people in the laser treatment area should be protected from flammable hazards associated with laser use.

Fire is a potential hazard of laser use.[3,4,8,11,33-35] The intense heat of laser beams can ignite combustible or flammable solids, liquids, and gases.[34] The presence of increased oxygen concentrations enhances combustion and leads to the rapid spread of flames.

VII.a. Fire safety measures should be followed when lasers are in use according to local, state, and federal regulations.[36,37]

Lasers are a potential ignition and fire source in the perioperative environment.[11]

VII.a.1. The laser should not be activated in the presence of flammable agents (eg, antimicrobial skin prep or hand antisepsis agents, tinctures, de-fatting agents, collodion, petroleum-based lubricants, phenol, aerosol adhesives, uncured methyl methacrylate) until the agents are dry and vapors have dissipated.[11,33,38-41]

Alcohol-based prep agents remain flammable until they are completely dry. Vapors occurring during evaporation also are flammable. Trapped solution or vapors under clear, adhesive, or surgical drapes increases the risk of fire or burn injury.[40] Alcohol-based skin prep agents are particularly hazardous because the surrounding hair or fabric can become saturated.

Pooling can occur in body folds and crevices (eg, umbilicus, sternal notch).

Ignition of flammable substances by lasers has caused fires and patient injuries. Flammable prep agents can be safely used by adhering to National Fire Protection Agency standards, local fire codes, and AORN recommendations and guidance statements.

Use of nonflammable prep agents will minimize this risk.[20,37,38,41]

VII.a.2. Caution should be used when using a laser in the presence of combustible anesthetic gases during surgery on the head, face, neck, and upper chest.[11,34,39,42]

The intense heat of laser beams can ignite combustible or flammable solids, liquids, and gases.[34] The presence of increased oxygen concentrations enhances combustion and leads to the rapid spread of flames.[42]

VII.a.3. When using a laser, sponges and drapes near the surgical site should be kept moist.[3,4,11,27,33,35,43,44]

In an oxygen-enriched environment, the high energy delivery of a laser will burn anything combustible or flammable.[11,44] The fire triangle requires an ignition source (eg, the laser); an oxidizer (eg, the oxygen enriched environment); and fuel (eg, surgical drapes). Moistening draping materials decreases the potential for fire.[4]

VII.a.4. During perineal surgery, moistened radiopaque sponges may be used for rectal packing or covering the anus.[1,4,7]

Moist packing prevents the release of methane gas from the rectum. Methane gas is highly flammable and potentially explosive.[3,4,7]

VII.b. Laser surgery should not be performed in an oxygen-enriched environment.[11,34]

An oxygen-enriched environment lowers the temperature and energy at which fuels will ignite.[8,33,40,42] Fires, including airway fires, have resulted from the laser sparking in the presence of concentrated oxygen.[8]

VII.b.1. The lowest possible oxygen concentration that provides adequate patient oxygen saturation should be used.[1,4,33,35,38,43,45-47]

Mixing oxygen with nonflammable gases such as medical air or helium reduces the risk of fire.[1,11,47,48]

VII.b.2. Surgical drapes should be arranged to minimize the buildup of oxidizers (eg, oxygen, nitrous oxide) under the drapes.[11,33,35,42,43]

VII.c. Personnel should be prepared to immediately extinguish flames should they occur.[11]

A small fire can progress to a life-threatening emergency in seconds. Lasers are a potential ignition source and a common cause of surgical fires and patient injury.[11]

VII.c.1. Wet towels and saline should be available on the sterile field to extinguish a fire should one occur.[4,6]

VII.d. Fuel risks should be minimized.[11]

Many of the materials and solutions used in the perioperative setting are potential fuel sources (eg, prepping agents, linens, dressings, ointments, anesthesia components).[11]

VII.d.1. Flammable prep solution should have enough time to evaporate before drapes are applied.[11,43]

Prep solutions can be absorbed into linens and body fibers (eg, hair). Alcohol-based skin prep vapors can become trapped under drapes and coverings, and the volatility of these vapors can increase the risk of surgical drape fires.[11]

VII.d.2. Pooled solutions should be removed or patted dry.[4,11]

VII.e. The LSO should determine the type of extinguisher needed for each specific laser based on manufacturers' suggestions.[44]

VII.e.1. Fire extinguishers and saline should be immediately available where lasers are used.[1,4,7]

Immediate action can reduce the magnitude of injury.[1]

VII.f. Laser-resistant endotracheal tubes should be used to minimize the potential for fire during laser procedures involving the patient's airway or aerodigestive tract.[1,7,8,10,11,34,35,42,43,49]

Polyvinylchloride (PVC), silicone, and red rubber endotracheal tubes are combustible.[1,4,8,34,49] Burned PVC produces hydrochloric acid and harmful vapors.[1,42] Burned red rubber tubes produce carbon monoxide.[1] An airway fire may result in damage to the trachea and lungs, severe injury, and death.[8,49]

VII.f.1. Endotracheal tube cuffs should be inflated with normal saline during laser procedures involving the patient's airway or aerodigestive tract.[1,4,8,11,43,49,50]

VII.f.2. Saline with dye (eg, methylene blue) in the endotracheal tube cuff should be used to enhance the detection of a cuff puncture.[4,8,11,42,43,49,50]

Using saline with dye in the endotracheal tube cuff helps perioperative personnel recognize punctures and take immediate action.[43,49,50] The saline also provides a means of heat transfer and fire suppression.[50]

VII.f.3. Moistened packs may be placed around the endotracheal tube. These packs should be kept moist throughout the procedure.[1,11,43]

VII.f.4. Health care personnel should be aware of other flammable items associated with endotracheal tube use during laser procedures. These include, but are not limited to,
- plastic items (eg, breathing circuit, airway, suction catheter);[11,34,49]
- adhesive tape;[11] and
- ointment or lubricant.[11,34,49]

VII.g. The airway fire management procedure should be posted in laser treatment areas.[49]

Immediate action is required if an airway fire occurs. An airway fire can damage a patient's lungs almost immediately.[49]

VII.h. Surgical fires should be reported as a sentinel event to the appropriate agency (eg, FDA, state health department, certifying body, local fire department, ECRI).[43,51]

Reporting surgical fires raises awareness about hazards and adds to the body of prevention knowledge.[52]

Recommendation VIII

Personnel working in laser environments should demonstrate competency commensurate with their responsibilities. Education programs should be specific to laser systems used and procedures performed in the facility.

Initial education on the underlying principles of laser safety and laser biophysics provides direction for personnel in providing a safe environment. Additionally, periodic educational programs provide reinforcement of principles of laser technology and new information on changes in technology, its application, compatibility of equipment and accessories, and potential hazards.

VIII.a. Personnel working in a laser environment should have knowledge of the established laser safety program.

The laser safety education program should provide health care personnel with a thorough understanding of laser procedures and the technology required for establishing and maintaining a safe environment during laser procedures. Laser education and training gives direction for personnel working in or near laser use areas and provides a safe environment for the patient and health care personnel.

VIII.a.1. Program criteria and content should be in accordance with applicable standards; the facility's policies and procedures; and federal, state, and local regulations.

VIII.a.2. Personnel should be required to demonstrate laser competency periodically and when new laser equipment, accessories, or safety equipment is purchased or brought into the practice environment.

VIII.a.3. The laser safety program should provide participants with a thorough understanding of laser procedures and the technology required for establishing and maintaining a safe environment during laser procedures.

VIII.b. The LSO should be qualified through education and experience to administer the laser safety program.[1]

Laser education and training gives direction for the LSO to provide a safe environment for the patient and health care personnel.

VIII.b.1. The LSO should have education and experience in laser operations, clinical applications, and safety.[5]

VIII.b.2. Laser safety officer education and preparation should include, but not be limited to,
- completion of a formal medical laser safety course,
- completion of a formal medical laser safety officer course,
- certification as a medical laser safety officer, and
- previous laser operator work experience.

VIII.c. The LSS and laser assistant (eg, laser nurse, technician) should be qualified by education and training.[1]

Laser education and training gives direction for the laser operator to provide a safe environment for patients and health care personnel.

VIII.c.1. Laser assistant training should include, but not be limited to,
- laser operation principles;[5]
- laser biophysics;
- clinical applications;[5]
- potential risks to the patient and health care personnel;[5]
- safety procedures;[3,5]
- care of the laser, safety equipment, and accessories;[5] and
- hands-on use of the laser (eg, set-up, testing, control panel use).[5]

VIII.d. Personnel using lasers should be knowledgeable about the fire hazards associated with laser use.[34]

Fire is a potential hazard of laser use.[8,11,33,35] The intense heat of laser beams can ignite combustible or flammable solids, liquids, and gases.[34] The presence of increased oxygen concentrations during surgery enhances combustion and leads to the rapid spread of flames.

Flammable and combustible items in the laser environment include
- liquids (eg, alcohol-based skin prep solutions);[11,44]
- ointments (eg, petroleum- or oil-based lubricants);[11,44]
- gases (eg, oxygen, methane, anesthetic agents, alcohol vapor);[11]
- plastics;[44]
- paper or gauze materials;[8]
- surgical drapes;[4,11,44]
- foam positioning devices;
- adhesive tape;[11] and
- endotracheal tubes.[8,11,34,44]

VIII.d.1. Emergency fire drills should be performed at least once a year with the entire perioperative team, including anesthesia care providers.[43,44] Airway fire management should be included in fire drills.[49] Fire extinguisher training should be included as part of the health care organization's fire plan.[44]

VIII.e. Administrative personnel should assess and document initial and annual competency of personnel in the safe use of lasers and the accessories for each type of laser used.[4]

A competency assessment provides a record that personnel have a basic understanding of laser technology, its risks, and appropriate corrective actions to take in the event of a fire or injury. This knowledge is essential to minimize the risks of equipment misuse and to provide a safe environment of care.

Recommendation IX

Policies and procedures for laser surgery should be developed, reviewed periodically, revised as necessary, and readily available in the practice setting.[5]

Policies and procedures assist in the development of patient safety protocols, as well as quality assessment and improvement activities. Policies and procedures establish authority, responsibility, and accountability within the facility. They also serve as operational guidelines that are used to minimize patient risk factors, standardize practice, direct staff members, and establish guidelines for continuous performance improvement activities.

IX.a. Policies and procedures for laser safety should be developed with regard to individual practice settings, applicable standards, and federal and state regulations.

Policies and procedures define administrative, engineering, and procedural control measures for beam and non-beam hazards.[1]

IX.a.1. Policies and procedures for laser use should include, but not be limited to, the following:
- equipment checks before initial use,[1]
- equipment maintenance schedules,
- safety features required on the laser,
- reporting and impounding malfunctioning equipment,[9]
- injury reporting,
- precautions during use,
- fire safety,
- laser sanitation, and
- documentation of laser procedure.

IX.b. The health care organization's policies and procedures for laser surgery must be in compliance with the Safe Medical Devices Act of 1990, as amended in March 2000.[5,53]

The Safe Medical Device Act requires personnel at the facility where the device is used to report deaths and serious injuries caused or contributed by a device, to establish and maintain adverse event files, and to submit follow-up and summary reports to the FDA.[53]

IX.b.1. Incidents of patient or personnel laser injury or equipment failure should be reported as required by regulation to federal, state, and local authorities and to the equipment manufacturer.[9] Device identification, maintenance and service information, and adverse event information should be included in the practice setting report.

Documentation of details of the laser equipment allows for retrievable information for investigation into an adverse event.[9]

IX.c. A written fire prevention and management policy and procedure should be developed by a multidisciplinary group that includes all categories of perioperative personnel.[37]

Fire is a risk to both patients and health care workers in the perioperative setting. Fire is a potential hazard of laser use.[4,8,11,33-35] The intense heat of laser beams can ignite combustible or flammable solids, liquids, and gases.[34] The presence of increased oxygen concentrations during surgery enhances combustion and leads to the rapid spread of flames.

IX.c.1. The policy and procedure should describe processes to be implemented to safely manage different fire scenarios.

IX.c.2. The policy and procedure should include the roles and responsibilities of the perioperative team responding to fire.[11,44]

IX.d. A health care organization-specific policy and procedure should be developed by a multidisciplinary team to describe actions to take in the event of an airway fire.[4,7,51]

Airway fires are life-threatening emergencies.[7] Quick action may minimize consequences.

IX.d.1. The airway fire policy and procedure should include, but not be limited to, the following actions:
- removing the endotracheal tube while simultaneously disconnecting the breathing circuit;[7,11,43]

- turning off the oxygen;[7,11,43]
- pouring saline into the airway;[43]
- removing all flammable and burning substances from the airway;[43,50]
- re-establishing the airway initially using air and then switching to oxygen when the anesthesia care provider determines there is no burning in the airway;[11]
- assessing the airway for damage with a bronchoscope;[7,11]
- performing a tracheostomy if the patient cannot be reintubated or as necessitated by the patient's condition;[7]
- assessing the patient for follow-up care (eg, admission to an intensive care unit for observation and further evaluation);[7,43] and
- saving all involved materials for investigation.[11]

Recommendation X

Documentation should be completed to enable the identification of trends and demonstrate compliance with regulatory and accrediting agency requirements.

Documentation of all nursing activities performed is legally and professionally important for clear communication and collaboration between health care team members and for continuity of patient care.

X.a. Documentation data elements regarding the laser procedure should include, but not be limited to, the following:
- patient information;[1]
- type of laser used (eg, wavelength, serial or biomedical number);
- laser settings and parameters;[1]
- safety measures implemented during laser use;[1]
- surgical procedure;[1]
- on/off laser activation and de-activation times for head, neck, and chest procedures; and
- patient protection (eg, eyewear, eye shield).[1]

Documentation provides communication among all care providers involved in planning and implementing patient care.

X.b. A laser safety checklist should be used.[1,5,7]

A laser safety checklist helps ensure that all safety measures have been implemented.[1,5,7]

X.b.1. A laser safety checklist includes, but is not limited to the following activities
- performing a laser self-test check before the patient is brought into the room,
- calibrating the laser if needed,
- conducting a test fire of the laser,
- posting "laser in use" signs at all entrances of the procedure room,
- providing appropriate eyewear,
- covering the windows of the procedure room as needed,[1]
- checking the availability of saline at the surgical field, and
- checking the appropriate type of fire extinguisher for the laser being used.

X.c. A laser log may be used as an adjunct to the perioperative documentation.

The laser log may serve as a reporting mechanism for
- collecting statistics,
- tracking types of procedures,
- identifying deviations from policies and procedures, and[1,7]
- usage trends.

X.c.1. Data that may be tracked with a laser log can include the
- individual patient's identification information;
- type of laser, its model number, serial number, and health care organization biomedical number;
- procedures performed with laser surgery;
- names of the personnel in the room;
- completed laser safety checklists;
- number of joules used;
- total energy used; and
- wattage used.[1,7]

X.d. Service and maintenance activities should be documented.

Documentation of actions taken to ensure the reliability and safe operation of lasers assists the LSO in maintaining a safe laser environment. Recurring problems can be detected and solved with appropriate follow-up.[1]

Recommendation XI

A quality assurance and performance improvement process should be in place to measure patient, process, and structural (eg, system) outcome indicators.

A fundamental precept of AORN is that it is the responsibility of professional perioperative RNs to provide safe, high-quality nursing care to patients undergoing operative and invasive procedures.[54]

XI.a. A laser safety audit of the health care organization and safety equipment should be completed at least annually or more frequently as determined by the LSO.[1]

A laser safety audit validates the testing of the equipment and the presence of protective safety measures (eg, glasses, smoke/plume evacuation, warning signs).[1]

XI.a.1. The safety audit should include, but not be limited to,
- examining all laser-related equipment and safety features (eg, eyewear, warning signs, smoke plume evacuation equipment, inspection stickers);[1]
- examining laser use areas;
- assessing staff members' knowledge of laser safety; and
- observing laser practices for compliance with the health care organization's written policies and procedures.

XI.a.2. The safety audit should be documented according to health care organizational policy.[1] The written report should include identified deficits and describe a proposed correction plan.

XI.b. A medical surveillance program should be established for health care personnel participating in laser use.

A medical surveillance program provides a baseline of visual acuity and documents physical changes that occurred after an abnormal exposure.[1]

XI.b.1. A physician should perform an examination of the affected body part as soon as possible after a suspected or confirmed laser-induced injury.[1]

XI.c. Incidents of failure to follow the health care organization's laser safety policy, laser and related equipment failure, and patient or personnel injury should be reported to the LSO and reviewed by the laser safety or safety committee.[1,9]

All laser accidents require reporting and follow-up.[1,53]

XI.d. Laser devices should be tested or assessed before initial use, inspected periodically, and undergo preventive maintenance by a designated, trained individual who is responsible for laser equipment maintenance (eg, biomedical engineering services personnel).[3]

Periodic preventive maintenance helps support continued safe operation of laser devices.[3,44]

Glossary

American National Standards Institute: Organization that provides guidance for the safe use of lasers for diagnostic and therapeutic uses in health care facilities. ANSI facilitates the development of consensus US standards and administers a system that assesses conformance to standards such as the ISO 9000 (quality) and ISO 14000 (environmental).

Anodized: A matte finish applied to metal surgical instruments to decrease reflectivity.

Authorized laser operator: A person educated and trained in laser safety and approved by the facility to operate the laser.

Class 3 laser: Lasers that are potentially hazardous for direct exposure to specular (ie, mirror-like) reflection.

Class 4 laser: Lasers that present significant skin and fire hazards. Most surgical lasers are class 4 lasers.

Controlled access area: The area where the laser is to be used. Access to this area is restricted to laser team members and/or those given permission to enter the area. Access is granted only to those who have been approved by the laser safety officer.

Corneal eye shield: A device placed over the eye to protect the cornea from self-induced trauma, such as rubbing, pressure, or excessive use.

Ebonized: A black finish applied to metal surgical instruments to decrease reflectivity.

Fire/flame retardant: A substance that by chemical or physical action reduces flammability of combustibles.

Health care laser system: A system used in health care applications that includes a delivery apparatus to direct the output of the laser, a power supply with control and calibration functions, a mechanical house with interlocks, and associated fluids and gases required for the operation of the laser.

High-efficiency particulate air filter (HEPA): Filters composed of a material of randomly arranged fibres having a filtration rating of 0.3 microns at 99.7% efficiency.

High filtration masks: Masks having a filtering capacity of particulate matter at 0.3 microns to 0.1 microns in size.

Laser: A device that produces an intense, coherent, directional beam of light by stimulating electronic or molecular transitions to lower energy levels. An acronym for "light amplification by stimulated emission of radiation."

Laser assistant: The person who sets up the laser and runs the laser console to control the laser parameters under the supervision of the laser user.

Laser-generated airborne contaminants: Particles, toxins, and steam produced by vaporization of target tissues.

Laser safety officer: Person responsible for effecting the knowledgeable evaluation of laser hazards and authorized and responsible for monitoring and overseeing the control of such laser hazards.

Laser safety specialist: The designated person responsible for oversight of safe laser use in each area where a laser is used. Synonym: laser resource nurse.

Laser treatment area: Area in which the laser is being operated.

Laser user: The person employing the laser for its intended purpose within the user's scope of practice, education, and experience. Synonym: laser operator.

Limiting-exposure duration: The length of time for which tissue can be exposed to the laser beam. This duration is determined by the design and/or intended use of the laser.

Maximum permissible exposure: The level of laser radiation to which a person may be exposed without hazardous effects of adverse biologic changes in his or her eyes or skin.

Nominal hazard zone: The space in which the level of direct, reflected, or scattered radiation used during normal laser operation exceeds the applicable maximum permissible exposure. Exposure levels beyond the boundary of the nominal hazard zone should be below the appropriate maximum permissible exposure level of the laser. Special eye and skin precautions must be enforced in the nominal hazard zone.

Optical density: Ability to absorb a specific laser wavelength.

Oxygen-enriched environment: Atmosphere containing more than 21% oxygen, frequently occurring in the oropharynx, trachea, lower respiratory tract, and near the head and neck during administration of oxygen to the patient.

Ultra low particulate air (ULPA) filter: Theoretically, a ULPA filter can remove from the air 99.9999% of bacteria, dust, pollen, mold, and particles with a size of 120 nanometers or larger.

REFERENCES

1. *Z136.3-2005: Safe Use of Lasers in Health Care Facilities*. Washington, DC: American National Standards Institute; 2005.

2. *Z136.1-2007: Safe Use of Lasers*. Washington, DC: American National Standards Institute; 2007.

3. Annex D. The safe use of high-frequency electricity in health care facilities. In: *Health Care Facilities Handbook*. 10th ed. Quincy, MA: National Fire Protection Association; 2005.

4. Houck PM. Comparison of operating room lasers: uses, hazards, guidelines. *Nurs Clin North Am*. 2006; 41(2):193-218, vi.

5. ECRI. Laser safety. *Healthcare Risk Control*. 2008;1(January):1-14.

6. Baxter DA. Laser safety in the operating room. *Insight*. 2006;31(4):13-14.

7. Andersen K. Safe use of lasers in the operating room—what perioperative nurses should know. *AORN J*. 2004;79(1):171-188.

8. Patient Safety Authority. Airway fires during surgery. *PA-PSRS Patient Safety Advisory*. 2007;4(1):1, 4-6.

9. ECRI. Investigating device-related skin "burns." *ORRM*. 2006;2(Quality Assurance/Risk Management 3): 1, 3-10.

10. Muller GJ, Berlien P, Scholz C. The medical laser. *Medical Laser Application*. 2006;21:99-108.

11. New clinical guide to surgical fire prevention. *Health Devices*. 2009;38(10):314-332.

12. Occupational Health and Safety Administration. 29 CFR § 1910.132-134: General requirements; eye and face protection; respiratory protection; 2008.

13. Medical surveillance (rationale). In: *Environmental Health Criteria 23: Lasers and Optical Radiation*. Geneva, Switzerland: World Health Organization;1982:132.

14. Suess MJ, Benwell-Morrison DA. *Nonionizing Radiation Protection*. 2nd ed. Copenhagen; Albany, N.Y.: World Health Organization, Regional Office for Europe; distributed by WHO Publications Centre USA; 1989.

15. Bigony L. Risks associated with exposure to surgical smoke plume: a review of the literature. *AORN J*. 2007;86(6):1013-20; quiz 1021-4.

16. ECRI Institute. Smoke evacuation systems, surgical. *Healthcare Product Comparison System*. November 2007.

17. NIOSH Hazard Control HC11: Control of smoke from laser/electric surgical procedures. *http://www.cdc.gov/niosh/hc11.html*. Accessed October 6, 2010.

18. Alp E, Bijl D, Bleichrodt RP, Hansson B, Voss A. Surgical smoke and infection control. *J Hosp Infect*. 2006;62(1):1-5.

19. Ulmer BC. The hazards of surgical smoke. *AORN J*. 2008;87(4):721-34, quiz 735-8.

20. Barker SJ, Polson JS. Fire in the operating room: a case report and laboratory study. *Anesth Analg*. 2001;93(4):960-965.

21. Hoglan M. Potential hazards from electrosurgery plume—recommendations for surgical smoke evacuation. *Can Oper Room Nurs J*. 1995;13(4):10-16.

22. Occupational Safety and Health Administration, Hospital eTool: Surgical Suite—Use of Medical Lasers. *http://www.osha.gov/SLTC/etools/hospital/surgical/lasers.html*. Accessed October 5, 2010.

23. Garden JM, O'Banion MK, Shelnitz LS, et al. Papillomavirus in the vapor of carbon dioxide laser-treated verrucae. *JAMA*. 1988;259(8):1199-1202.

24. Hallmo P, Naess O. Laryngeal papillomatosis with human papillomavirus DNA contracted by a laser surgeon. *Eur Arch Otorhinolaryngol*. 1991;248(7):425-427.

25. Occupational Safety and Health Act of 1970, S 2193, 91st Cong (1970). Pub L No. 91-596, 84 Stat 1590. Amended January 1, 2004.

26. Safety and health topics: laser hazards. *http://www.osha.gov/SLTC/laserhazards*. Accessed October 6, 2010.

27. Part 8: Guidelines for the safe use of laser beams on humans. In: *IEC TR 60825-8: Safety of Laser Products*. 2nd ed. Geneva, Switzerland: International Electrotechnical Commission; 2006.

28. Respirator trusted-source information page. National Institute for Occupational Safety and Health. *http://www.cdc.gov/niosh/npptl/topics/respirators/disp_part/RespSource.html*. Accessed October 6, 2010.

29. Oberg T, Brosseau LM. Surgical mask filter and fit performance. *Am J Infect Control*. 2008;36(4):276-282.

30. Derrick JL, Li PT, Tang SP, Gomersall CD. Protecting staff against airborne viral particles: in vivo efficiency of laser masks. *J Hosp Infect*. 2006;64(3):278-281.

31. Garden JM, O'Banion MK, Bakus AD, Olson C. Viral disease transmitted by laser-generated plume (aerosol). *Arch Dermatol*. 2002;138(10):1303-1307.

32. Siegel JD, Rinehard E, Jackson M, Chiarello L; the Healthcare Infection Control Practices Advisory Committee. *2007 Guideline for Isolation Precautions: Preventing Transmission of Infectious Agents in Healthcare Settings*. Atlanta, GA: Centers for Disease Control and Prevention; 2007. *http://www.cdc.gov/hicpac/pdf/isolation/Isolation2007.pdf*. Accessed October 6, 2010.

33. ECRI. Top 10 health technology hazards. *Health Devices*. 2008;November:343-350.

34. Rinder CS. Fire safety in the operating room. *Curr Opin Anaesthesiol*. 2008;21(6):790-795.

35. Daane SP, Toth BA. Fire in the operating room: principles and prevention. *Plast Reconstr Surg*. 2005;115(5):73e-75e.

36. AORN guidance statement: Fire prevention in the operating room. In: *Perioperative Standards and Recommended Practices*. Denver, CO: AORN, Inc; 2009: 195-203.

37. Recommended practices for a safe environment of care. In: *Perioperative Standards and Recommended Practices*. Denver, CO: AORN, Inc; 2010: 217-240.

38. Environment of care. In: *Comprehensive Accreditation Manual for Hospitals*. Oakbrook Terrace, IL: The Joint Commission; 2010.

39. Beesley J, Taylor L. Reducing the risk of surgical fires: are you assessing the risk? *J Perioper Pract*. 2006;16(12):591-597.

40. A clinician's guide to surgical fires. How they occur, how to prevent them, how to put them out. *Health Devices*. 2003;32(1):5-24.

41. *NFPA 99 Standard for Healthcare Facilities*. Quincy, MA: National Fire Protection Association; 2005: 13.4.1.2.2-A.

42. Sheinbein DS, Loeb RG. Laser surgery and fire hazards in ear, nose, and throat surgeries. *Anesthesiol Clin*. 2010;28(3):485-496.

43. American Society of Anesthesiologists Task Force on Operating Room Fires, Caplan RA, Barker SJ, et al. Practice advisory for the prevention and management of operating room fires. *Anesthesiology*. 2008;108(5):786-801, quiz 971-2.

44. National Fire Protection Association. *NFPA 115: Standard for Laser Fire Protection*. 2008 ed. Quincy, MA: National Fire Protection Association; 2008.

45. ECRI. Surgical fires. *ORRM*. 2006;2(Safety 1):1-18.

46. Bielen RP; National Fire Protection Association. Annex C: additional explanatory notes to chapters 1-20. In: *Health Care Facilities Handbook*. Quincy, MA: National Fire Protection Association; 2005:567-568.

47. Podnos Y, Irving CA, Williams R; American College of Surgeons Committee on Perioperative Care. Fires in the operating room. *http://www.facs.org/about/committees/cpc/oper0897.html*. Accessed October 5, 2010.

48. McHenry CR, Berguer R, Ortega RA, Yowler CJ. Recognition, management, and prevention of specific operating room catastrophes. *J Am Coll Surg*. 2004; 198(5):810-821.

49. ECRI. Fighting airway fires. *Healthcare Risk Control*. 2010;4(Surgery and Anesthesia 10):1-5.

50. ECRI. Selecting laser-resistant tracheal tubes [Membership required]. *https://members2.ecri.org/Components/HRC/Pages/SurgAnPol27.aspx*. Accessed April 22, 2010.

51. Beyea SC. Preventing fires in the OR. *AORN J*. 2003;78(4):664-666.

52. The Joint Commission. Preventing surgical fires. *Sentinel Event Alert*. June 24, 2003;29. *http://www.jointcommission.org/SentinelEvents/SentinelEventAlert/sea_29.htm*. Accessed October 5, 2010.

53. Food and Drug Administration. Medical device reporting: manufacturer reporting, importer reporting, user facility reporting, distributor reporting. *Fed Regist*. 2000;654112-4121.

54. Quality and performance improvement standards for perioperative nursing. In: *Perioperative Standards and Recommended Practices*. Denver, CO: AORN, Inc; 2010: 783-792.

Acknowledgements

LEAD AUTHORS

Mary Ogg, MSN, RN, CNOR
Perioperative Nursing Specialist
AORN Center for Nursing Practice
Denver, Colorado

Evangeline Dennis, RN, CNOR, CMLSO
Clinical Manager for Procedural Service
Gwinnett Medical Center
Duluth, Georgia

CONTRIBUTING AUTHORS

Carla M. McDermott, RN, CNOR
Staff Nurse
South Florida Baptist Hospital
Lakeland, Florida

David L. Feldman, MD, MBA, CPE, FACS
American College of Surgeons
Vice President Perioperative Services
Maimonides Medical Center
Brooklyn, New York

PUBLICATION HISTORY

Originally published November 1989, *AORN Journal*. Revised November 1993.

Revised November 1997; published January 1998, *AORN Journal*. Reformatted July 2000.

Revised November 2003; published in *Standards, Recommended Practices, and Guidelines*, 2004 edition. Reprinted April 2004, *AORN Journal*.

Revised October 2010 for online publication in *Perioperative Standards and Recommended Practices*.

The following Recommended Practices for Minimally Invasive Surgery were developed by the AORN Recommended Practices Committee and have been approved by the AORN Board of Directors. They were presented as proposed recommendations for comments by members and others. They are effective December 1, 2009. These recommended practices are intended as achievable recommendations representing what is believed to be an optimal level of practice. Policies and procedures will reflect variations in practice settings and/or clinical situations that determine the degree to which the recommended practices can be implemented. AORN recognizes the various settings in which perioperative nurses practice. These recommended practices are intended as guidelines adaptable to various practice settings. These practice settings include traditional operating rooms (ORs), ambulatory surgery centers, physicians' offices, cardiac catheterization laboratories, endoscopy suites, radiology departments, and all other areas where surgery and other invasive procedures may be performed.

Purpose

These recommended practices are intended to provide guidance to

- perioperative personnel to reduce risks to patients and the perioperative team during minimally invasive surgery (MIS) and computer-assisted technology procedures;
- perioperative registered nurses (RNs) to assist in managing distention media (eg, gas, fluid) and irrigation fluid; and
- health care administrators to identify considerations, including workplace safety and ergonomics, that need to be addressed when expanding services to accommodate new trends.

Flexible endoscopic gastrointestinal procedures are not addressed in these recommended practices. For information on the care and cleaning of instruments and related equipment, refer to the AORN "Recommended practices for care and cleaning of instruments and powered surgical equipment"[1] and "Recommended practices for cleaning and processing flexible endoscopes and endoscope accessories."[2] Implementing or expanding MIS and computer-assisted technologies often requires innovative problem solving, state-of-the art equipment, new relationships between diverse teams, and additional learning requirements for all members of the perioperative team. MIS techniques have evolved from diagnostic techniques to complex operative procedures, primarily because of the documented patient benefits compared to the conventional surgical procedures. Robotic and interventional radiology techniques are examples of computer-assisted trends that continue to evolve and integrate with conventional surgical procedures. Emerging technologies may require construction of new, or renovation of existing, facilities and also may include audio-visual technology transmission to settings outside the traditional walls of the OR.

Recommendation I

A multidisciplinary planning team should be established to develop the design of new construction or renovation of existing ORs to accommodate MIS, interventional radiology, or other computer-assisted technology equipment. The design considerations should include safety; long-term expansion of services; and compliance with federal, state, and local building regulations.

MIS and computer-assisted procedures are frequently performed in a low-light environment and may involve complex equipment interfaces that include numerous cords, plugs, foot switches, and video equipment. Additional equipment for distention media; fluid management systems; radiologic surveillance; and therapeutic applications (eg, lasers, lithotripsy devices, ultrasound) may contribute to distractions or miscommunications that could compromise safety for both the patient and the perioperative team. An effective OR design accommodates ergonomically safe and efficient use of MIS equipment and supplies, while enabling the perioperative clinical team adequate space to work.[3] Trends for technological expansion in perioperative settings often include complex electronic systems, including web-based information systems and robotic fixtures.[3,4] The goals for technological expansion usually include streamlined communications; better resolution and visualization (eg, augmented reality system, three-dimensional images); increased potential for delineating types of tissue (eg, benign, malignant); and a real-time histological analysis of tissues within the operating field.[5] Progressive nanotechnologies (eg, micro-electrical machinery) and miniaturization of robotic components (eg, intracorporeal mobile devices) open the potential for application of surgical procedures in restricted spaces, including single-cell surgery.[4,5] As design trends and MIS technology evolve toward smaller and more remote equipment, it could result in a reduction in the size of the traditional OR in the future.[6] However, in spite of rapid developments toward miniaturization for diagnostics, expansion to allow for oversized equipment is still a common consideration when planning construction or renovation in perioperative settings. Health care facilities may have a variety of reasons other than financial return for expanding to accommodate new technologies (eg, reputation in the community, growing demand from the public and surgeons to provide state-of-the-art minimally invasive techniques). A cost-benefit analysis for expansion to include robotic services may include the following considerations:

♦ Procedure times in the OR may increase initially due to the learning curve with robotic technologies, affecting OR utilization.

♦ Even in an established program, OR productivity may not show increases in efficiency, as robotic procedure times may be the same as conventional techniques.

♦ The benefits to the patient when a robotic system is used may include reduced blood loss, shortened hospitalization, less postoperative pain, and faster return to normal activities.[4,7,8]

♦ The benefits to the surgeon when a robotic system is used may include improved ergonomics, improved visualization including three-dimensional imaging, and stabilization of instruments.[9]

♦ The benefits to the health care organization may include a reduction in length of stay even for patients undergoing more complex procedures with increased patient acuity.

Planning for compliance with local building and zoning codes and state and federal regulations early in the planning stages of a construction or renovation project may prevent costly adjustments later in the project.

I.a. The physical design of the OR, interventional radiology suite, or hybrid OR should allow personnel access to the patient and the surgical field.

I.b. Potential ergonomic hazards specific to MIS and computer-assisted technology should be identified in the design phase of the construction project.[10,11]

Ergonomically positioned monitors help prevent fatigue and musculoskeletal disorders by limiting twisting motions and allowing neck and eye muscles to be relaxed.[12,13] An OR that is too small has restricted walking paths, which increase the risk of slipping, tripping, or falling for members of the perioperative team. An OR that is too large has an increased distance between the supply areas and the surgical field and puts perioperative team members at risk for slipping, tripping, or falling when they have to move quickly across long distances to retrieve supplies or equipment during the procedure.[14-19]

I.b.1. Provisions should be made for preventing slips, trips, and falls.

Floor incongruities of greater than one-fourth of an inch and cords and cables on the floor are factors that increase the risk of slipping, tripping, or falling for members of the perioperative team.[14-19]

I.b.2. Provisions should be made regarding height, hydraulic, or electric mobility and securing ceiling-suspended equipment (eg, booms) to reduce injury risk for the perioperative team.

MIS expansion projects often include physiologic monitors, camera control units, insufflators, and video recording units that are suspended from booms. This allows the premium space around the draped patient to be free of unsterile carts and improves the chances for ergonomic organization of equipment for the sterile surgical team members. Eliminating the need for video carts also allows the unsterile perioperative team members to have fewer obstacles on the floor space and may simplify room cleaning and turnover. The primary disadvantage is the decreased flexibility to move equipment to other rooms.[15,20] Video carts are heavy to move because they have several pieces of equipment on them, increasing the risk of back injury for perioperative team members.[10] Even when ceiling-mounted booms are installed, conventional monitors require heavy-duty booms and substantial physical strength to move.[17] New technologies (eg, flat screen monitors, hydraulic or electric carts and booms) help alleviate the physical strain of moving booms or carts. Securing the monitors to a boom or securing monitors and other equipment to a video cart may prevent injury to patients and personnel as well as damage to equipment.

I.b.3.   Provisions should be made for adequate lighting for the unsterile perioperative team to complete their responsibilities without risk of injury despite the low lighting that is required for optimum visualization for the sterile surgical team during MIS procedures.

Ambient blue or green light enhances the MIS screens and allows adequate visibility for other personnel in the room to work safely.[15] However, contrasts in lighting still may have negative consequences for the unsterile perioperative team when they have to adapt their vision between the amplified illumination of the surgical site and the overall dim OR lighting.[14] A wide range of lighting levels can be provided in the OR by using a ring of fluorescent lights around the diffusers and an outer ring of dimmable down-lights. The fluorescent lights can be designed to have two separate switches: one to control a set of white lights, the other to control a set of green lights that are designed to reduce glare.[15] Indirect or diffused lighting in the OR will provide the sterile surgical team with more flexibility in positioning monitors. Voice-activated switching systems also are available.[14]

I.b.4.   Video vendors and experts in the field of ergonomic safety should be consulted regarding lighting, optimal procedure table height, and location of booms and monitors.

Five design considerations are associated with non-neutral postures during MIS procedures: position of monitor, use of foot pedals, poorly adjusted table height, the hand-held design of laparoscopic instruments, and static body postures.[12] A study conducted in the Netherlands identified five ergonomically

optimal positions and the number of monitors needed for each position when two or three people were scrubbed for the procedure. Each position provided a monitor across from the surgical team member.[17] Ergonomically positioned monitors help prevent fatigue and musculoskeletal disorders by limiting twisting motions and allowing neck and eye muscles to be relaxed.[12,13] Ceiling-suspended monitors that allow monitors to be positioned apart from the rest of the laparoscopic equipment are more versatile when planning ergonomically optimal positions.[21] Research suggests optimal monitor positions include, but are not limited to, the following:

- For the horizontal plane, positioning the monitor straight ahead of the surgical team member, aligned with the forearm-instrument motor axis, will prevent the person from having axial rotation of the spine.
- For the sagittal plane, positioning the monitor lower than eye level, approximately 15 degrees downward, will prevent neck extension.
- For viewing distance, the position of the monitor will depend on the size of the screen. If the monitor is too close, the surgical team member's eyes may undergo extensive accommodation and conversion by the extraocular musculature. If the monitor is too far away, the person may be required to strain and may not be able to see detail.[21]

The amount of glare is another important consideration when positioning monitors. In addition to having high resolution and a high contrast ratio, quality monitors also have a surface material that minimizes the effects of reflected light. Changing the orientation of a monitor (eg, tilt, angle) can create or eliminate glare, which also may be a contributing factor for muscle strain.[14]

I.c.   The extent of OR integration and telecommunication technology should be determined and information system interface requirements identified (eg, compatibility between clinical computer-assisted technologies and administrative computer interfaces).

OR integration involves centralized control of audiovisual equipment and information, and is capable of controlling a variety of equipment and activities within the surgical suite.[20] The evolution of software and equipment integration capabilities may require architectural design adjustments or engineering retrofit to accommodate such things as a control desk and housing for the computer and other equipment. Moving the electronics outside the OR room itself frees up space inside the OR, removes a major source of heat from within the OR, and eliminates the need for electronics technicians to enter the sterile environment of an OR to service the equipment.[22] It can save money to install cabling and other infrastructure to accommodate OR integration during construction or renovation, even if a health care facility does not intend to implement OR integration in phase one of the MIS expansion project.[20]

A central database that allows continuous live feeds throughout the health care facility is another important component for ORs that are designed for MIS procedures. The live feed allows data retrieval after the procedure for educational or reporting purposes, including video clips or still images. Full integration of the entire surgical platform can accommodate coordinated scheduling and interfaces with the electronic medical record and monitoring systems.[22] The terms *integrated OR* or *digital OR* may be used for facilities designed with these capabilities.

Picture archiving and communication systems (PACS) monitors, touch-screen, and voice-activated controls are examples of trends that can be incorporated into an MIS expansion project.[15] The term *de-tethering* refers to wireless technology (eg, wireless communications, laptop computers, network portals, e-mail). Privacy, security, and reliability are issues associated with de-tethering.[23]

I.c.1. Planning should include collaboration with vendors to achieve medical device interoperability and upgrade potential.

Consumer electronics with "plug and play" capability have set an expectation that pieces of medical equipment from various manufacturers have the capacity to "talk to each other." The Center for Integration of Medicine and Innovative Technology (CIMIT) is an example of one nonprofit consortium that has established interdisciplinary teams in the Boston area who work toward this goal.[20]

I.c.2. Remote telecommunications technology requirements should be identified to meet the health care organization's strategic plan.

Robotic technology allows an experienced health care provider to gain physical telepresence to interact with patients or other health care providers in remote locations.[24,25] Telemedicine and telesurgery technology have potential for global application for disaster responses (eg, natural disaster, chemical, biological, nuclear attack, battlefields); regional application for providing expertise and access to rural areas to alleviate shortages in medical and surgical specialties; and intraoperative application for allowing anesthesiologists to provide remote support to nurse anesthetists.[25] Current limitations in wireless broadband requirements and the resulting latency in transmission may prevent broad applications of this technology, but the US Army's Telemedicine and Advanced Technology Research Center (TATRC) continues to fund research in this area.[26] Researchers in Canada have found telementoring and telerobotic technologies to be effective tools for providing care to rural areas; however, reimbursement and legal barriers contribute to delays in widespread application and the goal to achieve a uniform standard of care for MIS procedures in rural areas.[24,27]

I.c.3. Considerations to decrease traffic in teaching institutions should be anticipated (eg, integrated camera systems that provide for internal and external web casts).

Audiovisual components are used by OR staff members in providing patient care, but can also be wired to give interns, residents, and visitors a clear view of surgical procedures without requiring them to be in the room. Reducing traffic during patient care decreases the risk for infection and may reduce distraction and noise for the perioperative team.[20,28]

I.d. Work space and architectural and engineering structures should be designed to accommodate progressive technologies and strategic expansion of MIS and computer-assisted services.

Considering expansion (eg, voice-activated technology, centralized command consoles, two-way video and audio connections) and a progression for increased patient acuity and emergencies in the early stages of the design process can potentially increase the long-term value of the construction project and may prevent the necessity for future renovation.[3,20,29,30] Important considerations for MIS expansion projects include, but are not limited to,

- door placement in relation to the sterile field;
- a modular, structural, ceiling system with multiple mounting locations and a center mounting location reserved for a ceiling-mounted robotic arm;
- placement of the equipment boom(s) on the sterile core side of the room away from the OR door;
- placement of a seated workstation facing the procedure bed and adjacent to the door between the OR and the sterile core; and
- adequate expansion space for future robotic systems.[15]

Space planning advisors also may suggest moving the control desk away from the wall and reducing it in scale to accommodate only monitoring screens and keyboards or adding wheels to provide a movable workstation. This creates a peninsula that allows the perioperative RN to sit at one of the monitors on the desk facing the surgical team, providing more direct observation of all activity during the procedure. It also may allow room for another person to sit at a second monitor with touch-screen controls of the integration system or access to video systems.[22]

I.d.1. The perioperative administrator should investigate the feasibility of constructing a dedicated interventional radiology suite versus a hybrid OR.

A hybrid OR may be used for procedures requiring the combined efforts of a surgeon and an interventional radiologist or cardiologist.[31] They also are intended to improve patient care and efficiency by eliminating the need to transfer the patient from radiology or the cardiac catheterization laboratory to the OR when there is an urgent need for a more invasive surgery.[13] The size of a hybrid suite will depend on the required equipment and additional shielding that the equipment may require based on the manufacturer's specifications. Additional square footage will be needed for storage room (eg, perfusion supplies, cardiopulmonary bypass machine); radiology control room; electrical panels; and equipment cooling devices. Sufficient space and anticipated placement of anesthetic equipment may be required to accommodate modern procedure beds that have a movable table top. When the table top is moved longitudinally, away from the broad part of the procedure bed, the surgeon has better ergonomic access to the patient for an open procedure.[13]

I.d.2. A multidisciplinary team should be identified to delineate the procedures (eg, cardiac, neurological) to be performed in the expanded MIS construction project.

Considerations for composition of the team include, but are not limited to, perioperative RNs, physicians, infection preventionists, and staff member representatives from the appropriate service lines.

I.d.3. The multidisciplinary design team should evaluate the benefits of each type of imaging system (ie, portable versus fixed) when choosing a procedure-related imaging system.

A portable system is beneficial because it allows personnel to move the fluoroscopy unit away from the sterile field when the unit is not in use. A fixed system, however, may have better resolution.[13] The imaging system decision will affect all other decisions, including the equipment and the square footage required.[19]

I.d.4.   Staffing requirements for a hybrid OR should be considered during the design planning phase.

     The perioperative team in a hybrid OR may include the following personnel:

- perioperative circulating nurse,
- radiology circulating nurse,
- surgical scrub person,
- radiology scrub person,
- surgeon,
- surgical first assistant,
- anesthesia care provider(s),
- radiology technician,
- interventional radiologist,
- interventional cardiologist, and
- perfusionist.

     It may be necessary to have additional personnel present to provide safety and efficiency while interacting with multiple services. The surgeon and the interventional cardiologist or radiologist may work simultaneously; therefore, additional staff members may be necessary.[13,32]

I.e.   An infection control risk assessment should be completed before construction or renovation to determine any infection control risks.[33]

     An infection control risk assessment before constructing or remodeling existing health care facilities is a regulatory requirement in most states. MIS expansion projects may require specialized equipment that can raise room temperature and increase the risk of infection, and stakeholders may request that traffic patterns be varied from traditional ORs. It is important to continue thorough planning and coordination to minimize the risk for airborne infection both during and after the completion of the expansion project. An ongoing multidisciplinary team may be necessary to assess infection prevention, safety, and personnel implications.[28,30]

I.e.1.   The OR or procedure room size should be sufficient to accommodate all equipment and allow ease of movement of personnel without compromising the sterile field.

     Large equipment often is needed for MIS and other computer-assisted procedures, which may result in a crowded OR if adequate floor space is not identified in the planning phase of a construction project. The minimum recommended size of a traditional OR is 400 square feet, but this may not be sufficient for MIS rooms. Health care architects currently recommend MIS rooms be at least 600 square feet.[15] Procedures that include computer-assisted or imaging equipment may require an OR in the 750- to 800-square-foot range.[6]

I.e.2.   Manufacturers' recommendations for cleaning and disinfection should be considered when selecting equipment for the MIS expansion project.

     Liquid crystal diodes (LCD), recording devices, plasma video displays, and other electronic equipment may have specific instructions for cleaning from the manufacturer.

I.f.   New and existing air supply, exhaust, and domestic water systems should be assessed for effective adaptation to changing ventilation and fluid management needs in an MIS expansion project.

     Imaging systems and computer-assisted technology may require additional cooling systems. Fluid management systems may involve plumbing and additional specifications regarding waste removal.

I.f.1.   Electrical panels should be assessed and upgraded, as needed, to provide for the maximum possible concurrent use of advanced technologies.

I.f.2.   MIS expansion projects should be built to meet state building code criteria, including, but not limited to,

- air exchanges per hour,
- temperature and humidity control ranges, and
- air flow.

     Regulations for outpatient facilities may have different floor-to-floor height requirements when compared to hospital buildings. However, regulations for outpatient imaging centers may require floor-to-floor heights that are similar to hospital buildings. The same may be true for power; heating, ventilation, and air conditioning (HVAC); plumbing; and fire protection systems.[19] The number of air exchanges for interventional radiology suites, cardiac catheterization rooms, and ORs are required to be a minimum rate of 15 total air exchanges per hour with a recommended range of 20 to 25 air exchanges in ORs.[34]

I.f.3.   State regulations should be followed regarding radiation protection and building requirements for the walls of the entire suite.

The required radiation protection is based on the selected radiology system's specifications. Radiation protection must be built into the walls between the OR and the control room to protect the personnel working in the control room. If required by state regulations, radiation protection must be built into the walls of the entire suite.[34]

Recommendation II

Fluids that will be used for irrigation and as distention media at a temperature other than room temperature should be warmed or cooled and stored in a safe manner.

There is an increased risk for patient injury if fluid storage is not systematically monitored and rotated.[35] Solution stability may vary according to composition.[36] The storage container for the fluid also may undergo changes when stored at temperatures higher or lower than room temperature.[37] Intravenous (IV) bags are among the medical devices listed in a safety assessment from the US Food and Drug Administration regarding safe levels of exposure to di-(2-ethylhexyl)phthalate (DEHP), a compound used as a plasticizer to provide flexibility for polyvinyl chloride (PVC). Expert panels have not reached consensus about the toxic and carcinogenic effects of DEHP in humans exposed to devices that contain them. However, the scientific community does agree that DEHP and other phthalate esters produce adverse effects in experiments with animals.[37]

II.a.   Sterile water should be segregated from other irrigation solutions during storage.

The purpose of segregating sterile water and irrigation solutions is to reduce the risk for errors. Reports indicate IV bags of sterile water were stored near IV bags of 0.9% sodium chloride resulting in the incorrect administration of sterile water intravenously on a dialysis unit. The use of sterile water for continuous irrigation or as a distention media can cause hemolysis if it is absorbed into the bloodstream.[38]

II.b.   Written storage instructions for warming and storing fluids should be obtained from the manufacturer of the fluid and reviewed annually to maintain proper storage protocols.

The manufacturer of the fluid is the best source of information about the duration of time that a fluid can be stored at different temperatures. The expiration date on the solution indicates the duration during which the solution can be used if stored at room temperature. Manufacturers conduct studies to determine how long solutions can be stored at higher temperatures without altering the physical and chemical properties of the solution. The duration for flexible IV bags may be different than the duration for hard plastic pour bottles if DEHP is used in the production process.[37]

II.b.1.   Fluids kept in a warming cabinet should be labeled with an expiration date based on the manufacturer's recommendation for storage above room temperature.

Placing the warming expiration date on the fluid container facilitates communication. Adherence to the manufacturer's instructions for safe temperature ranges will provide stability of the solutions being stored.

II.b.2.   Fluids kept in a warming cabinet should be rotated on a first-in, first-out basis.

This process helps to facilitate turnover of inventory and increases the probability of using fluid containers before the expiration date.

II.b.3.   Unopened fluid containers should be removed from the warming cabinet when the expiration date has been reached.

After removal from the warming cabinet, the irrigation or distention fluid may be used at room temperature until the manufacturer's expiration date has been reached unless information from the manufacturer specifies otherwise.

II.b.4.   After the unopened fluid container is removed from the warming cabinet, a "do not re-warm" label should be applied to the fluid container, and the fluid should not be returned to the warming cabinet.

Heat and moisture enhance microbial growth. Temperature fluctuations may contribute to breakdown of the fluid container. Unless information from the manufacturer specifies otherwise, persistent exposure to heat and variations in temperature could increase the risk for contaminants and container breakdown. A "do not re-warm" label on the fluid container increases the probability of compliance among members of the perioperative team.

II.c. A warming cabinet that is designed to warm fluids and has temperature control settings should be used when it is necessary to store fluids for irrigation or distention media at a temperature higher than room temperature.

Using a warming cabinet designed to warm fluids allows for better monitoring of temperatures specific to the safe ranges identified for the fluids. Thermal injuries have occurred as a result of overheating irrigation fluid or IV fluids.[39,40]

II.c.1. Separate warming cabinets or separate compartments with individual temperature control should be designated for blankets and fluids used for irrigation or distention media.

When fluids are placed in warming cabinets with blankets, there is an increased risk that the fluid will be warmed to an unsafe temperature, especially if the blankets can be safely heated to higher temperatures than the fluids.[35]

II.c.2. The temperature in the warming cabinet should be maintained at the temperature range indicated by the fluid manufacturer.

II.c.3. The warming cabinet temperature should be checked at regular intervals per the organization's policy and documented.[41]

Temperature logs are an indicator that the warming cabinet is functioning properly and is warming fluids within the safe parameters indicated by the fluid manufacturer's specifications. Periodic biomedical inspections and regular preventive maintenance help to keep fluid warming devices in properly functioning condition. Cabinets that are overloaded may not warm fluids uniformly and may not function properly. Follow warming cabinet manufacturers' recommendations for appropriate volume of fluid to be stored.

II.c.4. The warming cabinet should be labeled with the safe temperature range settings for the fluids stored in the warming cabinet as determined by the fluid manufacturer.

Labeling the warming cabinet will help facilitate communication to the perioperative team members about the safe temperature range recommended by the fluid manufacturer.

II.c.5. A microwave or autoclave should not be used to heat irrigation fluids or fluids used for distention media.

Microwaves and autoclaves are uncontrolled methods of warming that could result in an unknown or uneven fluid temperature, increasing the risk of patient injury. Perioperative team members also may be at risk for burns from excessively heating the product or container. The composition of the solution or the container could be at risk when uncontrolled methods of warming are used.

II.d. Fluids used for irrigation should be cooled and stored in a safe manner that prevents contamination and degradation of the solution or container.

The composition of the fluid or container can change with fluctuations in temperature.

II.d.1. Written instructions for storage and cooling fluids should be obtained from the manufacturer of the fluid and reviewed annually.

II.d.2. A systematic rotation and expiration date labeling process should be defined for storing cooled fluids, based on the best available information.

Rotating inventory before the expiration date helps to reduce waste. Expiration dates defining safe duration of time a fluid can be cooled will help to maintain the integrity of the solution and the container and prevent waste.

II.d.3.   Fluids that are being cooled below room temperature should be stored in an area that is designated for patient care items and separate from food.[42]

II.e.   Fluid containers that have been opened and not completely used should be discarded and should not be returned to a storage area.

Opening a fluid container allows air and potential contaminants to enter the container. The edge of a container is considered contaminated after the contents have been poured; therefore, the sterility of the contents cannot be ensured if the cap is replaced or the seal to the IV bag has been broken.[43]

Recommendation III

During the preoperative nursing patient assessment, the perioperative RN should identify unique patient considerations that require additional precautions or contraindications related to MIS procedures, fluid management, and the medications that may be added to irrigation fluids.

Preoperative nursing assessment of patients for specific risk factors related to MIS patient positioning, fluid management, and medication sensitivities before the invasive procedure will facilitate safe patient care.

III.a.   The preoperative patient assessment should include identification of risk factors related to extreme patient positioning that may be required for MIS or computer-assisted procedures.

It is not unusual to have patients in the extreme Trendelenburg or reverse Trendelenburg positions for laparoscopic surgical procedures and procedures involving robotic equipment because the gravitational effect allows organs to move away from the surgical field.[44] The Trendelenburg position increases venous return and increases the risk for cardiac or respiratory congestion. The reverse Trendelenburg position reduces venous return and cardiac output, increases peripheral and pulmonary resistance, and has the potential for misalignment of the patient's extremities.[45]

III.a.1.   The preoperative nursing risk assessment related to positioning for MIS procedures should include, but not be limited to, the following:

- age-specific risk factors,
- cardiovascular compromise,
- respiratory compromise,
- pregnancy, and
- increased intraocular or intracranial pressure.

Older adults who have coexisting cardiac or pulmonary disease are at higher risk during laparoscopic procedures that require general anesthetics, pneumoperitoneum, and extreme positions.[46] Premature infants have compromised cardiovascular, respiratory, and thermoregulatory systems that may not tolerate increased intra-abdominal pressure or the Trendelenburg position.[47] Patients who have increased intracranial pressure, severe myopia, and/or retinal detachment are also at high risk during laparoscopic procedures performed using the Trendelenburg position. Patients who are pregnant, have bullous emphysema, or a history of spontaneous pneumothorax are also at higher risk.[45]

III.a.2.   The preoperative nursing risk assessment related to prevention of venous stasis should include, but not be limited to,

- the type of procedure,
- the position required,
- the length of procedure, and
- a patient history that reflects a need for increased surveillance for deep vein thrombosis (DVT).

Laparoscopic surgery patients who will be in the reverse Trendelenburg position and have pneumoperitoneum are at risk for venous stasis. Patients who are undergoing procedures lasting longer than 30 to 45 minutes are at risk for venous stasis, as are patients whose surgery involves the use of a tourniquet (eg, arthroscopy).[48,49] Patients who are scheduled for longer complex laparoscopic procedures (eg, laparoscopic Roux-en-Y gastric bypass patients) are at a higher risk for DVT.[50] Venous thromboembolism prophylaxis is indicated whenever major abdominal operations are performed; however, there are varying opinions about routine prophylaxis if the laparoscopic procedure does not involve stirrups and is expected to be brief, including cholecystectomy and herniorrhaphy.[51-53] Examples of medical history assessment findings that indicate a need for increased surveillance for DVT include, but are not limited to, the following:

- history or family history of thrombosis, coagulopathy blood clots, blood-clotting disorders, DVT, or pulmonary embolism;
- varicosities or leg swelling;
- smoking; or
- sedentary/nonambulatory lifestyle greater than 72 hours.[48]

III.b. The preoperative nursing risk assessment should include safety considerations for intraoperative magnetic resonance imaging (MRI) when applicable.

Physical contraindications for patients in the MRI environment include, but are not limited to, pacemakers, certain cranial aneurysm clips, and certain implants. Manufacturers of the implant can verify whether it is safe or not safe for the intraoperative MRI environment if there is a question.[32]

III.c. The preoperative nursing risk assessment related to fluid management should include, but not be limited to, the following:

- the patient's skin color and turgor,
- weight,
- allergies and sensitivities to medications,
- NPO status,
- patient conditions or diseases that predispose or exacerbate the seriousness of hyponatremia or hypervolemia, and
- medications that predispose or exacerbate the seriousness of hyponatremia or hypervolemia.

The use of improper or excessive amounts of fluid for irrigation or distention media can lead to hypervolemia and hyponatremia. Patients who have congestive heart failure, liver cirrhosis, and renal diseases are more susceptible to hypervolemia and hyponatremia. The main causes of hyponatremia in hypo-osmolar patients are inappropriate antidiuretic hormone secretion, renal disorders, endocrine deficiencies, and certain medications.[54] Medications that predispose or exacerbate the seriousness of hyponatremia and hypervolemia include, but are not limited to, the following:

- diuretics;
- anticonvulsants (eg, carbamazepine); and
- serotonin and norepinephrine reuptake inhibitors.[54]

Medications may be added to irrigation or fluid used for distention media. Identifying allergies and sensitivities in the preoperative phase of care will facilitate communications and decrease the risk of patient complications in the intraoperative and postoperative phases of care.

III.d. The perioperative RN should review preoperative laboratory tests (eg, electrolytes, coagulation studies) and report abnormalities to the surgeon and anesthesia care provider.

Surgeons or anesthesia care providers may order additional laboratory tests for patients who have identified risk factors related to fluid management or DVT. Identifying electrolyte imbalances, coagulopathy, or other unusual laboratory findings preoperatively provides an opportunity to implement corrective measures or postpone the operative or invasive procedure.

III.e. Fluid selection should be based on the individual patient assessment and the intended use.

The selection of fluid to be used for irrigation or distention media depends on the type of procedure being performed, the patient's condition, and the use of electrosurgery. Fluids are divided into electrolyte and nonelectrolyte media. Nonelectrolyte media can lead to hyponatremia when the irrigation or distention fluid is absorbed into the circulatory system[55] (**Table 1**).

III.e.1. Nonelectrolyte distention fluids should be used when monopolar electrosurgery is the planned equipment for the MIS procedure.

Electrolyte solutions conduct electricity and dissipate the energy transferred. This can result in ineffective hemostasis or collateral thermal tissue damage. When bipolar electrosurgery is used, electrolyte solutions can be used.[56]

III.e.2. Potential contraindications of fluid distention media should be reported to the surgeon and anesthesia care provider for evaluation of significance and appropriate actions to be taken.

Recommendation IV

Personnel should take additional precautions when using electrosurgery units (ESUs) during MIS and computer-assisted procedures.

MIS procedures using electrosurgery present unique patient safety risks, such as direct coupling of current, insulation failure, and capacitive coupling and tissue damage that may be out of the field of vision.[57]

IV.a.   ESUs and accessories should be selected that include technology that minimizes or eliminates the risk of insulation failure and capacitive-coupling injuries.

   During MIS procedures, alternate site injuries have resulted from insulation failure and capacitive coupling.[58-63] These injuries are far more serious than skin burns and have increased in number with the increase in MIS procedures.[64] The use of active electrode monitoring has minimized these risks.[61,63,65-68]

IV.b.   Personnel should verify the properties of the distention media to minimize risks related to electrosurgery.

   Collateral damage secondary to increased temperatures can occur if the distention media conducts current.

IV.b.1.   Personnel should verify that the insufflation gas is nonflammable (ie, carbon dioxide).

   Carbon dioxide is noncombustible and will not ignite if the active electrosurgical electrode sparks. Gases (eg, oxygen, nitrous oxide, air) are oxidizers that may support combustion. An oxidizer-enriched environment may enhance ignition and combustion.[69,70]

IV.b.2.   Nonelectrolyte distention fluids should be used when monopolar electrosurgery is used.

   Electrolyte solutions conduct electricity and dissipate the energy transferred. This can result in ineffective hemostasis or burns to internal tissue.

   Table 1 presents a comparison of the properties of various fluids used for distention media.

IV.c.   Conductive trocar systems should be used.

   Conductive trocar cannulas provide a means for the electrosurgical current to flow safely between the cannula and the abdominal wall. This reduces high density current concentration and heating of non-target tissue.[61,62,65,71,72]

IV.c.1.   Hybrid trocar (ie, combination plastic and metal) systems should not be used.

   Each trocar and cannula can act as an electrical conductor inducing an electrical current from one to the other potentially causing a capacitive-coupling injury.[71]

IV.d.   MIS electrodes should be examined for impaired insulation before use.

   Insulation failure of electrodes caused by damage during use or reprocessing provides an alternate pathway for the electrical current to leave the active electrode. Some insulation failures are not visible. This has resulted in serious patient injuries.[59,61,62,65-67,71-74]

IV.d.1.   Methods should be used to detect insulation failure, including, but not limited to,
- active electrode shielding and monitoring,[65,68]
- using active electrode indicator shafts that have two layers of insulation of different colors,[65]
- using active electrode insulation integrity testers that use high DC voltage to detect full thickness insulation breaks.[65]

   Active electrode shielding continuously monitors the endoscopic instruments to minimize the risks of insulation failure or capacitive-coupling injuries.[59,61-63,66-68,71,72] The inner layer of a different color is designed to show through the outer layer if there is an insulation break.[65] Testing the electrode before the procedure identifies damaged electrodes that should be taken out of service. Testing may be done in the sterile processing department, at the sterile field, or with the sterilizable probes and cables that will alert the surgeon of an insulation break during the procedure. The surgical wound can be explored and treated if an alert occurs during the procedure.[65,74]

IV.d.2.   The lowest power setting that achieves the desired result should be selected.[72]

Table 1

continued on next page

FLUIDS USED FOR IRRIGATION OR DISTENTION MEDIA				
Solution	Electrolyte Solution	Uses	Potential Contraindications	Adverse Reactions
0.9% Sodium Chloride[1]	YES	General irrigation, hysteroscopy, use with laser and bipolar electrosurgery, and urologic procedures[2,3]	Monopolar electrosurgery	Hypervolemia, pulmonary edema, abdominal cramping, nausea and vomiting, diarrhea
Ringer's Lactate[4]	YES	General irrigation	Monopolar electrosurgery	Fluid shift from intracellular to extracellular compartment, hypervolemia
Dextran[1]	NO	Hysteroscopy, volume generally limited to 300 mL and not to exceed 500 mL[5]	Allergy to beet sugar;[5] hypersensitivity to dextran or any component of the formulation; hemostatic defects (eg, thrombocytopenia, hypofibrinogenemia); cardiac decompensation; renal disease with severe oliguria or anuria; hepatic impairment	Plasma expander leading to fluid or solute overload; disseminated intravascular coagulation (DIC), for every 100 mL absorbed, the plasma volume expands by an additional 860 mL;[5] overdose, marked by pulmonary edema, increased bleeding time, and decreased platelet function
Glycine 1.5%[6]	NO	Urologic irrigation, hysteroscopy, and resectoscopy with monopolar electrosurgery[3]	Severe cardiopulmonary or renal dysfunction, decreased liver function; additives may be incompatible, consult with a pharmacist	Aggravated pre-existing hyponatremia caused by shifts from intracellular to extracellular compartment; fluid and electrolyte disturbances (eg, edema, marked diuresis, pulmonary congestion); impaired liver function leading to accumulation of ammonia in the blood; allergic reactions, which are rare
Mannitol 5%[7]	NO	Urologic irrigation; hysteroscopy and resectoscopy with monopolar electrosurgery[3]	Severe cardiopulmonary or renal dysfunction	Aggravated pre-existing hyponatremia caused by shifts from intracellular to extracellular compartment; fluid and electrolyte disturbances (eg, edema, marked diuresis, pulmonary congestion); hypernatremia caused by loss of water and excess of electrolytes from continuous administration

Editor's note: This table presents irrigation solutions that are in common use; however, it is not all-inclusive. Use of other irrigation solutions may be indicated in certain patient populations and for certain conditions.

Lower power settings for both cut and coagulation reduce the likelihood of insulation failure and capacitive-coupling injuries. Lower power settings also minimize damage from direct coupling when the active electrode is activated while in close proximity to another metal device inserted into an adjacent trocar port.[61,72]

IV.e. The active electrode should not be activated until it is in close proximity to the tissue.[61,62]

Activation only when in close proximity to the tissue minimizes the risk of current arcing and contacting unintended tissue.[61,62] Activating the electrode when it is not in very close proximity to the targeted tissue increases the risk of capacitive coupling. Capacitance is reduced during closed-circuit activation.

Table 1 *continued from previous page*

FLUIDS USED FOR IRRIGATION OR DISTENTION MEDIA

Solution	Electrolyte Solution	Uses	Potential Contraindications	Adverse Reactions
Sorbitol 3%[8]	NO	Urological irrigation	Severe cardiopulmonary or renal dysfunction, fructose intolerance	Aggravated pre-existing hyponatremia caused by shifts from intracellular to extracellular compartment; hypernatremia caused by loss of water and excess of electrolytes from continuous administration hyperglycemia in patients with diabetes mellitus; allergic reactions (eg, urticaria)
Sorbitol 3% / Mannitol 0.5%[9]	NO	Urologic irrigation	Severe cardiopulmonary or renal dysfunction; fructose intolerance	Aggravated pre-existing hyponatremia caused by shifts from intracellular to extracellular compartment; hypernatremia caused by loss of water and excess of electrolytes from continuous administration; hyperglycemia in patients with diabetes mellitus; hyperlactatemia in patients who are metabolically compromised caused by metabolism of sorbitol
Sterile Water[10]	NO	General irrigation, washing, rinsing, and dilution purposes; transurethral resection of prostate[11]	Continuous irrigation, as a distention medium; additives may be incompatible, consult with a pharmacist	Hemolysis when absorbed into the bloodstream

1. Lexi-Comp, Inc, AORN. *Drug Information Handbook for Perioperative Nursing.* Hudson, OH: Lexi-Comp; 2006.
2. Ho HS, Cheng CW. Bipolar transurethral resection of prostate: a new reference standard? *Curr Opin Urol.* 2008; 18(1):50-55.
3. ACOG Committee on Practice Bulletins. Endometrial ablation [ACOG Practice Bulletin: Clinical management guidelines for obstetrician-gynecologists, Number 81, May 2007]. *Obstet Gynecol.* 2007;109(5):1233-1248.
4. Lactated Ringer's irrigation [package insert]. Lake Forest, IL: Hospira; 2004.
5. American College of Obstetricians and Gynecologists. Hysteroscopy [ACOG technology assessment in obstetrics and gynecology, Number 4, August 2005]. *Obstet Gynecol.* 2005;106(2):439-442.
6. 1.5% glycine irrigation [package insert]. Lake Forest, IL: Hospira; 1999.
7. 5% mannitol irrigation [package insert]. Irvine, CA: B. Braun Medical, Inc; 2002.
8. 3% sorbitol urologic irrigating solution [package insert]. Deerfield, IL: Baxter Healthcare Corp; 2004.
9. Sorbitol-mannitol irrigation [package insert]. Lake Forest, IL: Hospira; 2004.
10. Sterile water for irrigation [package insert]. Lake Forest, IL: Hospira; 2004.
11. Moharari RS, Khajavi MR, Khademhosseini P, Hosseini SR, Najafi A. Sterile water as an irrigating fluid for transurethral resection of the prostate: anesthetical view of the records of 1600 cases. *South Med J.* 2008;101(4):373-375.

IV.f. Only the user of the active electrode should activate the device whether it is hand- or foot-controlled.[58]

Activation by the user of the active electrode prevents unintentional discharge of the device and minimizes the potential for patient and personnel injury.

IV.g. Bipolar active electrodes (eg, vessel occluding devices) should be used in a manner that minimizes the potential for injuries.

Unlike the monopolar ESU, bipolar technology incorporates an active electrode and a return electrode into a two-poled instrument, such as forceps or scissors.[60,75,76] Current flows only through the tissue contacted between two poles of instruments; thus, the need for a dispersive electrode is eliminated.[76] This also eliminates the chance of stray or alternate pathways for current flow.[76] The bipolar ESU provides precise hemostasis or dissection at the surgical site with less lower voltage and decreased thermal spread to nearby structures.[76]

IV.g.1.   When bipolar resection devices are used, electrolyte solutions should be used.

Bipolar resection devices need an electrolytic solution to conduct the electrical flow.[77]

IV.h.   Argon-enhanced coagulation (AEC) technology poses unique risks to patient and personnel safety and should be used in a manner that minimizes the potential for injury.[57]

Each type of AEC has specific manufacturer's written operating instructions describing safe operation of the unit. The AEC unit uses monopolar alternating current delivered to the tissue through ionized argon gas. The risks of monopolar electrosurgery are present.[78]

IV.h.1.   All safety measures for AEC technology outlined in the AORN "Recommended practices for electrosurgery" should be referenced when using AEC technology.[57]

Patient injury and death have occurred as a complication of argon-enhanced technology. There is a significant risk of gas embolism when AEC is used during laparoscopic procedures from abdominal over-pressurization and displacement of CO_2 by argon gas.[79-82] (See Recommendation VI.i.)

IV.i.   Patients should be instructed to immediately report any postoperative signs or symptoms of electrosurgical injury. Postoperative patient care instructions should include symptoms to look for, including, but not limited to,
- fever,
- inability to void,
- lower gastrointestinal bleeding,
- abdominal pain,
- abdominal distention,
- nausea,
- vomiting, and
- diarrhea.[62]

Symptoms of a minimally invasive electrosurgical injury can occur days after discharge from the perioperative setting and may include infection from an injured intestinal tract. Prompt reporting of electrosurgical injury symptoms ensures timely treatment and minimizes adverse outcomes.[62,73]

IV.j.   Potential hazards associated with surgical smoke generated in the practice setting should be identified, and safe practices established.[57]

Surgical smoke (ie, plume) is generated from use of heat-producing instruments such as electrosurgical devices. Airborne contaminants produced during electrosurgery have been analyzed. The electrosurgery plume contains toxic gas and vapors (eg, benzene, hydrogen cyanide, formaldehyde); bioaerosols; dead and living cell material including blood fragments; and viruses.[83,84] Many additional hazardous chemical compounds have been noted in surgical smoke.[85-89]

At some level, these contaminants have been shown to have an unpleasant odor, cause problems with visibility of the surgical site, cause ocular and upper respiratory tract irritation, and have demonstrated mutagenic and carcinogenic potential.[83] The possibility for bacterial and/or viral contamination of smoke plume remains controversial but has been highlighted by different studies.[90,91]

The National Institute of Occupational Safety and Health (NIOSH) recommends that smoke evacuation systems be used to reduce potential acute and chronic health risks to personnel and patients.[83] The Occupational Safety and Health Administration (OSHA) has no separate standard related to surgical smoke. OSHA addresses such safety hazards in the "General duty clause and bloodborne pathogens standard."[88]

IV.j.1.   Surgical smoke should be removed by use of a smoke evacuation system in both open and laparoscopic procedures.

Potential health and liability risks may be reduced by the evacuation of smoke plume.[92]

IV.j.2.   Surgical smoke should be evacuated and filtered during the laparoscopic procedure and at the end of the procedure when the pneumoperitoneum is released.

Smoke generated in the pneumoperitoneum may be more concentrated than smoke generated from an open surgical procedure if it accumulates in the closed cavity.[93] The risk to the patient due to the exposure to this concentrated smoke is not yet identified. One source reports suppressed cell-mediated intra-abdominal immunity during a laparoscopic procedure with pneumoperitoneum.[93] Port site metastasis, also known as the chimney effect, has been studied in an attempt to understand the capability of electrosurgical smoke serving as a vehicle for transplanting malignant cells to benign tissue.[86,93-95] At the end of the procedure, if the smoke in the pneumoperitoneum is released directly from a cannula and without a filter, the concentrated smoke can expose the perioperative team to contaminants.[86,93]

Recommendation V

Potential injuries and complications associated with MIS and computer-assisted procedures should be identified and practices should be established to reduce risk.

MIS and computer-assisted procedures often involve use and application of complex technologies that may require unique safety precautions.

V.a.   The perioperative team should determine what emergency supplies and equipment should be available before the procedure begins.[96]

In an analysis of complications from retroperitoneoscopic procedures of the urinary tract, researchers found that the rate of complications was dependent on the complexity of the procedure and the learning curve of the surgeon.[97] The risk of conversion from MIS to an open procedure may not always require a double setup for an open procedure. Conversion rates vary according to specific procedures and complexities, ranging from 4.6% to 7.4%.[7,97,98] Historically, 1.2% of the patients undergoing laparoscopic cholecystectomy required conversion to a laparotomy.[99] Injuries to bowel and major blood vessels in gynecology cases range in frequency from 0.05% to 0.14%.[100]

V.b.   Specific positioning devices should be provided to secure the patient and provide safety in accordance with the AORN "Recommended practices for positioning the patient in the perioperative practice setting."[101]

MIS surgery may require exaggerated patient positioning to displace viscera and enhance visibility for the surgical team. More complex procedures are being done with MIS and computer-assisted techniques, consequently the operating procedure time may be prolonged when compared to MIS procedures with lower acuity. Access to the patient may be limited by robotic surgical systems.[102] The patient also may be in extreme positions for extended periods of time, and when a robot is docked to the patient during the procedure, repositioning is improbable, if not impossible.[44,103] Restraints or methods to secure the patient to the procedure bed may be necessary if extreme Trendelenburg or reverse Trendelenburg positions are used.[44] The patient's position may be adjusted to facilitate the surgeon and assistant's view of the monitors and ergonomic access to laparoscopic instruments and accessories. One member of the surgical team may be positioned between the patient's legs when he or she is in the lithotomy position.[21] For surgical reasons, it may be necessary to tuck the patient's arms at his or her sides to make room for other assistants and to avoid moving the armboards to angles of more than 90 degrees.[104] The patient is at risk of injury to the brachial plexus caused by stretching if the arms are positioned in an exaggerated abduction raising them above the head.[105]

V.b.1.   The perioperative RN should initiate actions to reduce the risk of pressure on the patient during MIS and computer-assisted procedures.

There is increased risk of adding pressure on the patient when the robotic arms are brought into position and docked. Static positions are often required in MIS procedures, increasing the risk of personnel leaning on the patient during the procedure.

V.b.2.   The perioperative RN should ensure the patient is undocked from the robotic system before repositioning is initiated.

If the decision is made to reposition the patient during a long procedure using robotic systems, the patient is at risk for injury if proper procedures for docking and undocking are not followed.

V.c. Electrical cords and plugs should be handled in a manner that minimizes the potential for damage and subsequent patient or staff injuries.

Stress on cords that are too short may cause damage to the cord, posing an electrical hazard. Cords that are too short also increase the risk for tripping members of the perioperative team.[41]

V.c.1. Equipment should be placed near the sterile field, with cords reaching the wall or column outlet without stress on a cord.[41]

It may be necessary to consult with the manufacturer and biomedical personnel to change the cord lengths to avoid the use of extension cords. Cords that do not lie flat or are stretched create a risk for tripping, fraying of the cord, or accidental unplugging of the equipment. Use of extension cords can result in excessive current leakage and/or electrical-system overload.[41]

V.c.2. Cords should be free of kinks, knots, and bends that could damage the cord or cause leakage, current accumulation, and overheating of the cord's insulation.[41]

V.c.3. Cords should be removed from use if they are frayed or char debris is noted.

V.c.4. Cords should be kept away from fluids.

Fluids dripping onto the cord or connections cause electrical hazards.[106]

V.d. Protective measures should be implemented to prevent fire or thermal injury. Measures should include, but not be limited to, the following:
- Turn off light sources when they are not in use.
- Hold fiber-optic light cables away from drapes or place on a moist towel.
- Connect all fiber-optic light cables before activating the source.
- Place the light source on standby when disconnecting fiber-optic light cables.
- Allow all flammable prep solutions to dry fully before placing surgical drapes.[41,107]

The heat from fiber-optic light cables or endoscopes may burn the skin and may cause drapes to burn. Hot fiber-optic light cables increase the risk of fire when in contact with flammable materials. A moist towel can help to cool the light cable.[107]

V.e. Fiber-optic light cables should be inspected regularly for broken light bundles before use.

Broken light bundles will diminish the transmission of light and decrease visibility. Having sterile backup cables readily available decreases surgical delays.

V.e.1. Fiber-optic light cables should be long enough to reach from the surgical field to the equipment without undue stress.

Tension increases the risk that the fiber-optic light cables will become disconnected or break, thereby creating a safety hazard for patients and personnel.

V.e.2. A backup fiber-optic light cable should be available and used if broken light bundles are apparent.

V.f. Considerations to prevent surgical site infection should be implemented with all MIS and computer-assisted procedures.

Specialized cells line the peritoneal cavity and serve as the first line of defense for the immune system in the abdomen. This defense system of the peritoneum may be negatively affected by the pneumoperitoneum used in many MIS procedures. This is important because intra-abdominal infections often begin in the peritoneal cavity.[108] The mechanical distension changes the peritoneal microstructure allowing passage of bacteria. This systemic response coupled with the amount of tissue damage and the duration of the procedure may potentially lead to a higher risk for infection.[109]

Single port access laparoscopy and natural orifice transluminal endoscopic surgery (NOTES) are examples of new approaches for MIS procedures. It is important to clarify access points before the surgery to prepare the skin adequately for the incision and for any expanded incisions that might be necessary.[110-116]

V.f.1. Care should be taken when retrieving specimens to prevent cross contamination and ensure complete extraction.

Infection rates for laparoscopic cholecystectomies has been reported to be as low as 0.38 infections per 100 procedures.[117] However, other procedures may have a higher risk of infection from the extraction of an infected appendix or infected cysts through a small incision. In such procedures, there is a need for careful handling with atraumatic grasping forceps or specimen bags to avoid rupture and contamination into the peritoneal space.[118,119] Morcellators may be used to cut up and remove large specimens.[119,120] There is a potential for retained myomas or dissemination of various cancers when using a morcellator.[120]

V.g. Endoscopic trocars and Veress needles should be selected based on safety criteria established for the practice setting.

Catastrophic patient injuries may occur from excessive use of pressure during trocar insertion. Trocar injuries are grouped into three primary groups: vascular, visceral, or the anterior or posterior abdominal wall.[121] There are three techniques used for trocar insertion: direct or blind insertion, Veress needle technique, and the Hasson technique. Risks of gas embolism or formation of subcutaneous or subfascial emphysema are possible when using a Veress needle before insufflation and trocar insertion. The Hasson technique, also known as a "cut down" or "open" technique, exposes the fascia using a scalpel to make a 2-cm to 3-cm skin incision. Shielded trocars also may help to reduce the risk for trocar injuries.[121,122]

V.h. MIS and computer-assisted equipment and accessories should be used in a manner that minimizes the potential for injuries.

V.h.1. Instructions for MIS and computer-assisted equipment use, warranties, and a manual for maintenance and inspections should be obtained from the manufacturer and be readily available to users.

V.h.2. All MIS and computer-assisted equipment should be checked before use.

White balancing may be required for optimum video image for both traditional laparoscopic and robotic surgery. Appropriate lighting for cameras facilitates surgeon and surgical team visualization for the procedure. Voice-activated systems or other technologies that allow the surgeon to control settings may facilitate efficiency during the procedure.[123]

V.i. Data collected during the procedure should be monitored and retrieved before shutting down the video systems.

V.i.1. Video equipment should have adequate memory and retrieval capabilities throughout the procedure and for documentation.

V.j. Special considerations should be implemented for the intraoperative MRI environment.

V.j.1. Equipment and other items should be labeled as safe for use in the MRI environment or secured to minimize the risk for injury.

Metal objects (eg, oxygen tanks, stretchers, surgical instruments) can become projectiles in the MRI environment. It may be necessary to acquire equipment or other items that are composed of titanium, plastic, ceramic, aluminum, or a high-grade nonmagnetic stainless steel. Metal items that remain in an MRI environment can be tethered to the wall or secured in another way that has been tested to prevent patient or perioperative personnel risk for injury.[32]

V.j.2. When in an MRI environment, electrical cords should not cross each other or loop.

Patient burns may result if there is a coil or antenna placed on the patient over an electrical cord (eg, electrosurgical pad, rectal probe).[32]

Recommendation VI

Potential patient injuries and complications associated with gas distention media used during MIS procedures should be identified, and practices that reduce the risk of injuries and complications should be established.

Although endoscopic procedures are minimally invasive from the surgical perspective, the use of CO_2 to establish pneumoperitoneum increases the risk of hypercarbia, hypoxemia, subcutaneous emphysema, pneumothorax, and other hemodynamic changes depending on the patient's medical history.[45,46,124,125] End tidal CO_2 is closely monitored to detect the onset of hypercarbia, especially for patients with compromised pulmonary function.[126]

Nitrous oxide may be beneficial for patients who have depressed pulmonary function and may be advantageous over other gases if an IV embolization occurs.[45,124] The fear of combustion when using nitrous oxide was a topic studied in 1995. The researchers reported that the risk of combustion is low when using nitrous oxide for the pneumoperitoneum in gastrointestinal laparoscopic procedures because the mixture of methane and hydrogen were not in a high enough concentration for combustion to occur. They concluded nitrous oxide is an option not only for patients with cardiopulmonary and metabolic acidosis, but also for prolonged procedures and for pregnant patients because of the concern for fetal acidosis when using CO_2.[127]

Air and oxygen are not used for insufflations during laparoscopy because of the risk of combustion when electrosurgery or lasers are used. Helium and nitrogen are not used because they are not as soluble as CO_2, which increases the risk for more serious consequences in the event of a gas embolism. There are cost concerns with using helium. Argon has a negative effect on hepatic blood flow.[45]

Carbon dioxide insufflation is one cause of hypothermia because of the exposure of the peritoneal surface to a large volume of CO_2 gas that is insufflated at room temperature.[128] However, the other contributing factors of thermal loss include, but are not limited to,

♦ irrigation fluids or fluids as distention media,
♦ OR temperature,
♦ exposed body surface,
♦ procedure length, and
♦ the patient's age and medical condition.

Many studies have been conducted to investigate the potential benefits of heating CO_2 or adding humidity, not only for the prevention of hypothermia but also for the effect on postoperative pain.[128-134] Of the studies reviewed, only one reported a significant decrease in heat loss during the surgery and reduced postoperative shivering, pain, and analgesic requirement.[132] Most researchers report there is no difference in patient outcomes when the temperature or humidity for CO_2 insufflation is changed.[128-131,133,134] Two researchers reported they still prefer to use heated and/or humidified CO_2 for insufflation because it has a positive effect on the total OR time and decreased the amount of time the surgeon spent cleaning the scope and the need for changing the warm saline to prevent fogging.[131,134] Misplacement of the Veress nee-

dle directly into a vein or parenchymal organ can lead to a CO_2 gas embolism. Sixty percent (60%) of the symptomatic cases of gas embolism occur during initial insufflation.[124] Gasless laparoscopic techniques rely on an abdominal wall lift to create an intra-abdominal space at atmospheric pressure to eliminate the risk of hypercapnia and CO_2 embolization. This technique or a combination of abdominal wall lifting with low-pressure pneumoperitoneum may be a good alternative for laparoscopic cholecystectomy procedures for elderly patients or those with cardiopulmonary problems.[45] Researchers in Kentucky evaluated five different insufflation techniques from a retrospective analysis of more than 3,000 laparoscopic procedures over a 13-year period. The research findings revealed that certain laparoscopic methods were more appropriate for patients with particular characteristics (eg, previous surgery).[135] There is also a risk for CO_2 embolism during minimally invasive vein harvesting when CO_2 is used to create a closed tunnel to prepare and harvest the greater saphenous vein or radial artery.[136,137]

VI.a. The cylinder should be checked to verify that it contains the appropriate gas and that it is sufficiently full before starting the procedure.

Carbon dioxide is the most commonly used insufflation gas because it is readily absorbed by the body and excreted by the lungs, does not support combustion, and is commonly available.[45,124] Changing the gas tank when it is empty disrupts the gas flow and risks a decrease in the intra-abdominal pressure. In some cases, it also may cause a malfunction in the suction and pumping mechanism. This can lead to a risk of contamination from aspiration of fluids toward the insufflator.[138]

VI.a.1. Before use, gas cylinders should be checked for
• appropriate label,
• appropriate pin-index safety system connector,
• appropriate color coding, and
• volume.[41]

VI.b. The insufflator should be elevated above the level of the surgical cavity.

When the pressure on the patient side is higher than at the insufflator connecting point, body fluid or gas is allowed to flow up the trocar cannula through the insufflation tubing and into the insufflator. This may result in cross contamination or damage to the insufflating device.[138]

VI.c. The insufflator and insufflation tubing should be flushed with gas before personnel connect the tubing to the cannula (eg, Veress needle).

Flushing removes residual air from tubing, reducing the risk of air embolism. It also determines whether residues are present inside the insufflator.[138]

VI.d. Carbon dioxide insufflators should be filtered with a single-use hydrophobic filter that is compatible with the insufflator and impervious to fluids.

A filter helps prevent gas cylinder contaminants from flowing through the insufflator into the surgical cavity, prevents backflow of abdominal fluids and particulates that could contaminate the insufflator, and prevents cross contamination. When the filter is compatible with the insufflator, it does not interfere with flow rate.[138] Cylinders with nonferrous internal surfaces and surfaces incapable of creating residual material that could escape during the gaseous phase of delivery may be helpful in preventing the transfer of particulate matter.[139]

VI.e. Insufflators designed for laparoscopic procedures should not be substituted for insufflators designed for hysteroscopy procedures.

The American College of Obstetricians and Gynecologists recommend that insufflators designed for use with laparoscopic procedures are not to be used for hysteroscopy procedures.[56] Laparoscopic insufflators supply large volumes at low pressures. Hysteroscopic insufflators supply high pressures with low volume.

VI.f. Insufflator pressures should be monitored throughout the procedure.

Maintaining intra-abdominal pressure under 12 mmHg in adult patients reduces the risk of systemic hemodynamic changes.[124,138,140-142] For heavier or taller patients, an intra-abdominal pressure of 20 mmHg to 30 mmHg may be necessary to establish the appropriate pneumoperitoneum.[100] For pediatric patients, the insufflation pressures should be set as low as possible while creating the pneumoperitoneum; however, there are no known studies to define standard ranges.[47] Monitoring intra-uterine pressures to less than 100 mmHg helps minimize the risk of gas embolization.[56]

VI.f.1. A second CO_2 cylinder should be readily available for each procedure.

VI.f.2. The CO_2 cylinder should be replaced before it is empty.

Methods of monitoring the level of remaining gas in the cylinder include, but are not limited to, observing the insufflator gas cylinder gauge level, monitoring the refill history, and tracking cylinder use. The flow of contaminants occurs more readily when the volume of remaining gas in the cylinder is low. Replacing the primary cylinder before the gas level is low helps prevent contamination of the sterile field by particulate matter.[139]

VI.g. The insufflator tubing should be disconnected from the trocar cannula before personnel deactivate the insufflator.

VI.h. Endoscopic CO_2 insufflators should be equipped with alarms that cannot be deactivated.[41]

Alarms alert personnel to equipment malfunction.

VI.i. When using an AEC unit during MIS procedures, personnel should follow all safety measures identified for AEC technology.

AEC acts as a secondary source of pressurized argon gas that can cause the patient's intra-abdominal pressure to rise rapidly and exceed venous pressure, possibly creating argon-enriched gas emboli formation. This has resulted in gas emboli.[79,80]

VI.i.1. The active electrode and argon gas line should be purged according to the manufacturer's recommendations.[79]

VI.i.2. The patient's intra-abdominal cavity should be flushed with several liters of CO_2 between extended activation periods.[79]

Flushing the intra-abdominal cavity with several liters of CO_2 between extended periods of activation reduces the potential for argon gas emboli formation.[79]

VI.i.3. Patient monitoring should include devices that are considered effective for early detection of gas emboli (eg, end-tidal carbon dioxide).[78,79,81]

There is a significant risk of gas embolism when AEC is used during laparoscopic procedures from abdominal overpressurization and displacement of CO_2 by argon gas.[79-82]

Recommendation VII

Potential injuries and complications associated with fluid used for irrigation or as distention media during MIS and computer-assisted procedures should be identified and practices should be established to reduce risk.

Many MIS procedures require irrigation fluid to clear the operative field of blood and debris or fluid used as a distention media to create a broader visual operative field inside a cavity. Patient outcomes may not be optimal, if fluids used for irrigation or as distention media are not managed appropriately. Fluid extravasation, hyponatremia, hypervolemia, cardiovascular and peripheral vascular complications, pulmonary air or fluid emboli, and hypothermia are a few examples of complications resulting from mismanagement of distention media or irrigation fluids.[143,144] Monitoring and early recognition of the complications associated with the intraoperative use of distention media or irrigation fluids are keys to maintaining patient safety and quality control for MIS procedures.

VII.a. Perioperative registered nurses should be aware of uses, contraindications, and risk of fluids used for distention media.

The selection of fluid to be used for irrigation or distention media depends on the type of procedure being performed, the patient's condition, and the use of electrosurgery.

For example, for arthroscopy procedures normal saline (ie, 0.9% sodium chloride) is used unless monopolar electrosurgery is planned.

Normal saline and Lactated Ringer's solution are isotonic, electrolyte fluids. The American College of Obstetricians and Gynecologists consider these solutions to be the media of choice for diagnostic hysteroscopy or intraoperative hysteroscopy when mechanical, laser, or bipolar energy is used.[56] Low viscosity, hyperosmolar, electrolyte-poor fluids (glycine 1.5%, sorbitol 3%, and mannitol 5%)

are compatible with monopolar radiofrequency energy but can cause hyponatremia and decreased serum osmolality. Their absorption in excess can result in fatal complications such as cerebral edema and death. Mannitol 5% is isoosmolar and causes diuresis, which can lead to excessive absorption. Dextran 70 is a high-viscosity fluid and a potent plasma expander. Anaphylaxis and disseminated intravascular coagulopathy have occurred when Dextran 70 has been used for uterine distention. This solution crystallizes on instruments and is very difficult to remove. Dextran 70 is contraindicated for patients who are allergic to beet sugar.[56]

Nonelectrolyte solutions such as glycine, mannitol, or sorbitol often are used in urologic procedures when monopolar electrosurgical devices are used. These solutions do not dissipate the electrical current. Glycine is the fluid medium commonly used with monopolar electrosurgical technology.[145] The complication known as transurethral resection (TUR) syndrome may be observed when glycine is used as irrigating or distention media. Exposed blood vessels from tissue removal and elevated pressure being applied to the distention fluid enables intravasation (ie, distention fluid flows into the vascular system).[146] Monopolar electrosurgical energy can result in temperatures up to 400° C (752° F) because of the resistance with surrounding tissue.[147] Bipolar electrosurgical use has achieved similar clinical efficacy to monopolar procedures, but with shorter catheterization times and shorter hospital stays. For bipolar electrosurgical technology, normal saline, which reduces the occurrence of TUR syndrome, may be used as the fluid medium rather than glycine.[147]

VII.b. Fluids used for irrigation or as distention media should be contained.

Fluid that is not contained cannot be measured. It is important to measure fluids returned from irrigation or distention media to monitor for fluid deficit. Fluid standing on the floor can pose a fall risk to surgical team members. Fluid becomes an electrical hazard when it comes into contact with electrical equipment. Containing the fluid prevents environmental contamination.

VII.b.1. The patient should be draped in a manner that enables as much capture of fluid return as possible.

Drapes designed for collection facilitate the accurate measurement of fluid. Fluid absorption is determined through monitoring the volumetric fluid balance by subtracting the amount of fluid recovered from the amount of fluid instilled. The volumetric calculation does not take into consideration extraneous fluid losses (ie, fluid loss on the floor, on the drape, etc.), which cannot be accurately quantified, nor does it consider additives, such as blood.

VII.b.2. Fluid administered to the patient should be collected in a closed container system.

Using a suction canister or fluid collection system prevents the fluid from contaminating the environment and the clothing of personnel. Surgical drapes with fluid collection pouches may assist in preventing fluid from contaminating the floor. Fluid collection mats on the floor may assist with managing fluid that does contact the floor.

VII.b.3. Fluids used for irrigation or as distention media should be prevented from coming into contact with electrical equipment.

Containing fluid used during a procedure prevents contact with electrical outlets, switches, and the internal components of electrical equipment including electrosurgical electrodes. Preventing fluid contact with electrical equipment minimizes the risk of burns, fires, and damage to the equipment.

VII.b.4. Fluid used during a procedure must be handled and discarded as a biohazardous waste in a manner consistent with local, state, and federal regulations.

Fluid that has been used inside a patient's body is considered biohazardous. Management of biohazardous waste is regulated by federal, state, and local agencies.[148]

VII.c. Fluids used for irrigation or as distention media should be monitored for appropriate temperature.

Fluids that are too warm can cause burns.[39] Cool irrigation solutions in body cavities enhance heat transfer from the body core to the solution and increase the risk of heat loss. Perioperative hypothermia is associated with serious cardiac events.[144] Equipment is commercially available to warm irrigation fluid as it is administered.

Warming irrigation fluid to body temperature near 37° C (98.6° F) is an adjunct therapy to decrease heat loss but is insufficient alone to prevent hypothermia.[149] In a study of patients undergoing laparoscopy without forced air warming, patients receiving warmed irrigation solutions maintained higher core body temperatures than those receiving room temperature solutions. However, warmed irrigation fluids alone did not prevent hypothermia.[150] No improvement in body temperature was found when using warmed irrigation during arthroscopic surgery.[151]

The value of warming irrigation solutions during urologic procedures is controversial. The procedure associated with the greatest temperature drop is percutaneous lithotripsy.[152] The combination of warmed irrigation and IV fluids has been found to result in less of a temperature drop in patients undergoing TUR.[153] When active patient surface warming was used during TUR, patients remained normothermic when room temperature irrigation fluids were used. Researchers reported that the temperature of the irrigation fluid did not have as great an effect on the core body temperature as other factors, including ambient temperature of the OR, time spent in the OR, the resection time, and amount of irrigation fluid absorbed.[154]

Using warm distention media for hysteroscopy may dilate the vasculature and lead to intravasation.[155,156]

VII.d Fluid management systems should be used in a manner that minimizes potential for injury.

Automated fluid management systems calculate the amount of fluid dispensed to the patient and compare this with the amount returned to the system. The deficit is measured and an alarm alerts the user of potential fluid overload. This timely notification of a deficit provides an opportunity to take corrective action before physiologic compromise of the patient.

VII.d.1. The perioperative RN should follow the manufacturer's written instructions for use of fluid management systems.

VII.d.2. The fluid selected for the distention media should be consistent with the fluid management system and the endoscope manufacturer's written instructions.

VII.d.3. Accessories (eg, tubing, collection canisters) should be compatible with the fluid management system.

Fluid management system tubing has a transducer that works with the electronic equipment to measure input and output. Using incompatible tubing results in inaccurate fluid measurements.

VII.d.4. The perioperative RN should calibrate the fluid management system as per the manufacturer's instructions.

Proper calibration of the fluid management system will calculate instillation and total fluid deficit amounts accurately.

VII.d.5. A fluid management system designed for intrauterine distention should be used when distending the uterus with more than 1,000 mL of fluid.

The amount of fluid contained in an IV bag or bottle can be up to 3.3% to 10% more than the amount stated on the label.[157,158] The actual amount of fluid in collection canisters may be 20% more or less than the measured amount. When large volumes of fluid are instilled, this inaccuracy can result in unidentified fluid deficit.[157] This inaccuracy may not be clinically significant when small volumes (ie, less than 1,000 mL) are used.

VII.d.6. The perioperative RN should verify the volume setting for fluid distention with the surgeon before administration.

Volume settings are based on the procedure being done, the size of the patient, and the patient's condition. During operative endoscopic urologic procedures, large volumes of fluid are instilled to enhance visualization and evacuate tissue and blood clots. Irrigation fluid can be absorbed into the intravascular system by instrument perforation during tumor or fibroid resection, or forced into the intraperitoneal or retroperitoneal space. The amount of fluid absorbed increases with the extent of the resection and prolonged exposure.[143] Smoking is the only known risk factor for patients that is associated with an increase in fluid absorption.[159]

VII.e. The perioperative RN should monitor the amount of fluid dispensed and returned during the procedure.

Monitoring irrigation fluid use facilitates calculation of blood loss and determines existing fluid deficit, representing fluid that is being absorbed by the patient (ie, fluid intravasation). Dilutional hyponatremia is associated with intravasation of nonelectrolyte solutions. Rapid influx of hypotonic fluid increases circulation of free water and reduces the extracellular sodium concentration.[54,160] During hysteroscopy procedures, fluid is absorbed through the uterine vessels and the bowel if there is a perforation, or the fluid egresses through patent fallopian tubes. This can lead to serious complications. Measuring fluid volume deficit can prevent complications when identified early and the procedure is terminated.[56]

The critical volume of intravasation before symptoms are exhibited is not predictable.[161] The American College of Obstetricians and Gynecologists suggest that 750 mL of fluid absorption implies excessive intravasation. They further advise planning for terminating the procedure for patients who are elderly and for those with cardiovascular compromise when this occurs.[56]

The incidence and severity of fluid symptoms from increased amounts of intraoperative or postoperative absorbed fluid have been documented during TUR and endometrial ablation procedures. During TUR procedures where glycine was used as the fluid distention media, patients exhibited symptoms of excessive fluid absorption when 1 L to 2 L of fluid had been absorbed.[143]

VII.e.1. Fluid deficit amount should be reported to the anesthesia care provider and surgeon at regular intervals throughout the procedure.

Fluid absorption increases with increased length of the procedure. Completing procedures in one hour or less may help limit complications from fluid absorption.[143]

VII.e.2. The perioperative RN should initiate corrective action in response to audible alarms from the fluid management system and notify the surgeon and anesthesia care provider if corrective actions do not result in a decrease of fluid volume deficit to a safe level.

VII.e.3. The patient should be monitored for physiologic changes, including core temperature and potential fluid retention.

TUR syndrome, mild to moderately severe absorption of nonelectrolyte solution, occurs in up to 8% of patients undergoing TUR. Absorption of more than 1 L has been reported in 5% to 20% of TURs and results in symptoms.[143] The most serious adverse events occur when more than 3 L of fluid are absorbed.[143] Extravasation can occur during renal stone surgery or when instruments perforate the bladder or prostate capsule.[143] Glycine absorption causes circulatory (ie, chest pain, bradycardia, hypertension) and neurological (ie, blurred vision, nausea and vomiting, apprehension, confusion) symptoms.[143] In a recent study of patients undergoing transurethral resection of the prostate (TURP), glycine absorption was associated with echocardiogram changes and myocardial stress.[146] Physiological responses that can result from excessive fluid absorption include

- cardiac overload,
- cerebral edema,
- dilutional hyponatremia, and
- water intoxication.[143,146,162]

VII.e.4. The patient's neck and facial area should be assessed intraoperatively when volumetric fluid calculations are being performed.

Manual volumetric calculations made intraoperatively provide crude estimates only. Edema of the parotid area is a late sign of interstitial edema that develops as a result of a fluid deficit up to or greater than 1,000 mL. Manual calculation is a simple and inexpensive means to determine fluid deficit over 1,000 mL when accurate volumetric fluid balance calculations are hampered by extraneous fluid losses.[163]

VII.e.5. The nurse should be prepared to coordinate and report laboratory testing of serum electrolytes.

When the patient is at risk of hyponatremia, serum electrolyte or urine electrolyte testing often is performed. Normal serum sodium is 135 mmol/L to 145 mmol/L. Hyponatremia occurs when serum sodium levels fall below 135 mmol/L.[164,165]

VII.f. Patients should be monitored for adverse reactions when medications are added to fluids used for irrigation or distention media.

Antibiotics may be added to irrigation fluid for MIS procedures. For arthroscopy procedures, epinephrine may be added to the irrigation/distention fluid medium resulting in vasoconstriction and hemostasis with an increased visual field for the surgeon.

Recommendation VIII

The patient's physiologic response, including core temperature and potential fluid retention, should be evaluated postoperatively.

Nausea and vomiting are common postoperative complaints after laparoscopic surgery and can cause delays in the patient's discharge.[45] Signs and symptoms related to fluid and medication absorption can occur after the procedure. The most common signs and symptoms reported after a urologic procedure are nausea, hypotension, low urinary output, visual disturbances, and confusion. Abdominal pain accompanied by hypotension and poor urinary output may be an indication of extravasation of fluid.[143] Adverse events related to irrigation and distention fluid may occur postoperatively. Pulmonary edema in the postanesthesia care unit has been reported in healthy, young patients after orthopedic arthroscopy procedures.[166] The potential for complications related to extra-articular fluid migration is likely to increase in relation to the duration and complexity of the arthroscopic procedure. Prolonged use of high irrigation flow rates and pressures (eg,100 mmHg for 60 to 90 minutes) may increase the risk of complications.[167,168]

Recommendation IX

Personnel should receive initial and ongoing education and demonstrate competency in the perioperative nursing care of patients who undergo MIS and computer-assisted procedures and in the use of MIS and computer-assisted equipment.

Initial education on the nursing care of MIS patients, procedures, and related equipment provides direction for personnel in providing safe patient care. Additional periodic educational programs provide opportunities to reinforce previous learning, introduce new information on changes in technology, its application, compatibility of equipment and accessories, and potential hazards.

IX.a. An introduction and review of policies and procedures for MIS and computer-assisted procedures should be included in orientation and ongoing education of personnel.

Review of policies and procedures assists health care personnel in the development of knowledge, skills, and attitudes that affect patient outcomes.

IX.b. Perioperative RNs should be knowledgeable about new instrumentation; equipment; computer-assisted technology (eg, robotics, voice recognition software); and camera technologies being used in the health care organization.

Technology is continually evolving. Rapid technological advances require continuous learning and skills updating to maintain competency.

IX.b.1. Perioperative personnel should demonstrate competency in the use of MIS and computer-assisted equipment, following manufacturers' written instructions, before use.

Instruction and return demonstration in proper usage minimizes the risk of injury and extends the life of the equipment. Competencies based on the manufacturer's instructions ensure that personnel have the knowledge about the proper use of the fluid management system and other MIS equipment. Incorrect use can result in serious patient complications.

Equipment instruction manuals assist in developing operational, safety, and maintenance guidelines and serve as a reference for safe, appropriate use.

IX.b.2. Education and competency validation should include all components of the MIS and computer-assisted equipment including, but not limited to,
- equipment operation and safety considerations,
- computer system use,
- position of equipment for specific surgeries, and
- troubleshooting malfunctioning equipment.[3]

IX.b.3. The perioperative RN should be instructed in the safety considerations and risks of gas insufflation and demonstrate competency in the management of its risks.

IX.b.4. Personnel should be instructed in the safety considerations and risks of electrosurgery and demonstrate competency in the use of electrosurgery equipment and related accessories during MIS and computer-assisted procedures.[57]

IX.b.5. Personnel using AEC should be knowledgeable about signs, symptoms, and treatment of venous emboli.

There is a significant risk of gas embolism when AEC is used during laparoscopic procedures from abdominal over-pressurization and displacement of CO_2 by argon gas.[79-82]

IX.c. Personnel should receive education about the selection of fluids used for irrigation and distention media selection, fluid administration equipment and procedures, and fluid storage requirements.

IX.c.1. Education and competency validation should include, but not be limited to,
- fluid storage and fluid warming equipment,
- distention fluid selection,
- proper use of distention fluid management systems,
- patient assessments, and
- response to patient complications.

An understanding of appropriate use, risks, and precautions to minimize these risks provides the foundation for compliance with procedures and the delivery of safe patient care.

IX.d. Team training and team building should be implemented whenever new procedures or new team dynamics are introduced (eg, hybrid/integrated OR).

Creating a hybrid OR requires advanced education of perioperative team members that emphasizes teamwork and the importance of what each member of the team brings to total patient care. Some team members may be resistant to working together in a hybrid OR because of previous departmental borders. Techniques such as those described in the AORN Human Factors in Health Care Tool Kit may be useful for the education process.[169]

Recommendation X

The perioperative RN should document the care of patients undergoing MIS and computer-assisted procedures throughout the continuum of care.

Documentation of all nursing activities performed is legally and professionally important for clear communication and collaboration between health care team members and for continuity of patient care.

X.a. Documentation using the PNDS should include a patient assessment, a plan of care, nursing diagnoses, identification of desired outcomes, interventions, and an evaluation of the patient's response to the care provided.

Documentation provides communication among all care providers involved in planning and implementing patient care. Standardized documentation allows the potential for consistent data retrieval and comparison.

X.b. Documentation should be recorded in a manner consistent with the health care organization's policies and procedures.

X.b.1. Documentation for MIS procedures should include, but not be limited to,
- distention media used;
- equipment used for distention media administration, including the equipment identification number;
- quantity of fluid administered and flow rate;

- quantity of fluid returned, if applicable;
- urinary output;
- medication added to distention fluid; and
- relevant information about equipment used (eg, insufflation, electrosurgery, positioning).

Recommendation XI

Policies and procedures for MIS and computer-assisted procedures should be developed, reviewed periodically, and readily available in the practice setting.

Policies and procedures assist in the development of patient safety, quality assessment, and improvement activities. Policies and procedures establish authority, responsibility, and accountability with the organization. They also serve as operational guidelines that are used to minimize patient risk factors, standardize practice, direct staff members, and establish guidelines for continuous performance improvement activities.

XI.a. The health care organization's policies and procedures for MIS equipment must be in compliance with the Safe Medical Devices Act (SMDA) of 1990, as amended in March 2000.[170]

XI.a.1. When patient or personnel injuries or equipment failures occur, the equipment and associated device(s) should be removed from service and the associated devices retained if possible.

Identification and segregation of the complete system allows for a thorough evaluation and identification of the cause of the equipment failure.

XI.a.2. Incidents of patient or personnel injury or equipment failure should be reported as required by regulation to federal, state, and local authorities and to the equipment manufacturer. Device identification, maintenance and service information, and adverse event information should be included in the report from the practice setting.

Documentation of details of the involved equipment and associated devices allows for retrievable information for investigation into an adverse event.

XI.b. Policies and procedures must comply with the Standards of Privacy and Security of the Health Insurance Portability and Accountability Act of 1996 for the protection of health information.[171]

XI.b.1. MIS patient privacy policies and procedures should include, but not be limited to,
- disclosure of information,
- access to and use of databases,
- access to and use of digital images, and
- data security.

XI.c. Policies should be written and readily available in the practice setting.

XI.c.1. Policies regarding MIS and computer-assisted equipment should include, but not be limited to,
- required qualifications and credentials for operation of specific equipment or devices (eg, radiologic, MRI equipment);
- procedure scheduling related to equipment availability;
- equipment acquisition;
- personnel training and competency validation before use of equipment;
- equipment maintenance and repair;
- types of MIS procedures approved in the practice setting; and
- reporting of adverse events.
  Compromised patient safety, delay in care, or cancellation of the procedure may result when required equipment or qualified personnel are not available.[172]

XI.c.2. Policies and procedures regarding the selection, storage, administration, and required monitoring of fluid used for irrigation or distention media and gases used for distention media should include, but not be limited to,
- manufacturers' written instructions for storage, warming, and use of fluid administration or gas insufflation equipment;
- requirements of regulatory and accrediting agencies; and
- evidence from published scientific literature.

Recommendation XII

Quality assurance/performance improvement process should be in place that measures patient; process; and structural (eg, system) outcome indicators.

A fundamental precept of AORN is that it is the responsibility of professional perioperative RNs to ensure safe, high-quality nursing care to patients undergoing operative and other invasive procedures.[173]

XII.a. Structure, process, and clinical outcomes performance measures should be identified.
Performance measures can be used to improve patient care and monitor compliance with facility policy and procedure, national standards, and regulatory requirements.[173]

XII.a.1. Process indicators should be collected, analyzed, and used for performance improvement.[173] Indicators may include, but are not limited to information about adverse patient outcomes and near misses associated with electrosurgery or other MIS or computer-assisted equipment.

XII.b. Quality assurance/performance improvement processes should be in place to evaluate the safety of fluid management in the health care setting.
Quality control programs that enhance personnel performance and monitor fluid management efficacy are established to promote patient and employee safety.

XII.b.1. A quality management program should be in place to evaluate at least the following:
- daily temperature checks of fluid warming storage cabinets,
- temperature of warmed fluids at the point of use,
- bioengineering safety checks for fluid warming and administration equipment, and
- reporting mechanisms for adverse events and near misses related to fluid management.

XII.b.2. Adverse events and near misses related to fluid management or other MIS or computer-assisted equipment should be reported and investigated and corrective action taken.

Reporting adverse events and near misses through an adverse event reporting and investigation system provides a mechanism to determine trends, potential risk factors, and evaluate the effectiveness of corrective actions.

XII.c. Fluid management systems and other MIS and computer-assisted equipment should be evaluated and approved by the health care organization's biomedical personnel before use and assigned an identification or serial number for tracking.[41]

Hazards associated with medical equipment, if not corrected, may result in injury to patients, staff members, or visitors. The identification or serial number facilitates documenting maintenance performed on the individual system and tracking of problems when they occur. Endoscopic equipment manuals provide guidelines for developing operating, safety, and maintenance practices. Proper inspection, testing, use, and processing of equipment reduces the risk of adverse outcomes or damage to equipment. Equipment that functions correctly promotes patient safety and efficiency during the surgical procedure.[172]

XII.c.1. Correct control settings should be labeled on equipment and on a quick reference chart attached to the equipment.

Standardization of equipment allows for interchangeability in the event of equipment malfunction.

XII.c.2. The manufacturer's manual for maintenance and inspections for all MIS-related equipment, written instructions for reprocessing any supplies or accessories, and warranties should be easily retrievable for the clinical perioperative team.

Equipment instruction manuals assist in developing operational, safety, and maintenance guidelines and serve as a reference for safe, appropriate use.

XII.c.3. MIS equipment should have standard safety features including, but not limited to, appropriate alarm and monitoring systems. Clinical alarms should be audible and should not be disabled.[41]

Safety features include, but are not limited to, the following:

- audible alarms for absence of fluid in the dispensing tubing,
- audible alarms to indicate air in the fluid dispensing tubing,
- audible alarms to indicate fluid deficit,
- pressure regulated without fluctuation,
- accurate outflow measure,
- accurate measurement of fluid instilled and returned to the regulator,
- measurement of intrauterine pressure, and
- fluid management systems with accurate calculations of fluid volume deficit.

Glossary

Active electrode: The electrosurgical unit (ESU) accessory that directs current flow to the surgical site (eg, pencils, various pencil tips).

Active electrode indicator shaft: An active electrode composed of two layers of insulated material of different colors. The inner layer is a bright color, the outer layer is black. When the brightly colored inner layer is evident upon visual inspection, a break in the insulation is indicated.

Active-electrode insulation testing devices: Devices designed to test the integrity of the insulation surrounding the conductive shaft of laparoscopic electrosurgical active-electrode instruments. The devices detect full thickness breaks in the insulation layer.

Active electrode monitoring: A dynamic process of searching for insulation failures and capacitive coupling during monopolar surgery. If the monitor detects an unsafe level of stray energy, it signals the generator to deactivate.

Alternate site injury: Patient injury caused by an electrosurgical device that occurs away from the dispersive electrode site.

Argon-enhanced coagulation (AEC): Radiofrequency coagulation from an electrosurgical generator that is capable of delivering monopolar current through a flow of ionized argon gas.

Automated fluid management system: Mechanical medical devices designed to calculate the amount of fluid dispensed to the patient compared to the amount returned to the system; alarms alert the user to fluid deficit to prompt corrective action.

Bipolar resection devices: Mechanical medical devices that use an electrolytic solution to conduct electrical flow to resect tissue. Often used for hysteroscopy procedures.

Capacitance: Ability of an electrical circuit to transfer an electrical charge from one conductor to another, even when separated by an insulator.

Capacitive coupling: Transfer of electrical current from the active electrode through intact insulation to adjacent conductive items (eg, tissue, trocars).

Capacitors: Two conductors separated by an insulator (eg, insulated active electrode, trocar cannula); instrument for storing electricity.

Computer-assisted technologies: Robotic, interventional radiology, voice-recognition software, or other computer technologies used to enhance minimally invasive surgery.

Dilutional hyponatremia: A decrease in the serum sodium level caused by intravasation of fluids, which dilute the soluble components of the serum.

Digital OR: Technology that includes a centralized database that allows continuous live feeds throughout the health care facility, allowing data retrieval (eg, video clips, still images) after the procedure for educational or reporting purposes. Synonym: Integrated OR.

Direct coupling: The contact of an energized active electrode tip with another metal instrument or object within the surgical field.

Endoscopic surgery: A surgical technique using endoscopic instrumentation inserted through a natural orifice or through one or more small incisions.

Extravasation: To pass by infiltration or effusion from a proper vessel or channel (as a blood vessel) into surrounding tissue.

Fluid deficit: When the amount of fluid infused to the patient is more than the amount returned to suction or fluid management system.

Hybrid OR: An operating room designed with numerous imaging technologies (eg, 3D angiography, computed tomography, magnetic resonance imaging, positron-emission tomography, intravascular ultrasound) to support surgical procedures that require multiple care providers with varied expertise to provide patient care in one location.

Hyponatremia: An abnormally low concentration of sodium ions in circulating blood.

Hydrophobic insufflation filter: An in-line filter that retains a high percentage of particulates greater than a specified size. The hydrophobic media protects against fluid backflow into the insufflation gas.

Hypothermia: A decrease in core body temperature to a level below the normothermic range.

Hypervolemia: An excessive volume of fluid in the vascular space.

Hysteroscopy: Endoscopic visualization of the uterine cavity and tubal orifices.

Insufflate: The introduction of a flow of gas into a body cavity.

Insufflation: The act of blowing gas into a body cavity or the state of being distended with gas for the purpose of visual examination.

Integrated OR: An operating room equipped with technology that centralizes control of audiovideo equipment and information systems and is capable of controlling a variety of equipment and activities within the surgical suite. Synonym: digital OR.

Intracorporeal mobile devices: Minitiarized robotic devices designed to allow access to restricted spaces for surgical or diagnostic purposes.

Intravasation: The entrance of foreign material or solution into a blood vessel.

Light cable: Fiber-optic filaments joined into a cable used to transport light to the surgical field.

Minimally invasive surgery: Surgical procedures performed through one or more small incisions using endoscopic instruments, radiographic and magnetic resonance imaging, computer-assisted devices, robotics, and other emerging technologies.

Nanotechnologies: The science and technology of creating nanoparticles and of manufacturing machines that have sizes within the range of 0.1 to 100 nanometers. An advanced technology involving the fabrication and use of devices so small that the convenient unit of measurement is the nanometer (one billionth of a meter).

NOTES: Natural orifice transluminal endoscopic surgery.

Pneumoperitoneum: The presence of air or gas within the peritoneal cavity of the abdomen often induced for diagnostic purposes.

Single-port access laparoscopy: One incision is used, rather than several incisions, to insert laparoscopic instrumentation.

Telepresence: Robotic and computer technology that allows a health care provider to interact physically with patients or other health care providers in remote locations.

TUR syndrome: A mild to moderately severe absorption of nonelectrolye solution following transurethral resection.

Water intoxication: An increase in the volume of water in the body, resulting in dilutional hyponatremia.

White balancing: A part of the color balancing process that renders neutral color adjustment to achieve balanced intensities and avoid unrealistic color casts.

REFERENCES

1. Recommended practices for cleaning and care of surgical instruments and powered equipment. *Perioperative Standards and Recommended Practices*. Denver, CO: AORN, Inc; 2009:611-636.

2. Recommended practices for cleaning and processing flexible endoscopes and endoscope accessories. *Perioperative Standards and Recommended Practices*. Denver, CO: AORN, Inc; 2009:595-610.

3. Acevedo AL. Construction of an integrated surgical suite in a military treatment facility. *AORN J*. 2009; 89(1):151-159.

4. Cepolina F, Michelini RC. Review of robotic fixtures for minimally invasive surgery. *Int J Med Robot*. 2004;1(1):43-63.

5. Taylor GW, Jayne DG. Robotic applications in abdominal surgery: their limitations and future developments. *Int J Med Robot*. 2007;3:3-9.

6. Gordon D. Trends in surgery-suite design. Part I. *Healthcare Design*. 2007;6.

7. Burgess NA, Koo BC, Calvert RC, Hindmarsh A, Donaldson PJ, Rhodes M. Randomized trial of laparoscopic v open nephrectomy. *J Endourol*. 2007;21(6):610-613.

8. Sroga J, Patel S D, Falcone T. Robotics in reproductive medicine. *Front Biosci*. 2008;13:1308-1317.

9. Herron DM, Marohn M; SAGES-MIRA Robotic Surgery Consensus Group. A consensus document on robotic surgery. *Surg Endosc*. 2008;22(2):313-325.

10. Petersen C, ed. AORN Guidance Statement: *Safe Patient Handling and Movement in the Perioperative Setting*. Denver, CO: AORN, Inc; 2007.

11. AORN position statement on ergonomically healthy workplace practices. AORN, Inc. *http://www.aorn .org/PracticeResources/AORNPositionStatements /Position_Ergonomics/*. Accessed October 13, 2009.

12. van Veelen, Jakimowicz, Kazemier. Improved physical ergonomics of laparoscopic surgery. *Minim Invasive Ther Allied Technol*. 2004;13(3):161-166.

13. Sikkink C J, Reijnen M M, Zeebregts CJ. The creation of the optimal dedicated endovascular suite. *Eur J Vasc Endovasc Surg*. 2008;35(2):198-204.

14. Brogmus G, Leone W, Butler L, Hernandez E. Best practices in OR suite layout and equipment choices to reduce slips, trips, and falls. *AORN J*. 2007;86(3):384-398.

15. Mathur NS. The next generation of operating rooms. *Academy Journal*. 2005;8

16. Berguer R. Surgery and ergonomics. *Arch Surg*. 1999;134(9):1011-1016.

17. Albayrak, Kazemier, Meijer, Bonjer. Current state of ergonomics of operating rooms of Dutch hospitals in the endoscopic era. *Minim Invasive Ther Allied Technol*. 2004;13(3):156-160.

18. Sandberg WS, Daily B, Egan M, et al. Deliberate perioperative systems design improves operating room throughput. *Anesthesiology*. 2005;103(2):406-418.

19. Rostenberg B, Horii SC. *The Architecture of Medical Imaging: Designing Healthcare Facilities for Advanced Radiological Diagnostic and Therapeutic Techniques*. Hoboken, NJ: John Wiley & Sons; 2006.

20. ECRI. OR integration: what, why, and how? *Operating Room Risk Management*. 2008;17(4):1-6.

21. van Det MJ, Meijerink WJ, Hoff C, Totté ER, Pierie JP. Optimal ergonomics for laparoscopic surgery in minimally invasive surgery suites: a review and guidelines. *Surg Endosc*. 2009;23(6):1279-1285.

22. Gordon D. Trends in surgery-suite design. Part II. *Healthcare Design*. 2007;7(6):32-40.

23. Catalano K, Fickensscher K. Emerging technologies in the OR and their effect on perioperative professionals. *AORN J*. 2007;86(6):958-969.

24. Latifi R, Peck K, Satava R, Anvari M. Telepresence and telementoring in surgery. *Stud Health Technol Inform*. 2004;104:200-206.

25. Chung KK, Grathwohl KW, Poropatich RK, Wolf SE, Holcomb JB. Robotic telepresence: past, present, and future. *J Cardiothorac Vasc Anesth*. 2007;21(4):593-596.

26. Doarn CR, Hufford K, Low T, Rosen J, Hannaford B. Telesurgery and robotics. *Telemed J E Health*. 2007; 13(4):369-380.

27. Sebajang H, Trudeau P, Dougall A, Hegge S, McKinley C, Anvari M. The role of telementoring and telerobotic assistance in the provision of laparoscopic colorectal surgery in rural areas. *Surg Endosc*. 2006;20(9):1389-1393.

28. Recommended practices for traffic patterns in the perioperative practice setting. *Perioperative Standards and Recommended Practices*. Denver, CO: AORN, Inc; 2009: 327-330.

29. Lindeman WE. Design and construction of an ambulatory surgery center. *AORN J*. 2008;88(3):369-380.

30. Worley DJ, Hohler SE. OR construction project: from planning to execution. *AORN J*. 2008;88(6):917-941.

31. Jacob AL, Regazzoni P, Bilecen D, Rasmus M, Huegli RW, Messmer P. Medical technology integration: CT, angiography, imaging-capable OR-table, navigation and robotics in a multifunctional sterile suite. *Minim Invasive Ther Allied Technol*. 2007;16(4):205-211.

32. Russell L. Intraoperative magnetic resonance imaging safety considerations. *AORN J*. 2003;77(3):590-592.

33. Chapter 1.5: Planning, design, and construction. In: AIA Academy of Architecture for Health, Facilities Guidelines Institute, eds. *Guidelines for Design and Construction of Health Care Facilities*. Washington, DC: American Institute of Architects; 2006:26-30.

34. AIA Academy of Architecture for Health, Facilities Guidelines Institute. *Guidelines for Design and Construction of Health Care Facilities*. Washington, DC: American Institute of Architects; 2006.

35. ECRI Institute upholds recommendations on warming cabinet temperatures. *Risk Management Reporter*. 2007;26(2):9-10.

36. ECRI Institute. Hazard report update: Limiting the temperature of warming cabinets remains a good safety practice. *Health Devices*. 2006;35(12):458-461.

37. US Food and Drug Administration. Safety assessment of Di(2-ethylhexyl)phthalate (DEHP) released from PVC medical devices. 2001.

38. Avoiding mix-ups between sterile water and sodium chloride bags. *ISMP MedicationSafetyAlert*. 2007;12(25).

39. Huang S, Gateley D, Moss AL. Accidental burn injury during knee arthroscopy. *Arthroscopy*. 2007;23(12):1363.e1-1363.e3.

40. Kressin KA. Burn injury in the operating room: a closed claims analysis. *ASA Newsl*. 2004;68(6):9-11.

41. Recommended practices for a safe environment of care. In: *Perioperative Standards and Recommended Practices*. Denver, CO: AORN, Inc; 2009:415-438.

42. Recommended practices for prevention of transmissible infections in the perioperative practice setting. In: *Perioperative Standards and Recommended Practices*. Denver, CO: AORN, Inc; 2009:475-486.

43. Recommended practices for maintaining a sterile field. In: *Perioperative Standards and Recommended Practices*. Denver, CO: AORN, Inc; 2009:317-326.

44. Sullivan MJ, Frost EA, Lew MW. Anesthetic care of the patient for robotic surgery. *Middle East J Anesthesiol*. 2008;19(5):967-982.

45. Gerges FJ, Kanazi GE, Jabbour-Khoury SI. Anesthesia for laparoscopy: a review. *J Clin Anesth*. 2006;18(1):67-78.

46. Henny CP, Hofland J. Laparoscopic surgery: pitfalls due to anesthesia, positioning, and pneumoperitoneum. *Surg Endosc*. 2005;19(9):1163-1171.

47. Harrington S, Simmons K, Thomas C, Scully S. Pediatric laparoscopy. *AORN J*. 2008;88(2):211-236.

48. AORN guideline for prevention of venous stasis. In: *Perioperative Standards and Recommended Practices*. Denver, CO: AORN, Inc; 2009:165-182.

49. Cantrell SW, Ward KS, Van Wicklin SA. Translating research on venous thromboembolism into practice. *AORN J*. 2007;86(4):590-606.

50. Society of American Gastrointestinal and Endoscopic Surgeons (SAGES) Guidelines Committee. Guidelines for deep venous thrombosis prophylaxis during laparoscopic surgery. *Surg Endosc*. 2007;21(6):1007-1009.

51. Rasmussen MS. Is there a need for antithrombotic prophylaxis during laparoscopic surgery? Always. *J Thromb Haemost*. 2005;3(2):210-211.

52. Ljungstrom KG. Is there a need for antithromboembolic prophylaxis during laparoscopic surgery? Not always. *J Thromb Haemost*. 2005;3(2):212-213.

53. Goldfaden A, Birkmeyer JD. Evidence-based practice in laparoscopic surgery: perioperative care. *Surg Innov*. 2005;12(1):51-61.

54. Haskal R. Current issues for nurse practitioners: hyponatremia. *J Am Acad Nurse Pract*. 2007;19(11):563-579.

55. ACOG Committee on Practice Bulletins. Clinical management guidelines for obstetrician-gynecologists [ACOG Practice Bulletin. Number 81, May 2007]. *Obstet Gynecol*. 2007;109(5):1233-1248.

56. American College of Obstetricians and Gynecologists. ACOG technology assessment in obstetrics and gynecology, number 4, August 2005: hysteroscopy. *Obstet Gynecol*. 2005;106(2):439.

57. Recommended practices for electrosurgery. In: *Perioperative Standards and Recommended Practices*. Denver, CO: AORN, Inc; 2010. In press.

58. ECRI Institute. Electrosurgery. *Healthcare Risk Control*. 2007;4(Surgery and Anesthesia 16).

59. Odell RC. Pearls, pitfalls, and advancements in the delivery of electrosurgical energy during laparoscopy. *Problems in General Surgery*. 2002;19(2):5-17.

60. ECRI Institute. Operating room risk management: ORRM, Laparoscopic electrosurgery risks. *Operating Room Risk Management*. 1999;2(Surgery 19):1-11.

61. Guidance section: ensuring monopolar electrosurgical safety during laparoscopy. *Health Devices*. 1995;24(1):20-26.

62. Wu MP, Ou CS, Chen SL, Yen EY, Rowbotham R. Complications and recommended practices for electrosurgery in laparoscopy. *Am J Surg*. 2000;179(1):67-73.

63. Vilos GA, Newton DW, Odell RC, Abu-Rafea B, Vilos AG. Characterization and mitigation of stray radiofrequency currents during monopolar resectoscopic electrosurgery. *J Minim Invasive Gynecol*. 2006;13(2):134-140.

64. Physician Insurers Association of America, eds. *Laparoscopic Injury Study*. Rockville, MD: Physician Insurers Association of America; 2000:1-5.

65. ECRI Institute. Safety technologies for laparoscopic monopolar electrosurgery; devices for managing burn risks. *Health Devices*. 2005;34(8):259-272.

66. Evaluation of Electroscope Electroshield System. *Health Devices*. 1995;24(1):11-19.

67. Dennis V. Implementing active electrode monitoring: a perioperative call. *Ssm*. 2001;7(2):32-38.

68. Harrell GJ, Kopps DR. Minimizing patient risk during laparoscopic electrosurgery. *AORN J*. 1998;67(6):1194-1196.

69. Surgical fire safety. *Health Devices*. 2006;35(2):45-66.

70. Greilich PE, Greilich NB, Froelich EG. Intra-abdominal fire during laparoscopic cholecystectomy. *Anesthesiology*. 1995;83(4):871-874.

71. Tucker RD, Voyles CR, Silvis SE. Capacitive coupled stray currents during laparoscopic and endoscopic electrosurgical procedures. *Biomed Instrum Technol*. 1992;26(4):303-311.

72. Wang K, Advincula AP. "Current thoughts" in electrosurgery. *Int J Gynaecol Obstet*. 2007;97(3):245-250.

73. Shirk GJ, Johns A, Redwine DB. Complications of laparoscopic surgery: How to avoid them and how to repair them. *J Minim Invasive Gynecol*. 2006;13(4):352-359.

74. Yazdani A, Krause H. Laparoscopic instrument insulation failure: the hidden hazard. *J Minim Invasive Gynecol*. 2007;14(2):228-232.

75. Smith TL, Smith JM. Electrosurgery in otolaryngology-head and neck surgery: principles, advances, and complications. *Laryngoscope*. 2001;111(5):769-780.

76. NFPA 99 Standard for Health Care Facilities. Quincy, MA: National Fire Protection Association; 2002: Issue D.7.3:203.

77. Garuti G, Luerti M. Hysteroscopic bipolar surgery: a valuable progress or a technique under investigation? *Curr Opin Obstet Gynecol*. 2009;21(4):329-334.

78. Matthews K. Argon beam coagulation. New directions in surgery. *AORN J*. 1992;56(5):885-889.

79. Fatal gas embolism caused by overpressurization during laparoscopic use of argon enhanced coagulation. *Health Devices*. 1994;23(6):257-259.

80. Kizer N, Zighelboim I, Rader JS. Cardiac arrest during laparotomy with argon beam coagulation of metastatic ovarian cancer. *Int J Gynecol Cancer*. 2009;19(2):237-238.

81. Misra S, Kimball WR. Pneumothorax during argon beam-enhanced coagulation in laparoscopy. *J Clin Anesth*. 2006;18(6):446-448.

82. Sezeur A, Partensky C, Chipponi J, Duron JJ. Death during laparoscopy: can 1 gas push out another? Danger of argon electrocoagulation. *Surg Laparosc Endosc Percutan Tech*. 2008;18(4):395-397.

83. HC11: Control of smoke from laser/electric surgical procedures. *http://www.cdc.gov/niosh/hc11.html*. Accessed October 13, 2009.

84. Ball K. *Lasers: The Perioperative Challenge*. Denver, CO: AORN, Inc; 2004.

85. Barker SJ, Polson JS. Fire in the operating room: a case report and laboratory study. *Anesth Analg*. 2001; 93(4):960-965.

86. Ulmer BC. The hazards of surgical smoke. *AORN J*. 2008;87(4):721-738.

87. Hoglan M. Potential hazards from electrosurgery plume—recommendations for surgical smoke evacuation. *Can Oper Room Nurs J*. 1995;13(4):10-16.

88. Safety and health topics: laser/electrosurgery plume. US Department of Labor Occupational Safety and Health Administration. *http://www.osha.gov/SLTC/laserelectrosurgeryplume/index.html*. Accessed October 13, 2009.

89. Alp E, Bijl D, Bleichrodt RP, Hansson B, Voss A. Surgical smoke and infection control. *J Hosp Infect*. 2006;62(1):1-5.

90. Garden JM, O'Banion MK, Shelnitz LS, et al. Papillomavirus in the vapor of carbon dioxide laser-treated verrucae. *JAMA*. 1988;259(8):1199-1202.

91. Hallmo P, Naess O. Laryngeal papillomatosis with human papillomavirus DNA contracted by a laser surgeon. *Eur Arch Otorhinolaryngol*. 1991;248(7):425-427.

92. ECRI Institute. Smoke evacuation systems, surgical. *Healthcare Product Comparison System*. 2007; November.

93. Barrett WL, Garber SM. Surgical smoke: a review of the literature. Is this just a lot of hot air? *Surg Endosc*. 2003;17(6):979-987.

94. Alp E, Bijl D, Bleichrodt RP, Hansson B, Voss A. Surgical smoke and infection control. *J Hosp Infect*. 2006;62(1):1-5.

95. Bigony L. Risks associated with exposure to surgical smoke plume: a review of the literature. *AORN J*. 2007;86(6):1013-1024.

96. Recommended practices for transfer of patient care information. In: *Perioperative Standards and Recommended Practices*. Denver, CO: AORN, Inc; 2010. In press.

97. Liapis D, de la Taille A, Ploussard G, et al. Analysis of complications from 600 retroperitoneoscopic procedures of the upper urinary tract during the last 10 years. *World J Urol*. 2008;26(6):523-530.

98. Marakis GN, Pavlidis TE, Ballas K, et al. Major complications during laparoscopic cholecystectomy. *Int Surg*. 2007;92(3):142-146.

99. Deziel DJ, Millikan KW, Economou SG, Doolas A, Ko ST, Airan MC. Complications of laparoscopic cholecystectomy. a national survey of 4,292 hospitals and an analysis of 77,604 cases. *Am J Surg*. 1993;165(1):9-14.

100. Abu-Rafea B, Vilos GA, Vilos AG, Hollett-Caines J, Al-Omran M. Effect of body habitus and parity on insufflated CO_2 volume at various intraabdominal pressures during laparoscopic access in women. *J Minim Invasive Gynecol*. 2006;13(3):205-210.

101. Recommended practices for positioning the patient in the perioperative practice setting. In: *Perioperative Standards and Recommended Practices*. Denver, CO: AORN, Inc; 2009:525-548.

102. Underwood S. Reducing positioning changes during robotic lead placement. *AORN J*. 2006;83(2):399-401.

103. Ito F, Gould JC. Robotic foregut surgery. *Int J Med Robot*. 2006;2(4):287-292.

104. Barnett JC, Hurd WW, Rogers RM Jr, Williams NL, Shapiro SA. Laparoscopic positioning and nerve injuries. *J Minim Invasive Gynecol*. 2007;14(5):664-673.

105. Pillai AK, Ferral H, Desai S, Paruchuri S, Asselmeier S, Perez-Gautrin R. Brachial plexus injury related to patient positioning. *J Vasc Interv Radiol*. 2007;18(7):833-834.

106. AORN position statement on fire prevention. AORN, Inc. *http://www.aorn.org/PracticeResources/AORNPositionStatements/Position FirePrevention*. Accessed October 14, 2009.

107. Hazard report: Reducing the risk of burns from surgical light sources. Health devices 2009;38(9):304-305.

108. Whelan RL, Fleshman J, Fowler DL. *The SAGES Manual of Perioperative Care in Minimally Invasive Surgery*. New York, NY: Springer-Verlag; 2006.

109. Strickland AK, Martindale RG. The increased incidence of intraabdominal infections in laparoscopic procedures: potential causes, postoperative management, and prospective innovations. *Surg Endosc*. 2005;19(7):874-881.

110. Shafi BM, Mery CM, Binyamin G, Dutta S. Natural orifice translumenal endoscopic surgery (NOTES). *Semin Pediatr Surg*. 2006;15(4):251-258.

111. Willingham FF, Brugge WR. Taking NOTES: translumenal flexible endoscopy and endoscopic surgery. *Curr Opin Gastroenterol*. 2007;23(5):550-555.

112. Malik A, Mellinger JD, Hazey JW, Dunkin BJ, MacFadyen BV Jr. Endoluminal and transluminal surgery: current status and future possibilities. *Surg Endosc*. 2006;20(8):1179-1192.

113. Kantsevoy SV, Hu B, Jagannath SB, et al. Transgastric endoscopic splenectomy: is it possible?. *Surg Endosc*. 2006;20(3):522-525.

114. de la Fuente SG, Demaria EJ, Reynolds JD, Portenier DD, Pryor AD. New developments in surgery: Natural Orifice Transluminal Endoscopic Surgery (NOTES). *Arch Surg*. 2007;142(3):295-297.

115. Robinson TN, Stiegmann GV. Minimally invasive surgery. *Endoscopy*. 2007;39(1):21-23.

116. Jin J, Rosen M, Ponsky J. Minimally invasive surgery 2006-2007. *Endoscopy*. 2008;40(1):61-64.

117. Biscione FM, Couto RC, Pedrosa TM, Neto MC. Factors influencing the risk of surgical site infection following diagnostic exploration of the abdominal cavity. *J Infect*. 2007;55(4):317-323.

118. Gupta R, Sample C, Bamehriz F, Birch DW. Infectious complications following laparoscopic appendectomy. *Can J Surg*. 2006;49(6):397-400.

119. Miller CE. Methods of tissue extraction in advanced laparoscopy. *Curr Opin Obstet Gynecol*. 2001;13(4):399-405.

120. Milad MP, Sokol E. Laparoscopic morcellator-related injuries. *J Am Assoc Gynecol Laparosc*. 2003; 10(3):383-385.

121. ECRI Institute. Safe use and selection of trocars in laparoscopy. *Healthcare Risk Control*. 2006;4(Surgery and Anesthesia 25).

122. Vilos GA, Ternamian A, Dempster J, Laberge PY; The Society of Obstetricians and Gynaecologists of Canada. Laparoscopic entry: a review of techniques,

technologies, and complications. *J Obstet Gynaecol Can.* 2007;29(5):433-465.

123. Salama IA, Schwaitzberg SD. Utility of a voice-activated system in minimally invasive surgery. *J Laparoendosc Adv Surg Tech A.* 2005;15(5):443-446.

124. Gutt CN, Oniu T, Mehrabi A, et al. Circulatory and respiratory complications of carbon dioxide insufflation. *Dig Surg.* 2004;21(2):95-104.

125. Wadlund DL. Laparoscopy: risks, benefits and complications. *Nurs Clin North Am.* 2006;41(2):219-229.

126. Yoshida H, Kushikata T, Kabara S, Takase H, Ishihara H, Hirota K. Flat electroencephalogram caused by carbon dioxide pneumoperitoneum. *Anesth Analg.* 2007;105(6): 1749-1752.

127. Hunter JG, Staheli J, Oddsdottir M, Trus T. Nitrous oxide pneumoperitoneum revisited. Is there a risk of combustion? *Surg Endosc.* 1995;9(5):501-504.

128. Yeh CH, Kwok SY, Chan MK, Tjandra JJ. Prospective, case-matched study of heated and humidified carbon dioxide insufflation in laparoscopic colorectal surgery. *Colorectal Dis.* 2007;9(8):695-700.

129. Jacobs VR, Kiechle M, Morrison JE Jr. Carbon dioxide gas heating inside laparoscopic insufflators has no effect. *JSLS.* 2005;9(2):208-212.

130. Savel RH, Balasubramanya S, Lasheen S, et al. Beneficial effects of humidified, warmed carbon dioxide insufflation during laparoscopic bariatric surgery: a randomized clinical trial. *Obes Surg.* 2005;15(1):64-69.

131. Champion JK, Williams M. Prospective randomized trial of heated humidified versus cold dry carbon dioxide insufflation during laparoscopic gastric bypass. *Surg Obes Relat Dis.* 2006;2(4):445-450.

132. Hamza MA, Schneider BE, White PF, et al. Heated and humidified insufflation during laparoscopic gastric bypass surgery: effect on temperature, postoperative pain, and recovery outcomes. *J Laparoendosc Adv Surg Tech A.* 2005;15(1):6-12.

133. Farley DR, Greenlee SM, Larson DR, Harrington JR. Double-blind, prospective, randomized study of warmed, humidified carbon dioxide insufflation vs standard carbon dioxide for patients undergoing laparoscopic cholecystectomy. *Arch Surg.* 2004;139(7):739-744.

134. Barragan AB, Frezza EE. Impact of a warm gas insufflation on operating-room ergonometrics during laparoscopic gastric bypass: a pilot study. *Obes Surg.* 2005;15(1):70-72.

135. Pasic RP, Kantardzic M, Templeman C, Levine RL. Insufflation techniques in gynecologic laparoscopy. *Surg Laparosc Endosc Percutan Tech.* 2006;16(1):18-24.

136. Calcaterra D, Salerno TA. Venous gas embolization during endoscopic vein harvesting for coronary artery revascularization: a life-threatening event. *J Card Surg.* 2007;22(6):498-499.

137. Potapov EV, Buz S, Hetzer R. CO(2) embolism during minimally invasive vein harvesting. *Eur J Cardiothorac Surg.* 2007;31(5):944-945.

138. Jacobs VR, Morrison JE Jr, Kiechle M. Twenty-five simple ways to increase insufflation performance and patient safety in laparoscopy. *J Am Assoc Gynecol Laparosc.* 2004;11(3):410-423.

139. Entry of abdominal fluids into laparoscopic insufflators. *Health Devices.* 1992;21(5):180-181.

140. Mertens zur Borg IR, Lim A, Verbrugge SJ, IJzermans JN, Klein J. Effect of intraabdominal pressure elevation and positioning on hemodynamic responses during carbon dioxide pneumoperitoneum for laparoscopic donor nephrectomy: a prospective controlled clinical study. *Surg Endosc.* 2004;18(6):919-923.

141. Meierhenrich R, Gauss A, Vandenesch P, Georgieff M, Poch B, Schutz W. The effects of intraabdominally insufflated carbon dioxide on hepatic blood flow during laparoscopic surgery assessed by transesophageal echocardiography. *Anesth Analg.* 2005;100(2):340-347.

142. Koivusalo AM, Pere P, Valjus M, Scheinin T. Laparoscopic cholecystectomy with carbon dioxide pneumoperitoneum is safe even for high-risk patients. *Surg Endosc.* 2008;22(1):61-67.

143. Hahn RG. Fluid absorption in endoscopic surgery. *Br J Anaesth.* 2006;96(1):8-20.

144. Recommended practices for the prevention of unplanned perioperative hypothermia. In: *Perioperative Standards and Recommended Practices.* Denver, CO: AORN, Inc; 2009:491-504.

145. Moharari RS, Khajavi MR, Khademhosseini P, Hosseini SR, Najafi A. Sterile water as an irrigating fluid for transurethral resection of the prostate: anesthetical view of the records of 1600 cases. *South Med J.* 2008;101(4):373-375.

146. Collins JW, Macdermott S, Bradbrook RA, Drake B, Keeley FX, Timoney AG. The effect of the choice of irrigation fluid on cardiac stress during transurethral resection of the prostate: a comparison between 1.5% glycine and 5% glucose. *J Urol.* 2007;177(4):1369-1373.

147. Ho HS, Cheng CW. Bipolar transurethral resection of prostate: a new reference standard? *Curr Opin Urol.* 2008;18(1):50-55.

148. Recommended practices for environmental cleaning in the perioperative setting. In: *Perioperative Standards and Recommended Practices.* Denver, CO: AORN; 2009:439-453.

149. Sessler DI. Complications and treatment of mild hypothermia. *Anesthesiology.* 2001;95(2):531-543.

150. Moore SS, Green CR, Wang FL, Pandit SK, Hurd WW. The role of irrigation in the development of hypothermia during laparoscopic surgery. *Am J Obstet Gynecol.* 1997;176(3):598-602.

151. Kelly JA, Doughty JK, Hasselbeck AN, Vacchiano CA. The effect of arthroscopic irrigation fluid warming on body temperature. *J Perianesth Nurs.* 2000;15(4):245-252.

152. Mirza S, Panesar S, AuYong KJ, French J, Jones D, Akmal S. The effects of irrigation fluid on core temperature in endoscopic urological surgery. *J Perioper Pract.* 2007;17(10):494-503.

153. Okeke LI. Effect of warm intravenous and irrigating fluids on body temperature during transurethral resection of the prostate gland. *BMC Urol.* 2007;7:15.

154. Jaffe JS, McCullough TC, Harkaway RC, Ginsberg PC. Effects of irrigation fluid temperature on core body temperature during transurethral resection of the prostate. *Urology.* 2001;57(6):1078-1081.

155. Young EC. Hysteroscopy and fluid management. *Perioperative Nursing Clinics.* 2006;4(1):365-373.

156. de Freitas Fonseca M, Andrade CM Jr, Cardoso MJE, Crispi CP. Temperature of distention fluid and risk of overload in operative hysteroscopy. *J Minim Invasive Gynecol.* 2008;15(6):77S-78S.

157. Boyd HR, Stanley C. Sources of error when tracking irrigation fluids during hysteroscopic procedures. *J Am Assoc Gynecol Laparosc.* 2000;7(4):472-476.

158. Nezhat CH, Fisher DT, Datta S. Investigation of often-reported ten percent hysteroscopy fluid overfill: is this accurate? *J Minim Invasive Gynecol.* 2007;14(4):489-493.

159. Hahn RG. Smoking increases the risk of large scale fluid absorption during transurethral prostatic resection. *J Urol.* 2001;166(1):162-165.

160. Yeates KE, Singer M, Morton AR. Salt and water: a simple approach to hyponatremia. *CMAJ.* 2004;170(3):365-369.

161. Morrison DM. Management of hysteroscopic surgery complications. *AORN J.* 1999;69(1):194-221.

162. Bennett KL, Ohrmundt C, Maloni JA. Preventing intravasation In women undergoing hysteroscopic procedures. *AORN J.* 1996;64(5):792-799.

163. Sinha M, Hegde A, Sinha R, Goel S. Parotid area sign: a clinical test for the diagnosis of fluid overload in hysteroscopic surgery. *J Minim Invasive Gynecol.* 2007;14(2):161-168.

164. Singer GG, Brenner BM. Chapter 46: Fluid and electrolyte disturbances. In: Fauci AS, Braunwald E, Kasper DL, Hauser SL, Longo DL, Jameson JL, Loscalzo J, eds. *Harrison's Principles of Internal Medicine.* 17th ed. New York, NY: McGraw-Hill; 2008.

165. Kaye AD, Riopelle JM. Chapter 54: Intravascular fluid and electrolyte physiology. In: Miller RD, ed. *Miller's Anesthesia.* 7th ed. Edinburgh: Churchill Livingstone; 2009:1705-1737.

166. Ray JM, Conner J, Dillman G, Haynes WB, Lock R. Post-arthroscopic pulmonary edema in two healthy teenage athletes. *J Ky Med Assoc.* 1991;89(2):75-78.

167. Hynson JM, Tung A, Guevara JE, Katz JA, Glick JM, Shapiro WA. Complete airway obstruction during arthroscopic shoulder surgery. *Anesth Analg.* 1993;76(4):875-878.

168. Smith CD, Shah MM. Fluid gain during routine shoulder arthroscopy. *J Shoulder Elbow Surg.* 2008;17(3):415-417.

169. Human Factors in Health Care Tool Kit. AORN, Inc. http://www.aorn.org/PracticeResources/ToolKits/HumanFactorsInHealthCareToolKit. Accessed October 14, 2009.

170. Title 21, Pt. 803: Medical Device Reporting. In: *Code of Federal Regulations.* 2009.

171. HHS Office for Civil Rights. Standards for privacy of individually identifiable health information. Final rule. *Fed Regist.* 2002;67(157):53181-53273.

172. Wiegmann DA, ElBardissi AW, Dearani JA, Daly RC, Sundt TM 3rd. Disruptions in surgical flow and their relationship to surgical errors: an exploratory investigation. *Surgery.* 2007;142(5):658-665.

173. Quality and performance improvement standards for perioperative nursing. In: *Perioperative Standards and Recommended Practices.* Denver, CO: AORN, Inc; 2009:65-74.

Acknowledgements

LEAD AUTHOR
Bonnie Denholm, RN, MS, CNOR
Perioperative Nursing Specialist
AORN Center for Nursing Practice
Denver, Colorado

CONTRIBUTING AUTHORS
Sharon Van Wicklin, RN, MSN, CNOR, CRNFA
Educator/Staff Development
Williamson Medical Center
Franklin, Tennessee

Eileen C. Young, RN, CNOR
Senior Clinical Nurse Educator
Gyrus ACMI, an Olympus Company
Kutztown, Pennsylvania

Annette Wasielewski, BSN, RN, CNOR
Administrative Director Minimally Invasive Surgery, Robotics, Bariatrics
Hackensack University Medical Center
Hackensack, New Jersey

PUBLICATION HISTORY
Originally published as proposed recommended practices February 1994, *AORN Journal.*

Revised November 1998; published February 1999, *AORN Journal.* Reformatted July 2000.

Revised November 2004; published as "Recommended Practices for Endoscopic Minimally Invasive Surgery" in *Standards, Recommended Practices, and Guidelines,* 2005 edition. March 2005, *AORN Journal.*

Revised October 2009 for online publication in *Perioperative Standards and Recommended Practices.*

Recommended Practices for the Use of the Pneumatic Tourniquet in the Perioperative Practice Setting

The following recommended practices were developed by the AORN Recommended Practices Committee and have been approved by the AORN Board of Directors. They were presented as proposed recommended practices for comments by members and others. They are effective January 1, 2007.

These recommended practices are intended as achievable recommendations representing what is believed to be an optimal level of practice. Policies and procedures will reflect variations in practice settings and/or clinical situations that determine the degree to which the recommended practices can be implemented.

AORN recognizes the numerous settings in which perioperative nurses practice. These recommended practices are intended as guidelines adaptable to various practice settings. These practice settings include traditional operating rooms, ambulatory surgery centers, physicians' offices, radiology departments, and all other areas where operative and other invasive procedures may be performed.

Purpose

These recommended practices provide guidelines for use of pneumatic tourniquets, which are primarily used to occlude blood flow, obtain a near bloodless field for extremity surgery, and to confine a bolus of anesthetic in an extremity for intravenous regional anesthesia (IVRA; ie, Bier block). These recommended practices provide information for testing, applying, and cleaning pneumatic tourniquet equipment, and the patient care associated with the safe use of this equipment. Pneumatic tourniquet equipment consists of a pressure regulator with display, connective tubing, and an inflatable cuff. These recommended practices provide general guidelines for developing policies and procedures for safe use of a pneumatic tourniquet in the practice setting. Due to the variety and complexity of current pneumatic tourniquet equipment, policies and procedures should reflect considerations for the specific pneumatic tourniquet system being used.

Recommendation I

Patient safety should be the primary consideration in evaluation, selection, purchase, and use of the pneumatic tourniquet and accessories.

1. Equipment selected should include technology to determine cuff pressure during use.

2. The pressure regulator should be self-calibrating upon activation.

3. If electric, the regulator should have a backup battery for use during a power failure.

4. The pressure display should be visible whenever the cuff is inflated.

5. An audible activation indicator(s) and alarm(s) should be present and loud enough to be heard above other sounds in the OR to alert personnel to a change in pressure and lapse of a designated duration of inflation time.[1]

6. The pneumatic tourniquet electrical cord should be flexible and adequate in length to reach the electrical outlet without stress or require the use of an extension cord.

7. Tourniquet cuffs and tubing should be compatible with the tourniquet regulator and other accessories. The tourniquet tubing should be incompatible with other tubing (eg, intravenous) or labeled to clearly identify that it is part of the tourniquet system. Although the US Food and Drug Administration (FDA) has not received reports of misconnections involving tourniquet tubing, over 300 cases of misconnections of other types of tubing resulting in injury have been reported.[2] Many of these reports involved luer connections. The Joint Commission for the Accreditation of Healthcare Organizations (JCAHO) has received reports of eight deaths associated with misconnections of tubing.[2]

8. Tourniquet cuffs should be clean. If the cuffs are unable to be adequately cleaned, single-use cuffs should be selected.

9. A variety of sizes and shapes of tourniquet cuffs should be available to meet the needs of the patients treated in the health care organization. Contoured cuffs should be available for use on extremities of patients where there is a significant difference in circumference between the proximal and distal edges of the cuff (eg, those seen in obese patients). Pediatric cuffs should be available for children. Injuries can result from the use of an inappropriate size or shape of cuff.

10. Pneumatic tourniquet technology continues to evolve, changing the way in which limb blood

occlusion is achieved. Health care organizations and personnel should stay abreast of evolving technology and its effect on patient care and safety.

Recommendation II

The pneumatic tourniquet and its accessories should be inspected, tested, and maintained according to manufacturers' written instructions.

1. Instructions for pneumatic tourniquet use, warranties, and a manual for maintenance and inspections should be obtained from the manufacturer and be readily available to users. Equipment manuals assist in developing operational, safety, and maintenance guidelines, as well as serve as a reference for appropriate use.

2. A brief set of clearly readable operating instructions should be readily accessible with each tourniquet system. These instructions should be placed on or attached to each pneumatic tourniquet for quick reference.

3. Before initial use, designated personnel within the health care organization should evaluate the pneumatic tourniquet system for safety.

4. Each pneumatic tourniquet should be assigned an identification or serial number. This number facilitates documenting maintenance performed on individual pneumatic tourniquets and tracking of problems that occur.

5. Safety/warning alarms should be operational at all times. Lights should be operational and visible. The volume of the activation indicator should be maintained at an audible level to immediately alert personnel when the pneumatic tourniquet has detected a problem.

6. Before each use, the entire tourniquet system should be checked.
   ♦ If attached to a gas source, the source should be compatible with the equipment design and the connections secure.
   ♦ The cuff, tubing, connectors, gauges, and pressure source should be clean and kept in working order.
   ♦ The tourniquet should be tested for integrity and function. Assuring that the tourniquet functions properly before a procedure minimizes the risk of pressure loss or patient injury. Most electric tourniquets automatically self-test and calibrate upon activation.

♦ The cuff and tubing should be inspected for cracks, leaks, and the security of the closure mechanism. Unintentional pressure loss can result from loose tubing connectors, deteriorated tubing, or cuff bladder leaks, and may result in patient injury.[3]

7. The pneumatic tourniquet system should be evaluated for safe use by designated personnel (eg, biomedical engineering personnel) within the health care organization, at intervals consistent with the manufacturer's written instructions and policies of the health care organization. Nerve injuries have been reported when malfunctioning equipment has caused excessive pressure.[4]

8. A pneumatic tourniquet that is not working properly or is damaged should be removed from service immediately, along with all accessories, and reported to the designated individual responsible for equipment maintenance (eg, biomedical engineering personnel).

Recommendation III

The perioperative nurse should assess the patient preoperatively for risks and report potential contraindications to the surgeon.

Note: The operating physician determines use of a tourniquet, based upon the risks and benefits to the patient.

1. The perioperative nurse should assess the patient for considerations related to tourniquet use. This assessment should include, but not be limited to,
   ♦ planned location of the tourniquet;
   ♦ relative contraindications, including, but not limited to
     – extremity infection,[4,5]
     – open fracture,[4,5]
     – tumor distal to the tourniquet,[4,5]
     – sickle cell anemia,[4]
     – impaired circulation,[4-6]
     – previous revascularization of the extremity,[6]
     – extremities with dialysis access (eg, AV shunts, fistulas),
     – venous thromboembolism,[6]
     – increased intracranial pressure,[4,5] and
     – acidosis;[5]
   ♦ size and shape of the extremity.
   ♦ condition of skin under and distal to the cuff site; and
   ♦ peripheral pulses distal to the cuff.

2. Prophylactic antibiotics, when ordered, should be completely infused before tourniquet cuff inflation. Efficacy of the prophylactic antibiotics requires tissue perfusion of the surgical site. Optimum tissue concentrations have been found when antibiotics were administered 20 minutes before tourniquet inflation.[7,8]

Recommendation IV

The pneumatic tourniquet should be connected to the appropriate power/gas source in a manner that minimizes risk of patient injury.

1. The appropriate gas source should be selected according to manufacturers' written instructions. Tourniquet systems use compressed gas to apply a carefully controlled amount of tourniquet pressure. The design of the specific tourniquet system determines whether this gas is nitrogen or air. Gas (either nitrogen or compressed air) may be delivered from a portable canister, tank, or built-in system. Connection of the incorrect gas for inflation creates a fire hazard.[3]

2. Tourniquets should never be inflated with nitrous oxide or oxygen because of risk of fire.[3] Some tourniquets have an internal pump that compresses room air, eliminating the risk of erroneously connecting the system to an oxidizing gas.

Recommendation V

The components of the pneumatic tourniquet should be handled in a manner that minimizes the potential for damage and risk of subsequent patient injuries.

1. The pneumatic tourniquet regulator should be securely mounted on a fixed column or pole with a tip-resistant base. Applying tension on the electrical cord increases the risk that it will become disconnected, frayed, or move the equipment, which may result in injuries to patients and personnel.

2. The pneumatic tourniquet regulator should be placed near the point of use and the electrical cord should reach the wall or column outlet without stress on the cord and without blocking a traffic path. Stress on the cord may cause damage to the cord, posing a hazard. The electrical cord should be free of kinks, knots, and bends

that could damage the cord or cause leakage, current accumulation, and overheating of the cord's insulation.

3. The pneumatic tourniquet plug, not the cord, should be held when it is removed from the outlet. Pulling on the cord may cause cord breakage and poses a fire hazard.

4. Tourniquet cuffs should be handled carefully. Care should be taken to avoid puncturing the cuff. Towel clips used near the cuff should be carefully placed to avoid damage to the cuff.

5. Excessive compression of the tourniquet cuff by a limb-positioning device should be avoided.

6. The pneumatic tourniquet and electrical cord should be kept dry. Pooled fluids on the floor and fluids dripping into the pneumatic tourniquet regulator or electrical connections create an electrical hazard.

Recommendation VI

A pneumatic tourniquet cuff should be selected and applied in a manner to minimize the risk of injury to the patient.

Improper tourniquet cuff application may lead to venous congestion, bruising, blistering, pinching, ecchymosis, or necrosis of the skin.

1. The width of the tourniquet cuff should be individualized, with consideration to the size and shape of the patient's limb. The cuff should be wider than half the limb's diameter. Wider cuffs minimize the risk of injury to underlying tissue by dispersing pressure over a greater surface area. In clinical trials, using a wider cuff has been found consistently to occlude blood flow at a lower pressure in adult patients.[9-14] Similar results were found using wider cuffs in children.[15]

2. Wider, contoured tourniquet cuffs should be used for patient extremities in which there is a tapering of the extremity between the upper and lower edge of the cuff (eg, obese, very muscular). Contoured tourniquet cuffs have been found in clinical trials to occlude arterial flow at lower pressures than straight tourniquet cuffs of equal width.[11,13,14] Contoured tourniquet cuffs minimize the risk of excessive pressure on one edge of the cuff, migration of the cuff, and a shearing injury to underlying tissue.

3. The length of the tourniquet cuff should be individualized, taking into consideration the size and circumference of the patient's limb. The tourniquet cuff should overlap at least three inches but not more than six inches.[4] Too much overlap causes increased pressure and potential rolling or wrinkling of underlying soft tissue. Too small an overlap compromises effective tourniquet inflation and can result in unexpected release or inadequate constriction.

4. The correct surgical site should be verified before application of the tourniquet cuff.

5. A soft padding should be placed around the limb, being careful to stretch the padding so that it is wrinkle-free and does not pinch the skin. In a clinical trial, the overall skin complication rate was lower when padding was used.[16,17] Options include, but are not limited to, limb protection sleeves matched to the specific tourniquet cuff or two layers of stockinette stretched to fit the extremity. Materials that may shed loose fibers (eg, cotton cast padding, sheet padding) should be avoided. Lint from these materials can become embedded in the fasteners and reduce the effectiveness, possibly leading to an unexpected release of the cuff during the procedure.

6. Tourniquet cuffs should be applied to the verified operative extremity in a location with adequate muscle mass to protect nerves and vessels.
   - Upper arm and thigh tourniquets should be positioned on the limb at the point of maximum circumference proximal to the incision.[18,19]
   - Forearm tourniquets should be positioned mid-forearm.[18,19]
   - Calf tourniquets should be placed with the proximal edge on the largest area of calf circumference.[20]
   - Ankle tourniquets should be placed over the lower third of the lower leg, with the distal edge proximal to the malleoli.[20-23]

   There is a potential risk to superficial nerves in unprotected areas during cuff placement. When the tourniquet cuff is inflated, nerves and blood vessels are compressed.

7. To improve tourniquet cuff positioning on an obese patient's extremity, an assistant should manually grasp the adipose tissue of the extremity and gently apply and hold traction distal to the tourniquet site until the padding and cuff are placed. Traction should be maintained until the cuff is secured.[24]

8. The patient's skin under the tourniquet cuff should be protected to prevent fluid accumulation (eg, skin prep solutions, irrigation) under the cuff, which may cause skin injury.

9. The cuff should be applied in its final position. If at any time a cuff position change is necessary, the cuff should be removed and reapplied. Moving a cuff after placement may cause shearing of underlying tissues and subsequent injury.

10. The cuff tubing should be positioned on or near the lateral aspect of the extremity to avoid pressure on nerves and kinking of the tubing.

11. Reusable tourniquet cuffs should be protected from contamination by fluid, blood, and other potentially infectious material during surgery. Tourniquet protectors (eg, U-shaped drapes, adhesive drapes, tourniquet covers) should be used to minimize soiling.

12. The use of a single-use cuff should be considered when adequate protection of the cuff cannot be assured.

Recommendation VII

The extremity should be exsanguinated before inflation of the tourniquet.

1. The extremity should be elevated to allow venous blood to exit the limb.

2. An elastic wrap (eg, Esmarch's bandage) should be available for exsanguination.

   An elastic wrap compresses superficial blood vessels, forcing blood out of the extremity. The surgeon determines use of an elastic wrap with consideration to the risks and benefits to the patient.
   - Use of an elastic bandage for exsanguination enhances the bloodless field and may minimize the pain associated with tourniquet use.
   - Exsanguination using an elastic wrap may not be appropriate following traumatic injury or if the extremity has been in a cast. In these instances, thrombi in blood vessels may become dislodged, resulting in emboli. Fatal pulmonary emboli have been reported following exsanguinations of such extremities.[25-27]

♦ In the presence of infection, malignant tumor, or fractures in the extremity, exsanguination should be accomplished by extremity elevation alone. Infection as well as malignant cells can be forced into the torso during aggressive exsanguination. Additional tissue damage can result from compressing of fractures.

3. The anesthesia care provider should be alerted before wrapping the extremity. Notification of the anesthesia care provider facilitates monitoring for potential complications.

Recommendation VIII

Tourniquet inflation pressure should be kept to the minimum effective pressure.[4,11,28,29]

Overpressurization may cause pain at the tourniquet cuff site; muscle weakness; compression injuries to blood vessels, nerve, muscle, or skin; or extremity paralysis. Underpressurization may result in blood in the surgical field, passive congestion of the limb, shock, and hemorrhagic infiltration of a nerve.

1. Pressure settings should be based on limb occlusion pressure (LOP). Research studies have shown that occlusion can be achieved using a lower pressure when using a LOP method in conjunction with a wide tourniquet cuff in adult patients.[12,13,15,28,30,31] The same was found when studying children.[15] Applying lower pressure has been found to result in less postoperative pain.[11,31,32] Some tourniquet systems are designed to determine LOP automatically and add a safety margin to allow for fluctuations in blood pressure intraoperatively. If a standard tourniquet cuff is used, the LOP should be determined using the following steps.
   ♦ Apply the tourniquet cuff over the appropriate limb protection material.
   ♦ Using a Doppler stethoscope, locate an arterial pulse distal to the cuff. Normally, the radial artery is used on the arm and the posterior tibial artery is used on the leg. The dorsalis pedis artery may also be used for the leg.
   ♦ Slowly increase cuff pressure until the arterial pulse stops and remains stopped for several heartbeats.
   ♦ Note the cuff pressure. This is the LOP.
   ♦ Deflate the cuff and confirm that the distal pulse resumes.

♦ Before cuff inflation, adjust the cuff pressure setting by adding a safety margin to the LOP as follows:
   – add 40 mm Hg for LOP less than 130 mm Hg,
   – add 60 mm Hg for LOP between 131–190 mm Hg,
   – add 80 mm Hg for LOP greater than 190 mm Hg[33];
   – for pediatric patients, adding 50 mm Hg has been recommended.[34]

2. The LOP measurement should be made when the blood pressure is stabilized to the level expected during surgery. The LOP measurement may be completed before or after induction of anesthesia. Blood pressure at the time of LOP measurement should be documented.

3. The LOP and inflation pressure setting should be confirmed with the surgeon.

4. Inflation of the tourniquet cuff should be under the direction of the surgeon and coordinated with the anesthesia care provider.

5. After limb exsanguination and cuff inflation, there is an increase in blood volume to vital organs and a subsequent increase in systolic blood pressure.[4] Coordination with the anesthesia care provider facilitates management of the patient during this rapid physiologic change.

6. Pneumatic tourniquets should be inflated rapidly. Rapid tourniquet cuff inflation occludes arteries and veins almost simultaneously, preventing filling of superficial veins before occlusion of arterial blood flow.

7. While the tourniquet cuff is inflated, the pressure gauge or digital display should be clearly visible and monitored for excessive fluctuation. Nerve damage may result from excessive tourniquet pressure or uneven padding.[35] Catastrophic neurological complications (eg, permanent nerve palsy) can occur with excessive tourniquet inflation pressures.[36]

Recommendation IX

Pneumatic tourniquet inflation time should be kept to a minimum and deflation managed to minimize risks to the patient.

Excessive inflation time may result in venous engorgement, hyperemia, muscle weakness, ischemic injury, or extremity paralysis. Neurological complications have been found to be associated with longer inflation times.[37]

1. The surgeon should be informed of the duration of the tourniquet time at regular, established intervals. Use of a timer and audible alarm on the tourniquet regulator facilitates this communication. Serious patient injury, including extremity paralysis, may result from prolonged inflation of the tourniquet.[38-40] Safe tourniquet inflation time has not been precisely determined. The time varies with the patient's age, physical status, and the vascular supply to the extremity. There is general agreement that inflation time should not exceed 60 minutes for an upper extremity and 90 minutes for a lower extremity.[33] In pediatric patients, inflation times of less than 75 minutes for lower extremities has been recommended.[41]

2. When prolonged tourniquet time is desired, the tourniquet should be released for reperfusion of the limb every hour. The reperfusion time should be 15 minutes, after which the tourniquet may be reinflated for another full period as above. Reperfusion allows oxygenation and continued viability of the tissue. Fifteen minutes of reperfusion after one hour has been found to minimize the tissue inflammatory response and is recommended.[42-45]

3. Deflation of the tourniquet should be coordinated with the anesthesia care provider. Physiologic changes resulting from deflation of the tourniquet are dependent upon the relative size of the extremity, duration of tourniquet time, and overall physiologic status of the patient. A decrease in blood pressure occurs as blood is shunted to the extremity.[4] A significant decrease in core body temperature occurs upon deflation of a lower extremity cuff.[46,47] Products of anaerobic metabolism enter the circulation upon deflation of the cuff causing a transient hyperemia and a mixed respiratory/metabolic acidosis. This results in a decrease in oxygen saturation and increase in end-tidal carbon dioxide. In a study measuring emboli released upon cuff deflation, the highest number were released within one minute of deflation.[48] Coordination with the anesthesia care provider or perioperative registered nurse monitoring the patient facilitates management of

the patient's physiologic status during this rapid change.

4. Pneumatic tourniquets should be deflated as recommended by the manufacturer. The cuff and sleeve/padding should be removed from the extremity upon deflation of the tourniquet. Even the slight impedance of venous return by the padding or deflated cuff may lead to congestion and pooling of blood at the surgical site.[34]

Recommendation X

The patient should be monitored continuously with special consideration to pain and temperature while the tourniquet cuff is inflated.

1. Pain should be assessed and managed. After inflation of the pneumatic tourniquet for 30 to 60 minutes, patients may experience "tourniquet pain," accompanied by an increase in heart rate and blood pressure.[4,49]

2. The patient's temperature should be continuously monitored during use of a pneumatic tourniquet. In pediatric and adult patients, inflated tourniquets result in an increase in core body temperature.[41,50]

3. Care should be exercised to avoid overheating the patient while the tourniquet cuff is inflated, particularly in pediatric patients.[51,52]

Recommendation XI

The perioperative registered nurse should evaluate the outcome of the patient care at the end of the procedure.

1. The patient should be continuously monitored for 15 minutes after deflation of the pneumatic tourniquet.
   - A decrease in blood pressure occurs as blood is shunted to the extremity.
   - Products of anaerobic metabolism enter the circulation upon deflation of the tourniquet cuff, causing transient hyperemia and a mixed respiratory/metabolic acidosis. This results in a decrease in oxygen saturation.[41,49,53]
   - Increases in end-tidal carbon dioxide occur.[41,49,54-56] The time for clearance of the metabolites depends upon the patient's physiologic status, extremity involved, and duration of tourniquet inflation.

♦ A decrease in core body temperature typically occurs upon deflation of a lower extremity tourniquet cuff.[46,47,50]

♦ An increase in intracranial pressure can occur.[43,57]

♦ An embolism can be released from the extremity upon deflation of the tourniquet cuff.[58-62]

In a study of patients undergoing total knee arthroplasty, blood pressure dropped immediately upon tourniquet cuff deflation and remained depressed for 15 minutes. Metabolites were reabsorbed within 30 minutes of deflation.[54] The peak number of emboli released occurs within 60 seconds of tourniquet cuff deflation.[56]

2. The immediate postoperative evaluation should include, but not be limited to,
   ♦ vital signs, including oxygen saturation;
   ♦ skin condition under the tourniquet (eg, temperature, color, integrity);
   ♦ pulses distal to the tourniquet cuff; and
   ♦ temperature.

3. Use of the pneumatic tourniquet and patient outcomes should be reported during patient hand off to other caregivers.[63]

4. Any complications should be reported to the surgeon and anesthesia care provider and discussed during the hand off of care to other caregivers.

5. Potential complications include, but are not limited to,
   ♦ injury to skin, muscle, nerves, and vessels underneath the tourniquet cuff;
   ♦ hematoma;
   ♦ edema;
   ♦ circulatory impairment distal to the tourniquet cuff, venous congestion, or emboli;
   ♦ damage to nerves distal to the tourniquet cuff;[20,37,64]
   ♦ wound effusion;
   ♦ compartment syndrome;[65-68] and
   ♦ pulmonary embolism.[48,69-71]

Serious injuries due to the use of pneumatic tourniquets are uncommon, but the risk is present. The risk of pulmonary emboli has been found to be associated with duration of tourniquet time.[4,48] Neurological complications have also been found to be associated with longer tourniquet times.[37]

Recommendation XII

Additional care should be taken in procedures involving tourniquet control on two extremities because the risk of complications and the systemic effects of tourniquet use may be increased.

1. The perioperative registered nurse, surgical team, and anesthesia care provider should be familiar with the respective placement of the tourniquets when using tourniquets on more than one extremity. Labeling the tubing to each cuff minimizes the risk of inflating/deflating the wrong cuff.

2. Blood pressure should be closely monitored. Exsanguination and inflating the cuff on both extremities in rapid succession may cause a more pronounced blood pressure rise due to the sudden decrease in effective circulation system volume.

3. Temperature should be monitored and care should be taken not to overheat the patient with warming devices. In studies of children, the rise in core body temperature is significantly greater with bilateral tourniquets compared to a single tourniquet.[34,41]

4. When tourniquets are used on more than one extremity, the first tourniquet cuff inflated should be completely deflated (and the cuff and limb protection removed, if possible) to assure circulation in the first limb has been restored. Problems related to incomplete tourniquet deflation could go unnoticed throughout the second limb procedure.

5. If possible, tourniquet deflations should be staggered 30 to 45 minutes apart to reduce the rapid release of large amounts of metabolic byproducts into the vascular system. Tourniquet use causes anaerobic metabolism, which produces lactic acid and other metabolites. Lactic acidosis causes a decrease in vascular resistance and allows an increased blood flow when the tourniquet is deflated. The larger the muscle mass experiencing ischemia from the tourniquet, the greater the production of these metabolic byproducts. Sequential deflation lessens the potential for adverse patient reactions to these byproducts.[72] In children, when simultaneous deflation of bilateral tourniquets occurred, systolic blood pressure decreased 8–10 mm Hg and a greater decrease in pH was seen.[41]

Recommendation XIII

Potential patient injuries and complications associated with intravenous regional anesthesia (IVRA [ie, Bier block]) should be identified and safe practices should be established.

1. Tourniquet users should be familiar with the inflation-deflation sequence when using a dual-bladder cuff and when using two single-bladder cuffs together for IVRA. Severe injuries and deaths have occurred when the wrong cuff was deflated.[73]

2. Patient assessment and tourniquet application before IVRA should include, but not be limited to, allergies to local anesthetics.

3. The appropriate tourniquet cuff should be selected.
   - A dual-bladder tourniquet cuff and extra connective tubing are generally required.
   - A wider placement site is needed because of the additional width of the dual-bladder tourniquet cuff.
   - A higher pressure is generally required because each cuff bladder is narrower.

4. The tourniquet user should be fully aware of which cuff is proximal, which cuff is distal, and the inflation/deflation status of each at all times. Labeling or color-coding of the tubings to these cuffs facilitates identification.[2]

5. The tourniquet should be deflated gradually as determined by the physician to minimize the potential for an adverse reaction. As the tourniquet cuff deflates, the anesthetic agent is released into the circulatory system, causing systemic effects.

6. The perioperative registered nurse circulator should be aware of the patient's physiological status. Adverse reactions to local anesthetic agents are potential complications of IVRA. A bolus of local anesthesia entering the general circulation can occur when there is a sudden deflation of the tourniquet, from deflation soon after injection of local anesthetic, or if the bolus is released too rapidly at the end of the procedure. The sudden rush of anesthetic and metabolites into the circulatory system affects the central nervous system (eg, ringing in the ears, tingling, numbness, loss of consciousness, seizures) and the heart.

Recommendation XIV

The pneumatic tourniquet and accessories should be cleaned after each use.

1. After use, personnel should turn off the pneumatic tourniquet, clean all reusable parts, and inspect these parts according to the manufacturer's written instructions.

2. Reusable cuffs and bladders should be cleaned, rinsed, and dried between patients using a US Environmental Protection Agency (EPA) registered, intermediate-level, tuberculocidal disinfectant. The cuff and bladder should be rinsed thoroughly because cleaning solution residue may cause skin irritation, increase the chance of allergic reaction, and decrease the life of the cuff and bladder. If a cuff is unable to be cleaned adequately, it should be discarded in an appropriate receptacle.

3. All tubing should be cleaned, rinsed, and dried between patients and before storage, using an EPA-registered, detergent/intermediate-level disinfectant. Care must be taken to prevent introduction of solutions into the ports. Water in the ports contributes to microbial growth. Subsequent deflation of wet bladders may cause minute droplets of solution to be forced into the tourniquet regulating mechanism, causing damage.

4. Single-use cuffs should be discarded in an appropriate receptacle.

5. Tourniquet components contaminated with blood or other potentially infectious material should be cleaned with an enzymatic solution and an EPA-registered, intermediate-level disinfectant.

Recommendation XV

Patient assessments, the plan of care, interventions implemented, and evaluation of care related to use of a pneumatic tourniquet should be documented.

1. The Perioperative Nursing Data Set (PNDS), the uniform perioperative nursing vocabulary, should be used to document patient care and to develop policies and procedures related to pneumatic tourniquets on the intraoperative patient record. The expected outcomes of primary importance to these Recommended Practices are "The patient is free from signs or symptoms of injury due to equipment, instrumentation, sponges, or sharps"

(O2). This outcome falls within the domain of Safety (D1). The associated nursing diagnoses may include "ineffective tissue perfusion" (X61), "risk for impaired skin integrity" (X51), and "risk for impaired peripheral neurovascular function (X41). The associated interventions that may lead to the desired outcome may be "Implements protective measures to prevent skin/tissue injury due to mechanical sources" (I77), "Uses supplies and equipment within safe parameters" (I122), "Evaluates for signs and symptoms of physical injury to skin and tissue" (I152), "Identifies baseline tissue perfusion" (I60), "Assesses factors related to risks for ineffective tissue perfusion" (I15), and "Evaluates postoperative tissue perfusion" (I46).[74]

2. Documentation should include, but not be limited to,
   - pneumatic tourniquet system identification serial number (I122),
   - calibrations (I122),
   - cuff pressure (I77),
   - skin protection (I77),
   - location of tourniquet cuff (I143),
   - skin integrity under the cuff before and after use of the pneumatic tourniquet (I77),
   - person placing tourniquet cuff,
   - time of inflation and deflation, and
   - assessment and evaluation of the entire extremity (I77).

3. Documentation of tourniquet testing should reflect the biomedical equipment identification number and/or serial number date of inspection, preventive maintenance, and status of all equipment. Records of equipment failure and preventative maintenance assist in identifying equipment performance problems or hazards and minimize risk of patient injury and equipment failure.

Recommendation XVI

Education, competency assessment, and validation should be conducted before the perioperative registered nurse manages the care of a patient using a pneumatic tourniquet.

1. Education of personnel operating pneumatic tourniquets should include, but is not limited to,
   - indications and contraindications,
   - physiologic changes during and after tourniquet use,
   - risks to patients,
   - precautions to minimize these risks,
   - proper operation of the tourniquet regulator,
   - proper cuff application,
   - measurement of LOP,
   - documentation and communication,
   - corrective actions to employ in the event of a patient injury, and
   - proper care and handling of the tourniquet and accessories.

   Tourniquets and accessories have been associated with patient injuries. Education provides a foundation to guide safe patient care and minimize these risks.

2. Periodic educational programs should be provided as reinforcement of principles and introduction of new technology and procedures. This periodic education should include, but is not limited to,
   - changes in technology or procedures,
   - compatibility of equipment and accessories,
   - potential hazards, and
   - precautions to be taken.

4. Administrative personnel should ensure that assessment and documentation of initial and annual personnel competency in the safe use of pneumatic tourniquets and accessories is performed. Individual competency assessment should include, but is not limited to,
   - contraindications,
   - risks,
   - assessment of the skin under the cuff before and after use,
   - assessment of limb perfusion before and after use,
   - pre-use equipment checks,
   - appropriate gas source,
   - appropriate cuff selection,
   - appropriate cuff pressure,
   - approved duration and communication of tourniquet times, and
   - required documentation.

   Incorrect pneumatic tourniquet use can result in serious patient injury. Competency assurance verifies that personnel have knowledge of the use of the pneumatic tourniquet and appropriate corrective action taken in the event of a patient injury. This knowledge is essential to minimizing the risks of misuse of the equipment and providing a safe environment of care.

Recommendation XVII

Policies and procedures for pneumatic tourniquets should be developed, reviewed periodically, revised as necessary, and readily available in the practice setting.

1. Policies and procedures for the pneumatic tourniquet should include, but are not limited to,
   - safety features required on pneumatic tourniquets;
   - equipment maintenance programs;
   - supplemental safety monitors required;
   - equipment checks before initial use;
   - reporting and impounding malfunctioning equipment;
   - preoperative, intraoperative, and postoperative patient assessments;
   - responsibility for cuff application;
   - precautions during use;
   - reporting of injuries;
   - potential adverse events;
   - care and cleaning of the tourniquet after use; and
   - documentation.

2. The frequency, method, and criteria for pneumatic tourniquet testing should be established according to manufacturers' written instructions. A pneumatic tourniquet management program assists in identifying equipment problems that may have adverse effects on patient safety.

3. These recommended practices should be used as guidelines for developing policies and procedures in the practice setting. Policies and procedures establish authority, responsibility, and accountability. They also serve as operational guidelines and guide development of performance improvement activities.

Recommendation XVIII

The health care organization's quality management program should include investigation of adverse events and near misses associated with use of a pneumatic tourniquet.

1. Adverse patient outcomes and near misses associated with use of a pneumatic tourniquet should be collected, analyzed, and used for performance improvement as part of the health care organization's system-wide performance improvement program. To evaluate the quality of patient care and formulate plans for correc-

tive action, it is necessary to maintain a system of evaluation.

2. If a patient injury or equipment failure occurs, the pneumatic tourniquet system (eg, regulator, tubing, cuff) must be handled in accordance with the Safe Medical Devices Act of 1990, amended in March 2000.[75] Device identification, maintenance and service information, and adverse event information should be included in the report from the practice setting. Retaining the regulator, tubing, and cuff allows for a complete systems check to determine the tourniquet system integrity.

Glossary

Bier block: A regional anesthetic involving occluding blood flow to and from the extremity and infusing local anesthetic agent intravenously into the extremity.

Contoured cuff: A tourniquet cuff with a distal edge shorter than the proximal edge, creating a funnel-like shape when applied to an extremity.

Compartment syndrome: A pathologic condition caused by the progressive development of arterial compression and consequent reduction of blood supply. Clinical manifestations include swelling, restriction of movement, vascular compromise, and severe pain or lack of sensation.

Exsanguination: The process of forcible expulsion of blood from an extremity before tourniquet use. The term also means massive blood loss.

Limb occlusion pressure (LOP): The unique cuff pressure required to occlude arterial flow in the limb.

Pneumatic: Pertaining to gas or air; filled with compressed gas or air.

Regulator: The mechanical device controlling the inflation, deflation, cuff pressure, and alarms for a tourniquet.

Shearing: A sliding movement of skin and subcutaneous tissue that leaves the underlying muscle stationary.

REFERENCES

1. "2004 National Patient Safety Goals: Practical strategies and helpful solutions for meeting these goals," Joint Commission on Accreditation of Healthcare Organizations, *http://www.jointcommission.org/PatientSafety /NationalPatientSafetyGoals/04_npsgs.htm* (accessed 13 Sept 2006).

2. "Tubing misconnections—A persistent and potentially deadly occurrence," *Sentinel Event Alert* (April 3, 2006) 36.

3. ECRI, "Tourniquets, pneumatic," *Healthcare Product Comparison System* (Plymouth Meeting, Pa: ECRI, 1997) 2.

4. P C Kam, R Kavanagh, F F Yoong, "The arterial tourniquet: Pathophysiological consequences and anaesthetic implications," *Anaesthesia* 56 (June 2001) 534-545.

5. J P Estebe, "Recommandations pour le bon usage du garrot pneumatique en chirurgie," *Annales Francaises d'Anesthesie et de Reanimation* 25 (March 2006) 330-332.

6. T P Kalla et al, "Survey of tourniquet use in podiatric surgery," *Journal of Foot and Ankle Surgery* 42 (March/April 2003) 68-76.

7. E Dounis et al, "Effect of time interval on tissue concentrations of cephalosporins after tourniquet inflation. Highest levels achieved by administration 20 minutes before inflation," *Acta Orthopedica Scandinavica* 66 (April 1995) 158-160.

8. N Papaioannou et al, "Tissue concentrations of third-generation cephalosporins (ceftazidime and ceftriaxone) in lower extremity tissues using a tourniquet," *Archives of Orthopedic Trauma Surgery* 113 (April 1994) 167-169.

9. A G Crenshaw et al, "Wide tourniquet cuffs more effective at lower inflation pressures," *Acta Orthopedica Scandinavica* 59 (August 1988) 447-451.

10. M R Moore, S R Garfin, A R Hargens, "Wide tourniquets eliminate blood flow at low inflation pressures," *American Journal of Hand Surgery* 12 (November 1987) 1006-1011.

11. J P Estebe et al, "Tourniquet pain in a volunteer study: Effect of changes in cuff width and pressure," *Anaesthesia* 55 (January 2000) 21-26.

12. R A Pedowitz et al, "The use of lower tourniquet inflation pressures in extremity surgery facilitated by curved and wide tourniquets and an integrated cuff inflation system," *Clinical Orthopedics and Related Research* 287 (February 1993) 237-244.

13. A S Younger, J A McEwen, K Inkpen, "Wide contoured thigh cuffs and automated limb occlusion measurement allow lower tourniquet pressures," *Clinical Orthopedics and Related Research* 428 (November 2004) 286-293.

14. B Graham et al, "Occlusion of arterial flow in the extremities at subsystolic pressures through the use of wide tourniquet cuffs," *Clinical Orthopedics and Related Research* 286 (January 1993) 257-261.

15. J R Lieberman, L T Staheli, M C Dales, "Tourniquet pressures on pediatric patients: A clinical study," *Orthopedics* 20 (December 1997) 1143-1147.

16. C Olivecrona et al, "Skin protection underneath the pneumatic tourniquet during total knee arthroplasty: A randomized controlled trial of 92 patients," *Acta Orthopedica* 77 (June 2006) 19-523.

17. R Din, T Geddes, "Skin protection beneath the tourniquet a prospective randomized trial," *ANZ Journal of Surgery* 74 (September 2004) 721-722.

18. A C Maury, W S Roy, "A prospective, randomized, controlled trial of forearm versus upper arm tourniquet tolerance," *British Journal of Hand Surgery* 27 (August 2002) 359-360.

19. A Odinsson, V Finsen, "The position of the tourniquet on the upper limb," *British Journal of Bone Joint Surgery* 84 (March 2002) 202-204.

20. V Finsen, AM Kasseth, "Tourniquets in forefoot surgery: Less pain when placed at the ankle," *British Journal of Bone Joint Surgery*, 79 (January 1997) 99-101.

21. R Derner, J Buckholz, "Surgical hemostasis by pneumatic ankle tourniquet during 3027 podiatric operations," *Journal of Foot and Ankle Surgery* 34 (May/June 1995) 236-246.

22. N S Lichtenfeld, "The pneumatic ankle tourniquet with ankle block anesthesia for foot surgery," *Foot & Ankle* 13 (July/August 1992) 344-349.

23. A K Rudkin, G E Rudkin, G C Dracopoulos, "Acceptability of ankle tourniquet use in midfoot and forefoot surgery: Audit of 1000 cases," *Foot & Ankle International* 25 (November 2004) 788-794.

24. K A Krackow, "A maneuver for improved positioning of a tourniquet in the obese patient," *Clinical Orthopedics and Related Research* 168 (August 1982) 80-82.

25. R S Cajee, "Fatal thrombo-embolism after limb exsanguination: A case report," *South African Medical Journal* 68 (August 31 1985) 349-350.

26. S Darmanis, A Papanikolaou, D Pavlakis, "Fatal intra-operative pulmonary embolism following application of an Esmarch bandage," *Injury* 33 (November 2002) 761-764.

27. J G Boogaerts, "Fatal pulmonary embolism during limb exsanguination," (Letters to the Editor) *Canadian Journal of Anaesthesia* 45 (October 1998) 1031-1032.

28. J A McEwen et al, "Tourniquet safety in lower leg applications," *Orthopedic Nursing* 21 (September/October 2002) 55-62.

29. B Tuncali et al, "A new method for estimating arterial occlusion pressure in optimizing pneumatic tourniquet inflation pressure," *Anesthesia and Analgesia* 102 (June 2006) 1752-1757.

30. RR Hagenouw et al, "Tourniquet pain: A volunteer study," *Anesthesia and Analgesia* 65 (November 1986) 1175-1180.

31. R J Newman, A Muirhead, "A safe and effective low pressure tourniquet: A prospective evaluation," *British Journal of Bone and Joint Surgery* 68 (August 1986) 625-628.

32. R L Worland et al, "Thigh pain following tourniquet application in simultaneous bilateral total knee replacement arthroplasty," *Journal of Arthroplasty* 12 (December 1997) 848-852.

33. J A McEwen, "Tourniquet use and care," *http://www .interchg.ubc.ca/jamc/use_care.html* (accessed 20 Sept 2006).

34. S J Tredwell et al, "Pediatric tourniquets: Analysis of cuff and limb interface, current practice, and guidelines for use," *Journal of Pediatric Orthopedics* 21 (September/October 2001) 671-676.

35. A J Hodgson, "A proposed etiology for tourniquet-induced neuropathies," *Journal of Biomechanical Engineering* 116 (May 1994) 224-227.

36. M D Jacobson et al, "Muscle functional deficits after tourniquet ischemia," *American Journal of Sports Medicine* 22 (May-June 1994) 372-377.

37. T T Horlocker et al, "Anesthetic, patient, and surgical risk factors for neurologic complications after prolonged total tourniquet time during total knee arthroplasty," *Anesthesia and Analgesia* 102 (March 2006) 950-955.

38. A Y On, O Ozdemir, R Aksit, "Tourniquet paralysis after primary nerve repair," *American Journal of Physical Medicine & Rehabilitation* 79 (May/June 2000) 298-300.

39. ECRI, "Unintended inflation and deflation of Zimmer model ATS 1500 pneumatic tourniquet cuffs," *Health Devices* 26 (September/October 1997) 391-392.

40. K Aho et al, "Pneumatic tourniquet paralysis: Case report," *British Journal of Bone and Joint Surgery* 65 (August 1983) 441-443.

41. A M Lynn et al, "Systemic responses to tourniquet release in children," *Anesthesia and Analgesia* 65 (August 1986) 865-872.

42. P M Sutter et al, "Increased surface expression of CD18 and CD11b in leukocytes after tourniquet ischemia during elective hand surgery," *World Journal of Surgery* 21 (February 1997) 179-184, (Invited Commentary) 185.

43. J P Estebe, Y Malledant, "Le garrot pneumatique d'orthopedie (Pneumatic tourniquets in orthopedics)," *Annales Francaise d'Anesthesie et Reanimation* 15 (February 1996) 162-178.

44. J C Tsui et al, "Altered endothelin-1 levels in acute lower limb ischemia and reperfusion," *Angiology* 55 (September/October 2004) 533-539.

45. A Wakai et al, "Tourniquet-induced systemic inflammatory response in extremity surgery," *Journal of Trauma* 51 (November 2001) 922-926.

46. J P Estebe et al, "Use of a pneumatic tourniquet induces changes in central temperature," *British Journal of Anaesthesia* 77 (December 1996) 786-788.

47. B J Sanders, J G D'Alessio, J R Jernigan, "Intraoperative hypothermia associated with lower extremity tourniquet deflation," *Journal of Clinical Anesthesia* 8 (September 1996) 504-507.

48. K Hirota et al, "The relationship between pneumatic tourniquet time and the amount of pulmonary emboli in patients undergoing knee arthroscopic surgeries," *Anesthesia and Analgesia* 93 (September 2001) 776-780.

49. M Girardis et al, "The hemodynamic and metabolic effects of tourniquet application during knee surgery," *Anesthesia and Analgesia* 91 (September 2000) 727-731.

50. T Akata et al, "Changes in body temperature following deflation of limb pneumatic tourniquet," *Journal of Clinical Anesthesia* 10 (February 1998) 17-22.

51. E C Bloch et al, "Limb tourniquets and central temperature in anesthetized children," *Anesthesia and Analgesia* 74 (April 1992) 486-489.

52. E C Bloch, "Hyperthermia resulting from tourniquet application in children," *Annals of the Royal College of Surgeons of England* 68 (July 1986) 193-194.

53. D L Bourke et al, "Respiratory responses associated with release of intraoperative tourniquets," *Anesthesia and Analgesia* 69 (October 1989) 541-544.

54. H S Townsend et al, "Tourniquet release: Systemic and metabolic effects," *Acta Anaesthesiologica Scandinavica* 40 (November 1996) 1234-1237.

55. H Iwama et al, "Circulatory, respiratory and metabolic changes after thigh tourniquet release in combined epidural-propofol anaesthesia with preservation of spontaneous respiration," *Anaesthesia* 57 (June 2002) 588-592.

56. K Hirota et al, "Quantification and comparison of pulmonary emboli formation after pneumatic tourniquet release in patients undergoing reconstruction of anterior cruciate ligament and total knee arthroplasty," *Anesthesia and Analgesia* 94 (June 2002) 1633-1638.

57. K R Conaty, M S Klemm, "Severe increase of intracranial pressure after deflation of a pneumatic tourniquet," *Anesthesiology* 71 (August 1989) 294-295.

58. B J McGrath et al, "Venous embolization after deflation of lower extremity tourniquets," *Anesthesia and Analgesia* 78 (February 1994) 349-353.

59. J L Parmet et al, "The incidence of large venous emboli during total knee arthroplasty without pneumatic tourniquet use," *Anesthesia and Analgesia* 87 (August 1998) 439-444.

60. J L Parmet et al, "The incidence of venous emboli during extramedullary guided total knee arthroplasty," *Anesthesia and Analgesia* 81 (October 1995) 757-762.

61. J L Parmet et al, "Echogenic emboli upon tourniquet release during total knee arthroplasty: Pulmonary hemodynamic changes and embolic composition," *Anesthesia and Analgesia* 79 (November 1994) 940-945.

62. J L Parmet et al, "Thromboembolism coincident with tourniquet deflation during total knee arthroplasty," *Lancet* 341 (April 24, 1993) 1057-1058.

63. "2006 Critical Access Hospital and Hospital National Patient Safety Goals," Joint Commission on Accreditation of Healthcare Organizations, *http://www.jointcommission.org/PatientSafety/NationalPatientSafety Goals/06_npsg_cah.htm* (accessed 10 Aug 2006).

64. A S Younger et al, "Survey of tourniquet use in orthopaedic foot and ankle surgery," *Foot & Ankle International* 26 (March 2005) 208-217.

65. D O'Neil, J E Sheppard, "Transient compartment syndrome of the forearm resulting from venous congestion from a tourniquet," *American Journal of Hand Surgery* 14 (September 1989) 894-896.

66. Greene TL, Louis DS. Compartment syndrome of the arm—A complication of the pneumatic tourniquet: A case report," *American Journal of Bone and Joint Surgery* 65 (February 1983) 270-273.

67. F W Blaisdell, "The pathophysiology of skeletal muscle ischemia and the reperfusion syndrome: A review," *Cardiovascular Surgery* 10 (December 2002) 620-630.

68. A Wakai et al, "Pneumatic tourniquets in extremity surgery," *Journal of the American Academy of Orthopedic Surgery* 9 (September/October 2001) 345-351.

69. J D Cohen et al, "Massive pulmonary embolism and tourniquet deflation," *Anesthesia and Analgesia* 79 (September 1994) 583-585.

70. S Araki, M Uchiyama, "Fatal pulmonary embolism following tourniquet inflation: A case report," *Acta Orthopedica Scandinavica* 62 (October 1991) 488.

71. A T Berman et al, "Emboli observed with use of transesophageal echocardiography immediately after tourniquet release during total knee arthroplasty with cement," *American Journal of Bone and Joint Surgery* 80 (March 1998) 389-396.

72. J J Branson, W M Goldstein, "Sequential bilateral total knee arthroplasty," *AORN Journal* 73 (March 2001) 610-635.

73. "Pneumatic tourniquets used for regional anesthesia," *Health Devices* 12 (December 1982) 48-49.

74. S C Beyea, ed, *Perioperative Nursing Data Set: The Perioperative Vocabulary,* second ed, (Denver: AORN, Inc, 2002) 85-87.

75. "Medical device reporting: Manufacturer reporting, importer reporting, user facility reporting, distributor reporting," *Federal Register* 65 (Jan 26, 2000) 4112-4121.

PUBLICATION HISTORY

Originally published April 1984, *AORN Journal.* Revised November 1990.

Published as proposed recommended practices March 1994. Revised November 1998; published December 1998. Reformatted July 2000.

Revised November 2001; published February 2002, *AORN Journal.*

Revised 2006; published in *Standards, Recommended Practices, and Guidelines,* 2007 edition.

AORN Perioperative Standards and Recommended Practices, 2012 Edition

Recommended Practices for
Product Selection in Perioperative Practice Settings

The following Recommended Practices for Product Selection in Perioperative Practice Settings were developed by the AORN Recommended Practices Committee and have been approved by the AORN Board of Directors. They were presented as proposed recommendations for comments by members and others. They are effective March 1, 2010.

These recommended practices are intended as achievable recommendations representing what is believed to be an optimal level of practice. Policies and procedures will reflect variations in practice settings and/or clinical situations that determine the degree to which the recommended practices can be implemented.

AORN recognizes the various settings in which perioperative RNs practice. These recommended practices are intended as guidelines adaptable to various practice settings. These practice settings include traditional operating rooms (ORs), ambulatory surgery centers, physicians' offices, cardiac catheterization laboratories, endoscopy suites, radiology departments, and all other areas where surgery and other invasive procedures may be performed.

Purpose

These recommended practices provide guidelines for evaluating and purchasing medical devices and other products used in perioperative settings. Patient and worker safety, quality, and cost containment are primary concerns of perioperative RNs as they participate in evaluating and selecting medical devices and products for use in practice settings.[1] In this document, the term *product(s)* will be used to refer to all products, medical devices, and capital equipment unless otherwise stated.

Recommendation I

A mechanism for product selection should be developed.

A mechanism for product selection assists with consistently selecting functional and reliable products that are safe, cost effective, and environmentally friendly; promote quality care; and prevent duplication or rapid obsolescence.

I.a.   A multidisciplinary product evaluation and selection committee should be established.

Involvement of a multidisciplinary committee allows input from all departments where the product will be used and from personnel with expertise beyond clinical end users (eg, infection control, finance, materials management/purchasing).[2,3]

I.a.1.   The members of a multidisciplinary product evaluation and selection committee should be based on the size of the health care organization, the type of product, and the affected end users consisting of, but not limited to,[3,4]
- RNs;
- physicians;
- scrub personnel;
- central/sterile processing personnel;
- anesthesia care providers;
- infection preventionists;
- pharmacists;
- nurse educators; and
- material management/purchasing agents;

and, as applicable, liaisons from
- environmental services,
- administration,
- biomedical engineering,
- risk management,
- radiology,
- finance, and
- laboratory.

Adjusting the composition of the committee will allow health care organizations of various sizes to appoint a responsible individual with the competency and authority to fulfill more than one role (eg, perioperative RN functioning as an infection preventionist and nurse educator). There may be products that do not affect all departments, in which case only the specific end users or representatives from directly affected departments would need to be involved.

I.b.   Perioperative RNs should have an integral role in the evaluation and selection of surgical products.

The perioperative RN has a professional responsibility to consider "factors related to safety, effectiveness, efficiency, and the environment, as well as the cost in planning, delivering, and evaluating patient care."[1(p19)] Perioperative RNs play a crucial role in providing practical insight and expertise in the use and evaluation of surgical products.[5,6]

Recommendation II

The multidisciplinary committee should develop a process to guide product selection.

A standardized product selection process assists in the selection of functional and reliable products that are safe, cost-effective, and environmentally friendly and that promote quality care, as well as decrease duplication or rapid obsolescence.[3,7,8]

II.a.   The committee should gather information about new or existing products from professional resources and the manufacturer.

Manufacturers' representatives have access to information concerning products currently on the market. Manufacturers' representatives can provide both clinical and technical data related to product research, processing, packaging, disinfection, sterilization, and environmental conservation.[3]

II.b.   Consistent requirements should be identified for each product under evaluation.

The health care organization's multidisciplinary product evaluation and selection committee identifies the written objective, generic criteria specific to the desired product, and its ability to function as desired. Consistency in process requirements provide a reliable and valid means of evaluating the end results.[5,9]

II.b.1.   Product-specific requirements should include, but not be limited to,
   • contractual agreements (eg, warranties and maintenance agreements);[5]
   • required compatibility with new or existing products;
   • compatibility with existing disposal methods;
   • compatibility with existing reprocessing methods;
   • procedure-related requirements (eg, for a drape: resistance to penetration by blood and other body fluids, size, presence of adhesive apertures, low linting);
   • end-user preference and requirements (eg, for a surgical gown: comfort,

degree of protection from blood and body fluids, size, absence of toxic ingredients/allergens; for an instrument: ease of use, performance, the type of decontamination and sterilization process necessary);
   • patient-related requirements (eg, the size of the patient, presence of allergies or infectious diseases);
   • compliance with federal, state, and local regulatory agencies such as the Occupational Safety and Health Administration (OSHA) or the US Food and Drug Administration (FDA);[10-13] and
   • compliance with standards-setting bodies.

Contractual agreements are documents such as warranties and maintenance agreements that are stipulated before the time of evaluation assisting the manufacturer to be aware of the requirements of the health care organization.

Defining compatibility requirements assists in ensuring that the new product will be compatible with an existing product or if it is not compatible will clarify the need for additional adapters or other products.

The disposal method is considered to determine the effect of disposing of the product on the existing methods and to ensure the correct disposal method is available. For example, if the product is considered a hazardous material, consider whether a method exists for disposing of hazardous materials, including appropriate labeling and a company to remove the waste.

The list of products which the reprocessing company has obtained clearance to reprocess may not contain the product under consideration. An additional company may be required for reprocessing the product, if the product is on the FDA list of approved products to be reprocessed.[14]

Procedure-related requirements define what is required for the procedure or multiple procedures for which the product will be used. Some of these requirements can be determined by using a scale such as the ANSI/AAMI barrier performance scale.[15,16]

End-user-related requirements will vary depending on how the product is used and, when addressed, increase the compliance by the end-user.

Patient-related requirements define the ability of the product to adapt to individual patients.

Most standards-setting bodies use research to create standards, and some of the standards may be adopted for enforcement by regulatory agencies.[15,17-20]

II.c. A financial impact analysis should be performed on each product to be purchased.

A financial impact analysis can be used to clarify a choice between two different products with equivalent functionality.[3,5]

II.c.1. The financial impact analysis should include
- direct costs (eg, cost of the product, replacement strategy, associated equipment);
- indirect costs (eg, utilities, waste disposal, processing, training, storage, energy utilization, depreciation, retrofitting to existing equipment);[5]
- reimbursement potential; and
- group purchasing organization (GPO) contract pricing.

When a product is being replaced, the replacement strategy is a direct cost resulting from the need to dispose of the existing stock of the product being replaced. If the new product is being phased in and will replace the existing product after the current inventory is exhausted, then there will be no additional direct cost. The indirect costs are the costs associated with the use of the product after purchase. These costs may include electricity, decontamination and sterilization method, and disposal. The sum of the direct and indirect costs incurred over the product's lifetime is the complete cost for the product.[3,21] An example of a large indirect cost is energy, on which hospitals spend approximately $8.3 billion annually.[22]

The reimbursement potential is used in determining the impact on the profit margin of each procedure and will vary with each product.

Group purchasing organization contract pricing may determine the direct cost of the product by defining the quantities required, applicable time frames, and pricing on other products purchased.[5]

II.c.2. As appropriate, other health care organizations should be contacted based on contract terms and affiliations or working relationships regarding
- purchasing partial quantities of infrequently used supplies or
- creating a shared inventory.

Purchasing partial quantities of infrequently used supplies or using a shared inventory may assist with decreasing the amount of infrequently used inventory in stock, direct costs, and the amount of waste generated.

II.c.3. Vendors should be contacted regarding
- return of unopened, expired products;
- creation of a consigned inventory; and
- lowest unit of purchase.

Returning unopened, expired products may decrease the amount of infrequently used inventory in stock and the amount of waste generated. Expenses may be reduced based on the cost associated with restocking and freight for the return shipment. The up-front expense for consigned inventory may be less because the product is paid for at the time of use, and the product is frequently only a portion of the total inventory consigned. If the product was not consigned, the entire inventory would need to be purchased before use. Vendors may be willing to ship in small quantities to meet the needs of the health care organization that requires a low inventory because of low usage.

II.d. An interdepartmental and intradepartmental standardization initiative and plan should be developed and reviewed to determine the applicability for each product being evaluated.

Reports indicate that standardization can reduce costs and may improve inventory control and use of storage space. Standardization also decreases end user training and errors related to unfamiliarity with the product.[3,5,6,9] The perioperative RN is a qualified person to assist with standardization because of familiarity with the use of many products.

II.d.1. The plan should include a list of products requiring standardization and a process for determining which products will be standardized.

II.e. The product's environmental impact should be assessed by addressing the following criteria:
- Can the product be recycled?
- Is the product made of recycled materials?
- What method is used for disposal?

Using any or all of these criteria can help decrease the 6,600 tons of waste generated daily by US health care facilities.[23] Considering only one of the environmental impact criteria may not reveal other environmental benefits or negative effects of the product.[24] It is estimated that only 10% to 25% of hospital waste is regulated waste; the remainder is equivalent to household waste and can be recycled.[23,25,26] Recycling noninfectious waste materials has environmental and financial benefits that may include, but are not limited to,
- providing materials for remanufacture;
- limiting the expansion of landfills and incinerator use, thereby decreasing air and water pollution;
- conserving energy;
- preserving resources for future generations; and
- decreasing the cost of waste removal.[22,27,28]

The method of disposal is assessed to determine if the product can be disposed of by a method currently being used or if a new method needs to be introduced. For example, if the health care organization has never handled hazardous waste such as chemotherapy products, a method to dispose of this type of waste would be necessary before the product is introduced.

Products manufactured from recycled materials decrease the amount of waste created and natural resources utilized in creation of the product.[29]

Resources are available (eg, sample policies and procedures, contract language, a listing of environmentally friendly products)

to assist in determining the environmental impact of products.[30]

II.f. The following criteria should be considered when determining whether to purchase a single-use, reposable, or reusable product:
- the useful life of the product;
- the estimated use of the product;
- the availability of required decontamination and sterilization processes;
- if single-use, whether the product can be reprocessed;
- inventory required;
- storage facilities;
- knowledge of health care workers who use, maintain, and reprocess instruments and other equipment; and
- maintenance, repair, or restoration programs for instruments and equipment.

Purchasing reusable products demonstrates the health care organization's commitment to supply conservation and fiscal responsibility through conservation of resources and energy, optimization of resources, and reduction of the pollution that occurs with waste disposal. Health care organizations have reported a large reduction in the amount of waste generated annually by reusing, repairing, and refurbishing products.[22,31]

Pollution is reduced when a health care organization purchases a reposable or reusable product or reprocesses a single-use product because the final disposal of the product is delayed. Health care organizations have reported large monetary savings when using reusable products.[2,32] There are reports of original equipment manufacturers increasing the cost of products because a single-use product was reprocessed, which caused a decrease in the number of new products being purchased.[2]

Projecting the useful life of the product assists in maintaining an adequate inventory to allow for completion of scheduled maintenance and to reduce frequency of reprocessing and wear. When the product has a short life span, it may be more economical to consider a disposable option because the product may become outdated before use.

When a product has a very low usage, purchasing a disposable product may be more economical when compared to a reusable product that requires repeated sterilizations and other maintenance.

If the required decontamination and sterilization processes, including proper containment devices, are not available, the cost per use may increase.[33] Proper sterilization processes are required because to achieve a sterile product, the sterilizing agent must contact all surfaces.[34]

The amount of inventory directly affects the amount of storage space required, and reusable items may require less inventory and storage space.

If health care workers who use, maintain, and reprocess instruments and other equipment are knowledgeable of the processes involved, the life of the product will be extended.

Regular maintenance, repair, or remanufacturer programs for instruments and equipment will reduce malfunction and maintain function.[4]

II.g. When determining if a product labeled as a single-use device (SUD) should be reprocessed, consider
  - whether the product is listed on the FDA list of products approved for reprocessing,
  - the financial effect of the reprocessing program, and
  - whether the health care organization can accomplish the reprocessing with existing internal or external resources.

Certain SUDs are listed by the FDA as being acceptable for reprocessing.[14] The financial effect is determined by weighing the cost savings against the cost of initiating and maintaining the program. Some facilities report a cost savings from reprocessing some SUDs, a major reason for initiating a reprocessing program. The amount of cost savings depends on the size of the health care organization, the number of devices reprocessed, staff education, labor costs, and the health care organization's commitment to the program.[35,36] The FDA requires health care organizations and third parties that reprocess SUDs to adhere to the same regulations as the original equipment manufacturers. These regulations include
  - quality system regulations,[37]
  - medical device reporting,[38]
  - registration and listing,[39]
  - labeling,[40]
  - premarket approval and premarket notification,[41-43]
  - medical device corrections and removals,[44] and
  - medical device tracking.[45]

These regulations lead many health care organizations to hire a third party reprocessor.[2,35]

II.h. An evaluation process should be developed based on objective criteria specific to the product.

Using a consistent evaluation process assists with obtaining an objective review and analysis.[3,5,46]

II.h.1. A multidisciplinary evaluation team of end users and representatives from other departments affected by a product (eg, infection control, sterile processing) should be developed to participate in the clinical evaluation process.

Involvement of a multidisciplinary team allows input from departments with varying needs to select the most appropriate products to meet those needs.[2] Including all clinical areas in the evaluation process provides direct feedback from staff members whose practices will be affected by the product.[3,27] The team concept also allows input from departments that are not end users but can provide expert advice beyond the scope of the end users (eg, infection preventionists).

II.h.2. A product-specific evaluation tool should be developed using unique product-specific criteria, which may include, but is not limited to,
  • safety;
  • performance;
  • quality;
  • efficiency;
  • ease of use;
  • compatibility with other products;
  • effect on quality patient care and clinical outcomes;
  • evidence-based efficacy;
  • financial impact analysis;
  • compliance with GPO agreements;
  • sterilization/reprocessing parameters including degree of difficulty;

- liability (eg, for investigational products);
- federal, state, and local regulatory requirements;
- standardization;
- compatibility with new and existing products;
- environmental impact;
- availability and quality of service after purchase;
- amount of personnel training required; and
- the quality of the manufacturer's instructions.

Careful selection of criteria ensures the reliability and validity of trial evaluation results. A product-specific written or electronic evaluation tool facilitates an objective review and analysis.[46]

II.h.3.   Limits should be placed on the scope of the clinical evaluation. These limitations should include, but not be limited to,
- the number of users;
- cost;
- the number of products to be evaluated;
- time span;
- the number of departments and clinical areas involved;
- desired patient outcomes; and
- follow-up patient data, if indicated.

Placing limits on product evaluations increases the usefulness of user feedback. Allowing unlimited time to evaluate products may result in decreased evaluator input and enthusiasm.[5]

II.h.4.   The amount of end user education required regarding the use of the product being evaluated should be determined.

The amount of time required for education may differ between products based on the familiarity of personnel with one of the products compared to the other. The time required for education will affect the indirect cost of the product and the start time of the evaluation.

II.h.5.   Evaluation data should be analyzed to determine product purchase recommendations based on actual clinical performance compared to the predetermined, unique, product-specific criteria.

This information facilitates efficient and consistent decisions based on previously established criteria and an evidence-based product assessment.[5]

II.i.   After a product has been selected, a comprehensive plan for introduction and use should be developed and implemented to include, but not be limited to,
- education required to complete the end users' competencies in all departments involved,
- physician credentialing required before use,
- projected date of first use, and
- replacement strategy.

The development of a comprehensive plan for the introduction of a product will facilitate smooth implementation. The development of a replacement strategy also assists in decreasing inventory and dual educational needs. This strategy also may reduce the risk of making an unsatisfactory product selection.

Recommendation III

Perioperative RNs should demonstrate competency related to product evaluation and selection.

Ongoing competency validation and education provides the perioperative RN with the information required to take an active role and effectively influence the evaluation process and product selection.

III.a.   Educational programs should be provided regarding
- specific steps required for product selection;
- safe care and handling of products;
- selection of products;
- the environmental effects of health care, new environmental conditions, and appropriate green responses;[27]
- governmental regulations regarding purchasing and product requirements;
- reprocessing, repair, recycling, and refurbishing initiatives of the health care organization;[2,47] and
- how to evaluate and provide objective input on the product's appropriateness and effectiveness.

Staff members should be educated about manufacturers' various methods of designating specific product characteristics, such as using color-coded labels to signify a sterile gown's level of protection.[48,49]

Education increases the perioperative RN's active participation in decreasing the environmental impact of health care.[27,47]

III.b. Demonstration and instruction on the use of the products should be conducted before the clinical evaluation and before initiating general use.

Instructing all individuals involved in the clinical evaluation facilitates safe clinical practice and helps establish validity of the product evaluation.[5]

Recommendation IV

The product selection process and any product-specific information should be documented.

Documentation of this information provides retrievable records to answer potential questions regarding the justification for purchasing a specific product and for future purchasing decisions.

IV.a. Documentation of the product-selection process using a specific product-related evaluation tool[5] or meeting minutes should include, but not be limited to,
- the names of the committee participants,
- generic product performance requirements,
- requirements for standardization,
- the environmental impact,
- results of the financial impact analysis,
- evaluation methods to include the tools and the results of the evaluations,
- a comparative listing of products evaluated,
- justification for purchasing single-use versus reusable products,
- an implementation plan, and
- the final decision.

Recommendation V

Policies and procedures for evaluating and selecting products should be developed, reviewed periodically, revised as necessary, and readily available in the practice setting.

Policies and procedures assist in the development of patient and worker safety, quality assessment, and improvement activities. Policies and procedures establish authority, responsibility, and accountability within the facility. They also serve as operational guidelines that are used to minimize patient and worker risk factors, standardize practice, direct staff members, and establish guidelines for continuous performance improvement activities.

V.a. Policies and procedures should encompass all aspects of the product selection process to include
- the composition of the multidisciplinary committee members,
- product performance requirements to include patient and worker safety requirements,
- standardization process,
- the environmental impact assessment,
- the financial impact assessment,
- utilization of evaluation methods,
- components of an implementation plan,
- authorization and approval process,
- how products are introduced and the role of the health care industry representative,
- the role and responsibility of the health care industry representative,[50]
- the process to request and initiate a product review, and
- steps to take if an injury occurs during trial or use as described in the Safe Medical Devices Act of 1990.[51]

Recommendation VI

A quality assurance/performance improvement process should be established to measure product performance to include post-purchase cost effectiveness and user satisfaction.

This evaluation helps to ensure that new products are meeting expected performance criteria (eg, cost-effectiveness, product life span) and that the pre-selection evaluation process has met its objectives.

VI.a. New product performance and user satisfaction should be evaluated at planned intervals.

Establishing intervals for measurement assists in ensuring all products are evaluated and inventories can be adjusted as necessary to eliminate ineffective products.

VI.b. Quality programs should include monitoring of reprocessing and recycling efforts to include review of additional opportunities to minimize environmental impact.

Monitoring of reprocessing and recycling efforts provides the data to assess operational errors and noncompliance, quality and effectiveness of the product, and financial impact.[2]

VI.c. The quality program must describe required actions necessary for compliance with the Safe Medical Devices Act of 1990.[51]

VI.d. After a product has been selected, a comprehensive plan for evaluation of the product should be developed and implemented to include, but not be limited to, frequency and criteria for reevaluation.

Glossary

Process: "A goal-directed, interrelated series of actions, events, mechanisms, or steps. An interrelated series of events, activities, actions, mechanisms, or steps that transforms inputs into outputs." (Source: Joint Commission on Accreditation of Healthcare Organizations. Glossary. In: *Hospital Accreditation Standards*. Oakbrook Terrace, IL: Joint Commission on Accreditation of Healthcare Organizations; 2002:331, 346, 354, 360.)

Reposable: An instrument that has limited use or an instrument with a combination of reusable and disposable components.

Reprocessing: Includes all operations to render a contaminated reusable or single-use device patient ready. Single-use devices to be reprocessed may be either used or unused. Reprocessing steps include cleaning, decontamination, functional testing, repackaging, relabeling, and sterilization/disinfection.

Reusable: Any product or piece of equipment intended by the manufacturer for multiple uses. As appropriate to each item, the manufacturer is to provide instructions for reprocessing, care, and/or maintenance of the item.

Reuse: The repeated or multiple uses of any medical device whether marketed as reusable or single-use. Repeated/multiple use may be on the same patient or on different patients with applicable reprocessing of the device between uses.

Useful life: Length of time, as determined by the manufacturer, for which a product maintains acceptable safety and performance characteristics. The manufacturer should provide data to support useful life of the material. Useful life is affected by the number of sterilization processing and washing cycles a product can endure and yet maintain an acceptable barrier capability.

REFERENCES

1. Standards of perioperative nursing. In: *Perioperative Standards and Recommended Practices*. Denver, CO: AORN, Inc; 2010:9-62.
2. Flynn AB, Knishinsky R. A matter of reprocessing. *Mater Manag Health Care*. 2005;14(10):32-35.
3. Barlow RD. Infusing value analysis in contracting strategies: it's not just a pricing or product evaluation and selection game. *Healthc Purchasing News*. 2008;32(10):62.
4. DeMeo M. Understanding the elements of reprocessing surgical instrumentation for clinically safer and financially sound outcomes. *Infection Control Today*. 2009;13(5):24-26.
5. Halvorson CK, Chinnes LF. Collaborative leadership in product evaluation. *AORN J*. 2007;85(2):334-352.
6. Greene J. Value analysis team guides OR purchasing. *OR Manager*. 2006;22(11):19, 21.
7. Adler S, Scherrer M, Ruckauer KD, Daschner FD. Comparison of economic and environmental impacts between disposable and reusable instruments used for laparoscopic cholecystectomy. *Surg Endosc*. 2005;19(2):268-272.
8. Howes BW. The reliability of laryngoscope lights. *Anaesthesia*. 2006;61(5):488-491.
9. Hupp D. A strategy for review of new products. *OR Manager*. 2005;21(11):23-24.
10. Medical gloves and gowns. US Food and Drug Administration Center for Devices and Radiological Health. *http://www.fda.gov/MedicalDevices/ProductsandMedicalProcedures/MedicalToolsandSupplies/PersonalProtectiveEquipment/ucm056077.htm*. Accessed February 10, 2010.
11. Siegel JD, Rhinehart E, Jackson M, Chiarello L; the Healthcare Infection Control Practices Advisory Committee. *2007 Guideline for Isolation Precautions: Preventing Transmission of Infectious Agents in Healthcare Settings*. *http://www.cdc.gov/hicpac/2007IP/2007isolationPrecautions.html*. Accessed February 10, 2010.
12. FDA-cleared surgical drapes. US Food and Drug Administration Center for Devices and Radiological Health, 2003-2008. *http://www.accessdata.fda.gov/scripts/cdrh/devicesatfda/index.cfm*. Accessed February 10, 2010.
13. US Occupational Health and Safety Administration. Bloodborne pathogens. 29 CFR 1910.1030. Revised July 1, 2009. *http://edocket.access.gpo.gov/cfr_2009/julqtr/pdf/29cfr1910.1030.pdf*. Accessed February 10, 2010.
14. FDA's web site for cleared reprocessed single-use devices. US Department of Health and Human Services. *http://www.fda.gov/MedicalDevices/DeviceRegulationandGuidance/ReprocessingofSingle-UseDevices/ucm121197.htm*. Accessed February 10, 2010.
15. AAMI. *Technical Information Report 11: Selection and Use of Protective Apparel and Surgical Drapes in Health Care Facilities*. Arlington, VA: Association for the Advancement of Medical Instrumentation; 2005.
16. AAMI. *PB70:2003: Liquid Barrier Performance and Classification of Protective Apparel and Drapes Intended for Use in Health Care Facilities*. Arlington, VA: Association for the Advancement of Medical Instrumentation; 2003.

17. ANSI. *Z136.3-2005: Safe Use of Lasers in Health Care Facilities*. New York, NY: American National Standards Institute; 2005.

18. Recommended practices for laser safety in practice settings. In: *Perioperative Standards and Recommended Practices*. Denver, CO: AORN, Inc; 2010:133-138.

19. Recommended practices for electrosurgery. In: *Perioperative Standards and Recommended Practices*. Denver, CO: AORN, Inc; 2010:105-126.

20. ASTM International. *ASTM F2407: Standard Specification for Surgical Gowns Intended for Use in Healthcare Facilities*. West Conshohocken, PA: ASTM International; 2006.

21. Carter S. How to evaluate and justify the implementation of disposal products in your facility. *Infection Control Today*. 2009;13(6):80.

22. Serb C. Think green. *Hosp Health Netw*. 2008; 82(8):22-6, 35.

23. Waste management. Practice Greenhealth. *http://www.practicegreenhealth.org/educate/operations /waste*. Accessed February 10, 2010.

24. Davis MR. Environmental impacts of surgical draping and gowning systems: results of a Life Cycle Analysis. *ACORN*. 2005;18(4):16-17, 21-24.

25. Chaerul M, Tanaka M, Shekdar AV. A system dynamics approach for hospital waste management. *Waste Manag*. 2008;28(2):442-449.

26. Cheng YW, Sung FC, Yang Y, Lo YH, Chung YT, Li KC. Medical waste production at hospitals and associated factors. *Waste Manag*. 2009;29(1):440-444.

27. McGain F, Clark M, Williams T, Wardlaw T. Recycling plastics from the operating suite. *Anaesth Intensive Care*. 2008;36(6):913-914.

28. Ogden J. Blue wrap recycling: it can be done! *AORN J*. 2009;89(4):739-743.

29. Environmentally preferable purchasing. Environmental Protection Agency. *http://www.epa.gov/epp/*. Accessed February 10, 2010.

30. Environmental purchasing. Practice Greenhealth. *http://www.practicegreenhealth.org/educate/purchasing*. Accessed February 10, 2010.

31. Birk S. An issue that can't be contained. *Mater Manag Health Care*. 2008;17(5):42-44.

32. Texas health system identifies numerous cost-savings opportunities. *Hosp Mater Manage*. 2007; 32(4):1-3.

33. Recommended practices for sterilization in the perioperative practice setting. In: *Perioperative Standards and Recommended Practices*. Denver, CO: AORN, Inc; 2010:457-480.

34. AAMI. *ST65: Processing of Reusable Surgical Textiles for Use in Health Care Facilities*. Arlington, VA: Association for the Advancement of Medical Instrumentation; 2000.

35. Follow expert insight to launch a successful reprocessing program. *Hosp Mater Manage*. 2008;33(3):1-4.

36. DiConsiglio J. Reprocessing SUDs reduces waste, costs. *Mater Manag Health Care*. 2008;17(9):40-42.

37. US Food and Drug Administration. Definitions. 21 CFR 820.3. Revised April 1, 2008. *http://edocket.access .gpo.gov/cfr_2008/aprqtr/pdf/21cfr820.3.pdf*. Accessed February 10, 2010.

38. How to report a problem (medical devices). US Food and Drug Administration. *http://www.fda.gov/cdrh /mdr/mdr-general.html*. Accessed February 10, 2010.

39. US Food and Drug Administration. 21 CFR 807. Establishment registration and device listing for manufacturers and initial importers of devices. Revised April 1, 2008. *http://www.access.gpo.gov/nara/cfr/waisidx 08 /21cfr807_08.html*. Accessed February 10, 2010.

40. US Food and Drug Administration. Labeling. 21 CFR 801. Revised April 1, 2008. *http://www.access.gpo .gov/nara/cfr/waisidx_08/21cfr801_08.html*. Accessed February 10, 2010.

41. US Food and Drug Administration. Exemptions for device establishments. 21 CFR 807.65. Revised April 1, 2008. *http://edocket.access.gpo.gov/cfr_2008/aprqtr /pdf/21cfr807.65.pdf*. Accessed February 10, 2010.

42. US Food and Drug Administration. Premarket approval of medical devices. 21 CFR 814. Revised April 1, 2008. *http://www.access.gpo.gov/nara/cfr/waisidx _08/21cfr814_08.html*. Accessed February 10, 2010.

43. US Food and Drug Administration. Investigational device exemptions. 21 CFR 812. Revised April 1, 2008. *http://www.access.gpo.gov/nara/cfr/waisidx_08/21cfr81 2_08.html*. Accessed February 10, 2010.

44. US Food and Drug Administration. Definitions. 21 CFR 806.2. Revised April 1, 2008. *http://edocket.access .gpo.gov/cfr_2008/aprqtr/pdf/21cfr806.2.pdf*. Accessed February 10, 2010.

45. US Food and Drug Administration. Medical device reporting. 21 CFR 803. Revised April 1, 2009. *http://www .access.gpo.gov/nara/cfr/waisidx_09/21cfr803_09.html*. Accessed February 10, 2010.

46. Akridge J. Softer, stronger fabrics enhance gowns and drapes. *Healthc Purchasing News*. 2009;33(4):14-19.

47. Topf M. Psychological explanations and interventions for indifference to greening hospitals. *Healthc Manage Rev*. 2005;30(1):2-8.

48. Williamson JE. New gown, drape features have O.R. staff covered. *Healthc Purchasing News*. 2005; 29(9):22, 24, 26 assm.

49. Akridge J. Task-specific surgical apparel balances comfort with protection. *Healthc Purchasing News*. 2008;32(10):28.

50. AORN guidance statement: The role of the health care industry representative in the perioperative setting. In: *Perioperative Standards and Recommended Practices*. Denver, CO: AORN, Inc; 2010:657-660.

51. Medical device reporting: manufacturer reporting, importer reporting, user facility reporting, distributor reporting. Food and Drug Administration, HHS. Final rule. *Fed Reg*. 2000;65(17):4112-4121.

Acknowledgements

LEAD AUTHORS

Byron Burlingame, RN, MS, CNOR
Perioperative Nursing Specialist
AORN Center for Nursing Practice
Denver, Colorado

George Allen, PhD, RN, CNOR, CIC
Director of Infection Control
Downstate Medical Center
Brooklyn, New York

CONTRIBUTING AUTHORS

Josette Coicou-Brioche, RN, MSN, CNOR
Associate Director of Perioperative Services
Kings County Hospital Center
Brooklyn, New York

Nancy B. Bjerke, RN, MPH, CIC
Health Care Consultant
San Antonio, Texas

PUBLICATION HISTORY

Originally published April 1989, *AORN Journal.* Revised August 1993.

Revised November 1997; published January 1998, *AORN Journal.* Reformatted July 2000.

Revised November 2003; published in *Standards, Recommended Practices, and Guidelines,* 2004 edition. Reprinted March 2004, *AORN Journal.*

Revised January 2010 for online publication in *Perioperative Standards and Recommended Practices.*

Recommended Practices
for Surgical Tissue Banking

The following recommended practices were developed by the AORN Recommended Practices Committee and have been approved by the AORN Board of Directors. They were presented as proposed recommended practices for comments by members and others. They are effective January 1, 2006.

These recommended practices are intended as achievable recommendations representing what is believed to be an optimal level of practice. Policies and procedures will reflect variations in practice settings and/or clinical situations that determine the degree to which the recommended practices can be implemented.

AORN recognizes the numerous settings in which perioperative nurses practice. These recommended practices are intended as guidelines adaptable to various practice settings. These practice settings include traditional operating rooms, ambulatory surgery centers, physicians' offices, cardiac catheterization suites, endoscopy suites, radiology departments, and all other areas where operative and other invasive procedures may be performed.

Purpose

Surgical tissue banking encompasses procuring, processing, preserving, and/or storing selected human cells and tissue. Human tissue includes, but is not limited to, bone, cartilage, ligaments, tendons, fascia, dura mater, sclera, corneas, heart valves/conduits, bone marrow, vessels, and skin. It is beyond the scope of these recommended practices to address all areas of tissue banking, solid organ transplantation, or nonhuman tissue. These recommended practices provide guidance for developing organizational policies and procedures that are specific to the needs of surgical patients and address the perioperative practice setting and expertise required of personnel.

A tissue bank should be established only where a need exists. Before the decision is made to establish a tissue bank, consideration should be given to personnel, equipment, and practical operational requirements for providing safe, reliable, and biologically useful products.

In 1997, the US Food and Drug Administration (FDA) announced a program for comprehensive regulatory oversight of tissue banking.[1] In support of this program, the FDA has published proposed guidance documents that were later clarified as final rules.[2-6] The agency intends to propose more regulations in the future in the form of guidance documents. Adherence to these regulations is required during the development and ongoing operation of a human tissue bank. In addition, the standards published by the American Association of Tissue Banks (AATB)[7] should be referred to for additional direction.

Effective July 1, 2005, the Joint Commission on Accreditation of Healthcare Organizations (JCAHO) standards for tissue banking have been updated in the laboratory accreditation program and additionally applied to ambulatory care, critical access hospital and hospital accreditation programs, and office-based surgery practices. The standards apply to organizations that store or issue human, nonhuman, and synthetic tissue, including surgery and outpatient centers.[8]

Recommendation I

Facilities procuring, processing, and/or preserving tissue, and facilities storing tissue for potential transfer to a different facility, must register as tissue banks with the FDA.[4]

1. A list of types of human cells, tissue, and cellular and tissue-based products must be submitted with the application to the FDA.[4] Facilities that recover, screen, test, process, label, package, and/or distribute human cells or tissue for implantation, transplantation, or infusion must register with the FDA. The registration form includes a list of tissues and cells to be used in this process.[4] Facilities must register within five days after beginning operations, notify the FDA within six months of changes in products, and update the registration annually in December. Facilities storing only purchased tissue for use within the same facility, or those who recover autologous skin or skull bone flaps for later reimplantation into the same patient, are not required to register as tissue banks. Additional clarification is available from the FDA.

2. Facilities should verify that tissue and cells acquired from outside sources have been procured, processed, stored, and distributed by tissue banks registered with the FDA and licensed by state agencies.[8] Depending on the type of tissue being acquired, outside sources of cells or

tissues also should be accredited by the AATB, the Eye Bank Association of America (EBAA), or the AABB (formerly known as the American Association of Blood Banks). Accreditation by any of these agencies demonstrates that these sources periodically pass inspections by the accrediting agency and provides minimum assurance of quality control for the recovery, screening, testing, processing, storage, and distribution of the tissue. Some tissue banks purchase tissue procured or processed by other tissue banks and have limited registration or accreditation. All tissue banks involved in handling the tissue must be registered and should be accredited. Copies of current certificates should be requested annually and kept on file.

Recommendation II

Facilities procuring, processing, preserving, storing, or distributing tissue to other facilities should have defined oversight with authority and accountability for all activities performed.[8]

1. A facility performing any tissue-banking activities should appoint an administrator or oversight group accountable for these activities. The administrator of a tissue bank is accountable for all aspects of the tissue bank's activities, including compliance with regulations. This role requires a broad understanding of the processes and responsibilities involved.

2. Administrative personnel should be knowledgeable about
   - all applicable federal, state, and local regulations;
   - applicable standards of the AATB, EBAA, and AABB;
   - accrediting agency requirements;
   - screening and testing criteria;
   - the grieving process;
   - aspects of informed consent;
   - donor and recipient rights;
   - quality control;
   - documentation and record-keeping requirements;
   - confidentiality and release of information;
   - requirements for release of tissue;
   - adverse event reporting; and
   - ethical considerations.

3. A physician or medical advisory committee should be available to provide direction for

medical decisions. The AATB recommends that a medical director be appointed.[7]

4. Tissue ordering and receiving, procuring, processing, preserving, storing, and distributing should be coordinated throughout the health care facility.[8] Centralized oversight of all aspects of tissue banking is necessary to ensure that all tissue received and stored is safe for implantation, that processes are validated and monitored on an ongoing basis, and that all tissue can be traced back to the source or easily recalled if necessary.

Recommendation III

Surgical tissue bank personnel must be knowledgeable about the aspects of tissue banking in which they participate.[6]

1. Personnel should be knowledgeable about the importance of the tissue bank's products and services. An understanding of the importance of tissue bank activities instills an attitude of attention to detail and may minimize errors.

2. Personnel soliciting tissue donations must be knowledgeable about
   - federal and state regulations,
   - screening and testing criteria,
   - the grieving process,
   - aspects of informed consent,
   - donor and recipient rights, and
   - ethical considerations.

   Requesting authorization for donation of tissue requires unique interpersonal communication skills to ensure that donations are legally and ethically solicited and accepted.

3. Personnel screening potential donors must be knowledgeable about
   - the grieving process;
   - screening and testing criteria;
   - sources of information for screening (eg, relevant medical records, knowledgeable historian);
   - techniques to obtain accurate and complete information; and
   - resources and options available when screening results are ambiguous or unclear.

   Screening requires specific training to learn the best sources of medical history and behavioral risk assessment information. This source may be friends rather than family members. Obtaining the most accurate information requires strategies for interviewing. At times, the results of screening may not be clear. The screening individual needs to know what resources are available to assist with the determination of suitability.

4. Personnel processing and/or packaging tissue must be knowledgeable about
   - environmental conditions required,
   - steps in the processing procedures,
   - labeling requirements,
   - packaging,
   - documentation,
   - appropriate measures to be taken when tissue is compromised, and
   - disposal of unsuitable tissue.

   Understanding the steps of tissue processing is essential to preventing errors that may alter the integrity and/or function of the tissue, contaminate it, or negatively affect the outcomes of transplantation. Disposal of human tissue must be done in compliance with federal and state regulations. Complete and accurate documentation for tracing tissue disposition is required by the FDA.

5. Administrators should ensure that initial and ongoing educational opportunities are provided to meet the needs of personnel who perform tasks within the surgical tissue bank. Regulations and standards affecting tissue bank activities are evolving. Initial education provides a baseline to support a beginning level of job performance. Ongoing education offers personnel an opportunity to enhance skills and learn about changes in regulations and standards. An introduction and review of tissue banking policies and procedures should be included in the orientation and ongoing education of personnel to assist in the development of knowledge, skills, and attitudes that positively affect patient outcomes.

6. Administrators should ensure that the employees performing tasks within the surgical tissue bank are competent to perform these tasks. Competency assurance is essential because errors may cause breaches in regulations, compromise the integrity or function of the tissue, contaminate it, and/or lead to negative outcomes of transplantation.

Recommendation IV

Potential donors, their families, and recipients of tissue should be treated with respect, dignity, and sensitivity, and their rights should be protected.

1. Personnel approaching living donors or families of potential deceased donors to request consent for donation should be sensitive to the level of distress the situation may cause and respect the individual's rights. Tissue donation is frequently requested at the time of an unexpected death. This event creates distress in the survivors and is emotionally charged. Sensitivity to the needs of the survivors is essential to a successful donation. Perioperative personnel also should recognize that the deceased donor is an individual with the same rights that would be afforded to any other patient. At times, donation is requested of a living relative. This situation also may trigger strong emotions and ethical dilemmas. The person's rights should be honored.

2. Personnel should obtain informed consent from the donor or donor's responsible party before tissue recovery. Permission to retrieve tissue from nonliving donors should be sought from next of kin in order of legal precedence. If the next of kin is unavailable, local, state, and federal regulations should be followed. The Uniform Anatomical Gift Act (UAGA) of 1968, passed in all 50 states, provides guidelines within which consent may be obtained upon death of the donor, including an order of priority for the potential donor's next of kin. Additional guidelines concerning donations appear in the 1987 amendments to the UAGA and were clarified in 2001 by the US Department of Health and Human Services.[9] Individual state laws may vary. Some states expressly honor the donor's documented wishes (eg, donor registry, driver's license, donor card or directive) as legal consent in lieu of obtaining additional authorization from the next of kin. Key elements of an informed consent include
   - identification of tissues to be recovered;
   - explanation of the potential uses of the tissue (eg, transplantation, research, education);
   - a general description of the recovery process; and
   - explanations that the family may limit or restrict the use of the tissue.[9]

3. Personnel should provide the family with written materials disclosing the intended uses of the tissue and the nature of the donation, including
   ♦ a copy of the signed consent form,
   ♦ instructions on how to follow up with the tissue bank should concerns arise,
   ♦ a description of the uses for which donated tissue may be applied, and
   ♦ a list and description of other companies and entities with which the tissue bank has relationships for processing and distributing tissue.

   The tissue bank is responsible for ensuring that accurate, sensitive, and appropriate information is shared with the person giving consent. Using written materials ensures consistency and allows the person providing consent an opportunity to review the material again.[2]

4. Allograft donations from living donors should be accepted only if the medical, legal, and ethical conditions surrounding the donations meet approved criteria. Questionable conditions include undue medical risk to the donor, coercion, promises of monetary gain, and the diminished capacity of the donor to evaluate the medical or surgical risks.[7]

5. Informed consent should be obtained from patients receiving tissue transplants, following a discussion of the risks, benefits, and alternatives.

Recommendation V

Tissue for transplantation must be recovered only from suitable donors.

1. A responsible individual(s) must determine allograft donor suitability based on results of required screening and testing for risk factors or the presence of relevant communicable disease agents and diseases.[5,7] Individuals making the determination of donor suitability must be knowledgeable about the legal requirements and medical risks involved and must have the formal authority to make this determination. This responsibility may rest with a medical director or a medical advisory committee.

2. A responsible individual should screen donors of allografts for risk factors and clinical evidence of relevant infectious agents and diseases before recovery of tissues. Screening includes documenting the review of relevant medical records, performing a strict physical assessment, and conducting detailed interviews with a knowledgeable historian. Donor screening minimizes the risk of transmission of infectious agents and diseases to the recipient and minimizes the risk of retrieving tissue that is not suitable for transplantation.

3. Allograft donor exclusion criteria include the following:
   ♦ active systemic viral, bacterial, or fungal infection;
   ♦ disease history of unknown etiology;
   ♦ risk associated with human transmissible spongiform encephalopathy (eg, Creutzfeldt-Jakob disease [CJD], a blood relative with noniatrogenic CJD, rapidly progressive dementia, receipt of human pituitary-derived hormones, receipt of human dura mater grafts, travel/residency risks associated with variant CJD);
   ♦ certain autoimmune diseases;
   ♦ fever associated with a possible infectious etiology; and
   ♦ meeting any of the high-risk criteria for relevant communicable disease agents identified by the FDA, including
     – physical evidence for risk of sexually transmitted diseases such as genital ulcerative disease, herpes simplex, syphilis, chancroid;
     – for a male donor, physical evidence of anal intercourse, including perianal condyloma;
     – physical evidence of nonmedical percutaneous drug use, such as needle tracks, (note any tattoos that may be covering needle tracks);
     – physical evidence of recent tattooing, ear piercing, or body piercing;
     – disseminated lymphadenopathy;
     – oral thrush;
     – blue or purple spots consistent with Kaposi's sarcoma;
     – unexplained jaundice, hepatomegaly, or icterus (note that hepatomegaly may not be apparent in a physical assessment unless an autopsy is performed);
     – physical evidence of sepsis, such as unexplained generalized rash;
     – large scab consistent with recent smallpox immunization;
     – eczema vaccinatum;
     – generalized vesicular rash (ie, generalized vaccinia);

- severely necrotic lesion consistent with vaccinia necrosum; and/or

- corneal scarring consistent with vaccinial keratitis.[10]

The medical director or medical advisory committee should evaluate potential donors with metabolic or bone disease, malignancy or malignant neoplasm, or disease of unknown etiology on a case-by-case basis. Some diseases have a range of severity that may cause the tissue to be appropriate or inappropriate for donation. A physician with knowledge and oversight responsibilities should evaluate these potential donors and make this determination. Potential donors are screened to minimize the risk of transmission of infection or disease. Recipients of pituitary-derived human growth hormone, human dura mater, or gonadotropin, as well as those who meet the travel/residency parameters associated with an increased exposure risk to the human form of bovine spongiform encephalopathy (BSE), may be at risk of carrying the agent causing CJD or variant CJD and should be excluded from consideration for tissue procurement.[5,10] Xenotransplantation recipients and their intimate contacts should be excluded from potential transplantation because xenotransplants may harbor infectious agents from the donor animal. These infectious agents also may have been transmitted to intimate contacts of the xenotransplant recipient. The FDA considers these individuals not to be suitable donors.[5,10]

Donor screening minimizes the risk of transmitting infectious agents and diseases to tissue recipients through transplantation.[10] Contraindications and exclusion criteria are evolving as new knowledge is gained and infectious disease threats are identified. Tissue bank administrations should remain informed of changes in the recommendations of the Centers for Disease Control and Prevention (CDC), FDA, and AATB and incorporate these changes into screening criteria.

4. Donors of allografts must be tested with FDA-approved, cleared, or licensed tests by laboratories compliant with the Clinical Laboratory Improvement Amendments of 1988 and found negative for relevant infectious agents and diseases, including, but not limited to

  - HIV type 1 and type 2 (anti-HIV-1 and anti-HIV-2);

  - hepatitis B virus (HBV) surface antigen (HBsAg);

  - total antibody to hepatitis B core antigen (antiHBc)—(IgG+IgM);

  - hepatitis C virus (HCV) (anti-HCV);

  - *Treponema pallidum* (syphilis) confirmatory test;

  - human T-lymphotropic virus (Types I and II); and

  - cytomegalovirus.[5]

Living donors should be tested for hepatitis HBc core antibody (anti-HBc) and should be retested 180 days after recovery before tissues are released for allogenic use. Testing for these infectious agents minimizes the risk of transmission and is required by the FDA final rule.[3] Donors of dura mater grafts also must be tested for the infectious agent that causes CJD; this includes a recommendation that a qualified pathologist perform an examination of the donor's entire brain.[5]

Recommendation VI

Tissue must be recovered, processed, and transplanted in clean, controlled environments appropriate for sterile surgical procedures.

1. Traffic patterns should be established and maintained in accordance with AORN's "Recommended practices for traffic patterns in the perioperative practice setting."[11] Traffic control in the OR minimizes the potential for contamination of the tissue retrieved. Eyes usually are procured with intact corneas in less controlled environments; however, the corneas should be removed from the eyes, processed, and transplanted in an OR-type environment.

2. The environment should be cleaned in accordance with AORN's "Recommended practices for environmental cleaning in the surgical practice setting."[12] Cleaning should be performed on a routine basis and as needed to reduce the amount of organic and inorganic debris and microbial load that can potentially contaminate the tissue. The FDA requires that the facility for tissue recovery be controlled to minimize the risk for contamination or cross-contamination through the introduction or transmission of communicable disease.[6(p68683)]

3. Surgical attire should be worn during recovery and transplantation of tissue in accordance

with AORN's "Recommended practices for surgical attire."[13] Clean surgical attire minimizes contamination of the tissue.

4. Only powder-free gloves should be used. Glove powder is aerosolized when powdered gloves are used.[14] Powder can contaminate recovered tissue and may lead to adverse reactions or rejections of the tissue by the recipient.[15-23]

5. When it is known that the potential tissue recipient has antibodies to natural rubber proteins, the tissue should be recovered with latex-free supplies in accordance with the "AORN latex guideline."[24] Transplanting tissue with an antigen to which the recipient is allergic can lead to adverse outcomes, including tissue rejection, impaired healing, and allergic reaction.

Recommendation VII

Tissue must be recovered and processed in a manner that minimizes microbial growth, contamination, and cross-contamination.[6(p68681)]

1. Postmortem donors should be placed in refrigeration within 12 hours of asystole, and tissue should be procured within 24 hours of asystole. Refrigeration minimizes cell oxygen consumption and microbial growth. Prolonged times between cell ischemia and tissue recovery provides an opportunity for microbial proliferation. Recommendations for maximum duration of time between recovery and transplantation have been established by the AATB.[7]

2. A sterile field should be established and maintained in accordance with AORN's "Recommended practices for maintaining a sterile field."[25] Aseptic practices are used to prevent contamination of the tissue and minimize the risk of subsequent infection. Sterile surgical drapes provide a barrier to minimize contamination of the recovered tissue.

3. The donor site and operative site should be prepared in accordance with AORN's "Recommended practices for skin preparation of patients."[26] Adequate skin preparation reduces the microbial count of the skin that can lead to contamination of recovered tissue.

4. The surgical team should perform surgical hand antisepsis and wear sterile gowns and gloves during recovery of tissue, in accordance with AORN's "Recommended practices for surgical hand antisepsis/hand scrubs."[27] Surgical hand antisepsis reduces microbial flora and may reduce the contamination of the tissue. Gowns and gloves provide a barrier to microbial contamination. When corneas are recovered, the sterile field is very small, and gowns may not be necessary.

5. Transplantation of tissue has resulted in transmission of viral, bacterial, and fungal infections. Inadequate tissue processing and quality controls have resulted in postoperative infections and graft failures.[6(p68651)] In 2002, the CDC published an investigation of 26 reported cases of allograft-associated infections.[28] During an investigation of voluntary reports, the FDA identified failure to validate procedures to prevent contamination and cross-contamination during processing in more than half of reported adverse events.[6(p68652)] Proper processing and quality controls minimize the risk of adverse events associated with transplanted tissue.

Recommendation VIII

Tissue must be prepared, processed, and preserved in a manner that minimizes microbial growth and optimizes the condition of the tissue for transplantation.[6(p68681)]

1. Aerobic and anaerobic tissue cultures should be collected when tissue is retrieved. Culture results may identify tissue that is inappropriate for transplantation and also provide a baseline for evaluation of processing and storage.

2. Tissue that will not undergo a sterilization process should be aseptically prepared and transferred to a sterile storage container. Aseptic technique is used to prevent contamination of tissue.

3. The package or container selected should provide an adequate barrier to microbial contamination and should be compatible with the type of sterilization, preservation, and storage conditions. Packages of refrigerated and frozen tissue become wet during storage and form condensation upon removal from storage. Containers should be impervious to moisture.

4. For sterilization of tissue, FDA-approved technology should be used in accordance with the FDA current good tissue practices[6] and AATB

standards for guidance. The FDA regulations and recommendations are evolving as new knowledge is gained. The AATB periodically reviews and revises the standards for tissue banking. It is important to review information from these sources to minimize risks of tissue processing.

5. Pooling (ie, commingling) of tissue from two or more donors must not occur.[6(p68684)]

6. When processing dura mater, a validated procedure must be used to minimize the risk of transmitting human transmissible spongiform encephalopathy (eg, prion disease, CJD).[6(p68683)] Transplantation of contaminated tissue has resulted in transmission of viral, bacterial, and fungal infections.[6] Proper processing and quality controls minimize the risk of adverse events associated with transplanted tissue.

Recommendation IX

Tissue must be labeled in a manner that provides direction for preparation and implantation and minimizes the risk of errors.[6,7]

1. Proper labeling of tissue minimizes the risk of errors. The allograft package/storage container should be labeled with the following information:
   ◆ tissue identification number (this may include a bar code);
   ◆ description of the tissue;
   ◆ name, address, and telephone number of the tissue bank responsible for determining donor suitability, processing, storage, and distribution of the allograft;
   ◆ recovery or distribution center that is responsible for determining donor suitability, processing, and distribution;
   ◆ recovery date and time;
   ◆ expiration date, if applicable, including the month and year;
   ◆ acceptable storage conditions, including recommended storage temperature and acceptable storage temperature range;
   ◆ the disinfection or sterilization method used, if applicable;
   ◆ if not sterilized, whether the tissue was procured and prepared under aseptic conditions;
   ◆ quantity of tissue expressed as volume, weight, dimensions, or a combination of these units of measure, if applicable;

   ◆ potential residues of processing agents and solutions (eg, antibiotics, ethanol, ethylene oxide, dimethyl sulfoxide); and
   ◆ package inserts containing instructions for use, indications and contraindications, preparation of tissue for use, expiration dates, and specific tests performed on tissues, warnings and potential adverse reactions, and instructions for opening packages or containers.[6,7]

2. The autograft package/storage container should be labeled with the following information:
   ◆ name, address, and telephone number of the tissue bank responsible for processing, storing, and distributing the autograft;
   ◆ the statements "For Autologous Use Only" and "Autologous Donation";[7(p86)]
   ◆ disinfection/sterilization method, if used;
   ◆ if not sterilized, whether the tissue was recovered and prepared under aseptic conditions;
   ◆ the warning "Not Evaluated For Infectious Substances" if infectious disease testing has not been performed;
   ◆ the warning "Biohazard" if infectious disease tests were performed and found to be positive;
   ◆ two unique identifiers of the donor/ recipient (eg, name, medical records number), including bar code;
   ◆ description of the tissue;
   ◆ recovery date and time;
   ◆ expiration date, if applicable, including the month and year;
   ◆ acceptable storage conditions, including recommended storage temperature and acceptable storage temperature range;
   ◆ method of preservation, if applicable; and
   ◆ potential residues of processing agents and solutions (eg, antibiotics, ethanol, ethylene oxide, dimethyl sulfoxide).[6,7] This information is necessary for release of the autograft for reimplantation only into the same donor/ patient, quality control, and appropriate tissue preparation for implantation.

   This documentation is required for certification by the AATB. Some of the information also is required by the FDA. Autografts have not undergone testing for infectious agents and diseases and must be released only to the donor. Release to another recipient may cause serious injury. Using two unique donor/recipient identifiers is consistent with JCAHO's safety goal of patient identification.[29] The application of bar code labeling facilitates matching of tissue to the desired recipient and accurate record keeping. These strategies minimize the potential for errors. The FDA requires that a procedure be maintained to verify the accuracy of labels when labeling human tissue.[6(p68684)]

Recommendation X

Allograft tissue obtained from an outside tissue bank should be handled in a manner consistent with the source facility's or manufacturer's written instructions.

1. Incoming tissue should be recorded, including the unique identifiers of the tissue and expiration date, the identification of the person accepting the tissue, and the date and time of receipt.

2. The packaging and transport conditions of incoming tissue should be examined to verify that the tissue integrity and temperature are acceptable and have been maintained during transport.

3. The tissue should be transferred to storage in manner consistent with the source facility's and manufacturer's written instructions.

Recommendation XI

Tissue is transported and stored in a manner that minimizes the risk of compromise or contamination.[6]

1. Containers for transporting and/or temporarily storing tissue must protect the tissue from contamination and maintain tissue at appropriate temperatures during transport.[6(p68660), 8(PC.17.10.C)]

2. Tissue for transplantation at a later date should be contained and frozen as soon as possible after recovery. Warm tissue is a medium for microbial growth. Tissue contamination may be multifactorial, and no finite time frame has been established. Institutions should determine this time frame with consideration of the type of tissue and recovery conditions.

3. Tissue must be stored in a secure area, with access restricted to authorized personnel, to minimize the risk of mix-ups, contamination, or improper distribution of tissue.[6(p68685)]

4. Temperatures selected for storage should be consistent with the AATB standards.[7]
   - Lyophilized or dehydrated musculoskeletal tissue should be stored at ambient temperature or cooler (but not be frozen).
   - Refrigerated musculoskeletal and osteoarticular tissue should be aseptically recovered, stored in an isotonic solution containing suitable antibiotics, and stored at 33.8° F (1° C) to 50° F (10° C).
   - Refrigerated skin should be stored at 33.8° F (1° C) to 50° F (10° C).
   - Frozen musculoskeletal and osteoarticular tissue should be processed and stored at −40° F (−40° C) or colder for long-term storage; and between −4° F (−20° C) to −40° F (−40° C) for short-term storage (fewer than six months).
   - Frozen or cryopreserved skin should be stored at −40° F (−40° C) or colder.
   - Frozen, cryopreserved cardiovascular tissue should be stored at −148° F (−100° C) or colder.
   - Reproductive cells should be frozen and cryopreserved in a liquid nitrogen freezer. Storage may be in either the liquid or vapor phase.
   - Refrigeration minimizes oxygen consumption of cells and prolongs their life. Dead cells provide a medium for microbial growth. Refrigeration minimizes microbial growth.

5. Autologous tissue should be segregated from allografts.[7] Autologous tissue usually has not undergone testing for infectious diseases or suitability screening for use for other patients, and its use is restricted to the donor only. Segregation minimizes the risk of error that may result in a negative outcome to a tissue recipient.

6. An expiration date for each tissue must be assigned. This expiration date must be based on tissue type, processing, preservation, storage, and packaging.[6(p68683)] The expiration time of tissue should not exceed the following recommendations of the AATB:[7]
   - refrigerated musculoskeletal tissue: five days;
   - refrigerated skin: 14 days;
   - frozen and cryopreserved cells and tissue (−40° F [−40° C] or colder): five years; and
   - lyophilized or dehydrated tissue: five years.

   Safe duration of storage of autografts may be influenced by processing and packaging methods and should be defined by the facility, not to exceed the recommendations of the AATB listed above. A process should be in place to minimize the number of autografts in storage to those that will be reimplanted. This is facilitated by periodic communication with surgeons or review of medical records to determine whether patients have survived.

7. Refrigerator and freezer units used for storing tissue should
   ◆ be monitored and daily temperature checks recorded,
   ◆ have annual calibration checks, and
   ◆ have an alarm system that is continuously monitored and that sounds when the temperature is not within the acceptable range.

   Restricted access is required to verify the safety and security of tissues. Maintenance of temperatures within the refrigerator or freezer unit ensures tissue integrity. Acceptable temperature range limits for the storage of tissue at each phase of the operation should be set in accordance with established standards and federal and state regulations. Temperature fluctuations outside the recommended temperature range may render tissue unsafe for patient use. The source facility should be consulted if this occurs. The alarm should sound in an area where an individual is present at all times to initiate immediate corrective action.

8. Personnel should have a specific contingency plan for refrigerator or freezer malfunction. Storage freezers and refrigerators should be attached to an emergency power system. In the event of failure of a refrigerator or freezer, the temperature of tissue should be monitored and maintained to prevent compromise of the tissue. All events should be properly documented.

Recommendation XII

Tissue should be quarantined until all steps of the tissue banking process have been reviewed and found acceptable.

1. Allografts should be segregated and not released until all screening, testing, processing, labeling, and storage criteria have been reviewed and determined to be satisfactory. The tissue should remain in an area segregated from available tissue until this review has been completed and the tissue is available for implantation. Segregation minimizes the risk of implanting unsuitable tissue. A checklist of criteria for release provides a standardized method of verifying release criteria and minimizes the potential for errors.

2. Autografts should be segregated and not released until all processing, labeling, and storage criteria have been reviewed and determined to be satisfactory. Segregation minimizes the risk of implanting unsuitable tissue. A checklist of criteria for release provides a standardized method of verifying release criteria and minimizes the potential for errors.

3. Autografts meeting all criteria for release should be released only for reimplantation in the autologous donor. Two unique identifiers (eg, donor name, medical record number) should be used for release of autografts. Autografts usually have not undergone testing for infectious agents and diseases and must be released only for reimplantation in the donor. Release to another recipient may cause serious injury. Using two unique donor identifiers is in accordance with the Joint Commission's safety goal of patient identification.[29] This strategy minimizes the potential for errors.

4. Tissue not meeting the release criteria should be considered compromised and should be destroyed in accordance with state and federal regulations. Regulations addressing human tissue disposal vary from state to state. Tissue that has not undergone sterilization is considered biohazardous.

5. Before dispensing tissue from the tissue bank, the processes used should be reviewed, and the suitability of the tissue for implantation should be determined. A standardized process should be in place to verify the donor tissue and recipient match, when applicable.

6. Verification of tissue availability should be incorporated into the verification process used to ensure the correct patient, procedure, site, position, and implants.[30]

7. The contents of the package, expiration date, and other pertinent information should be read back and verified before the tissue is dispensed onto the sterile field. Use of bar coding technology facilitates matching tissue to the desired recipient and keeping accurate records.

Recommendation XIII

Each tissue bank must maintain donor, tissue, and recipient records to ensure that pertinent data are retrievable.

1. The surgical tissue bank should have a tissue identification system that allows for tracking of tissues from the donor source to the recipient patient or institution, and vice versa.[6] Quality control issues and infections from implanted tissue have been reported. An identification system provides a means to determine what tissue is affected, rapidly quarantine the tissue, and follow up with affected recipients to ensure timely intervention to minimize morbidity.

2. Surgical tissue banks procuring, processing, distributing, and storing tissues should keep accurate records of the distribution of each tissue according to donor identification number, tissue type and identifying number, and identifying information for the receiving center, along with the dates of recovery and distribution.[6] This information provides a means to recall tissue that may be compromised.

3. Records should be developed and maintained according to the recommendations of AATB and in compliance with FDA rules. Records should include the following information:
   - FDA registration, if applicable;
   - copies of FDA registration and AATB accreditation of outside vendors from whom tissue is obtained (EBAA for ocular tissue, AABB for stem cells);
   - listing of all tissue products ordered, stored, and used;
   - informed consent documents;
   - donor suitability assessment criteria;
   - recovery;
   - processing;
   - preservation;
   - labeling;
   - storage;
   - quarantining;
   - testing record review;
   - releasing;
   - distribution;
   - ordering and receipt of tissue acquired from other sources:
     - package integrity upon receipt,
     - transport temperature-controlled and acceptable, and
     - source facility and unique identifier of the tissue;
   - instructions/procedures for reconstitution;
   - identity of personnel preparing, accepting, and issuing tissue;
   - dates and times of preparing, accepting, and issuing tissue;
   - documentation in the recipient's health record of the unique identifier of the tissue;
   - quality management records;
   - recall criteria and procedures; and
   - disposal of tissue.

   For tissue obtained from outside tissue banks, copies of pertinent records should be forwarded to the source facility. Documentation assists in clinical evaluation and in tracking recipients if an adverse event is identified.[6]

4. Records must be maintained for 10 years after tissue is dispensed or the tissue expiration date is reached, whichever is longer.[6] Tissue may be used years after recovery. For that reason, the FDA requires that records must be maintained for 10 years.

Recommendation XIV

A quality management program must be in place to evaluate the structure, processes, and outcomes of tissue bank services.[6(p68682)]

1. An initial program review should be performed by a multidisciplinary committee, comparing procedures with regulations and standards. Program review should be done annually to ensure ongoing compliance with regulations and ensure safe tissue banking practices.

2. Quality indicators should include, but not be limited to,
   - donor screening and testing;
   - tissue processing procedures;
   - labeling procedures;
   - storage requirements;
   - criteria for release of tissue;
   - the use of two unique donor identifiers for release of autografts; and
   - adverse events (including posttransplantation infections), corrective action, and evaluation.

   Tissue bank services involve significant risks to recipients if errors are made. The FDA requires any facility performing tissue banking to maintain a quality management program intended to prevent the introduction, transmission, or spread of communicable disease for every step of tissue banking performed.[6(p68682)] Ongoing quality management involves verifying that these steps are done in a safe, efficacious manner. These quality indicators address specific issues that may compromise the tissue. Specific quality indicators will depend on the services provided.

3. The FDA final rule for current good tissue practices requires the following aspects of quality management:[6]
   ◆ ensuring that required procedures are established and maintained;
   ◆ ensuring the appropriate analysis and sharing of information that could affect the potential contamination of the product or the potential transmission of communicable disease by the product;
   ◆ ensuring that appropriate corrective actions are taken and documented;
   ◆ ensuring proper training and education of personnel;
   ◆ establishing and maintaining appropriate monitoring systems;
   ◆ establishing and maintaining a system of records;
   ◆ investigating and documenting product deviations and making certain required reports; and
   ◆ conducting evaluations, investigations, audits, and other actions necessary to ensure compliance with the regulations.[6]

This quality framework is required by the FDA. Administrative personnel should be familiar with this requirement and its application to the components of tissue banking performed.

4. Facilities should report adverse events, including infections for which there is a reasonable possibility that the transplanted tissue caused the event. The tissue bank manufacturing the tissue is required to report adverse events to the FDA.[6] These reports are submitted through MedWatch at *http://www.fda.gov/medwatch/report/instruc.htm*. For events that result from tissue acquired from an outside tissue vendor, the report should be sent to the vendor and also may be submitted to the FDA.

Recommendation XV

Policies and procedures for preserving, storing, and maintaining tissue should be established, reviewed annually, and readily available in the practice setting.

1. Policies establishing authority, responsibility, and accountability for tissue handling and appropriate donor testing within the practice setting must be established and maintained for all steps performed by the facility.[6(p68683)] These policies may include, but are not limited to,
   ◆ authority and accountability for processes;
   ◆ screening and testing criteria;
   ◆ obtaining informed consent from the donor;
   ◆ providing information and obtaining informed consent from the allograft recipient;
   ◆ evaluating culture and serology tests with appropriate interventions for positive results;
   ◆ processing and preserving tissue;
   ◆ packaging and labeling tissue;
   ◆ sterilizing processes, if applicable;
   ◆ monitoring temperature during storage;
   ◆ maximum storage duration;
   ◆ handling frozen tissue if there is a freezer malfunction or power outage;
   ◆ warming or reconstituting preserved tissue;
   ◆ rinsing solutions from tissues;
   ◆ criteria for return of unused tissue into inventory;
   ◆ disposal of tissue;
   ◆ documenting implanted and discarded tissue in a retrievable format, and notifying recipients or recalling released tissues;
   ◆ responses to adverse events; and
   ◆ responses to recalls of tissue from tissue vendors.

2. Before implementation, procedures must be approved by the responsible authority within the health care organization.[6(p68683)] Institutional policies and procedures may seriously affect patient safety and should be reviewed by designated authorities within the facility (eg, infection control committee, pathology department). Tissue may be used years after recovery. For that reason, the FDA final rule for good tissue practices requires that policies and procedures be reviewed periodically, be readily available in the practice setting, and be archived for 10 years after recovery or the expiration date of the tissue, whichever is longer.[6(p68685)] These recommended practices should be used as guidelines, along with the standards of the AATB and regulations and recommendations of the FDA, for the development of policies and procedures for surgical tissue banking in the practice setting. Policies and procedures establish authority,

responsibility, and accountability and serve as operational guidelines.

3. The uniform perioperative nursing vocabulary should be used to document perioperative nursing care of the transplant donor and recipient on the intraoperative patient record. The perioperative nursing vocabulary is a clinically relevant and empirically validated standardized nursing language. This standardized language consists of the Perioperative Nursing Data Set (PNDS) and includes perioperative nursing diagnoses, interventions, and outcomes. The expected outcome of primary importance to these recommended practices is outcome O10, "The patient is free from signs and symptoms of infection." This outcome falls within the domain of Safety (D1). Interventions that might lead to the desired outcome include I98, "Protects from cross-contamination"; I121, "Assesses susceptibility for infection"; and I188, "Monitors for signs and symptoms of infection."[31]

Editor's note: The American Association of Tissue Banks can be reached at 1320 Old Chain Bridge Road, Suite 450, McLean, VA 22101; telephone (703) 827-9582.

Glossary

Allografts: Grafts taken from a living or nonliving donor for transplantation to a different individual.

American Association of Tissue Banks (AATB): A nonprofit organization that defines the standards for tissue banking.

Autografts: Tissue derived from an individual for implantation exclusively on or in the same individual.

Donor screening: Review of the donor's relevant medical records and physical assessment for evidence of past or present risk factors for relevant infectious agents or disease.

Donor testing: Laboratory tests on blood specimens collected from a potential donor.

Prion diseases: A classification of infectious diseases, including Creutzfeldt-Jakob disease (CJD), caused by a unique proteinaceous agent.

Tissue bank: A facility that participates in procuring, processing, preserving, and/or storing human cells and tissue for transplantation.

Xenotransplant: Cells or tissue from a nonhuman animal source that are transplanted, implanted, or infused into a human.

Xenotransplantation: Any procedure that involves the transplantation, implantation, or infusion into a human recipient of either (a) live cells, tissues, or organs from a nonhuman animal source (eg, bovine heart valves); or (b) human body fluids, cells, tissues, or organs that have had ex vivo contact with live nonhuman animal cells, tissues, or organs.

REFERENCES

1. US Food and Drug Administration, *Proposed Approach to Regulation of Cellular and Tissue-Based Products* (Rockville, Md: US Food and Drug Administration, Feb 28, 1997) 1-37.

2. US Food and Drug Administration, "Current good tissue practice for manufacturers of human cellular and tissue-based products; inspection and enforcement; proposed rule," *Federal Register* 66 (January 8, 2001) 1507-1559. Also available at *http://www.fda.gov/OHRMS /DOCKETS/98fr/010801c.pdf* (accessed 13 Sept 2005).

3. US Food and Drug Administration, "Suitability determination for donors of human cellular and tissue-based products; proposed rule," *Federal Register* 64 (Sept 30, 1999) 52696-52718. Also available at *http:// www.fda.gov/OHRMS/DOCKETS/98fr/093099a.pdf* (accessed 13 Sept 2005).

4. US Food and Drug Administration, "Human cells, tissues, and cellular and tissue-based products; establishment registration and listing; final rule," *Federal Register* 66 (Jan 19, 2001) 5447-5469. Also available at *http:// www.fda.gov/OHRMS/DOCKETS /98fr/011901a.pdf* (accessed 13 Sept 2005).

5. US Food and Drug Administration, "Eligibility determination for donors of human cells, tissues, and cellular and tissue-based products; final rule and notice," *Federal Register* 69 (May 25, 2004) 29785-29834. Also available at *http://www.fda.gov/OHRMS/DOCKETS /98fr/04-11245.pdf* (accessed 13 Sept 2005).

6. US Food and Drug Administration, "Current good tissue practice for human cell, tissue, and cellular and tissue-based product establishments; inspection and enforcement; final rule," *Federal Register* 69 (Nov 24, 2004) 68612-68688.

7. American Association of Tissue Banks, *Standards for Tissue Banking,* 10th ed (McLean, Va: American Association of Tissue Banks, 2002).

8. Joint Commission on Accreditation of Healthcare Organizations, "Standards approved for transplant and implant tissue storage and issuance," *Joint Commission Perspectives* (February 2005) 8-11.

9. Office of Inspector General, *Informed Consent in Tissue Donation: Expectations and Realities,* publ OEI-01-00-00440 (Boston: US Department of Health and Human Services, January 2001).

10. US Food and Drug Administration, *Guidance for Industry: Eligibility Determination for Donors of Human Cells, Tissues, and Cellular and Tissue-Based Products (HCT/Ps): Draft Guidance* (Rockville, Md: US Food and Drug Administration, May 2004) 1-52.

11. "Recommended practices for traffic patterns in the perioperative practice setting," in *Standards, Recommended*

Practices, and Guidelines (Denver: AORN, Inc, 2005) 483-485.

12. "Recommended practices for environmental cleaning in the surgical practice setting," in *Standards, Recommended Practices, and Guidelines* (Denver: AORN, Inc, 2005) 361-366.

13. "Recommended practices for surgical attire," in *Standards, Recommended Practices, and Guidelines* (Denver: AORN, Inc, 2005) 299-305.

14. D Beezhold, D Kostyal, J Wiseman, "The transfer of protein allergens from latex gloves: A study of influencing factors," *AORN Journal* 59 (March 1994) 605-613.

15. D Abeck et al, "Latex allergy and repeated graft rejections," *The Lancet* 339 (June 27, 1992) 1609.

16. D Beezhold, W Beck, "The absorbability and immunology of starch glove powders," *Complications in Surgery* (July/August 1992) 36-40.

17. C Bene, G Kranias, "Possible intraocular lens contamination by surgical glove powder," *Ophthalmic Surgery* 17 (May 1986) 290-291.

18. I Singh, W L Chow, L V Chablani, "Synovial reaction to glove powder," *Clinical Orthopaedics and Related Research* 99 (March/April 1974) 285-292.

19. P H McKee, E F McKeown, "Starch granulomata of the endocardium," *Journal of Pathology* 126 (October 1978) 103-105.

20. S Moriber-Katz et al, "Contamination of perfused donor kidneys by starch from surgical gloves," *American Journal of Clinical Pathology* 90 (July 1988) 81-84.

21. D I Vâge et al, "Elutable factors from latex-containing materials activate complement and inhibit cell proliferation. An in vitro biocompatibility study of medical devices," *Complement Inflammation* 7 (January-February 1990) 63-70.

22. C M Ruhl et al, "A new hazard of cornstarch, an absorbable dusting powder," *The Journal of Emergency Medicine* 12 (January/February 1994)11-14.

23. D A A Verkuyl, "Glove powder introduced in the circulation by autotransfusion and severe cardiac failure," *The Lancet* 340 (Aug 29, 1992) 550.

24. "AORN latex guideline," in *Standards, Recommended Practices, and Guidelines* (Denver: AORN, Inc, 2005) 117-132.

25. "Recommended practices for maintaining a sterile field," in *Standards, Recommended Practices, and Guidelines* (Denver: AORN, Inc, 2005) 453-457.

26. "Recommended practices for skin preparation of patients," in *Standards, Recommended Practices, and Guidelines* (Denver: AORN, Inc, 2005) 443-446.

27. "Recommended practices for surgical hand antisepsis/hand scrubs," in *Standards, Recommended*

Practices, and Guidelines (Denver: AORN, Inc, 2005) 377-385.

28. Centers for Disease Control and Prevention, "Update: Allograft-associated bacterial infections—United States," *Morbidity and Mortality Weekly Report* 51 (March 15, 2002) 207-210. Also available at *http://www.cdc.gov /mmwr/preview/mmwrhtml/mm5110a2 .htm* (accessed 13 Sept 2005).

29. "2005 Hospitals' National Patient Safety Goals," Joint Commission on Accreditation of Health Care Organizations, *http://www.jcaho.org/accredited+organizations /patient\safety/05\npsg/05npsghap.htm* (accessed 13 Sept 2005).

30. "Universal protocol for preventing wrong site, wrong procedure, wrong person surgery," Joint Commission on Accreditation of Health Care Organizations, *http://www.jcaho.org/accredited+organizations/patient +safety/universal+protocol/universal_protocol.pdf* (accessed 13 Sept 2005).

31. S C Beyea, ed, *Perioperative Nursing Data Set: The Perioperative Nursing Vocabulary*, second ed (Denver: AORN, Inc, 2002).

RESOURCES

Bren, L. "Keeping human tissue transplants safe," *FDA Consumer Magazine* 39 (May/June 2005) 30-36.

Verble, M; Worth, J. "Cultural sensitivity in the donation discussion," *Progress in Transplantation* 13 (March 2003) 33-37.

Verble, M; Worth, J. "Fears and concerns expressed by families in the donation discussion," *Progress in Transplantation* 10 (March 2000) 48-55.

PUBLICATION HISTORY

Originally published September 1984, *AORN Journal*. Revised April 1991.

Published as proposed recommended practices, February 1994.

Revised November 1998; published March 1999, *AORN Journal*. Reformatted July 2000.

Revised November 2003; published February 2004, *AORN Journal*.

Revised November 2005; published in *Standards, Recommended Practices, and Guidelines*, 2006 edition. Reprinted February 2006, *AORN Journal*.

AORN Perioperative Standards and
Recommended Practices, 2012 Edition

Customizable tools for your facility!

Implement recommended practices more easily!

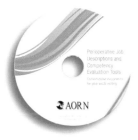

Perioperative Job Descriptions and Competency Evaluation Tools

These tools will help you meet the expectations of your facility, regulators, and, most importantly, your patients. Included in this CD:

- 14 perioperative job descriptions
- 11 role-specific evaluation tools
- 31 evaluation tools based on AORN's recommended practices
- Perioperative Staff RN Core Competencies Crosswalk

All documents included are customizable, with the exception of the Competencies Crosswalk.

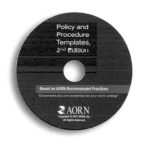

Policy & Procedure Templates, 2nd Edition

This CD provides you with a collection of sample policies and customizable templates based on AORN's *Perioperative Standards and Recommended Practices.* All are customizable to your facility.

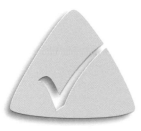

AORN Tool Kits *(free member benefit)*

AORN's award-winning Took Kits address critical issues impacting perioperative nurses and patient safety. Access a wealth of resources and education tools that may be customized to fit the needs of your facility. Tool Kits may include the following:

- AORN Position Statements
- Sample Policies and Procedures
- Case Studies and Scenarios
- Educational Training Presentations
- References and Resources

Not a member, yet? Enroll today at www.aorn.org

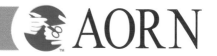

Education Resources

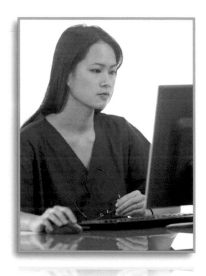

Periop 101: A Core Curriculum™

We set the standard so you can raise the bar.

Periop 101 is a program used by educators to train new perioperative nurses and consists of 25 online learning modules, delivered through AORN's e-learning platform. Each learning module includes required reading and suggested videos from AORN's Perioperative Nursing Video Library. Periop 101 is designed as a blended program to be given in conjunction with a clinical preceptorship.

Periop 101 is available for individual purchase and facility subscription.

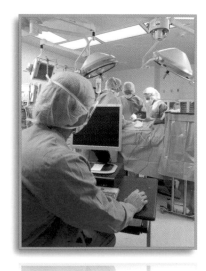

AORN Confidence-Based Learning (CBL)

When you make a critical decision in your OR, how confident are you that your decision is correct?

Patient safety depends upon making accurate, knowledgeable, and confident decisions, but many times your level of knowledge and confidence in accuracy are not the same. AORN's Confidence-Based Learning (CBL) meets that challenge by creating a mastery of knowledge so that you can confidently make correct decisions. CBL modules are based on AORN's *Perioperative Standards and Recommended Practices*.

CBL is available for individual purchase and facility subscription.

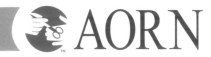

The following recommended practices for maintaining a safe environment of care were developed by the AORN Recommended Practices Committee and have been approved by the AORN Board of Directors. They were presented as proposed recommendations for comments by members and others. They are effective December 1, 2009.

These recommended practices are intended as achievable recommendations representing what is believed to be an optimal level of practice. Policies and procedures will reflect variations in practice settings and/or clinical situations that determine the degree to which the recommended practices can be implemented.

AORN recognizes the various settings in which perioperative nurses practice. These recommended practices are intended as guidelines adaptable to various practice settings. These practice settings include traditional operating rooms, ambulatory surgery centers, physician's offices, cardiac catheterization laboratories, endoscopy suites, radiology departments, and all other areas where surgery may be performed.

References to nursing interventions (I) used in the Perioperative Nursing Data Set, second edition, (PNDS) are noted in parentheses when a recommended practice corresponds to a PNDS intervention.[1] The reader is referred to the PNDS for further explanation of nursing diagnoses, interventions, and outcomes.[1]

Purpose

These recommended practices provide guidance for providing a safe environment of care and assist perioperative registered nurses in the identification of potential hazards in the practice setting. They include information on
- security;
- privacy rules;
- workplace ergonomics;
- electrical safety;
- heating, ventilation, air conditioning (HVAC);
- medical equipment;
- clinical alarms;
- blanket- and solution- warming cabinets;
- fire safety;
- medical gases;
- anesthesia gas systems;
- surgical smoke plume;
- chemicals;
- methyl methacrylate bone cement;

- chemotherapeutic agents;
- tubing connections; and
- hazardous upon disposal waste.

They are not intended to cover aspects of perioperative patient care addressed in other recommended practices.

Recommendation I

Potential security risks associated with the perioperative environment should be identified and safe practices should be established.

A security program helps to promote the
- safety of patients,
- safety of staff members,
- safety of visitors,
- prevention of drug diversion,
- theft, and
- protection of patient information.

I.a. A risk assessment should be conducted by an interdisciplinary committee at least annually, to identify potential security issues. The interdisciplinary committee members provide various areas of expertise and the resources necessary to evaluate the entire scope of security issues.

I.a.1. Occurrence reports regarding security-related incidents should be reviewed along with electronic surveillance records and logs to determine the numbers, seriousness, and types of issues.

I.a.2. Potential resolutions should be determined, based upon this risk assessment.[2,3]

I.b. An identification process should be in place to identify all persons entering the perioperative suite or the ambulatory surgery center.
Access to the perioperative environment should be limited to those who have authorized access verified by proper identification.[2,4]

I.b.1. Photo identification badges should be
- worn by all authorized personnel,
- worn on the upper body, and
- be visible.[5]

I.b.2. Anyone without an authorized badge should be stopped and questioned to assure the appropriateness of their presence in the facility.[5]

I.b.3. Individuals with limited or temporary access to the perioperative environment (eg, students, health care industry representatives, parents of pediatric patients) should be identified as visitors.

I.b.4. Visitors should wear temporary identification badges.

I.c. Tracking systems should be in place to identify who is present in the perioperative suite, (eg, electronic ID access tracking systems, visitor logs). In case of fire, disaster, evacuation, or other emergency, the identity of those present in the perioperative suite is necessary to assure that everyone has been evacuated and accounted for.

I.d. Door security systems should be used to restrict traffic.

I.e. Video surveillance should be used to monitor access. Video surveillance provides monitoring of entry areas during off-shift hours.

I.f. A written management plan should be created describing security management activities to include:
- employee and visitor badges;
- security cameras;
- alarm systems;
- emergency alert devices (eg, panic buttons);
- security illumination;
- restricted access to the facility during off hours; and
- restricted access to departments (eg, OR, postanesthesia care unit [PACU], endoscopy suites) or areas (eg, medication storage areas, medical records, sterile supply/equipment storage areas).[2-4]

Recommendation II

The perioperative environment must provide for the privacy of patients and patient information, including their identity and reason for hospitalization.[6,7] (PNDS: I151)

The Health Insurance Portability and Accountability Act of 1996 establishes guidelines for the safe communication of paper, electronic, and oral patient information and must be followed.[6,7]

II.a. Perioperative registered nurses must share only the information necessary to provide safe care (eg, surgery schedules, hand-off report tools) and only if appropriate to their job role.[6-8] (PNDS: I116)

Information is necessary to enable care to be delivered and continued safely.

II.b. Protected health information should be shared only with individuals (eg, family members, significant others) the patient has identified as being able to receive this information. (PNDS: I116)

II.b.1. Visitors may be assigned a number or pager to ensure that information is shared with the correct person.

II.c. Patient names may be listed on a display board in the restricted area.[7,8] (PNDS: I116)

II.d. Copies of personal health information including, but not limited to,
- surgery schedules,
- identification labels,
- identification/stamp plates,
- forms with patient identification, and
- photographs
should be shredded. (PNDS: I116)

II.d.1. Paper shredders or secured disposal containers (eg, shredding bins) should be readily available for proper disposal of hard copy or paper copies of personal health information. (PNDS: I151)

Recommendation III

Potential ergonomic hazards associated with the perioperative environment should be identified, and safe practices should be established.

Ergonomic hazards are found throughout the perioperative environment and are created by patient and equipment handling or the physical environment and, if not corrected, can cause injury to staff members.[9,10]

III.a. Perioperative staff members should follow the algorithms outlined in the AORN guidance statement *Safe Patient Handling and Movement in the Perioperative Setting*[10] and their organization's policies and procedures while completing activities including
- lateral transfer from stretcher to OR bed;
- positioning or repositioning the patient on the OR bed;
- lifting and holding extremities and heads for prepping;

- prolonged standing while holding retractors;
- retraction of tissue;
- lifting and carrying supplies or equipment; and
- pushing, pulling, and moving equipment on wheels.[10]

These activities can create ergonomic stressors that, if not recognized, can cause injury to staff members. Ergonomic stressors can be defined as tasks which include, but are not limited to,

- forceful tasks (eg, pushing a stretcher and patient up a ramp);
- repetitive motion (eg, passing instruments, opening suture packets, tying suture);
- static posture (eg, standing for long periods of time in one position);
- moving or lifting patients or equipment;
- carrying heavy instruments or equipment; and
- overexertion (eg, protecting a combative patient emerging from anesthesia).[10]

III.b. The physical environment should be designed to minimize the risk of ergonomic injury (eg, adequate room lighting, adequate storage to eliminate clutter).[9,10]

III.b.1. During the design phase of construction, provisions should be made to minimize hazards (eg, head injuries) to staff members in operating rooms which will contain ceiling-suspended equipment (eg, booms).[10]

III.b.2. Ceiling-, floor-, or wall-mounted booms should be hydraulic or electric and provide for ease of movement.[10]

III.c. Adequate staff members and equipment should be available and used to decrease risks due to ergonomic hazards.[11]

Appropriate mechanical devices should be used to reduce the risk of strain when moving a large or unconscious patient or a patient's large extremities.[11,12]

Recommendation IV

Potential hazards associated with the use of electrical equipment in the practice setting should be identified, and safe practices should be established. (PNDS: I138)

Electrical hazards in the operating room may lead to fires, burns, and electric shocks. These injuries result from electric current flowing through inappropriate pathways.

IV.a. The electrical supply should be reliable and consistent with the needs of the operating room.[13,14] (PNDS: I122)

IV.b. Electrical access panels or circuit breaker panels should be
- located on the same floor they serve,
- easily accessible, and
- not obstructed by equipment or carts.[15]

IV.c. Isolated power systems should be considered for operating rooms, which may be considered wet locations.[16] (PNDS: I138)

Adequate grounding provides protection from electric shock and fire hazards.[16]

IV.d. Line-isolation monitors should be provided for each isolated power system to indicate possible leakage or faulty currents.[16,17]

Line-isolation monitoring systems or ground-fault interrupting systems provide for continuous monitoring of current leakage. Systems that monitor current leakage and ground integrity reduce the hazards of shock, cardiac fibrillation, or burns produced by electrical current flowing through the patient's body to ground.[16,17]

IV.e. General lighting and specialty lighting, such as operating room overhead lights, should be on separate circuits.[15,18]

IV.f. Lighting should be in working order and adequate for illuminating the surgical field, monitoring the patient, and performing perioperative duties. (PNDS: I138)

Adequate lighting is necessary to perform the planned invasive procedure and to evaluate the patient.

IV.f.1. The light over the surgical field should be equipped with an automatic switch to the emergency power source for use if the usual power supply fails.[19] (PNDS: I138)

IV.f.2. Surgical lights should produce a minimum of radiant heat to reduce damage to exposed tissues and discomfort to the surgical team.[18] (PNDS: I138)

IV.f.3. Minimally invasive surgical suites (MIS), gastrointestinal endoscopy suites, and other procedure rooms should provide the low lighting required for optimum surgical visibility while providing adequate lighting for the perioperative team to complete their responsibilities without risk of injury from tripping, slipping, or falling.

Ambient blue or green light enhances the MIS screens and allows adequate visibility for other personnel in the room to work safely.[20]

IV.f.4. Video vendors and the personnel responsible for the organization's lighting should be consulted regarding lighting options and placement.

IV.g. Alternate sources of lighting and electrical power should be available when normal power is interrupted.[15,21]

Battery-powered emergency lights provide immediate lighting in a power failure, which decreases the potential negative effect of a total power interruption.[19]

IV.g.1. Batteries should be labeled with their expiration date and replaced as needed.[19]

IV.h. The emergency/alternate power source should begin operating within 10 seconds and have the capacity to operate equipment for monitoring, anesthesia delivery, and surgical equipment for a minimum of two hours.[14,22]

IV.h.1. Emergency power should be tested per local, state, and federal regulations.[19]

IV.h.2. All emergency electrical outlets should be tested, including those on booms.

IV.h.3. If the testing fails, the organization should implement interim measures, make necessary repairs, and perform a retest.[23]

IV.h.4. Electrical receptacle cover plates should be distinctly colored or marked if supplied by the emergency backup system.[13,15]

IV.i. Life-sustaining medical equipment should have battery backup, and backup supplies should be immediately available.[13]

IV.j. Clinical contingency plans should be developed for periods of loss of emergency power.[21]

Recommendation V

Potential hazards associated with HVAC systems in the practice setting should be identified, and safe practices should be established. (PNDS: I98, I21)

Air in the perioperative environment contains microbial-laden dust, lint, skin squames, and respiratory droplets.[24] The number of microorganisms in the air in an operating room is directly proportional to the number of personnel moving in and around the room. Outbreaks of surgical-site infections have been traced to airborne contamination from colonized health care workers.[24] Heating, ventilation, and air conditioning systems dilute and remove contaminants from the air and control airflow patterns. Key components of an effective HVAC system are proper air quality, air volume changes, and air flow direction. In an operating room or procedural area, proper functioning of these components minimizes the contamination of the sterile field and risk of infection to the patient. A properly functioning HVAC system carries microbial-laden skin squames, dust, and lint away from the sterile field, and removes these contaminants through the exhaust ducts at the periphery.

V.a. The quality of air entering the operating rooms should be carefully controlled. (PNDS: I98)

V.a.1. The air should be sequentially filtered through two filters. The first filter should be rated as 30% efficient and the second should be 90% efficient.[15,22]

V.a.2. A minimum of 20% of the incoming air (ie, three air changes per hour) should be from the outdoors.[15,24]

Filtered outdoor air minimizes the recirculation of indoor contaminants within the perioperative area.

V.b. Relative humidity should be maintained between 30% and 60% within the perioperative suite, including operating rooms, recovery area, cardiac catheterization rooms, endoscopy rooms, instrument processing areas, and sterilizing areas and should be maintained below 70% in sterile storage areas.[14,15] (PNDS: I98)

Low humidity increases the risk of electrostatic charges, which pose a fire hazard in an oxygen-enriched environment or when flammable agents are in use and increases the potential for dust. High humidity increases the risk of microbial growth in areas where sterile supplies are stored or procedures are performed.

V.b.1. Free-standing humidifiers should not be used because they can harbor microorganisms in fluid reservoirs and aerosolize these microorganisms into the clean environment.

V.b.2. Humidity should be monitored and recorded daily using a log format or documentation provided by the HVAC system.[25]

V.c. Temperature should be monitored and recorded daily using a log format or documentation provided by the HVAC system.[25] (PNDS: I128)

V.c.1. Temperature should be maintained between 68° F to 73° F (20° C to 23° C) within the operating room suite and general work areas in sterile processing.[15]

Self-regulating, area-specific chiller units may be required because operating rooms are filled with personnel and heat-emitting equipment; therefore, achieving the low end of this range can be difficult.

V.c.2. The decontamination area temperature should be maintained between 60° F to 65° F (16° C to 18° C).[15]

V.c.3. A temperature of 70° F to 75° F (21° C to 24° C) should be maintained in recovery areas and cardiac catheterization rooms.[15]

V.d. The air-exchange rate in the perioperative area should be carefully controlled. (PNDS: I98, I128)

The number of air changes per hour is based upon the need to remove microbiological or chemical contaminants from the environment.

V.d.1. The minimum rate of total air exchanges per hour should be maintained at a constant level as follows.
- **Operating room:** minimum of 15 air exchanges per hour with a recommended range of 20 to 25 air exchanges.
- **Cardiac catheterization rooms:** 15 air exchanges per hour.

- **Postanesthesia care unit:** six air exchanges per hour.
- **Compressed-gas storage area:** eight air exchanges per hour.
- **Sterile storage area:** four air exchanges per hour.[15]

V.d.2. Air exchanges per hour should be monitored per the organization's policy. (PNDS: I128)

V.e. Air-flow patterns within the perioperative setting should be controlled and uninterrupted. (PNDS: I81, I98, I128)

Air-flow patterns are architecturally designed and engineered to minimize contamination of the sterile field. Disruptions in the air-flow patterns within the operating room can redirect contaminants onto the sterile field, increasing the risk of surgical site infection.

V.e.1. The pressure gradient in the operating room should be positive to outer corridors at all times.[16,25]

V.e.2. Doors to the operating room or invasive procedure room should remain closed except when patients, personnel, and supplies are being actively moved in and out of the room.[26] (PNDS: I81)

V.e.3. Equipment and supplies should be located away from exhaust ducts to allow directed air flow out of the room.

V.e.4. Free-standing fans, humidifiers, or dehumidifiers should not be used in the operating room or sterile processing areas.[22,25,27]

Free-standing fans can disrupt the air-flow patterns, resulting in contamination of the sterile field.

V.f. In the event of a failure of the HVAC system,
- surgeries presently in progress should be completed,
- elective procedures should not be started until the HVAC system is functioning correctly,
- procedures should be redirected to areas of the surgical suite where the HVAC system is functioning or postponed until the problem has been corrected, and
- the event should be reported through the organization event-reporting system.

V.g. Preventive maintenance, including regular inspection, should be performed on HVAC systems (ie, changing filters on a routinely scheduled basis).

A properly functioning HVAC system minimizes the risk of contamination to the sterile field and is an essential component to infection prevention. Failure of the system poses an unnecessary risk for the elective surgical patient.

Recommendation VI

Potential hazards associated with the use of medical equipment in the practice setting should be identified, and safe practices should be established.

Hazards associated with medical equipment may be caused by frayed cords, damaged outlets, or extension cords and, if not corrected, may result in injury of patients, staff members, or visitors.

VI.a. Equipment should be inspected periodically by a qualified biomedical technician or engineer.[17,23,28] (PNDS: I138)

VI.a.1. All electrical equipment should be inspected before use. Inspection should include, but not be limited to
- new equipment before it is introduced into the practice setting,[23]
- checking power cords and plugs for fraying or other damage, and
- checking outlets and switch plates for damage.

VI.a.2. Damaged power cords or outlets can result in excessive current being delivered to the patient and/or staff members.

VI.b. Hospital-grade plugs are recommended when available, but plugs with adequate strain relief also may be used.[16,23] (PNDS: I138)

VI.c. Device cord length should be appropriate for the intended use of the equipment. (PNDS: I138)

Cords that do not lie flat create a risk for tripping or accidental unplugging of the equipment.

VI.c.1. Cords should be secured in a safe manner. An electrically safe, cleanable, or disposable device should be used to decrease the potential of tripping by personnel.

VI.c.2. Extension cords should be avoided unless used to decrease the potential for tripping.

Use of extension cords can result in excessive current leakage and/or electrical-system overload.

VI.c.3. Biomedical personnel should change cords of inadequate length to longer cord lengths to eliminate the need for extension cords and decrease the risk of tripping.

VI.d. Equipment found to be in disrepair should be immediately removed from service. (PNDS: I122)

VI.d.1. Organizational policy and procedure should be followed regarding routing of equipment in need of repair.

VI.e. A written plan should be developed describing the processes to be implemented to effectively manage medical equipment including selection, purchase, inspection, and maintenance.

Recommendation VII

Clinical alarms should be audible and should not be disabled. (PNDS: I122)

A clinical alarm is an alarm that is patient specific and used for the purpose of alerting staff members to a patient emergency.[29]

VII.a. An environmental assessment of every piece of equipment in the clinical setting should be conducted. (PNDS: I122)

VII.a.1. The assessment should
- be developed as a collaborative effort between clinical engineering and nursing; and
- include a list of those devices with alarms, including but not limited to
  - electrosurgery units (ESUs),
  - pneumatic tourniquets,
  - cardiac monitors,
  - carbon dioxide (CO_2) insufflators,
  - anesthesia equipment, and
  - infusion pumps.

VII.b. Alarms should be sufficiently audible to allow them to be heard at reasonable distances and above competing noise. (PNDS: I122)

RECOMMENDED HVAC SETTINGS[1,2,3]

Hospital area/Agency Recommendations	Temperature	Air flow	Humidity	Exchanges per hour	Outdoor air exchanges per hour	Recirculated by room unit (eg, fans)	Exhaust directed outside
Operating room			N/D = Not designated				
American Institute of Architects (AIA)	68°-73° F (20°-23° C)	Positive	30% to 60%	Minimum 15	3	No	N/D
American Association for the Advancement of Medical Instrumentation (AAMI)	N/D	N/D	N/D	N/D	N/D	N/D	N/D
National Fire Protection Association			35%				
Anesthesia gas storage							
AIA	N/D	Negative	N/D	8	N/D	N/D	Yes
AAMI	N/D	N/D	N/D	N/D	N/D	N/D	N/D
Postanesthesia care unit							
AIA	70°-75° F (21°-24° C)	N/D	30% to 60%	6	2	No	N/D
AAMI	N/D	N/D	N/D	N/D	N/D	N/D	N/D
Soiled decontamination							
AIA	68°-73° F (20°-23° C)	Negative	N/D	10	N/D	No	Yes
AAMI	60°-65° F (16°-18° C)	Negative	30% to 60%	10	N/D	N/D	Yes
Sterilizer equipment access							
AIA	N/D	Negative	N/D	10	N/D	N/D	Yes
AAMI	75°-85° F (21°-29° C)	Negative	N/D	10	N/D	N/D	Yes
Sterilizer loading/unloading							
AIA	N/D	N/D	N/D	N/D	N/D	N/D	N/D
AAMI	68°-73° F (20°-23° C)	Positive	30% to 60%	10	N/D	N/D	Yes
Restroom/housekeeping							
AIA	N/D	N/D	N/D	10	N/D	N/D	N/D
AAMI	< 75° F (< 24° C)	Negative	30% to 60%	10	N/D	N/D	Yes
Preparation and packaging							
AIA	75° F (24° C)	Positive	30% to 60%	4	N/D	No	N/D
AAMI	68°-73° F (20°-23° C)	Positive	35% to 50%	10	N/D	N/D	No
Textile packaging room							
AIA	N/D	N/D	N/D	N/D	N/D	N/D	N/D
AAMI	68°-73° F (20°-23° C)	Positive	30% to 60%	10	N/D	N/D	No
Clean/sterile storage							
AIA	75° F (24° C)	Positive	30% to 60%	4	N/D	No	N/D
AAMI	< 75° F (< 24° C)	Positive	< 70%	4	N/D	N/D	No

1. *American Institute of Architects.* Guideline for Design and Construction of Hospitals and Health Care Facilities, 2006. *Washington DC: American Institute of Architects Press; 2006:130-131.*

2. *Association for Advancement of Medical Instrumentation.* Comprehensive Guide to Steam Sterilization and Sterility Assurance in Health Care Facilities, 2006. *Arlington, VA: Association for Advancement of Medical Instrumentation; 2006:24.*

3. *Bielen RP, ed.* Health Care Facilities Handbook, 2005. *Quincy, MA: National Fire Protection Association, 2005:290.*

VII.c. Alarms should be checked
- upon initial setup,
- when connecting or reconnecting a device,
- before transporting a patient, and
- after transporting a patient.[30] (PNDS: I122)

VII.d. Alert alarms (eg, medical gas alarms, code blue alarms) should be tested according to organizational policy and procedure.

Recommendation VIII

Blanket- and solution-warming cabinet temperatures should be controlled.

The danger of thermal burns from heated blankets or solutions is increased in the perioperative setting because patients are unconscious or sedated and cannot feel the increase in temperature or communicate their discomfort. Attention to the temperature of warming cabinets is important. Even when solutions and blankets do not feel warm to staff members, heat continues to build up in these items and can be transferred to the patient.[31]

VIII.a. The warming cabinet temperature should be checked at regular intervals per the organization's policy and documented on a temperature log or recorded on a record provided by an electronic recording system.[31-33] (PNDS: I122)

VIII.a.1. The responsibility for setting, maintaining, and monitoring warmers should be assigned to specific personnel (eg, delegated assistive staff members).

VIII.a.2. If solution is stored in the warming cabinet, the cabinet should be labeled with safe temperature range settings as determined by the solution manufacturer.

VIII.a.3. Cabinet temperature above the safe range should be reported to clinical engineering for maintenance.[31-33]

VIII.a.4. Dual cabinets should have dual controls for accurate regulation of both cabinets.

VIII.a.5. Blanket-warming cabinet temperatures should not exceed 130° F (54° C).[34]

VIII.a.6. Blankets should be rotated on a first-in, first-out basis.

VIII.b. Solution-warming cabinet temperatures should be limited to the solution manufactur-

er's specifications for warming.[32] The fluid manufacturer's recommendations should be obtained and followed for the maximum temperature and length of time fluids should remain in the warming cabinet. (PNDS: I122)

Solution stability may vary according to the type of solution and storage container.

VIII.b.1. Fluids kept in fluid warmers should be labeled with the date they should be removed or the date when they were placed in the warmer.

VIII.b.2. Solutions should be rotated on a first-in, first-out basis.

VIII.b.3. IV solutions should only be warmed using technology designed for this purpose.[35]

VIII.c. Intravenous (IV) fluid or irrigation fluid bags should not be used for patient warming devices. (PNDS: I122)

Warmed IV bags used as warming devices have led to patient burns.[36] In a closed claims study of intraoperative patient burns, the most common device causing the burn was either heated IV bags or bottles of irrigation fluids.[33]

VIII.d. Fluids used for intracorporeal irrigation should not exceed 98.6° F (37° C) or approximate normal body temperature.[35,37,38]

VIII.d.1. The temperature of fluid on the sterile field should be measured using a sterile thermometer or a commercially available intraoperative irrigation warming bath to ensure it does not exceed 98.6° F (37° C).[35,38] (PNDS: I76)

VIII.d.2. Solutions warmed to higher temperatures should be cooled to normal body temperature before use inside body cavities.

VIII.e. Surgical skin prep solutions should not be warmed in warming cabinets unless stated as allowable in the manufacturer's directions. (PNDS: I122)

Recommendation IX

Potential hazards associated with fire safety in the practice setting should be identified, and safe practices should be established.

Fire is always a risk to both patients and healthcare workers in the operating room.

IX.a. A written fire prevention and management plan should be developed by a multidisciplinary group and include all categories of perioperative personnel.

IX.a.1. The plan should describe processes to be implemented to safely manage different fire scenarios.[39]

IX.b. Ignition sources should be controlled. (PNDS: I72, I73, I77)

IX.b.1. The active electrode tip of the ESU should be kept clean and in a holster when not in use.

IX.b.2. Electrosurgical units provide an ignition source when not used according to manufacturers' recommendations and when active electrodes are used in the presence of oxidizers, flammable solutions, and volatile or combustible chemicals or liquids.

IX.b.3. Lasers should be used with wet towels placed around the surgical site and after flammable prep solutions have dried.[40]

IX.b.4. The ends of an active fiber-optic light cable should not come in contact with surgical drapes.

Fiber-optic light cables provide an ignition source if they are disconnected from the working element or light source and allowed to contact drapes, sponges, or other fuel sources.

IX.b.5. Light cables should be connected before activating the light source.

IX.b.6. The light source should be placed into a stand-by mode when not in use to prevent ignition.

Backing into the light source or turning the fiber-optic light cable toward the body may cause surgical attire to ignite.[41]

IX.c. Personnel should move any equipment that emits smoke at any time, whether in use or not, to a safe area.[42]

IX.d. Fuel sources should be controlled. (PNDS: I72, I73)

IX.d.1 Waterless, brushless, surgical-scrub solutions should be allowed to dry completely to decrease the potential to produce ignition by static electricity or sparks.

IX.d.2. Local and state fire regulations regarding storage of alcohol-based, surgical-scrub solutions and hand sanitizers should be followed.[14]

IX.d.3. Provide adequate time for the flammable surgical prep solution to dry completely and any fumes to dissipate before applying surgical drapes, using an active electrode or laser, or activating a fiber-optic light cable.[43-45]

IX.d.4. Prevent prep solutions from pooling, or soaking into the table linens or the patient's hair by
- using reusable or disposable sterile towels to absorb drips and excess solutions during the skin prep application,
- removing materials saturated with prep solution before draping the patient,[14] and
- wicking excess solution with a sterile towel to facilitate the surgical prep area drying completely.[14,16,47]

IX.d.5. Drapes should not be applied until prep solutions are dry, to prevent the accumulation of volatile fumes beneath them.

IX.d.6. Surgical skin preparations with clear instructions for use, preferably with unit dosed applicators should be used.[14,46]

IX.d.7. Gowns and drapes should not be exposed to ignition sources.

IX.e. Oxidizers should be controlled. (PNDS: I72, I73)

IX.e.1. Oxygen and nitrous oxide should be used with caution in the presence of any ignition or fuel sources.

IX.e.2. Oxygen-enriched environments are created when the oxygen concentration is greater than 21%. This lowers the temperature and energy at which fuels will ignite.[48,49]

IX.e.3. Anesthesia circuits should be free of leaks.

IX.e.4. Electrosurgical units and lasers should be used with caution where oxygen is flowing.

IX.e.5. Suction should be used to evacuate anesthetic gas accumulation.

IX.e.6. When using a laser, only laser-resistant endotracheal tubes should be used for upper airway procedures or procedures near the trachea.[40,48]

IX.e.7. For surgeries involving the head and neck, water-soluble substances should be used to cover facial hair.[50]

IX.e.8. Oxygen concentration under drapes should be minimized by
• tenting of drapes, and
• using the lowest possible oxygen concentration that provides adequate patient oxygen saturation.[14,40,48,51,52]
Mixing oxygen with nonflammable gases such as medical air reduces the risk of fire.[17,40,50]

IX.e.9. Precautions should be taken when operating in the gastrointestinal tract because hydrogen and methane, which are flammable gases, may be present.[50]

IX.e.10. Nitrous oxide should be considered an oxidizer, and the same precautions that are used with oxygen should be observed.[42]

IX.f. Risk of airway fires should be minimized by
– using radiopaque wet sponges in the back of the throat to prevent or decrease oxygen leaks;
– inflating endotracheal tube cuffs with tinted solutions to improve visibility in the event of a cuff rupture;
– using suction to evacuate oxygen buildup;
– tenting drapes to prevent the accumulation of gases; and
– using pulse oximetry to evaluate the patient's optimal oxygen saturation level.[17,40,50] (PNDS: I73)

IX.g. Processes should be in place to regularly inspect, test, and maintain fire extinguishing equipment and supplies.

IX.h. Fire extinguishers should be selected according to standards established by the National Fire Protection Association (NFPA) and the local authority having jurisdiction, and be immediately available for every operating and procedural room.[14,48,53] (PNDS: I72, I73)

IX.h.1. The NFPA recommends either a water mist or CO_2 extinguisher be used in the operating room.[53]
Water mist extinguishers are rated Class 2A: C.[53]

IX.h.2. The ECRI Institute recommends CO_2 extinguishers because the spray has a cooling effect, does not leave residue, and is not likely to injure patients or personnel.[48,53]
Carbon dioxide extinguishers are rated Class B and C, but may also be used for Class A fires.[53]

IX.i. Fire blankets should not be used in an operating room.[41] (PNDS: I72, I73)
Fire blankets may trap fire next to or under the patient and cause more harm. Fire blankets can burn in an oxygen-enriched environment. Fire blankets are less effective in controlling a fire on a patient than other methods. Usage can lead to wound contamination or spread the fire.

IX.j. Specific evacuation routes should be established for the perioperative environment and developed in collaboration with local authorities and guided by NFPA regulations.[14]

IX.j.1. Personnel and emergency responders should be educated about how to implement the evacuation plan.

IX.j.2. Evacuation routes should be clearly displayed in multiple locations throughout the practice setting.

IX.k. All personnel should recognize medical, gas-control valves and have the ability to shut down medical gases in the event of a fire.[48, 54]

IX.l. All personnel should receive instructions on how to contact the local fire department.[42]

Recommendation X

Potential hazards associated with medical gases in the practice setting should be identified, and safe practices should be established. (PNDS: I122)

The US Food and Drug Administration (FDA) considers compressed medical gases to be prescription drugs that must be dispensed by prescription only. Therefore, these gases should be stored in a secure area with controlled access.[13,55]

X.a. Medical gases should be stored in a secure area, separate from industrial gases. (PNDS: I122)

X.a.1. Full cylinders should be segregated from empty cylinders.[55]

Segregating full cylinders from empty cylinders minimizes the risk of connection to an empty cylinder and a delay in administration of vital gases.

X.b. Medical gas cylinders stored indoors should be in a room with a minimum one-hour fire resistance rating.[14,23]

X.c. Gas cylinders should be stored in a well-ventilated room in a holder or storage rack, away from heat sources.[14]

Securing cylinders with a chain-like device or in racks prevents the cylinders from falling out of the holder or rack.

X.d. Cylinders should not be stored in an egress hallway.[14]

Cylinders and carts directly associated with a currently present patient are considered "in use." Cylinders and carts not directly associated with a specific patient for 30 minutes or more are considered not in use or in storage. These cylinders and carts should be removed from corridors and properly stored.[14]

X.e. Gas cylinder valves should be closed properly to avoid leakage during storage.

X.f. Gas cylinders should be transported in a carrier designed to prevent tipping, dropping, or damage to the cylinder and not carried by hand. Carrying a cylinder by hand poses a risk of dropping the cylinder and causing sudden release of the compressed gas, which can cause propulsion of the cylinder and subsequent injury.

X.g. Gas cylinders used during patient transport should be secured to the transport cart or bed in holders designed for this purpose and not placed on top of the bed or cart next to the patient.

Holders minimize the risk of the cylinder falling. Transport carts are available with built-in holders.

The maximum amount of oxygen stored inside a health care institution is 566,335 L or 20,000 cubic feet.[14,15] Reserve cylinders provide an emergency backup for use in a medical gas failure.

X.h. Gas cylinders and gas lines must clearly identify the medical gas contained or delivered by the color of the cylinder/line, written labels, and a unique pin-index safety system connector.

The FDA has approved standardized colors for identification of different medical gases (eg, green indicates oxygen).[56,57] The pin-index safety system connector for different medical gases prevents connecting the wrong gas to the delivery system.

Serious injuries and deaths have resulted when an incorrectly identified medical gas has been used. Reliance on the color of the cylinder alone does not differentiate between single gases and combinations of gases that may be contained in a cylinder. In one instance, insufflation of a combination of oxygen and carbon dioxide from a blue cylinder into a patient's abdomen resulted in that patient's death.[55]

X.h.1. Before use, gas cylinders should be checked for
- appropriate label,
- appropriate pin-index safety system connector, and
- appropriate color coding.

X.h.2. When opening a cylinder valve, a small amount of gas should be released before attaching the regulator.[14]

X.h.3. Compressed medical gas tank valves should be opened fully during use to prevent excessive heat buildup through the regulator. Temperatures can increase more quickly if the valve is only partially opened. A flash fire may occur if combustible materials such as dirt or oil are present at the gas outlet.[58]

X.i. Fittings on medical gas cylinders and hoses should not be altered under any circumstances.[59,60] Serious injuries and deaths have resulted when personnel have altered the pin-index safety system, permitting delivery of an incorrect gas into the system.

X.i.1. If the fitting does not easily connect, the label on the gas cylinder or hose should be checked to verify that it is correct.

X.i.2. If the label is correct, the cylinder should be returned to the distributor for examination.[60]

X.i.3. If the label is incorrect; the cylinder should be replaced with a correctly labeled gas cylinder.

X.j. Shut-off valves must be identified with the name of the gas, the location served, and a caution to avoid closing the valve except in emergency situations.[14]

X.j.1. Responsibility and authority for valve shut-off should be defined in the health care organization policy and procedure, but all staff members should be knowledgeable about the procedure.

X.k. Vacuum systems should exhaust outdoors, away from windows, doors, and air intakes.[14]

Exhausting vacuum systems outdoors away from windows, doors, and air intakes will help to prevent contamination of the facility or environment.[14]

X.l. Liquid oxygen tanks must be handled, filled, stored, and transported according to state and federal regulations.[61]

X.l.1. Gloves and personal protective equipment (PPE) must be worn and the tanks held an elbow-length away from the body at filling stations.[61]

X.l.2. Liquid oxygen containers should be stored in a cool, dry place outside of the building or in a separate building.[14]

X.l.3. Liquid oxygen containers should have product identification visible from all sides with a 360-degree label and two-inch high letters.[14]

X.l.4. Liquid oxygen container contents should be verified before use.[14]

X.m. Manufacturer recommendations for attaching regulators to oxygen tanks should be followed.

X.m.1. The sealing gasket specified by the regulator company should be used.

X.m.2. The regulator, gasket, and washers should be inspected before use.

X.m.3. Washers present on oxygen cylinder yokes should be removed before installing the oxygen regulator.

X.m.4. The regulator should be tightened with a T-handle until it is firmly in place.

X.m.5. The valve should be opened slowly to determine if there is a leak, and the valve should be closed quickly if a leak is found.[59,61]

X.m.6. Reusable gaskets on oxygen regulators should be checked regularly and at least with each cylinder change for failure to seal properly.[62]

X.m.7. Reusable gaskets should be discarded if deformed or leaking.[62]

X.m.8. Fluorocarbon, elastomer, and brass gaskets should be used because of their low ignition potential.[62]

X.m.9. An adequate emergency supply of oxygen should be stored at the facility to provide an uninterrupted supply for one day.

Recommendation XI

Potential hazards associated with the use of anesthetic gases in the practice setting should be identified, and safe practices should be established.[13,14]

The level of occupational risk associated with exposure to trace anesthetic gases is unclear. Uncontrolled, retrospective studies conducted in the 1970s found an increase in the incidence of spontaneous abortion and development of congenital abnormalities in offspring among OR personnel.[63-65] Researchers found a relationship between anesthetic gases and chromosome deformities after prolonged exposure.[66] In a prospective study, researchers found no relationship between trace anesthetic gas exposure and adverse health effects.[67] Subjects exposed to sevoflurane concentrations below the National Institute for Occupational Safety and Health (NIOSH) recommended limits showed no kidney damage, in another study.[68,69]

Delivering nitrous oxide through an open system has been found to result in high concentrations of nitrous oxide in the air and is associated with reduced fertility and spontaneous abortion in female dental assistants.[70]

The level of risk from occupational exposure to halogenated anesthetic agents has not been thoroughly studied.[71] Therefore; it remains prudent to limit the amount of waste anesthetic gases in the perioperative environment.

XI.a. The health care organization should establish a waste anesthetic gas management program that minimizes the exposure of health care workers to waste anesthetic gases.

The NIOSH standard for nitrous oxide levels is no more than 25 parts per million (ppm) over an eight-hour period and no more than 2 ppm of any halogenated anesthetic agent over one hour.[68] When scavenging systems are not used, levels can exceed 1000 ppm.[70]

XI.a.1. Air sampling for the most frequently used anesthetic gases should be conducted every six months to evaluate occupational exposures and the effectiveness of control measures.[71]

XI.a.2. Gas monitoring should occur at the organization's defined scheduled intervals for nitrous oxide and other inhalation anesthetics using dosimeters or analyzers.[71]

XI.b. A scavenging system should be used to remove waste anesthetic gases.

XI.b.1. The scavenger system connections should be intact and functioning.[15]

XI.b.2. Scavenging systems should be tested when installed and at three-month intervals for leaks and compliance documentation maintained.[68]

XI.b.3. The scavenger system should be vented directly to the outside of the building.[15]

XI.c. Anesthesia delivery systems should be in proper working order and maintained on a regularly scheduled basis, consistent with the manufacturer's written instructions and the organization's policies.

XI.d. Anesthesia equipment located in areas other than the surgical suite should be included in the safety program.

Recommendation XII

Potential hazards associated with surgical smoke generated in the practice setting should be identified, and safe practices should be established.

Surgical smoke (ie, plume) is generated from use of heat producing instruments such as electrosurgical devices and lasers. This plume has been found to contain toxic gases and vapors (eg benzene, hydrogen cyanide, formaldehyde) that produce an offensive odor; bio-aerosols, including blood fragments; and viruses.[72] Experts have noted that there may be more than 600 chemical compounds that exist in surgical smoke.[73] In high concentrations, surgical smoke causes ocular and upper respiratory tract irritation in health care personnel.[74] The smoke generated from electrosurgery and laser contain chemical by-products.[74-77]

The NIOSH recommends that smoke evacuation systems be used to reduce potential acute and chronic health risks to personnel and patients.[74] The Occupational Safety and Health Administration (OSHA) has no separate standard related to surgical smoke. The OSHA addresses such safety hazards in the General Duty Clause and Bloodborne Pathogen Standard.[75]

XII.a. Smoke plume should be removed by use of a smoke evacuation system in both open and laparoscopic procedures.

XII.a.1. The suction wand of the smoke evacuation system should be placed as close to the source of the smoke generation as possible to maximize particulate matter and odor capture and enhance visibility at the surgical site.[78]

XII.a.2. In situations in which minimal plume is generated, a central suction system with an in-line filter may be used to evacuate the plume. The in-line filter is placed between the suction wall/ceiling connection and the suction canister.[78,79]

Central wall suction units are designed to capture liquids, making the use of in-line filters necessary. Low suction rates associated with wall suction units limit their efficacy in evacuating plume, making them suitable for minimal plume evacuation only.[79] A centralized system dedicated for smoke evacuation may be available.

XII.a.3. Care should be taken to flush the smoke evacuator lines, according to the manufacturer's instructions, to ensure particulate matter build-up does not occur.

XII.a.4. The risk of patient and caregiver exposure to surgical smoke during laparoscopic procedures should be minimized.

- by continuous venting of the smoke from the pneumoperitoneum using a filtering device (eg, an attachment to the cannula), and

- when exhausting the pneumoperitoneum the cannula should be pointed away from all personnel.[76,77]

The continuous venting of the pneumoperitoneum the through filter attachment decreases the amount of particulate matter released, decreases the amount of absorption by the patient, and improves the surgeon's vision during the procedure. Pointing the cannula away from all personnel when exhausting the pneumoperitoneum decreases the amount of particulate matter inhaled by the personnel.

XII.a.5. In circumstances in which large amounts of plume are generated, an individual smoke evacuation unit with an ultra-low penetration air filter should be used to remove smoke plume. Smoke evacuation systems, individual units, and accessories should be used according to manufacturers' written instructions. Filters should be changed as recommended by the manufacturer.[78,79]

XII.a.6. Smoke evacuation systems and accessories should be used according to manufacturers' written instructions.

Detectable odor during the use of a smoke evacuation system is a signal that

- smoke is not being captured at the site where the plume is being generated,

- inefficient air movement through the suction or smoke evacuation wand is occurring, or

- the filter has exceeded its usefulness and should be replaced.[79]

XII.b. Standard precautions should be used when changing smoke evacuation system filters.[78]

Airborne contaminants produced during electrosurgery or laser procedures have been analyzed and are shown to contain gaseous toxic compounds, bioaerosols, and dead and living cell material. At some level, these contaminants have been shown to have an unpleasant odor, cause visual problems for physicians, cause ocular and upper respiratory tract irritation, and have demonstrated mutagenic and carcinogenic potential.[78] The possibility for bacterial and/or viral contamination of smoke plume remains controversial but has been highlighted by different studies.[80,81]

XII.c. Personnel should wear high-filtration surgical masks during procedures that generate surgical smoke.

High-filtration masks are specially designed to filter particulate matter that is 0.1 micron in size and larger and help filter particulate matter found in surgical smoke plume.[82] These masks should not be viewed as absolute protection from chemical or particulate contaminants and should not be used as the first line of protection against surgical smoke inhalation.[78]

Recommendation XIII

Potential hazards associated with the use of chemicals, including methyl methacrylate, in the practice setting should be identified, and safe practices should be established.

Improper handling of chemicals can result in injury to health care workers and patients. Injuries may result from exposure to any portion of the body, including the integumentary or respiratory systems.

XIII.a. Material safety data sheet (MSDS) information for every potentially hazardous chemical must be readily accessible to employees within the practice setting. This information includes identification of hazards, precautions or special handling, signs and symptoms of toxic exposure, and first aid treatments for exposure.[83]

XIII.b. When using chemicals, personnel should read and follow all instructions provided on the container label or found on the MSDS provided by the manufacturer of the chemical. (PNDS: I122)

XIII.b.1. All chemicals should be handled according to their respective MSDS sheets, including, but not limited to,

- disinfectants and sterilants (eg, glutaraldehyde, ortho-phthalaldehyde, ethylene oxide, hydrogen peroxide, peracetic acid);

- tissue preservatives (ie, formalin); and
- antiseptic agents such as hand hygiene products and surgical prep solutions.[84,85]

XIII.c. Chemicals should not be combined unless safe outcomes can be ensured.

Mixing chemicals can result in unsafe substances that are unstable and/or caustic.

XIII.d. Chemicals should be stored according to
- MSDS sheets;
- manufacturer's directions;
- flammability;
- patient and staff safety requirements; and
- local, state, and federal regulations. (PNDS: I122)

XIII.e. Safe practices should be established for the use of methyl methacrylate bone cement. (PNDS: I75)

Methyl methacrylate is a respiratory, eye, and skin irritant. The fumes contain carbon monoxide, hydrogen, and methane, which can cause personnel to experience vertigo, difficulty breathing, and nausea. All of these symptoms are short-term and are relieved once the fumes dissipate.[86] The OSHA permissible exposure limit for methyl methacrylate for general industry is 100 ppm or a time-weighted average of 410 mg/m³.[86]

XIII.e.1. Methyl methacrylate fumes should be extracted from the environment and the fumes exhausted to the outside air or absorbed through activated charcoal.

XIII.e.2. Vacuum mixers with fume extraction should be used to reduce the fume levels users are exposed to.[85,87]

XIII.e.3. Eye protection should be worn to prevent contact with eyes.[86]

Methyl methacrylate fumes may produce an adverse reaction with soft contact lenses leading to irritation and possible corneal ulceration. There is no documented evidence of problems with hard contact lenses.

XIII.e.4. Manufacturer's recommendations should be followed for mixing and required PPE.[86,88]

XIII.e.5. A second pair of gloves should be worn when handling methyl methacrylate and should be discarded after use.[86] Manufacturer's instructions should be followed regarding the composition of the second pair of gloves.[88]

Methyl methacrylate may be absorbed through the skin and penetrate many plastic and latex compounds, leading to dermatitis.[85] The liquid portion should not come in contact with gloves.[88]

XIII.e.6. A cement gun or mixing system should be used to reduce handling of the product, instead of hand mixing.[85,89] The cement mixture should not be touched until it is the consistency of dough.[88]

XIII.e.7. For spills of methyl methacrylate
- the spill area should be ventilated until odor has dissipated,
- all sources of ignition should be removed,
- appropriate PPE should be worn during clean up,
- the spill area should be isolated,
- the liquid should be covered with an activated charcoal absorbent, and
- the waste product should be disposed of in a hazardous waste container.[90]

XIII.e.8. Methyl methacrylate is hazardous waste and should be disposed of per state, local, and federal requirements.[90]

Recommendation XIV

Hazards associated with chemotherapeutic (eg, cytotoxic) agents used in the practice setting should be identified, and safe practices should be established.

Cytotoxic drugs have the potential to cause serious health risks to health care workers exposed to them. These risks may include carcinogenicity, teratogenicity, reproductive toxicity, organ or tissue damage, and chromosomal damage. Occupational Safety and Health Administration has not determined safe levels of exposure to these drugs and no reliable system is available to monitor exposure levels.[91,92]

XIV.a. Health care organizations should develop a plan for medical surveillance of personnel handling cytotoxic agents.[91]

XIV.b. A current MSDS sheet must be kept on all cytotoxic agents used in the workplace.[92]

XIV.c. Cytotoxic agents should be transported in sealed containers with Luer caps and no needles attached.[93] (PNDS: I122)

XIV.c.1. The transport container should be
- leak proof,
- resistant to breakage, and
- labeled with warning labels to alert personnel that contents are hazardous.[93]

XIV.d. Personnel handling cytotoxic agents should wear PPE consistent with the type of exposure that can reasonably be anticipated.

XIV.d.1. When administering or handling open containers of chemotherapy drugs, personnel should double-glove and change the outer glove after contact with the cytotoxic agent.[93]

Gloves to be worn for chemotherapy administration should meet the American Society for Testing and Materials D 6978 standards.[94] This information should be received from the glove manufacturers before using the gloves for chemotherapy administration.

XIV.d.2. An impervious or chemotherapy-rated gown should be worn when arms and torso skin contact may occur.[91]

XIV.d.3. Face shields should be worn when the potential for splashing or splattering exists. Face shields protect against mucous membrane and skin exposure. Some cytotoxic agents may cause corneal damage.[93]

XIV.e. Chemotherapy spill kits should be available to contain accidental spills.[93]

XIV.f. Unused chemotherapy agents must be disposed of in accordance with federal, state, and local laws.[89]

Items contaminated with small amounts of chemotherapy agents should be disposed of according to written instructions from the health care organization's waste management vendor.

XIV.g. Manufacturer's recommendations for use of the chemotherapeutic agent should be followed regarding requirements for cleaning and handling of instrumentation exposed to the chemotherapeutic agent.

Some chemotherapeutic agents leave a residue on instruments and require specific PPE and cleaning techniques.

XIV.h. Staff members involved in handling cytotoxic agents should be educated regarding the hazards involved, exposure prevention, and management of spills.[93]

XIV.i. Recommendations from the manufacturer of the chemotherapeutic agent should be followed regarding requirements for disposal of body fluids of patients receiving chemotherapeutic agents (eg, flushing the toilet/hopper twice for disposing of body fluids up to 48 hours after chemotherapeutic agent infusion).

Recommendation XV

Waste that is hazardous upon disposal must be identified and disposed of in manner consistent with federal, state, and local laws.[95]

Waste classified by the Environmental Protection Agency (EPA) as hazardous upon disposal (eg, hazardous, acutely hazardous, flammable chemicals, acids and bases, heavy metals) is regulated under the Resource Conservation and Recovery Act and must be managed in a way that minimizes environmental effects.[95,96]

XV.a. Chemicals considered hazardous upon disposal must be placed in hazardous waste containers at the point of use to alert handlers to take precautions upon its disposal.[95,97] State and local laws also may apply and may be more stringent.

XV.a.1. Flammable liquids (eg, alcohol, benzoin, collodion, formalin, methyl methacrylate, silver nitrate) must be contained and placed into a hazardous waste receptacle for disposal.[98] These chemicals pose a fire and environmental hazard if discarded in the regular waste stream.

XV.b. The use of mercury-containing devices should be eliminated in the practice setting.[97,99]

Alternative non-mercury products (eg, thermometers, manometers) are available. Mercury poses a serious contamination risk to wildlife and to people, who may eat contaminated fish or game.[100]

Recommendation XVI

Potential hazards associated with misconnections of tubing and lines should be identified and safe practices established. (PNDS: I138)

Multiple cases of tubing which has been incorrectly connected (ie, blood pressure monitors to needleless IV ports; oxygen tubing to needleless IV ports) have led to patient injuries. This has occurred due to Luer connectors that allow different equipment to be connected if a female and male Luer connection are present.[101]

XVI.a. Safe practices should be established when using Luer connectors. (PNDS: I122)

XVI.a.1. When purchasing equipment with Luer connectors, the connector should not be compatible with IV Luer connectors.[102]

XVI.a.2. When connecting two or more lengths of tubing, the tubing should be traced to the point of origin.[103]

XVI.a.3. During the hand-off process, all tubing should be traced to the point of origin.[102]

XVI.a.4. Indirect caregivers, patients, and families should be instructed to obtain help before connecting or disconnecting tubing.[103]

XVI.a.5. Tubing used for high-risk catheters should be labeled and should not have injection ports.[103]

XVI.a.6. Tubing and catheters should be routed to avoid tangling and facilitate easy identification.[101]

XVI.a.7. Standard Luer syringes should not be used for oral medications or enteric feedings.[101]

Recommendation XVII

Competency
Personnel should receive initial education and competency validation and at least annual updates on new regulations, equipment, and procedures.

Ongoing education of perioperative personnel facilitates the development of knowledge, skills, and attitudes that affect patient and worker safety.

XVII.a. An introduction and review of policies and procedures should be included in orientation to the perioperative setting for personnel and observers. Continuing education should be provided when new elements in the environment of care are introduced.

XVII.a.1. Education should include, but not be limited to,
- potential security and other hazards in the environment along with methods of protection;[3,4]
- how to implement the evacuation plan;
- patient privacy policy;[7]
- available ergonomic equipment and safe lifting/moving practices;
- safe use of electrical equipment in the practice setting;
- the location of ventilation and electrical systems and who is permitted to shut them off in the event of an emergency;
- environmental controls, including air exchange rate, temperature, and humidity parameters;
- the safe use of medical equipment in the perioperative environment;
- appropriate responses to clinical alarms;
- the safe use of blanket- and solution-warming cabinets;
- fire prevention education and fire drills, which should be conducted regularly as per the AORN guidance statement, federal, state, local regulations, and accrediting agency standards;
- the safe use and handling of medical and anesthetic gases;
- the location and operation of medical gas shut-off panels;
- the procedures involved in maintaining a safe environment of care; and
- the correct procedures involved to avoid tubing misconnections.[101]

XVII.a.2. Employers must provide training and competency validation of staff members who work with chemicals and other agents in the workplace.[92] Training should include, but is not limited to, the safe handling of
- methyl methacrylate bone cement;
- chemicals (eg, disinfectants, sterilants, formalin);
- cytotoxic agents, the hazards involved, exposure prevention, and management of spills;
- hazardous wastes and their disposal; and
- handling of instruments exposed to chemotherapeutic agents.

Recommendation XVIII

Documentation
Records should be maintained for a time period specified by the health care organization and in compliance with local, state, and federal regulations.

Accurate records are necessary for identifying trends, and demonstrating compliance with regulatory and accrediting agency requirements.

XVIII.a. The following items should be documented per organization policy, including but not limited to
  - daily operating room HVAC system function (eg, air exchange rate, temperature, humidity);[25]
  - blanket/fluid warming cabinet temperature;
  - testing of anesthesia waste gas scavenging systems;[66] and
  - employee health records.

Recommendation XIX

Policies and Procedures
Polices and procedures for the provision of a safe environment of care should be developed, reviewed periodically, revised as necessary, and readily available in the practice setting.

Policies and procedures serve as operational guidelines and establish authority, responsibility, and accountability within the organization. Policies and procedures also assist in the development of patient safety, quality assessment, and improvement activities.

XIX.a. The policies and procedures should include, but not be limited to,
  - safe patient handling and movement in the perioperative setting;
  - description of security management activities, including access control;
  - action to be taken during periods of loss of usual and emergency power;[21]
  - monitoring of environmental controls including air exchanges per hour, temperature, and humidity;
  - describing the processes to be implemented to effectively manage medical equipment, including selection, purchase, inspection, and maintenance processes;
  - monitoring and recording the temperature of warming cabinets;
  - inspection, testing, and maintenance of fire extinguishing equipment and supplies;
  - defining responsibility and authority for gas valve shut-off;
  - monitoring of nitrous oxide and other inhalation anesthetics;
  - schedule and criteria for maintenance of anesthesia delivery systems;

  - medical surveillance of personnel handling cytotoxic agents;
  - storage of chemicals according to manufacturer's directions, MSDS sheets, flammability, patient and staff safety requirements and local, state, and federal regulations; and
  - other policies as dictated by applicable local, state, and federal regulations.

Recommendation XX

Quality
The health care organization's quality management program should evaluate the environment of care to improve patient safety.

XX.a. Personnel in the perioperative setting should
  - identify safety hazards,
  - take appropriate corrective actions, and
  - report hazards per organizational policy.

XX.b. A quality-management plan should be developed by a team involving representatives from all types of positions within the perioperative area. The quality management plan should include
  - critiquing of fire drills by a team that includes members from all perioperative departments and categories of personnel to identify deficiencies and opportunities for improvement;
  - collecting and analyzing information about adverse outcomes associated with the environment of care as a part of the institution-wide performance improvement program that addresses adverse events and near misses;[24]
  - creation of a patient safety culture, to include policies and procedures supporting that culture;
  - the creation of a patient safety culture that will foster reporting of adverse events and near misses;[104]
  - monitoring of actual and potential risks in each of the environment of care areas, to be completed on a regular basis (eg, at least monthly environment of care rounds by a team that includes clinicians, administrators, support personnel);[24]
  - developing a process to monitor and report incidents of equipment malfunction leading to patient harm as outlined in the Safe Medical Devices Act of 1990;[105]

- developing a plan to monitor compliance with safe handling of chemicals, cytotoxic agents, and hazardous waste in the workplace;
- conducting scheduled "walk-around" safety rounds to test clinical alarms and to observe staff members' response to the alarms;
- developing an organization-wide event reporting system for HVAC failures and power interruptions;[29]
- developing processes to regularly inspect, test, and maintain fire extinguishing equipment and supplies; and
- a mechanism for reporting work-related health problems.

Glossary

Clinical alarms: Alarm systems that are patient specific and are used for the purpose of alerting staff members to a patient emergency.

Compressed medical gas (CMG): A liquefied or vaporized gas alone, or in combination with other gases, that is a drug as defined by the FDA (eg, oxygen, nitrogen, nitric oxide, nitrous oxide, carbon dioxide, helium, medical air).

Container: A metal container designed to contain either liquefied or vaporized CMG.

Cylinder: A metal container designed to contain CMG at a high pressure.

Ground-fault circuit interrupter: A device that senses a significant flow of leakage current and interrupts the flow of electricity to prevent electric shock.

Hazardous upon disposal waste: Certain pharmaceutical and chemical products, as determined by the EPA, become hazardous waste when discarded. The residual in the container after use is considered hazardous. Hazardous wastes can be liquids, solids, or contained gases.

Line-isolation monitor: A device used to continuously monitor an ungrounded power system that is isolated from the commercial power supply received from the utility company. Isolated ungrounded power systems may allow leakage currents, also known as hazard currents, to flow from the power system to ground. This leakage current may flow through a person's body and presents a shock hazard to that person. Standards for the maximum allowed leakage current have been established. The line isolation monitor displays the calculated level of leakage current and sounds an alarm if the current exceeds the predetermined level.

Pin-index safety system: A safeguard to eliminate cylinder interchanging and the possibility of accidentally placing the incorrect gas on a yoke designed to accommodate another gas. Two pins on the yoke are arranged so that they project into the cylinder valve. Each gas or combination of gases has a specific pin arrangement.

Teratogenicity: The ability of a substance to cause the development of abnormal structures in an embryo or fetus exposed to that substance during gestation.

Warming device: A device used in the perioperative setting to assist with the control of body temperature and prevent hypothermia.

Wet locations: Patient care areas where procedures are performed that are normally subject to wet conditions, including standing fluids on the floor or drenching of the work area, while patients are present.

REFERENCES

1. Beyea SC, ed. *Perioperative Nursing Data Set.* Rev 2nd ed. Denver CO: AORN, Inc; 2007.

2. Occupational Safety and Health Administration. Guidelines for preventing workplace violence for health care and social service workers. http://www.osha.gov/Publications/OSHA3148/osha3148.html. Accessed June 27, 2007.

3. Joint Commission Resources. Protecting your health care workers from violence in the workplace. *The Source.* 2006; 4:1-10.

4. Centers for Disease Control and Prevention. Developing and implementing a workplace violence prevention program and policy. http://www.cdc.gov/niosh/violcohnt.html. Accessed June 27, 2007.

5. Krozek C, Scoggins A. Meeting Environment of Care Standards on the Patient Care Unit: Part I. http://gateway.ut.ovid.com/gw1/ovidweb.cgi. Accessed August 22, 2007.

6. Department of Health and Human Services. Rules and regulations, 45 CFR part 162: HIPAA administrative simplification: standard unique health identifier for health care providers; final rule. *Federal Register.* 2004;69: 3434-3469.

7. Standards for Privacy of Individually Identifiable Health Information. http://www.hipaaadvisory.com/regs/finalprivacy. Accessed August 22, 2007.

8. Standards of perioperative professional practice. In: *Standards, Recommended Practices, and Guidelines.* Denver, CO: AORN, Inc;2007:433-436.

9. AORN position statement on ergonomically healthy workplace practices. In: *Standards, Recommended Practices, and Guidelines.* Denver, CO: AORN, Inc; 2007:382-384.

10. Peterson, C, ed. *Safe Patient Handling and Movement in the Perioperative Setting.* Denver, CO: AORN, Inc; 2007.

11. Nelson A, Fragala G, Menzel N. Myths and facts about back injuries in nursing. *American Journal of Nursing.* 2003;103:32-41.

12. AORN position statement: statement on workplace safety. In: *Standards, Recommended Practices, and Guidelines.* Denver, CO: AORN, Inc; 2007:416-417.

13. National Fire Protection Association, *National Electrical Code Handbook (NFPA 70)*. 10th ed. Quincy, MA; National Fire Protection Association; 2005:408-425.

14. Bielen RP, ed. *Health Care Facilities Handbook, 2005*. Quincy, MA: National Fire Protection Association, 2005:567-568.

15. American Institute of Architects. Ventilation requirements for areas affecting patient care in hospitals and outpatient facilities. In: *Guidelines for Design and Construction of Hospitals and Health Care Facilities, 2001*. Washington, DC: American Institute of Architects Press; 2001:79-80.

16. Electrical safety Q&A: a reference guide for the clinical engineer. *Health Devices*. 2005;34:58-75.

17. McHenry C, Bergue R, Ortega RA, Yowler CJ. Recognition, management, and prevention of specific operating room catastrophes. *Journal American College of Surgeons*. 2004;198:810-821.

18. Illuminating Engineering Society of North America Committee for Health Care Facilities. Recommended practice-29-95. In: *Lighting for Hospitals and Health Care Facilities*. New York, NY; Illuminating Engineering Society of North America;1995:1-75.

19. National Fire Protection Association, *NFPA 110 Standard for Emergency and Standby Power Systems*. 2005 Ed. Quincy, MA; National Fire Protection Association; 2005.

20. American Institute of Architects. The next generation of operating rooms. *http://www.aia.org/nwsltr_print .cfm?pagename=aah_jrnl_20051019_ORs*. The American Institute of Architects. Accessed August 22, 2007.

21. The Joint Commission. Preventing adverse events caused by emergency electrical power system failures. *Sentinel Event Alert*: 2006: 37, *http://www.jointcommission .org/SentinelEvents/SentinelEventAlert/sea_37.htm*. Accessed August 22, 2007.

22. *Standards and Checklist for Accreditation of Ambulatory Surgery Facilities*. Mundelein, IL: American Association for Accreditation of Ambulatory Surgery Facilities, Inc; 2005:4–17.

23. The Joint Commission. Management of the environment of care. In: *Comprehensive Accreditation Manual for Hospitals: The Official Handbook*. Oakbrook Terrace, IL: The Joint Commission; 2006:EC1-EC30.

24. Mangram A, Horan TC, Pearson ML, Silver LC, Jarvis WR. Guideline for prevention of surgical site infection, 1999. Hospital Infection Control Advisory Committee. *Infection Control and Hospital Epidemiology*.1999;20:250-278.

25. Association for Advancement of Medical Instrumentation. *Comprehensive Guide to Steam Sterilization and Sterility Assurance in Health Care Facilities*, 2006. Arlington, VA. Association for Advancement of Medical Instrumentation; 2006:24.

26. Recommended practices for traffic patterns in the perioperative practice setting. In: *Standards, Recommended Practices, and Guidelines*. Denver, CO: AORN, Inc; 2007:703-706.

27. American Society of Heating, Refrigerating and Air-Conditioning Engineers. *HVAC Design Manual for Hospitals and Clinics*. Atlanta, GA: American Society of Heating, Refrigerating and Air-Conditioning Engineers, Inc; 2003:37.

28. Centers for Disease Control and Prevention. Guidelines for Environmental Infection Control in Health-Care Facilities. *http://www.cdc.gov/ncidod/dhqp/pdf/guide lines/Enviro_guide_03.pdf*. Accessed July 24, 2007.

29. Surgical and related services. In: *Accreditation Handbook for Ambulatory Health Care*. Wilmette, IL: Accreditation Association for Ambulatory Health Care; 2006: 48-51.

30. Phillips J, Barnsteiner JH. Clinical alarms: improving efficiency and effectiveness. *Critical Care Nursing Quarterly*. 2005;28:317-323.

31. Williams JS. Meeting the challenge: how hospitals comply with new clinical alarms requirement. *Biomedical Instrumentation and Technology*. 2003;37:319-328.

32. ECRI. *Operating Room Risk Management. http:// www.ecri.org/MarketingDocs/0306news.pdf*. Accessed May 25, 2007.

33. Kressin KA. Burn injury in the operating room: a closed claims analysis. *ASA Newsletter*. 2004;68:9-11.

34. Hazard report update: ECRI Institute revises its recommendation for temperature limits on blanket warmers. *Health Devices*. 2009;38:230-231.

35. Limiting temperature settings on blanket and solution warming cabinets can prevent patient burns. [Problem Reports]. *Health Devices*. 2005;34:168-171.

36. Bonati, et al. *Ex vivo* testing of a temperature- and pressure-controlled amino-irrigator for fetoscopic surgery. *J of Ped Surgery*. 2002;37:18-24.

37. Recommended practices for prevention of unplanned perioperative hypothermia. In: *Standards, Recommended Practices, and Guidelines*. Denver, CO: AORN, Inc; 2008:407-420.

38. Moore SS, Green CR, Wang FL, Pandit SK, Hurd WW. The role of irrigation in the development of hypothermia during laparoscopic surgery. *Am J Obstet Gynecol*. 1997;176:598-601.

39. AORN position statement: statement on fire prevention. In: *Standards, Recommended Practices, and Guidelines*. Denver, CO: AORN, Inc; 2007:385-386.

40. American National Standards Institute. Fire and explosive hazards. In: *American National Standard for Safe Use of Lasers in Health Care Facilities; Standard Z136.3*. Orlando, FL: American National Standards Institute, Inc; 2005:19-20.

41. A clinician's guide to surgical fires: how they occur, how to prevent them, how to put them out. *Health Devices*. 2003;32:5-24.

42. AORN guidance statement: fire prevention in the operating room. In: *Standards, Recommended Practices, and Guidelines*. Denver, CO: AORN, Inc; 2007:259-267.

43. Recommended practices for skin preparation of patients. In: *Standards, Recommended Practices, and Guidelines*. Denver, CO: AORN, Inc; 2007:653-606.

44. Recommended practices for electrosurgery. In: *Standards, Recommended Practices, and Guidelines*. Denver, CO: AORN, Inc; 2007:515-530.

45. Recommended practices for laser safety in practice settings. In: *Standards, Recommended Practices, and Guidelines*. Denver, CO: AORN, Inc; 2007:593-598.

46. NFPA accepts ASHE's amendment to NFPA 99 on alcohol based surgical prep solutions. American Society for Healthcare Engineering of the American Hospital Association. *http://www.ashe.org/ashe/codes/nfpa/nfpa099 _proposeamend_absp.html*. Accessed August 22, 2007.

47. Improper use of alcohol-based skin preps can cause surgical fires. [Hazard Report]. *Health Devices*. 2003;32:441-43.

48. Surgical fires. In: *Operating Room Risk Management*. Plymouth Meeting, PA: ECRI; 2006:2.

49. Guidance article: surgical fire safety. *Health Devices*. 2006;35: 45-66.

50. Podnos Y, Irving CA, Williams R. Fires in the operating room. American College of Surgeons Committee on Perioperative Care available at *http://www.facs.org/about/committees/cpc/oper0897.html*. Accessed June 25, 2007.

51. Rationale and interpretive guidelines for the 2005 National Patient Safety Goals. *Joint Commission Perspectives on Patient Safety*. 2004;I4:3-4.

52. Pollock G. Eliminating surgical fires: a team approach. *AANA Journal*. 2004;72:293–297.

53. National Fire Protection Association, *NFPA 10—Standard for Portable Fire Extinguishers, 2005 Edition*. Quincy, MA: National Fire Protection Association; 2005.8,29-43.

54. Medical gas fires: does your staff know how to recognize and extinguish them? [Problem Reports]. *Health Devices*. 2003;32:39–40.

55. Guidance for hospitals, nursing homes, and other health care facilities. FDA public health advisory. US Department of Health and Human Services, Food and Drug Administration, Center for Drug Evaluation and Research. *http://www.fda.gov/cder/guidance/4341fnl.pdf*. Accessed August 22, 2007.

56. US Department of Health and Human Services, Food and Drug Administration, Center for Drug Evaluation and Research. Compressed Medical Gases Guidelines. *http://www.fda.gov/cder/guidance/cmgg89.htm*. Accessed August 22, 2007.

57. Compressed Gas Association. *Standard Color Marking of Compressed Gas Cylinders Intended for Medical Use in the United States*. Arlington, VA: Compressed Gas Association; 1998.

58. Giarrizzo-Wilson S. Postoperative vision loss; cellular telephones; medical gas handling; roller latches. [Clinical Issues]. *AORN Journal*. 2006; 84:107-108,111-114.

59. Questions and Answers on the Proposed Rule for Medical Gas Containers. US Department of Health and Human Services, Food and Drug Administration, Center for Drug Evaluation and Research. *http://www.fda.gov/cder/dmpq/MedGas_QA_20060410.htm*. Accessed August 22, 2007.

60. Medical Gas Containers and Closures; Current Good Manufacturing Practice Requirements. US Department of Health and Human Services, Food and Drug Administration. *http://www.fda.gov/OHRMSDOCKETS/98fr/06-3370.htm*. Accessed August 22, 2007.

61. Regulations (Standards-29CFR) Oxygen—1910.104. US Department of Labor, Occupational Safety and Health Administration. *http://www.osha.gov/pls/oshaweb/owadisp.show_document?p_id=9750&p_table=STANDARDS*. Accessed August 22, 2007.

62. Reusable gaskets on oxygen regulators will wear out. [Hazard Reports]. *Health Devices*. 2003;32:39-40.

63. Askrog V, Harvald B. Teratogenic effects of inhalation anesthetics. [Danish]. *Nord Med*. 1970;83:498-500.

64. Cohen EN, Bellville JW, Brown BW, Jr. Anesthesia, pregnancy, and miscarriage: a study of operating room nurses and anesthetists. *Anesthesiology*. 1971;35:343-347.

65. Knill-Jones RP, Rodrigues LV, Moir DD, Spence AA. Anaesthetic practice and pregnancy: controlled survey of women anaesthetists in the United Kingdom. *Lancet*. 1972;1: 1326-1328.

66. Bilban M, Jakopin CB, Ogrinc D. Cytogenetic tests performed on operating room personnel (the use of anaesthetic gases). *International Archives of Occupational & Environmental Health*. 2005;78:60-64.

67. Spence AA. Environmental pollution by inhalation anaesthetics. *British Journal of Anaesthesiology*. 1987;59:96-103.

68. National Institute for Occupational Safety and Health. *Occupational Exposure to Waste Anesthetic Gases and Vapors: Criteria for a Recommended Standard*. [Publication DHEW (NIOSH)]. Cincinnati, OH: US Dept of Health, Education, and Welfare, Public Health Service, Center for Disease Control, National Institute for Occupational Safety and Health; 1977;77-140.

69. Trevisan A, Venturini MB, Carrieri M, et al. Biological indices of kidney involvement in personnel exposed to sevoflurane in surgical areas. *Am J Ind Med*. 2003; 44:474-480.

70. Rowland A.S, Baird DD, Weinberg CR, Shore DL, Shy CM, Wilcox AJ. Reduced fertility among women employed as dental assistants exposed to high levels of nitrous oxide. *N Engl J Med*. 1992;327:993–997.

71. Anesthetic Gases: Guidelines for Workplace Exposures. US Department of Labor, Occupational Safety and Health Administration. *http://www.osha.gov/dts/osta/anestheticgases/index.html*. Accessed August 22, 2007.

72. Ball KA. *Lasers: The Perioperative Challenge*. 3rd ed. Denver, CO: AORN, Inc; 2004.

73. Hoglan M. Potential hazards from electrosurgery plume: recommendations for surgical smoke evacuation. *Canadian Operating Room Nursing Journal*. 1995;13:10-16.

74. NIOSH Hazard Controls. Control of Smoke from Laser/Electric Surgical Procedures-HC11. Available at: *http://www.cdc.gov/niosh/hc11.html*. Accessed August 22, 2007.

75. US Department of Labor, Occupational Safety, and Health Administration. Safety and Health Topics: Laser/Electrosurgery Plume. Available at: *http://www.osha.gov/SLTC/laserelectrosurgeryplume/index.html*. Accessed August 22, 2007.

76. Barret W.L, Garber SM. Surgical smoke: a review of the literature: is this just a lot of hot air? *Surgical Endoscopy*. 2003;17:979-987.

77. Alp E, Bijl D, Bleichrodt RP, Hansson B, Voss A. Surgical smoke and infection control. *Journal of Hospital Infection*. 2006; 62:1-5.

78. American National Standards Institute. *American National Standard for Safe Use of Lasers in Health Care Facilities*. Orlando, FL: Laser Institute of America; 2005:19-20.

79. ECRI Institute. Smoke evacuation systems, surgical, *Healthcare Product Comparison System*. Plymouth Meeting, PA: ECRI Institute; March 2002:1-3.

80. Garden JM, O'Banion MK, Shelnitz LS, et al. Papillomavirus in the vapor of carbon dioxide laser-treated verrucae. *JAMA*. 1988; 259:1199-1202.

81. Hallmo P, Naess O. Laryngeal papillomatosis with human papillomavirus DNA contracted by a laser surgeon.

European Archives of Oto-Rhino-Laryngology. 1991; 248:425-7.

82. Romig Cl, Smalley PJ. Regulation of surgical smoke plume. Health Policy Issues. *AORN J.* 1997;65:824-828.

83. Hazard Communication OSHA Standards. US Department of Labor, Occupational Safety and Health Administration. *http://osha.gov/SLTC/hazardcommunications/standards.html.* Accessed October 6, 2007.

84. Recommended practices for surgical hand antisepsis/hand scrubs. In: *Standards, Recommended Practices and Guidelines.* Denver, CO: AORN, Inc; 2007:565-574.

85. McHugh E. The principles of mixing and handling to minimise potential hazards of methyl methacrylate bone cement. *British Journal of Theatre Nursing.* 1998;7:9-12.

86. Chemical Sampling Information: Methyl methacrylate. US Department of Labor, Occupational Safety and Health Administration. *http://osha.gov/dts/chemical sampling/data/CH_254400.html.* Accessed July 16, 2007.

87. Eveleigh R. Fume levels during bone cement mixing. *British Journal of Perioperative Nursing.* 2002; 12:145-150.

88. Medical Devices; Reclassification of Polymethylmethacrylate (PMMA) Bone Cement. Environmental Protection Agency. *http://www.epa.gov/fedrgstr/EPA-IMPACT/2002/July/Day-17/i18036.htm.* Accessed September 26, 2007.

89. Schlegel UJ, Sturm M, Ewerbeck V, Breusch SJ. Efficacy of vacuum bone cement mixing systems in reducing methylmethacrylate fume exposure: comparison of 7 different mixing devices and handmixing. *Acta Orthop Scandinavica.* 2004;75:559-566.

90. Methyl methacrylate MSDS. *http://www.cdc.gov/niosh/ipcsneng/neng0300.html.* Accessed June 25, 2007.

91. Polovich M, White JM, Kelleher LO. Fundamentals of administration. In: *Chemotherapy and Biotherapy Guidelines and Recommendations for Practice.* 2nd ed. Pittsburg, PA: Oncology Nursing Society, 2005:53-62.

92. OSHA Technical Manual. Controlling Occupational Exposure to Hazardous Drugs. *http://www.osha.gov/dts/osta/otm/otm_vi/otm_vi_2.html.* Accessed August 22, 2007.

93. Preventing Occupational Exposure to Antineoplastic and Other Hazardous Drugs in Health Care Settings. NIOSH alert Jan 21, 2005. *http://www.cdc.gov/niosh/docs/2004-165/pdfs/2004-165.pdf.* Accessed August 22, 2007.

94. American Society for Testing and Materials International, ed. *Standard Practice for Assessment of Resistance of Medical Gloves to Permeation by Chemotherapy Drugs, Standard D 6978-05.* West Conshohocken, PA: American Society for Testing and Materials, International; 2005.

95. Laws and Regulations, Chapter 1 – Environmental Protection Agency, Subchapter 1—Solid Wastes, parts 260-270. Environmental Protection Agency. *http://www.epa.gov/docs/epacfr40/chapt-I.info.* Accessed August 22, 2007.

96. AORN guidance statement: environmental responsibility. In: *Standards, Recommended Practices and Guidelines.* Denver, CO: AORN, Inc; 2007:251-258.

97. Environmental Protection Agency. Wastes. *http://www.epa.gov/epaoswer/osw.* Accessed August 20, 2007.

98. Environmental Protection Agency. Sloan-Kettering fined for failure to properly manage hazardous waste. (January 27, 2004). *http://www.epa.gov/region02/healthcare.* Accessed August 22, 2007, 2007.

99. World Health Organization. Mercury in Health Care. Policy Paper. August, 2005. *http://www.healthcarewaste.org.* Accessed August 22, 2007.

100. Health Care Without Harm. Making Medicine Mercury-free: A Resource Guide for Mercury-free Medicine. Available at: *http://www.noharm.org/library/docs/Going_Green_Making_Medicine_Mercury_Free.pdf.* Accessed August 21, 2007.

101. Joint Commission on the Accreditation of Health Care Organizations. Tubing Misconnections – A Persistent and Potentially Deadly Occurrence. [Sentinel Event Alert]. Issue 36 (April 3, 2006). *http://www.jointcommission.org/SentinelEvents/SentinelEventAlert/sea_36.htm.* Accessed August 22, 2007.

102. Paparella S. Inadvertent attachment of a blood pressure device to a needless "y-site": surprising, fatal connections. *Journal Emergency Nursing.* 2005; 31:180-182.

103. Institute for Safe Medical Practices. Medication Safety Alert. June 17, 2004. *http://www.ismp.org/MSA articles?tubingprint.htm.* Accessed August 21, 2007.

104. AORN guidance statement: creating a patient safety culture. In: *Standards, Recommended Practices and Guidelines.* Denver, CO: AORN, Inc; 2007:305-310.

105. US Department of Health and Human Services, Public Health Service/Food and Drug Administration Center of Devices and Radiological Health. *The Safe Medical Devices Act 1990 and The Medical Device Amendments of 1992* HHS Publication FDA 93-4243.Washington DC: US Department of Health and Human Services, 1992.

PUBLICATION HISTORY

Originally published February 1988, *AORN Journal,* as "Recommended practices for safe care through identification of potential hazards in the surgical environment." Revised March 1992.

Revised November 1995; published March 1996, *AORN Journal.* Reformatted July 2000.

Revised; published March 2003, *AORN Journal.*

Revised 2007; published in *Perioperative Standards and Recommended Practices,* 2008 edition, as "Recommended practices for a safe environment of care."

Revised November 2009 for online publication in *Perioperative Standards and Recommended Practices.*

Minor editing revisions made in November 2010 for publication in *Perioperative Standards and Recommended Practices,* 2011 edition.

Recommended Practices for Environmental Cleaning in the Perioperative Setting

The following recommended practices for environmental cleaning in the perioperative setting were developed by the AORN Recommended Practices Committee and have been approved by the AORN Board of Directors. They were presented as proposed recommendations for comments by members and others. They are effective January 1, 2008.

These recommended practices are intended as achievable recommendations representing what is believed to be an optimal level of practice. Policies and procedures will reflect variations in practice settings and/or clinical situations that determine the degree to which the recommended practices can be implemented.

AORN recognizes the numerous types of settings in which perioperative nurses practice. These recommended practices are intended as guidelines adaptable to various practice settings. These practice settings include traditional ORs, ambulatory surgery units, physicians' offices, cardiac catheterization suites, endoscopy suites, radiology departments, and all other areas where operative and other invasive procedures may be performed.

References to nursing interventions (I) used in the Perioperative Nursing Data Set, second edition, (PNDS) are noted in parentheses when a recommended practice corresponds to a PNDS intervention.[1] The reader is referred to the PNDS for further explanation of nursing diagnoses, interventions, and outcomes.

Purpose

These recommended practices provide guidance for environmental cleaning and disinfection in the surgical practice setting. Conscientious application of these recommended practices should result in a clean environment for surgical patients and minimize the exposure risk of health care personnel and patients to potentially infectious microorganisms. Potentially, any patient could be infected with bloodborne or other pathogens; therefore, all surgical procedures should be considered potentially infectious.

Recommendation I

The patient should be provided a clean, safe environment.

Exogenous sources for pathogens that may cause a surgical site infection (SSI) include surgical personnel; the operating room environment (including the air); and all tools, instruments, and supplies brought to the sterile field during the procedure. Exogenous flora are mainly aerobes.[2] Health care-associated infections have been linked to external sources, which can include environmental surfaces.[3] The risk of infection from pathogenic organisms on environmental surfaces is due not only to their presence, but to their ability to survive on and be transferred to many surfaces.[4]

I.a. The perioperative registered nurse should assess the perioperative environment frequently for cleanliness and take action to implement cleaning and disinfection procedures if needed.[5] (PNDS: I98) Cleanliness means the absence of visible dust, debris, soil, or body substances.

Environmental cleaning and disinfection is a team effort involving surgical personnel and environmental services personnel. The responsibility for verifying a clean surgical environment rests with perioperative nurses. (PNDS: I98)

I.a.1. Preparation of the OR should include visual inspection for cleanliness before case carts, supplies, equipment, and instrument sets are brought into the room.

I.b. All horizontal surfaces in the OR (eg, furniture, surgical lights, booms, equipment) should be damp dusted before the first scheduled surgical procedure of the day.[2] Plasma and monitor screens should be cleaned according to manufacturers' instructions.

Dust is known to contain human skin and hair, fabric fibers, pollens, mold, fungi, insect parts, glove powder, and paper fibers among other things.[6-8] Airborne particles range in size from 0.001 microns to several hundred microns. Contamination from particles can come from an external source (eg, ventilation, doors) or an internal source (eg, equipment, personnel activity).[9] (PNDS: I98)

In settings with dry conditions, gram-positive cocci (eg, coagulase negative *Staphylococcus* species) found in dust may persist; in settings with surfaces that are moist and soiled, the growth of gram-negative bacilli may persist.[10] Fungi, which favor moist, fibrous material, also are found in dust. Damp dusting prevents microbial-laden dust from being dispersed throughout the environment.[8] (PNDS: I98)

I.b.1. Equipment from areas outside the restricted area of the OR should be cleaned before being brought into an OR.

I.b.2. A clean, lint-free cloth moistened with an Environmental Protection Agency (EPA)-registered hospital detergent/disinfectant should be used to damp-dust. (PNDS: I98)

I.b.3. Cleaning and disinfection methods that produce mist, aerosols, or dust (eg, spray bottles containing disinfectant) should not be used.[11]

I.b.4. Gloves used for environmental cleaning and disinfection should be made of natural rubber latex, nitrile, chloroprene blends, or butyl rubber.[12] Vinyl gloves should not be used in environmental cleaning and disinfection. Vinyl glove barrier protection failure rates can be very high.[13]

I.c. Environmental Protection Agency-registered disinfectants should be used to clean floors, noncritical equipment, and other surfaces.[8] (PNDS: I98) Material safety data sheets (MSDSs) should be available and reviewed for each disinfectant used in the perioperative setting.

Environmental surfaces that touch intact skin are considered noncritical items requiring low-level disinfection. Environmental surfaces can serve as a means of secondary transmission by providing a reservoir for infectious organisms that can contaminate the hands of health care personnel. This is known as surface-to-hand transfer of bacteria.[3,14-16] Field and laboratory studies have shown the importance of environmental cleaning and disinfection as part of an infection prevention process in reducing microbial bioburden in the environment, thereby interrupting microorganism transmission.[4] One study has shown that vancomycin-resistant enterococci species (VRE) can be transmitted by a contaminated surface.[17] Another study has shown that a persistence of pathogens can survive on fabrics and plastics.[18] (PNDS: I98)

I.c.1. Reusable string and microfiber mops and cleaning cloths should be changed after each use.[8,19] Used cleaning mops or cloths should not be returned to the cleaning solution container.

I.c.2. Single-use disposable mop heads and cloths may be used.[8]

I.c.3. Mops that dispense cleaning disinfectant may be used.

Cleaned and dried mop heads and cleaning cloths decrease the level of contamination.[20] Microfiber mops are an option for mopping floors because

- they can withstand up to 300 launderings;
- the microfiber particles are positively charged and draw negatively charged particles (ie, dirt);
- traditional string mops weigh about 10 pounds while microfiber mops weigh about two pounds; and
- lighter mops may reduce personnel injuries.[19]

Mops that dispense cleaning fluid eliminate the risk of contamination of multi-use containers of cleaning solution and reduce the risk of chemical splashes.

I.d. Measures should be taken to prevent vermin infestation of the perioperative environment.[8,21]

Insects and rodents can carry pathogens that cause disease (eg, flies carrying *Shigella* which can cause diarrhea by contaminating food).[22] Food left out in staff member lounges for long periods of time may be a focus of fly infestation.

I.d.1. To prevent vermin infestations, the following steps should be taken:

- remove food sources and any environment that attracts pests; and
- keep windows and doors closed.[21]

I.d.2. If prevention measures fail, a credentialed pest control specialist should be contacted to eliminate the cause of the infestation.[8,21]

Recommendation II

A safe, clean environment should be reestablished after each surgical procedure.

Routine cleaning and disinfection reduces the amount of dust, organic debris, and microbial load in the environment. Following scientifically based recommendations for cleaning and disinfection practices in health care organizations helps to reduce infections associated with contaminated items. Many studies have documented that failure to comply with scientifically based recommendations has led to infection outbreaks.[14]

II.a. Operating rooms should be cleaned after each surgical or invasive procedure with a lint-free or microfiber cloth moistened with a detergent/disinfectant and water.[2,8,19]

II.a.1. When feasible, products that are environmentally friendly should be considered when selecting a disinfectant.[23-25]

II.a.2. Detergent and EPA-registered disinfectant solutions should be prepared daily or as needed according to manufacturers' instructions.[8]

II.a.3. Chemicals placed into a secondary container must be labeled with the chemical and the solution's concentration.[26]

II.a.4. High-level disinfectants or liquid chemical sterilants should not be used for cleaning and disinfection environmental surfaces or noncritical devices.[8]

II.a.5. Alcohol should not be used to clean large environmental surfaces.[8]
Alcohol is not an EPA-registered disinfectant. Alcohol does not remove soil or debris. Alcohol is a flammable antiseptic which must be used with caution in the surgical setting.[27,28]

II.b. Mattresses and padded positioning device surfaces (eg, OR beds, arm boards, patient transport carts) should be moisture-resistant and intact.

II.b.1. Nonporous surfaces such as mattress covers, pneumatic tourniquet cuffs, blood pressure cuffs, and other patient equipment should be cleaned and disinfected with an EPA-registered hospital disinfectant between patient use.[8]

II.b.2. Manufacturers' instructions for cleaning and disinfection specialized beds should be followed.

II.b.3. Damaged or worn coverings should be replaced.

II.b.4. Fabric coverings should be changed and laundered after each patient use.

II.b.5. Penetration of the cover by needles and other sharp items should be avoided.[8,29]

II.c. Patient transport vehicles including straps and attachments should be cleaned after each patient use.[30]

II.c.1. Single-use straps should be discarded after one use.

II.d. All receptacles (eg, bins, kick buckets, pails), work surfaces, and tables should be cleaned and disinfected.[5,8]

II.e. Contaminated laundry should be handled as little as possible.[8]
Handling contaminated laundry with a minimum of agitation avoids contamination of air, surfaces, and personnel.[5,8]

II.e.1. Contaminated laundry should be placed in leak-proof containers or bags and labeled appropriately at the location where it was used.[5,8]

II.e.2. Linen should be laundered in a designated, organization-approved and monitored laundry facility.

II.f. Laundry chutes in the perioperative setting should be designed to enable cleaning and disinfection and maintenance on a regular basis.[8,31,32]
Laundry bags travel through a laundry chute with a back-and-forth motion that can disperse airborne pathogens throughout a health care facility.[33] Maintaining negative pressure in the chute prevents the spread of pathogens from one floor to the next.[34] (PNDS: I98)

II.g. Manufacturers' cleaning recommendations should be consulted before cleaning computer keyboards, monitor screens, telephones, and other electronic devices. If appropriate, these items should be cleaned with a detergent- and water-moistened lint-free cloth. If the item cannot be cleaned, it should be covered with a moisture-impervious protective covering that can be cleaned or discarded after each use.[8,35]

Computers and other sensitive electronic devices are likely to become contaminated and may be difficult to clean.[8] Sensitive computer components such as monitor screens may be damaged by cleaning disinfectants.[5]

II.h.   Tacky mats should not be used.[8]

Tacky mats have not been shown to reduce the number of organisms on shoes or equipment wheels, nor do they reduce the risk of SSIs. An exception to not using tacky mats would be their use inside the entry of cordoned-off construction areas within the health care facility as a means to contain dust and debris.[8]

II.i.   Neonatal patient contact with wet environmental disinfectants should be avoided.[8]

After cleaning and disinfection, all surfaces should be dry before patient contact. Chemical residue may remain on the bassinet or the incubator if not thoroughly dried.[8]

II.i.1.   Incubators or bassinets should not be cleaned when the neonate is in the incubator, warming bed, or bassinet. The neonate should be moved to another incubator or bassinet that is clean and dry.[8,36]

II.i.2.   An EPA-registered germicide, in the concentration indicated in the manufacturers guideline for nurseries and neonates, should be used.[8,36]

Recommendation III

Contaminated disposable and reusable items should be handled safely according to state and federal regulations.

Disposable and reusable items may be classified as either potentially infectious or noninfectious. Strategies for handling these items help promote a safe and healthy environment.[25]

III.a.   Disposable items contaminated with blood and/or tissue that would release blood or other infectious materials in a liquid or semi-liquid state if compressed, or items that are caked with dried blood or other potentially infectious material, must be placed in closable, leak-proof containers or bags that are color coded, labeled, or tagged for easy identification as biohazardous waste.[5]

Leak-proof containers prevent exposure of personnel to blood, tissue, and body fluids and prevent contamination of the environment. Color coding and/or labeling alert personnel and others to the presence of items potentially contaminated with infectious microorganisms, prevent exposure of personnel to infectious waste, and prevent contamination of the environments.[5] (PNDS: I98)

Contaminated disposable items may include gowns; gloves; sponges, procedural drapes; suction tubing, liners, and canisters; and opened or used supplies.

III.a.1.   Disposable items that do not release blood and/or other infectious material in a liquid or semi-liquid state if compressed, or that are not caked with dried blood or other potentially infectious materials, are considered noninfectious and should be placed in a separate receptacle designated for noninfectious waste.[5]

III.b.   Regulated waste should be stored in an area with a floor drain, cleanable floor and wall surfaces, lighting, and exhaust ventilation and should be safe from weather, insects, animals, and unauthorized entry until transportation for treatment and or disposal.[5]

III.c.   Containers or bags containing regulated medical waste should be transported according to state regulations. Containers or bags containing regulated medical waste may be required to be transported in washable and closed or covered carts or vehicles.[5]

III.d.   Reusable items contaminated with blood and/or tissue that would release blood or other infectious materials in a liquid or semi-liquid state if compressed, or items that are caked with dried blood or other potentially infectious materials, must be placed in closable, leak-proof containers and labeled as infectious.

Leak-proof containers prevent exposure of personnel to blood, tissue, and body fluids and prevent contamination of the environment. Color coding and/or labeling alert personnel and others to the presence of items potentially contaminated with infectious microorganisms, prevent exposure of personnel to infectious items, and prevent contamination of the environment.[5] (PNDS: I98)

III.e. Personal protective equipment (PPE) must be worn to prevent a splash or splatter when disposing of liquid waste.[37]

III.e.1. Liquid waste may be disposed of according to state regulations including, but not limited to the following methods:
- adding a solidifying powder to the liquid,
- using a medical liquid waste disposal system, or
- pouring the liquid down a sanitary sewer.[37]

Recommendation IV

Surgical and invasive procedure rooms and scrub/utility areas should be terminally cleaned daily.

Terminal cleaning and disinfection of the perioperative environment decreases the number of pathogens, dust, and debris that is created during the day.[2,4]

IV.a. Terminal cleaning and disinfection of operating and invasive procedure rooms should be done
- when the scheduled procedures are completed for the day, and
- each 24-hour period during the regular work week.[2,8]

IV.a.1. Unused rooms should be cleaned once during each 24-hour period during the regularly scheduled work week.[8]
Personnel enter unused rooms and move equipment and supplies in and out of the room.

IV.a.2. Floors should be wet-vacuumed with an EPA-registered disinfectant after scheduled cases are completed.[8]

IV.a.3. Other areas requiring cleaning and disinfection include, but are not limited to,
- all horizontal surfaces (eg, cabinet tops, tops of sterilizers, solution/blanket warmers);
- hallways and floors;
- substerile areas;
- scrub/utility areas; and
- sterile storage areas.

IV.b. Cleaning equipment should be disassembled, cleaned, disinfected with an EPA-registered disinfectant, and dried before reuse and storage.[8]

Equipment is cleaned to prevent the growth of microorganisms during storage and to prevent subsequent contamination of the perioperative area.

IV.c. Refillable liquid hand soap dispensers should not be used.[38,39]
Refillable liquid soap dispensers can become contaminated and serve as reservoirs for microorganisms. Prolonged use of a multi-use container, transferring solutions to secondary containers, and refilling containers such as povidone iodine dispensers has resulted in contamination of the antiseptic with *Pseudomonas aeruginosa*.[40]

Recommendation V

All areas and equipment in the surgical practice setting should be cleaned according to an established schedule.

A clean environment will reduce the numbers of microorganisms present.[2,4]

V.a. A cleaning schedule for areas and equipment that should be cleaned on a daily, weekly, or monthly basis should be established. The schedule should be developed by a multi-disciplinary team to determine appropriate cleaning and disinfection and maintenance frequencies.

V.a.1. Areas and equipment that should be cleaned on a weekly or monthly basis should include, but are not limited to,
- heating and air-conditioning equipment;
- pneumatic tubes and carriers;
- sterilizers and their loading carts/carriages;
- clean and soiled storage areas;
- walls and ceilings;
- unrestricted areas (eg, offices, waiting rooms, lounges, lavatories, and locker rooms).[41]

V.b. Ventilation ducts should be cleaned and filters changed on a regularly scheduled basis.

V.c. All refrigerators and ice machines should be cleaned on a routine basis.

V.c.1. Patient refrigerators should be cleaned weekly and outdated food removed.

Cleaning and disinfection should be logged on log sheet.

V.c.2. Ice scoops should not be kept in the ice compartment.

V.c.3. Ice scoops should be cleaned on a weekly basis.[8] Ice machines with a dispenser are preferable to ones that require the use of scoops.

V.d. After cleaning, an EPA-registered disinfectant should be used to disinfect scrub sinks and wash basins following a regular schedule.[8]

An example of a pathogen known to cause health care-associated infection outbreaks is *Pseudomonas aeruginosa,* which thrives in moist and humid environments such as sinks. *Pseudomonas aeruginosa* do not need many nutrients and can grow in large numbers.[33,42] (PNDS: I98)

V.d.1. Aerators on faucets should be cleaned and disinfected weekly by removing the aerator, scrubbing it with a detergent and a brush reserved for this purpose, and immersing it in a disinfectant.[43]

V.e. Eye wash stations should be cleaned and checked weekly to ensure that they are in working order.[5]

Recommendation VI

All personnel should take precautionary measures to limit transmission of microorganisms when performing routine environmental cleaning and disinfection activities.

Federal regulations for bloodborne pathogen standards were first published by the Occupational Safety and Health Administration (OSHA) in 1991 to protect health care workers from exposure to bloodborne infections. The Needlestick Safety and Prevention Act was passed by Congress in 2000 and enacted in 2001 to protect health care workers from contaminated sharps injury.[44]

VI.a. All personnel must comply with OSHA's bloodborne pathogen standards when performing cleaning and disinfection procedures involving contact with blood and other potentially infectious materials.[5]

Following bloodborne pathogen precautions can reduce health risks for personnel who may be exposed to blood and other potentially infectious material. Approximately 8,700 health care personnel are infected with hepatitis B annually, resulting in 200 deaths. Wearing PPE can reduce the risk of becoming infected with HIV/AIDS and hepatitis C as well.[5]

VI.b. Health care personnel must follow standard precautions to prevent contact with blood or other potentially infectious material.[5]

All body fluids (eg, semen, vaginal secretions, cerebrospinal fluid, synovial fluid, pleural fluid, pericardial fluid, peritoneal fluid, amniotic fluid, saliva,) except sweat are potentially infectious.[5] (PNDS: I98)

VI.c. Health care personnel handling contaminated items must wear appropriate PPE to reduce the risk of exposure to bloodborne or other potentially infectious microorganisms and hazardous materials.[4]

VI.c.1. Gloves must be worn when it is reasonably anticipated that personnel may have contact with blood or other potentially infectious materials while handling or touching contaminated items or surfaces.[5,8]

VI.c.2. Masks, eye protection, and face shields must be worn whenever contact with splashes, spray, splatter, or droplets of blood or other potentially infectious material is anticipated.[5,8]

VI.d. Hand hygiene should be performed when gloves are removed and as soon as possible when hands are soiled.[16]

VI.e. When visible soiling by blood or other potentially infectious materials appear on OR surfaces or equipment during or after a surgical procedure, an EPA-registered detergent/disinfectant should be used to clean those areas as soon as possible.[5,8]

VI.f. Spills that contain blood or other potentially infectious material should be removed with an absorbent material as soon as possible, then the area should be disinfected with an EPA-registered disinfectant to confine and contain the spill.[5,8]

VI.f.1. When cleaning spills of blood, other potentially infectious material, or hazardous materials, PPE must be worn. This includes the use of gloves, and may include gown, mask, and eye protection.[5]

VI.f.2. The contaminated absorbent cleaning material used to clean a spill must be disposed of in a designated biohazardous waste receptacle.

VI.g. Items that are in a semi-liquid state when compressed or that are caked with blood must be placed in a biohazardous waste container.[5]

VI.h. Contaminated sharps (eg, needles, blades, sharp disposable instruments) must be immediately discarded in a closable, puncture-resistant, leak-proof (on both sides and bottom) receptacle. The receptacle must be marked with a biohazard label that meets OSHA bloodborne pathogen standards.[5,8]

VI.i. Broken glassware should not be handled directly with unprotected hands.[5]

Recommendation VII

Procedures for environmental cleaning and disinfection and PPE use should be established for circumstances that may require contact or airborne precautions.

In health care organizations, pathogens may be disseminated by person-to-person, direct or indirect contact via a contaminated environmental surfaces or fomites; airborne transmission; fecal-oral transmission; or percutaneous exposure.[45] These pathogens may result in morbidity and mortality for patients and personnel. Standard precautions and disinfection procedures are adequate for most, but not all, of these circumstances.[14] The incidence of multi-drug resistant organisms has risen steadily in hospitals over the past few decades.[46] Both methicillin-resistant *Staphylococcus epidermidis* (MRSE) and VRE have been found to survive for long periods of time on environmental surfaces and fabrics. Methicillin-resistant *Staphylococcus epidermidis* and VRE can survive longer than 90 days on fabrics and plastics.[18] (PNDS: I98)

Prions present unique infection prevention and control challenges. Prions are proteinaceous, infectious agents containing no DNA or RNA and may be transmitted iatrogenically by direct inoculation. Prions cause transmissible spongiform encephalopathies including Creutzfeldt-Jakob disease (CJD). Prions are resistant to traditional chemical and physical decontamination methods.[45,46] (PNDS: I98)

VII.a. Extraordinary cleaning procedures or closure of operating rooms following procedures identified as contaminated or dirty-infected (Class III or IV) is not necessary, with the exception of cases involving patients suspected of having CJD.[8]

VII.b. Appropriate cleaning and disinfection methods should be enforced following care of patients infected or colonized with
- methicillin-resistant *Staphylococcus aureus;*
- VRE;
- any multi-drug-resistant pathogen, including vancomycin-intermediate enterococcus;
- vancomycin-resistant *Staphylococcus aureus;*
- extended spectrum β-lactamases;
- multi-drug-resistant gram-negative bacteria; and
- resistant *Streptococcus pneumoniae.* (PNDS: I98)

Although cleaning and disinfection is appropriate for removal of infectious agents, one study found that VRE was recovered from 50% of inadequately cleaned surfaces after inoculation.[47] Conscientious adherence to approved cleaning and disinfection procedures is crucial for the prevention of antibiotic-resistant organism transmission.

VII.b.1. Closure of the room or extraordinary cleaning and disinfection procedures are not required.[8]

VII.b.2. Contact precautions should be instituted when performing environmental cleaning and disinfection of rooms used to care for patients colonized or infected with drug resistant pathogens.[45,46]

VII.b.3. When providing environmental cleaning and disinfection for patients in contact isolation, all health care personnel should wear isolation gowns and gloves. If splash or splatter is anticipated, a mask with a face shield or a mask and goggles must be worn.[5,45]

Personal protective equipment is required by OSHA to protect mucous membranes, airways, skin, and clothing from exposure to potentially infectious material.[5,45]

VII.c. An EPA-registered, hypochlorite-based disinfectant should be used to clean a patient area when the patient is diagnosed or suspected of infection with *Clostridium difficile (C. difficile)*.[5,14,48]

Clostridium difficile is transmitted via fecal-oral exposure. In health care settings this primarily occurs when there is hand contact with fecally contaminated surfaces that is then transferred from hands to mouth or by unknowingly inserting fecally contaminated thermometers or other devices into the mouth.

In its spore form, *C. difficile* can survive up to five months in the environment and can be transmitted from person-to-person via fecal-oral transmission as well as by touching surfaces and objects contaminated by feces and placing fingers in the mouth. In the health care setting, *C. difficile* has been cultured in rooms occupied by infected patients up to 40 days after their discharge.[48] (PNDS: I98)

VII.c.1. When performing environmental cleaning and disinfection, all health care personnel should wear isolation gowns and gloves. If splash or splatter is anticipated, a mask with a face shield or a mask and goggles must be worn.[5,45]

Personal protective equipment is required by OSHA to protect mucous membranes, airways, skin, and clothing from exposure to potentially infectious material.[5,45]

VII.d. Personnel performing environmental cleaning and disinfection in the room of a patient who has an airborne disease (ie, rubeola, varicella, tuberculosis [TB]), must use a properly fit-tested N95 mask or powered air purifying respirator until complete air exchange has been achieved.[49]

VII.d.1. Environmental cleaning and disinfection may proceed without respiratory PPE after a complete air exchange has been achieved. The period of time required for the ventilation system to achieve a 99.9% air exchange should be noted (eg, 28 minutes for a 15-air-exchanges-per-hour cycle).[49] Testing of air exchanges should be done according to AORN's "Recommended practices for a safe environment of care"[50] (**Table 1**).

VII.d.2. Access to the room should be restricted until the 99.9% air exchange has been completed. Any personnel entering the room before the air exchange has been completed must wear a fit-tested N95 mask or powered air-purifying respirator.

VII.d.3. An EPA-registered germicide disinfectant with a label claim for tuberculocidal activity (ie, intermediate-level disinfectant) may be used for cleaning and disinfection. Floors, walls, or surfaces with minimal hand contact do not need to be cleaned with a tuberculocidal germicide disinfectant. This activity assures that pathogens with less resistance than TB also will be killed.[49]

VII.e. Special cleaning and decontamination procedures should be used after a surgical procedure involving high risk tissue (ie, brain, spinal cord, eye tissue) on a patient who has been diagnosed or is suspected of having CJD.[8]

VII.e.1. Disposable linens should be used when the patient is suspected of having CJD. Before the procedure begins, personnel should cover work surfaces with a disposable, impervious material that can be removed and incinerated after the procedure.

Use of disposable linens minimizes contamination of the room and decreases the need for environmental cleaning and disinfection of these surfaces.

VII.e.2. Reusable linens may be used in cases where the patient is suspected of having CJD. The linen may be laundered as per routine laundering processes if not contaminated with high infectivity tissue (eg, spinal fluid, central nervous system tissue). If such contamination occurs, the contaminated linen should be incinerated.

Chemicals used in hospital laundry are not effective in deactivation of prions. More information on this subject is available in AORN's "Recommended practices for cleaning and care of instruments and powered equipment."[51]

VII.e.3. Environmental surfaces (ie, noncritical surfaces) contaminated with high-risk tissues

Table 1

AIR CHANGES PER HOUR AND TIME REQUIRED FOR AIRBORNE CONTAMINANT REMOVAL EFFICIENCIES OF 99% AND 99.9%*[1]		
Air Changes per Hour (ACH)	Minutes Required for 99% Removal Efficiency†	Minutes Required for 99.9% Removal Efficiency†
2	138	207
4	69	104
6	46	69
12	23	35
15	18	28
20	7	14
50	3	6
400	<1	1

* This table can be used to estimate the time necessary to clear the air of airborne *Mycobacterium tuberculosis* after the source patient leaves the area or when aerosol-producing procedures are complete.
† Time in minutes to reduce the airborne concentration by 99% or 99.9%.

REFERENCE

1. Jensen PA, Lambert LA, Iademarco MF, Ridzon R. Guidelines for preventing the transmission of Mycobacterium tuberculosis *in health care settings, 2005.* Morbidity & Mortality Weekly Review. *[Recommendations and Reports]. 2005; 54 (RR17): 1-141.*

(ie, brain, spinal cord, eye tissue) should be cleaned and then decontaminated with a solution of sodium hypochlorite (1 part chlorine bleach to 5 parts diluent) or sodium hydroxide (1 Normal or 1 Molar).

- Sodium hypochlorite solution should be prepared daily. Health care facilities without a hood should not mix sodium hydroxide.
- Sodium hydroxide is commercially available in solution. The MSDSs for both sodium hypochlorite and sodium hydroxide should be reviewed. The contact time for both sodium hypochlorite and sodium hydroxide should be 30 to 60 minutes.[8]

No transmissions of prion diseases from environmental surfaces have been reported; however, it remains prudent to eliminate highly infectious material from the operating room surfaces that are contacted during subsequent surgeries.

VII.e.4. Single use disposable gowns, gloves, masks, and eyewear should be worn for environmental cleaning and disinfection.

VII.e.5. Contaminated disposable supplies should be incinerated following the procedure.[52]

Splashing of mucous membranes (eg, eyes, mouth) and accidental ingestion may be considered a risk for incurring prion diseases. The highest potential risk for occupational exposure to high-risk tissue is through needlestick injuries.[52,53] (PNDS: I98)

Prions have been experimentally transmitted by conjunctival instillation of inoculum.[54] There is a theoretical risk that a mucous membrane splash of prion-contaminated fluid could lead to transmission.

VII.e.6. All disposable instruments placed in biohazard sharps boxes should be marked for incineration as well.[52] (PNDS: I98)

VII.e.7. Liquids used in cleaning and disinfection should be solidified and incinerated.

Recommendation VIII

A containment, cleaning and disinfection, and surveillance process should be in place during construction, renovation, remediation, repair, or demolition.

It is important that the environment not serve as a source of pathogens. Fungi such as *Aspergillus* are an example of pathogens that can be released and dispersed as a result of damage to a water pipe in a ceiling or demolition of a wall.[55] (PNDS: I98)

VIII.a. Protective barriers should be maintained to protect patients and personnel from dust and debris. Pathogens may be released into the environment during construction (eg, *Aspergillus*).[55]

VIII.b. Areas within and adjacent to the construction site should be cleaned on an ongoing basis whenever debris or dust is present.[55]

VIII.c. Particle counts should be done adjacent to barriers at seams, joints, and entry/exits into the construction zone to ensure that dust and debris are adequately contained.[56]

VIII.d. Air sampling done in the contaminated room, and adjacent areas may be used to establish whether fungi (ie, *Aspergillus*) are present in the area.[56-58]

VIII.d.1. Air sampling should be done before construction begins, after demolition occurs, and at the end of the project.[56-58]

VIII.d.2. If *Aspergillus* is found in the area, dust and debris first must be cleaned with detergent. The walls and ceilings then should be decontaminated by using copper-8-quinolinolate or other EPA-registered fungicide.[55] Personnel trained to do this should wear the appropriate PPE when cleaning and decontaminating the area.

VIII.e. Terminal cleaning and disinfection should be performed before placing equipment and supplies in the area when the construction, renovation, remediation, repair, or demolition is completed.[58]

VIII.f. The health care organization's procedure for preventing risks to patients, health care personnel, and visitors during construction should be documented and shared with employee health, risk management, and plant operations personnel.[55]

Recommendation IX

Competency
Personnel should receive initial education, training, and competency validation on proper environmental cleaning and disinfection methods, agent selection, and safety precautions.

The Occupational Health and Safety Act of 1970 (Public Law 91) mandates employers to provide programs for the education and training of employees in the recognition, avoidance, and prevention of unsafe or unhealthful working conditions.[59]

IX.a. Employees should receive initial education, and competency validation on regulations, equipment, chemicals, and safety procedures.

IX.b. Employees should be provided additional training when procedures or supplies and equipment change.

IX.c. Training materials should be appropriate in content, vocabulary level, literacy, and language of the target personnel.[5]

IX.d. Training content should include, at a minimum,
 – an accessible copy of the regulatory text;
 – explanation of signs and labels and/or color coding required for contaminated items;
 – the employer's exposure control plan and the means for personnel to obtain a copy;
 – methods to recognize tasks and other activities that may involve occupational exposure;
 – location and use of eye wash stations;
 – use and limitations of engineering controls, work practices, and PPE;
 – information on the types, proper selection, proper use, location, removal, handling, decontamination, and disposal of PPE;
 – information on hepatitis B vaccination; and
 – location of MSDSs.

Recommendation X

Policies and Procedures
Policies and procedures for environmental cleaning and disinfection should be written, reviewed annually, and readily available in surgical practice settings.

Policies and procedures establish authority, responsibility, and accountability and serve as operational guidelines. Policies and procedures also assist in the development of patient safety, quality assessment, and improvement activities. Practices and policies and procedures are subject to change with the advent of new technologies.

X.a. Policies and procedures for environmental cleaning and disinfection should include, but not be limited to,
- identification of responsible personnel;
- competency validation;
- standard cleaning and disinfection procedures;
- frequency of cleaning and disinfection;
- chemicals approved for use;
- labeling of secondary containers;
- required PPE; and
- cleaning and disinfection procedures for special cases (ie, transmissible diseases).

X.b. An introduction and review of policies and procedures should be included in orientation and ongoing education of perioperative personnel to assist them in obtaining knowledge and developing skills and attitudes that affect patient outcomes.

Recommendation XI

Quality

A quality management program should be in place to evaluate products, processes, and outcomes of the environmental cleaning and disinfection program.

Quality and performance improvement functions ensure that organizations design processes well and systematically monitor, analyze, and improve their outcomes.[60,61]

XI.a. A multidisciplinary committee involved with the quality management program should include, at a minimum, perioperative, infection control, and environmental services personnel.

XI.b. Quality indicators should include, but not be limited to,
- compliance with regulatory standards;
- review of products and manufacturer directions for use;
- procedures;
- monitoring cleaning and disinfection practices; and
- reporting and investigation of adverse events (ie, outbreaks, product issues, corrective actions, evaluation).

Glossary

Aspergillosis: An opportunistic disease, usually respiratory, that may be life threatening and is caused by *Aspergillus*, a fungi. *Aspergillus* may be aerosolized when building structure, plumbing, and surrounding soil is disturbed.

Clean: The absence of visible dust, soil, debris, blood, or other potentially infectious material.

Cleaning: A process using friction, detergent, and water to remove organic debris; the process by which any type of soil, including organic debris, is removed. Cleaning removes rather than kills microorganisms.

Confine and contain: A principle that recommends prompt cleanup of items contaminated with blood, tissue, or body fluids.

Contaminated: The presence of potentially infectious pathogenic microorganisms (eg, blood, other potentially infectious material) on or in animate or inanimate objects.

Decontamination: Any physical or chemical process that removes or reduces the number of microorganisms or infectious agents and renders reusable medical products or equipment safe for handling or disposal; the process by which contaminants are removed, either by hand cleaning or mechanical means, using specific solutions capable of rendering blood and debris harmless and removing them from the surface of an object or instrument.

Disinfection: A process that kills most forms of microorganisms on inanimate surfaces. Disinfection destroys pathogenic organisms (excluding bacterial spores) or their toxins or vectors by direct exposure to chemical or physical means.

End-of-procedure cleaning: Cleaning that is performed at the end of one surgical procedure and before the start of another surgical procedure in the same room.

Endogenous. A source from the patient (eg, skin).

Environmentally friendly products: Products that contribute to better air quality and are less toxic to patients, visitors, and health care personnel.

EPA-registered agent: A microorganism-killing agent registered with the Environmental Protection Agency (EPA). The EPA classifies germicides as sporicides, general disinfectants, hospital disinfectants, detergents, sanitizers, and others.

Exogenous: From a source other than the patient (eg, personnel, equipment, the environment, instruments, supplies).

Fomites: Inanimate objects which, when contaminated with a viable pathogen (eg, bacterium, virus), can transfer the pathogen to a host.

High-level disinfection: A process that kills all microorganisms with the exception of high numbers of bacterial spores and prions. High-level disinfectants have the capability to inactivate the hepatitis B virus, HIV, and *Mycobacterium tuberculosis,* but do not inactivate the prion that causes Creutzfeld-Jacob disease. Government-registered high-level disinfection agents kill vegetative bacteria, tubercle bacilli, some spores and fungi, and lipid and nonlipid viruses, given appropriate concentration, submersion, and contact time.

Iatrogenic: A response to a medical or surgical treatment which results in a poor outcome.

Intermediate-level disinfection: A process that kills *Mycobacterium tuberculosis,* vegetative bacteria, most viruses, and most fungi but does not necessarily kill bacterial spores.

Low-level disinfection: A process by which most bacteria, some viruses, and some fungi are killed. This process cannot be relied on to kill resistant microorganisms such as *Mycobacterium tuberculosis* or bacterial spores.

Molarity: The number of moles of solute per solution.

Molar solutions: Denoting a concentration of 1 gram molecular weight (1 mol) of solute per liter of solution, the common unit of concentration in chemistry.

Normal solutions: Denotes a solution containing 1 equivalent of replaceable hydrogen ions or hydroxyl per liter (eg, 1 mol/L HCL is 1 N) or a solution containing 1 gram of a substance or its equivalent in hydrogen ions. Normality is a ratio which relates the amount of solute to the total volume of a solution.

Organic debris: Blood, tissue, and body fluids.

Personal protective equipment (PPE): Specialized equipment or clothing for eyes, face, head, body, and extremities; protective clothing; respiratory devices; and protective shields and barriers designed to protect the worker from injury or exposure to a patient's blood, tissue, or body fluids. Used by health care workers and others whenever necessary to protect themselves from the hazards of processes or environments, chemical hazards, or mechanical irritants encountered in a manner capable of causing injury or impairment in the function of any part of the body through absorption, inhalation, or physical contact.

Regulated medical waste: Liquid or semi-liquid blood or other potentially infectious materials; contaminated items that would release blood or other potentially infectious materials in a liquid or semi-liquid state if compressed; items that are caked with dried blood or other potentially infectious materials and are capable of releasing these materials during handling; contaminated sharps; and pathological and microbiological wastes containing blood or other potentially infectious materials.

Reusable: Any product or piece of equipment intended by the manufacturer for multiple uses. As appropriate to each item, the manufacturer is to provide instructions for reprocessing, care, and/or maintenance of the item.

Terminal cleaning: Cleaning that is performed at the completion of surgical practice settings' daily surgery schedules. Terminal cleaning is performed in surgical procedure rooms and scrub/utility areas and includes, but is not limited to, surgical lights and external tracks; fixed and ceiling-mounted equipment; all furniture, including wheels and casters; equipment; handles of cabinets and push plates; ventilation faceplates; horizontal surfaces (eg, tops of counters, sterilizers, fixed shelving); the entire floor; kick buckets; and scrub sinks.

Used items: Items that are opened for a surgical procedure that may or may not have come in contact with a patient's blood, tissue, or body fluids.

REFERENCES

1. Petersen C, ed. *Perioperative Nursing Data Set.* Rev 2nd ed. Denver, CO: AORN, Inc; 2007.

2. Mangram AJ, Horan TC, Pearson ML, Silver LC, Jarvis WR. Guideline for prevention of surgical site infection, 1999. *Infect Control and Hosp Epidemiol.* 1999:20: 250-278.

3. Rutala WA, Weber DJ. Surface disinfection: should we do it? *J Hosp Infect Control.* 2001;48(Suppl A):S64-68.

4. Cozad A, Jones RD. Disinfection and the prevention of infectious disease. *Am J of Infect Control.* 2003;31:243-54.

5. US Department of Labor, Occupational Safety and Health Administration. Final Rule on Occupational Exposure to Bloodborne Pathogens,1910.1030. *http://www .osha.gov /pls/oshaweb/owadisp.show_document?p_table= STANDARDS&p_id=100.* Accessed October 26, 2007.

6. AORN latex guideline. In: *Standards, Recommended Practices, and Guidelines.* Denver, CO: AORN, Inc; 2007:203-218.

7. Bray WJ. What is everyday dust made of? MadSci Network: Environment and Ecology. 2007. *http://www.madsci .org /posts/archives/dec98/912530774.En.r.html.* Accessed October 26, 2007.

8. Sehulster L, Chinn RY. Centers for Disease Control and Prevention, Health care Infection Control Practices

Advisory Committee (HIPCPAC). Guidelines for environmental infection control in health-care facilities. 2003. *MMWR Morb Mortal Wkly Rep.* 2003;52[RR-10]:1-44.

9. Air Crafters. Clean Room Concepts: Airborne particulate control. *http://www.air-crafters.com/concepts2.html.* Accessed October 26, 2007.

10. Dancer SJ. Mopping up infection. *J Hosp Infect.* 1999;43:85-100.

11. Centers for Disease Control and Prevention. *Guidelines for Environmental Infection Control in Health-Care Facilities.* Atlanta, GA: Centers for Disease Control and Prevention; 2003:134.

12. Centers for Disease Control and Prevention. Infection Control in Dental Settings. Personal Protective Equipment (Masks, Protective Eyewear, Protective Apparel, Gloves). *http://www.cdc.gov/OralHealth/infectioncontrol/faq/protective_equipment.* Accessed October 29, 2007.

13. Rego A, Roley L. In-use barrier integrity of gloves: latex and nitrile superior to vinyl. *Am J Infect Control.* 1997;27:405-410.

14. Rutala WA, Weber DJ. Cleaning, disinfection and sterilization in health care facilities. In: *APIC Text of Infection Control and Epidemiology.* 2nd ed. Washington, DC: Association for Professionals in Infection Control and Epidemiology; 2005: 21.1-21.12.

15. Association for Professionals in Infection Control and Epidemiology. Disinfection and Sterilization Principles. *http://www.apic.org/AM/AMTemplate.cfm?Section=Brochures&Template=/CM/ContentDisplay.cfm&ContentFileID-2558.* Accessed October 26, 2007.

16. Recommended practices for surgical hand antisepsis/ hand scrubs. In: *Standards, Recommended Practices, and Guidelines.* Denver, CO: AORN, Inc; 2007:565-574.

17. Rutala WA, Weber DJ, Gergen MF. Studies on the disinfection of VRE-contaminated surfaces. *Infection Control & Epidemiology.* 2000;21:548.

18. Neely AN, Maley MP. Survival of enterococci and staphylococci on hospital fabrics and plastic. *J of Clin Microbiol.* 2000;38:274-726.

19. Rutala, WA, Weber, DJ. Surface disinfection: new processes and products. In: *Disinfection, Sterilization and Antisepsis Principals, Practices, Current Issues, and New Research.* Rutala WA, ed. Washington, DC: Association for Infection Control Practitioners; 2007:97-106.

20. Scott E, Bloomfield SF. Investigations of the effectiveness of detergent washing, drying, and chemical disinfection on contamination of cleaning cloths. *J Appl Bacteriol.* 1990;68:279-83.

21. Chou T. Environmental services. In: Association for Professionals in Infection Control and Epidemiology, eds. *APIC Text of Infection Control and Epidemiology.* 2nd ed. Washington, DC: Association for Professionals in Infection Control and Epidemiology; 2005:102-1-102-12.

22. Graczyk TK, Knight R, Tamang L, Pandalai SG. Filth, flies, and human diseases. *Recent Res Devel Applied Biotechnol.* 2005;2:21-31.

23. Health Care Without Harm. Cleaning. Chemical Use Hospital Fact Sheet 2004. *http://www.noharm.org/details.cfm?ID=606&type=document.* Accessed October 10, 2007.

24. Cleaning for Health: Products and Practices for a Safer Environment, 2002. *http://www.informinc.org/reportpdfs/chp/CleaningForHealth.pdf.* Accessed October 11, 2007.

25. Guidance statement on environmental responsibility. In: *Standards, Recommended Practices, and Guidelines.* Denver, CO: AORN, Inc; 2007:251-258.

26. US Department of Labor, Occupational Safety and Health Administration. [Hazard Communication]. Labels and other forms of warning. In: *29CFR 1910-1200 Toxic and Hazardous Substances.* Washington, DC: US Department of Labor, Occupational Safety and Health Administration; 2007:460-482.

27. Molinari, JA, Harte, JA. Dental services. In: *Association for Infection Control Practitioners Text of Infection Control and Epidemiology.* Washington, DC: Association for Infection Control Practitioners; 2005:51 1-16.

28. ECRI. A team approach to surgical fire prevention. Understanding the fire triangle. *Health Devices.* 2006;35:56.

29. Fogg D. Mattress disinfection; hand hygiene; latex safety; abdominal-perineal preps; hand rub characteristics; radiopaque packing. *AORN J.* 2004;79:645-652, 651-652.

30. Friedman C, Petersen KH. Ambulatory surgery. In: *Infection Control in Ambulatory Care.* Boston, MA: Jones and Bartlett Publishers; 2004:64.

31. American National Standards Institute, Association for Advancement of Medical Instrumentation. *Processing of Reusable Surgical Textiles for Use in Health Care Facilities. ANSI/AAMI ST65:2000.* Arlington, VA: Association for the Advancement of Medical Instrumentation; 2005:1-49.

32. Michaelsen GS. Designing linen chutes to reduce spread of infectious organisms. *Hospitals JAHA.* 1965; 39:116-9.

33. Ortolano G, McAlister MB, Angelbeck JA, et al. Hospital water point-of-use filtration. a complementary strategy to reduce the risk of nosocomial infection. *Am J Infect Control.* 2005; 33(Suppl):S1-S19.

34. Whyte W, Baird G, Annand R. Bacterial contamination on the surface of hospital linen chutes. *J Hyg.* [London]. 1969;67:427-35.

35. Public Notification from FDA, CDC, EPA, and OSHA: Avoiding Hazards with Using Cleaners and Disinfectants on Electronic Medical Equipment. US Food and Drug Administration Center for Devices and Radiological Health. October 3, 20007:1-9. *http://www.fda.gov/cdrh/safety.html.* Accessed November 27, 2007.

36. Academy of Pediatrics. The American College of Obstetricians and Gynecologists. Infection control. In: *Guidelines for Perinatal Care.* 5th ed. American Academy of Pediatrics. Washington, DC: The American College of Obstetricians and Gynecologists; 2002:349-350.

37. Ticer J. Choosing and implementing proper storage and disposal for your facility. Medical waste management. In: *Medical Construction and Design.* Scottsdale, AZ: Inform Publications; 2007(3):24-25.

38. Archibald LK, Corl A, Shah B, et al. *Serratia marcescens* outbreak associated with extrinsic contamination of 1% chlorxylenol soap. *Infect Control Hosp Epidemiol.* 1997;18:704-709.

39. Grohskopf LA, Roth VR, Felkins DR, et al. *Serratia liquefaciens* bloodstream infections from contamination of epoetin alfa at a hemodialysis center. *N Engl J Med.* 2001;344:1491-1497.

40. Anderson RI, Vess RW, Panlillo AL, Favero MS. Prolonged survival of *Pseudomonas cepacia* in commercially manufactured povidone–iodine. *Applied Environmental Microbiology*. 1990;56:3598-3600.

41. Lafreniere R, Berguer R, Seifert PC, et al. Preparation of the operating room. In: *American College of Surgeons ACS Surgery: Principles & Practice 2004*. New York, NY: WebMD Professional Publications; 2004:3-16.

42. Trautman M, Lepper PM, Haller M. Ecology of *Pseudomonas aeruginosa* in the intensive care unit and the evolving role of water outlets as a reservoir of the organism. *Am J of Infect Control*. 2005;33(Suppl 1):S41-49.

43. Schraag J. Waterborne pathogens: what's lurking in your facility's pipes? *Infect Control Today*. 2005; 9:14-19.

44. Occupational Safety and Health Administration. 29 CFR Part 1910: Occupational exposure to bloodborne pathogens; needlestick and other sharps injuries. Final rule. *Federal Register*. Jan 18, 2001:5318-5325.

45. Siegel JD, Rhinehart E, Jackson M, Chiarello L, the Health care Infection Control Practices Advisory Committee. CDC. Guideline for Isolation Precautions: Preventing Transmission of Infectious Agents in Healthcare Settings 2007.1-219. *http://www.cdc.gov/ncidod/dhqp/pdf/guidelines/Isolation2007.pdf*. Accessed October 26, 2007.

46. Siegel JD, Rhinehart E, Jackson M, Chiarello L. Management of Multidrug–Resistant Organisms in Healthcare Settings, 2006: CDC and the Health care Infection Control Practices Advisory Committee. Atlanta, GA. *http://www.cdc.gov/ncidod/dhqp/pdf/ar/MDRO Guideline2006.pdf*. Accessed October 29, 2007.

47. Langford MG, Collins S, Youngberg L, Rooney DM, Warren JR, Noskins GA. Assessment of materials commonly utilized in health care: implications for bacterial survival and transmission. *AJIC*. 2006; 34:258-263.

48. *Clostridium difficile*: a sometimes fatal complication of antibiotic use. *Patient Safety Advisory*. 2005;2:1-8.

49. Jensen PA, Lambert LA, Iademarco MF, Ridzon R. Guidelines for preventing the transmission of *Mycobacterium tuberculosis* in health-care settings, 2005. *MMWR Morb Mortal Wkly Rept*. 2005;54:(RR-17):1-102.

50. Recommended practices for a safe environment of care. In: *Standards, Recommended Practices, and Guidelines*. Denver, CO, AORN, Inc: 2008;351-374.

51. Recommended practice for cleaning and care of instruments and powered equipment. In: *Standards, Recommended Practices, and Guidelines*. Denver, CO, AORN, Inc: 2008; 421-445.

52. World Health Organization. WHO Infection Control Guidelines for Transmissible Spongiform Encephalopathies. *http:/whqlibdoc.who.int/hq/2000/WHO_CDS_CSR_APH_2000.3.pdf*. Accessed October 26, 2007.

53. Rutala WA, Weber DJ. Creutzfeldt-Jakob disease: recommendations for disinfection and sterilization. *Clin Dis Inf*. 2001;32:1348-1356.

54. Scott JR, Foster JD, Fraser H. Conjunctival instillation of scrapies in mice can produce disease. *Vet Microbiol*. 1993;934:305-309.

55. Bartley J. Construction and renovation. In: Association for Professionals in Infection Control and Epidemiology, eds. *APIC Text of Infection Control and Epidemiology*. 2nd ed. Washington, DC: Association for Professionals in Infection Control and Epidemiology; 2005:108-1-108-16.

56. Streifel AJ. Design and maintenance of hospital ventilation systems and the prevention of airborne nosocomial infections. In: *Hospital Epidemiology and Infection Control*. 3rd ed. Philadelphia, PA: Lippincott Williams & Wilkins; 2004:1579-1589.

57. Cosgrove SE, Perl TM. Infection control and prevention in hematopoietic stem cell transplant patients. In: *Hospital Epidemiology and Infection Control*. 3rd ed. Philadelphia, PA: Lippincott Williams & Wilkins; 2004: 1019-1023.

58. Bartley J. Prevention of infections related to construction, renovation, and demolition. In: *Hospital Epidemiology and Infection Control*. 3rd ed. Philadelphia, PA: Lippincott Williams & Wilkins; 2004:1549-1575.

59. US Department of Labor, Occupational Safety and Health Administration. OSHA Act of 1970, Pub.L.105.97, Sec 21. *http://www.osha.gov/pls/oshaweb/owadisp.show _document?p_table=STANDARDS&p_id=10051*. Accessed October 26, 2007.

60. AORN quality and performance improvement standards for perioperative nursing. In: *Standards, Recommended Practices, and Guidelines*. Denver, CO: AORN, Inc; 2007:437-446.

61. Joint Commission on Accreditation of Health care Organizations. Improving organization performance. In: *Comprehensive Accreditation Manual for Hospitals*. Oak Brook Terrace, IL: The Joint Commission;2007 PI-1–PI-10.

RESOURCE

Center for Infection Control and Prevention Questions and answers: Creutzfeldt-Jocob Disease Infection Control Practices. *http://www.cdc.gov/ncidod/dvrd/ cjd/infection_control_cjd.htm*. Accessed November 26, 2007.

PUBLICATION HISTORY

Originally published June 1975, *AORN Journal*, as "Recommended practices for sanitation in the surgical practice setting."

Format revised March 1978; March 1982; July 1982. Revised April 1984; November 1988; December 1992.

Revised June 1996; published October 1996, *AORN Journal*. Reformatted July 2000.

Revised; published December 2002, *AORN Journal*.

Revised 2007; published in *Perioperative Standards and Recommended Practices*, 2008 edition.

Recommended Practices for Medication Safety

The following Recommended Practices for Medication Safety have been approved by the AORN Recommended Practices Advisory Board. They were presented as proposed recommendations for comments by members and others. They are effective December 1, 2011. These recommended practices are intended as achievable recommendations representing what is believed to be an optimal level of practice. Policies and procedures will reflect variations in practice settings and/or clinical situations that determine the degree to which the recommended practices can be implemented. AORN recognizes the various settings in which perioperative nurses practice. These recommended practices are intended as guidelines adaptable to various practice settings. These practice settings include traditional operating rooms (ORs), ambulatory surgery centers, physicians' offices, cardiac catheterization laboratories, endoscopy suites, radiology departments, and all other areas where surgery and other invasive procedures may be performed.

Purpose

These recommended practices are intended to provide guidance to perioperative RNs to develop, implement, and evaluate safe medication management practices specific to the perioperative setting. Evidence-based approaches to medication safety in perioperative settings are not well established; therefore, guidance emerges from broad knowledge of adverse events and strategies to prevent medication errors identified in other settings.[1-3] Medication errors may go undetected, but when they are reported, the sources of the errors are multidisciplinary and multifactorial. Results of medication errors can include substantial threats to patients, increased health care costs, and compromised patient confidence in the health care system.[4,5]

Awareness of medication errors increased after the 1999 Institute of Medicine report *To Err Is Human: Building a Better Health System* stated that "medication errors account for one out of 131 outpatient deaths and one out of 854 inpatient deaths."[6] Since that time, the Joint Commission's *Sentinel Event Alert* reports have indicated that medication errors resulting in death or permanent loss of function continue to occur each year.[7]

The recommendations that follow are consistent with the six phases of the medication use process, including procuring, prescribing, transcribing, dispensing, administering, and monitoring.[4] Medication errors can originate at any point in the medication use process and affect patients of all ages. Perioperative settings present additional challenges for safe medication practices. Factors affecting the medication process in the perioperative environment include, but are not limited to,

- the aseptic transfer of medications onto the sterile field,
- the presence of an intermediary who is in sterile attire to receive and transfer dispensed medications to the licensed independent practitioner who is in sterile attire (eg, surgeon),
- time-sensitive conditions, and
- sensory distractions intrinsic to the environment.

Potential risks associated with medication errors in the perioperative setting include, but are not limited to,

- inconsistent communication of current and previous medication regimens (ie, medication reconciliation);
- confusion in the medication order (eg, name, strength, dose) caused by muffled verbal orders delivered through surgical masks;
- incomplete, ambiguous, incorrect, or illegible written or spoken orders;
- inaccurate, illegible, or outdated surgical preference cards;
- medication that is removed from the original manufacturer's packaging to aseptically deliver contents onto the sterile field;
- allied heath professionals in sterile attire who receive medications onto the sterile field having limited knowledge of medications;
- inconsistent labeling of medications on and off the sterile field;
- medication dispensed to the sterile field that may be handled by multiple individuals before reaching the licensed individual administering the medication;
- medication preparations without a pharmacist in the setting to perform or oversee the preparation or provide consultation;
- high-alert medications that are available in multiple dose forms and concentrations;

- look-alike and sound-alike medications stored in close proximity;
- patient care complexity that requires rapid perioperative interventions;
- extended work hours leading to health care worker fatigue;
- care provided by multiple health care providers simultaneously;
- multiple patient hand offs between care providers; and
- misuse or failure of medical devices used to store, dispense, or administer medications.

Safe medication practices require open, honest, and clear communication throughout the medication use process and the perioperative continuum of care. The following recommendations for perioperative settings are consistent with established professional standards of care for the medication use process. In addition, these recommendations provide guidance for the comprehensive planning required for managing medication inventory across the medication use process. Perioperative administrators can use these evidence-based recommendations to facilitate policy development and provide a foundation for creating quality-improvement and process-improvement monitors. For the purposes of this document, medication includes prescription products, IV and irrigation fluids, medication patches, implanted devices that contain or deliver medication, medical gases, herbal and dietary supplements, and over-the-counter agents.

Recommendation I

A multidisciplinary team approach for medication management and the prevention of medication errors should be used throughout the phases of perioperative care.

Involving all health care professionals who participate in the medication use process assists with identifying medication error risk factors from a variety of perspectives. In many settings, the nurse may be the primary person administering medications. However, there is still a need for collaboration between all stakeholders (eg, nurse, physician, pharmacist) to address issues relating to the medication management plan and to ensure that the plan is effective.[8] In the perioperative setting, there are medication hand offs among perioperative team members, and medications may be given concurrently by the sterile team members and

anesthesia professionals, which adds further justification for collaborating to prevent medication errors. Creating quality improvement teams that include stakeholders relevant to this patient safety issue was among the recommendations identified in a report from the Agency for Healthcare Research and Quality describing successful initiatives nurses can use to guide efforts to improve quality.[9]

I.a. A pharmacy and therapeutics committee or medication safety committee should be established.[5]

A committee that is focused on medication safety issues helps to ensure ongoing interaction among health care providers. The American Society of Health-System Pharmacists states that it is a minimum standard in both hospital and ambulatory settings to have a multidisciplinary team for medication-use policy development and to make decisions concerning medication use.[10,11] A multidisciplinary approach may help balance pharmaceutical cost containment and the risk of adverse drug events in patient settings.[12]

I.a.1. The medication safety committee should include key stakeholders (eg, nurses, physicians, anesthesia professionals, pharmacists, risk management personnel, purchasing personnel, administrators) who participate in the medication use process.

I.b. A medication management plan should be developed by a multidisciplinary team to identify risk-reduction strategies for each of the six phases of the medication use process, including procuring, prescribing, transcribing, dispensing, administering, and monitoring. The medication management plan should be communicated to all members of the perioperative team and implemented consistently in all perioperative practice settings (eg, preoperative, intraoperative, day surgery, postoperative).

Developing a medication management plan that incorporates structures, processes, and professional responsibilities into each of the six phases of the medication use process allows for identification of latent and active failures. The medication error can be associated with the point of origin in the medication use process and targeted interventions can be identified.[4]

Increasing the perioperative team's awareness of the health care organization's medication management plan disseminates a broader picture of medication risk-reduction strategies and can help communicate the interdependency of the team's actions to provide safe medication practices. Promoting effective team functioning is among the five principles for creating safe systems of health care delivery reported in the Institute of Medicine report on medical errors.[6] Involving key people is among the strategies for developing a strategic plan for medication safety in the 2002 Pathways for Medication Safety report developed by the Institute for Safe Medication Practices (ISMP) in a partnership with American Hospital Association and the Health Research and Educational Trust.[13] The report indicated that involvement of informal leaders from the front line, senior administrative leaders, physicians, and managers helps garner support and enthusiasm, nurtures broad networks, and provides feedback about levels of support needed to ensure a meaningful and effective medication management plan.[13] Although there are not many quantitative research findings that document the relationship between team behaviors and outcomes in health care, research supports developing surgical teams to focus on sharing potential problems, inquiries, and briefings.[14,15]

Consistent implementation of the medication management plan across all phases of perioperative patient care establishes clarity and decreases ambiguity. Consistency between perioperative practice settings establishes the same standard of care for patients regardless of where a surgical or other invasive procedure is performed.

I.b.1. Nurses, prescribers, and pharmacists should collaborate with each other and assess the needs of patients and their designated support persons to develop a structured and systematic approach to the medication management plan.[16,17]

A systems approach to patient-centered medication administration includes interprofessional collaboration.[8] A model strategic plan for medication safety also may include involvement from patients, people who are designated to support patients, and community leaders to promote community medication safety initiatives and medication self-management programs.[13] Multidisciplinary and patient collaboration to enhance the effectiveness of medication reconciliation was identified as a primary medication error risk-reduction strategy based on a review of eight studies focusing on prescribing and medication reconciliation.[16]

I.b.2. Pharmacists should be involved in the planning, development, and continuous evaluation of the medication management plan.

Pharmacists are trained to detect potential medication errors and to identify contraindications of medications and drug-drug interactions.[4,18,19] One of the roles of the pharmacist is to prepare and present drug product evaluation reports that consider all aspects of safety, effectiveness, and cost to the pharmacy and therapeutics committee to evaluate the need for policy development or revisions to existing medication-use policies.[10]

I.b.3. The medication management plan should promote the use of integrated technology whenever possible during the medication use process. Medication technology may include, but is not limited to,
- automated dispensing storage systems that have patient profiles and drug formularies,
- smart infusion pumps,
- electronic medical record systems that contain decision support systems,
- automated medication dosage calculations, and
- bar-coding technology.

The Institute of Medicine identified the use of well-designed technologies as a priority for health care organizations for the delivery of safe medication care.[17] Researchers who conducted a review reported evidence that information technology has been used to facilitate medication reconciliation activities including obtaining medication information, comparing medications, and clarifying discrepancies (eg, duplication, appropriateness).[20]

An interdisciplinary group of practitioners convened in 2007 to identify medication error risk-reduction strategies. The strategies identified include positioning computer monitors or a means to access drug information resources and the medical administration record in close proximity to an automated dispensing storage system or medication storage.[21] The group also identified profiled automated dispensing storage systems as a strategy that can be implemented to comply with the Joint Commission medication management accreditation requirement that specifies that a pharmacist should review all new orders before they are available for selection and administration by the nurse, respiratory therapist, or physician.[21,22]

One study showed a substantial reduction in medication errors at patient admission after implementation of a process that mapped data between a medication reconciliation system and a computerized-provider order (CPOE) entry system.[23] Another study showed a reduction in potential adverse medication events after an information technology application designed to facilitate medication reconciliation was integrated into the CPOE system.[24] Clinical decision support systems alert the perioperative team member administering the medication to possible out-of-range doses or contraindications with other medications to help identify and avert medication errors.[24-26] When fully implemented, use of bar-code technolo-gies during medication administration provides a way for the perioperative team member who is administering the medication to confirm patient identification, dose, and product, and it allows pharmacy personnel to confirm order verification.[27,28]

I.b.4. The medication management plan should include strategies for providing immediate access (preferably electronic information resources) to current medication information resources for perioperative personnel who administer medications. Current medication information resources should be available for all new medications and acceptable concentrations that will be dispensed or accessible.

Health care organizations have the responsibility to provide easily accessible and current information resources to assist perioperative personnel who administer medications.[17] Important information includes, but is not limited to, nutrition and herbal supplement interactions (eg, calcium channel blockers and grapefruit) and medication allergies or side effects associated with other medications (eg, amoxicillin and cephalexin). Dose errors or omissions may occur in printed medication references or the information provided may not match the medication concentrations that are acceptable for use in critical care settings.[29] Newly released medications present risk for error because nurses are less likely to be familiar with them and information often cannot be found in printed medication references.[29]

I.c. Pharmacists should be available for consultation with members of the perioperative team in all facilities, including ambulatory surgery centers and office-based surgery facilities, and at each phase of the medication use process.[30]

Errors may be more likely to occur when medication products and dosing strengths are available without pharmacist review. Collaboration between pharmacists and members of the perioperative team to determine special considerations for medications (eg, temperature ranges for medication storage, disposal of medications) or patient conditions (eg, medication reconciliation, allergies, weight-based dosing, side effect management) decreases the opportunity for medication errors.

Recommendation II

Medications, chemicals, reagents, and related supplies should be procured and stored in a manner that facilitates safe and efficient delivery to the patient.

Medication errors have been traced back to procurement, the first phase of the medication use process.[1] Risk for errors at this phase can be reduced by making proactive decisions about unit-of-use versus multidose containers, shelf life, and the general supply chain (ie, medication availability, delivery, and protection during transit from the wholesaler to the end user).[4]

II.a.   The health care organization's medication management plan should incorporate considerations for procurement including, but not limited to,

- obtaining medications from manufacturers or suppliers with established quality programs;
- developing procedures for current or potential product shortages, discontinuations, and recalls;
- implementing procedures for verifying accuracy of medications upon receipt; and
- implementing processes that promote accurate medication stocking and restocking.

Medication manufacturers and suppliers that define target product profiles relating to quality, safety, and efficacy (eg, dosage form, bioavailability, strength, stability) and identify critical quality attributes are more likely to provide timely notification of recalls or shortages.[31] An investigation of a multi-state outbreak of *Serratia marcescens* related to contaminated prefilled syringes revealed poor compliance with Food and Drug Administration (FDA) Good Manufacturing Practices and quality system

regulations.[32] The same investigation also revealed that National Drug Codes are the most reliable method for identifying potentially contaminated syringes because some had gone through three distribution steps before reaching the end user and others bore the name of a subsidiary company to the original manufacturer.[32]

Errors at the procurement phase have been reported when medications that are received are not verified with what was ordered before they are stocked. The Pennsylvania Patient Safety Authority reports two circumstances involving errors in stocking 1,000 mL bags of IV solutions. One involved 1,000 mL of sterile water for injection that was mistakenly dispensed and stored on a dialysis unit instead of 0.9% saline solution. The other involved a wholesaler who mistakenly delivered 1,000 mL of sterile water for injection instead of 5% dextrose solution.[33]

II.a.1.   Medications in perioperative storage areas should be rotated based on the expiration date indicated on the medication label.

Medication storage areas that are organized to avoid outdated items helps to reduce the risk of administering expired medications to patients. Medications that are stored on emergency or special procedure carts may not be used frequently and have increased risk of becoming outdated before they are used. Rotating low volume medications back through a central or regional pharmacy or through vendor agreements may save money in spite of potential restocking fees and also reduces potential environmental pharmaceutical waste.

II.a.2.   Processes should be implemented when stocked medications are not available because of shortages, discontinuations, or recalls. Processes should include, but not be limited to,

- removing recalled items from storage and returning them to the appropriate location,
- procuring substitutions, and

reduction practices at the administration end of the medication use process. In spite of standardization through automated dispensing storage systems, there have been reports of errors such as a nurse retrieving phenylephrine from an adjacent compartment when the intent was to obtain an antiemetic agent. The wrong medication was administered and caused the patient to spend additional time in the postanesthesia care unit (PACU) to manage the effects of the phenylephrine.[18]

II.f.1.   Nursing and pharmacy personnel should collaborate to establish, monitor, and periodically review medications that are routinely stocked at par level in various bins or drawers in all medication storage areas (eg, automated dispensing storage systems, refrigerated areas, anesthesia carts, emergency carts).

Collaboration between nursing and pharmacy personnel may help to identify changes in storage that will reduce errors related to the wrong medication being retrieved for the procedure case cart. When perioperative RNs and surgical technologists implement the medication orders as specified on surgeon preference cards, they may identify areas of potential confusion and have recommendations for standardizing units of use and concentrations. Sharing information with pharmacists that will contribute to changes relating to procurement and storage is one way that front-line practitioners can help to ensure the safe delivery of medications to patients.[1]

II.f.2.   Medications in the storage area should be organized using safety considerations including, but not limited to,
- separating medications by generic name and packaging;
- separating look-alike, sound-alike medications;
- separating high-alert medications;
- providing separate bins or dividers for all medications in storage;

- labeling storage bins, using enhanced lettering when possible, with both the medication's generic and brand names;
- positioning medication containers so that their labels are visible; and
- avoiding alphabetical storage.[35,51-57]

More than 1,400 medications (ie, 57% brand or proprietary names, 43% generic names) have been involved in look-alike, sound-alike medication errors. Almost 800 medications have been identified as a distinct pair, meaning look-alike, sound-alike errors were associated with only one other product. More than 600 medications were paired with two or more distinct medications.[46] Even though the largest percentage of look-alike, sound-alike medication errors originated in the dispensing phase of the medication use process,[46] obtaining the wrong medication from a storage area has resulted in patient injury or death.[46] Anticipating a look-alike, sound-alike medication error and adjusting the organization of the medication storage area accordingly is an effective medication error risk-reduction strategy.

II.f.3.   Medications and related supplies stored on anesthesia carts should be standardized within perioperative areas and, if possible, in the community when anesthesia professionals rotate between multiple health care organizations. Medications should be organized according to order of use, frequency of use, similarity of action, severity of harm from misuse, and lack of similar appearance.[58]

The Anesthesia Patient Safety Foundation identified standardization within all anesthesia workstations in an institution as a risk-reduction strategy for medication errors related to anesthesia medication administration.[25] When anesthesia professionals rotate from one facility to another within the community, standardized anesthesia carts provide consistency and may reduce human factor errors. Studies of human error show that many errors involve deviation from routine practice. Standardization of equipment and problems with medication stock control, including delivery to and from storage, were among the unsafe acts described in a classic paper about the nature and likelihood of anesthesia errors.[59] A case report described an incident of unexplained apnea during surgery caused by a mix-up with cefazolin and vecuronium located in adjacent compartments in the anesthesia drawer.[60]

II.f.4. Medications and related supplies stored in emergency and specialty carts in perioperative areas should be standardized and be available in unit-dose, age-specific, and ready-to-use forms.

Consistency between emergency carts will facilitate efficiency in the medication use process and reduce the risk of error. Studies of human error show that many errors involve deviation from routine practice.[59]

II.g. Medications should be procured in limited varieties of concentrations and dosages and standardized in all perioperative medication storage areas.

Standardizing medication concentrations and dosing is a strategy that can be implemented to ensure that excessive amounts of medication are not available. This creates a forcing function intended to promote patient safety. Safety principles include restricting access to high concentrations of heparin (eg, 10,000 units per mL). Another example may be to have morphine routinely available in doses smaller than 10 mg/mL (eg, 2 mg or 4 mg), which would still allow for dose titration.[18]

Epinephrine in concentrations of 1:1,000 is a high-alert medication that has been reported to cause harm when it is not diluted.[61] Warning labels may help to reduce confusion when a high-alert medication requires dilution, but it may be more effective to store the vials in the pharmacy to reduce the risk of error.[61]

Toxic dose calculations for pediatric and adult dosages can be clarified more easily when there is a standardization and limited number of medications in the storage area.[62] Drug libraries for infusion pumps serve as a resource for toxic dose calculations but cannot be established without standardizing the medications on hand.[50]

II.g.1. Concentrated electrolytes including, but not limited to, sodium chloride solutions more concentrated than 0.9%, potassium chloride, and potassium phosphate should be ordered from the pharmacy when needed rather than stored at the unit level or in ambulatory surgery centers.[63]

Mortality has been reported as a result of concentrated electrolytes being mistakenly administered too rapidly and without proper dilution.[63] A neonate died as a result of a nurse mistakenly removing a vial of concentrated (23.4%) sodium chloride from the unit medication storage area and administering the solution intravenously, instead of administering normal saline (0.9% sodium chloride) flush.[63]

II.h. Perioperative RNs should collaborate with pharmacists to procure and store single-dose vials rather than multidose vials.

Multidose vials of medication contain a preservative to help prevent bacterial growth, single-use vials do not.[64] There may be viral contamination of multidose vials because the preservative may be effective only for inhibiting bacterial growth.[65] With some multidose vials, the preservative may not become entirely effective until two hours after it has been opened, which leaves the possibility of the presence of bacterial organisms in the meantime.[66]

Nurses can provide practical insight by investigating ways to decrease the use of multidose vials.[67] The rationale for stocking multidose vials may be related to cost savings or because there is a short supply of the medication available on the market. When medications are supplied in quantities that exceed the amount typically given, health care workers may be at risk of misinterpreting the amount in the vial, or may use the vial for more than one patient in an effort to avoid waste.[66]

Primary safety concerns related to the use of multidose vials include, but are not limited to, potential

- cross contamination from one patient to another,[65]
- risk of administering too much medication,
- confusion in labeling and expiration dates with open vials, and
- issues of proper disposal of unused pharmaceuticals and inconsistent documentation of waste.[68-71]

II.h.1. Medications labeled as single-use vials that are found opened should not be used and should be discarded.

II.h.2. Opened multidose medication containers must be dated to indicate expiration within 28 days of opening and should be discarded immediately upon expiration.[30] When a product has been opened or a vial cap has been punctured or removed, the manufacturer's expiration date is no longer valid and should be replaced with a new date.

The Centers for Medicare & Medicaid Services requires that over-the-counter medications, including cough and pediatric elixirs, be disposed of within 28 days of breaking the label regardless of manufacturer's printed expiration date on the multidose container.[30]

The manufacturer's labeled expiration date represents the beyond-use date for a product that has not been opened. The effectiveness of the bacteriostatic agent used in the multidose vial is only tested by the manufacturer of the product for a period of 28 days. There is increased risk for bacterial growth the longer the seal is broken and a container is open.

II.h.3. Multidose medications used for more than one patient should not be stored in the immediate area where direct patient contact occurs and should be separated from single-dose vials in the storage area.[30]

There is an increased risk for a dosage medication error if multidose medications are stored in the same area as single-dose vials. Expiration dates on multidose medications that are opened are likely to be shorter than the single-dose vials, which increases the risk that an expired medication could be administered. Separating opened multidose vials in the storage area facilitates checking for outdated stock.

II.i. Nonmedication solutions and chemicals should not be stored in medication storage areas.

Storing bleach, formaldehyde, cleaning products, and other chemicals in areas where medications are stored may increase the risk of mistaking the solution as a medication.

II.i.1. Chemicals and reagents (eg, formalin, Lugol's solution, radiopaque dyes, glutaraldehyde) should be procured and stored with the same care and caution as medications.

Nonmedication solutions may be packaged in containers that look similar and can be confused with medications or confused with each other. One incident of acetone being mistaken for an ingestible solution has been published.[72] Other examples of confusion have occurred with hydrogen peroxide/denatured ethyl alcohol and hydrogen peroxide/ethanol. Both solutions have been reported to be mistaken for eye drops because the containers are similar in size and shape.[63]

II.i.2. Chemicals and reagents should be stored in their original containers with the original labels.

Errors resulting in patient injury have been reported as a consequence of chemicals being stored in unlabeled containers.[73]

II.i.3. Potential hazards associated with medical gases in the practice setting should be identified, and safe practices should be established. Medical gases should be stored separately from industrial gases in a secure area with controlled access.[74]

The FDA considers compressed medical gases to be prescription drugs that can only be dispensed by prescription.[75] According to FDA reports, medical gas mix-ups have resulted in at least seven deaths and 15 serious injuries.[74,76]

Recommendation III

Prescribing personnel should provide clear, unambiguous, and accurate medication orders.

Medication errors can occur at the point of prescribing.[4,18] In perioperative settings, surgeons, anesthesia professionals, and advanced practice nurses are examples of prescribers who are licensed to write orders, give verbal orders, or verify standing orders. Having three distinct prescribing processes rather than one contributes to the complexity of the prescription process in perioperative areas. Complex processes open more opportunities for errors related to increased variables and breakdowns in communication.[9,77]

III.a.   Prescribers should have access to all pertinent patient data and reference material.

Medication errors have occurred because prescribers have insufficient patient data (eg, allergy information, current medications) or medication information (eg, indications for special populations, laboratory parameters).[51,78-82] Not having access to patient information has led to errors across the perioperative continuum, with a larger percentage of prescribing errors occurring in the outpatient setting.[4] Researchers of one study reported that higher rates of prescribing errors occurred with less frequently prescribed analgesics, new medications when they are first introduced to the organization, and older medications that are used in new or uncommon ways.[79]

Preference cards are not directly linked to patient data, but rather are related to systems level data (eg, type of procedure). This can increase the risk for error when patient information is not integrated into the care plan on the day of surgery.

III.b.   Prescribers should incorporate the Beers criteria or other tools for identifying potentially inappropriate medication use for special populations.

The Beers criteria identify appropriate medications for adult patients who are older than 65 years of age and calls to attention medications that are inappropriate because of the heightened risk for adverse outcomes.[83] Application of the Beers criteria and other tools enables prescribers to carefully weigh the benefits against the risks of using such medications.[83,84] Prescribing approaches that apply to younger adult patients and guidelines for patients with specific chronic disorders may not be effective or safe for frail, elderly patients.[85] Older patients, patients with multiple health conditions, and pediatric patients often are excluded from evidence-generating, randomized, controlled trials.[85-87] A study of the frequency of off-label prescribing to children showed that the majority of pediatric outpatient visits involve off-label prescribing. The researchers concluded that up-to-date tools for pediatric prescribing information should be included as a priority for medication safety.[86]

III.c.   Medication orders that appear in preprinted forms, standing orders, and preference cards should be reviewed annually by perioperative team members including perioperative RNs, prescribers, and pharmacists.

Medications listed on preference cards are not considered to be standing orders unless they have been reviewed and signed by the prescriber. Annually reviewing medication orders allows prescribers and pharmacists to collaborate with other members of the perioperative team to confirm or update all forms and documents associated with perioperative care.[4,88-90]

III.c.1.   Evidence of the review should be documented on the preprinted forms, standing orders, and preference cards, as should the adoption date and subsequent revision dates.

III.c.2.   Standing orders should be reviewed and approved by the prescriber when they are created and whenever changes are made.

Researchers of one study reported that changes made to preference cards by perioperative nurses are not always verified and approved by the prescriber. In addition, researchers found that medication orders on preference cards were outdated or missing information, or were not what the surgeon intended to use.[91]

III.d. Verbal medication orders should be limited,[92] especially with medications identified as high risk for sound-alike errors or for having commonly confused names.[93]

Verbal orders can be misinterpreted for a number of reasons including, but not limited to, regional dialects, background noise, muffled voices behind surgical masks, and orders involving sound-alike or commonly confused medication names.[4,94,95] Verbal orders have been the source of medication errors.[4,94] In one study aimed at understanding the content and context of verbal orders, researchers reported that 80% of the verbal orders given by physicians and received by nurses included medication-related orders. Further examination revealed that 20% of the orders that matched medications listed on the ISMP's list of commonly confused medications were verbal orders involving fentanyl, furosemide, lidocaine 1% injection, midazolam, or dextrose 50% syringe. Of the medication orders that involved high-alert medications, 20% were verbal orders involving narcotic medicines, sedating agents, anticoagulants, and low-molecular-weight heparin. The risk of verbal orders may be further compounded because commonly confused medications and high-alert medications are often involved.[95]

III.d.1. When verbal orders are necessary, they should be received and carried out only by persons who are authorized to do so and consistent with federal and state law and the health care organization policy and procedures.[92]

Medication use is included in the professional licensing process. State regulations identify the scope of practice for unlicensed personnel related to participation in medication administration.

III.d.2. Perioperative RNs should confirm verbal medication orders by reading back the order to the prescriber digit by digit and spelling out the medication name, if necessary.

Verification of critical components of perioperative verbal orders, before the implementation of the order, affords an opportunity to confirm the accuracy of the verbal order.[5,77,94,96]

III.d.3. Perioperative RNs should immediately record verbal medication orders in the patient's record.

Immediate documentation of verbal orders in the patient's record increases accuracy and allows the recipient of the order to read it back to the prescriber for confirmation.

III.d.4. Prescribers should review, validate, and sign the transcribed verbal medication order on the patient's record as close as possible to the time of the medication administration.

Verifying the accuracy of the documented verbal order allows for confirmation that the intended medication order matches what is administered to the patient.[96] Verifying the verbal order as close as possible to the time the medication is administered allows timely corrective action to be taken if a medication error is discovered.

III.e. When available, prescribers should use CPOE systems.

Computerized-provider order entry systems, especially those with clinical rule-based decision support aids, have reduced opportunity for errors.[97,98] Between April and August 2008, researchers used a simulation tool to assess 62 hospitals, representing about 8% of US hospitals with CPOE systems, and found wide variation in the type of decision support aids used to provide alerts and advice for medication orders that have a high risk of resulting in harm to patients. This study showed that the hospitals had higher scores for basic clinical decision support, and the most reliably detected adverse drug event was a drug-to-allergy contraindication. This study also showed that drug-to-diagnosis contraindications, including pregnancy, were only detected 15% of the time, leading the researchers to emphasize the importance of pharmacy and nursing review processes to intercept medication errors until advanced clinical decision support tools can be integrated into CPOE systems.[80]

Providers who use CPOE systems support pay-for-performance initiatives and quality outcomes that are clinically driven.[4] Computerized provider order entry systems allow for an electronic record of medication administration and decrease the risk for misinterpretation of medication orders from illegible handwriting or misunderstood verbal orders.[99] When studying the characteristics of verbal orders at a tertiary children's hospital, researchers found that CPOE system implementation reduced verbal orders and unsigned verbal orders.[100]

III.e.1. Computerized-provider order entry systems should be designed with prescriber input and evaluated continually for effectiveness.

The authors of one systematic review noted that continual evaluation of the CPOE system is necessary to study the interfaces of CPOE systems with the normal flow of actions in the prescribing processes and other subtle design features (eg, inconvenient logging procedures may encourage physicians to order medications at computer terminals not yet "logged out" by other physicians if the log-out time is slow).[101] Authors of another systematic review noted the substantial difference in how studies on CPOE systems are conducted in terms of setting, design, quality, and definition of the measured outcome variable and noted that electronic prescribing systems could increase the number of medication errors if the system is not designed and implemented appropriately.[102]

Recommendation IV

Safe medication order transcribing processes should be implemented.

Transcribing is the point in the medication use process that involves anything related to the act of recording or transferring an order by someone other than the prescriber for order processing.[1] When inaccuracies occur during the transcribing process, there is a risk for medication error (eg, medication given to the wrong patient) at the administering phase of the medication use process or omission errors may occur (eg, medication is not transcribed, so the patient misses the dose that was ordered).[4]

IV.a. Perioperative RNs should be alert to potential transcribing errors throughout each phase of perioperative care.

Medication errors attributed to the transcribing phase are reported to occur less frequently than other phases in the medication use process.[4] However, case studies and data analysis reports reflect errors in perioperative settings. Examples include an outpatient setting where a staff nurse incorrectly stamped the wrong patient name on a hand-written medication order, resulting in the wrong patient receiving a medication;[4] an omission error in the PACU where a patient did not receive a calcium replacement because postoperative orders were not transcribed;[4] and an error with transcription during the medication reconciliation process that resulted in an overdose of blood pressure medication being administered, resulting in the patient developing asystole while in the OR.[103]

Recommendation V

Pharmacists should be actively involved in dispensing aspects of perioperative medication use across all perioperative settings.

Dispensing is the fourth phase of the medication use process. This phase begins with a pharmacist's assessment of a medication order and continues to the point of release of the product for use by another health care professional.[1] When pharmacists identify prescribing errors at the dispensing phase of the medication use process, it reduces the risk of errors at the administration phase of the medication use process.

Regulatory agencies, accreditation, and standards-setting organizations recommend pharmacy oversight of the medication management practices.[5,30]

V.a.   Pharmacists should review medication orders before administration. In perioperative settings, this review should include standing orders (eg, preference cards).

Pharmacists are trained to detect errors, contraindications of medications, and drug-drug interactions.[4,5] When a pharmacist reviews medication orders, it increases the potential of identifying errors in prescribing early in the medication use process.[5]

V.b.   The health care organization should comply with local, state, and federal regulations for pharmacy resources and ensure solutions are prepared according to national standard specified in *The United States Pharmacopeia,* Chapter <797>.[104]

The Centers for Medicare & Medicaid Services regulations specify that hospitals must have pharmaceutical services that meet the needs of patients and that all compounding, packaging, and dispensing of medications must be under the supervision of a pharmacist and performed consistently with state and federal laws.[105] The regulation does not require a pharmacist to be on site unless an ambulatory surgery center is in a state that has passed a law that requires a licensed pharmacist to provide oversight or consultation for pharmaceutical services.[30] The federal regulations for ambulatory surgery centers state that a designated licensed health care professional must be "routinely present during regular business hours."[30]

The United States Pharmacopeia, Chapter <797>, addresses sterile parental products.[104] Sterile preparations reduce microbial contamination.[106] When perioperative nurses are mixing, diluting, or compounding medications, they bypass the dispensing function of the pharmacy oversight that is intended to ensure the correct ingredient identity, purity, strength, and sterility in addition to accurate labeling on the appropriate type of container.[106,107]

V.c.   Perioperative administrators should investigate the feasibility of implementing a decentralized perioperative pharmacy located within the perioperative suite.[4]

Decentralized (eg, satellite) pharmacies provide support to perioperative staff members with mixing, diluting, and compounding medications to ensure compliance with the specific national standard that pertains to sterility of parenteral products.[25,107]

V.d.   Pharmacists should provide oversight of automated dispensing storage system processes.

Automated dispensing storage systems are an extension of the pharmacy department; therefore, these systems fall under their jurisdiction.[106] The safe use of automated dispensing storage systems is dependent on cooperation between nursing and pharmacy personnel.[21] Automated dispensing storage systems are complex and have design and function variations that require specific maintenance and education. When these systems are not used appropriately, there can be a compromise in patient safety.[106]

Recommendation VI

The perioperative RN should assess the patient and review the patient's record to confirm the patient's metric weight, medication history, and current medication orders before administering medications.

Medication administration is the fifth phase of the medication use process.[1] This phase begins with nursing assessment and continues through planning and intervention. Coupling the medication use process with the nursing process allows risk-reduction strategies to be identified at each step of each process across all phases of perioperative care. Thorough nursing assessment and patient record review is the foundation for planning and implementing the nursing medication plan.[108]

VI.a.   The perioperative RN should confirm that the patient's weight is documented accurately in both pounds and kilograms in the patient's record.

Many medication dosages are calculated according to a patient's weight. There is an increased risk for dosage medication error when the patient's weight is not documented or is inaccurately documented, or when the health care worker estimates the patient's weight.[109] According to the Pennsylvania Patient Safety Authority Advisory,

479 medication error events between June 2004 and November 2008 were associated with inaccurate patient weights with approximately 65% of those reported resulting in an over- or under-dose of the medication ordered.[110,111]

VI.a.1. Electronic or paper patient record forms should be designed to clearly reflect weight in both metric (eg, kilograms) and English (eg, pounds) measurements.

VI.b. The perioperative RN should collaborate with personnel in other disciplines and participate in medication reconciliation activities.

Medication reconciliation is a strategy to promote safe patient outcomes by facilitating patient-centered care, providing insight into preexisting disease processes, reducing opportunities for errors, and detecting duplicate therapies.[3,17,112-114] Medication errors related to transcribing and prescribing may be prevented through the medication reconciliation process.[81,115]

Identifying home medication bottles accurately and collaborating with pharmacists to review home medications may help to identify transcribing errors. In a case report analysis where 75 mg of metoprolol was mistakenly identified as a daily dose on the patient's list of home medications, the author identified the pharmacist as the one more likely to point out that metoprolol is only available in 25-mg or 50-mg tablets.[103] The patient received a fourfold overdose of the medication when the dose was increased from 75 mg to 100 mg. The prescriber's intent was to increase the home dose by 25 mg, but because of a transcribing error, he did not realize that the home dose was 25 mg per day as opposed to 75 mg per day.[103]

VI.b.1. The perioperative RN should actively involve the patient or authorized representative in obtaining a complete list of the patient's current medications, including dietary supplements and over-the-counter products as well as dosages and allergies to the same.[17,103,116]

Researchers from one study in an ambulatory setting found that the accuracy of medication lists improved from 23.1% to 37.7% when perioperative staff members called patients the day before their appointments and reminded them to bring their original medication containers or an updated list of medications for their appointment.[117]

VI.b.2. When compiling information from the medication history during the preoperative assessment, the perioperative RN should collaborate with pharmacy personnel to investigate medications identified by the patient that have no corresponding disease or condition in the patient's record.

Researchers who conducted one study found that medication-condition matching may decrease unnecessary medication use in older adult populations and allow prescribers to make more educated decisions about continuing or discontinuing home medications at the time of patient discharge.[118] In another study, researchers found that it may be useful to identify patients ahead of time who have a higher risk of medication reconciliation errors so that proactive arrangements can be made for pharmacy personnel involvement during transitions in patient care (eg, medication histories upon admission, medication counseling at discharge).[114]

VI.b.3. The perioperative RN should confirm with the patient routes of administration for every product identified during the medication reconciliation process. When they are providing their medication history, patients should be reminded to include all medications they are taking, not just oral medications, injections, or those taken regularly, but also those only taken PRN.

Reports indicate patient injury has resulted from fentanyl and nitroglycerin skin patches when they are not removed before clinical interventions.[119,120] Transdermal patches may contain aluminum or other metals that can overheat during a magnetic resonance imaging (MRI) scan and cause skin burns in the immediate area of the patch.[121]

VI.b.4. Perioperative RNs should use a standardized, multidisciplinary medication reconciliation format that is readily available for review at every transition of patient information.[114,122]

A retrospective chart review revealed that the most accurate method of obtaining complete medication lists at the time of hospital admission is a combination of techniques including compiling a list of medication names and strengths from admission patient interviews as well as from a pharmacy claims database.[123]

VI.c. In the preoperative phase of care, the perioperative RN should confirm that medications and herbal supplements were taken as prescribed or discontinued on the day of surgery or the designated number of days before surgery as per physician orders.

Pharmacokinetic information is not available for most herbs and, therefore, it is not known how long it takes for most herbal products to be cleared from the body. Patients are often instructed to discontinue herbal products five to seven days before surgery.[124] Herbs that are known to affect clotting include bromelain, cayenne pepper, chamomile, cinchona bark, dong quai, fenugreek, feverfew, garlic, ginger, ginkgo, ginseng, guggul, horse chestnut, vitamin E (ie, more than 1,200 IU), and willow bark.[124] Fish oil, glucosamine, flax seed, saw palmetto, chondroitin, mild thistle, and green tea are other examples of natural products that may need to be discontinued two to three weeks before surgery, but the guidelines for discontinuation are not well defined.[125] Researchers report that aspirin may not need to be stopped before surgical or invasive procedures unless the risk of bleeding exceeds the thrombotic risk from withholding the medication.[126]

VI.d. Medication allergy and reaction information should be obtained from patients, family members, legal guardians, and/or previous medical records and should be documented clearly in the patients' records.

In a two-year period, researchers reported 35 incidents in a surgical setting involving medications that were prescribed for or administered to elective surgery patients who had a previous allergy to that medication or a related medication.[127] The Pennsylvania Patient Safety Authority identified documenting allergies and the reaction that a patient experiences to the medication upon admission to a health care facility as an important risk-reduction strategy.[128]

Recommendation VII

Across all phases of care and in all perioperative settings, the perioperative RN should develop a nursing medication plan.

The administering phase of the medication use process requires perioperative RNs to use their knowledge of pharmacology and the patient's condition to establish an individualized medication plan before obtaining or giving medications to the patient.[107,129]

VII.a. The nursing medication plan should include, but not be limited to,
- incorporating findings from the medication history and medication reconciliation process,
- verifying medication orders associated with the patient's planned surgical or other invasive procedure, and
- collaborating with other professionals to resolve discrepancies.

Interpreting and comparing the findings from the medication reconciliation with medication plans outlined for the scheduled surgical or invasive procedure allows communication and revisions to the plan early in the patient's encounter if revisions to the plan are determined to be necessary.[129] Verifying medication orders and seeking pharmacy consultation to confirm contraindications, drug-drug interactions, or specific medication information for special populations are examples of action items in the medication planning stage of the nursing process. Collaborating with other professionals to resolve discrepancies and clarify medication orders is a risk-reduction strategy for establishing an individualized medication care plan that produces maximum benefit from the medications and minimizes harm.[108,129]

VII.a.1. The perioperative RN should contact the prescriber when clarification is needed for medication orders, including medications specified on surgeon preference cards as standing or preprinted orders.

VII.a.2. The perioperative RN should collaborate with the pharmacist when it is necessary to obtain unique medications that are not in the standardized department inventory.

VII.b. The nursing medication plan should include verifying high-risk medications and toxic dosage ranges for products with a narrow therapeutic range, especially in pediatric patients, older adults, and patients who are pregnant, to decrease the risk for adverse effects.

Reports indicate a higher frequency of medication errors or more harm resulting from medication errors for pediatric patients and older adults.[4,83,130,131] Patients who are pregnant are at risk for potentially narrow therapeutic ranges and teratogenic medications.[132]

VII.b.1. Perioperative team members should not be interrupted when verifying an independent dose confirmation of high-alert medications or medications intended for pediatric use.

High-alert medications have a higher risk of causing harm when an error occurs.[13] Most medications administered to pediatric patients have a narrow therapeutic range.[130] Medication calculation errors are five times more likely to occur with pediatric patients.[4,130]

Distractions are a contributing factor in all phases of perioperative care.[4] The presence of interruptions and the frequency of interruptions have been found to be a contributing factor to medication errors,[133] with more interruptions resulting in a greater severity of error.[47] Environments that promote safe medication use are described as locations where the potential for distraction or interruption can be minimized.[134]

VII.b.2. Perioperative team members should use specific weight-based conversion charts or other technological devices for each of the major error-prone medications identified for the population at risk.

VII.b.3. When possible, pharmacists should be consulted to oversee calculations.

Recommendation VIII

The perioperative RN should implement the medication care plan by using safe medication practices to obtain, verify, prepare, and administer medications throughout all phases of perioperative care and in all perioperative settings.

Failure to follow current medication safety practices can lead to adverse effects.[4,9] Medication administration is performed at the intervention level of the nursing process. Medication administration is the point where the medication interfaces with the patient.[1] This phase is the point in the medication use process that represents the last opportunity to detect an error to avoid potential harm to the patient.

VIII.a. The perioperative RN should retrieve medications for only one patient at a time from storage bins or automated dispensing storage systems.

Retrieving medications for more than one patient at a time increases the risk for error.[135] Medication administration errors have occurred because a perioperative nurse retrieved the wrong product from an automated dispensing system.[18] If a restocking error has occurred, it is more likely to be caught if the nurse is focused on each medication required for the individual patient at the time the medication is being retrieved.

VIII.b. The perioperative RN should verify all medications retrieved against the original medication order or preference card.

The original medication order, including preprinted order forms, prescriptions, or preference cards, establishes what

dose errors can result from illegible hand-writing and incorrect placement of decimal points.[130] Wrong dose errors include either too much (ie, excessive) or too little of the intended medication. The most serious errors that have been reported in the OR include an excessive dose (20-fold extra) of heparin administered during a plastic surgery case, leading to loss of soft tissues, and a tenfold overdose of digoxin administered to an infant, resulting in cardiac toxicity and death.[4] In the outpatient setting, 3.3% of wrong-dose errors resulted in patient harm.[4]

Wrong time errors are defined as medication administration outside of the health care organization's parameters. A reported example involved a mannitol order that was delayed 5.5 hours from the time ordered postoperatively, resulting in increased intracranial pressure.[18]

Wrong route errors are defined as the medication being administered via a route other than intended. Wrong route errors are the second most commonly reported type of harmful medication errors.[4] Tubing misconnections often contribute to wrong route errors and have serious outcomes.[18,142] Examples of wrong route errors include antimicrobial agents intended for parenteral administration (eg, IV piggyback) being connected and infused through epidural or intrathecal catheters, and epidural medication infusions being connected to IV catheters. Other wrong route errors included IV fluids connected to indwelling catheters as bladder irrigants and a harmful case in which an antimicrobial agent delivered via IV piggyback was mistakenly connected to an external ventricular drain.[18] Cases also have been reported where magnesium sulfate was infused through epidural catheters instead of the intended mixture of local anesthetic and narcotic analgesics.[143]

VIII.h.1.   Perioperative personnel who administer medications should verify patient identification using at least two patient identifiers before administering medication.

VIII.h.2.   Perioperative personnel who administer medications should verify all medications just before administration, giving special consideration (eg, independent double check) to high-alert medications[82,144,145] and products that have been identified as high risk because they sound-alike or look-alike.

VIII.h.3.   Perioperative personnel who administer medications should verify the correct dose of the medication before administration. Medication dose verification should include, but not be limited to,
- confirming doses to be administered to vulnerable populations;
- using caution with medications that are available in multiple strengths or concentrations;
- using caution to draw up the proper dose of a medication that is packaged in a multidose container;
- using dosage conversion charts or electronic aids to calculate maximum dose limits, especially for high-alert medications;
- identifying out of range or toxic limits;
- confirming correct standard infusion pump settings; and
- recognizing special circumstances that require checks by two individuals, such as independent verification of high-alert doses and pain-controlled-analgesia pump settings, or that require independent confirmation of calculations for weight-based medications.

VIII.h.4.   Perioperative personnel who administer medications should verify the right medication administration time. Medication timing should include, but not be limited to,
- verifying the timing of antibiotic administration and
- collaborating with members of the perioperative team on what medications have been or are about to be administered.

VIII.h.5.   Perioperative personnel who administer medications should administer the medication via the right route. Considerations for the right medication route should include, but not be limited to,

- labeling multiple lines, catheters, and connection ports (eg, spinal, parenteral, drains, indwelling catheters);
- confirming the potential for adverse effects related to medication administration that is not consistent with manufacturer's recommendation (eg, rapid vancomycin infusion);[146] and
- verifying the integrity of the parenteral site.

VIII.h.6. Perioperative personnel who administer medications should have knowledge about the medication's intent for use and any contraindications. In confirming the right indication, perioperative personnel should identify considerations including, but not limited to,
- abnormal renal and hepatic function,
- off-label use for special populations (eg, pediatric use, pregnancy), and
- triggering agents for patients who are known to be susceptible to malignant hyperthermia.

VIII.h.7. Medications should be documented in the patient record as close as possible to the time they were administered.

VIII.i. Perioperative personnel who administer medications should follow the medication manufacturer's directions for use.

All medication products have an FDA-approved package insert with instructions for dosage and administration. Some medications have specific timing for administration.[146] Medication errors have been reported as a result of failure to follow manufacturer directions for administration.[4]

VIII.j. Perioperative personnel who administer medications should comply with constraints and forcing functions that have been initiated to minimize risks related to medication administration.

Constraints and forcing functions are human factors-proven interventions that reduce risk and are deployed at the sharp end of patient care.[6] Constraints are approaches that make a medication error difficult. Examples include dose limit protocols, automatic stop orders, redundant checks, and labeling all medications that are removed from their original containers. Another example of a constraint would be obtaining medication packaged in the final unit of use (ie, single-dose preparations). When there is extra product in the container, it increases the potential for the practitioner to draw up the entire amount, risking an overdose.

Forcing functions are approaches that reduce the potential for medication errors and are set around processes put into place that minimize opportunity for workarounds. Examples include removing certain medications (eg, cytotoxic agents, concentrations of saline higher than 0.9%) from the OR. Other examples include medical gas connectors (eg, oxygen versus nitrous) that are not interchangeable and password-protected access to electronic equipment or storage devices.[75]

VIII.k. Perioperative team members should implement known safe practices when identifying conditions related to medication administration that have been associated with adverse effects (eg, multiple tubings, potential confusion with patient names, equipment risks, handling sharps).

Multiple patient injuries have been caused by incorrect tubing connections. Tubing connections errors include
- blood pressure monitors connected to needleless IV ports,
- oxygen tubing connected to needleless IV ports, and
- enteral feeding systems connected to an IV catheter, peritoneal catheter, tracheostomy tube cuff, or medical gas tubing.[37-39]

Medication errors and omissions have been reported in association with medication-related equipment and sharps.[4,147]

VIII.k.1. Perioperative personnel who administer medications should implement known safe practices that minimize the risks associated with tubing including, but not limited to,
- tracing all tubing to the point of origin and point of insertion,
- labeling all tubing and injection ports,

- avoiding use of y-port extension tubing,
- aligning tubing to avoid tangling and to facilitate easy identification, and
- avoiding use of standard Luer-lock syringes for medications intended for oral or enteric administration.

VIII.k.2. Perioperative team members should implement safety practices that minimize the risk of administering medications to the wrong patient because of patients who have the same or similar names.

Implementing safety measures for patients who have the same or similar names is a risk-reduction strategy that has prevented a medication being administered to the wrong patient on several occasions.[148]

VIII.k.3. Perioperative team members should implement safety practices that minimize the risk from equipment including, but not limited to,
- eliminating free-flow IV tubing,
- programming non-smart IV pumps (eg, key-bounce errors),
- avoiding work-arounds associated with automated dispensing storage systems and other technologies,
- ensuring activation of all medication reconstitution devices (eg, planned IV piggybacks), and
- complying with sharps safety guidelines.

Recommendation IX

Safe medication practices should be used when transferring medications to, handling medications on, and administrating medications from the sterile field.

Transferring medications to the sterile field poses increased risks for contamination of the medication, the sterile field, or both. Information is displaced and verification processes are different because the medications are removed from their original containers.

Safe practices include accurately labeling medications in their new sterile containers to provide consistency for communication when handing off medications that will be administered on the sterile field. Hand offs involving multiple personnel increase the risk for miscommunication. Enhancing communication among the perioperative team has been recognized as a strategy to reduce medication errors.[4]

IX.a. Aseptic technique should be used when transferring medications to the sterile field.

Medication vials are not designed to aseptically pour the contents into a secondary container on the sterile field. Transfer devices are designed to minimize splashing, spilling, and the need to reach over the sterile field, which could cause contamination of the sterile field.

IX.a.1. The RN circulator should obtain commercially available sterile transfer devices (eg, sterile vial spike, filter straw, plastic catheter) to prepare products for aseptic presentation to the sterile field.

IX.a.2. Stoppers should not be removed from vials for the purpose of pouring medications.

IX.a.3. The RN circulator should check the expiration date and visually inspect the medication for any indication that the medication was compromised during the storage process (eg, particulates, discoloration) before transferring the medication to the sterile field. If there is any question of compromise, the item should not be transferred to the sterile field.

Medications that have signs of being compromised may have reduced effectiveness or could be contaminated.

IX.b. The RN circulator should transfer one medication at a time to the sterile field in an environment without distraction or interruption.

Focusing on transferring one medication at a time without distraction or interruption facilitates performance of aseptic technique and accurate identification of the medication being transferred.

IX.b.1. The RN circulator should confirm dose limits previously established before he or she transfers the medication to the sterile field.

IX.b.2. The RN circulator transferring the medication to the sterile field and the perioperative team member receiving the medication should concurrently verify the medication name, strength, dosage, and expiration date.

IX.b.3. If there is no designated scrub person, the RN circulator should confirm the medication visually and verbally with the licensed independent professional performing the procedure.

IX.c. Immediately upon receipt of the medication to the sterile field, the person receiving the medication should label the medication container. The label should include, at a minimum, the medication name, strength, and concentration.[149,150]

Fatal errors directly related to unlabeled containers of medication have been reported.[4,151-156] One study suggests that scrub personnel are more likely to label medications and medication-delivery devices when preprinted labels are provided.[150]

IX.c.1. The label should be confirmed by both the RN circulator and the scrub person.

IX.c.2. Any solution or medication found on the sterile field without an identification label should be discarded.

IX.d. Verbal confirmation should be given when handing medications to the licensed independent practitioner for subsequent administration, even when only one medication is on the sterile field.

A standardized method of communication helps reduce the risk of error involving medications on the sterile field.[4]

IX.e. All medications on the sterile field should be verified with the relief person during any personnel changes (eg, shift relief, breaks).

A standardized method of communication helps to reduce the risk of error involving medications on the sterile field.[4]

IX.f. Perioperative team members should use safe injection practices (eg, one syringe and one needle) when infiltrating medications (eg, local anesthetics) to multiple areas within the same surgical site.

Using needles and syringes more than once increases the risk of infection.

IX.f.1. A syringe and needle should be used only once to administer a medication to a single patient, after which the syringe and needle should be discarded. When administering incremental doses to a single patient from the same syringe is an integral part of the procedure, the same syringe and needle may be reused, with strict adherence to aseptic technique, for the same patient as part of a single procedure. The syringe should never be left unattended and should be discarded immediately at the end of the procedure.

IX.g. Perioperative team members should retain and isolate all delivery devices and original medication containers for medications that have been delivered to the sterile field until the end of the procedure.

The practice of maintaining possession of delivery devices and medication containers until the patient leaves the OR or invasive procedure room is important in the event of a medication-related error or adverse reaction.[153] Maintaining possession of these containers may facilitate the root cause analysis of an adverse event. Isolating broken ampoules or other glass containers may reduce the risk of sharps injuries.

IX.h. Unused, opened irrigation or IV solutions should be discarded at the end of the procedure.

Irrigation and IV containers and supplies are considered single-patient use. Using surplus volume from any irrigation or IV solution containers or supplies for more than one patient increases the risk of cross contamination.

Recommendation X

Perioperative team members should monitor the patient for therapeutic effect or adverse reactions to medications.

Evaluating and documenting the patient's physical, emotional, or psychological response to medications is part of the monitoring phase of the medication use process, which is the sixth and final phase. This phase allows an opportunity to detect both therapeutic and adverse effects of products, as well as detect errors.[1,4]

X.a. Perioperative team members should observe the patient for effectiveness of medications that are administered.

Monitoring the patient for effects of medications is a core principle of pharmacotherapy and is consistent with professional standards associated with the medication use process.[108,129]

X.a.1. Perioperative personnel should document patient responses as close as possible to the time the medication was administered and the response is observed.

X.a.2. As appropriate to their roles, perioperative team members should reevaluate ineffective responses to determine whether further investigation is warranted.

Reports indicate that health care professionals may divert pain medications and the patient may receive a replacement of lesser or no strength.[44,48,157] By evaluating the effectiveness for pain management and sedation (eg, amount given and expected response), perioperative team members may be able to correlate findings from patient assessment data with inventory management documents.

X.b. Perioperative team members should observe the patient for adverse reactions to medication and should document patient responses as close as possible to the time the response is observed.

Assessing and documenting the patient's response to medication provides vital information related to dose effectiveness and the presence of a potential medication-related adverse effect. Adverse effects of medication use include allergy (eg, anaphylaxis), toxicity, oversedation, and underusage.[4,18,151-156,158]

Immediate documentation of untoward effects is a medicolegal standard and contributes to planning, intervening, and supporting continuity of care. Documentation also serves as a means for systems review to improve processes related to medication use.

X.c. Perioperative team members should implement role-appropriate processes to detect and report potential hazards and near-misses, as well as actual medication errors.

Medication errors (eg, adverse effects) may occur earlier in the medication use process but can be detected in the monitoring phase.[4]

X.c.1. In the event of unexpected patient responses, all pertinent data and all the steps of the medication use process should be reviewed to determine a plausible explanation.

Recommendation XI

In final phases of the postanesthesia care (eg, phase 2 recovery), the perioperative RN should coordinate patient education plans that are focused on discharge and aftercare instructions related to medication use.

Clearly delineated postprocedural orders provide the basis for patient safety after the patient leaves the health care organization. Adherence to aftercare instructions is an essential component to facilitate recovery and prevent complications. After discharge, patients and their designated support person(s) are often responsible for incorporating new postprocedure medications into their old medication regimens and identifying symptoms of reactions and monitoring for effectiveness.[159] Effective communication between the patient, designated support person(s), and perioperative team members enhances the patient's capacity for medication self-management after discharge.[17,160]

XI.a. The perioperative RN should review postprocedure physician medication orders, resolve any discrepancies, and plan care accordingly.

Reviewing the medication orders before the patient is discharged is a strategy to reduce medication errors or omissions after the patient leaves the health care organization.

XI.a.1. When reviewing patient medications after a surgical or other invasive procedure, the perioperative RN should understand the procedure performed and the patient's preexisting conditions before he or she compares those considerations with the medications prescribers have initiated, resumed, or discontinued to verify medications are consistent with the therapeutic objective and relevant medical history.

XI.a.2. Perioperative RNs should clarify medication orders that are not specific including, but not limited to, "resume previous orders."

The Joint Commission discourages prescribers from resuming previous orders.[161] Improving communication between physicians who are writing discharge orders and patients' primary care physicians has been identified as a key issue for promoting effective transitions of care at discharge.[159]

XI.b. Using the medication reconciliation process, the perioperative RN should collaborate with physicians and pharmacists to develop effective medication plans for educating patients and their designated support persons at the time of discharge.

Discrepancies found through the medication reconciliation process often occur at the discharge phase of care.[162] Effective medication reconciliation is a strategy to promote safe patient outcomes by reducing opportunities for errors and detecting duplicate therapies.[112,163,164] Researchers have reported that patients whose medications are electronically reconciled have a greater understanding of medication administration and the potential adverse effects of the medications they are taking at the time of hospital discharge.[165] Some medications (eg, oral antidiabetic agent metformin) cause complications (eg, contrast-induced nephropathy) if resumed too soon after the procedure.[166,167] Researchers report that patients who have a prescription to take warfarin are more likely to discontinue the medication after

an overnight hospitalization for elective surgery or an ambulatory procedure compared with the general population.[168] There is a need for active communication between patients and their prescribers about when to resume anticoagulation therapy because there is increased potential for miscommunication when the prescriber discontinuing the medication therapy is different from the prescriber expected to write the order for resuming the therapy.[168]

Patients and the people who support them may be at risk for medication errors or less effective treatment when they have limited health literacy that influences their ability to understand instructions on prescription medication labels.[169,170] Using appropriate teaching strategies based on the patient's needs (eg, learning readiness, language preference, cognitive ability) and adjusting teaching strategies based on feedback are key components of the AORN "Standards of perioperative nursing" that can be applied at the time of patient discharge.[108]

XI.b.1. The discharge medication plan should include instructions for the patient to follow up with the primary care provider to determine when to resume maintenance medications (eg, medications for blood pressure, diabetes).

XI.b.2. The discharge medication plan should include follow-up instructions regarding laboratory tests that may be needed to assess levels of medications.

XI.b.3. The discharge medication plan should specify when to discontinue medications.

XI.b.4. The discharge medication plan should include provisions for patients and their designated support persons who cannot read or when English is the second language.

XI.c. The perioperative RN should use the discharge medication plan to educate patients and their designated support persons about how to implement the plan in their aftercare setting.

Patient-centered care is facilitated by linking the procedure just performed and preexisting conditions to the medication plan. Teaching enhances compliance with the medication plan.[17,49,171]

Because medication labels and the medication package inserts are often confusing, patients and the people who support them in aftercare need access to up-to-date information (eg, patient education fact sheets, online resources) about how to use their medications safely.[5,51]

XI.c.1. The perioperative RN should instruct patients and their designated support persons regarding medication use in the aftercare setting.[164,170] Instructions should include, but not be limited to,

- emphasizing the importance of carrying a medication list that has up-to-date information, including prescriptions, over-the-counter medications, and dietary supplements[17] and

- explaining how to schedule, administer, and use adjunct equipment and supplies.

XI.d. The perioperative RN should be familiar with state pharmacy laws regarding dispensing medications.

State pharmacy laws vary regarding dispensing medications for patient use. Pharmacists are accountable for ensuring compliance with state laws pertaining to dispensing medications for aftercare use.[10,11]

XI.d.1. Facility-based pharmacists should be available if any medications or pharmaceutical products are to be sent home with the patient from the perioperative area. Partially used solutions (eg, ear drops, eye drops) should only be sent home with the patient after being properly labeled by a pharmacist in a manner that is consistent with state pharmacy laws regarding dispensing.

XI.e. The perioperative RN should coordinate medication orders, written or electronic, with third-party providers.

The complexity of aftercare requires coordination with third-party providers (eg, pharmacy, durable medical equipment, home health agencies) to ensure appropriate medications, equipment (eg, patient-controlled analgesia pump), and supplies are available for aftercare use by patients or their designated support persons.

XI.f. The perioperative RN should perform an aftercare assessment (eg, telephone call).

Aftercare patient assessment is a safety strategy that can identify patient status, response to medications, actual adverse conditions (eg, nausea, vomiting, ineffective pain control, inability to perform activities of daily living), and knowledge and compliance with the medication plan. Additional elements (eg, infection prevention, wound care/management, patient satisfaction) also can be collected during the aftercare assessment.[160]

XI.f.1. The perioperative RN performing the aftercare patient assessment should document the findings as soon as possible and take action as appropriate.

XI.g. Perioperative RNs and pharmacists should be involved in developing suitable aftercare medication written instruction forms that take into consideration age-specific requirements (eg, large print), special populations (eg, readability and suitability, language requirements), and health literacy.[10,11,17]

Enhancing communication about medications and enabling patients to better understand their medications can be accomplished by creating a patient-friendly medication schedule tool.[116] Safety issues (eg, incorrect dispensing of eardrops instead of eyedrops; patient self administering with glaucoma eye drops instead of anti-inflammatory eye drops) have been reported with look-alike, sound-alike ophthalmic medications.[172] Patients who have limited or impaired vision may need additional care to encourage them to verify labels on medications that will be used at home after discharge. Including direct caregivers in the development of patient teaching tools enhances the effectiveness of the tools because they can supply information based on patient feedback.[116]

Recommendation XII

A comprehensive safety program should be developed to identify special care and handling of hazardous medications that are used in perioperative environments.

To be in compliance with the Occupational Safety and Health Administration (OSHA) hazard communication standard, health care organizations are required to have practice-specific assessments for hazardous medications that are used within the organization.[173,174]

XII.a. The health care organization must have a hazard communication program that identifies a continually updated list of hazardous medications that may be encountered by perioperative staff members. The list of hazardous medications must be posted to ensure worker safety.[173,174]

Hazard communication programs help inform health care workers about the risk of exposure to medications that are defined as hazardous but that have dosage formulations that are solid or intact (eg, coated tablets or capsules) and may not pose a significant risk of direct occupational exposure unless they are altered (eg, crushing tablets, making solutions from capsules outside of a ventilated cabinet).[174]

XII.a.1. A current material safety data sheet must be immediately available for all hazardous medications that are used in the workplace.[173,175]

XII.b. Hazardous medications or solutions should be stored in segregated areas with clear signage and warning labels.

Clear signage and warning labels in storage areas separate from other medications helps to reduce the risk of errors in medication administration and the risk of injury to the health care worker. Immediately available spill kits and waste containers facilitates containment of spilled hazardous substances and reduces the risk of injury to persons in the area.[176,177]

XII.b.1. Spill kits and waste containers for hazardous medications should be stored with hazardous medications or solutions in the storage area.

XII.c. Hazardous medications should be transported in sealed containers with Luer caps and no needles attached. The transport container should be
- leak proof,
- resistant to breakage, and
- labeled with warning labels to alert personnel that contents are hazardous.[174,178]

XII.d. Personnel handling hazardous medications should wear personal protective equipment (PPE) consistent with the type of exposure that can reasonably be anticipated. Personal protective equipment should include the following:
- chemical protective gowns and two pairs of gloves when handling hazardous medications in the storage area or transporting hazardous medications to the point of use,[176,178]
- face shields when there is a potential for splashing or splattering, and
- gloves.

An impervious or chemotherapy-rated gown protects perioperative team members' skin, especially on the arms and torso, from exposure to the hazardous medication when reconstituting or admixing medications.[174,170]

Face shields protect mucous membranes, skin, and eyes from injury that can be caused by some cytotoxic agents.[174]

Double-gloving and changing the outer glove after contact with hazardous medications protects perioperative team members from exposure when administering or handling open containers of chemotherapy drugs.[174]

XII.d.1. Gloves worn for chemotherapy administration should meet the American Society for Testing and Materials D 6978 standards.[179]

XII.e. Perioperative team members should follow the medication manufacturer's recommendations for cleaning and handling of instrumentation exposed to the chemotherapeutic agent, for disposal of body fluids of patients receiving chemotherapeutic agents, and for disposal of unused medication.

Some cytotoxic agents leave a residue on instruments and require specific PPE and cleaning techniques. Traces of the medication may be retained in body fluids, making special disposal considerations necessary. Hazardous medications may have different disposal requirements than other medications.

XII.f. The hazardous medication safety plan should include medical surveillance of personnel who handle cytotoxic agents.

Cytotoxic drugs have the potential to cause serious health risks to health care workers who are exposed to them.[176] These medications are often mutagenic, carcinogenic, and teratogenic and may cause local injury when they come into direct contact with skin, eyes, or mucous membranes.[180] Safe levels of exposure to these drugs have not been determined by OSHA, and no reliable system is currently available to monitor exposure levels.[175]

Recommendation XIII

Medications should be disposed of according to local, state, and federal regulations; manufacturer's instructions; and health care organization policy.

A medication may be classified as a controlled substance or a medical hazardous waste and have federal, state, or local requirements for disposal. Factors influencing the decision for how to dispose of medication waste include the ease of, access to, and cost of disposal.[181]

The Resource Conservation and Recovery Act is the federal law for management and disposal of solid and hazardous waste.[69,182] Hazardous and non-hazardous waste regulations are defined by the Environmental Protection Agency and enforced at both the federal and state levels.[183]

The FDA web site is a source for information on medications that are safe to be flushed. Restrictions on flushing pharmaceuticals and related waste can be found in the federal Clean Water Act,[184] as well as in state and local regulations. Fines and warnings of future penalties may be issued for failure to comply with restrictions for disposing of pharmaceutical waste into waterways.[69]

XIII.a. Perioperative RNs should collaborate with pharmacists to determine compliance with federal, state, or local regulations and man-

ufacturer recommendations for disposal of hazardous medications or solutions.

In general, about 5% of pharmaceuticals are considered hazardous because they have one or more of the following characteristics: waste ignitability, corrosivity, reactivity, or toxicity.[69,182,183] Hormonal agents and hazardous medications may not be identified as hazardous waste at the federal level but may be managed as hazardous waste at the state level.[178] Because of the complexity of hazardous pharmaceutical waste disposal, pharmacy consultation may be necessary to determine compliance.[183]

XIII.a.1. Medications should be disposed of by one of the following methods:
- returning to the manufacturer,
- donating the unused portion for reuse,
- flushing down the drain,
- disposing into a landfill, or
- incinerating.[181]

XIII.a.2. Medication disposal should be performed in a manner that does not contaminate the water supply. When prescription medications are not labeled as safe for flushing, pharmacists should advise health care workers as to the appropriate method for disposal at the point of use or if the item should be returned to the pharmacy for proper disposal.[69]

XIII.b. Perioperative RNs should collaborate with pharmacy personnel to develop processes for determining the proper methods of disposal and how unused and unopened medications in the medication storage areas are to be returned to the pharmacy.

Medication storage and control are important components of the medication management system.[43] Returning medications to pharmacies increases the accuracy for accounting for unused medications. Returning unopened medications to pharmacies may increase the chances for exchanging the medications to avoid outdates and consequent waste.

XIII.c. Perioperative personnel who administer medications or handle medications within their scope of practice must follow established practices to validate controlled substance (Schedule II to IV) waste.

Licensed individuals are accountable for adhering to the Controlled Substance Act. Such adherence extends to retrieving and administering medication, and documenting the wasting of unused products.[45]

XIII.c.1. Licensed perioperative team members should participate in inventory management of controlled substances.

XIII.c.2. Licensed perioperative team members should waste unused scheduled medications in accordance with federal regulations and health care organization policy.

Recommendation XIV

Perioperative personnel should receive initial and ongoing education and demonstrate competency in the performance of safe medication practices at least on an annual basis.

Initial and periodic education on safe medication practices provides direction for personnel in providing safe patient care. Additional periodic educational programs provide opportunities to reinforce previous learning and introduce new information on adjunct technology, its use, and potential risks. Competency validation serves as an indicator that personnel have an understanding of safe medication practices. Evolving technology interfaces associated with infusion pumps, computerized order entry, and automated dispensing systems require initial and ongoing training to achieve the benefit of equipment designed to reduce medication errors.[21,25,185]

XIV.a. An introduction to and review of policies and procedures for safe medication practices should be included in orientation and ongoing education of personnel.

Reviewing policies and procedures assists health care personnel in developing knowledge, skills, and attitudes that affect patient outcomes.

XIV.b. At a minimum, education, training, and competency validation should address the following areas:
- the medication use process;

- at-risk behaviors in perioperative settings;
- the nurse's role in medication reconciliation;
- medications associated with emergency care;
- education tools for patients and their support persons about prescribed medications;
- pharmaceutical waste; and
- new regulations, technology, and procedures relevant to safe medication practices.

XIV.b.1. Competency validation should be documented.

Documented competency validation serves as a basis for staff development, quality improvement, and performance evaluation. Documentation tools facilitate objectivity and consistency and remove subjectivity from the validation process.

XIV.c. Perioperative team members who handle medication products should demonstrate competency in the procuring process.

Product shortages occur in the procuring phase of the medication use process. Automatically substituting other medication products increases the risk for human errors.[186] When perioperative team members understand the medication purchasing process for perioperative patient care areas and participate in or serve on medication safety committees, more clinically relevant decisions can be made to reduce the risk for human errors.

XIV.c.1. Education should include product packaging considerations (eg, single-dose, multidose vials, inner sterile wrap), bioequivalent issues, and pharmacotherapeutic issues that potentially increase the risk for error.

XIV.c.2. Education and competency validation should include safety considerations related to medication inventory and par levels including, but not limited to,
- standardizing strength and concentration,

- identifying distinct pairs for look-alike, sound-alike medication products,
- separating look-alike medication products, and
- disseminating information about product shortages and recalls.

XIV.c.3. Education should include risk-reduction strategies for inventory management including, but not limited to,
- establishing temperature control for medications,
- rotating stock,
- processing product returns, including outdated medications, and
- securing medication inventory (ie, both scheduled and non-scheduled products).

XIV.d. Education and competency validation should include barriers to successful prescribing including, but not limited to,
- determining scope of practice boundaries;
- recognizing what constitutes prescribing;
- receiving and processing verbal, written, or electronic orders; and
- maintaining preference cards and standing order forms.

Educating perioperative team members about the parameters of the perioperative prescribing process is a strategy designed to reduce opportunities for adverse events. By establishing a broad understanding and appreciation of how their role supports accuracy in the prescribing process, perioperative team members are more likely to be accountable for ensuring the accuracy of verbal and standing orders.

XIV.e. Education should include the risks inherent to the transcribing process.

From a national perspective, approximately 22% of the reported errors occurred at the point of transcribing.[4]

XIV.f. Education and competency validation should include barriers to successful dispensing.

There are variations in dispensing processes across perioperative settings. Educating perioperative team members about safety parameters that are designed into the dispensing phase of the medication use process is a strategy intended to improve compliance with medication verification and accuracy before the medication intersects with direct patient care.

XIV.f.1. Education and competency validation should include retrieving or returning medications from automated dispensing storage systems or medication storage areas.

XIV.f.2. Education should include the pharmacist's role regarding safety parameters in the dispensing process.

In the dispensing process, pharmacists review medication orders, prepare products for perioperative use, serve as consultants to perioperative team members, and participate in inventory management with automatic dispensing systems. Some perioperative settings do not have a direct opportunity for pharmacists' participation and, therefore, have reduced support in the dispensing process. Educating perioperative team members about pharmacists' contributions at the dispensing phase will increase their awareness of safety parameters that are necessary to build into safe medication practices in perioperative settings.

XIV.g. Perioperative team members should demonstrate competency appropriate to their roles in the perioperative medication administration process.

Through education, perioperative RNs are able to exercise critical judgment in administering medications with the intent to reduce infections and adverse medication events. Licensed individuals other than RNs have multiple ways to demonstrate competency, such as medical staff appointment processes (eg, credentialing process), peer review, and quality reports. Through education, unlicensed personnel are able to demonstrate appropriate handling of medications (eg, labeling, handing off).

Medication errors occur at the administration phase and across all phases of care in perioperative settings.[4] Knowledge and performance deficits and calculation errors have been reported among the five leading causes of pediatric medication errors.[130] Effective training, education, and support are identified as key elements to the success of using computer-entry systems to reduce medication errors.[185]

XIV.g.1. Perioperative RNs should demonstrate age-specific competencies in obtaining, preparing, and administering medications.

XIV.g.2. Perioperative team members should demonstrate competency in aseptic technique when preparing, handling, and administering medications.

XIV.g.3. Perioperative team members should demonstrate competency appropriate to their roles regarding recommended safety practices for medication administration including, but not limited to,
- confirming the medication with visual and verbal validation,
- labeling medications on the sterile field,
- labeling medications when outside of their original container regardless of the perioperative setting, and
- confirming safe dosage limits and dosage calculations.

XIV.g.4. Perioperative team members should demonstrate competency appropriate to their roles related to safe injection practices including, but not limited to,
- using one needle per injection,
- using one syringe per injection, and
- complying with sharps safety measures.

XIV.g.5. Perioperative team members should demonstrate competency appropriate to their roles related to the use of medication containers, adjunct equipment, and supplies including, but not limited to,
- ampoules;
- filtered needles for use with ampoules;
- devices used to transfer medications to the sterile field;
- infusion pumps;
- volume injectors;

- IV and irrigation tubing and connectors; and
- syringes, needles, stopcocks, and sharp-safety systems.

XIV.g.6. Perioperative team members should demonstrate competency appropriate to their roles related to documenting medication administration.

XIV.g.7. Perioperative team members should be able to describe how the following conditions act as barriers to successful medications administration:
- hand off, shift relief, and breaks;
- noise;
- distractions;
- lighting;
- interruptions;
- muffled voices through masks;
- regional dialects; and
- staff member age-related sensory changes (eg, hearing, vision).

XIV.g.8. Perioperative team members should demonstrate safe handling of hazardous medications and solutions (eg, cytotoxic and chemotherapeutic agents) including, but not limited to,
- preventing exposure,
- managing spills,
- disposing of hazardous wastes, and
- handling of instruments that are exposed to chemotherapeutic agents. Education and competency validation of the perioperative team members who work with the hazardous agents are essential to minimize exposure and promote workplace safety.[174,175]

XIV.h. Perioperative team members should demonstrate competency appropriate to their roles in monitoring patients' responses to medications including, but not limited to, recognizing
- effectiveness,
- ineffective responses, and
- adverse reactions to medications.

Education helps to support perioperative team members in exercising critical judgment in evaluating patients' physical, emotional, or psychological responses to the medication and recording such findings.[46]

XIV.h.1. Perioperative team members should demonstrate competency appropriate to their roles related to documenting patients' responses to medications.

XIV.h.2. Perioperative team members should be able to describe how the following conditions act as barriers to successful monitoring:
- shift changes,
- interruptions,
- noise,
- distractions, and
- patient transfers to other phases of perioperative care.

XIV.i. Perioperative team members should demonstrate competency in emergency medication administration and management (eg, malignant hyperthermia, cardiac arrest, respiratory depression).

XIV.i.1. Education should include mock drills for malignant hyperthermia, cardiac arrest, and other emergencies related to adverse medication responses.

Mock drills help perioperative team members develop critical thinking skills.

XIV.j. Education sessions for perioperative team members should be initiated when new regulations, technologies, and procedures related to safe medication practices become available.

Regulations regarding pharmaceutical waste and safe medication administration continue to be updated. Technologies and new procedures relating to safe medication practices continue to evolve. When perioperative team members are up to date on recent regulatory developments and new equipment or product trends, they will be better prepared to comply with regulations, identify safety issues, and take appropriate actions.

Recommendation XV

Perioperative team members, consistent with their roles, should document all activities related to the medication use process throughout all phases of perioperative patient care.

Documentation throughout the medication use process is a professional medicolegal standard. Documentation is applicable at the systems level and the patient care level. At the systems level, documentation serves as basis for monitoring compliance and measuring performance. At the patient care level, documentation facilitates continuity of patient care through clear communication and supports collaboration between health care team members.

XV.a. Perioperative team member participation in the procuring process should be documented in a retrievable manner (eg, committee minutes, logs, reports).

Documentation serves as the medicolegal standard to measure adherence with safety practices including, but not limited to,
- selecting standardized products for use;
- rotating stock;
- returning products, including outdated medications;
- securing medication inventory (ie, both scheduled and non-scheduled products);
- reversing distribution or disposing of unused medications; and
- controlling temperature for temperature-sensitive medications.

XV.b. Perioperative team members' involvement in the prescribing process should be documented in a manner that is consistent with their roles and scopes of practice.

Documentation serves as the medicolegal standard to measure adherence with prescribing processes.

XV.b.1. Medication orders, regardless of origin (eg, standing, verbal, written, electronic), should be documented and signed by the prescriber.

XV.b.2. Medication orders should be legible and reflect legible signatures of the prescriber initiating the order and the caregiver transcribing the verbal order.

It is the responsibility of the health care practitioner, in concert with the health care organization, to ensure that documentation clearly and unambiguously reflects the individualized treatment of the patient. Having all health care providers use block print and sign their names to all written and verbal orders is one risk-reduction strategy designed to improve communication among caregivers. The extra step of block-printing the name of the prescriber affords the caregiver an opportunity to contact the provider if a question, concern, or issue were to arise related to the written order. If the receiver of the order is unable to hear the order correctly or the caregiver is unable to read the written order, confusion or misinterpretation could result and lead to an adverse patient event.[4]

XV.b.3. Verbal and telephone orders should be authenticated with the prescriber's signature and date and time.

XV.b.4. Standing medication orders should contain evidence of periodic review for accuracy.

Medication errors can occur from a failure to update standing orders or to individualize patient care by assessing the standing order for appropriateness to a specific patient condition or clinical situation.[3] One study revealed that intraoperative standing orders in the form of preference cards increased the risk of potential medication errors.[91] The following were among the major concerns from the study findings:

• Surgeons were not double-checking changes made to the preference cards.

• Medications listed on the preference cards were not what the surgeon wanted or intended to use.[91]

In another study, researchers implemented preprinted physician orders for pediatric procedural sedation and reported an increase in documentation compliance (ie, legibility, completeness) and a decrease in medication ordering errors.[89]

XV.c. Perioperative team members' involvement in the transcribing process should be docu-

mented in a manner that is consistent with their roles.

Documentation serves as the medicolegal standard to measure adherence with transcribing processes.

XV.d. Perioperative team members' involvement in the dispensing process should be documented in a manner that is consistent with their roles and scopes of practice.

Documentation serves as the medicolegal standard to measure adherence with dispensing processes.

XV.d.1. Documentation should reflect a pharmacist's review of all medication orders. Automated dispensing systems and pharmacy computer systems may be used to document pharmacist validation of medication orders.[21]

XV.e. Medications administered should be documented in a manner that
– is legible and easily accessible,
– is free of unapproved abbreviations and acronyms,
– is timely,
– identifies the concentrations of the medication and solutions administered and the route of administration,
– identifies the person who administered the medication, and
– indicates total amounts administered when there are multiple injections of the same medication (eg, lidocaine) administered during a procedure.

Documentation serves as the medicolegal standard to measure adherence with administering processes. Documenting the total amount of medication administered when a medication is administered repeatedly over a course of time decreases the risk of injecting medications at toxic levels.

XV.e.1 Documentation should reflect that Schedule II through V products that were not administered to the patient were disposed of in accordance with local, state, and federal law, as well as with the health care organization's policy.

XV.f. Documentation should reflect patient responses to administered medications.

Documentation serves as the medico-legal standard to measure adherence with monitoring processes.

XV.f.1. In the presence of ineffective response or adverse events, documentation should reflect actions initiated or interventions that were implemented.

XV.g. Documentation should reflect the discharge process related to medication reconciliation and the instructions presented to patients and their designated support persons for medications.[187]

Documentation serves as the medico-legal standard to measure adherence with medication reconciliation processes and to reflect the patient's or designated support person's response to the instructions given about medications.

XV.h. Documentation should reflect the aftercare process including, but not limited to, a nursing evaluation of the patient's postprocedure progress and follow-up activities that are deemed necessary based on the aftercare phone call.

Documentation serves as the medicolegal standard to measure adherence to aftercare processes.

XV.i. Medication documentation should include correct placement of zeroes and be free of unapproved abbreviations, acronyms, symbols, and dose designations.

Confusing or easily misinterpreted abbreviations, acronyms, or symbols put caregivers at risk of making errors and compromising patient safety.[188] A misplaced decimal point, a "U" interpreted as a "0" (zero), "QOD" confused with "QID," or "AS" misinterpreted as "OS" puts patients at risk for medical errors with potentially serious results (eg, overdose, inadequate dose, omission due to laterality error, wrong medication administered, error in frequency of administration). Improving communication by reducing abbreviations, acronyms, and symbols is a significant step toward reducing the occurrence of errors related to the inability to accurately read and interpret written medical orders and transcribed verbal orders.[189]

Computer systems designed for medication documentation may increase the risk of errors when their programs include
– abbreviated medication names because of character length limitations,
– medication names listed in alphabetical order without mixed-case lettering or alternating colored lines as differentiators, or
– unclear expressions of drug dosages (eg, 40000 versus 40,000).[185]

XV.i.1. Documentation should reflect that the minimally required list of do-not-use items in the health care organization's policy has been augmented to include problem-prone, high-risk, and high-volume abbreviations, acronyms, and symbols that are unique to medications in the perioperative practice setting.

XV.i.2. Abbreviations related to laterality should not be used when documenting activities related to medications.

XV.i.3. Documentation should include leading zeroes (eg, 0.X mg rather than .X mg) and be free of trailing zeroes (eg, X mg rather than X.0 mg).

XV.i.4. Medication orders should not be numbered.

XV.j. Across all perioperative settings and all phases of the medication use process, perioperative RNs should incorporate the Perioperative Nursing Data Set (PNDS) taxonomy when documenting medications whenever possible.

The PNDS is the standardized perioperative nursing vocabulary.[190] Standardized documentation promotes nursing research.

Recommendation XVI

Policies and procedures for safe medication practices should be developed, readily available in the practice setting, and reviewed periodically, and they should address direct patient care situations as well as organizational level situations.

Policies and procedures are the operational guidelines that can be used to minimize patient risk factors while strategically linking the health care organization's mission to its day-to-day operations. Policies and procedures establish authority, responsibility, and accountability within the organization. Policies and procedures assist perioperative team members in developing guidelines for continuous performance improvement and activities that support patient safety.

In addition to dosing errors and miscommunication, ineffective policies have been reported as one of the main categories associated with causes of error.[130] Policies are needed in perioperative settings to help clarify the increased complexities that occur at several points in the medication use process, including communications related to verbal orders, medications removed from original containers, and sensory distractions.[130] In addition, policies may help with improving inconsistent practices for communicating current and previous medication regimens (ie, medication reconciliation) and reporting drug diversion in perioperative settings.[44,130] Administrative policies that are developed with participation from a variety of perspectives are more likely to provide guidance at the point of care, including education and training and appropriate documentation, as well as to provide for workplace safety and to set the tone for a culture of safety.

XVI.a. Policies and procedures should be developed collaboratively by stakeholders who are knowledgeable and are willing to advocate for safe practices in the various phases of the medication use process.

Involving all stakeholders in the process strengthens policies and procedures, contributes to interprofessional respect, and enhances teamwork and, therefore, compliance.

XVI.a.1. Stakeholders who are involved in policy and procedure development should be willing to advocate for culturally sensitive medication practices within the communities served including, but not limited to,
- age-specific populations,
- special populations (eg, women's services, ophthalmology, oncology), and
- ethnically diverse populations.

XVI.a.2. Stakeholders should help identify the types of resources that should be provided to the perioperative team via policies and procedures. Examples include, but are not limited to,
- up-to-date online reference materials,
- access to Drug Information Centers, and
- defined parameters for supplemental staff members (eg, agency nurse, consulting pharmacist).

XVI.a.3. Stakeholders in the medication use process should identify barriers and solutions to achieving immediate access to medication safety policies and procedures at the time needed regardless of setting.

Ready access to policies and procedures provides clarity and guidance and reduces variance across the medication use process.

XVI.b. Perioperative administrators should conduct a periodic review of the policies and procedures for the health care organization's medication use process that is specific enough to consider external changes in medication safety best practices and the regulatory landscape in which the organization must comply.

Periodic reviews identify new knowledge, new regulatory guidelines, and internal limitations or weaknesses that may exist in the medication use process, as well as determine continued relevance to setting.

XVI.c. Policies and procedures should promote safe medication practices throughout the medication use process and establish authority, responsibility, and accountability at the point of care.

Establishing authority, responsibility, and accountability for medication use at the point of care is a risk-reduction strategy that supports patient safety by facilitating development of quality assessment measures and guidelines for continuous performance improvement. The framework created through the health care organization's policies and procedures pertaining to medication-use-process activities contributes to patient safety by aligning perioperative team members' roles and responsibilities with their respective scopes of practice.

XVI.c.1. Policies and procedures for procuring medications should include, but not be limited to,
- therapeutic considerations for formulary management (eg, generation of antibiotics, addition of new products to formulary);
- packaging considerations (eg, standardization, look-alike, sound-alike, unit of use);
- security for medication inventory (ie, both scheduled and non-scheduled products);
- rotation of stock (eg, first in, first out);
- plans for medication disposal (eg, unused, outdated) and product returns; and
- standardization of all locations where medications are stored including, but not limited to,
  - anesthesia carts,
  - emergency medication carts,
  - refrigerators, freezers, or warmers,
  - automated dispensing storage systems,
  - satellite pharmacies,
  - storage areas with controlled access, and
  - storage devices associated with scheduled substances.

XVI.c.2. Policies and procedures for prescribing medications should include, but not be limited to,
- what constitutes prescribing;
- parameters regarding who can prescribe;
- the format (eg, verbal, written, electronic) for medication prescribing;
- clear medication orders (eg, no unapproved abbreviations);
- a process for creating, maintaining, and reviewing preference cards and standing order forms;
- verbal order verification (eg, read back, whiteboard);
- environmental conditions that interfere with successful prescribing (eg, noise, interruptions);[134] and
- forcing functions and constraints when appropriate.

When the health care organization has an electronic environment for prescribing medications (eg, CPOE system), the policies and procedures should be consistent with information technology policies for user verification and password security.

XVI.c.3. Policies and procedures for transcribing medications should include, but not be limited to,
- the roles and responsibilities of the person involved in transcribing;
- the health care organization's specific forms (eg, medication administration record);
- a process for verifying accurate patient identification on all forms;
- the process for documenting that the order has been transcribed; and
- how to transmit the order to the pharmacy for processing, if appropriate.

XVI.c.4. Policies and procedures for dispensing medications should include, but not be limited to,
- what constitutes dispensing;
- parameters regarding who can dispense;
- pharmacy or a comparable type of oversight for medication management processes;
- par levels of medications in storage areas, including automated dispensing storage systems;
- a process for retrieving or returning medications from automated dispensing storage systems or medication storage areas;
- a process for how medications are prepared (eg, compliance with *The United States Pharmacopeia* Chapter <797> guidelines[104]);
- forcing functions for certain medications; and
- a process for restocking medication storage areas, including automated dispensing storage systems (ie, replenishment).

XVI.c.5. Policies and procedures for administering medications should include, but not be limited to,
- what constitutes medication administering;
- parameters regarding who can administer what medications;
- forcing functions and constraints when appropriate;
- weight-based dose conversion charts into practice;
- practices that incorporate the use of at least two patient identifiers to medication order;
- competencies and verification processes for administering medications;
- use of labels when medications are removed from their original containers;
- guidelines for holding all containers until the end of the procedure;
- disposal of unused medications and containers;
- compliance with federal regulations (eg, Controlled Substances Act[45] Resource Conservation and Recovery Act[182]); and
- documentation of all medications administered, including compliance with documentation standards and do-not-use abbreviations and symbols.

XVI.c.6. Policies and procedures should define the role of perioperative team members with regard to monitoring patients' responses to medications. Considerations should include, but not be limited to,
- parameters (eg, how long, how often) for observing patients' responses to medications,
- competencies for monitoring patients' responses to medications, and
- documentation of nursing activities related to the monitoring process (eg, evaluation findings, steps taken for adverse reactions).

XVI.d. Policies and procedures should establish authority, responsibility, and accountability, consistent with scope of practice boundaries, for safe medication practices and should be standardized across all phases of perioperative patient care.

Standardizing the process for transfer of medication information with the broader process for transferring perioperative patient care information provides consistency and improves the accuracy, reliability, and quality of the information reported.[191]

XVI.d.1. Policies and procedures should define the roles of perioperative team members with regard to the medication reconciliation, discharge, and aftercare processes.

In addition to policies for the medication use process, policies for other processes that involve medications (eg, medication reconciliation, discharge, aftercare, transfer of information) provide a framework for safe patient care.[192]

XVI.d.2. Contents of the medication transfer-of-patient-information report for each phase of perioperative care should include, but not be limited to, the following:

Preoperative phase:
- medication allergies;
- medication side effects;
- vital signs (eg, temperature, pulse, respiration, blood pressure);
- pain assessment; and
- medication profile, including preoperative medications.

Intraoperative phase:
- medication allergies;
- medication side effects;
- anesthesia type and route;
- current or pending laboratory or other test results that relate to medications;
- medications administered, including dose and time; and
- administered IV and irrigation fluids.

Postoperative phase:
- anesthesia type and route;
- anesthesia professional's orders related to IV medications;
- infusion pump settings;

procurement process to examine areas including, but not limited to,

- identifying inventory items with sound-alike, look-alike drug names;
- identifying inventory items with similar packaging;
- restricting types of medications and concentrations based on pharmacy and therapeutics committee recommendations;
- defining processes for product shortage situations;
- defining processes for determining replacement systems when recalls or system malfunction trends are identified; and
- defining processes for reverse distribution of unopened, unused, or expired products.

XVII.a.2. Perioperative prescribers should develop proactive risk-reduction strategies for the prescribing process including, but not limited to,

- adopting electronic health records,
- avoiding verbal orders,
- using clear handwriting without abbreviations,
- standardizing forms, and
- using Beers criteria.

XVII.a.3. Perioperative team members should develop risk-reduction strategies for the transcribing process including, but not limited to,

- clearly communicating medication orders in the medication administration record or the perioperative record and
- minimizing manual order transcription.

XVII.a.4. Perioperative team members should develop risk-reduction strategies for the dispensing process including, but not limited to,

- controlling and recording access to inventory management when perioperative staff members obtain medications,
- developing a methodology for accurate replenishing of automated dis-

pensing storage systems within an established time frame, and

- implementing processes for irrigant and solution preparation by pharmacy staff members.

XVII.a.5. Perioperative team members should develop risk-reduction strategies for the administering process including, but not limited to,

- increasing the use of technology (eg, bar coding, dose confirmation software),
- standardizing and simplifying dosing charts,
- reporting medication allergies and medication contraindications,
- verifying timing of prophylactic antibiotics, and
- ensuring timely and adequate documentation.

XVII.a.6. Perioperative team members should develop risk-reduction strategies for the monitoring process including, but not limited to,

- auditing for documentation of the effects of medications and
- selecting appropriate equipment for use in the medication use process (eg, smart infusion pumps, adjunct equipment).

XVII.a.7. When making financial investments for performance-improvement strategies related to computer-entry or computer-related errors, considerations should include

- training programs for health care practitioners about how to use computer systems effectively,
- robust clinical decision-support databases, and
- full integration and connectivity with other key information systems (eg, laboratory, pharmacy).[185]

Bar-code technology and computer documentation are examples of performance-improvement strategies designed to increase compliance with documentation for medication administration. One study revealed a 21.7% increase in the number of medications documented per cardiac surgery case when a bar-code medication administration system was used by anesthesia professionals.[210] Another practice report discussed findings that revealed new opportunities for wrong dose or wrong drug errors when computer systems were used depending on the configuration of how medication names and dosages were displayed on the computer screen.[185]

Training programs increase familiarity with new systems. Robust clinical decision-support databases are designed to alert users about computer-entry errors to allow correction before the error is made.

XVII.b. Perioperative team members should develop processes for monitoring the medication management system to identify risk factors associated with medication errors and to strive for compliance with safety measures.

Monitoring provides a means to identify medication errors at the time or before the time they occur. Monitoring compliance with safety measures provides a means to correct situations at the time of occurrence and collect data for use in process-improvement projects. As a system, monitoring in the medication use process allows for process improvement and compliance with regulatory standards.

XVII.b.1. The health care organization should include a variety of error-detection strategies in the monitoring process including, but not limited to,
- spontaneous reports;
- computerized triggers;
- random chart reviews, including medication audits; and
- a classification reporting system, such as one endorsed by the World Health Organization (eg, Eindhoven Classification Model).[211,212]

Using more than one strategy facilitates identification of errors and risks for errors from multiple perspectives.

XVII.b.2. Perioperative team members should observe each other at various points in the medication use process to monitor for processes that inhibit safe medication use, including safe injection practices.

Observing interactions between working conditions, equipment, and people may reveal vulnerability for medication errors and opportunities for spontaneous coaching interactions to engage staff members in identifying risks (eg, discussion with a staff member not responding to clinical alarms).

XVII.b.3. Perioperative team members should monitor aftercare processes.

XVII.b.4. Perioperative team members should monitor compliance with safe handling of chemicals, cytotoxic agents, and hazardous waste in the workplace.

XVII.b.5. When observing for potential risks where medications are stored or used, perioperative team members should address environmental conditions including, but not limited to,
- space,
- illumination,
- noise, and
- interruptions.

XVII.b.6. Perioperative team members should monitor for potential risks for medication errors related to equipment including, but not limited to,
- equipment alarms (eg, temperature, pumps),
- infusion pumps,
- tubing interconnectivity, and
- hood or ventilation requirements for compounding irrigants.

XVII.b.7. Perioperative team members should actively participate in monitoring the health care organization's medication management system.

Given that there are numerous failures in medication management systems,[6] perioperative team members bear the responsibility for actively identifying system level barriers that impede safe medication use.[17] Actively participating in the improvement process requires monitoring of the medication use process to identify patterns and trends. Armed with such information, perioperative team members can close the divide between expected care and actual care that is delivered.[213]

XVII.b.8. Perioperative team members should monitor for a blame-free culture.

A culture of safety provides an atmosphere where perioperative team members can openly discuss errors, process improvements, or system issues without fear of reprisal.

XVII.c. The quality improvement/process improvement (QI/PI) program should include a routine review and update of all performance improvement activities.

Reviewing the established QI/PI program may identify failure points contributing to medication errors and may aid in improving patient safety.

XVII.c.1. The perioperative QI/PI program should include periodic evaluation of the medication management process; for example, a routine review and update of all preprinted order sheets and facility-approved standing orders for clarity of
- medication choice,
- dose, and
- delivery method.

XVII.c.2. The PNDS should be used to establish guidelines to monitor and manage institutional improvements with regard to medication safety and to identify desired outcomes including, but not limited to,
- the patient receives appropriate prescribed medication(s) safely administered during the perioperative period,
- the patient demonstrates knowledge of medication management, and
- the patient demonstrates knowledge of pain management.[190]

XVII.c.3. Medication performance improvement indicators should include structure, process, and outcome metrics. A baseline and a target should be used for routine reviews of performance indicators including, but not limited to,

- reducing the number of preoperative antibiotics administered outside of the acceptable time frame;
- eliminating the number of medication range orders without specification;
- reducing the number of medications drawn up in unlabeled syringes;
- reducing the number of outdated medications found;
- reducing the number of clinical staff members who do not demonstrate knowledge of the proper verbal order process, including "read back;"
- reducing the number of times unapproved abbreviations occur in nursing documentation; and
- reducing the number of illegible entries of medications that occur in nursing documentation.[49]

XVII.c.4. Standardized medication safety event measurements should be incorporated into performance improvement reviews. Measurements should include, but not be limited to,
- event definitions,
- event severity classification,
- event preventability criteria,
- control event capture,
- standardized recording tools, and
- rater training and ongoing inter-rater reliability evaluation.[214]

XVII.d. Quality improvement activities (eg, root cause analysis) should be used to investigate and document all actual or potential (eg, near miss) medication errors across the medication use process.

Quality improvement activities are expectations for all professionals within the health care team.[215] Documenting such activities fulfills regulatory and accreditation requirements.

XVII.e. Health care organizations should adopt a standardized approach to reporting (eg, incident report, hotline) errors and near misses related to medications and medication administration equipment.

Standardization helps to achieve consistency in reporting.

XVII.e.1. Perioperative team members should actively participate in error reporting regardless of where the error originates within the medication use process and regardless of whether patient harm results from the error.

Information from near-miss and medication error reports can be used to identify trends, develop new safety measures, and educate members of the perioperative team to increase awareness of and improve compliance with safe medication practices.

XVII.e.2. Health care organizations should participate in a national medication error reporting program.

Participation in national medication error programs (eg, ISMP National Medication Error Reporting Program) and state reporting programs will enhance the data available to identify trends for medication errors in perioperative settings. The information collected by the national medication error programs is used to educate regulatory agencies, professional organizations, frontline practitioners, consumers, and the pharmaceutical industry about preventing future adverse drug events.[1]

XVII.e.3. Health care organizations should have a process to monitor and report incidents of equipment malfunction that lead to patient harm as outlined in the Safe Medical Devices Act of 1990.[216]

XVII.e.4. Health care organizations should have a process to report serious adverse events, product quality problems, or product use errors to the ISMP and FDA through the MedWatch web site.

The data from these reports are used to maintain safety surveillance of products associated with medication administration and may be used to prompt a modification in use or design of the product to improve its safety profile and patient safety.[51]

XVII.f. Perioperative team members who serve on their organization's quality improvement committee or root cause analysis group should be included when analyzing findings from medication error reports and planning corrective interventions.

XVII.f.1. When a medication error or near-miss occurs, perioperative administrators should collaborate with the health care organization's quality improvement committee members regarding disclosure of medication errors to patients and their designated support persons.

Glossary

Compounding: The process of combining two or more different medications. Compounding does not include mixing, reconstituting, or similar acts that are performed in accordance with the directions contained on approved labeling that is provided by the product's manufacturer or other manufacturer directions consistent with that labeling.

Multidose vial: Defined by the Safe Injection Practices Coalition (SIPC) as a bottle of injectable medication that contains more than one dose of medication and has a label to indicate approval by the US Food and Drug Administration for use on more than one person.

Par level: Minimum inventory level that has been identified to match the volume typically used within a specified time frame to promote rotation of stock and avoid outdates.

REFERENCES
1. Wanzer LJ, Hicks RW, Goeckner B, Cole L. A focused review: perioperative safe medication use. *Perioper Nurs Clin.* 2008;3(4):305-316. doi:10.1016/j.cpen.2008.08.001.
2. Wanzer LJ, Hicks RW. Medication safety within the perioperative environment. *Annu Rev Nurs Res.* 2006;24:127-155.
3. Beyea S. Safe medication practices in perioperative settings. *Perioper Nurs Clin.* 2006;1(3):283-288.
4. Hicks RW, Becker SC, Cousins DD. *MEDMARX Data Report: A Chartbook of Medication Error Findings from the Perioperative Settings from 1998-2005.* Rockville, MD: US Center for the Advancement of Patient Safety; 2006.
5. ASHP guidelines on preventing medication errors in hospitals. In: *Best Practices for Hospital & Health-System Pharmacy: Position & Guidance Documents of ASHP.* Bethesda, MD: American Society of Health-System Pharmacists; 2009:178-186.
6. Kohn LT, Corrigan JM, Donaldson MS, eds. *To Err Is Human: Building a Safer Health System.* Washington, DC: National Academy Press; 1999. *http://www*

.nap.edu/openbook.php?record_id=9728. Accessed September 27, 2011.

7. Sentinel event data: event type by year, 1995-third quarter 2010. The Joint Commission. http://www.jointcommission.org/se_data_event_type_by_year_/. Accessed September 9, 2011.

8. Macdonald M. Patient safety: examining the adequacy of the 5 rights of medication administration. Clin Nurse Spec. 2010;24(4):196-201. doi:10.1097/NUR.0b013e3181e3605f.

9. Hughes RG. Tools and strategies for quality improvement and patient safety. In: Hughes RG, Smith JD, Jones RA, eds. Patient Safety and Quality: An Evidence-Based Handbook for Nurses; volume 3. Rockville, MD: Agency for Healthcare Research and Quality; 2008:22-43.

10. ASHP guidelines: minimum standard for pharmaceutical services in ambulatory care. In: Best Practices for Hospital & Health-System Pharmacy: Position & Guidance Documents of ASHP. Bethesda, MD: American Society of Health-System Pharmacists; 2009:392-400.

11. ASHP guidelines: minimum standard for pharmacies in hospitals. In: Best Practices for Hospital & Health-System Pharmacy: Position & Guidance Documents of ASHP. Bethesda, MD: American Society of Health-System Pharmacists; 2009:401-406.

12. ASHP guidelines on medication cost management strategies for hospitals and health systems. In: Best Practices for Hospital & Health-System Pharmacy: Position & Guidance Documents of ASHP. Bethesda, MD: American Society of Health-System Pharmacists; 2009:314-328.

13. American Hospital Association, Health Research & Educational Trust, Institute for Safe Medication Practices. Pathways for Medication Safety: Leading a Strategic Planning Effort. Chicago, IL: Health Research and Educational Trust; 2002.

14. Mazzocco K, Petitti DB, Fong KT, et al. Surgical team behaviors and patient outcomes. Am J Surg. 2009;197(5):678-685. doi:10.1016/j.amjsurg.2008.03.002.

15. Neily J, Mills PD, Young-Xu Y, et al. Association between implementation of a medical team training program and surgical mortality. JAMA. 2010;304(15):1693-1700. doi:10.1001/jama.2010.1506.

16. Brady AM, Malone AM, Fleming S. A literature review of the individual and systems factors that contribute to medication errors in nursing practice. J Nurs Manag. 2009;17(6):679-697. doi:10.1111/j.1365-2834.2009.00995.x.

17. Institute of Medicine. Preventing Medication Errors: The Quality Chasm Series. Washington, DC: The National Academies Press; 2006. http://books.nap.edu/openbook.php?record_id=11623. Accessed September 27, 2011.

18. Hicks RW, Becker SC, Windle PE, Krenzischek DA. Medication errors in the PACU. J Perianesth Nurs. 2007;22(6):413-419. doi:10.1016/j.jopan.2007.08.002.

19. ASHP statement on standards-based pharmacy practice in hospitals and health system. In: Best Practices for Hospital & Health-System Pharmacy: Position & Guidance Documents of ASHP. Bethesda, MD: American Society of Health-System Pharmacists; 2009:312-313.

20. Bassi J, Lau F, Bardal S. Use of information technology in medication reconciliation: a scoping review. Ann Pharmacother. 2010;44(5):885-897. doi:10.1345/aph.1M699.

21. Guidance on the Interdisciplinary Safe Use of Automated Dispensing Cabinets. Horsham, PA: Institute for Safe Medication Practices; 2008. http://www.ismp.org/tools/guidelines/ADC_Guidelines_Final.pdf. Accessed September 27, 2011.

22. Medication management. In: Comprehensive Accreditation Manual for Hospitals. E-dition v3.6.0.0. Oakbrook Terrace, IL: Joint Commission Resources; 2011.

23. Agrawal A, Wu WY. National patient safety goals. Reducing medication errors and improving systems reliability using an electronic medication reconciliation system. Joint Comm J Qual Patient Saf. 2009;35(2):106-114.

24. Schnipper JL, Hamann C, Ndumele CD, et al. Effect of an electronic medication reconciliation application and process redesign on potential adverse drug events: a cluster-randomized trial. Arch Intern Med. 2009;169(8):771-780. doi:10.1001/archinternmed.2009.51.

25. Eichhorn JH. APSF hosts medication safety conference: consensus group defines challenges and opportunities for improved practice. APSF Newsletter. 2010;25(1):1, 3-8.

26. Medication safety. Healthcare Risk Control. 2011;4(Pharmacy and Medications 1):1-32.

27. Poon EG, Keohane CA, Yoon CS, et al. Effect of bar-code technology on the safety of medication administration. N Engl J Med. 2010;362(18):1698-1707. doi:10.1056/NEJMsa0907115.

28. Cochran GL, Jones KJ, Brockman J, Skinner A, Hicks RW. USP medical safety forum. Errors prevented by and associated with bar-code medication administration systems. Joint Comm J Qual Patient Saf. 2007;33(5):293-301.

29. Paparella S. Drug information resources: essential but may be error prone. J Emerg Nurs. 2010;36(3):250-252. doi:10.1016/j.jen.2010.01.012.

30. Appendix L: Guidance for surveyors: Ambulatory surgical centers [Rev. 56, 12-30-09]. In: State Operations Manual. Washington, DC: Centers for Medicare & Medicaid Services; 2009

31. Guidance for Industry: Q8(R2) Pharmaceutical Development. Rev. 2. Washington, DC: Food and Drug Administration; 2009.

32. Blossom D, Noble-Wang J, Su J, et al. Multistate outbreak of Serratia marcescens bloodstream infections caused by contamination of prefilled heparin and isotonic sodium chloride solution syringes. Arch Intern Med. 2009;169(18):1705-1711. doi:10.1001/archinternmed.2009.290.

33. Sterile water should not be given "freely." Pa Patient Saf Advis. 2008;5(2):53-56.

34. ISMP's List of Confused Drug Names. Horsham, PA: Institute for Safe Medication Practices; 2009.

35. FDA Name Differentiation Project. http://www.fda.gov/Drugs/DrugSafety/MedicationErrors/ucm164587.htm. Updated June 18, 2009. Accessed September 27, 2011.

36. Kelly WN, Grissinger M, Shaw Phillips M. Look-alike drug name errors: is enhanced lettering the answer? *Patient Saf Qual Healthc.* 2010;July/August:22-26.

37. Preventing misconnections of lines and cables. *Health Devices.* 2006;35(3):81-95.

38. Beyea SC, Simmons D, Hicks RW. Caution: tubing misconnections can be deadly. *AORN J.* 2007;85(3):633-635.

39. Guenter P, Hicks RW, Simmons D, et al. Enteral feeding misconnections: a consortium position statement. *Jt Comm J Qual Patient Saf.* 2008;34(5):285-292, 245.

40. Simmons D, Graves K. Tubing misconnections—a systems failure with human factors: lessons for nursing practice. *Urol Nurs.* 2008;28(6):460-464.

41. Simmons D, Phillips MS, Grissinger M, Becker SC; USP Safe Medication Use Expert Committee. Error-avoidance recommendations for tubing misconnections when using Luer-tip connectors: a statement by the USP Safe Medication Use Expert Committee. *Jt Comm J Qual Patient Saf.* 2008;34(5):293-6, 245.

42. *Guideline for Industry: Quality of Biotechnological Products: Stability Testing of Biotechnological/ Biological Products.* Food and Drug Administration; 1996.

43. ASHP technical assistance bulletin on hospital drug distribution and control. *Am J Hosp Pharm.* 1980;37:1097-1103.

44. Drug diversion in healthcare: risks and prevention. *Risk Management Reporter.* 2007;26(5):1, 3-10.

45. Controlled Substance Act, 21 USC §801-971 (2006).

46. Hicks RW, Becker SC, Cousins DD, eds. *MEDMARX Data Report: A Report on the Relationship of Drug Names and Medication Errors in Response to the Institute of Medicine's Call for Action.* Rockville, MD: Center for the Advancement of Patient Safety, US Pharmacopeia; 2008.

47. Westbrook JI, Woods A, Rob MI, Dunsmuir WT, Day RO. Association of interruptions with an increased risk and severity of medication administration errors. *Arch Intern Med.* 2010;170(8):683-690. doi:10.1001/archinternmed.2010.65.

48. Bryson EO, Silverstein JH. Addiction and substance abuse in anesthesiology. *Anesthesiology.* 2008;109(5):905-917. doi:10.1097/ALN.0b013e3181895bc1.

49. Burden N. A comprehensive medication management program in the ambulatory surgery setting. *J Perianesth Nurs.* 2007;22(1):40-46. doi:10.1016/j.jopan.2006.12.002.

50. *Infusing Patients Safely: Priority Issues From the AAMI/FDA Infusion Device Summit.* Arlington, VA: Association for the Advancement of Medical Instrumentation; 2010. http://www.aami.org/infusionsummit/AAMI_FDA_Summit_Report.pdf. Accessed September 28, 2011.

51. *FDA's Safe Use Initiative: Collaborating to Reduce Preventable Harm from Medications.* Silver Spring, MD: Food and Drug Administration; 2009. http://www.fda.gov/downloads/Drugs/DrugSafety/UCM188961.pdf. Accessed September 30, 2011.

52. Labeling Issuance, 21 CFR §211.125 (2010). http://edocket.access.gpo.gov/cfr_2005/aprqtr/pdf/21cfr211.130.pdf. Accessed September 30, 2011.

53. Garnerin P, Perneger T, Chopard P, et al. Drug selection errors in relation to medication labels: a simulation study. *Anaesthesia.* 2007;62(11):1090-1094. doi:10.1111/j.1365-2044.2007.05198.x.

54. Santell JP, Cousins DD. Medication errors related to product names. *Jt Comm J Qual Patient Saf.* 2005;31(11):649-654.

55. McCoy LK. Look-alike, sound-alike drugs review: include look-alike packaging as an additional safety check. *Jt Comm J Qual Patient Saf.* 2005;31(1):47-53.

56. Gabriele S. The role of typography in differentiating look-alike/sound-alike drug names. *Healthc Q.* 2006;9 Spec No:88-95.

57. High-alert medications. *Healthc Risk Control.* 2004;4(Pharmacy and Medications 1.4):1-7.

58. Shultz J, Davies JM, Caird J, Chisholm S, Ruggles K, Puls R. Standardizing anesthesia medication drawers using human factors and quality assurance methods. *Can J Anaesth.* 2010;57(5):490-499. doi:10.1007/s12630-010-9274-8.

59. Reason J. Safety in the operating theatre—part 2: human error and organisational failure. *Qual Saf Health Care.* 2005;14(1):56-60.

60. Girard NJ. Unexplained apnea during surgery. *AORN J.* 2008;87(6):1288, 1216.

61. Paparella S. Fatal confusion with epinephrine: 1:1,000 is not 1:10,000. *J Emerg Nurs.* 2005;31(1):86-88. doi:10.1016/j.jen.2004.09.016.

62. Bullock J, Jordan D, Gawlinski A, Henneman FA. Standardizing IV infusion medication concentrations to reduce variability in medication errors. *Crit Care Nurs Clin North Am.* 2006;18(4):515-521. doi:10.1016/j.ccell.2006.08.008.

63. Smetzer JL, Cohen MR. Preventing drug administration errors. In: Cohen MR, ed. *Medication Errors.* 2nd ed. Washington, DC: American Pharmacists Association; 2007:235-274.

64. Paparella S. The risks associated with the use of multidose vials. *J Emerg Nurs.* 2006;32(5):428-430. doi:10.1016/j.jen.2006.05.016.

65. Perz JF, Thompson ND, Schaefer MK, Patel PR. US outbreak investigations highlight the need for safe injection practices and basic infection control. *Clin Liver Dis.* 2010;14(1):137-151. doi:10.1016/j.cld.2009.11.004.

66. Pugliese G, Gosnell C, Bartley JM, Robinson S. Injection practices among clinicians in United States health care settings. *Am J Infect Control.* 2010;38(10):789-798. doi:10.1016/j.ajic.2010.09.003.

67. Recommended practices for product selection in perioperative practice settings. In: *Perioperative Standards and Recommended Practices.* Denver, CO: AORN, Inc; 2011: 191-200.

68. Dangers associated with shared multidose vials. *Pa Patient Saf Advis.* 2008;5(2):68.

69. Pharmaceutical waste disposal practices get legal evil eye. *Environ Care Lead.* 2010;15(3):1, 5-6.

70. Dolan SA, Felizardo G, Barnes S, et al. APIC position paper: safe injection, infusion, and medica-

tion vial practices in health care. *Am J Infect Control.* 2010;38(3):167-172. doi:10.1016/j.ajic.2010.01.001.

71. Vonberg R, Gastmeier P. Hospital-acquired infections related to contaminated substances. *J Hosp Infect.* 2007;65(1):15-23.

72. Kushakovskyy V. Acetone on the labour ward: an accident waiting to happen. *Int J Obstet Anesth.* 2008;17(3):285-286. doi:10.1016/j.ijoa.2008.02.002.

73. Smędra-Kaźmirska A, Żydek L, Barzdo M, Machała W, Berent J. Accidental intravenous injection of formalin. *Anaesthesiol Intensive Ther.* 2009;XLI(3):133-135.

74. Feigal DW Jr, Woodock J. FDA public health advisory: potential for injury from medical gas misconnections of cryogenic vessels [medical device safety: alerts and notices]. Silver Spring, MD: US Food and Drug Administration; July 20, 2001. *http://www.fda.gov/MedicalDevices/Safety/AlertsandNotices/PublicHealthNotifications/ucm062189.htm.* Accessed September 28, 2011.

75. Center for Drug Evaluation and Research, Food and Drug Administration. Compressed medical gases guideline. *http://www.fda.gov/Drugs/GuidanceComplianceRegulatoryInformation/Guidances/ucm124716.htm.* Updated February 1989. Accessed September 28, 2011.

76. Medical gas errors. *Practitioners' Reporting News.* June 19, 2001.

77. Greenberg CC, Regenbogen SE, Studdert DM, et al. Patterns of communication breakdowns resulting in injury to surgical patients. *J Am Coll Surg.* 2007;204(4):533-540. doi:10.1016/j.jamcollsurg.2007.01.010.

78. Engum SA, Breckler FD. An evaluation of medication errors—the pediatric surgical service experience. *J Pediatr Surg.* 2008;43(2):348-352. doi:10.1016/j.jpedsurg.2007.10.042.

79. Smith HS, Lesar TS. Analgesic prescribing errors and associated medication characteristics. *J Pain.* 2011;12(1):29-40. doi:10.1016/j.jpain.2010.04.007.

80. Metzger J, Welebob E, Bates DW, Lipsitz S, Classen DC. Mixed results in the safety performance of computerized physician order entry. *Health Aff (Millwood).* 2010;29(4):655-663.

81. Picone DM, Titler MG, Dochterman J, et al. Predictors of medication errors among elderly hospitalized patients. *Am J Med Qual.* 2008;23(2):115-127. doi:10.1177/1062860607313143.

82. Grissinger MC, Hicks RW, Keroack MA, Marella WM, Vaida AJ. Harmful medication errors involving unfractionated and low-molecular-weight heparin in three patient safety reporting programs. *Jt Comm J Qual Patient Saf.* 2010;36(5):195-202.

83. Fick DM, Cooper JW, Wade WE, Waller JL, Maclean JR, Beers MH. Updating the Beers criteria for potentially inappropriate medication use in older adults: results of a US consensus panel of experts. *Arch Intern Med.* 2003;163(22):2716-2724. doi:10.1001/archinte.163.22.2716.

84. Stefanacci RG, Cavallaro E, Beers MH, Fick DM. Developing explicit positive Beers criteria for preferred central nervous system medications in older adults. *Consult Pharm.* 2009;24(8):601-610.

85. Kaur S, Mitchell G, Vitetta L, Roberts MS. Interventions that can reduce inappropriate prescribing in the elderly: a systematic review. *Drugs Aging.* 2009;26(12):1013-1028. doi:10.2165/11318890-000000000-00000; 10.2165/11318890-000000000-00000.

86. Bazzano ATF, Mangione-Smith R, Schonlau M, Suttorp MJ, Brook RH. Off-label prescribing to children in the United States outpatient setting. *Acad Pediatr.* 2009;9(2):81-88.

87. Woo T. Pharmacology of cough and cold medicines. *J Pediatr Health Care.* 2008;22(2):73-82. doi:10.1016/j.pedhc.2007.12.007.

88. Hamilton T. "Standing orders" in hospitals—revisions to S&C memoranda [memorandum]. Baltimore, MD: Department of Health & Human Services; 2008. Ref: S&C-09-10.

89. Broussard M, Bass PF III, Arnold CL, McLarty JW, Bocchini JA Jr. Preprinted order sets as a safety intervention in pediatric sedation. *J Pediatr.* 2009;154(6):865-868. doi:10.1016/j.jpeds.2008.12.022.

90. Straube BM. Letter to David T. Tayloe Jr. [written communication]. Baltimore, MD: Department of Health & Human Services; 2010. *http://practice.aap.org/public/Straube%20Letter%20to%20Tayloe.PDF.* Accessed September 30, 2011.

91. Dawson A, Orsini MJ, Cooper MR, Wollenburg K. Medication safety—reliability of preference cards. *AORN J.* 2005;82(3):399-414.

92. Medicare and Medicaid programs; hospital conditions of participation: requirements for history and physical examinations; authentication of verbal orders; securing medications; and postanesthesia evaluations. Final rule. *Fed Regist.* 2006;71(227):68671-68695. *http://edocket.access.gpo.gov/2006/pdf/E6-19957.pdf.* Accessed September 30, 2011.

93. Recommendations to reduce medication errors associated with verbal medication orders and prescriptions. National Coordinating Council for Medication Error Reporting and Prevention. *http://www.nccmerp.org/council/council2001-02-20.html.* Published February 20, 2001. Updated February 24, 2006. Accessed September 28, 2011.

94. Lambert BL, Dickey LW, Fisher WM, et al. Listen carefully: the risk of error in spoken medication orders. *Soc Sci Med.* 2010;70(10):1599-1608. doi:10.1016/j.socscimed.2010.01.042.

95. Wakefield DS, Brokel J, Ward MM, et al. An exploratory study measuring verbal order content and context. *Qual Saf Health Care.* 2009;18(3):169-173.

96. Wakefield DS, Wakefield BJ. Are verbal orders a threat to patient safety? *Postgrad Med J.* 2009;85(1007):460-463. doi:10.1136/qshc.2009.034041.

97. Kaushal R, Goldmann DA, Keohane CA, et al. Medication errors in paediatric outpatients. *Qual Saf Health Care.* 2010;19(6):e30. doi:10.1136/qshc.2008.031179.

98. Bates DW, Leape LL, Cullen DJ, et al. Effect of computerized physician order entry and a team intervention on prevention of serious medication errors. *JAMA.* 1998;280(15):1311-1316.

99. Computerized provider order-entry systems. *Healthcare Risk Control.* 2002;suppl A(Pharmacy and Medications 6):1-21.

100. Kaplan JM, Ancheta R, Jacobs BR. Inpatient verbal orders and the impact of computerized provider order entry. *J Pediatr.* 2006;149(4):461-467.

101. Khajouei R, Jaspers MW. The impact of CPOE medication systems' design aspects on usability, workflow and medication orders: a systematic review. *Methods Inf Med.* 2010;49(1):3-19. doi:10.3414/ME0630.

102. Ammenwerth E, Schnell-Inderst P, Machan C, Siebert U. The effect of electronic prescribing on medication errors and adverse drug events: a systematic review. *J Am Med Inform Assoc.* 2008;15(5):585-600. doi:10.1197/jamia.M2667.

103. Weber RJ. Medication reconciliation pitfalls. *AHRQ WebM&M* [serial online]. February 2010. *http://www.webmm.ahrq.gov/case.aspx?caseID=213.* Accessed September 28, 2011.

104. United States Pharmacopeia Convention. Committee of Revision. Pharmaceutical compounding—sterile preparations. In: *The United States Pharmacopeia.* 27th ed. Rockville, MD: United States Pharmacopeial Convention, Inc; 2009:318-354.

105. Centers for Medicare & Medicaid Services, US Department of Health and Human Services. Condition of Participation: Pharmaceutical Services. 42 CFR §482.25 (2009). *http://edocket.access.gpo.gov/cfr_2010/octqtr/pdf/42cfr482.25.pdf.* Revised November 27, 2006. Accessed September 12, 2011.

106. ASHP guidelines on quality assurance for pharmacy-prepared sterile products. In: *Best Practices for Hospital & Health-System Pharmacy: Position & Guidance Documents of ASHP.* Bethesda, MD: American Society of Health-System Pharmacists; 2009:71-89.

107. Hicks RW, Wanzer L, Goeckner B. Perioperative pharmacology: a framework for perioperative medication safety. *AORN J.* 2011;93(1):136-145. doi:10.1016/j.aorn.2010.08.020.

108. Standards of perioperative nursing. In: *Perioperative Standards and Recommended Practices.* Denver, CO: AORN, Inc; 2011:3-20.

109. Hicks RW, Becker SC, Cousins DD. Harmful medication errors in children: a 5-year analysis of data from the USP's MEDMARX program. *J Pediatr Nurs.* 2006;21(4):290-298. doi:10.1016/j.pedn.2006.02.002.

110. Annual Report 2009. Pennsylvania Patient Safety Authority. April 28, 2010. *http://patientsafetyauthority.org/PatientSafetyAuthority/Documents/Annual_Report_2009.pdf.* Accessed September 12, 2011.

111. Medication errors: significance of accurate patient weights. *Pa Patient Saf Advis.* 2009;6(1):10-15.

112. Murphy EM, Oxencis CJ, Klauck JA, Meyer DA, Zimmerman JM. Medication reconciliation at an academic medical center: implementation of a comprehensive program from admission to discharge. *Am J Health Syst Pharm.* 2009;66(23):2126-2131. doi:10.2146/ajhp080552.

113. Schwarz M, Wyskiel R. Medication reconciliation: developing and implementing a program. *Crit Care Nurs Clin North Am.* 2006;18(4):503-507. doi:10.1016/j.ccell.2006.09.003.

114. Pippins JR, Gandhi TK, Hamann C, et al. Classifying and predicting errors of inpatient medication reconciliation. *J Gen Intern Med.* 2008;23(9):1414-1422. doi:10.1007/s11606-008-0687-9.

115. Boockvar KS, Carlson LaCorte H, Giambanco V, Fridman B, Siu A. Medication reconciliation for reducing drug-discrepancy adverse events. *Am J Geriatr Pharmacother.* 2006;4(3):236-243. doi:10.1016/j.amjopharm.2006.09.003.

116. Fredericks JE, Bunting RF Jr. Implementation of a patient-friendly medication schedule to improve patient safety within a healthcare system. *J Healthc Risk Manag.* 2010;29(4):22-27. doi:10.1002/jhrm.20030.

117. Nassaralla CI, Naessens JM, Hunt VL, et al. Medication reconciliation in ambulatory care: attempts at improvement. *Qual Saf Health Care.* 2009;18(5):402-407. doi:10.1136/qshc.2007.024513.

118. Gizzi LA, Slain D, Hare JT, Sager R, Briggs F III, Palmer CH. Assessment of a safety enhancement to the hospital medication reconciliation process for elderly patients. *Am J Geriatr Pharmacother.* 2010;8(2):127-135. doi:10.1016/j.amjopharm.2010.03.004.

119. Frolich MA, Giannotti A, Modell JH. Opioid overdose in a patient using a fentanyl patch during treatment with a warming blanket. *Anesth Analg.* 2001;93(3):647-648.

120. Wrenn K. The hazards of defibrillation through nitroglycerin patches. *Ann Emerg Med.* 1990;19(11):1327-1328.

121. Public health advisory: risk of burns during MRI scans from transdermal drug patches with metallic backings. US Food and Drug Administration. *http://www.fda.gov/Drugs/DrugSafety/PostmarketDrugSafetyInformationforPatientsandProviders/DrugSafetyInformationforHeathcareProfessionals/PublicHealthAdvisories/ucm111313.htm.* Published March 5, 2009. Updated June 23, 2010. Accessed September 30, 2011.

122. Sullivan C, Gleason KM, Rooney D, Groszek JM, Barnard C. Medication reconciliation in the acute care setting: opportunity and challenge for nursing. *J Nurs Care Qual.* 2005;20(2):95-98.

123. Warholak TL, McCulloch M, Baumgart A, Smith M, Fink W, Fritz W. An exploratory comparison of medication lists at hospital admission with administrative database records. *J Manag Care Pharm.* 2009;15(9):751-758.

124. Kuhn MA. Herbal remedies: drug-herb interactions. *Crit Care Nurse.* 2002;22(2):22-35.

125. King AR, Russell FS, Generali JA, Grauer DW. Evaluation and implications of natural product use in preoperative patients: a retrospective review. *BMC Complement Altern Med.* 2009;9:38. doi:10.1186/1472-6882-9-38.

126. O'Riordan JM, Margey RJ, Blake G, O'Connell PR. Antiplatelet agents in the perioperative period. *Arch Surg.* 2009;144(1):69-76. doi:10.1001/archsurg.144.1.69.

127. Farooq M, Kirke C, Foley K. Documentation of drug allergy on drug chart in patients presenting for surgery. *Ir J Med Sci.* 2008;177(3):243-245. doi:10.1007/s11845-008-0166-7.

128. Medication errors associated with documented allergies. *Pa Patient Saf Advis.* 2008;5(3):75-80.

129. Lehne RA. Application of pharmacology in nursing practice. In: *Pharmacology for Nursing Care.* 7th ed. St Louis, MO: Saunders/Elsevier; 2010:5-14.

130. Payne CH, Smith CR, Newkirk LE, Hicks RW. Pediatric medication errors in the postanesthesia care unit: analysis of MEDMARX data. *AORN J.* 2007;85(4):731-744. doi:10.1016/S0001-2092(07)60147-1.

131. Chuo J, Hicks RW. Computer-related medication errors in neonatal intensive care units. *Clin Perinatol.* 2008;35(1):119-139. doi:10.1016/j.clp.2007.11.005.

132. Kfuri TA, Morlock L, Hicks RW, Shore AD. Medication errors in obstetrics. *Clin Perinatol.* 2008;35(1):101-117. doi:10.1016/j.clp.2007.11.015.

133. Ozkan S, Kocaman G, Ozturk C, Seren S. Frequency of pediatric medication administration errors and contributing factors. *J Nurs Care Qual.* 2011;26(2):136-143. doi:10.1097/NCQ.0b013e3182031006.

134. <1066> Physical environments that promote safe medication use. *USP Revision Bull.* October 2010:1-6.

135. ISMP Guidelines for Standard Order Sets. Institute for Safe Medication Practices. *http://www.ismp.org/tools/guidelines/StandardOrderSets.pdf.* Published 2010. Accessed September 28, 2011.

136. Hicks RW, Sikirica V, Nelson W, Schein JR, Cousins DD. Medication errors involving patient-controlled analgesia. *Am J Health Syst Pharm.* 2008;65(5):429-440. doi:10.2146/ajhp070194.

137. Biron AD, Loiselle CG, Lavoie-Tremblay M. Work interruptions and their contribution to medication administration errors: an evidence review. *Worldviews Evid Based Nurs.* 2009;6(2):70-86. doi:10.1111/j.1741-6787.2009.00151.x.

138. Biron AD, Lavoie-Tremblay M, Loiselle CG. Characteristics of work interruptions during medication administration. *J Nurs Scholarsh.* 2009;41(4):330-336. doi:10.1111/j.1547-5069.2009.01300.x.

139. Smetzer J, Baker C, Byrne FD, Cohen MR. Shaping systems for better behavioral choices: lessons learned from a fatal medication error. *Jt Comm J Qual Patient Saf.* 2010;36(4):152-163.

140. Best practices for safe medication administration. *AORN J.* 2006;84(Suppl 1):S45-S56.

141. *Schroeder v. Northwest Community Hospital,* NE 2d, 2006 WL 3615559 (Ill App, December 12, 2006).

142. Hicks RW, Becker SC, Jackson DG. Understanding medication errors: discussion of a case involving a urinary catheter implicated in a wrong route error. *Urol Nurs.* 2008;28(6):454-459.

143. Goodman EJ, Haas AJ, Kantor GS. Inadvertent administration of magnesium sulfate through the epidural catheter: report and analysis of a drug error. *Int J Obstet Anesth.* 2006;15(1):63-67. doi:10.1016/j.ijoa.2005.06.009.

144. Otoya M. Heparin safety in the neonatal intensive care unit: are we learning from mistakes of others? *Newborn Infant Nurs Rev.* 2009;9(1):53-61. doi:10.1053/j.nainr.2008.12.007.

145. Medication errors with the dosing of insulin: problems across the continuum. *Pa Patient Saf Advis.* 2010;7(1):9-17.

146. Vancomycin [package insert]. Lake Forest, IL: Akorn-Strides, LLC; July 2009.

147. AORN guidance statement: Sharps injury prevention in the perioperative setting. In: *Perioperative Standards and Recommended Practices.* Denver, CO: AORN, Inc; 2011:639-644.

148. Lee ACW, Leung M, So KT. Managing patients with identical names in the same ward. *Int J Health Care Qual Assur.* 2005;18(1):15-23.

149. Seitz IA, Tojo D, Schechter LS. Anatomy of a medication error: inadvertent subcutaneous injection of neosynephrine during nasal surgery. *Plast Reconstr Surg.* 2010;125(3):113e-114e. doi:10.1097/PRS.0b013e3181cb68f9.

150. Jennings J, Foster J. Medication safety: just a label away. *AORN J.* 2007;86(4):618-625. doi:10.1016/j.aorn.2007.04.003.

151. Haas D. In memory of Ben. *Risk Management Reports.* 1998;12.

152. Cohen MR, Smetzer JL. Unlabeled containers lead to patient's death. *Jt Comm J Qual Patient Saf.* 2005;31(7):414-417.

153. Case update: epinephrine death in Florida. *ISMP Medication Safety Alert!.* December 4, 1996.

154. Hass D. Moving beyond blame to create an environment that rewards reporting. In: Youngberg BJ, Hatlie MJ, eds. *Patient Safety Handbook.* Sudbury, MA: Jones and Bartlett Publishers; 2004:415-421.

155. Loud wake-up call: Unlabeled containers lead to patient's death. *ISMP Medication Safety Alert!.* December 2, 2004.

156. Fatal outcome after inadvertent injection of topical EPINEPHrine. *ISMP Medication Safety Alert!.* March 26, 2009.

157. McCormick CG, Henningfield JE, Haddox JD, et al. Case histories in pharmaceutical risk management. *Drug Alcohol Depend.* 2009;105(Suppl 1):S42-S55. doi:10.1016/j.drugalcdep.2009.08.003.

158. Devlin JW, Mallow-Corbett S, Riker RR. Adverse drug events associated with the use of analgesics, sedatives, and antipsychotics in the intensive care unit. *Crit Care Med.* 2010;38(Suppl 6):S231-S243. doi:10.1097/CCM.0b013e3181de125a.

159. Kripalani S, Jackson AT, Schnipper JL, Coleman EA. Promoting effective transitions of care at hospital discharge: a review of key issues for hospitalists. *J Hosp Med.* 2007;2(5):314-323. doi:10.1002/jhm.228.

160. Zavala S, Shaffer C. Do patients understand discharge instructions? *J Emerg Nurs.* In press. doi:10.1016/j.jen.2009.11.008.

161. Joint Commission. MM.04.01.01: Medication orders are clear and accurate. In: *Comprehensive Accreditation Manual for Hospitals.* E-dition v3.6.0.0. Oakbrook Terrace, IL: Joint Commission Resources; 2011.

162. Varkey P, Cunningham J, O'Meara J, Bonacci R, Desai N, Sheeler R. Multidisciplinary approach to inpatient medication reconciliation in an academic

setting. *Am J Health Syst Pharm.* 2007;64(8):850-854. doi:10.2146/ajhp060314.

163. Unroe KT, Pfeiffenberger T, Riegelhaupt S, Jastrzembski J, Lokhnygina Y, Colon-Emeric C. Inpatient medication reconciliation at admission and discharge: A retrospective cohort study of age and other risk factors for medication discrepancies. *Am J Geriatr Pharmacother.* 2010;8(2):115-126. doi:10.1016/j.amjopharm.2010.04.002.

164. Davis TC, Federman AD, Bass PF 3rd, et al. Improving patient understanding of prescription drug label instructions. *J Gen Intern Med.* 2009;24(1):57-62. doi:10.1007/s11606-008-0833-4.

165. Kramer JS, Hopkins PJ, Rosendale JC, et al. Implementation of an electronic system for medication reconciliation. *Am J Health Syst Pharm.* 2007;64(4):404-422. doi:10.2146/ajhp060506.

166. Schweiger MJ, Chambers CE, Davidson CJ, et al. Prevention of contrast induced nephropathy: recommendations for the high risk patient undergoing cardiovascular procedures. *Catheter Cardiovasc Interv.* 2007;69(1):135-140. doi:10.1002/ccd.20964.

167. Glucophage, Glucophage XR [package insert]. Princeton, NJ: Bristol-Myers Squibb Company; January 2009.

168. Bell CM, Bajcar J, Bierman AS, Li P, Mamdani MM, Urbach DR. Potentially unintended discontinuation of long-term medication use after elective surgical procedures. *Arch Intern Med.* 2006;166(22):2525-2531. doi:10.1001/archinte.166.22.2525.

169. Persell SD, Osborn CY, Richard R, Skripkauskas S, Wolf MS. Limited health literacy is a barrier to medication reconciliation in ambulatory care. *J Gen Intern Med.* 2007;22(11):1523-1526. doi:10.1007/s11606-007-0334-x.

170. Wolf MS, Davis TC, Bass PF, et al. Improving prescription drug warnings to promote patient comprehension. *Arch Intern Med.* 2010;170(1):50-56. doi:10.1001/archinternmed.2009.454.

171. National Patient Safety Agency. *Safety in Doses: Improving the Use of Medicines in the NHS.* London, England: National Health Service; 2009. *http://www.nrls.npsa.nhs.uk/resources/?entryid45=61625.* Accessed September 29, 2011.

172. Betz R. Letter to Margaret Hamburg [written communication]. Arlington, VA: American Association of Eye and Ear Centers of Excellence. January 11, 2010.

173. Hazard Communication, 29 CFR §1910.1200 (2010). *http://www.osha.gov/pls/oshaweb/owadisp.show_document?p_table=standards&p_id=10099.* Accessed September 29, 2011.

174. National Institute for Occupational Safety and Health. *Preventing Occupational Exposure to Antineoplastic and Other Hazardous Drugs in Health Care Settings.* Cincinnati, OH: US Department of Health and Human Services; 2004. NIOSH Alert; publication No. 2004-165.

175. Occupational Safety and Health Administration. Controlling occupational exposure to hazardous drugs. In: *OSHA Technical Manual.* Washington, DC: US Department of Labor; 1999. *http://www.osha.gov/dts/*

osta/otm/otm_vi/otm_vi_2.html. Accessed September 29, 2011.

176. Huber C. The safe handling of hazardous drugs. *Am J Nurs.* 2010;110(10):61-63. doi:10.1097/01.NAJ.0000389679.57273.c1.

177. Hazardous spills: the safe handling of hazardous drugs. *Pa Patient Saf Advis.* 2008;5(3):96-99.

178. ASHP guidelines on handling hazardous drugs. In: *Best Practices for Hospital & Health-System Pharmacy: Position & Guidance Documents of ASHP.* Bethesda, MD: American Society of Health-System Pharmacists; 2009:49-68.

179. *ASTM D6978-05 Standard Practice for Assessment of Resistance of Medical Gloves to Permeation by Chemotherapy Drugs.* West Conshohocken, PA: ASTM International; 2005.

180. Lehne RA. Anticancer drugs I: cytotoxic agents. In: *Pharmacology for Nursing Care.* 7th ed. St Louis, MO: Saunders/Elsevier; 2010: 1181-1196.

181. *Unused Pharmaceuticals in the Health Care Industry: Interim Report.* Washington, DC: Environmental Protection Agency; 2008. *http://water.epa.gov/scitech/swguidance/ppcp/upload/2010_1_11_ppcp_hcioutreach.pdf.* Accessed September 29, 2011.

182. Solid Waste Disposal Act (Resource Conservation and Recovery Act): as amended through P.L. 107–377, 42 USC §6901–6992k (2002). *http://epw.senate.gov/rcra.pdf.* Accessed September 29, 2011.

183. Managing pharmaceutical waste. *Healthcare Hazard Control.* 2005;(Waste Management 7):1-9.

184. Federal Water Pollution Control Act (Clean Water Act): as amended through P.L. 107–303, November 27, 2002, 33 USC §1251-1387 (2002). *http://epw.senate.gov/water.pdf.* Accessed September 29, 2011.

185. Santell JP, Kowiatek JG, Weber RJ, Hicks RW, Sirio CA. Medication errors resulting from computer entry by nonprescribers. *Am J Health Syst Pharm.* 2009;66(9):843-853. doi:10.2146/ajhp080208.

186. Hicks RW, Becker SC. An overview of intravenous-related medication administration errors as reported to MEDMARX, a national medication error-reporting program. *J Infus Nurs.* 2006;29(1):20-27.

187. Lafata JE, Simpkins J, Kaatz S, et al. What do medical records tell us about potentially harmful co-prescribing?. *Joint Comm J Qual Patient Saf.* 2007;33(7):395-400.

188. Brunetti L, Santell JP, Hicks RW. The impact of abbreviations on patient safety. *Jt Comm J Qual Patient Saf.* 2007;33(9):576-583.

189. Medical abbreviations. *Healthcare Risk Control.* 2010;2(Medical Records 2):1-9.

190. Petersen C. *Perioperative Nursing Data Set.* 3rd ed. Denver, CO: AORN, Inc;2011.

191. Recommended practices for transfer of patient care information. In: *Perioperative Standards and Recommended Practices.* Denver, CO: AORN, Inc; 2011: 381-387.

192. Paparella S. Choosing the right strategy for medication error prevention—part II. *J Emerg Nurs.* 2008;34(3):238-240. doi:10.1016/j.jen.2008.01.011.

193. Bloodborne Pathogens, 29 CFR §1910.1030 (2010). *http://www.osha.gov/pls/oshaweb/owadisp*

Lasers, which are recognized to be nonionizing radiation, are not within the scope of these recommended practices. These recommended practices provide guidance for developing institutional policies and procedures that can be used collaboratively by personnel in the radiology and surgical services departments and by the facility radiation safety officer.

The primary nursing diagnosis applicable in this recommended practice is the risk for impaired skin integrity from the effects of gamma radiation. To ensure optimal outcomes, the perioperative nurse should assess the patient at the end of the procedure to ensure that the patient's skin remains smooth, intact, and free from unexpected redness, blistering, or tenderness.[6] Each of the following recommended practices is a nursing intervention intended to protect the patient and staff members and ensure optimal outcomes.

Recommendation I

The patient's exposure to radiation should be minimized.

1. The patient's exposure to radiation should be limited to situations in which it is medically indicated and to the anatomical structures being treated. Fluoroscopy delivers some of the largest doses of radiation to patients.[7] Serious skin injuries to patients undergoing certain fluoroscopic procedures have been reported. The greatest dose of radiation to the patient occurs on the patient's skin, where the beam enters the body. The decision to use fluoroscopy during medical or surgical procedures should be approached with caution, weighing the benefits afforded by the technology against the need to keep radiation exposure limited.[7]

2. The perioperative registered nurse should review the patient record for relevant history involving radiation exposure and record study parameters such as fluoroscopy time and area irradiated. He or she also should advise the treating physician of any pertinent information that would be important in reducing patient risk.

3. The perioperative registered nurse should assess the patient for any previous procedure involving radioactive material (ie, nuclear medicine, radiation oncology). It may be necessary to delay the procedure if there is significant radioactive material remaining in the patient. The physician responsible for the radi-

ation treatment or diagnostic procedure should be consulted to determine exposure levels.

4. All reasonable means of reconciling an incorrect sponge, needle, or instrument count should be attempted before using a radiological examination to locate a sponge, sharp, or instrument that may be missing. Certain procedures, because of the complexity of the number of instruments used, may necessitate a postoperative x-ray as stated in the "Recommended practices for sponge, sharp, and instrument counts."[8] Controlling the amount of total fluoroscopic beam "on" time for these procedures through judicious control of the exposure time may help ensure that radiation exposure is as low as reasonably achievable.[4]

Recommendation II

The patient should be protected from unnecessary radiation exposure.

1. Care should be taken to keep extraneous body parts out of the radiation beam to prevent injury. Reports have shown that arms and breast tissue have been injured as a result of increased unintended radiation.[6] Parts of the patient's body not included in the intended radiation field that are located on the x-ray tube side can accumulate dose rapidly.[4] Implementing protective measures (eg, protective lead shielding) helps to prevent injury from radiation sources.[1] Lead shielding should be placed between the patient and the source of radiation.[9] Shielding placed on the wrong side (ie, away from the source) can actually increase the dose to the patient. Lead shielding should not be in the beam in fluoroscopic procedures (eg, hand surgery).

2. Lead shielding should be used, when possible, to protect the thyroid during x-ray studies of the upper extremities, trunk, and head. Thyroid and lymphoid tissues are shown to be sensitive to radiation exposure.[9]

3. Lead shielding should be used, when possible, to protect the patient's ovaries or testes (ie, gonads) during x-ray studies, including those performed on the hips and upper legs.

4. Female patients of childbearing age should be questioned about the possibility of pregnancy.

- If the possibility of pregnancy exists, the surgeon should be notified to determine the advisability of continuing or postponing the procedure.
- Lead shielding should be used to protect the fetus when other areas of a pregnant woman's body are x-rayed. The fetus is highly sensitive to ionizing radiation. Scatter radiation may expose the fetus to low-level radiation. Radiation to the abdomen and pelvis in women who are pregnant or may be pregnant poses an increased risk to the fetus and may result in childhood cancers.[10,11] Proper safety measures minimize the actual risk. The perioperative nurse should assess the history of all premenopausal women to ensure that they are aware of radiation exposure risks during pregnancy.[6]

Recommendation III

Occupational exposure to radiation should be minimized.

Guidelines for radiation safety are based on the principles of time, distance, and shielding. When exposed to radiation at a constant rate, the total dose equivalent received depends on the length of time exposed. If the distance from the point source of radiation is doubled, the exposure is quartered.[1] Radiation that scatters as the x-ray beam passes through the patient is the main source of radiation exposure. Passage through materials reduces the amount of radiation. State and government regulations that stipulate the dose limits for occupational exposure are described in the glossary.

1. Warning signs should be posted to alert personnel to potential radiation hazards at entrances to ORs and procedure rooms where radiological equipment is in use, as required by state regulations. State regulations provide requirements for posting warning signs at entrances to rooms where radiation is a potential hazard. These requirements apply equally to all areas where radiological equipment is used. Applicable state regulations should be followed.

2. Personnel should limit the amount of time spent in close proximity to the radiation source when exposure to radiation is possible.[12] Minimizing beam "on" time during fluoroscopic procedures by using the last-image hold fea-

ture may decrease the dose of radiation to the patient and personnel.[4,7]

3. The radiation equipment operator should notify personnel present in the treatment room before activating the equipment.[12]

4. During intracoronary brachytherapy, close contact with the patient should be limited to less than five minutes whenever possible. An authorized user, medical physicist, or radiation safety officer should be present before the therapy is initiated to ensure staff member safety. Designated safe areas should be determined before initiating treatment to allow staff members to distance themselves from exposure to increased radiation levels.[13]

5. Personnel should be aware of scatter radiation that is emitted from the patient in all directions in both radiological and fluoroscopic procedures.[13] Scatter radiation is a significant hazard to personnel, especially in fluoroscopic procedures. Variability exists as to the total amount of radiation that is emitted due to the intensity of the radiation primary beam, the size of the beam area, and the patient's dimensions. Larger patients may require greater radiation beam intensity in order to produce greater image quality, which may result in greater radiation scatter.[12]

6. During fluoroscopic procedures, personnel should keep the patient as close as possible to the image intensifier side of the fluoroscopic unit and away from the tube side of the unit. Keeping the patient close to the image intensifier side lowers the dose required to produce an image, decreases the amount of radiation scatter, and decreases the amount of radiation emitted to the personnel assisting with the procedure. Doubling the distance from the source of emitting radiation reduces the intensity of the radiation by a factor of four.[12]

7. To reduce exposure, personnel involved in fluoroscopic procedures should stand on the image intensifier side of the fluoroscopic unit whenever possible.[14] Using fluoroscopy in lateral views tends to produce greater radiation scatter from the patient. Personnel standing on the same side as the image intensifier experience a decrease in radiation intensity.[3,12]

8. Personnel assisting with radiological procedures should not hold the patient manually for

a study because of the risk of exposure by the direct beam.[12] Slings, traction devices, and sandbags should be used to maintain patient position during radiation exposure. Cassette holders should be used to position films. If manual holding cannot be avoided, the individual should be protected from the primary x-ray beam. A 0.5 mm lead-equivalent shield or apron should be worn.

9. Whenever possible, shielding should be employed to provide attenuation of the radiation being delivered to the personnel potentially exposed.[14] Types of shielding available to personnel may include, but are not limited to,
   ♦ walls, windows, control booths, and doors;
   ♦ mobile rigid shields on wheels for transport to various areas;
   ♦ ceiling-suspended transparent barriers;
   ♦ flexible aprons (eg, wraparound, open backs), vests, skirts, thyroid shields, and gloves; and
   ♦ leaded safety eyeglasses with side shields.

10. Personnel who may have to stand with their backs to the radiation beam should wear wraparound aprons to decrease the risk of exposure. It is important to note, however, that wraparound aprons may not provide the same level of protection to both sides of the staff member because the front of the apron usually is double in thickness.[3] Personnel should turn toward the radiation beam when possible to minimize the dose of radiation during a procedure and maximize safety. Light-weight aprons that meet the thickness requirements should be considered for comfort and user compliance.

11. Shielding of the upper legs of personnel near the radiation beam (eg, oblique imaging with the x-ray tube in close proximity to the lower body of the operator) should be initiated to protect the long bones and bone marrow from increased doses of radiation. Aprons should be as long and as wide as needed to provide protection.[12]

12. Shielding of the upper chest and neck of personnel nearest the x-ray tube (eg, oblique imaging with the x-ray tube in close proximity to the upper chest of the operator) may reduce radiation risk. Thyroid shields should be worn to protect the thyroid whenever the likelihood of the procedure (eg, orthopedic spinal fixation procedures) places the operator at higher risk because

of increased exposure.[15] Females should protect their breasts from radiation exposure and aprons should cover the area completely.[3]

13. Some individuals who will be farther away from the x-ray beam may choose to wear aprons with less protection because they are lighter and cause less muscle strain. If aprons with different levels of protection are stored in the same area, the aprons that have less protection should be easily identified to avoid confusion as to the level of safety afforded to the personnel who are wearing them. State regulations should be followed concerning the minimum thickness required for aprons in the facility.[3]

14. Shielding the lens of the eye by using leaded face shields or leaded eyeglasses with wraparound side shields should be used to reduce scatter radiation to the operator when it is anticipated that increased fluoroscopic time may be necessary. Repeated exposure of the eyes over time can produce ulceration of the cornea and cataracts.[16] Leaded eyewear is recommended for personnel who are likely to receive levels of radiation measured by collar badge readings above 15,000 millirem roentgen equivalent unit (mrem) per year annually. Side eye shields also may be beneficial for personnel who perform procedures during which it is necessary to turn away from the radiation beam.[12]

15. Personnel participating in fluoroscopic procedures during which they are less than 24 inches (ie, 70 cm) away from the x-ray beam may consider routinely wearing a thyroid shield and leaded eyeglasses especially during procedures where increased time/dose to the patient are performed.[17]

16. In general, no part of the operator's body should be in the direct x-ray beam. If the operator's hand will be in the direct beam, radiation attenuation gloves should be considered. These gloves afford some protection and may be of benefit in reducing the amount of radiation exposure during a procedure. Most radiation attenuation gloves provide only 33% to 35% safety attenuation.[15] Outside the direct beam, protective gloves are very cumbersome and the inconvenience may outweigh any protective advantage. Even if protective gloves are worn, hands still should be kept out of the x-ray beam as much as possible. Remote handling devices

(eg, forceps) should be used whenever possible to minimize the need for the operator's hand to be exposed to radiation.[12]

17. Occupational exposure should be minimized during sentinel node biopsy. Sentinel node biopsy is useful in demonstrating evidence of micrometastatic disease. A gamma-emitting radiocolloid (ie, technetium-99m) can be injected into the patient's tissue to find the sentinel node.[18] The use of time, distance, and shielding should be employed during these procedures to limit personnel exposure to the radioactive isotope. The risk of radiation exposure in these procedures is minimal. Sentinel nodes demonstrating radioactivity should be labeled as radioactive before transporting the specimens from the OR.

18. Personnel with known or suspected pregnancy should declare this condition to the radiation safety officer or other appropriate facility channels. State regulations vary regarding pregnant personnel and radiation safety. State guidelines are based upon the US Nuclear Regulatory Commission (NRC) guidelines regarding confidentiality in the pregnant worker. Disclosure of the pregnancy, even if it is obvious, is not required. A written, voluntary, official declaration that includes the estimated date of conception may be used to base the total dose limit to the pregnant person.[3] The NRC guidelines include the following.

♦ Occupational dose to the embryo or fetus of an occupationally exposed staff member who has declared her pregnancy must not exceed 0.5 rem during the entire gestational period.

♦ Dose should be uniform over time and not all at once (ie, at one point in the gestational period).

♦ Deep-dose equivalent of the declared pregnant worker must be used as the dose to the embryo or fetus. The dosimeter should be worn at the waist under the apron shield.[3] Radiation must pass through several layers of tissue before reaching the fetus; therefore, this dosimeter reading does not reflect the amount of radiation reaching the fetus. Leaded shielding will attenuate 95% to 98% of the radiation.

19. State regulations regarding the monitoring of radiation in pregnant workers may monitor radiation differently as evidenced by the number of dosimeters worn, the area(s) the dosimeters are placed on the body, and whether the dosimeters are placed under or over shielding during the procedure.[3]

20. Maternity aprons may be worn to decrease the amount of radiation to the embryo or fetus. Although there is double thickness in the area where most pregnant workers need the protection, caution should be used by the pregnant worker when turning away from the x-ray beam. Most aprons do not shield the back of the pregnant worker.[3] These aprons are heavier and may be more difficult to wear, placing extra strain on the shoulders of the pregnant worker. Organizations may decide to purchase these aprons for pregnant workers and should mark the aprons to make the aprons easy to identify and ensure that they will be available for those who choose to wear them.

Recommendation IV

Shielding devices should be handled carefully, visually examined before use, and x-rayed at least annually to detect and prevent damage that could diminish their effectiveness.

1. Newly purchased leaded protective devices should be tested for attenuation and for shielding properties to check for cracks and holes in shipping before use. Subsequently, all leaded protective devices should be checked for defects and wear at least annually and whenever damage is suspected.[3] The frequency of testing is dependent upon the type of device used and the care that the device receives as it is used because excessive misuse can increase the risk of cracks and damage.[19,20]

2. Leaded aprons and thyroid shields should be stored flat or hung vertically and should not be folded. Leaded aprons and shields are susceptible to cracking, which can reduce the apron's effectiveness as a shielding barrier.

3. Testing documentation of all leaded protective devices should be maintained in the radiology department or in the facility safety office. Areas that purchase new aprons should notify the department where the testing is performed so records are kept up-to-date and accurate. All aprons should be labeled or numbered so that each apron can be tracked if necessary.

4. Protective devices should be cleaned with an EPA-registered hospital disinfectant after every use.

Recommendation V

Individuals should be protected from exposure to patients who have received diagnostic or therapeutic radionuclides that may pose a radiation risk.

1. Facilities that use therapeutic radionuclides should employ a radiation safety officer. This individual should determine specific organizational policies and procedures. The primary function of the radiation safety officer is supervision of the daily operation of the radiation safety program to ensure that individuals are protected from radiation. The radiation safety officer should determine which individuals are in frequent proximity to radiation, which should wear monitoring devices, and how occupational exposure is monitored and recorded.

2. Personnel should use the principles of time, distance, and shielding when caring for patients who have received therapeutic radionuclides. Radionuclide materials are absorbed by the body and safety precautions are required depending on the absorption and excretion of the radionuclide.[3] Patients who have received radionuclides emit radiation until the nuclide has decayed or has been eliminated.[20] Body fluids and tissue removed from patients who have undergone recent diagnostic nuclear medicine studies should be handled according to radiation safety procedures and standard precautions and should be labeled radioactive. These procedures should be based on government regulations and recommendations.

3. Contamination-control measures should be applied to the use of unsealed radioactive materials.[1] When transferring patients who received therapeutic radionuclides in the OR, perioperative personnel should notify personnel receiving the patients of the radiation source and anatomical location before patient transfer. All radiation precautions should be observed during transfer of the patient from one area or unit to another. The radiation safety officer should establish policies concerning how patients are transferred after receiving therapeutic radionuclides to minimize exposure to staff

members. Advance communication allows personnel time to protect themselves, the patient's visitors and family members, and other patients from unnecessary exposure to radiation.[5]

4. Preparation of sealed radionuclides, such as prostatic seeds, may require sterilization before use. Manufacturers' written instructions should be followed for sterilization. Sealed radionuclides requiring sterilization should be packaged and sterilized according to the "Recommended practices for sterilization in perioperative practice settings."[21] Prevacuum sterilization cycles should not be used because the vacuum may displace the seeds and potentially cause a radiation hazard to personnel.[22] Flash sterilization of the seeds should be avoided. Implantable medical devices should not be flash sterilized because of possible patient complications and because it is difficult to ensure aseptic delivery and personnel safety. Varying sterilization times have been cited in the literature. Health care facilities may wish to purchase pre-sterilized seeds or needles to minimize the risk to personnel who have to prepare these devices for use.[23]

5. Manufacturers' written instructions for preparation of eye plaques should be followed. Eye plaques are a form of brachytherapy used for treatment of choroidal melanoma.[24] Radionuclide seeds are placed in silicone tubes and secured to gold discs sutured next to the tumor. Gold is used to decrease the amount of scatter radiation to the adjacent retina, choroid, and optic nerve. The same guidelines should be used as for other types of radioactive seeds. The radiation safety officer or a designee should ensure containment of the seeds.

6. The radiation safety officer or a designee should ensure compliance with NRC regulations when prostatic radionuclides are sterilized and used in the OR. This person should control and maintain strict surveillance of the radionuclides that are in controlled or unrestricted areas and that are not in storage.[25]

7. If radionuclide seeds such as prostate seeds are processed for use in a central processing department, the seeds must remain in constant surveillance during the entire processing period and delivery to the OR.[25] Central processing supervisors should consult the radiation safety officer for questions concerning dose limits and

surveillance in central processing. Dosimeter monitoring and specific training may be required to ensure that dose limits fall within the established guidelines. Staff members who sterilize prostatic seeds should receive training from the radiation safety officer that includes techniques for

- handling radioactive nuclides;
- minimizing exposure to radiation (ie, as low as reasonably achievable);
- controlling and providing security for the material (ie, constant surveillance); and
- emergency response to spills of radioactive material.[23]

Recommendation VI

Radiation monitors or dosimeters should be worn by personnel who are in frequent proximity to radiation as determined by the radiation safety officer.

1. Individuals must comply with state regulations concerning placement of the monitors worn. Personnel who routinely are involved in fluoroscopic procedures should wear at least one radiation monitor approved by the National Voluntary Laboratory Accreditation Program.[26] When single monitoring devices are used, they should be worn on the same area of the body by all health care personnel. Radiation monitoring devices are the principal mechanism for monitoring radiation exposure of the personnel on a day-to-day basis and, therefore, should be used consistently by health care personnel working with radiation.[14]

2. State regulations for radiation monitoring must be followed. When two monitoring devices are used, one usually is worn at the neckline outside the leaded apron and the other inside the leaded apron. The monitor worn under the apron measures whole-body levels, while the one at the neckline measures head, neck, and lens of the eye exposure.[26] The radiation safety officer may require that the monitors be worn at other sites depending on the dose information desired. Personnel monitoring is required for individuals who have a reasonable probability of exceeding 10% of the occupational dose equivalent limit of 0.05 Sievert (Sv) (ie, 5 rem) per year.[27] Practitioners who perform interventional vascular, biliary tract, or genitourinary tract procedures should wear a finger monitor in the same location for every procedure.[26]

3. Radiation monitors or radiation dosimeters should be worn at the waist for all pregnant personnel and read monthly, not quarterly.[1]

4. Radiation monitoring devices or dosimeters should be removed and stored at the facility at the end of every workday. Radiation monitoring devices should not be removed and taken home because the device will collect ionizing radiation from other sources (eg, sun, soil, airport scanners). Documentation of the readings of the dosimeters should be kept in the facility's safety office.

Recommendation VII

Therapeutic radiation sources should be handled minimally to minimize exposure. Protective measures are implemented to prevent injury.[2,6]

1. Radioactive materials always should be used under direct supervision of the radiation safety officer or an authorized user. Radioactive materials should be kept in a protective container. The container reduces, but does not eliminate, exposure to radiation. Radioactive sources should never be left unattended when not in use.[1] Transport containers should remain under the direct supervision of the radiation safety officer or authorized user, or locked in a safe storage area.[13] Radioactive waste should never be placed in a nonradioactive waste container.

2. Radioactive sealed sources (eg, capsules, seeds, needles) should be handled with forceps, tongs, or tube racks. Forceps are used to increase the distance between the health care worker and the radiation source. Health care workers should never handle a sealed source with hands or fingers. Radiation protective gloves and aprons do not provide adequate shielding of therapeutic radionuclides; their inconvenience precludes their use for therapy. Examination gloves do not provide radiation shielding. They serve to control contamination if the radionuclide is a liquid or an unsealed source.[1]

3. Radioactive spills must be contained and disposed of in accordance with state and federal regulations. The source should be contained and completely removed, and the area cleaned thoroughly to remove any residual contamination. The area should be tested to verify that all radioactive material has been removed. Supplies used for cleanup should be discarded as

radioactive waste. Perioperative registered nurses who work in this environment must receive training from the radiation safety officer or designee annually.[1]

4. An appropriate label (ie, radioactive waste label) must be placed on all radioactive waste. Such labels should include at least
   ◆ radioisotope name,
   ◆ activity,
   ◆ date of disposal, and
   ◆ radiation personnel's/authorized user's full name and contact information.[1]

Recommendation VIII

Measures taken to protect patients during the procedure from the risks of direct and indirect radiation exposure should be documented on the perioperative nursing record.

1. Perioperative nursing documentation should include the type of patient protection and the area(s) protected. Documentation of nursing interventions promotes continuity of patient care, improves communication among health care team members, and serves as a medical legal record of patient care.[28] Documentation of the protective measures used is necessary to track outcomes and ensure safety of the patient and staff members.

2. Documentation should include the perioperative nurse's patient skin assessment, including signs and symptoms of injury to the skin and tissue as evidenced by
   ◆ redness,
   ◆ abrasions,
   ◆ bruising,
   ◆ blistering, or
   ◆ edema.[2]

3. The Perioperative Nursing Data Set (PNDS), the uniform perioperative nursing vocabulary, should be used to document patient care and to develop policies and procedures related to radiological safety. The expected outcome of primary importance to this recommended practice is "The patient is free from signs and symptoms of radiation injury" (O7). This outcome falls within the domain of Safety (D1). The associated nursing diagnosis is "Risk of impaired skin integrity" (X51). The associated interventions that may lead to the desired outcome may be "Assesses history

of previous radiation exposure" (142); "Verifies operative procedure, surgical site, and laterality" (143); and "Implements protective measures to prevent injury due to radiation sources" (174).[6]

Recommendation IX

Policies and procedures regarding radiation exposure should be written, reviewed periodically, and readily available within the practice setting.

1. Policies and procedures should be developed collaboratively and approved by perioperative personnel, the radiation safety officer, or the director of the radiology department in cooperation with safety committee members or the radiation safety expert in accordance with government regulations. Polices and procedures should be reviewed by a medical radiation physicist. Collaboration should ensure compliance with current radiation safety policies and contribute to quality patient care.[1]

2. Polices and procedures should include, but are not limited to,
   ◆ establishing authority, responsibility, and accountability for radiation safety;
   ◆ identifying measures for protecting patients and personnel from unnecessary exposure to ionizing radiation;
   ◆ developing procedures for handling and disposing of body fluids and tissue that may be radioactive;
   ◆ ensuring that appropriate personnel wear radiation monitoring devices; and
   ◆ scheduling radiographic testing of leaded protective devices.

3. Policies and procedures should be established in conjunction with the radiation safety officer for radiation safety training and competency in special handling techniques for personnel in the central processing department if sterilization of radiation seeds is performed there.

Recommendation X

Personnel should receive initial education, training, and competency validation and at least annual updates on new regulations and procedures.

1. All authorized users and radiation workers should complete initial training to include
   ◆ radiation safety (eg, risk, hazards, spill containment);

- biological effects of radiation;
- regulatory requirements; and
- environmental workplace techniques and procedures.

2. Documentation of training should include the above components and be maintained by the radiation safety officer.[1] Personnel who have not been involved in radiation procedures during the preceding two-year period should complete a refresher education and training program.

3. The radiation safety officer should provide annual competency validation, to include
   - a refresher course and testing for radiation safety and
   - a review of new regulations or procedures.

4. Educational programs should be developed to enhance knowledge that minimizes patient, personnel, and public risk of unnecessary exposure.

Recommendation XI

Only personnel who have received specific state-approved radiological training may be permitted to operate radiographic equipment.[26]

1. State-specific regulations must be followed regarding who may operate radiographic equipment. Legislation has been issued in various states restricting the use of this equipment to specific personnel who have demonstrated successful completion of formal education and training.

2. Operators of miniature mobile fluoroscopy units must adhere to the same state and federal regulations as all other radiological sources. The manufacturer's safety recommendations for the use of the device should be used when writing policies and procedures for the facility.

Glossary

Absorbed dose: The energy imparted to matter by ionizing radiation per unit mass of irradiated material at the place of interest. The special units of absorbed dose are the radiation absorbed dose (rad) (ie, 0.01 joule per kilogram) and gray (gy) (ie, one joule per kilogram), which is equal to 100 rads). The units for biological effective dose are the rem and sievert (sv).

Attenuation: The process by which a beam of radiation is reduced in intensity when passing through some material.

Authorized user: A physician or someone who has received special training or is credentialed to use radioactive materials and understands radiation physics, radiobiology, radiation safety, and radiation management.

Beam: A unidirectional flow of particle or electromagnetic radiation.

Conference of Radiation Control Program Directors (CRCPD): A nonregulatory organization that is a 501(c)(3) nonprofit, nongovernmental, professional organization dedicated to radiation protection.

Deep dose equivalent: The dose equivalent at a tissue depth of 1 cm; applies to the external whole body exposure.

Distance: The physical space between a source of radiation and its target (or the distance away from a source of radiation). The greater the distance an individual or target is from the source of radiation, the less the amount of radiation exposure. The inverse-square law applies—at a 4-ft distance from the source, the exposure received is approximately one quarter of that received at a 2-ft distance. Likewise, at a 6-ft distance the radiation is one ninth that received at a 2-ft distance.

Dosimeter: A device that is used to determine the external radiation dose that a person has received.

Equipment operator: A person with demonstrated qualifications and competency to operate a fluoroscopic system while exposing a patient to radiation. According to the American College of Radiology technical standard, only a physician is qualified to hold this title. Registered and/or licensed radiologic technologists or radiation therapists may perform fluoroscopic procedures if they are monitored by a supervising physician who is readily available.

Exposure: A measure of the total quantity of radiation reaching a specific point measured in the air. The unit of measure is based on the amount of ionization produced in air by a specified amount of x-ray energy. Radiation exposure is controlled in three ways—time, distance, and shielding.

External dose: That portion of the dose equivalent received from radiation sources outside the body.

Fluoroscopy: Observation of the internal features of an object by means of the fluorescence produced on a screen by x-rays transmitted through the object.

Gamma radiation: The emission of electromagnetic energy from the nucleus of an atom.

Gonad: Ovary or testis.

Gonad shield: A leaded device used to reduce x-ray exposure to the reproductive organs.

High radiation area: An area in which radiation levels could result in an individual receiving a dose equivalent in excess of 100 mrem per hour.

Internal dose: That portion of the dose equivalent received from radioactive material taken into the body.

Ionizing radiation: Electromagnetic radiation (eg, x-rays, gamma rays) that yields ions as it passes through an absorbing material (eg, air, tissue). The ions produce chemical reactions that are responsible for the biological expression of radiation (eg, cancer).

Leaded apron: A leaded-rubber material worn to protect personnel from scatter radiation.

Occupational dose: Annual exposure limits that took effect in 1994.[11]

- ◆ Total effective dose equivalent (TEDE) to radiation workers—5 rem.
- ◆ Dose equivalent to the eye—15 rem.
- ◆ Shallow dose equivalent to the skin, extremities—50 rem.
- ◆ TEDE to any other individual organ—50 rem.
- ◆ TEDE to an embryo or fetus of declared pregnant woman—0.5 rem.
- ◆ Minors—10% of worker limit.
- ◆ Members of the public—0.1 rem.

Quantify amount: A millirem is one one-thousandth of a rem.

Rad: Radiation absorbed dose.

Radioactivity: The property, possessed by certain nuclides, of spontaneously emitting particles of gamma radiation or of emitting radiation after orbital electron capture or spontaneous fission.

Radionuclide: A radioactive atom used in nuclear medicine that shows radioactive disintegration and emits alpha and beta particles or gamma rays. Some radionuclides are used for diagnostic studies to trace the function and structure of most organs. Those emitting beta particles are used primarily for treating malignant tumors.

Rem: A special unit of dose equivalent. The dose equivalent in rems is numerically equal to the absorbed dose in rads multiplied by the quality factor, which for most medical radiation is one.

Scatter radiation: Radiation is scattered when an x-ray beam strikes a patient's body, as it passes through the patient's body, and as it strikes surrounding structures (eg, walls, OR furniture).

Sealed and unsealed sources: Many radioactive pharmaceuticals come in the form of liquids or capsules and are administered orally. These are classified as unsealed sources. Some radioactive materials are sealed in small containment vessels, such as seeds, for implanting into tumors. These are classified as sealed sources.

Shallow dose equivalent: The dose equivalent at a tissue depth of 0.007 cm averaged over an area of 1 cm.[1]

Shielding: Radiation interacts with any type of material, and the amount of radiation is reduced during passage through materials. A thin layer of lead can absorb most scattered diagnostic x-rays. Gamma radiation from medically useful radionuclides is substantially attenuated by 1 to 2 inches of lead.

Time factor: The less time a person is exposed to radiation, the less radiation one absorbs. Remaining close to a source of radiation for 15 minutes, an individual receives one-half the radiation dose received if the exposure time was 30 minutes.

Total effective dose equivalent: The sum of deep-dose equivalent (ie, external exposures) and the committed effective dose equivalent (ie, internal exposures).

US Nuclear Regulatory Commission (NRC): A government group that regulates use of nuclear materials and assists with formulation of regulations that protect workers, the public, and the environment. The NRC also regulates nuclear materials that are used in science, medicine, and industry. The NRC issues licenses to those who operate power plants or use nuclear materials and conducts inspections to make sure these facilities are following established regulations.

X-ray intensifier: The radiation detector that produces the image in fluoroscopy.

X-ray tube: The radiation sources for x-ray and fluoroscopic machine.

REFERENCES

1. "Radiation safety manual," (August 1999) Centers for Disease Control and Prevention Radiation Safety Committee, *http://www.cdc.gov/od/ohs/manual/radman .htm* (accessed 23 May 2004).

2. "Radiation safety guide, chapter 11: Permissible exposure levels (dose limits)," (May 14, 2004) National Institute of Environmental Health Sciences, *http://www .niehs.nih.gov/odhsb/radhyg/radguide/sectxi.htm* (accessed 12 Dec 2006).

3. L Brateman, "The AAPM/RSNA physics tutorial for residents: Radiation safety considerations for diagnostic radiology personnel," (May 11, 1999) RadioGraphics, *http://radiographics.rsnajnls.org/cgi/content/full/19/4/1037* (accessed 1 Sept 2006).

4. L Strangio, "Interventional uroradiologic procedures," *AORN Journal* 66 (August 1997) 286-294.

5. "ACR practice guideline for the performance of low-dose-rate brachytherapy," (Jan 1, 2001) American

College of Radiology, http://www.acr.org/s_acr/bin.asp?CID =0&DID=12243&DOC=FILE.PDF (accessed 30 Aug 2006).

6. S C Beyea, ed, *Perioperative Nursing Data Set: The Perioperative Nursing Vocabulary,* second ed (Denver: AORN, Inc, 2002) 100-101.

7. T G Norris, "Radiation safety in fluoroscopy," *Radiologic Technology* 73 no 6 (July-August, 2002) 511-533.

8. "Recommended practices for sponge, sharp, and instrument counts," in *Standards, Recommended Practices, and Guidelines* (Denver: AORN, Inc. 2006) 459-468.

9. L K Otto, S Davidson, "Radiation exposure of certified registered nurse anesthetists during ureteroscopic procedures using fluoroscopy," *Journal of the American Association of Nurse Anesthetists* 67 (February 1999) 53-58.

10. D Gilmour, "Risks for the new or expectant mother," *British Journal of Perioperative Nursing* 10 (June 2000) 306-310.

11. US Nuclear Regulatory Commission, Office of Nuclear Regulatory Research, *Instruction Concerning Prenatal Radiation Exposure,* Regulatory Guide 8.13, Revision 3 (June 1999) 8.13.11- 8.13.12.

12. S M Fishman et al, "Radiation safety in pain medicine," *Regional Anesthesia and Pain Medicine* 27 (May/June 2002) 296-305.

13. B G Bass, "How to maximize safety and minimize radiation exposure for cath lab personnel," *Cardiovascular Disease Management/COR Healthcare Resources* 7 (March 2001) 5-7.

14. J Newman, "Radiation protection for radiologic technologists," *Radiologic Technology* 71 no 3 (2000) 273-286.

15. Y R Rampersaud, K T Foley, A C Shen, et al "Radiation exposure to the spine surgeon during fluoroscopically assisted pedicle screw insertion," *Spine* 25 no 20 (2000) 2637-2645.

16. E Brailsford, P L Williams, "Evidence based practice: An experimental study to determine how different working practice affects eye radiation dose during cardiac catheterization," *Radiography* 7 no 1 (2000) 21-30.

17. C T Mehlman, T G DiPasquale, "Radiation exposure to the orthopaedic surgical team during fluoroscopy: How far away is far enough?" *Journal of Orthopaedic Trauma* 11 no 6 (1997) 392-398.

18. "Practice guideline for breast conservation therapy in the management of invasive breast carcinoma," (January 1, 2002) American College of Radiology, http://www.acr.org/s_acr/bin.asp?CID=0&DID=12238&DOC=FILE.PDF (accessed 30 Aug 30, 2006).

19. "Testing of lead aprons for QA," Pulse Medical, Inc, http://www.rci-pulsemed.com (accessed 30 Aug 2006).

20. "Recommended guidelines for controlling noninfectious health hazards in hospitals," Standard 5.2.3.6, in *Guidelines for Protecting the Safety and Health of Health Care Workers,* National Institute for Occupational Safety and Health, http://www.cdc.gov/niosh/hcwold5d.html (accessed 30 Aug 2006).

21. "Recommended practices for sterilization in the perioperative practice setting," in *Standards, Recommended Practices, and Guidelines* (Denver: AORN, Inc, 2006) 629-643.

22. Y Yu et al, "Permanent prostate seed implant brachytherapy: Report of the American Association of Physicists in Medicine task group No. 64," *Medical Physics* 26 (October 1999) 2054-2076.

23. T Lembcke, "Sterile loading of radioactive materials into needles," in *Trans-Rectal Ultrasound Guided Trans-Perineal Implants of the Prostate Using* ^{125}I and ^{103}P and $HDR(^{192}Ir)$, Oconee Regional Cancer Center, http://www.oconeecancercenter.com/prostate/prosbk10.htm (accessed 30 Aug 2006).

24. J I Hui, T G Murray, "Radioactive plaque therapy," *International Ophthalmology Clinics* 46 no 1 (Winter 2006) 51-68.

25. "What are safe and legal options for radioactive source security during sterilization?" answer to question #212 submitted to "Ask the experts," Health Physics Society, http://www.hps.org/publicinformation/ate/q212.html (accessed 30 August 2006).

26. "ACR technical standard for management of the use of radiation in fluoroscopic procedures," (Jan 1, 2003) *Management of Fluoroscopic Procedures,* American College of Radiology, http://www.acr.org/s_acr/bin.asp?CID=0&DID=12244&DOC=FILE.PDF (accessed 30 Aug 2006).

27. E C Lipsitz et al, "Does the endovascular repair of aortoiliac aneurysms pose a radiation safety hazard to vascular surgeons?" *Journal of Vascular Surgery* 32 (October 2000) 704-710.

28. "Recommended practices for documentation of perioperative nursing care," in *Standards, Recommended Practices, and Guidelines* (Denver: AORN, Inc, 2006) 477-479.

PUBLICATION HISTORY

Originally published October 1989, *AORN Journal.* Published as proposed recommended practices September 1993.

Revised and reformatted; published January 2001, *AORN Journal.*

Revised 2006; published in *Standards, Recommended Practices, and Guidelines,* 2007 edition.

AORN Perioperative Standards and Recommended Practices, 2012 Edition

Recommended Practices for Prevention of Retained Surgical Items

The following Recommended Practices for Prevention of Retained Surgical Items were developed by the AORN Recommended Practices Committee and have been approved by the AORN Board of Directors. They were presented as proposed recommendations for comments by members and others. They are effective July 15, 2010.

These recommended practices are intended as achievable recommendations representing what is believed to be an optimal level of practice. Policies and procedures will reflect variations in practice settings and/or clinical situations that determine the degree to which the recommended practices can be implemented.

AORN recognizes the various settings in which perioperative nurses practice. These recommended practices are intended as guidelines adaptable to various practice settings. These practice settings include traditional operating rooms (ORs), ambulatory surgery centers, physicians' offices, cardiac catheterization laboratories, endoscopy suites, radiology departments, and all other areas where surgery and other invasive procedures may be performed.

Purpose

These recommended practices (formerly titled "Recommended practices for sponge, sharp, and instrument counts") provide guidance to perioperative registered nurses (RNs) in preventing retained surgical items (RSIs) in patients undergoing surgical and other invasive procedures. Avoiding injuries from the care that is intended to help patients was identified by the Institute of Medicine as one of six goals to achieve a better health care system.[1] Counts for soft goods (eg, radiopaque sponges, radiopaque towels); sharps; and instruments are performed to account for all items used on the surgical field and to lessen the potential for injury to the patient as a result of an RSI. Health care organizations are responsible for employing standardized, transparent, verifiable, reliable practices to account for all surgical items used during a procedure to lessen the potential for patient harm as a result of retention. There is a potential for inaccurate counts with both current variable manual counting practices and the use of adjunct technology.[2-7] Therefore, behavioral change and an understanding of risk reduction strategies unique to each setting should be employed when adopting system(s) to account for all surgical items. A reliable system to account for all surgical items includes, but is not limited to, complete and accurate counting, radiological confirmation, and the use of adjunct technology, to promote optimal perioperative patient outcomes.

Current law does not prescribe what methodologies should be used, who should use them, or even that they need to be used. It does, however, require that surgical items not intended to remain in the patient be removed. The doctrine of res ipsa loquitur (ie, "the thing speaks for itself") is most applicable in RSI incidents. Therefore, the time and effort in legal tort cases is spent assigning blame or fault for the act because it is not always necessary to prove negligence. The "captain of the ship" doctrine is no longer assumed to be true, and members of the entire surgical team can be held liable in litigation for RSIs.[8-10]

Retained surgical items are considered a preventable occurrence. Many states require public reporting when these events occur. Federal and state agencies, accrediting bodies, third-party payers, and professional associations consider an RSI a sentinel event or "never event." Health care organizations and providers will not be reimbursed for additional care provided as a result of "never events."[8,11-15]

The incidence of RSIs is well-documented in the literature dating as early as the 1800s.[2,3,5-7,16-18] There is immense variability, however, in the occurrence rates and identified risks. In a study of retained foreign items, 52% were radiopaque sponges and 43% were instruments.[7] The RSIs in this study were associated with multiple major procedures being performed at the same time. Another study reported count discrepancies in 29 procedures (ie, 45% for radiopaque sponges, 34% for instruments, 21% for needles).[5] The study suggests that emergency procedures and unexpected changes in procedures correlated to an increased risk of RSIs. Closed claim studies conducted between 1985 and 2001 demonstrated that roughly 69% of reported cases of RSIs involved radiopaque sponges.[2]

Although the majority of retained radiopaque sponges are found in the abdomen and pelvis, there are reports in the literature discussing retained radiopaque sponges in the vagina, thorax, spinal canal, face, brain, and extremities.[2,6,8] The risk exists for RSIs even in the smallest of incisions.[3] A general strategy for preventing RSIs is to account for all items opened or used in a procedure at the end of the procedure because the potential risk for retention cannot always be predicted.

Common strategies in the literature that have been used to mitigate the incidence of RSIs include development of standardized procedures combined with manual counting; enhanced communication; multidisciplinary teamwork; radiological verification; and use of adjuncts (eg, count bags, technology to supplement manual sponge count procedures). Health care organizations are responsible for drafting policies and procedures applicable to their practice setting. It is imperative to value teamwork and hold all perioperative personnel accountable for the adoption, implementation, and review of their designated procedures and practices.

Recommendation I

A consistent multidisciplinary approach for preventing RSIs should be used during all surgical and invasive procedures.

Retained surgical items are preventable events that can be reduced by implementing multidisciplinary system and team interventions.[12,19,20] Retained surgical items may result in morbidity and mortality for the patient and prove to be costly to health care organizations.[3,13,14,21]

Establishing a system that accounts for all surgical items opened and used during a procedure constitutes a primary and proactive injury-prevention strategy. Performing surgical item counts is one RSI-prevention strategy. Accounting systems that involve counting and detection are, at a minimum, team-based activities composed of input from multiple team members. The practices employed should be standardized, transparent, verifiable, and reliable. All items need to be accounted for at the end of a procedure so that all team members can be sure that a surgical item is not left in the patient.[22]

I.a. All perioperative team members should be responsible for the prevention of RSIs.

I.a.1. Any individual who observes an item dropped from the surgical field should immediately inform the RN circulator and other members of the perioperative team.[3]

I.a.2. Any perioperative team member (eg, anesthesia care provider, float RN) who assists the surgical team by opening sterile items such as extra sutures or radiopaque sponges onto the sterile field should
- count the items with the scrub person;

- add the counted items to the count documentation (ie, count sheet, whiteboard); and
- promptly inform the RN circulator about what was added.[3,23]

Other team members may be asked to open supplies while the RN circulator is occupied with other patient care activities. Opening extra supplies without properly adding them to the count sheet or whiteboard may lead to a discrepancy at the end of the procedure.

I.a.3. A count may be initiated by any member of the perioperative team involved in the counting process.

I.a.4. Unnecessary activity and distractions should be curtailed during the counting process to allow the scrub person and RN circulator to focus on counting tasks.

An environment that is filled with noise and distractions is likely to result in ineffective communication.[19,24-26] Distractions during counting can lead to incorrect counts.[4,27,28] Distractions may include excessive noise (eg, radio, equipment, pagers, telephones); multi-tasking (eg, patient care, charting, retrieving supplies, adding surgical items to the field); and interruptions or breaks in attention (eg, conversations not related to patient care).[24,29,30] It is unlikely that all activities can be eliminated during the counting process; however, communication can be enhanced with reliable team-based practices that withstand the interruptions and conflicting activities that are part of the surgical environment.

I.a.5. Counts and events that would require a count (eg, relief of scrub person or RN circulator) should not be performed during critical portions of the procedure.

I.b. The RN circulator should actively participate in safety measures to prevent RSIs during all phases of a procedure and observe the sterile field to assist in the reduction of RSIs.

Accurately accounting for items used during a surgical procedure is a primary responsibility of the RN circulator and the perioperative team members.[31] The RN circulator plays a leading role in implementing measures to account for surgical items.

I.b.1.   The RN circulator should facilitate the count process by initiating the count, performing count procedures in concert with the perioperative team, documenting count reconciliation activities, and reporting any count discrepancy. (See Recommendation VI.)

I.c.   The scrub person and the RN circulator should perform standardized procedures when accounting for all surgical items opened or used during a procedure as required by the health care organization's policy.

Reason's study of human error has shown that errors involve some kind of deviation from routine practice.[32] Deliberate, consistent application and adherence to standardized procedures are necessary to prevent the retention of surgical items.[2-4,7,28,33-36]

I.c.1.   The scrub person should maintain an organized sterile field with minimal variation between scrub persons.

Maintaining an organized sterile field facilitates accounting for all objects during and after the operative procedure. Standardized sterile setups established by the health care organization's policy reduce variation and may lessen risk of error.

I.c.2.   Sharps should be confined and contained in specified areas of the sterile field or within a sharps containment device.

I.c.3.   The scrub person should maintain awareness of the location of soft goods (eg, radiopaque sponges, towels, textiles); miscellaneous items; and instruments on the sterile field during the course of the procedure. It is the scrub person's responsibility to

- know the character and configuration of soft goods, instruments, and devices that are used by the surgeons and first assistants;
- verify the integrity and completeness of soft goods when they are counted;
- ensure that the RN circulator sees surgical items being counted;
- confirm that instruments or devices that are returned from the operative site are intact; and
- speak up when a discrepancy exists.

A standardized, transparent, verifiable, reliable process of accounting for soft goods, sharps, needles, instruments, and small items may decrease the incidence of RSIs. Although there is a greater incidence of RSIs for soft goods, the risk also exists for retained instruments and device fragments.[3,5,7,37]

I.d.   Surgeons should engage in safe practices that support prevention of RSIs.

The American College of Surgeons recognizes patient safety as "the highest priority and strongly urges individual hospitals and healthcare organizations to take all reasonable measures to prevent the retention of foreign bodies in the surgical wound."[36] It is the responsibility of all perioperative team members to engage in safe practices for the prevention of RSIs.

I.d.1.   The surgeon(s) and surgical first assistant(s) should maintain awareness of all soft goods, instruments, and sharps used in the surgical wound during the course of the procedure. The surgeon does not perform the count but should facilitate the count process by

- using only radiopaque surgical items in the wound;
- communicating placement of surgical items in the wound to the perioperative team for notation (eg, whiteboard);
- acknowledging awareness of the start of the count process;
- removing unneeded soft goods and instrumentation from the surgical field at the initiation of the count process;
- performing a methodical wound exploration when closing counts are initiated;
- accounting for and communicating about surgical items in the surgical field; and
- notifying the scrub person and RN circulator about surgical items returned to the surgical field after the count.

I.e.   Anesthesia care providers should maintain situational awareness and engage in safe practices that support the prevention of RSIs.

Situational awareness is the process of recognizing a threat and taking steps to avoid the threat.

I.e.1.   Anesthesia care providers should plan anesthetic milestone actions so that these actions do not pressure the perioperative team to perform insufficient accounting practices.[3]

Completion of the proper counting procedures is the responsibility of the entire perioperative team.

I.e.2.   Anesthesia care providers should not use counted items.

I.e.3.   Anesthesia care providers should verify that throat packs, bite blocks, and other similar devices are removed from the oropharynx and communicate to the perioperative team when these items are inserted and removed.

I.f.   Complete and detailed communication between OR personnel and radiologic technologists and radiologists should occur when requesting radiological support to prevent RSIs. (See Recommendation VI.)

These activities focus the radiologist's view and aid in the best chance of being able to see the surgical items on the radiograph. Radiological imaging along with other perioperative activities may mitigate the risk of RSIs.[38]

Recommendation II

Radiopaque surgical soft goods (eg, sponges, towels, textiles) opened onto the sterile field should be accounted for during all procedures for which soft goods are used.

Accurately accounting for radiopaque sponges throughout a surgical procedure should be a priority and requires a multidisciplinary effort.[22,39-41]

Reports in surgical literature document that gossypiboma (ie, the unintentional retention of soft goods) can occur after a wide variety of surgical procedures.[2,37,42,43] Clinical presentation of gossypiboma is either acute or delayed. Acute presentations generally follow a septic course with abscess and/or granuloma formation. Delayed presentations may occur months or years after the original surgical intervention, with adhesion formation and encapsulation.[3,4,36,37,41,44-46]

II.a.   Initial counts of radiopaque soft goods should be performed and recorded for all surgical procedures.

Performing and recording initial counts establishes a baseline for subsequent counts on all procedures. Deliberate, consistent application and adherence to standardized procedures are necessary to prevent the retention of surgical items.[2-4,7,28,33-36]

II.b.   Counts of soft goods should be performed
- before the procedure to establish a baseline and identify manufacturing packaging errors (ie, initial count);
- when new items are added to the field;
- before closure of a cavity within a cavity (eg, uterus);
- when wound closure begins;
- at skin closure at the end of the procedure or at the end of the procedure when counted items are no longer in use (ie, final count); and
- at the time of permanent relief of either the scrub person or the RN circulator, although direct visualization of all items may not be possible.

Deliberate, consistent application and adherence to standardized procedures are necessary to prevent RSIs.[2-4,7,28,33-36] A standardized count procedure assists in achieving accuracy, efficiency, and continuity among perioperative team members. Studies of human error have shown that many errors involve some kind of deviation from routine practice.[32]

II.c.   Radiopaque sponges should be completely separated, viewed concurrently by two individuals, one of whom should be an RN circulator, and counted audibly.

Concurrent verification of counts by two individuals may lessen the risk of inaccurate counts. Separating radiopaque sponges during the initial baseline count helps to determine whether a sponge has been added to or removed from a sterilized package and that a radiopaque marker or identifying tag is present on each surgical sponge.

II.c.1.   Packages containing an incorrect number of radiopaque sponges or a manufacturing defect should be removed from the field, bagged, labeled, isolated from the rest of the radiopaque sponges in the OR, and excluded from the count. Packages containing an incorrect number of radiopaque sponges may be removed from the room before the patient's entry.

The initial sponge count is performed to determine that all packages of radiopaque sponges contain the correct number and the appropriate radiopaque marker or identification bar code, tag, or chip. Incorrect numbers of items or product defects within a package do occur.

Isolating the entire package containing an incorrect number of sponges may help reduce the potential for error in subsequent counts. Packages containing an incorrect number of radiopaque sponges may be removed from the room before the patient's entry to decrease confusion and the likelihood of error.

II.c.2. If the surgical sponge package is banded, the band should be broken and discarded before counting.

Leaving the package band in place may prevent the ability of each individual to see the sponges and allow one or more sponges to be undetected.

II.d. Additional radiopaque sponges added to the field should be counted at that time and recorded as part of the count documentation.

Counting and recording radiopaque sponges as they are added to the field is required to account for all items at the conclusion of the procedure.

II.e. Sponges should be left in their original configuration and should not be cut or altered in any way.

Altering a sponge by cutting or removing radiopaque portions invalidates counts and increases the risk of a portion being retained in the wound.

II.f. Soft goods counts should be conducted in the same sequence each time as defined by the health care organization. The counting sequence should be in a logical progression (eg, large to small item size, proximal to distal from the wound).

A standardized count procedure (ie, following the same sequence) assists in achieving accuracy, efficiency, and continuity among perioperative team members.[7,36] Studies of human error have shown that many errors involve some kind of deviation from routine practice.[32]

II.g. All soft goods used in the surgical wound should be radiopaque and easily differentiated from non-radiopaque soft goods (eg, sponges, towels).

Radiopaque indicators facilitate locating by radiograph an item presumed lost or left in the surgical field when a count discrepancy occurs.

Retained surgical towels have resulted in patient injury.[3,20,47,48] Surgical towels found in the abdomen and chest have been reported, as have instances of surgical towels found at autopsy or as a retained item after root cause analysis or focused case review.[49,50] When placed in a body cavity, an unmarked towel not included in the count may not be detected and increases the possibility of an RSI.

II.g.1. Non-radiopaque sponges used for skin preps that have a similar appearance to counted radiopaque sponges should be isolated before beginning the procedure to avoid possible confusion with the counted radiopaque sponges.

II.g.2. Radiopaque sponges should not be used as postoperative wound dressings.

The use of radiopaque sponges as surface dressings may invalidate subsequent counts if the patient is returned to the OR. The use of surgical sponges as surface dressings may appear as foreign items on postoperative radiographs and suggest a retained item.[51,52]

II.g.3. Non-radiopaque gauze dressing materials should be withheld from the field until the final count is conducted.

Separating dressing materials from the actual counted radiopaque sponges may help prevent intermingling with the sponges used in the procedure.

II.g.4. Dressing sponges included in custom packs should remain sealed and isolated on the field until the final count is resolved.

II.h. The final count should not be considered complete until all sponges used in closing the wound are removed from the wound and returned to the scrub person.

Sponges used in closing the wound could be left in the wound.

II.i. All counted radiopaque sponges should remain within the OR or procedure room during the procedure.

Confining all counted radiopaque sponges to the OR may help eliminate the possibility of a count discrepancy and aid in the disposal of all the radiopaque sponges to prevent carryover to subsequent procedures.

II.i.1. Pocketed sponge bags or similar systems should be used on all procedures where a soft goods count is performed.

Using a pocketed bag or other system for separating used radiopaque sponges facilitates the ability to see sponges for counting. Separating radiopaque sponges after use minimizes errors caused by sponges sticking together.

Draping used surgical sponges over the sides of the kick bucket is discouraged because it may be difficult for all team members to see each individual sponge. Wet, used sponges may drip blood and other potentially infectious fluids on the floor.

II.i.2. If a sponge is passed or dropped from the sterile field, the RN circulator should retrieve it using standard precautions, show it to the scrub person, isolate it from the field, and include it in the final count.

II.i.3. Linen and waste containers should not be removed from the OR or procedure room until all counts are completed and reconciled and the patient has been transferred out of the room.

II.i.4. Radiopaque surgical sponges should be disposed of and removed from the OR or procedure room at the end of the procedure after the patient has left the room.

Removing soft goods from the room at the end of the procedure may prevent potential count discrepancies between patients.

II.j. When soft goods are used as therapeutic packing (eg, intracavity, oral) and the patient leaves the OR with this packing in place, a standardized procedure should be defined and implemented to communicate the location of packing and the plan for eventual removal of the items.

II.j.1. When soft goods are intentionally used as therapeutic packing and the patient leaves the OR with this packing in place, the number and types of items placed should be documented in the medical record
- as reconciled and confirmed by the surgeon when this information is known with certainty, or
- as incorrect if the number and type of sponges used for therapeutic packing is not known with certainty.

II.j.2. The number and types of soft goods used for therapeutic packing should be included and communicated as part of the transfer of patient care information.[53]

II.j.3. When the patient is returned to the OR for a subsequent procedure or to remove therapeutic packing,
- the number and type of radiopaque soft goods removed should be documented in the medical record,
- the radiopaque sponges removed should be isolated and not included in the counts for the removal procedure,
- the surgeon and the surgical team should perform a methodical wound examination and consider taking an intraoperative radiograph, and
- the count on the removal procedure should be noted as reconciled if all radiopaque soft goods have been accounted for.

Additional safety measures may help to ensure that no soft goods remain in the patient when the number and type of radiopaque soft goods used for therapeutic packing is not known.

II.j.4. The surgeon should inform the patient of any soft good(s) purposely left in the wound at the end of the procedure and the plan for removing the item.[54]

Recommendation III

Sharps and other miscellaneous items that are opened onto the sterile field should be accounted for during all procedures for which sharps and miscellaneous item are used.

Needles may account for up to 50% of identified RSIs.[55] Miscellaneous items may be non-radiopaque and unintentionally retained in the surgical wound. Accurately accounting for sharps and other miscellaneous items during a surgical procedure is a primary responsibility of the RN circulator and the perioperative team members.

III.a. Initial sharps (eg, scalpels, needles) counts should be performed and recorded for all surgical procedures.

Performing and recording initial counts establishes a baseline for subsequent counts on all procedures. Deliberate, consistent application and adherence to standardized procedures is necessary to prevent the retention of surgical items.[2-4,7,28,33-36]

III.a.1. Standardized practices, manual counting procedures, and containment devices for sharps and needles should be employed to prevent needle miscounts, needle loss, and needlestick injuries.

Counting sharps and miscellaneous items is important to prevent item retention and reduce the risk of injuries to health care personnel and patients.[56] Operating room, sterile processing, housekeeping, laundry, and morgue personnel are at an increased risk for needlestick injury resulting in undue exposure to transmissible infections.[33,57] There are multiple reported cases of needlestick-associated injuries to health care personnel.[58-60] A standardized count procedure (ie, following the same sequence) assists in achieving accuracy, efficiency, and continuity among perioperative team members. Studies of human error have shown that many errors involve some kind of deviation from routine practice.[32]

III.a.2. All suture needles, regardless of size, should be counted for all surgical procedures.

Even small needles left in the patient may cause injury. Needles less than 10 mm, however, may be difficult to see radiographically when retention is suspected.[3,5,60] One study showed that radiologists inconsistently see small needles on intraoperative imaging studies.[55]

III.b. Counts of sharps and miscellaneous items should be performed

– before the procedure to establish a baseline and identify manufacturing packaging errors (ie, initial count);
– when new items are added to the field;
– before closure of a cavity within a cavity (eg, uterus);
– when wound closure begins;
– at skin closure at the end of the procedure or at the end of the procedure when counted items are no longer in use (ie, final count); and
– at the time of permanent relief of either the scrub person or the RN circulator, although the ability to directly see all items may not be possible.

III.b.1. Miscellaneous items that should be accounted for include, but are not limited to,
- defogger solution bottle, bottle cap, and associated accessories (eg, wipe, sponge);
- electrosurgery active electrode blades;
- electrosurgery scratch pads;
- endostaple reload cartridges;
- laparotomy sponge rings;
- Raney clips;
- trocar sealing caps;
- umbilical and hernia tapes;
- vascular inserts;
- vessel clip bars; and
- vessel loops.

III.c. Sharps and miscellaneous items should be counted audibly and viewed concurrently by two individuals, one of whom should be an RN circulator.

Concurrent verification of counts by two individuals may lessen the risk for count discrepancies.

III.d. Additional sharps and miscellaneous items added to the field should be counted when they are added and recorded as part of the count documentation.

Counting and recording sharps and miscellaneous items as they are added to the field may reduce the risk of error and may prevent an inaccurate count at the conclusion of the procedure.

III.e. Suture needles should be counted when the package is opened, verified by the scrub person, and recorded.

Viewing each needle will help ensure an accurate needle count.

III.e.1.   Empty suture packages should not be used to rectify a discrepancy in a closing needle count.

   The actual number of needles may not be the same as the number of empty packages.

III.f.   The scrub person should account for and confine all sharps on the sterile field until the final count is reconciled.

   Unconfined sharps remaining on the sterile field may be unintentionally introduced into the incision, dropped on the floor, or penetrate barriers. Confinement and containment of sharps may minimize the risk of needlestick injury to personnel as well as RSIs.

III.f.1.   Used sharps on the sterile field should be kept in a puncture-resistant container.

   Collecting used needles in a puncture-resistant container helps ensure their containment on the sterile field and assists in counting at the conclusion of the procedure.

III.g.   Sharps counts should be conducted in the same sequence each time as defined by the health care organization. The counting sequence should be in a logical progression (eg, sterile field to table to off the field).

   A standardized count procedure (ie, following the same sequence) assists in achieving accuracy, efficiency, and continuity among perioperative team members. Studies of human error have shown that many errors involve some kind of deviation from routine practice.[32]

III.h.   The scrub person should assess the condition of sharps or other items and verify that they are intact when returned from the operative site.

   Breakage or separation of parts can occur during open and minimally invasive surgical procedures. Verifying that all broken parts are present or accounted for helps prevent RSIs within the patient.[61,62]

III.h.1.   If a broken or separated item is returned from the operative site, the scrub person should immediately notify the perioperative team.

III.i.   The final count should not be considered complete until all the sharps used in closing the wound are removed from the wound and returned to the scrub person.

   Suture needles and other sharp items used in closing the wound could be left in the wound.

III.j.   All counted sharps should remain within the OR or procedure room during the procedure.

   Confining all sharps to the OR or procedure room helps minimize the possibility of a count discrepancy.

III.j.1.   If a sharp is passed or dropped from the sterile field, the RN circulator should retrieve it using standardized precautions, show it to the scrub person, isolate it from the field, and include it in the final count.

III.j.2.   Linen or waste containers should not be removed from the OR or procedure room until all counts are completed and reconciled and the patient has been transferred out of the room.

Recommendation IV

Instruments should be accounted for on all procedures in which the likelihood exists that an instrument could be retained.

Instrument counts protect the patient by reducing the likelihood that an instrument will be retained in the patient, including during minimally invasive procedures (eg, laparoscopy, thoracoscopy). Instrument counts are a proactive injury-prevention strategy. Retention of surgical instruments accounts for approximately one-third of retained item case reports.[5] Case studies demonstrate that many types and sizes of retained instruments have been found, ranging from small serrafine clamps to moderately sized hemostats (ie, 6 to 10 inches) to 13-inch-long retractors.[3,4]

IV.a.   Counts of instruments should be performed
   – before the procedure to establish a baseline (ie, initial count);
   – when new instruments are added to the field;
   – at wound closure or at the end of the procedure when counted items are no longer in use (ie, final count); and

   – at the time of permanent relief of either the scrub person or the RN circulator, although the ability to directly see all items may not be possible.

Deliberate, consistent application and adherence to standardized procedures are necessary to prevent RSIs (eg, surgical instruments).[2-4,7,28,33-36]

IV.a.1. Instruments should be counted when sets are assembled for sterilization.

A count of the instruments at assembly of the instrument set provides a basic inventory reference for the instrument set but is not considered the initial count before the surgical procedure. A count performed outside of the OR that is considered an initial count increases the number of variables that can contribute to a count discrepancy and unnecessarily extends responsibility to personnel not involved in direct patient care.

IV.b. The health care organization's policy should clearly define circumstances in which the instrument count may be waived.

Procedures in which accurate instrument counts may not be achievable or practical include, but are not limited to,
- complex procedures involving large numbers of instruments (eg, anterior-posterior spinal procedures);[6]
- trauma;[2,45,63]
- procedures that require complex instruments with numerous small parts; and
- procedures where the width and depth of the incision is too small to retain an instrument.

IV.c. Instruments should be counted audibly and viewed concurrently by two individuals, one of whom should be the RN circulator.

Concurrent verification of counts by two individuals assists in ensuring accurate counts.

IV.d. Individual pieces of assembled instruments (eg, suction tips, wing nuts, blades, sheaths) should be accounted for separately and documented on the count sheet.

Counting individual pieces of assembled instruments before and after a procedure reduces the risk of leaving a piece behind if the instrument becomes disassembled for any reason. Removable instrument parts can be purposefully removed or become loose and fall into the wound or onto or off of the sterile field.[61]

IV.e. Additional instruments should be counted and recorded as part of the count documentation when they are added to the sterile field.

Counting and recording instruments as they are added to the sterile field may prevent an inaccurate count at the conclusion of the procedure.

IV.f. Members of the surgical team should account for instruments in their entirety that may have broken or become separated within the confines of the surgical site.

Breakage or separation of parts can occur during open or minimally invasive surgical procedures. Verifying that the instrument is intact or that all broken parts are present and accounted for helps prevent RSIs within the patient.[61,62]

IV.g. Instrument counts should be conducted in the same sequence each time as defined by the health care organization. The counting sequence should be in a logical progression (eg, large to small item size, proximal to distal from the wound).

A standardized count procedure (ie, following the same sequence) assists in achieving accuracy, efficiency, and continuity among perioperative team members. Studies of human error have shown that many errors involve some kind of deviation from routine practice.[32]

IV.h. The final instrument count should not be considered complete until those instruments used in closing the wound (eg, malleable retractors, needle holders, scissors) are removed from the wound and returned to the scrub person.

Incidents of retained surgical instruments used in closing the wound have been reported.[64,65]

IV.i. All counted instruments should remain within the OR or procedure room during the procedure until all counts are completed and resolved.

Confining all counted instruments to the room helps eliminate the possibility of a count discrepancy.

IV.i.1.   Counted items either passed off or dropped from the sterile field should be retrieved by the RN circulator, isolated, and included in the final count.

IV.j.   All instruments should be accounted for and removed from the room during end-of-procedure cleanup.

Accounting for all instruments facilitates inventory control, as well as patient and personnel safety. Removing all instruments from the room helps prevent potential count discrepancies during subsequent procedures.

IV.k.   Preprinted count sheets should be used to record the counted instruments.

Preprinted count sheets provide organization and efficiency, which are key to preventing retained surgical instruments.

IV.k.1.   The circulating nurse should record only the number of instruments opened for the procedure.

IV.l.   Instrument sets should be standardized with the minimum number and variety of instruments needed for the procedure.

Reducing the number and types of instruments and streamlining standardized sets improves ease and efficiency of counting.

IV.l.1.   Instruments that are not routinely used on procedures should be removed from sets.

Specialty instruments, if needed, can be opened and added to the count at the time of the procedure.

Recommendation V

Measures should be taken to identify and reduce the risks associated with unretrieved device fragments.

Each year, the US Food and Drug Administration (FDA) Center for Devices and Radiological Health receives nearly 1,000 adverse event reports related to unretrieved device fragments. Serious adverse events have been associated with unretrieved device fragments. The FDA defines an unretrieved device fragment as "a fragment of a medical device that has separated unintentionally and remains in the patient after a procedure."[66]

V.a.   In the event that an unretrieved device fragment is left in the surgical wound (eg, broken instrument tip), the surgeon should inform the patient of the nature of the item and the risks associated with leaving it in the wound.

Health care professionals are encouraged to maintain public confidence by communicating with patients regarding their treatment and outcomes. Organizations are held accountable for informing patients of their rights when they enter the health care system.[54]

V.a.1.   Information provided to the patient should include, but is not limited to,
- material composition of the fragment (if known);
- size of the fragment (if known);
- location of the fragment;
- potential mechanisms for injury (eg, migration, infection);
- procedures or treatments that should be avoided, such as magnetic resonance imaging (MRI) examinations in the case of ferrous metallic fragments, which may help reduce the possibility of a serious injury from the fragment; and
- risks and benefits of retrieving the fragment as opposed to leaving it in the wound.

Recommendation VI

Standardized measures for investigation and reconciliation of count discrepancies should be taken during the closing count and before the end of surgery. When a discrepancy in the count(s) is identified, the surgical team should carry out steps to locate the missing item.[27,67]

Rapid intervention when an incorrect count is identified may reduce procedural time. Assessing the surgical site before closure decreases the time a patient remains under anesthesia and the risk of extended surgical time if the wound has to be reopened.[5] Early identification of RSIs decreases the likelihood that a surgical wound would need to be reopened and reduces or eliminates the need for radiographs to detect an RSI.[8]

VI.a.   The RN circulator should inform and receive verbal acknowledgment from the surgeon and surgical team as soon as a discrepancy in a surgical count is identified.[5,68]

The RN circulator has a responsibility and ethical obligation to speak up promptly when a discrepancy is identified. Clear and timely communication reinforces a safe patient culture.[3,31,69] A count discrepancy is a potential RSI incident.[70]

VI.a.1. The RN circulator should visually inspect the area surrounding the surgical field, including the floor, kick buckets, and linen and trash receptacles in an effort to locate the missing surgical item.

VI.a.2. The scrub person should assist with visual inspection of the area surrounding the sterile field when there is a count discrepancy.

VI.b. When a discrepancy in the count is identified, the surgeon(s) should
- suspend closure of the wound if the patient's condition permits,
- perform a methodical wound examination by actively looking for the missing item,
- cooperate in the attainment of radiographs or other modalities as indicated to find the missing item, and
- remain in the OR until the item is found or it is determined with certainty not to be in the patient.[3,4]

VI.c. If a missing item is not recovered, intraoperative imaging should be performed to rule out a retained item before final closure of the wound if the patient's condition permits. If the patient's condition is unstable, a radiograph should be taken as soon as possible in the next phase of care.[3,60]

Obtaining a radiograph when all other efforts have failed and before the patient's wound is closed allows the surgical team to remove a potential RSI before the wound is closed completely. In some jurisdictions, this also will prevent the necessity of reporting an RSI.

VI.c.1. In situations when accurate counting of surgical items is not possible, intraoperative imaging should be performed before the patient is transferred from the OR.[3,17,27,34]

VI.c.2. If intraoperative imaging is not available, the health care organization should have a policy and procedure describing the actions and communication required between referring and receiving organizations.

VI.c.3. A radiograph to locate a possible retained item may be waived under certain circumstances as defined in the health care organization's policy and procedure.

There are situations when it may be medically appropriate for the surgeon to determine it is not in the individual patient's best interest to perform an intraoperative radiograph to locate a potential RSI.

VI.c.4. Complete and detailed communication between OR personnel and radiologic technologists and radiologists should occur when requesting radiological support to prevent RSIs. The OR radiology request should include standardized information about the missing surgical item, including, but not limited to,
- the room where the procedure is being performed or the patient is located,
- the type of radiograph and views needed,
- a description of the missing surgical item,
- the operation performed, and
- the surgical site.[21,38]

These activities focus the radiologist's attention and aid in his or her ability to see the surgical items on the radiograph. Radiological imaging along with other perioperative activities may mitigate the risk of RSIs.[38]

VI.c.5. The radiologic technologist should be called promptly and respond expeditiously when an incorrect count occurs in the OR.[21]

VI.c.6. Intraoperative imaging should provide coverage of the surgical site and should include any views deemed necessary by the surgeon or radiologist to exclude the potential for RSIs. Radiological views should be obtained using recommended techniques and quality films or digital images to capture the full extent of the wound.

Progressive radiological techniques are recommended for successful identification of RSIs, including, but not limited to, multiple images, which may be necessary for full coverage. Images may include

- initial portable anterior and posterior (A&P) views followed by an oblique view if the A&P is negative;
- fluoroscopy, which may be used as an alternative technique if the RSI cannot be excluded with the intraoperative study; and
- unenhanced computerized tomography (CT), which should be considered if previous techniques are negative and a high suspicion remains for an RSI.[38]

VI.c.7. The radiologist should be consulted for guidance on the most appropriate available radiographic equipment to use to maximize the opportunity to identify a missing surgical item.[3,38]

Although some literature suggests that a radiograph taken in a radiology suite may be of better quality than a portable film taken in an OR, this would preclude finding a potential RSI before the wound is closed and the patient is taken out of the OR.[3,35,71] There is no evidence to support the use of a portable radiograph versus an image intensifier (ie, fluoroscopy). Portable radiographs have limitations, such as lower tube power; reduced ability to determine the character (eg, needle size and type) of an RSI; and limited placement options for film cassettes.[71]

VI.c.8. Intraoperative imaging for RSIs should be read by a radiologist and the results communicated directly to the surgeon in a timely manner.[3,38] Interpretation of intraoperative films should be communicated by direct report to the OR with read-back verbal confirmation between the radiologist and the surgeon.[21,38]

VI.c.9. Health care organizations should define needle size limit criteria where radiographs will effectively assist in identifying retained needles.

There is no definitive evidence to indicate how effective radiographs are in detecting small suture needles. Recent studies have demonstrated that needles 10 mm and smaller may not be consistently visible on a radiograph.[3,59,72,73] There is conflicting evidence regarding the visibility of 10-mm to 13-mm needles on radiographs.[3,19,20,35,55,60,72,73]

VI.c.10. The surgeon should inform the patient of the possibility of a retained needle as a result of an unresolved needle count and counsel the patient on the possible risks.

Recommendation VII

Perioperative staff members may consider the use of adjunct technologies to supplement manual count procedures.

Soft goods, such as radiopaque sponges and towels, represent the majority of RSIs. Paradoxically, studies suggest that the final count was documented as correct in 62% to 88% of RSI cases.[2,8,22,70,74] Manual counts can result in errors, especially during emergencies and unexpected surgical events. Intraoperative radiographs also are not always effective in identifying RSIs. In one study, 67% of intraoperative radiographs were read as negative when an RSI actually was present.[17]

Technologies have recently become available that are designed to supplement manual counting of soft goods, primarily radiopaque sponges, in an attempt to reduce RSIs.[20,75,76] Early identification of a retained sponge reduces the likelihood of delaying patient care; requiring additional measures, such as intraoperative radiographs to locate and retrieve the retained sponge; having to reopen the wound; or returning the patient to surgery for removal of the retained item at a later date. Use of this technology may allow timely detection of retained sponges even when a manual sponge count does not reveal a missing sponge. These technologies can be classified as count, detect, or count and detect.[20,70,75,77-81] In the future, adjunct technologies for accounting of needles and instruments may become available as well.

VII.a. A mechanism for evaluating and selecting existing and emerging adjunct technology products should be implemented.[82]

Patient safety is a primary concern of perioperative personnel. Safety concerns are the impetus for perioperative personnel as they participate in evaluating and selecting medical devices and products for use in practice settings.

VII.a.1. Perioperative RNs, physicians, and other health care providers involved in the use of products and medical devices for prevention of RSIs should be part of a multidisciplinary product evaluation and selection committee when the health care organization is evaluating the purchase of adjunct technology.[82]

VII.a.2. Perioperative personnel should evaluate existing and emerging adjunct technology to determine the application that may be most suitable in their setting.

Several adjunct technology products are currently available, and the technology is rapidly evolving.[44,75-77,79]

VII.a.3. Technology product standardization and value analysis processes should reflect functional and reliable products that are safe, cost-effective, environmentally friendly, and that promote quality patient care.[77,81,83]

VII.b. Adjunct technology may be used, where available, as an extra measure of safety to verify count accuracy throughout the reconciliation process.

The literature suggests that a combination of standardized procedures with manual counting; enhanced communication; multidisciplinary teamwork; radiological verification; and the use of adjuncts (eg, count bags, technology to supplement manual sponge count procedures) may decrease the incidence of RSIs.[2-4,7,17,19,44,48]

VII.b.1. Perioperative personnel should be aware of and competent in the proper use and application of adjunct technologies if used within the health care organization.[77]

Technological systems are dependent on proper usage and technique.

Recommendation VIII

Personnel should receive initial and ongoing education and demonstrate competency in the performance of standardized measures to prevent RSIs.

Initial and periodic education on practices for the prevention of RSIs provides direction for personnel in providing safe patient care. Additional periodic educational programs provide opportunities to reinforce previous learning and introduce new information on adjunct technology, its use, and potential risks. Competency validation serves as an indicator that personnel have an understanding of safe practices for the prevention of RSIs; the risks of injury (eg, needlesticks) to the patient and to health care personnel; and corrective actions that should be implemented when a process failure occurs.

VIII.a. An introduction and review of policies and procedures for prevention of RSIs should be included in orientation and ongoing education of personnel.

Reviewing policies and procedures assists health care personnel in developing knowledge, skills, and attitudes that affect patient outcomes.

VIII.b. Perioperative personnel should be knowledgeable about all accounting procedures, equipment, and technology used in the health care organization.

Rapid advances in clinical evidence and technology require continuous learning and skills updates to maintain competency.

VIII.b.1. Perioperative personnel should receive education and demonstrate competency in, but not limited to, the following:
- the performance of manual count procedures (eg, soft goods, instruments, sharps, miscellaneous items);
- the use of adjunct technology, following manufacturers' written instructions, if available;
- the roles, responsibilities, and accountability of each perioperative team member;
- measures for reconciliation of count discrepancies; and
- reporting of known or suspected RSIs.

Instruction and return demonstration in proper manual counting procedures and adjunct technology usage minimizes the risk of error. Competencies based on manufacturers' instructions provide personnel with information regarding the proper use of adjunct technologies. Incorrect use can result in

RSIs and serious patient injury. Equipment instruction manuals assist in developing operational, safety, and maintenance guidelines and serve as a reference for safe, appropriate use.

Recommendation IX

Measures taken for the prevention of RSIs should be documented in the patient's medical record.

Documentation of all nursing activities performed is legally and professionally important for clear communication and collaboration between health care team members and for continuity of patient care.[84]

IX.a. Sponge, sharp, and instrument counts should be documented on the patient's intraoperative record by the RN circulator.[84]

IX.b. Documentation of measures taken for the prevention of RSIs should include, but not be limited to,
- types of counts (eg, radiopaque sponges, sharps, instruments, miscellaneous items);
- number of counts;
- names and titles of personnel performing the counts;
- results of surgical item counts;
- surgeon notification of count results;
- any adjunct technology that was used and any associated records;
- an explanation for any waived counts;
- number and location of any instruments intentionally remaining with the patient or radiopaque sponges intentionally retained as therapeutic packing;
- unretrieved device fragments left in the wound, including
  - material composition,
  - size,
  - location (if known), and
  - manufacturer;
- actions taken if count discrepancies occur, including all measures taken to recover the missing item or device fragment and any communication regarding the outcome;
- rationale if counts are not performed or completed as prescribed by policy; and
- the outcome of actions taken.

Documentation of nursing activities related to the patient's perioperative care provides an account of the nursing care administered and provides a mechanism for comparing actual versus expected outcomes.[84] Such documentation is considered sound professional practice and demonstrates that all reasonable efforts were made to protect the patient's safety.[1] Extreme patient emergencies and certain individual patient considerations may necessitate waived counts to preserve a patient's life or limb. Documenting the rationale for waived counts and for variation in standard practice provides a record of the occurrence and an alert to subsequent caregivers that the patient may be at an increased risk for an RSI.

Recommendation X

Policies and procedures for the prevention of RSIs and unretrieved device fragments should be developed, reviewed periodically, revised as necessary, and readily available in the practice setting.

Policies and procedures establish authority, responsibility, and accountability. Policies and procedures assist in the development of patient safety, quality assessment, and quality improvement (QI) activities.[1] They also serve as operational guidelines that are used to minimize patient risk factors, standardize practice, direct staff members, and establish guidelines for continuous performance improvement activities. Best practices are subject to change with the emergence of new evidence and the advent of new technologies; therefore, periodic review and revision of the health care organization's policy is needed.

X.a. A multidisciplinary team should establish a policy and procedure for prevention of RSIs.[2,3,36,85] These policies and procedures should include, but not be limited to,
- items to be counted;
- directions for performing counts (eg, sequence, item grouping);
- waived count procedures in which baseline and/or subsequent counts may be exempt;
- alternative or additional safety measures for special circumstances;
- use of adjunct technology;
- measures necessary to reduce the risk of unretrieved device fragments including, but not limited to,

- use of the medical device in accordance with its labeled indications and the manufacturer's instructions for use, especially during insertion and removal,
- inspection of the medical device before use for damage during shipment or storage, as well as any out-of-box defects that could increase the likelihood of fragmentation during a procedure,
- inspection of the medical device immediately after removal from the patient for any signs of breakage or fragmentation, and
- retention of any damaged medical device to assist with the manufacturer's analysis of the event;
- the multidisciplinary team actions and procedures for count discrepancy reconciliation;
- when radiographic screening should be used in accounting for surgical items;
- documentation and reporting procedures for removal of RSIs; and
- competency validation.

All perioperative team members should be committed to and involved in establishing meaningful policies and procedures related to the prevention of RSIs. Detailed, clear, and concise policies provide consistent, standardized direction for the team. In situations with increased risk for RSIs, radiographic screening has been identified as an excellent method for improving early identification.[3,6,45]

X.a.1.   Polices and procedures should meet the requirements of regulatory and accrediting agencies.

X.a.2.   A policy and procedure for reporting product packaging defects to manufacturers should be established.

X.a.3.   Policies and procedures related to the use of adjunct technology should be based on the manufacturer's written instructions for use.

X.a.4.   If intraoperative imaging is not available, the health care organization should have a policy and procedure describing actions necessary and communication required between referring and receiving organizations.

X.b.   Based on risk analysis, the health care organization should establish policies that define when additional measures for prevention of RSIs must be performed or when they may be waived (eg, trauma, cystoscopy, ophthalmology).

Even in the smallest of incisions, the risk exists for RSIs.[3] The size of a pediatric patient may dictate a correspondingly small incision that would make retention of an instrument in the surgical wound unlikely; however, RSIs can occur in the smallest of incisions.[3] Careful consideration should be given when establishing a policy for waived counts for the pediatric patient because it is difficult to determine whether there is no risk of an RSI.

Some situations that have been identified as potentially contributing to the risk for RSI include,
- the emergent nature of a procedure;[8,63]
- an unexpected change in the procedure;[2]
- patient obesity;[2,7,8,44,45]
- multiple surgical teams;
- shift changes;[7]
- pressure to increase throughput (ie, reduce operating time);[44] and
- staff member inexperience.[86]

X.c.   Policies and procedures should include RSI prevention measures for organ procurement procedures.

Counted items that are sent with the donated organ(s) increase the risk for RSIs for the organ recipient. Counted sharps and instruments that are retained in the donor may contribute to inventory loss or injury to other health care workers. Counted items left in the OR or procedure room may increase the risk of inaccuracy in subsequent procedure counts or create sharps injury hazards for personnel.[87]

Recommendation XI

A quality assurance/performance improvement process should be in place to evaluate the incidence and risks of RSIs and to improve patient safety.

Quality and performance improvement functions may ensure that organizations design processes well and systematically monitor, analyze, and improve outcomes.[3,12,88-90] Continuous QI opportunities arise from documented and structured quality processes and measures that can define and resolve problems.

XI.a. A multiphase, multidisciplinary process improvement program should be implemented, including, but not limited to,
- an ongoing risk assessment and review (eg, failure mode effect analysis);
- policy design and review;
- a review of published evidence, internal data collection, and data analysis; and
- plans for the ongoing monitoring and analysis of processes, near misses, and adverse events related to the prevention of RSIs.

A comprehensive QI program may identify opportunities for minimizing the risk of RSI events.

XI.b. A critical investigation should be conducted regarding any adverse event or near miss related to RSIs.[1]

Error and near miss reporting are the first steps to addressing error reduction.[89,91] The distraction-prone environment of the perioperative practice setting makes it more likely that errors can be made during routine tasks, including surgical counts.[3,6] Errors can be divided into two categories: those at the human interface in a complex system (ie, active), and those representing a failed system design (ie, latent). There are a number of analysis methods (eg, root cause analysis, appreciative inquiry) available to health care organizations that may be used to conduct a critical investigation of adverse events.[7,12,90,92]

XI.b.1. Multidisciplinary teams should be involved in the review process and address any changes in policy that can improve patient safety.[1]

XI.c. Reporting mechanisms for adverse events and near misses related to RSIs should be established.

Many states require public reporting when these events occur. Federal and state agencies, accrediting bodies, third-party payers, and professional associations consider RSIs a sentinel event or "never event," which should be reported and investigated.[12-14,93-100]

XI.c.1. Events that necessitate reopening a wound to retrieve an RSI should be reported in compliance with health care organizational policy, as well as local, state, and federal regulatory agencies.

XI.d. Health care organizations should value learning and respond to errors with a focus on process improvement rather than individual blame.[69]

Systematic performance measures (ie, indicators) and/or priority areas are identified as opportunities for improvement based on the functions and processes of the perioperative episode.[51,89-91,101] Each perioperative team member has an ethical obligation to perform his or her role and responsibilities with appropriate competence and the highest level of personal integrity.[31]

XI.d.1. Errors should be evaluated in such a manner that contributing factors are first reviewed and then accountability is determined in relation to actions.

Continuous QI opportunities arise from documented and structured quality processes and measures that can define and resolve problems.

XI.d.2. Personnel should identify and respond to opportunities for improvement.

To evaluate the quality of patient care and formulate plans for corrective action, it is necessary to maintain a system of evaluation.

Glossary

Baseline: "A set of critical observations or data used for comparison or a control." (Source: Association for the Advancement of Medical Instrumentation. *Comprehensive Guide to Steam Sterilization and Sterility Assurance in Health Care Facilities; ANSI/AAMI ST79:2006.* Arlington, VA: Association for the Advancement of Medical Instrumentation; 2006:54-111.)

Gossypiboma: Surgical sponge or towel unintentionally retained in the body following surgery. Synonym: Textiloma.

Instruments: Surgical tools or devices designed to perform a specific function, such as cutting, dissecting, grasping, holding, retracting, or suturing.

Minimally invasive surgery: Surgical procedures performed through one or more small incisions using endoscopic instruments, radiographic and magnetic resonance imaging, computer-assisted devices, robotics, and other emerging technologies.

Miscellaneous items: In relation to items on the sterile field that require counting, this may include vessel clip bars, vessel loops, umbilical and hernia tapes, vascular inserts, electrosurgery scratch pads, trocar sealing caps, and any other small items that have the potential for being retained in a surgical wound.

Near miss: An occurrence that could have resulted in an accident, injury, or illness but did not by chance, skillful management, or timely intervention. "Any process variation that did not affect the outcome (for the patient or personnel), but for which a recurrence carries a significant chance of a serious adverse outcome. Such a near miss falls within the scope of the definition of a sentinel event, but those outside the scope of sentinel events that are subject to review by the Joint Commission under its Sentinel Event Policy." (Source: Glossary. In: *Hospital Accreditation Standards*. Oak Brook Terrace, IL: Joint Commission on Accreditation of Healthcare Organizations; 2002:331, 345, 351, 354, 360.)

Radio frequency identification (RFID): A system that transmits the identity (in the form of a unique serial number) of an object wirelessly using radio waves.

Root cause analysis: A retrospective approach to error analysis that focuses on failures of system design as related to common root causes of adverse events. "A process for identifying the basic or causal factors that underlie variation in performance, including the occurrence or a sentinel event. A root cause analysis focuses primarily on systems and processes, not individual performance. It progresses from special causes in clinical processes to common causes in organizational processes and identifies potential improvements in processes or systems that would tend to decrease the likelihood of such events in the future, or determines, after analysis that no such improvement opportunities exist " (Source: Sentinel events. In: *Hospital Accreditation Standards*. Oak Brook Terrace, IL: Joint Commission on Accreditation of Healthcare Organizations; 2002:51-52.)

Sentinel event: "An unexpected occurrence involving death or serious physical or psychological injury, or the risk thereof. Serious injury specifically includes loss of limb or function. The phrase 'or the risk thereof' includes any process variation for which a recurrence would carry a significant chance of a serious adverse outcome. Such events are called 'sentinel' because they signal the need for immediate investigation and response." (Source: Official accreditation policies and procedures. In: *Hospital Accreditation Standards*. Oak Brook Terrace, IL: Joint Commission on Accreditation of Healthcare Organizations; 2002:48-49.)

Sharps: Items with edges or points capable of cutting or puncturing through other items. In the context of surgery, items include, but are not limited to, suture needles, scalpel blades, hypodermic needles, electrosurgical needles and blades, instruments with sharp edges or points, and safety pins.

Sponges: Soft goods (eg, gauze pads, cottonoids, peanuts, dissectors, tonsil/laparotomy sponges) used to absorb fluids, protect tissues, or apply pressure or traction.

Waived count: Surgical procedures in which accurate accounting for sponges, instruments, and miscellaneous items is determined to be unachievable or in situations in which the time required to perform the count may present an unacceptable delay in patient care (eg, trauma procedures, anterior-posterior spinal procedures).

REFERENCES

1. Institute of Medicine Committee on Quality of Health Care in America. *Crossing the Quality Chasm: A New Health System for the 21st Century*. Washington, DC: National Academy Press; 2001.
2. Gawande AA, Studdert DM, Orav EJ, Brennan TA, Zinner MJ. Risk factors for retained instruments and sponges after surgery. *N Engl J Med*. 2003;348(3):229-235.
3. Gibbs VC, Coakley FD, Reines HD. Preventable errors in the operating room: retained foreign bodies after surgery—part I. *Curr Probl Surg*. 2007;44(5):281-337.
4. Gibbs VC. Patient safety practices in the operating room: correct-site surgery and nothing left behind. *Surg Clin North Am*. 2005;85(6):1307-1319.
5. Greenberg CC, Regenbogen SE, Lipsitz SR, Diaz-Flores R, Gawande AA. The frequency and significance of discrepancies in the surgical count. *Ann Surg*. 2008; 248(2):337-341.
6. Egorova NN, Moskowitz A, Gelijns A, et al. Managing the prevention of retained surgical instruments: what is the value of counting? *Ann Surg*. 2008;247(1):13-18.
7. Lincourt AE, Harrell A, Cristiano J, Sechrist C, Kercher K, Heniford BT. Retained foreign bodies after surgery. *J Surg Res*. 2007;138(2):170-174.
8. ECRI. Sponge, sharp, and instrument counts. *Healthcare Risk Control*. 2003;4(Surgery and Anesthesia 5):1-7.
9. Murphy EK. "Captain of the ship" doctrine continues to take on water. *AORN J*. 2001;74(4):525-528.
10. Surgical nurses: sponge count is strictly nurses' responsibility, court rules. *Legal Eagle Eye Newsl Nurs Prof*. 2000;8(9):2.
11. Focus on five. Preventing retained foreign objects: improving safety after surgery. *Joint Comm Perspect Patient Saf*. 2006;6(3):11.

12. Sentinel event policy and procedures. The Joint Commission. *http://www.jointcommission.org/Sen tinelEvents/PolicyandProcedures/*. Updated July 2007. Accessed July 1, 2010.

13. Centers for Medicare & Medicaid Services (CMS) HHS. Medicare program: changes to the hospital outpatient prospective payment system and CY 2008 payment rates, the ambulatory surgical center payment system and CY 2008 payment rates, the hospital inpatient prospective payment system and FY 2008 payment rates; and payments for graduate medical education for affiliated teaching hospitals in certain emergency situations Medicare and Medicaid programs: hospital conditions of participation; necessary provider designations of critical access hospitals. Interim and final rule with comment period. *Fed Regist*. 2007;72(227):66579-67226.

14. Centers for Medicare & Medicaid Services (CMS) HHS. Medicare program; proposed changes to the hospital inpatient prospective payment systems and fiscal year 2009 rates; proposed changes to disclosure of physician ownership in hospitals and physician self-referral rules; proposed collection of information regarding financial relationships between hospitals and physicians; proposed rule. *Fed Regist*. 2008;73(84):23527-23938.

15. Rosenthal MB. Nonpayment for performance? Medicare's new reimbursement rule. *N Engl J Med*. 2007;357(16):1573-1575.

16. Wilson C. Foreign bodies left in the abdomen after laparotomy. *Trans Am Gynecol Soc*. 1884;9:109-112.

17. Cima RR, Kollengode A, Garnatz J, Storsveen A, Weisbrod C, Deschamps C. Incidence and characteristics of potential and actual retained foreign object events in surgical patients. *J Am Coll Surg*. 2008;207(1):80-87.

18. Bani-Hani KE, Gharaibeh KA, Yaghan RJ. Retained surgical sponges (gossypiboma). *Asian J Surg*. 2005; 28(2):109-115.

19. Joint Commission Resources Inc. Preventing retention of foreign bodies after surgery. In: *Safety in the Operating Room*. Oakbrook Terrace, IL: Joint Commission on Accreditation of Healthcare Organizations; 2006:105-110.

20. Beyond the count: preventing retention of foreign objects. *Pa Patient Saf Advis*. 2009;6(2):39-45.

21. Retained surgical instruments and other items. NoThing Left Behind®. *http://www.nothingleftbehind .org/Instruments.html*. Accessed July 1, 2010.

22. Cima RR, Kollengode A, Storsveen AS, et al. A multidisciplinary team approach to retained foreign objects. *Jt Comm J Qual Patient Saf*. 2009;35(3):123-132.

23. *Implementation Manual Surgical Safety Checklist*. 1st ed. Geneva, Switzerland: World Health Organization; 2008. *http://www.who.int/patientsafety/safesurgery /tools_resources/SSSL_Manual_finalJun08.pdf*. Accessed July 6, 2010.

24. Sevdalis N, Healey AN, Vincent CA. Distracting communications in the operating theatre. *J Eval Clin Pract*. 2007;13(3):390-394.

25. Kracht JM, Busch-Vishniac IJ, West JE. Noise in the operating rooms of Johns Hopkins Hospital. *J Acoust Soc Am*. 2007;121(5 Pt1):2673-2680.

26. Joint Commission Resources Inc. Improving communication and avoiding distractions. In: *Safety in the Operating Room*. Oakbrook Terrace, IL: Joint Commission on Accreditation of Healthcare Organizations; 2006:3-19.

27. Jackson S, Brady S. Counting difficulties: retained instruments, sponges, and needles. *AORN J*. 2008; 87(2):315-321.

28. Best practices for preventing a retained foreign body. *AORN J*. 2006;84(Suppl 1):S30-S36, S58-S60.

29. Healey AN, Primus CP, Koutantji M. Quantifying distraction and interruption in urological surgery. *Qual Saf Health Care*. 2007;16(2):135-139.

30. Healey AN, Sevdalis N, Vincent CA. Measuring intra-operative interference from distraction and interruption observed in the operating theatre. *Ergonomics*. 2006;49(5-6):589-604.

31. Standards of perioperative nursing. In: *Perioperative Standards and Recommended Practices*. Denver, CO: AORN, Inc; 2010:9-62.

32. Reason J. Safety in the operating theatre—part 2: human error and organisational failure. *Qual Saf Health Care*. 2005;14(1):56-60.

33. Brown J, Feather D. Surgical equipment and materials left in patients. *Br J Perioper Nurs*. 2005;15(6):259-262.

34. Porteous J. Surgical counts can be risky business! *Can Oper Room Nurs J*. 2004;22(4):6-8.

35. VHA Directive 2006-030. *Prevention of Retained Surgical Items* [corrected copy]. Washington, DC: Department of Veterans Affairs; May 17, 2006.

36. Statement on the prevention of retained foreign bodies after surgery. American College of Surgeons. *http:// www.facs.org/fellows_info/statements/st-51.html*. Accessed July 1, 2010.

37. Kernagis LY, Siegelman ES, Torigian DA. Case 145: retained sponge. *Radiology*. 2009;251(2):608-611.

38. Whang G, Mogel GT, Tsai J, Palmer SL. Left behind: unintentionally retained surgically placed foreign bodies and how to reduce their incidence—pictorial review. *AJR Am J Roentgenol*. 2009;193(6 Suppl):S79-S89.

39. Catalano K. Knowledge is power: averting safety-compromising events in the OR. *AORN J*. 2008;88(6): 987-995.

40. Murphy EK. Protecting patients from potential injuries OR Nursing Law. *AORN J*. 2004;79(5):1013-1016.

41. Kim CK, Park BK, Ha H. Gossypiboma in abdomen and pelvis: MRI findings in four patients. *AJR Am J Roentgenol*. 2007;189(4):814-817.

42. Tammelleo AD. Gauze pad left in pt. during reversal of tubal ligation surgery. *Nurs Law Regan Rep*. 2004;45(7):4.

43. Is M, Karatas A, Akgul M, Yildirim U, Gezen F. A retained surgical sponge (gossypiboma) mimicking a paraspinal abscess. *Br J Neurosurg*. 2007;21(3):307-308.

44. Berkowitz S, Marshall H, Charles A. Retained intra-abdominal surgical instruments: time to use nascent technology? *Am Surg*. 2007;73(11):1083-1085.

45. Teixeira PG, Inaba K, Salim A, et al. Retained foreign bodies after emergent trauma surgery: incidence after 2526 cavitary explorations. *Am Surg*. 2007;73(10):1031-1034.

46. Tandon A, Bhargava SK, Gupta A, Bhatt S. Spontaneous transmural migration of retained surgical textile into both small and large bowel: a rare cause of intestinal obstruction. *Br J Radiol*. 2009;82(976):e72-e75.

47. Whang G, Mogel GT, Tsai J, Palmer SL. Left behind: unintentionally retained surgically placed foreign bodies and how to reduce their incidence—self-assessment module. *AJR Am J Roentgenol*. 2009;193(6 Suppl):S90-S93.

48. Camazine B. The persistent problem of the retained foreign body. *Contemp Surg*. 2005;8:398-400.

49. Wells J. Hospitals must disclose doctor errors. Oversight panel seeks to cut preventable patient injuries. *San Francisco Chronicle*. December 24, 2000;A:1.

50. Hartlaub P. S.F. settles suit over a painful pair of surgeries. Towel, tubing left inside woman. *San Francisco Chronicle*. June 28, 2001;A:13.

51. Retained surgical sponges. New York State Department of Health - NYPORTS. *NYPORTS News & Alert*. Department of Health, Issue 11. September 2002. *http://www.health.state.ny.us/nysdoh/hospital/nyports /annual_report/2000-2001/news_and_alerts.htm*. Accessed July 1, 2010.

52. Gencosmanoglu R, Inceoglu R. An unusual cause of small bowel obstruction: gossypiboma—case report. *BMC Surg*. 2003;3:6.

53. Recommended practices for transfer of patient care information. In: *Perioperative Standards and Recommended Practices*. Denver, CO: AORN, Inc; 2010: 371-378.

54. Rights and Responsibilities of the Individual: RI.01.01.03: The hospital respects the patient's right to receive information in a manner he or she understand. In: *2010 Comprehensive Accreditation Manual for Hospitals*. Oak Brook, IL: Joint Commission Resources; 2010.

55. Use of x-rays for incorrect needle counts. *Pa Patient Saf Advis*. 2004;1(2):5-6.

56. Dagi TF, Berguer R, Moore S, Reines HD. Preventable errors in the operating room—part 2: retained foreign objects, sharps injuries, and wrong site surgery. *Curr Probl Surg*. 2007;44(6):352-381.

57. Perry J, Parker G, Jagger J. FPINet report: 2001 percutaneous injury rates. *Adv Expo Prev*. 2003;6(3):32-36.

58. Jagger J, Berguer R, Phillips EK, Parker G, Gomaa AE. Increase in sharps injuries in surgical settings versus nonsurgical settings after passage of national needlestick legislation. *J Am Coll Surg*. 2010;210(4):496-502.

59. Berguer R, Heller PJ. Preventing sharps injuries in the operating room. *J Am Coll Surg*. 2004;199(3):462-467.

60. Ponrartana S, Coakley FV, Yeh BM, et al. Accuracy of plain abdominal radiographs in the detection of retained surgical needles in the peritoneal cavity. *Ann Surg*. 2008;247(1):8-12.

61. Thomas EJ, Moore FA. The missing suction tip [Case & Commentary]. *Morbidity & Mortality Rounds on the Web*. Surgery/Anesthesia. November 2003. *http:// www.webmm.ahrq.gov/case.aspx?caseID=37*. Accessed July 1, 2010.

62. Milankov M, Savic D, Miljkovic N. Broken blade in the knee: a complication of arthroscopic meniscectomy. *Arthroscopy*. 2002;18(1):E4.

63. Murdock D. Trauma: when there's no time to count. *AORN J*. 2008;87(2):322-328.

64. Retained surgical retractor. Closed claim studies—general surgery. Texas Medical Liability Trust. *http:// www.tmlt.org/newscenter/closedclaims/general surgery.html?x=1*. Accessed July 1, 2010.

65. Abdomen: retained retractor bolt on plain film. Lieberman's Classics Collections in Radiology. *http:// eradiology.bidmc.harvard.edu/Classics/item.aspx?sec tion=Patient+Safety+-+Retained+Surgical+Devices &labelpk=9e5a943e-3b2e-415e-82d8-e364853cf0a8 &pk=ec2ea0b8-4c64-4c71-b2af-f00f047c673f*. Accessed July 1, 2010.

66. Public health notification: unretrieved device fragments. US Food and Drug Administration. *http://www.fda .gov/cdrh/safety/011508-udf.html*. Accessed July 1, 2010.

67. Beyea SC. Counting instruments and sponges. *AORN J*. 2003;78(2):290, 293-294.

68. Eskreis-Nelson T. Nursing case law update. Medical errors and the need for nurses' continuing education. *J Nurs Law*. 2000;7(3):49-59.

69. AORN guidance statement: creating a patient safety culture. In: *Perioperative Standards and Recommended Practices*. Denver, CO: AORN, Inc; 2010:523-528.

70. Greenberg CC, Diaz-Flores R, Lipsitz SR, et al. Barcoding surgical sponges to improve safety: a randomized controlled trial. *Ann Surg*. 2008;247(4):612-616.

71. *Health Care Protocol: Prevention of Unintentionally Retained Foreign Objects During Vaginal Deliveries*. 2nd ed. Bloomington, MN: Institute for Clinical Systems Improvement; 2008.

72. Barrow CJ. Use of x-ray in the presence of an incorrect needle count. *AORN J*. 2001;74(1):80-81.

73. Macilquham MD, Riley RG, Grossberg P. Identifying lost surgical needles using radiographic techniques. *AORN J*. 2003;78(1):73-78.

74. Pelter MM, Stephens KE, Loranger D. An evaluation of a numbered surgical sponge product. *AORN J*. 2007;85(5):931-936.

75. Rogers A, Jones E, Oleynikov D. Radio frequency identification (RFID) applied to surgical sponges. *Surg Endosc*. 2007;21(7):1235-1237.

76. Regenbogen SE, Greenberg CC, Resch SC, et al. Prevention of retained surgical sponges: a decision-analytic model predicting relative cost-effectiveness. *Surgery*. 2009;145(5):527-535.

77. ECRI. Radio-frequency surgical sponge detection: a new way to lower the odds of leaving sponges (and similar items) in patients. *Health Devices*. 2008;37(7):193-203.

78. Fabian CE. Electronic tagging of surgical sponges to prevent their accidental retention. *Surgery*. 2005; 137(3):298-301.

79. Macario A, Morris D, Morris S. Initial clinical evaluation of a handheld device for detecting retained surgical gauze sponges using radiofrequency identification technology. *Arch Surg*. 2006;141(7):659-662.

80. Shojania KG, Duncan BW, McDonald KM, Wachter RM, eds. *Making Health Care Safer: A Critical Analysis of Patient Safety Practices*. Evidence Report/ Technology Assessment Number 43. Rockville, MD: Agency for Healthcare Research and Quality; 2001.

81. RF surgical sponge detection: lowering the odds of retention. *ORRM Newsletter*. 2009;18(2).

82. Recommended practices for product selection in the perioperative practice setting. In: *Perioperative Standards and Recommended Practices*. Denver, CO: AORN, Inc; 2010:189-192.

83. Van der Togt R, Van Lieshout EJ, Hensbroek R, Beinat E, Binnekade JM, Bakker PJ. Electromagnetic interference from radio frequency identification inducing potentially hazardous incidents in critical care medical equipment. *JAMA*. 2008;299(24):2884-2890.

84. Recommended practices for documentation of perioperative nursing care. In: *Perioperative Standards and*

Recommended Practices. Denver, CO: AORN, Inc; 2010:289-292.

85. Perioperative nursing: sponge inside patient, nurses faulted, but consequences disputed. *Legal Eagle Eye Newsl Nurs Prof*. 2004;12(7):8.

86. Riley R, Manias E, Polglase A. Governing the surgical count through communication interactions: implications for patient safety. *Qual Saf Health Care*. 2006; 15(5):369-374.

87. Burton JL. Health and safety at necropsy. *J Clin Pathol*. 2003;56(4):254-260.

88. Berryman R. Why count instruments and sponges in the operating room? Stories from home and abroad. *ACORN*. 2004;17(4):20, 22-4.

89. Dunn D. Incident reports—their purpose and scope. *AORN J*. 2003;78(1):45-66.

90. Root cause analysis. United States Department of Veterans Affairs. *http://www.patientsafety.gov/rca.html*. Accessed July 1, 2010.

91. Liang BA. The adverse event of unaddressed medical error: identifying and filling the holes in the health-care and legal systems. *J Law Med Ethics*. 2001;29(3-4):346-368.

92. Shendell-Falik N, Feinson M, Mohr BJ. Enhancing patient safety: improving the patient handoff process through appreciative inquiry. *J Nurs Adm*. 2007; 37(2):95-104.

93. Incorporating selected national quality forum and never events into Medicares list of hospital-acquired conditions [fact sheet]. Baltimore, MD: Centers for Medicare & Medicaid Services; April 14, 2008. *http://www.cms.hhs.gov/apps/media/press/factsheet.asp?Counter=3043&intNumPerPage=10&checkDate=&checkKey=&srchType=1&numDays=3500&srchOpt=0&srchData=&keywordType=All&chkNewsType=6&intPage=&showAll=&pYear=&year=&desc=false&cboOrder=date*. Accessed July 1, 2010.

94. Department of Health and Human Services, Office of the Inspector General. *Adverse Events in Hospitals: State Reporting Systems*. Washington, DC: HHS; 2008.

95. Hospital medical error reporting rule. 410 Indiana Administrative Code 15-1.4-2 (2009).

96. *Clinical Definitions Manual*. Version 4. Albany, NY: New York Patient Occurrence and Tracking System; 2005.

97. *Patient Safety Act*. New Jersey PL 2004 c. 9 26:2H-12.23-12.25.

98. California Health and Safety Code. Section 1275-1289.5.

99. Facility requirements to report, analyze, and correct. Minnesota statutes 144.7065 (2009).

100. *National Integrated Accreditation for Healthcare Organizations (NIAHO) Interpretive Guidelines and Surveyor Guidance*. Revision 8.0. Cincinnati, OH: DNV Healthcare Inc; 2009.

101. Sentinel event statistics. The Joint Commission. *http://www.jointcommission.org/SentinelEvents/Statistics/*. Accessed July 1, 2010.

Acknowledgements

LEAD AUTHORS
Sheila Mitchell, RN, BSN, MS, CNOR
Perioperative Nursing Specialist
AORN Center for Nursing Practice
Denver, Colorado

Judith L. Goldberg, RN, MSN, CNOR
Clinical Director, Sterile Processing Department
The William W. Backus Hospital
Norwich, Connecticut

CONTRIBUTING AUTHORS
Maria C. Arcilla, RN, BSN, CNOR
Education Coordinator
Texas Childrens Hospital
Houston, Texas

David L. Feldman, MD, MBA, CPE, FACS
Vice President, Perioperative Services
Maimonides Medical Center
Brooklyn, New York

PUBLICATION HISTORY
Originally published May 1976, *AORN Journal*, as "Standards for sponge, needle, and instrument procedures." Format revision March 1978, July 1982.

Revised March 1984, March 1990.

Revised November 1995; published October 1996, *AORN Journal*.

Revised; published December 1999, *AORN Journal*. Reformatted July 2000.

Revised November 2005; published as "Recommended practices for sponge, sharp, and instrument counts" in *Standards, Recommended Practices, and Guidelines*, 2006 edition. Reprinted February 2006, *AORN Journal*.

Revised July 2010 for online publication in *Perioperative Standards and Recommended Practices*.

Recommended Practices for the Care and Handling of Specimens in the Perioperative Environment

The following recommended practices were developed by the AORN Recommended Practices Committee and have been approved by the AORN Board of Directors. They were presented as proposed recommended practices for comments by members and others. They are effective January 1, 2006.

These recommended practices are intended as achievable recommendations representing what is believed to be an optimal level of practice. Policies and procedures will reflect variations in practice settings and/or clinical situations that determine the degree to which the recommended practices can be implemented.

AORN recognizes the numerous types of settings in which perioperative nurses practice. These recommended practices are intended as guidelines adaptable to various practice settings. These practice settings include traditional operating rooms, ambulatory surgery centers, physicians' offices, cardiac catheterization suites, endoscopy suites, radiology departments, and all other areas where operative and other invasive procedures may be performed.

Purpose

These recommended practices provide guidance for the implementation of containment, identification, labeling, preservation, transfer, transport, and disposition of surgical specimens. *Specimens* in this document include tissue, blood, body fluids, or foreign bodies (eg, plates, screws) removed from a patient for pathological, microbiological, or gross examination. Specimen identification, collection, and handling are multidisciplinary tasks that require vigilant attention to detail so that each person in the chain of custody understands the patient's needs and is aware of information about the specimen. Mishandling or misidentification of specimens can lead to inaccurate or incomplete diagnosis or the need for additional procedures.[1,2] These recommended practices are not intended to address aspects of perioperative patient care addressed in other recommended practices.

Recommendation I

Assessment of specimen collection and special handling needs should begin when the procedure is scheduled.

1. Specimen handling should be assessed and planned before the procedure. This assessment includes persons and departments to be notified (eg, pathology for frozen section); supplies needed for transfer or transport; availability of personnel; or specific requirements necessary for collection or handling of the specimen (eg, timing of transfer, solution, container). Early patient assessment and preplanning minimizes the time required during the surgical procedure and reduces the potential for mishandling specimens.

2. Containers and collection devices of appropriate size and type, with correct preservatives should be determined and obtained before the procedure. Containers should be large enough to safely secure the specimen and fluids, if used, to prevent leakage and unnecessary exposure of personnel or others handling the container or its contents. The container and collection device also should be of a size appropriate to allow the preservatives or solutions, if used, to contact all surfaces of the specimen. Collection containers may be sterile or clean, depending on collection requirements.

3. The patient's cultural considerations should be assessed to determine appropriate handling and disposal of specimens. Circumstances may require that specimens be handled or disposed of differently than routine requirements. The patient's written permission may be needed in advance for special requests.

Recommendation II

Procedures for correct patient and specimen identification should be implemented, including confirmation of consistent and accurate patient information on labels and forms.

1. Patient identification should be confirmed using two unique identifiers according to health care organization policy at the time the specimen is removed from the patient and when it is placed in the container for transfer and transport. Two unique patient identifiers should be used to minimize the risk of misidentification. Misidentification of a specimen, margins, or other information about a specimen can result in adverse outcomes, delay, error in diagnosis or treatment, or the need for an additional procedure.[2]

2. Specimen identification should begin at the time the specimen is removed from the patient with both verbal and written communication to confirm information. Communication should include a "read back" verification of the information. Using a "write down, read back" process to confirm the communication minimizes the risk of miscommunication.

3. Identification of the specimen should be confirmed verbally between the surgeon and registered nurse circulator and documented completely on the appropriate form(s). Identification should include, but is not limited to,
   ◆ originating source of specimen (eg, site or side),
   ◆ type of tissue,
   ◆ clinical diagnosis, and
   ◆ pertinent clinical information.

   Specific types of specimens may require additional information (eg, breast masses, which may include tissue markers of various types and suture tags for orientation).

4. Each specimen removed for examination should be clearly documented on the specimen container, operative record, and pathology documents.

5. Specimens should be protected and secured on the sterile field to maintain the integrity of the specimen. Specimens should be passed off the sterile field as soon as possible. Specimens that must be kept on the surgical field before transfer should be maintained and labeled appropriately to prevent loss, damage, or mishandling.

6. Specimens transferred from the sterile field should be visibly labeled by the scrub person to prevent errors and misidentification, following verbal communication and verification (ie, "write down, read back") of the information. Written communication about the specimen at the time of removal, confirmed with the surgeon, minimizes opportunities for errors during the transfer/transport process.

Recommendation III

Collection and handling of a specimen should be completed in a manner that protects and secures the specimen and prevents contamination of personnel handling the specimen.

1. Specimens secured on the sterile field before transfer should be maintained in a manner to prevent misidentification or mishandling. The method of maintaining the tissue should be consistent with the specimen type; this often requires that tissue remain moistened with sterile saline to prevent drying.

2. The specimen should be contained and labeled immediately to prevent mishandling and errors. Securing specimens at the point of removal (eg, specimen cup) prevents damage and minimizes the risk of mishandling.

   Specimens and containers removed from the surgical field should be handled using standard precautions. The sterility (if indicated) and integrity of the specimen should be maintained during transfer from the sterile field to the container. Clean secondary packaging should be used to prevent contamination of personnel and the environment during transport of specimens.

3. Specimen containers containing a preservative or anticoagulant should be mixed thoroughly before the specimen is placed in the container. The use of preservatives or chemical additives for tissue preservation should be confirmed with the physician. Personnel should practice safety and protective precautions when working with chemical agents.[3]

4. Specimens removed from the procedural area should be secured in an impervious container. The size or type of container is dependent on size of the specimen, timing of the specimen review, preservatives, and containment for transport of the specimen. Containers and collection devices should allow for transfer and transport of biohazardous material without leaking or spilling. Containers should be rigid, leak-proof, sturdy, and nonreactive to fixative solutions such as formalin and alcohol. Lids should fit tightly to prevent spillage.[4]

5. Syringes used for specimen collection and containment should be capped without needles. Needles should not be left on syringes that will be transported. Needles create an unnecessary hazard to those transporting and receiving specimens and may invalidate results due to exposure to air.

6. Caution should be used when handling or dispensing formalin. It can be absorbed through the

skin and nasal passages, splashed in the eyes, and ingested. Exposure can result in irritation, burns, and allergic reactions.[5]

♦ All formalin in the OR should be stored in one location, along with a material safety data sheet. Storage and use of formalin is regulated by the Occupational Safety and Health Administration and other federal and state health regulatory agencies.[6]

♦ Personnel handling formalin should wear appropriate personal protective equipment, which includes face and eye shields, gloves, and other protective garments.[5-7]

♦ Formalin should be dispensed and stored in an area other than the OR. The room should have a ventilation system incorporating negative pressure and an exhaust hood.[7]

♦ Policies and procedures should be established for safe storage and dispensing of formalin in the surgical environment.

♦ Personnel should be educated about the safe handling of formalin, including containment and cleanup of spills, and other measures to minimize risk of exposure.

♦ Formalin should be disposed of according to state and local regulations. Formalin is a U-listed chemical, hazardous upon disposal, and regulated by the US Environmental Protection Agency.[8]

Recommendation IV

Specimen containers should be labeled to communicate patient, specimen, preservative, and biohazard information.

1. Two unique identifiers should be used to identify the patient reference. Information on the label should include, but not be limited to,
   ♦ specimen type and site,
   ♦ health care organization-defined unique identifiers (eg, patient name and hospital number), and
   ♦ current date and time.

   Dark, indelible ink should be used. The label or tag should be secured on the specimen container.

2. Containers should be labeled to indicate that a biohazardous material is being transported to prevent contamination of personnel transporting or receiving the specimen.[4]

3. If chemical preservatives are used, the label should clearly identify these additives.

4. The label should be placed on the container, not the lid. This prevents the loss of appropriate identification after the container is opened for processing.

Recommendation V

Tissue specimens should be designated for routine pathological exam, gross identification only, or disposal according to health care organizational policies.

1. All tissue must be disposed of in a manner consistent with state and federal guidelines, whether or not it needs pathological examination.[2]

2. Health care organizations should develop policies and procedures regarding which tissues require only gross identification or disposal.[9-11]

3. The pathologist has the ultimate responsibility for making decisions about the extent of the examination of the tissue.

Recommendation VI

Health care organizations should establish communication and documentation methods regarding specimen accountability and accurate documentation.

1. Documentation should include, but not be limited to,
   ♦ type of specimen;
   ♦ patient name, age, gender, health care organization, history, and diagnosis;
   ♦ studies required;
   ♦ date and time of collection;
   ♦ information pertinent to the specimen or source;
   ♦ surgeon's name and contact number; and
   ♦ the registered nurse doing the preparation and documentation of the specimen for transport.

2. Documentation via printed tools should be used to minimize errors related to handwriting and inaccuracies. When handwritten documentation is required, it should be accurate and legible. Common reasons for pathology errors are unlabeled containers, insufficient patient identification, and incomplete or illegible information.

Technology applications, such as bar coding, may be used to minimize errors.[12]

3. Specimen identification and requisition forms should accompany the specimen in a manner that protects the form and keeps it secured with the specimen.

4. Documentation should establish the chain of custody from the point of removal until pathological examination. Chain of custody is required for tissue specimens as well as material removed for forensic examination (see Recommendation IX).

5. Methods should be implemented to accurately record critical information such as tissue margins or orientation of the tissue as it relates to the anatomy, special tests requested, or disposition of the specimen. Requests for other than routine handling should be noted (eg, decalcification, x-ray, freezing). Delays or misdiagnosis can occur when the information is not accurately or completely communicated for the examination.[1]

6. Criteria for verbal and written specimen identification should be established to prevent misinformation. Commonly used methods include "write down, read back" verification of verbal communication. Communication should include, but not be limited to,
   ♦ physician to physician,
   ♦ physician to scrub person,
   ♦ scrub person to registered nurse circulator, and
   ♦ physician to registered nurse circulator.

7. Any communication between physicians, such as pathologist and surgeon, should be direct (ie, not through an intermediary) when it relates to diagnosis or specific diagnostic information about the specimen. A record of communication should be documented in the patient's record, such as the direct report of frozen section results to the surgeon. If communication directly between physicians is not possible, it should be written, marked with the date and time, and included in the patient's record.

8. If the patient requests to keep a removed item (eg, implanted medical device), the nurse should follow procedures for identification and standard precaution guidelines per health care organization policy.

9. Requests for specimens to be returned to the patient should follow health care organization policy after the pathology examination is complete.

10. Disposition of all tissue, devices, and implants removed should be documented on the operative record according to health care organization policy or state guidelines.

Recommendation VII

Explanted defective medical devices must be reported to the manufacturer.[13]

1. Medical devices removed due to apparent failure of the device must be retained by the facility. All portions of the device should be retained together, as well as the packaging, if available.

2. Defective explanted medical devices should be sent for pathology examination for identification purposes.

3. The removed medical device should not be decontaminated or sterilized before it is transported from the surgical suite.

4. A risk management report should be completed regarding the defective device, per health care organization policy, and reported to the manufacturer.

5. Documentation should include the reason for removal, if known.

Recommendation VIII

Transfer and transport methods and processes should be established by the health care organization according to the specimen type and diagnostic requirements.

1. Procedures should be established to prevent mishandling of specimens by verifying patient and specimen information before transfer, and by transport personnel at each point of exchange. Proper documentation allows tracking of the specimen from its source to its final disposition. A logbook should be used to record specimen, date, time, and the name of each person involved in each transfer process.

2. All specimens must be identified as biohazardous and transported in a manner that prevents contamination by chemical, blood, and other

potentially infectious material to personnel and the environment.[3]

3. Containers with chemicals must have proper identifiers and labeling.[3]

4. Accompanying documents should be protected from contamination.

5. Specimens should be transferred and transported in a manner that protects their viability. This may include, but is not limited to, protective packaging, temperature control, adequate fluids, or culture media.

6. Specimens that will not be transported immediately to the laboratory should be temporarily stored to maintain integrity for examination. Appropriate equipment with a biohazard sign should be available for holding specimens at the correct temperature until transport can take place according to the guidelines of the Clinical Laboratory Improvement Act.[14]

7. Specimens should be transported in a manner that ensures confidentiality of personal health information and minimizes visibility of the specimen.[15]

8. Documentation should be completed to establish the chain of custody from the point of removal until examination. Chain of custody is required for tissue specimens as well as materials removed for forensic examination.

Recommendation IX

Forensic specimens should be handled in a manner that preserves the condition of the evidence and verifies that the evidence has been in secure possession at all times.

1. The surgeon should place the evidence directly into a designated envelope or bag. The contents should be listed and described on the appropriate form (eg, "Release of Evidence" or similar form) and attached to the envelope or bag. The evidence envelope or bag should be labeled with the patient's identification, collection date and time, and name of collector.

2. The sealed evidence envelope should be given to the responsible law enforcement officer. If the law enforcement officer is not immediately available, the health care organization's policy for disposition of a sealed evidence envelope

and attached documentation should be followed. Documentation in the operative record should include, but not be limited to,
- description of the removed item,
- area of the anatomy from which it was removed, and
- disposition.

3. Bullets should not be handled with metal instruments, if possible, because these may scratch the bullet surface.[16] After the bullet is removed, it should be placed into a nonmetal container and sealed evidence envelope. Bullets should be submitted per local and state law enforcement requirements.

4. In cases involving an ongoing criminal investigation, all of the patient's clothes and belongings should be secured as evidence, regardless of condition. Clothing removed from the patient should be cut along the seams or around bullet or stab wound holes. Items should be placed in a paper bag with the patient's identification, then into a personal belongings bag with the patient's identification. Plastic bags trap moisture and may facilitate growth of mold, which could destroy evidence. After collecting objects in appropriate paper containers, place heavily saturated objects in plastic to avoid leakage of fluids and contamination to evidence collectors.[17] Disposition must be completed per local and state law enforcement requirements.

5. Informational evidence (eg, patient statements, appearance, behavior, bodily marks) should be documented in detail.

6. Documentation should be completed to establish the chain of custody from the point of removal until examination.[18] Chain of custody is required for tissue specimens as well as clothing and other personal items removed for forensic examination.

Recommendation X

Each health care organization should develop written procedures for handling radioactive pathology specimens. These procedures should include, but are not limited to, specimen handling, labeling, transportation, storage, and disposal. The procedures should keep radiation exposure to hospital workers as low as reasonably achievable.[19,20]

1. Procedures should be developed in conjunction with the health care organization's radiation safety officer.

2. Policies should describe how specimen containers are labeled.[21]

3. Specimens containing radioactive materials should be promptly transported from the OR to the pathology department in properly labeled and sealed containers.

4. The health care organization should validate competencies of all personnel handling radioactive specimens.

Recommendation XI

Policies and procedures related to the collection and handling of specimens and establishment of safe practices should be developed, reviewed periodically, revised as necessary, and readily available in the practice setting.

1. Policies and procedures for the collection and handling of specimens should be written and approved by the disciplines responsible for collecting, handling, examining, storing, and transporting specimens and other related activities. Policies and procedures establish authority, responsibility, and accountability and serve as operational guidelines. Policies and procedures also assist in the development of patient and health care worker safety, quality assessment, and improvement activities. Nurses should collaborate with all members of the health care team and related law enforcement agencies to develop policies that address collection and handling of surgical or forensic specimens. Multidisciplinary review of policies and procedures ensures that specimen collection and handling policies are based on current knowledge and legal requirements. Applicable state and federal regulations must be followed.

2. Elements for safe specimen handling should include, but are not limited to,
   - containers, collection devices, and preservatives for each specimen type;
   - specimen, tissue, and patient identification;
   - labeling;
   - transfer and transport;
   - maintenance of the specimen;
   - documentation and communication of test ordered;
   - chain of custody;
   - patient requests or needs;
   - specimen disposition; and
   - communication of test results.

3. Education, competency assessment, and validation should be conducted at the time of employment. This includes, but is not limited to,
   - roles, responsibilities, and methods of communication required when specimens are removed;
   - methods and materials used for various types of specimen collection and handling;
   - regulatory guidelines related to specimen collection and handling; and
   - safety practices that ensure proper collection and handling.

4. Policies and procedures establish authority, responsibility, and accountability and serve as operational guidelines. Introduction and review of policies and procedures should be included in orientation and ongoing education of personnel to assist in the development of knowledge, skills, and attitudes that affect patient care. Policies and procedures also assist in development of performance improvement activities.

5. The uniform perioperative nursing vocabulary should be used to document specimens on the intraoperative patient record. The perioperative nursing vocabulary is a clinically relevant, empirically validated, standardized language describing perioperative nursing care. This standardized language consists of a collection of data elements, the Perioperative Nursing Data Set (PNDS), and includes perioperative nursing diagnoses, interventions, and outcomes. The expected outcomes of primary importance to these recommended practices are outcome 24 (O24), "The patient's care is consistent with the perioperative plan of care," and outcome 28 (O28), "The patient's value system, life-style, ethnicity, and culture are considered, respected, and incorporated in the perioperative plan of care as appropriate." The intervention specific to the domain of Safety is intervention 84 (I84), "Manages specimen handling and disposition."[22]

6. Quality monitoring of specimen collection processes, handling, and transport should be established to identify trends or near misses. A focus on error reduction should be developed. Methods of root cause analysis should

be used to examine near misses or specimen handling errors to identify opportunities for improvement.

7. Packaging and handling of specimens should follow policies and procedures developed by the health care organization (**Table 1**).

Glossary

Chain of custody: A legal term that refers to the ability to guarantee the identity and integrity of the specimen from collection through to reporting of the test results. A process used to maintain, secure, and document the chronological history of the evidence.[24]

Cytology: The study of cells, including their formation, origin, structure, function, biochemical activities, and pathologic characteristics.

Forensic evidence: Evidence for use in legal or criminal proceedings.

Frozen section: A method used in preparing a selected portion of tissue for pathologic examination. The tissue is moistened and, fixed or unfixed, is rapidly frozen and cut by a microtome in a cryostat. This method is very rapid, allowing the pathologist to examine the specimen during a surgical procedure.[23]

Microbiology: The study of microorganisms, including bacteria, fungus, algae, and protozoa.

Specimen: Tissue or body substance removed for study.

REFERENCES

1. R E Nakhleh, G Gephardt, R J Zarbo, "Necessity of clinical information in surgical pathology: A College of American Pathologists Q-probes study of 771,475 surgical pathology cases from 341 institutions," *Archives of Pathology and Laboratory Medicine* 123 (July 1999) 615-619.

Table 1

SAMPLE POLICIES AND PROCEDURES FOR PACKAGING AND HANDLING SPECIMENS[1]	
Aerobic culture	Minimize swab exposure to air.
Anaerobic culture	Should be collected via a closed system from deep sites, bypassing normal flora. The best method is an anaerobic tube or sterile container. Do not add fluid. Swabs are the least effective. Tissue or fluid specimens are the best; fluid must be in a capped syringe without air. Tube contains transport medium, and tissue/swab should be imbedded in transport medium. Send to laboratory within 30 minutes. Large specimens may be collected in a closed, sterile container, as they retain anaerobic conditions within the tissue.
Biopsy	Usually sent fresh, no preservative; taken to pathology immediately.
Cultures	Maintain sterility of container when placing specimen.
Cytology	For sputum, bronchial, or peritoneal washings. Saline or heparin may be added to some types.
Frozen section	No fixative, kept moist. Intended for immediate transport to pathology department for a special freezing and slicing process for a tentative diagnostic reading.
Fungal	Examination done on a culture specimen.
Gram stain	Sent with a culture specimen. May request anaerobic or aerobic testing.
Pap smear	A type of cytology in a special pap fixative (99% alcohol).
Routine tissue specimen	Kept moist and placed in a container to protect integrity of tissue. Generally placed in refrigerator for pathology pickup within a few hours or overnight.
Stones	Stones may be placed in a dry specimen container. Tissue specimens that contain stones should be placed in buffered formalin (eg, gallbladder with stones).
Swab	Place in an approved swab transport device.
Urine	Place in a sterile container.

1. "Specimen collection guide," *University of Washington Department of Laboratory Medicine,* http://depts .washington.edu/labweb/PatientCare/Clinical/Specimen.htm *(accessed 12 Jan 2006).*

2. L Slavin, M A Best, D C Aron, "Gone but not forgotten: The search for the lost surgical specimens; Application of quality improvement techniques in reducing medical error," *Quality Management in Health Care* 10 no 1 (2001) 45-53.

3. "Occupational exposure to hazardous chemicals in laboratories," 29 CFR 1910.1450, Occupational Safety and Health Administration, *http://www.osha.gov/pls /oshaweb/owadisp.show_document?p_table =STANDARDS&p_id=10106* (accessed 13 Oct 2005).

4. "Guidelines for the safe transport of infectious substances and diagnostic specimens," publ WHO/EMC/97.3 (1997), World Health Organization, *http://www.who.int /csr/emc97_3.pdf* (accessed 29 Nov 2005).

5. "Material safety data sheet: Formalin solution 5%," Science Stuff, Inc, *http://www.sciencestuff.com/msds /C1776.html* (accessed 11 Aug 2005).

6. "Substance technical guidelines for formalin," 29 CFR 1910.1048 App A, Occupational Safety and Health Administration, *http://www.osha.gov/pls/oshaweb /owadisp.show_document?p_table=STANDARDS&p_id= 10076* (accessed 13 Oct 2005).

7. "Recommended guidelines for controlling noninfectious health hazards in hospitals (continued)," National Institute for Occupational Safety and Health, *http://www.cdc.gov/niosh/hcwold5a.html* (accessed 29 Nov 2005).

8. "Introduction to hazardous waste identification," 40 CFR Parts 261 (September 2003), US Environmental Protection Agency, *http://www.epa.gov/epaoswer /hotline/training/hwid05.pdf* (accessed 29 Nov 2005).

9. R Zarbo, R Nakhleh, "Surgical pathology specimens for gross examination only and exempt from submission," *Archives of Pathology and Laboratory Medicine* 123 (February 1999) 133-139.

10. P Fitzgibbons, K Cleary, "CAP offers recommendations on selecting surgical specimens for examination," *CAP Today* 10 (July 1996) 40.

11. "College of American Pathologists policy on surgical specimens to be submitted to pathology for examination," (1999) College of American Pathologists, *http://www.cap .org/apps/docs/laboratory_accreditation/surgical _specimens.pdf* (accessed 19 Oct 2005).

12. P N Valenstein, R L Sirota, "Identification errors in pathology and laboratory medicine," *Clinical Laboratory Medicine* 24 (December 2004) 979-996.

13. "Medical device tracking requirements," 21 CFR 821 (April 1, 2005), US Food and Drug Administration, *http://www.accessdata.fda.gov /scripts/cdrh/cfdocs /cfcfr/CFRSearch.cfm?CFRPart=821&showFR=1* (accessed 13 Oct 2005).

14. "CLIA Subpart K—Quality systems for nonwaived testing," Centers for Medicare and Medicaid Services, Clinical Laboratory Improvement Amendments, *http://www.phppo.cdc.gov/clia/regs/subpart_k .aspx#493.1240* (accessed 29 Oct 2005).

15. "Summary of the HIPAA privacy rule," US Department of Health and Human Services, *http://www.hhs.gov /ocr/privacysummary.pdf* (accessed 29 Oct 2005).

16. S L Hanshaw, "Bullet retrieval in the operating room," *Seminars in Perioperative Nursing* 3 (October 1994) 232-236.

17. G A Muro, C R Easter, "Clinical forensics for perioperative nurses," *AORN Journal* 60 (October 1994) 585-593.

18. M M Evans, P A Stagner, "Maintaining the chain of custody: Evidence handling in forensic cases," *AORN Journal* 78 (October 2003) 563-569.

19. P Fitzgibbons, V LiVolsi, et al, "Recommendations for handling radioactive specimens obtained by sentinel lymphadenectomy," *American Journal of Surgical Pathology* 24 (November 2000) 1549-1551.

20. M Cibull, "Handling sentinel lymph node biopsy specimens: A work in progress," *Archives of Pathology and Laboratory Medicine* 123 (July 1999) 620-621.

21. "Exemptions to labeling requirements," 10 CFR 20.1905, Nuclear Regulatory Commission, *http://a257 .g.akamaitech.net/7/257/2422/14mar20010800/edocket .access.gpo.gov/cfr_2002/janqtr/10cfr20.1905.htm* (accessed 13 Oct 2005).

22. S C Beyea, ed, *Perioperative Nursing Data Set: The Perioperative Nursing Vocabulary*, second ed (Denver: AORN, Inc, 2002).

23. *Mosby's Medical, Nursing, and Allied Health Dictionary*, sixth ed (St Louis: Mosby, 2002) 710.

24. "Glossary: Chain of custody," Peace-Officers.com, *http://peace-officers.com/content/glossary/def-chain .shtml* (accessed 29 Oct 2005).

PUBLICATION HISTORY

Originally approved November 2005, AORN Board of Directors. Published in *Standards, Recommended Practices, and Guidelines*, 2006 edition. Reprinted March 2006, *AORN Journal*.

Recommended Practices for Prevention of Transmissible Infections in the Perioperative Practice Setting

The following recommended practices were developed by the AORN Recommended Practices Committee and have been approved by the AORN Board of Directors. They were presented as proposed recommended practices for comments by members and others. They are effective January 1, 2007.

These recommended practices are intended as achievable recommendations representing what is believed to be an optimal level of practice. Policies and procedures will reflect variations in practice settings and/or clinical situations that determine the degree to which the recommended practices can be implemented.

AORN recognizes the numerous types of settings in which perioperative nurses practice. These recommended practices are intended as guidelines adaptable to various practice settings. These practice settings include traditional operating rooms, ambulatory surgery centers, physicians' offices, cardiac catheterization suites, endoscopy suites, radiology departments, and all other areas where operative and other invasive procedures may be performed.

Purpose

The rapidly changing health care environment presents health care workers with continuing challenges in the form of newly recognized pathogens and well known microorganisms that have become more resistant to today's therapeutic modalities. Protecting patients and safeguarding health care workers from potentially infectious agent transmission continues to be a primary focus of perioperative registered nurses.

Recommendation I

Health care workers should use standard precautions when caring for all patients in the perioperative setting.

1. Standard precautions should be applied across all aspects of health care delivery.[1] Any individual (eg, patient, family member, significant other, visitor, or health care provider) may be transiently or chronically colonized with pathogenic microorganisms and may be asymptomatic, display active infection, or be in the incubation period of the infectious disease.[1]

2. Additional precautions may be needed for specific organisms encountered, but at a minimum, standard precautions should be used for all surgical patients.
   - Standard precautions apply to exposure or the potential for exposure to blood and all body fluids, secretions, and excretions (except perspiration) whether or not they contain visible blood; nonintact skin; and mucous membranes. Standard precautions are designed to protect patients and health care workers from contact with recognized and unrecognized sources of infectious agents.[1]
   - Infectious agents can be transmitted via direct and indirect contact, respiratory droplets, and airborne aerosols.

3. Exposure to potentially infectious agents should be minimized by the use of personal protective equipment (PPE) (eg, gloves, gowns, aprons), work practices, engineering controls, and other measures tailored to the specific work environment.[2]

Recommendation II

Hand hygiene should be performed before and after each patient contact.

1. All personnel should practice general hand hygiene. Prompt and frequent hand antisepsis is the single most important measure to reduce the spread of microorganisms.[1-3] Hand hygiene should be performed
   - at the beginning of a work shift,
   - before and after patient contact,
   - after removing gloves,
   - before and after eating,
   - before and after using the restroom,
   - any time there is a possibility that there has been contact with blood or other potentially infectious materials, and
   - any time when hands may have been soiled or any time the practitioner believes his or her hands may have been soiled.

2. An appropriate alcohol-based hand antiseptic agent should be available in convenient locations (eg, wall, bedside).[3] Frequency of health care providers' hand hygiene can be increased by convenient access to hand wash sinks or hand sanitation stations.[4]

Recommendation III

Protective barriers must be used to reduce the risk of skin and mucous membrane exposure to potentially infectious materials.

Personal protective barriers are required when it can be reasonably anticipated that a health care worker will be exposed to blood and body fluids or other potentially infectious materials.[2]

1. Gloves selected for use should provide an effective barrier against infectious materials (eg, blood, body fluids) and any anticipated chemicals to which the gloves may come in contact. Some chemicals may cause the breakdown of the glove material.

2. Use of polyvinyl chloride (PVC) or vinyl gloves should be limited to brief, low-risk exposures.[5-11] Research has shown that PVC and vinyl gloves have a high failure rate in use.

3. Users should refer to the glove manufacturer's written instructions for use with chemicals (eg, glutaraldehyde, peracetic acid, methyl methacrylate). When handling glutaraldehyde solutions, gloves that are impervious to glutaraldehyde should be worn.[12] Gloves should be changed immediately following direct contact with uncured methyl methacrylate (ie, bone cement). Exposure to uncured methyl methacrylate places the wearer at risk for direct contact with and skin absorption of the methyl methacrylate because it permeates the glove material. Users should contact the specific glove manufacturer and request written reports on specific glove styles and materials for the intrinsic ability of the glove to protect the wearer when exposed to chemotherapeutics, chemical agents, and bloodborne pathogens.

4. Exam gloves should be inspected upon donning, and changed after each patient contact, or when
   ♦ a visible defect is noted,
   ♦ perforation is suspected, and
   ♦ according to organizational policy.

5. Sterile surgical gloves should be inspected immediately upon donning and before contact with sterile supplies and tissue.[13] Sterile gloves should be changed
   ♦ after each patient contact;
   ♦ when a visible defect is noted;
   ♦ when suspected or actual contamination occurs;
   ♦ when a suspected or actual perforation from a needle, suture, bone, or other event occurs;
   ♦ immediately following direct contact with uncured methyl methacrylate because the wearer is at risk for direct contact and skin absorption of the methyl methacrylate via penetration of the glove material;[14]
   ♦ when an unintentional electrical shock from an electrosurgical unit (ESU) is received to the hand(s) of the user;[15]
   ♦ when gloves begin to swell, expand, and become loose on the wearer's hands, as a result of the material's absorption (ie, hydration) of fluid and fats; and
   ♦ according to organizational policy.

6. All end users should be familiar with the intended use and the limitations of each glove material.[16] Each surgical glove material has specific characteristics (eg, latex, polyisoprene, chloroprene) that affect the performance and intended use of the glove.

7. Gloves should not be washed between patient contacts or uses. Research has found that pathogens are not effectively removed from gloves by washing.[4] Washing gloves is not a substitute for hand washing.

8. Health care workers must wear masks to protect the mucous membranes of the nose and mouth during procedures and activities that generate splashes, splatters, sprays, or aerosols of blood or other potentially infectious materials.[2]

9. Health care workers must wear protective eyewear when splatter is anticipated.[2]

10. Health care workers must wear a face shield if a splash is anticipated.[2]

11. Health care workers must wear fluid-resistant attire to protect skin and clothing during activities that generate splashes, splatters, sprays, or aerosols of blood or other potentially infectious materials. Personal protective equipment is required and must be used whenever exposure to potentially infectious materials is anticipated. The type of PPE required depends upon the type of exposure anticipated. Work garments, such as scrub attire and warm-up jackets, are not considered PPE because they are not impervious to strike-through of hazardous materials.[2]

Recommendation IV

Health care practitioners should double-glove during invasive procedures.

1. Health care practitioners should wear two pairs of gloves, one over the other, during invasive procedures. A systematic review of 18 clinical trials of gloving practices clearly demonstrates that double-gloving minimizes the risk of exposure of health care workers to blood during invasive procedures. Meta-analyses of nine of these studies demonstrate the following.

   ♦ Perforation rates of the glove closest to the skin are significantly less when wearing double gloves compared to single gloves ($P < 0.00001$).

   ♦ Perforation rates are no different when wearing single gloves compared to the outer glove when two pairs of gloves are worn ($P = 0.3$).

   ♦ More glove perforations are detected when using a colored under-glove indicator system when compared to two pairs of standard latex gloves ($P = 0.002$).[17]

   This systematic review also included clinical trials addressing other aspects of gloving practices. These studies found the following.

   ♦ Wearing two pairs of gloves (ie, double-gloving) significantly reduces the number of perforations to the innermost glove, when compared to the outer glove or single gloves.[17]

   ♦ Wearing two pairs of gloves does not increase the likelihood of increased perforations to the outermost glove.[17]

   ♦ Wearing one pair of standard thickness gloves on top of a pair of standard thickness colored gloves facilitates the wearer's rapid recognition of perforations to the outer glove.[17]

   ♦ Wearing a single pair of orthopedic gloves (ie, thicker latex gloves) provides the same protection from perforations as does two pairs of standard latex gloves.[18]

   ♦ Wearing two layers of colored gloves does not assist in recognizing breaches to the glove closest to the wearer's skin.[19-21]

   ♦ Wearing a glove liner between two layers of gloves does reduce perforations to the innermost glove during orthopedic surgical procedures.[22,23]

   ♦ Wearing cloth outer gloves during orthopedic surgical procedures does decrease the number of perforations to the innermost glove when compared to double-glove layers.[24,25]

   ♦ Wearing steel weave outer gloves during orthopedic surgery does not reduce the number of perforations to the innermost gloves when compared to double gloves.[26]

   The Centers for Disease Control and Prevention (CDC), the American College of Surgeons, and the American Academy of Orthopedic Surgeons, support double-gloving during invasive procedures.[27-29]

2. Upon completion of the invasive procedure, both pairs of gloves should be discarded and hand hygiene should be performed.[3]

Recommendation V

Contact precautions should be used when providing care for patients who are known or suspected to be infected or colonized with microorganisms that are transmitted by direct or indirect contact with patients or items and surfaces in patients' environments (eg, herpes simplex, impetigo, infectious diarrhea, smallpox, methicillin-resistant *Staphylococcus aureus* [MRSA], and vancomycin-resistant enterococci [VRE]).

1. Contact precautions include many of the same elements found in the standard precautions requirements. These include

   ♦ wearing gloves when caring for patients or coming in contact with items that may contain high concentrations of microorganisms (eg, fecal material, blood, wound drainage), noting that gloves should be changed after contact with body fluids;

   ♦ wearing gowns when it is anticipated that clothing will have contact with infectious patients or items in the patients' environment (eg, transporting, transferring patient to a bed/cart, positioning);[30]

   ♦ wearing a mask when it is anticipated that aerosolized exposure to infectious microorganisms is possible;

   ♦ face protection (eg, goggles, face shield) when it is anticipated that splash or sneezing exposure to microorganisms is possible;

   ♦ ensuring that precautions are maintained during transport; and

   ♦ adequately cleaning and disinfecting patient care equipment and items before use with each patient.

2. When patient transport is necessary, barriers (eg, gown, gloves) should be used to reduce the opportunity for transmission of microorganisms to other patients, personnel, and visitors and to reduce contamination of the environment.[1]

3. Noncritical equipment (eg, equipment that touches intact skin) contaminated with blood, body fluids, secretions, or excretions should be cleaned and disinfected after each use, according to the organization's written policy.[1] The use of dedicated patient equipment may be indicated in some situations (eg, anesthesia, post-anesthesia care unit).

4. Routine cleaning of environmental surfaces (eg, floors and walls) is adequate for inactivation of MRSA, vancomycin intermediate resistant *Staphylococcus aureus* (VISA), and VRE.

5. When additional measures are indicated to prevent the spread of highly transmissible or epidemiologically important infectious organisms, an infection control professional should be consulted for guidance.[1]

Recommendation VI

Droplet precautions should be used when caring for patients who are known or suspected to be infected with microorganisms that can be transmitted by infectious large particle droplets (ie, larger than 5 microns in size) and generally travel short distances of three feet or less (eg, diphtheria, pertussis, influenza, mumps, pneumonic plague).

1. Droplet precautions include
   ◆ wearing a mask when within three feet of infectious patients,
   ◆ positioning patients at a distance of at least three feet from other patients, and
   ◆ placing surgical masks on patients during transport.

2. When patient transport is necessary, barriers should be used to reduce the opportunity for transmission of microorganisms to other patients, personnel, and visitors and to reduce contamination of the environment.

3. Noncritical equipment (eg, equipment that touches intact skin) contaminated with blood or other potentially infectious materials should be cleaned and disinfected after use.[1]

4. When additional measures are indicated to prevent the spread of highly transmissible or epidemiologically important infectious organisms, an infection control professional should be consulted for guidance.[1]

5. Droplets are generated from the source person primarily during coughing, sneezing, or talking. Transmission via droplet requires close contact between patients and personnel; droplets do not remain suspended in the air and generally travel short distances (eg, three feet or less).[1]

Recommendation VII

Airborne precautions should be used when caring for patients who are known or suspected to be infected with microorganisms that can be transmitted by the airborne route (eg, rubeola, varicella, tuberculosis [TB], and smallpox).

Microorganisms carried by airborne transmission (eg, droplet nuclei or dust particles) can be dispersed widely by air currents, remain suspended in the air for extended periods, and may become inhaled by a susceptible host within the same room or over a longer distance from the source patient.[1]

1. Airborne precautions should include
   ◆ National Institute of Occupational Safety and Health (NIOSH)–approved N95 mask worn by health care personnel,[1]
   ◆ placing surgical masks on patients during transport,
   ◆ airborne isolation rooms with special air handling, and
   ◆ ventilation for areas outside the surgical suite.

2. Additional perioperative considerations for patients known or suspected to have airborne diseases include the following.
   ◆ Elective surgical procedures on patients requiring airborne isolation precautions, such as TB, should be delayed until the patient is no longer infectious.
   ◆ Attempts should be made to perform procedures on patients requiring airborne isolation precautions at times when other patients are not present in the surgical suite and when a minimum number of personnel are present (eg, at the end of the day).
   ◆ Placing a bacterial filter on endotracheal tubes when operating on patients who have confirmed or suspected TB may help reduce

the risk for contaminating anesthesia equipment or discharging tubercle bacilli into the ambient air.[31]

♦ Strict traffic control should be enforced.

♦ After the patient leaves the room, the room should remain closed and not used until the air in the room has completely changed (eg, 15 air changes per hour requires 28 minutes for a 99.9% removal efficiency).[32]

♦ Health care personnel entering the OR suite immediately following a patient on airborne precautions should use an N95 mask and use proper PPE.

3. When surgical procedures are performed on patients who may have infectious TB, respiratory protection worn by personnel protects the sterile field from the respiratory secretions of the health care worker and protects the health care worker from the infectious droplets generated by patients.[32]

Recommendation VIII

Health care workers should be immunized against epidemiologically important agents according to CDC recommendations.

1. All health care workers must receive hepatitis B virus (HBV) immunizations unless medically contraindicated. Immunization against HBV is effective in preventing the disease and should be given before occupational exposure occurs. Information about HBV infection must be provided to employees within 10 days of hire, and informed consent should be given before employees accept HBV immunizations. Health care workers may decline the vaccine but shall do so by signing a declaration statement that declines the vaccine. Vaccination should remain available after this declaration in the event the employee changes his or her mind.[2]

2. Health care workers should be immunized against other communicable and infectious agents.[33,34]

Recommendation IX

Work practices must be designed to minimize risk of exposure to pathogens.

1. Work practice controls must be implemented to reduce the risk of exposure to bloodborne

pathogens, based upon input from nonmanagement staff members.[2] Activities involving hand-to-hand, hand-to-skin, hand-to-nose, hand-to-mouth, or hand-to-eye action can contribute to direct or indirect transmission via inanimate surfaces and should be prohibited in the work area.[1] These prohibited activities include, but are not limited to,

♦ eating,

♦ drinking,

♦ smoking,

♦ applying cosmetics or lip balm, and

♦ handling contact lenses.[2]

Strict adherence to standard precautions minimizes the risk of cross contamination among health care workers, patients, and their environment.

2. Food and drink should not be stored where the potential for exposure to blood or other potentially infectious materials could occur (eg, refrigerators, shelves, countertops, and cabinets).

3. Food and drink should not be present in the restricted and semirestricted areas of the surgical suite.

4. The environment should be kept in a clean and sanitary condition by cleaning and decontaminating all equipment and environmental surfaces between procedures.[26] Microbes such as HBV and VRE are known to remain viable on environmental surfaces for seven days or longer.[35-38]

Recommendation X

Personnel must take precautions to prevent injuries caused by needles, scalpels, and other sharp instruments.

1. Health care organizations must have a comprehensive exposure control plan that includes engineering and work practice controls.[2,39] Health care organizations must

♦ document in the exposure control plan that they have evaluated and implemented safety-engineered sharp devices and needleless systems;

♦ review and update changes in the exposure control plan at least annually to reflect changes in sharps safety technology;

♦ maintain a sharps injury log with detailed information about percutaneous injuries;

- solicit and document in the exposure control plan input from nonmanagerial health care workers when identifying, evaluating, and selecting safety engineered sharp devices; and
- provide engineering controls to include devices with engineered sharps injury protection.[2]

2. Perioperative registered nurses should be familiar with federal, state, and local regulations that mandate the use of needleless systems and sharps safety devices.

3. Sharps with engineering controls must be used when deemed acceptable.
   - Exposure to infectious material and the frequency of sharps injuries can be reduced through the use of safe needle devices and other technologies to minimize contact with sharp instruments.[2]
   - The use of blunt suture needles, when clinically indicated, can reduce the occurrence of glove perforations, needle sticks, and exposures to blood and other potentially infectious materials and are therefore recommended to be used in the perioperative setting as a method for reducing injuries.[29,40-46]
   - The use of a safety scalpel is recommended.[2]

4. Work practice controls must be in place to minimize health care worker exposure when handling sharps.
   - Surgical team members should use a neutral zone or hands-free technique for passing sharp instruments, blades, and needles whenever possible and practical.[16] Studies show that most sharps injuries occur when suture needles or sharps are passed between perioperative team members. Changes in surgical practice to minimize manual manipulation of sharps (ie, neutral zone or no-touch techniques) can have a major effect on these injuries. Creation of a neutral zone (ie, where instruments are put down and picked up, rather than passed hand-to-hand) may decrease injuries from sharp instruments.[2]
   - All sharps must be handled, removed, and disposed of properly. Contaminated sharps should be disposed of in a puncture-resistant, labeled, color-coded, leak-proof container.[2,29] This type of container helps prevent injuries to personnel cleaning the room or equipment after use. Used needles must not be sheared, bent, broken, recapped, or reshanthed by hand. If recapping is required, mechanical devices or the one-hand technique must be used.[2] Removable knife blades should be handled using an instrument or device.
   - Reusable sharps must be handled, removed, and sequestered at the end of the procedure in a labeled, puncture-resistant, closed transportation container. Removable, reusable sharps should be handled using an instrument or device.

Recommendation XI

Activities of personnel with infections, exudative lesions, nonintact skin, and/or bloodborne diseases should be restricted when these activities pose a risk of transmission of infection to patients and other health care workers. Identification, evaluation by a physician, and assessment of fitness for work performance in the perioperative setting should be required.

1. Health care workers infected with a bloodborne disease (eg, HIV, HBV, hepatitis C virus [HCV]) should use measures to protect themselves and others. The HIV-infected health care worker who carries out invasive procedures should double-glove during all procedures.[47] Case reports have demonstrated the nosocomial transmission of HBV, HCV, and other potentially infectious materials from health care professionals to patients during invasive procedures.[48-54]

2. Health care workers who have exudative lesions or weeping dermatitis should refrain from providing direct patient care or handling medical devices used in performing invasive procedures. Restricting personnel who have exudative lesions, nonintact skin, or weeping dermatitis reduces the risk of transmission of bloodborne and other pathogens between workers and patients.[1]

3. Health care workers should follow the organization's written policy regarding reporting potentially infectious conditions.

4. Health care workers should consult with the organization's designated health care provider (ie, employee or occupational health department physician) for assessment, treatment, and limits to perioperative practice, if indicated. The organization's written guidelines should be

followed with respect to the worker's ability to perform required job functions in the organization, especially in high-risk environments.

Recommendation XII

Policies and procedures that address responses to threats of intentionally released pathogens (eg, anthrax, botulism) should be written, reviewed periodically, and readily available within the practice setting.

1. Health care workers should follow the organization's emergency preparedness plan as modified from published CDC guidelines for treating patients exposed to a biological agent in the event of an actual or suspected biological agent release (eg, anthrax, botulism, plague, smallpox). The CDC guidelines, available at *http://www.bt.cdc.gov,* outline transmission precautions for each organism and define those recommendations. The current CDC guidelines should be consulted in conjunction with the organization's infection control practitioner.[55]

2. Perioperative registered nurses should actively participate in the organization's emergency preparedness plan for responding to an intentionally released biological pathogen.

Recommendation XIII

Policies and procedures that address responses to epidemic or pandemic pathogens (eg, severe acute respiratory syndrome [SARS], avian flu, influenza) should be written, reviewed periodically, and readily available within the practice setting.

1. Personnel should follow the organization's infection control plan for epidemics based on published CDC guidelines for treating patients exposed to organisms considered high public health risks. The CDC outlines precautions for each organism on its Web site at *http://www.cdc.gov.*[55] The organization's infection control practitioner should be consulted regarding additional specific precautions in the perioperative arena.

2. Perioperative registered nurses should create and maintain an optimal health environment for patients with human and avian influenza and SARS.[56]

3. Perioperative registered nurses should actively participate in the organization's emergency preparedness plan for responding to an epidemic or pandemic.

Recommendation XIV

Personnel should demonstrate competence in the prevention of transmissible infections.

1. Personnel should be knowledgeable about the principles of infection transmission, risks to patients and personnel, measures to minimize these risks, and actions to be taken in the event of an exposure.

2. Personnel must be instructed in the proper use of PPE and other measures to prevent transmission of infectious agents. Initial education must take place within 90 days of new hire according to the Occupational Safety and Health Administration regulations and updated at least annually.[2]

3. Health care personnel should be educated on the underlying principles of infection control, which provide direction for personnel in providing direct and indirect patient care. Additional periodic educational programs provide reinforcement of principles of infection control, new evidence on risks and preventive measures, and changes in technology and regulations.

4. Administrative personnel should assess and document initial and annual competency of personnel in the safe use of standard and transmission-based precautions, according to organization and department policy. Incorrect use can result in serious injury to patients and personnel. Competency validation assures that personnel have an understanding of risks and appropriate preventive actions. This knowledge is essential to minimizing the risks of transmission of infectious agents from health care personnel to patients and patients to health care personnel.

Recommendation XV

Policies and procedures should be written, reviewed periodically, and readily available within the practice setting.

1. Personnel should report all exposure incidents (eg, needle sticks, blood exposures); infections; or communicable disease to the health care

organization according to organization policy. Prompt reporting enables employers to provide timely and confidential postexposure evaluation, intervention, testing, or appropriate prophylaxis.[2]

2. An introduction and review of policies and procedures for infection prevention, exposure mitigation, and emergency response plans should be included in orientation and ongoing education of personnel to assist in the development of knowledge, skills, and attitudes that affect safety and surgical outcomes. Policies and procedures also assist in the development of quality assessment and improvement activities.

3. The uniform perioperative nursing vocabulary should be used to document patient care related to prevention of transmissible infections on the intraoperative patient record. The perioperative nursing vocabulary is a clinically relevant and empirically validated standardized nursing language. This standardized language consists of the Perioperative Nursing Data Set and includes perioperative nursing diagnoses, interventions, and outcomes. The expected outcome of primary import to this recommended practice document is Outcome 10 (O10), "The patient is free of signs and symptoms of infection." This outcome falls within the domain of Physiologic Responses (D2). The associated nursing diagnosis is (X28): "Risk for infection." The associated interventions that may lead to the desired outcome include (I98) "Protects from cross-contamination."[57]

4. Information about adverse events and near misses should be collected, analyzed, and used for performance improvement as part of the institution-wide performance improvement program. To evaluate the quality of patient care and to formulate plans for corrective action, it is necessary to maintain a system of evaluation.

5. Organizational policies and procedures that address occupational exposure to pathogens must be consistent with federal, state, and local rules and regulations that govern occupational exposure to bloodborne pathogens.

6. These recommendations should be used as guidelines for developing policies and procedures within the practice setting. Policies and procedures establish authority, responsibility, and accountability, and serve as operational guidelines.

Glossary

Airborne precautions: Precautions that reduce the risk of an airborne transmission of infectious airborne droplet nuclei (ie, small particle residue 5 microns or smaller). Airborne transmission refers to contact with infectious airborne droplet nuclei that can remain suspended in the air for extended periods of time or infectious dust particles that can be circulated by air currents.

Anthrax: An acute infectious disease caused by *Bacillus anthracis*. Exposure (ie, skin contact, ingestion, or inhalation) to *Bacillus anthracis* spores from infected animals or animal products can produce infection in humans. Routes of exposure include pulmonary (bioterrorism threat through aerosolization of spores), cutaneous, or gastrointestinal. Person-to-person transmission is not known to occur with inhalation or GI anthrax route of exposure.

Botulism: An acute infectious disease caused by *Clostridium botulinum*. Exposure can occur through contaminated food or aerosolization (ie, inhalation) of *Clostridium botulinum* spores. Person-to-person transmission is not known to occur.

Colonized: The presence of microorganisms that reproduce on tissue without invading tissue or causing disease or infections.

Contact precautions: Precautions designed to reduce the risk of transmission of epidemiologically important microorganisms by direct or indirect contact.

Direct contact: Person-to-person contact resulting in physical transfer of infectious microorganisms between an infected or colonized person and a susceptible host.

Droplet precautions: Precautions that reduce the risk of large particle droplet (ie, 5 microns or larger) transmission of infectious agents.

Droplet transmission: The transfer of infectious microorganisms by contact with conjunctival, nasal, or oral mucosa droplets (eg, coughing, sneezing, talking, suctioning). Viral particles can be acquired from environmental surfaces and transmitted to mucous membranes.

Exam glove: Intended for short duration use, size specific (eg, small, medium, large), can be either nonsterile or can be made sterile by the manufacturer, provided in pairs or singles, made from several materials (eg, latex, PVC, nitrile, chloroprene), but are not intended for invasive surgical procedures because of their lower acceptable quality limit (AQL).

Exposure incident to pathogens: Exposure via specific eye, mouth, or other mucous membranes; nonintact skin; or parenteral contact with blood or other potentially infectious materials that results from the performance of an employee's duties.

Indirect contact: Contact of a susceptible host to a contaminated object (instruments, bed rails, linens, equipment).

Invasive procedures: The surgical entry into tissues, cavities, or organs or repair of major traumatic injuries.

Multi-drug resistant organisms (MDRO): Bacteria that may be resistant to one or more antibiotics (eg, MRSA, VRE).

Neutral zone (synonym: hands-free technique): A safe work practice control technique used to ensure that the surgeon and scrubbed person do not touch the same sharp instrument at the same time. This technique is accomplished by establishing a designated neutral zone on the sterile field and placing sharp items within the zone for transfer of the item between scrubbed personnel.

Personal protective equipment: Protective equipment (eg, masks, gloves, fluid-resistant gowns, goggles, and face shields) for eyes, face, head, and extremities; protective clothing; respiratory devices; and protective shields and barriers designed to protect the wearer from injury. Used wherever it is necessary by reason of hazards of processes or environment, chemical hazards, radiological hazards, or mechanical irritants encountered in a manner capable of causing injury or impairment in the function of any part of the body through absorption, inhalation, or physical contact.

Personnel: Paid or unpaid health care workers, students, volunteers, physicians, and others who may have direct patient contact or opportunity for exposure to patients or devices, supplies, or equipment used for patients.

Plague: An acute, gram-negative, bacterial disease caused by *Yesinia pestis.* Bubonic and septicemic plague transmission is primarily from infected fleas, although pneumonic plague aerosolization of bacteria can result from bioterrorism-related acts. Person-to-person transmission usually occurs through large aerosol droplets of saliva during face-to-face contact (ie, coughing or sneezing).

Potentially infectious material: Blood; all body fluids, secretions, and excretions (except sweat), regardless of whether they contain visible blood; nonintact skin; mucous membranes; and airborne, droplet, and contact-transmitted epidemiologically important pathogens.

Sharps: Sharps include, but are not limited to, suture needles, scalpel blades, hypodermic needles, electrosurgical needles and blades, safety pins, and instruments with sharp edges or points.

Smallpox: An acute, highly contagious viral illness caused by the variola virus. It is transmitted through airborne or droplet exposure (ie, coughing, speaking) and skin contact with skin lesions and secretions. Once exposed, the patient is contagious from the onset of rash until scabs separate (ie, approximately three weeks).

Standard precautions: The primary strategy for successful infection control and reduction of worker exposure. Precautions used for care of all patients regardless of their diagnosis or presumed infectious status.

Surgical glove: Intended for invasive surgical procedures. Size and hand specific (eg, 5½ to 9, right or left). Manufactured to higher AQL for holes than exam gloves.

Transmission-based precautions (enhanced): Second tier of precautions designed to be used with patients known or suspected to be infected or colonized with highly transmissible or epidemiologically important pathogens for which additional precautions are needed to prevent transmission in the practice setting.

REFERENCES

1. Centers for Disease Control and Prevention, "Guideline for isolation precautions in hospitals," *Infection Control and Epidemiology* 17 (January 1996) 53-80.

2. Occupational and Safety and Health Administration, "Bloodborne pathogens" in *Code of Federal Regulations* (CFR) 29: Part 1910.1030.

3. "Recommended practices for surgical hand antisepsis/hand scrubs," in *Standards, Recommended Practices, and Guidelines* (Denver: AORN, Inc, 2006) 537-546.

4. Centers for Disease Control and Prevention, "Guideline for hand hygiene in health-care settings: Recommendations of the healthcare infection control practices advisory committee and the HICPAC/SHEA/APIC/IDSA Hand Hygiene Task Force," *Morbidity and Mortality Weekly Report* 51, No RR-16 (Oct 25, 2002).

5. R C Klein et al, "Bio diagnostics report: Virus penetration of examination gloves," *BioTechniques* 9 no 2 (1990) 196-199.

6. A Douglas et al, "Barrier durability of latex and vinyl medical gloves in clinical settings," *American Industrial Hygiene Association Journal* 58 (September 1997) 672-8.

7. R J Olsen et al, "Examination gloves as barriers to hand contamination in clinical practice," *Journal of the American Medical Association* 270 (July 21, 1993) 350-353.

8. D M Korniewicz et al, "Leakage of latex and vinyl exam gloves in high and low risk clinical settings," *American Industrial Hygiene Association Journal* 54 (January 1993) 22-26.

9. D M Korniewicz et al, "Barrier protection with examination gloves: Double versus single," *American Journal of Infection Control* 22 no 1 (1994) 12-15.

10. A Rego, L Roley, "In-use barrier integrity of gloves: Latex and nitrile superior to vinyl," *American Journal of Infection Control* 27 (October 1999) 405-410.

11. D M Korniewicz et al, "Performance of latex and non-latex medical examination gloves during simulated use," *American Journal of Infection Control* 30 (April 2002) 133-138.

12. "Use of latex surgical exam gloves for protection from glutaraldehyde," Occupational Safety and Health Administration, *http://www.osha.gov* (accessed 24 May 2006).

13. "Recommended practices for maintaining a sterile field," in *Standards, Recommended Practices, and Guidelines* (Denver: AORN, Inc, 2006) 621-628.

14. T H Waegermaekers et al, "Permeability of surgeons' gloves to methyl methacrylate," *Acta Orthopaedica Scandinavia* 54 (December 1983) 790-795.

15. "Recommended practices for electrosurgery," in *Standards, Recommended Practices, and Guidelines* (Denver: AORN, Inc, 2006) 481-496.

16. P Graves "Gloves: How do the pieces of the puzzle fit together?" *Infection Control Today* (September 2001) *http://www.infectioncontroltoday.com/articles/191feat1.htm* (accessed 29 Jan 2005).

17. J Tanner, H Parkinson, "Double gloving to reduce surgical cross-infection," (Cochrane Review) *The Cochrane Library,* Issue 3 (Oxford: John Wilson & Sons, 2003).

18. M Turnquist et al, "Perforation rate using a single pair of orthopedic gloves vs. a double pair of gloves in obstetric cases," *Journal of Maternal-Fetal Medicine* 5 no 6 (November-December 1996) 362-365.

19. C M E Avery, J Taylor, P A Johnson, "Double gloving and a system for identifying glove perforations in maxillofacial trauma surgery," B*ritish Journal of Oral and Maxillofacial Surgery* 4 (August 1999) 316-319.

20. J J Duron et al, "Efficacy of double gloving with a coloured inner pair for immediate detection of operative glove perforations," *European Journal of Surgery* 162 (December 1996) 941-944.

21. P Nicolai, C H Aldam, P W Allen, "Increased awareness of glove perforation in major joint replacement," *Journal of Bone and Joint Surgery,* British Volume 79 (May 1997) 371-373.

22. E J Sebold, L R Jordan, "Intraoperative glove perforation: A comparative analysis," *Clinical Orthopaedics and Related Research* 297 (December 1993) 242-244.

23. P M Sutton, T Greene, F R Howell, "The protective effect of a cut-resistant glove liner," *Journal of Bone and Joint Surgery* 80-B (May 1998) 411-413.

24. R Sanders et al, "Outer gloves in orthopaedic procedures," *Journal of Bone and Joint Surgery* 72 (July 1990) 914-917.

25. M J Underwood et al, "Prevalence and prevention of glove perforation during cardiac operation," (Letters to the Editor) *Journal of Thoracic and Cardiovascular Surgery* 106 (August 1993) 375-377.

26. S S Louis et al, "Outer gloves in orthopaedic procedures: A polyester/stainless steel wire weave glove liner compared with latex," *Journal of Orthopaedic Trauma* 12 (February 1998) 101-105.

27. "Advisory statement: Preventing the transmission of bloodborne pathogens," American Academy of Orthopedic Surgeons, *http://www.aaos.org/wordhtml/papers/advistmt/1018.htm* (accessed 24 May 2006).

28. Centers for Disease Control and Prevention, "Guideline for prevention of surgical site infection, 1999," *Infection Control and Hospital Epidemiology* 20 (April 1999) 247-277.

29. R Berguer, P J Heller, "Preventing sharps injuries in the operating room," *American College of Surgeons* 199 (Sept 2004) 462-467.

30. "Recommended practices for use and selection of barrier materials for surgical gowns and drapes," in *Standards, Recommended Practices, and Guidelines* (Denver: AORN, Inc, 2006) 531-536.

31. "Recommended practices for cleaning, handling, and processing anesthesia equipment," in *Standards, Recommended Practices, and Guidelines* (Denver: AORN, Inc, 2006) 441-450.

32. Centers for Disease Control and Prevention, "Guidelines for preventing the transmission of mycobacterium tuberculosis in health-care settings, 2005," *Morbidity and Mortality Weekly Report* 54 no RR 17 (Dec 30, 2005) 1-141.

33. Centers for Disease Control and Prevention, "Immunization of health-care workers," *Morbidity and Mortality Weekly Report* 46 no RR-18 (Dec 26, 1997) 1-42.

34. Centers for Disease Control and Prevention, "Influenza vaccination of health-care personnel," *Morbidity and Mortality Weekly Report* Early Release 55 (Feb 9, 2006) 1-16.

35. "Recommended practice for environmental cleaning in the surgical practice setting," in *Standards, Recommended Practices, and Guidelines* (Denver: AORN, Inc, 2006) 517-524.

36. G A Noskin et al, "Recovery of vancomycin-resistant enterococci on fingertips and environmental surfaces," *Infection Control and Hospital Epidemiology* 16 (October 1995) 577-581.

37. M J Boyce et al, "Controlling vancomycin-resistant enterococci," *Infection Control and Hospital Epidemiology* 16 (November 1995) 634-637.

38. H F Bonilla et al, "Long-term survival of vancomycin-resistant enterococci faecium on a contaminated surface," (Letters to the Editor) *Infection Control and Hospital Epidemiology* 17 (December 1996) 771-772.

39. "Needlestick safety and prevention act," Public Law 106-430, 106th Congress, *http://frwebgate.access.gpo.gov/cgi-bin/getdoc.cgi?dbname=106_cong_public_laws&docid=f:publ430.106* (accessed 24 May 2006).

40. J Jagger, M Bentley, P Tereskerz, "A study of patterns and prevention of blood exposures in OR personnel," *AORN Journal* 67 (1998) 979-984.

41. K U Wright, C G Moran, P J Briggs, "Glove perforation during hip arthroplasty: A randomized prospective study of a new taper point needle," *Journal of Bone and Joint Surgery* 75 B (November 1993) 918-920.

42. A Mingoli et al, "Influence of blunt needles on surgical glove perforation and safety for the surgeon," *American Journal of Surgery* 172 (November 1996) 512-517.

43. J J Rice et al, "Needlestick injury: Reducing the risk," *International Orthopaedics* 20 no 3 (1996) 132-133.

44. J E Hartley et al, "Randomized trial of blunt-tipped versus cutting needle to reduce glove puncture during mass closure of the abdomen," *British Journal of Surgery* 83 (August 1996) 1156-1157.

45. M I Dauleh, A D Irving, N H Townell, "Needle prick injury to the surgeon—Do we need sharp needles?" *Journal of the Royal College of Surgeons of Edinburgh* 39 (October 1994) 310-311.

46. F J Montz et al, "Blunt needles in fascial closure," (The Surgeon At Work) *Surgery, Gynecology, and Obstetrics* 173 (August 1991) 147-148.

47. "Policies and position statements, Guidelines: HIV and AIDS in the workplace," American College of Occupational and Environmental Medicine, *http://www.acoem.org* (accessed 24 May 2006).

48. "Transmission of Hepatitis B to patients from four infected surgeons without hepatitis B e antigen: The incident investigation teams and others," *The New England Journal of Medicine* 336 (Jan 16, 1997) 178-84.

49. B C Gartner et al, "High prevalence of hepatitis G (HGV) infections in dialysis staff," *Nephrology Dialysis Transplantation* 14 no 2 (February 1999) 406 8.

50. J L Esteban et al, "Transmission of hepatitis C virus by a cardiac surgeon," *The New England Journal of Medicine* 334 (Feb 9, 1996) 555-560.

51. R Harpaz et al, "Transmission of hepatitis B virus to multiple patients from a surgeon without evidence of inadequate infection control," *The New England Journal of Medicine* 334 (Feb 29, 1996) 549-554.

52. S A McNeil et al, "Outbreak of sternal surgical site infections due to *Pseudomonas aeruginosa* traced to a scrub nurse with onychomycosis," *Clinical Infectious Disease* 33 (Aug 1, 2001) 317-323.

53. P J van der Broek et al, "Epidemic of prosthetic valve endocarditis caused by *Staphlyococcus epidermis,*" *British Medical Journal* 291 (October 5, 1985) 949-950.

54. D L Wooster, R E Louch, S Krajden, "Intraoperative bacterial contamination of vascular grafts: A prospective study," *Canadian Journal of Surgery* 28 (September 1985) 407-409.

55. "Emergency preparedness & response: Bioterrorism agents/diseases," Centers for Disease Control and Prevention, *http://www.bt.cdc.gov/agent/agentlist.asp* (accessed 24 May 2006).

56. "Guidance statement: Human and avian influenza and severe acute respiratory syndrome," in *Standards, Recommended Practices, and Guidelines* (Denver: AORN, Inc, 2006) 225-237.

57. S C Beyea, ed, *Perioperative Nursing Data Set: The Perioperative Nursing Vocabulary,* second ed (Denver: AORN, Inc, 2002).

PUBLICATION HISTORY

Originally published February 1993, *AORN Journal,* as "Recommended practices for universal precautions in the perioperative practice setting."

Revised November 1998 as "Recommended practices for standard and transmission-based precautions in the perioperative practice setting"; published February 1999, *AORN Journal.* Reformatted July 2000.

Approved June 2006, AORN Board of Directors, as "Recommended practices for prevention of transmissible infections in perioperative practice settings." Published in *Standards, Recommended Practices, and Guidelines,* 2007 edition.

AORN Perioperative Standards and Recommended Practices, 2012 Edition

Recommended Practices for Prevention of Deep Vein Thrombosis

The following Recommended Practices for Prevention of Deep Vein Thrombosis were developed by the AORN Recommended Practices Committee and have been approved by the AORN Board of Directors. They were presented as proposed recommendations for comments by members and others. They are effective March 1, 2011.

These recommended practices are intended as achievable recommendations representing what is believed to be an optimal level of practice. Policies and procedures will reflect variations in practice settings and/or clinical situations that determine the degree to which the recommended practices can be implemented.

AORN recognizes the various settings in which perioperative nurses practice. These recommended practices are intended as guidelines adaptable to various practice settings. These practice settings include traditional operating rooms (ORs), ambulatory surgery centers, physicians' offices, cardiac catheterization laboratories, endoscopy suites, radiology departments, and all other areas where surgery and other invasive procedures may be performed.

Purpose

The purpose of these recommended practices is to guide perioperative RNs by providing a framework for developing a protocol for deep vein thrombosis (DVT) prevention. These recommended practices provide guidance for administering pharmacologic and/or mechanical DVT prophylaxis and patient and health care personnel education. Although the prevention of DVT and pulmonary embolism (PE) should be a priority of the entire health care organization, the particular risks facing perioperative patients makes it imperative that perioperative RNs take an active role in DVT prevention. The patient in the perioperative environment may present with or encounter one or more of the three primary causative factors of DVT formation (ie, venous stasis, vessel wall injury, hypercoagulability).[1] The risk for DVT may be elevated for all perioperative patients, including children, because of immobility, tissue trauma, and surgical positioning requirements.[1-8] Deep vein thrombosis usually occurs in the lower extremities but also may occur in the upper extremities.[9] Prevention of DVT reduces the potential for associated complications such as post-thrombotic syndrome and PE.[10,11]

The perioperative nursing care interventions related to the treatment of complications of DVT (eg, venous stasis ulcers or their postoperative treatment, post-thrombotic syndrome, PE) are beyond the scope of this document. The choice of DVT prophylaxis is a medical decision and is beyond the scope of this document.

Recommendation I

A health care organization-wide protocol for the prevention of DVT that includes care of the perioperative patient should be developed and implemented.[12,13]

Using an organization-wide protocol developed from evidence-based, professional guidelines and providing alternative treatment considerations prompts health care providers to give consistent and appropriate DVT prophylactic care.[13] In a study of 150 hospitals, Maynard concluded that a protocol including a risk assessment and physician orders for venous thromboembolism (VTE) prevention accelerated improvements in VTE prophylaxis efforts.[14] Integration of the health care organization's protocol into all physician orders provides consistency between all care providers and increases use of the protocol.[12,13,15]

I.a. The health care organization-wide DVT protocol should be developed by a multidisciplinary team that includes key stakeholders including, but not limited to,
- RNs;
- physicians;
- anesthesia professionals;
- pharmacists; and
- personnel from
  - quality/risk management,
  - information technology (IT), and
  - administration.[13]

Key stakeholders' acceptance of the protocol is improved if they are involved in the decision-making process.[13] Each key stakeholder provides knowledge and expertise according to his or her area of practice and responsibility. The perioperative RN is a key stakeholder as a primary professional involved in implementing the protocol in the perioperative area and provides evidence-based references related to the safety, effectiveness, efficiency, and financial considerations of DVT prophylactic measures.[16,17] Physicians representing each medical specialty can be resources for the evidence-based DVT prevention protocols developed by their medical specialty organizations.[8,14,18-20] Representatives from IT provide expertise in using technology to gather necessary data for use in the quality improvement program and by creating electronic programs that support protocol implementation. Administrative representatives approve the financial resources necessary to support the measures used in the protocol.

I.b.   The DVT protocol should
- be supported by an evidence-based model (eg, risk-based, group-specific);
- be accessible to all health care providers;
- contain links to evidence-based treatment options;
- provide alternatives to suggested treatment;
- list contraindications;
- be simple to apply; and
- apply to all patients within the health care organization's scope of service. [12-14,17]

A standardized protocol can be easier to approve, put into action, and modify as necessary.[13] Use of an evidence-based model (eg, risk-based, group-specific) facilitates consistency in treatment and promotes adherence to the protocol.[12] An evidence-based model is based on validated research studies and links patient-related criteria (eg, patient-specific risk factors, the reason for admission) to the preferred prophylactic method.[13,14,17] One example of a risk-based protocol defines a value for each prophylactic measure and a value for each patient-specific risk factor. The appropriate prophylactic measure is determined by summing the patient-specific risk factors values and connecting that number to the value assigned to the prophylactic measure.[21] Another risk-based protocol groups predetermined risk factors into categories such as a level one, two, or three. The appropriate prophylactic measure is determined by placing the patient into the appropriate group based on the patient's risk factors.[22] A group-specific

protocol initially determines the type of prophylaxis based on the reason for hospitalization. This initial determination may be changed when other risk factors identified during the assessment are included.[12]

I.b.1.   The DVT protocol should include the use of a computer-generated alert identifying the patient at risk for developing a DVT. The alert is created by compiling the information from the patient assessment to produce a clinical decision support tool. When computerized documentation is not available, the patient assessment form should highlight those items, or groups of items, that indicate risk for developing a DVT and a consistent order set should be used.

The computer-generated alert was shown in one study to improve the rate of prophylaxis from 1.5% to 10% for mechanical and from 13% to 23.6% for pharmacological prophylaxis. The population in this study consisted of 1,255 patients in the intervention group and 1,251 patients in the control group.[15]

O'Connor et al compared the number of patients receiving DVT prophylaxis when hand-written orders were used compared to when order sets were used. A random review of charts during an eight-month period (N = 291) showed that DVT prophylaxis was ordered for 35.6% of patients when order sets were used compared to 10% of patients when hand-written orders were used.[23]

Maynard et al demonstrated in a sample of 30,850 admissions that adequate prophylaxis improved from 58% in 2005 to 93% in 2007 with the use of a standardized prevention protocol and order set.[22] A review of the literature by Maynard et al also supported the effectiveness of a computer-generated alert and a consistent order set.[14]

The American College of Chest Physicians' evidence-based recommendations include the use of a computer decision support system.[12]

I.b.2.   The DVT protocol should include a start time (eg, upon admission, preoperatively, postoperatively) for all types of prophylaxis based on the clinical condition of the patient.

Preoperative initiation of DVT prophylaxis is listed as criteria in clinical trials and listed as a requirement in evidence-based guidance statements.[12,24-27] The risk of DVT formation begins with preoperative immobility and continues throughout the intraoperative phase of care and is decreased by preoperative initiation of DVT prophylaxis. Some prophylactic measures, such as pharmacological methods, may be contraindicated because of the increased risk of bleeding and may need to be started postoperatively.[12]

I.c. The organization-wide protocol should include specific DVT prevention measures that address perioperative-associated DVT risk factors including, but not limited to,
- positioning;
- compression of tissue caused by retraction; and
- use of a pneumatic tourniquet, especially during prolonged periods of inflation.

Specific DVT prevention measures are needed during the perioperative patient care period, which may not be applicable to other areas of the organization. Patient positioning for the surgical procedure, such as the reverse Trendelenburg position (ie, the patient's head is positioned above heart level) and other positions that cause flexion and internal rotation of the hip and knee, can cause venous stasis. Venous stasis also can be caused by tissue compression resulting from retraction.[2,12,28] Tourniquet pressure can cause venous stasis or congestion by prohibiting venous return.[29]

Recommendation II

The perioperative RN should complete a preoperative patient assessment to determine DVT risk factors.

The preoperative nursing assessment provides information necessary to determine the individual patient risk factors for DVT and identify the appropriate DVT prophylaxis measures.

II.a. The preoperative patient DVT risk factor assessment should include, but not be limited to, the following:[12,17,30]

- Venous stasis:
  - age greater than 40 years;
  - cancer (eg, active or occult) and associated therapy;
  - history of cardiac disease;
  - obesity;
  - pregnancy and the postpartum period;
  - prolonged bed rest or immobilization;
  - prolonged travel (ie, between four to 10 hours within the previous eight weeks);
  - surgery lasting longer than 30 minutes; and
  - varicose veins.

- Vessel wall injury:
  - cancer (eg, active or occult) and associated therapy;
  - central venous catheters;
  - extensive burns;
  - previous history of DVT or stroke;
  - surgery; and
  - trauma (eg, major trauma, lower-extremity injury).

- Hypercoagulability:
  - cancer (eg, active or occult) and associated therapy;
  - inherited or acquired thrombophilia (ie, conditions in which the blood coagulates faster than normal);
  - oral contraceptive use or hormone replacement therapy;
  - pregnancy and the postpartum period; and
  - trauma (eg, major trauma, lower-extremity injury).

- Other:
  - acute medical illness,
  - acute infectious processes,
  - inflammatory conditions, and
  - smoking.

The risk factor grouping of venous stasis, vessel wall injury, and hypercoagulability is frequently referred to in the literature as Virchow's Triad. Published reviews of the literature have indicated that patients with these risk factors exhibit a greater potential for DVT formation.[1,12,17,30,31]

II.b. The perioperative RN should consult and collaborate with surgical team members and members of other disciplines as appropriate regarding the need for and selection of prophylaxis based on the organizational protocol and the individual patient's DVT risk factor assessment.

The perioperative RN has a professional responsibility to advocate for the patient during the entire perioperative period by consulting and collaborating with other professional colleagues regarding patient care.[16,17]

Recommendation III

The perioperative RN should implement specific interventions when the patient is receiving mechanical DVT prophylaxis.

Mechanical prophylaxis may be used throughout the perioperative period for various procedures, and specific interventions are necessary to decrease potential complications. Mechanical prophylaxis includes early ambulation, active and passive foot and ankle exercises, and the use of graduated compression stockings and intermittent pneumatic compression devices.[17] *The American College of Chest Physicians Evidence-Based Clinical Based Guidelines,* 8th edition, states that mechanical prophylaxis has been shown to reduce the risk of DVT, may improve the effectiveness of pharmacological prophylaxis, may be used in patients with a high risk of bleeding, and may reduce leg swelling.[12]

III.a.   The perioperative RN should instruct the patient to perform foot and ankle exercises preoperatively.

Foot and ankle exercises create natural muscle compression of the venous system of the legs, decreasing venous stasis.

III.b.   The perioperative RN should implement specific activities when the patient is receiving mechanical DVT prophylaxis using intermittent pneumatic compression devices.

Researchers suggest that intermittent pneumatic compression devices reduce venous stasis by improving venous return from the lower extremities.[24] Several intermittent pneumatic compression devices, with a wide variety of design features providing inflation on the foot, calf, or entire leg have been cleared by the US Food and Drug Administration. The devices generally consist of wraps (eg, thigh- or knee-length,

foot sleeves) that are placed on the legs or feet; tubing that connects the wrap to the pump; and a pump. The wrap may consist of single or multiple chambers. The chambers may be inflated as a single unit or sequentially and may be cycled using a preset timing device or manual timing device. The compression system also may feature technology allowing the inflation to be synchronized to the patient's respiration-related venous phasic flow, or customized inflation based on the patient's individual venous refill time.[32] The pump may be mobile or stationary.[24]

Foot inflation devices simulate natural walking by providing compression to the plantar venous plexus. Calf and thigh devices work via a milking action that increases the velocity of venous return, enhances fibrinolysis, and increases the release of endothelial-derived relaxing factors and urokinase.[7,12,24] These relaxing factors and urokinase assist in preventing or inhibiting thrombosis development and enhance thrombolysis (ie, clot destruction) during thrombosis formation.[24]

In a study of 502 total hip arthroplasties, Hooker et al concluded that intraoperative and postoperative thigh-high intermittent pneumatic compression is an effective prophylactic measure.[33] Woolson studied 322 patients and came to a similar conclusion.[34] In another study (N = 3016), Sugano et al concluded that mechanical DVT prophylaxis is safe and effective for elective hip surgeries.[35]

III.b.1.   The perioperative RN should assess the patient for and report to the physician any contraindications or possible complications related to use of the intermittent pneumatic compression device.

Contraindications include, but are not limited to,
- conditions affecting the lower extremity (eg, dermatitis, gangrene, extreme leg deformity, untreated infected wounds, injuries, or surgical sites);
- conditions compromising lower extremity venous flow (eg, severe arteriosclerosis, other ischemic vascular disease, massive leg edema);
- sensitivity to latex, unless wraps and tubing are latex free; and
- severe congestive heart failure.[36]

Complications include, but are not limited to,

- compartment syndrome;
- latex sensitivity or allergy, unless the wraps and tubing are latex-free;
- peroneal nerve palsy; and
- skin injury.[24]

III.b.2. Intermittent pneumatic compression wraps should be applied according to the manufacturer's written instructions.

III.b.3. When the manufacturer's written instructions for use require the use of stockinet, elastic hose, or other material under the device wraps, the material should be wrinkle-free when applied to the skin.

Stockinet, elastic hose, or other materials may be recommended by some manufacturers for skin protection under the device wraps. Smooth, wrinkle-free under-wrap material may reduce the risk of skin injury.

III.b.4. During application, the device or wrap tubing should be placed external to the wrap and away from locations that may create a pressure injury.

Placement of the device or wrap tubing between the patient's skin and the device wrap may lead to a pressure injury.

III.b.5. The perioperative RN should re-assess and verify that the intermittent pneumatic compression device and wraps are operating and are positioned properly after the patient is transferred to the OR bed.

III.b.6. The perioperative RN should re-assess the wraps for proper placement if the patient's position is changed during the surgical procedure.

Reassessment of proper placement of wraps after the patient's position is changed is needed to verify proper device placement and correct function.

III.b.7. The intermittent pneumatic compression device should remain on during the intraoperative and immediate postoperative period except for very brief periods of time, when removal is necessitated by patient care needs.[12]

III.b.8. The DVT protocol should specify when the wraps should be disconnected from the pump and when a patient skin assessment should be performed (eg, ambulation, before discharge, transfer of care). If evidence of complications is present, the perioperative RN should document the information and report it to the physician.

III.c. The perioperative RN should implement specific activities when the patient is receiving mechanical DVT prophylaxis using graduated compression stockings.

Graduated compression stockings, either thigh-high or knee-high in length, are frequently used intraoperatively and postoperatively. The stockings are thought to work by applying a constant graduated pressure to the leg, thereby reducing the venous diameter and venous stasis.[37,38] Conflicting evidence exists regarding which length of stocking, thigh- or knee-length, provides the greatest efficacy.[26,38-42]

III.c.1. The perioperative RN should assess the patient for contraindications or possible complications related to the use of graduated compression stockings.

Contraindications include, but are not limited to,

- ankle-brachial pressure index < 0.8 mm Hg;
- arteriosclerosis;
- cellulitis in lower extremities;
- dermatitis in lower extremities;
- latex allergy or sensitivity, unless stockings are latex-free;
- leg edema;
- leg ulcers;
- peripheral vascular disease;
- presence of infectious processes;
- recent surgical graft;
- severe peripheral neuropathy; and
- thigh circumference exceeds the limit defined by the stocking manufacturer directions for use.[38,42,43]

Complications include, but are not limited to,

- ischemia;
- latex allergy or sensitivity, unless stockings are latex-free;
- numbness and tingling; and
- skin injury.[42,43]

III.c.2. Graduated compression stockings should be properly fitted to the individual patient. The patient's legs should be measured separately and according to the manufacturer's instructions.[42,44]

When stockings are too tight, venous return may be decreased and lead to venous pooling and clot formation. In addition, stockings that are too tight may cause the development of peroneal nerve palsy associated with increased direct pressure on the peroneal nerve.[45] When stockings are too loose, they may not provide the effective gradient compression required for DVT prevention. Measuring each of the patient's legs is necessary because there may be enough variability in circumference to require a different stocking size for each leg.[44]

III.c.3. Graduated compression stockings should be applied according to the manufacturer's written instructions, which may include verifying that the

- stockings are not rolled up or down;
- stockings are smooth when fitted;
- toe holes lie underneath the toes;
- heel patches are in the correct position; and
- thigh gussets are positioned on the patient's inner thighs.[42,43,45]

Skin breakdown or a tourniquet effect can be created by graduated compression stockings, if not applied correctly.[42-45]

III.c.4. The perioperative RN should verify that the graduated compression stockings have not rolled up the foot or down the leg during transfer to and from the OR bed or during procedural positioning.

When the graduated compression stockings are allowed to roll up the foot or down the patient's leg, a tourniquet effect can be created and may lead to the formation of a DVT, arterial ischemia, gangrene, and necrosis by constricting blood flow.[42,45]

III.d. As soon as possible postoperatively, the perioperative RN should assist the patient with ambulation if appropriate and should assist with foot and ankle exercises for the patient who is unable to ambulate.

Early ambulation and foot and ankle exercises create natural compression of the venous system and decrease venous stasis. These exercises alone are not adequate to prevent venous stasis in most hospitalized patients; therefore, supplemental mechanical or pharmacological prophylaxis may be required.[12]

Recommendation IV

The perioperative RN should implement specific interventions when the patient is receiving pharmacologic DVT prophylaxis.

Specific interventions are necessary to decrease the risk of potential complications from pharmacologic prophylaxis that may be used throughout the perioperative period. Pharmacologic prophylaxis consists of anticoagulant medications that inhibit blood clotting. The pharmacologic regimen may consist of medications such as warfarin; synthetic pentasacchride (ie, foundaparinux); low molecular weight heparin; and low-dose heparin.

IV.a. The perioperative RN should assess the patient for contraindications or the risk of possible complications related to pharmacologic DVT prophylaxis.

Contraindications include, but are not limited to,

- complex trauma injuries;
- hemorrhage;
- infective endocarditis;
- neurosurgery;
- ocular surgery;
- pregnancy;
- recent intracranial, gastric, or genitourinary bleeding;
- recent surgery (ie, within two days); and
- recent lumbar puncture or neuraxial (ie, spinal, epidural) anesthesia or analgesia (ie, within 24 hours).[12,46-48]

Complications include, but are not limited to,

- bleeding;
- compartment syndrome;
- hematoma formation;
- heparin-induced thrombocytopenia;
- osteoporosis and osteopenia;
- skin necrosis;
- thrombocytopenia; and
- urticaria at injection sites.[4,12]

IV.b.   Pharmacologic DVT prophylaxis should be administered in accordance with the "AORN guidance statement: Safe medication practices in perioperative settings across the life span."[49]

Recommendation V

The perioperative RN should provide the patient and his or her designated caregiver(s) instructions regarding prevention of DVT and the prescribed prophylactic measures.

Education related to DVT prevention and the prescribed prophylactic measures may improve patient compliance and acceptance.[17,30,42,50]

V.a.   The patient receiving mechanical prophylaxis and his or her designated caregiver(s) should receive preoperative and postoperative instructions including, but not limited to, the following topics
- the mechanism of mechanical prophylaxis;
- the importance of compliance;
- the importance of wearing properly sized, graduated compression stockings;
- removal and proper reapplication of the intermittent compression device immediately after ambulation; and
- proper application, removal, and reapplication of graduated compression stockings.[17,42-44]

Education assists the patient in understanding the potential complications of mechanical prophylaxis, as well as the importance of compliance with its correct use.[42,45,50]

V.b.   The patient receiving pharmacologic prophylaxis and his or her designated caregiver(s) should receive preoperative and postoperative instructions including, but not limited to, the importance of:
- follow-up appointments, including where and when they should occur;
- continuing medication post-discharge for the duration prescribed;
- following through with laboratory work at periodic intervals;
- avoiding certain activities (eg, contact sports);
- not using over-the-counter medications (eg, aspirin, ibuprofen);
- using a soft toothbrush;
- using an electric razor;
- reporting any unusual bruising;
- obtaining a medical alert bracelet;
- being aware of medication and food interactions, including herbal and other over-the-counter preparations (eg, ginger, ginkgo biloba, ginseng, feverfew, St. John's wort, green tea); and
- informing health care workers about pharmacologic prophylaxis before undergoing any procedures (eg, dental work, laboratory tests).[17,51]

V.c.   Before a patient is discharged, the perioperative RN should provide the patient and his or her designated caregiver(s) with instructions on the prevention of DVT including, but not limited to,
- current and future risk factors;
- maintaining adequate hydration;
- common signs and symptoms of DVT or PE (eg, leg pain, swelling, unexplained shortness of breath, wheezing, chest pain, palpitations, anxiety, sweating, coughing up blood);
- avoiding clothing that constricts the lower extremities;
- participating in physical exercise as indicated;
- performing active and passive range of motion, especially of the lower extremities, as indicated;
- avoiding sitting with knees bent or legs crossed for long periods of time;
- elevating legs when sitting;
- avoiding sitting or standing for long periods of time;
- complying with all forms of DVT prophylaxis;
- performing frequent coughing and deep breathing exercises and changing position when in bed;
- avoiding raising the knee gatch of the bed during inpatient care;
- alerting other patient care providers to the patient's history of DVT and current prophylactic measures; and
- the physiology of blood flow and clot formation.[17,52]

Education provides the patient with an awareness of DVT prevention measures and the signs and symptoms of DVT that should be reported to the physician.[17,53] Deep vein thrombosis frequently develops or becomes evident after the patient is discharged. This is supported by a study of 5,451 patients with DVT, nearly half of whom were diagnosed as outpatients, which indicates that more than half of those patients waited three or more days after the onset of symptoms to seek treatment.[52]

Recommendation VI

Personnel should receive initial education and competency validation, as applicable to their roles, on patient care measures to prevent DVT.

Initial and ongoing education of perioperative personnel on the prevention of DVT, the risk to the patient, and appropriate methods of prophylaxis facilitates the development of knowledge, skills, and attitudes that affect safe patient care.

VI.a. Perioperative RNs and all patient care personnel should receive initial education, competency validation, and current information on
- DVT prevention protocols and updates;
- DVT prevention policies and procedures and updates;
- DVT risk factors;
- perioperative-specific preventive measures; and
- the correct application and use of mechanical prophylactic measures (eg, contraindications, signs and symptoms of complications).

VI.b. Perioperative RNs should receive initial education and competency validation, as well as seek evidence-based knowledge, on
- the pathophysiology of DVT and PE;
- contraindications and complications for each category of prophylaxis;
- the selection of prophylactic measures; and
- the administration of pharmacologic prophylaxis.
  Perioperative RNs have a professional responsibility to incorporate research findings into practice.[16] Methods of DVT prophylaxis are evolving and new information is being published periodically.

Recommendation VII

Documentation should include a patient assessment, plan of care, nursing diagnoses, and identi-fication of desired outcomes and interventions, as well as an evaluation of the patient's response to the care provided.**

Documentation serves as a method of communication among all care providers involved in planning, implementing, and evaluating patient care. Documenting nursing activities provides a description of the perioperative nursing care administered and the status of patient outcomes on transfer of care.

VII.a. Documentation should be recorded in a manner consistent with the health care organization's policies and procedures and should include, but not be limited to,
- results of the nursing assessment including risk factors and complications, if present;
- application and removal times for all mechanical prophylactic measures;
- the type and size of wrap or graduated compression stockings applied;
- the identifier and settings of the mechanical unit, if applicable;
- the time, route, and dosage of all pharmacologic prophylaxis;
- the reason for any variance from the protocol; and
- responses to complications, if present.

Recommendation VIII

Policies and procedures for DVT prophylaxis should be developed, reviewed periodically, revised as necessary, and readily available in the practice setting.

Policies and procedures assist in the development of patient safety, quality assessment, and improvement activities. Policies and procedures establish authority, responsibility, and accountability within the facility. They also serve as operational guidelines that are used to minimize patient risk factors for complications, standardize practice, direct staff members, and establish continuous performance improvement programs.

VIII.a. The health care organization's policies and procedures regarding use of mechanical prophylaxis units must be in compliance with the Safe Medical Devices Act of 1990, as amended in March 2000.[54]

VIII.a.1. When patient or personnel injuries or equipment failures occur, the mechanical prophylaxis unit and its components should be removed from service and all components retained, if possible.

Retaining the unit and its components allows for a complete systems check to determine possible reasons for the failure.

VIII.b. Policies and procedures for preventing DVT should include the steps required for initiating and implementing the DVT protocol and reporting and responding to adverse events.[49]

Recommendation IX

A quality improvement program should be in place to evaluate the outcomes of DVT prophylaxis (eg, DVT rate) and protocol compliance.

The Agency for Healthcare Research and Quality states that quality and performance improvement programs assist in evaluating the quality of patient care and the formulation of plans for corrective actions. These programs provide data that may be used to determine whether an individual organization is within benchmark goals and, if not, identify areas that may require corrective actions.[13]

IX.a. The quality improvement program should include a study time frame (eg, six months before and six months after a change has been instituted) and should
- compare the health care organization's DVT prevention protocol to current research and established, research-based guidelines;
- determine the health care organization's DVT prevention protocol rate of use;
- determine and explore barriers to the use of the protocol; and
- determine the rate of readmissions for DVT or complications related to DVT.[13,14]

Establishing a time frame assists in determining a baseline for comparison. Measuring the rate of readmissions helps to determine the effectiveness of the DVT prevention protocol. Determining the rate of use and the barriers to use assists with refinement of the protocol and ideally leads to an increase in protocol compliance and an improvement in patient outcomes.[13,14]

REFERENCES

1. Ahonen J. Day surgery and thromboembolic complications: time for structured assessment and prophylaxis. *Curr Opin Anaesthesiol.* 2007;20(6):535-539.

2. Heck CA, Brown CR, Richardson WJ. Venous thromboembolism in spine surgery. *J Am Acad Orthop Surg.* 2008;16(11):656-664.

3. Osborne NH, Wakefield TW, Henke PK. Venous thromboembolism in cancer patients undergoing major surgery. *Ann Surg Oncol.* 2008;15(12):3567-3578.

4. Rawat A, Huynh TT, Peden EK, Kougias P, Lin PH. Primary prophylaxis of venous thromboembolism in surgical patients. *Vasc Endovascular Surg.* 2008;42(3):205-216.

5. Jackson PC, Morgan JM. Perioperative thromboprophylaxis in children: development of a guideline for management. *Paediatr Anaesth.* 2008;18(6):478-487.

6. Squizzato A, Venco A. Thromboprophylaxis in day surgery. *Int J Surg.* 2008;6 Suppl 1:S29-30.

7. Mayle RE Jr, DiGiovanni CW, Lin SS, Tabrizi P, Chou LB. Current concepts review: venous thromboembolic disease in foot and ankle surgery. *Foot Ankle Int.* 2007;28(11):1207-1216.

8. Forrest JB, Clemens JQ, Finamore P, et al. AUA Best Practice Statement for the prevention of deep vein thrombosis in patients undergoing urologic surgery. *J Urol.* 2009;181(3):1170-1177.

9. Arnhjort T, Persson LM, Rosfors S, Ludwigs U, Larfars G. Primary deep vein thrombosis in the upper limb: A retrospective study with emphasis on pathogenesis and late sequelae. *Eur J Intern Med.* 2007;18(4):304-308.

10. Prandoni P, Kahn SR. Post-thrombotic syndrome: prevalence, prognostication and need for progress. *Br J Haematol.* 2009;145(3):286-295.

11. Wille-Jorgensen P, Jorgensen LN, Crawford M. Asymptomatic postoperative deep vein thrombosis and the development of postthrombotic syndrome. A systematic review and meta-analysis. *Thromb Haemost.* 2005;93(2):236-241.

12. Geerts WH, Bergqvist D, Pineo G F, et al. Prevention of venous thromboembolism: American College of Chest Physicians Evidence-Based Clinical Practice Guidelines (8th Edition). *Chest.* 2008;133(6 Suppl):381S-453S.

13. Preventing hospital-acquired venous thromboembolism: a guide for effective quality improvement. Agency for Healthcare Research and Quality. *http://www.ahrq.gov/QUAL/vtguide/.* Accessed February 14, 2011.

14. Maynard G, Stein J. Designing and implementing effective venous thromboembolism prevention protocols: lessons from collaborative efforts. *J Thromb Thrombolysis.* 2010;29(2):159-166.

15. Kucher N, Koo S, Quiroz R, et al. Electronic alerts to prevent venous thromboembolism among hospitalized patients. *N Engl J Med.* 2005;352(10):969-977.

16. Standards of perioperative nursing. In: *Perioperative Standards and Recommended Practices.* Denver, CO: AORN, Inc; 2010: 9-27.

17. Barnett JS, DeCarlo LJ. Incidence of deep venous thrombosis in the surgical patient population and prophylactic measures to reduce occurrence. *Perioper Nurs Clin.* 2008;3(4):367-382.

18. Committee on Practice Bulletins—Gynecology American College of Obstetricians and Gynecologists.

ACOG practice bulletin No. 84: prevention of deep vein thrombosis and pulmonary embolism. *Obstet Gynecol.* 2007;110(2 Pt 1):429-440.

19. Richardson W, Apelgren K, Earle D, Fanelli R. Guidelines for deep venous thrombosis prophylaxis during laparoscopic surgery. *Surg Endosc.* 2007;21(12): 2331-2334.

20. Parvizi J, Azzam K, Rothman RH. Deep venous thrombosis prophylaxis for total joint arthroplasty: American Academy of Orthopaedic Surgeons guidelines. *J Arthroplasty.* 2008;23(7 Suppl):2-5.

21. Caprini JA. Risk assessment as a guide to thrombosis prophylaxis. *Curr Opin Pulm Med.* 2010;16(5):448-452.

22. Maynard GA, Morris TA, Jenkins IH, et al. Optimizing prevention of hospital-acquired venous thromboembolism (VTE): prospective validation of a VTE risk assessment model. *J Hosp Med.* 2010;5(1):10-18.

23. O'Connor C, Adhikari NK, DeCaire K, Friedrich JO. Medical admission order sets to improve deep vein thrombosis prophylaxis rates and other outcomes. *J Hosp Med.* 2009;41(2):81-89.

24. Colwell CW Jr, Froimson MI, Mont MA, et al. Thrombosis prevention after total hip arthroplasty: a prospective, randomized trial comparing a mobile compression device with low-molecular-weight heparin. *J Bone Joint Surg Am.* 2010;92(3):527-535.

25. Johanson NA, Lachiewicz PF, Lieberman J R, et al. Prevention of symptomatic pulmonary embolism in patients undergoing total hip or knee arthroplasty. *J Am Acad Orthop Surg.* 2009;17(3):183-196.

26. Venous thromboembolism: reducing the risk of venous thromboembolism (deep vein thrombosis and pulmonary embolism) in inpatients undergoing surgery. National Institute for Helth and Clinical Excellence. *http://guidance.nice.org.uk/CG46.* Accessed February 14, 2011.

27. National Quality Forum. National Voluntary Consensus Standards for Prevention and Care of Venous Thromboembolism: Additional Performance Measures. 2008.

28. Recommended practices for positioning the patient in the perioperative practice setting. In: *Perioperative Standards and Recommended Practices.* Denver, CO: AORN, Inc; 2010: 327-350.

29. Recommended practices for the use of the pneumatic tourniquet in the perioperative practice setting. In: *Perioperative Standards and Recommended Practices.* Denver, CO: AORN, Inc; 2010: 175-188.

30. Kehl-Pruett W. Deep vein thrombosis in hospitalized patients: a review of evidence-based guidelines for prevention. *Dimens Crit Care Nurs.* 2006;25(2):53-59.

31. Acute Pulmonary Embolism (Helical CT): eMedicine. *http://emedicine.medscape.com/article/361131-overview.* Accessed February 14, 2011.

32. Intermittent pneumatic compression devices. *Health Devices.* 2007;36(6):177-204.

33. Hooker JA, Lachiewicz PF, Kelley SS. Efficacy of prophylaxis against thromboembolism with intermittent pneumatic compression after primary and revision total hip arthroplasty. *J Bone Joint Surg Am.* 1999;81(5):690-696.

34. Woolson ST. Intermittent pneumatic compression prophylaxis for proximal deep venous thrombosis after total hip replacement. *J Bone Joint Surg Am.* 1996; 78(11):1735-1740.

35. Sugano N, Miki H, Nakamura N, Aihara M, Yamamoto K, Ohzono K. Clinical efficacy of mechanical thromboprophylaxis without anticoagulant drugs for elective hip surgery in an Asian population. *J Arthroplasty.* 2009;24(8):1254-1257.

36. Bonner L, Coker E, Wood L. Preventing venous thromboembolism through risk assessment approaches. *Br J Nurs.* 2008;17(12):778-782.

37. Morris RJ, Woodcock JP. Intermittent pneumatic compression or graduated compression stockings for deep vein thrombosis prophylaxis? A systematic review of direct clinical comparisons. *Ann Surg.* 2010;251(3):393-396.

38. Autar R. A review of the evidence for the efficacy of anti-embolism stockings (AES) in venous thromboembolism (VTE) prevention. *J Orthop Nurs.* 2009;13(1):41-49.

39. The CLOTS (Clots in Legs Or sTockings after Stroke) trial collaboration. Thigh-length versus below-knee stockings for deep venous thrombosis prophylaxis after stroke: a randomized trial. *Ann Intern Med.* 2010;153(9):553-562.

40. Morris RJ, Woodcock JP. Evidence-based compression: prevention of stasis and deep vein thrombosis. *Ann Surg.* 2004;239(2):162-171.

41. Sajid MS, Tai NR, Goli G, Morris RW, Baker DM, Hamilton G. Knee versus thigh length graduated compression stockings for prevention of deep venous thrombosis: a systematic review. *Eur J Vasc Endovasc Surg.* 2006;32(6):730-736.

42. Winslow EH, Brosz DL. Graduated compression stockings in hospitalized postoperative patients: correctness of usage and size. *Am J Nurs.* 2008;108(9):40-51.

43. Welch E. The assessment and management of venous thromboembolism. *Nurs Stand.* 2006;20(28): 58-66.

44. Walker L, Lamont S. Graduated compression stockings to prevent deep vein thrombosis. *Nurs Stand.* 2008;22(40):35-38.

45. Van Wicklin SA, Ward KS, Cantrell SW. Implementing a research utilization plan for prevention of deep vein thrombosis. *AORN J.* 2006;83(6):1353-1368.

46. Horlocker TT, Wedel DJ, Rowlingson JC, et al. Regional anesthesia in the patient receiving antithrombotic or thrombolytic therapy: American Society of Regional Anesthesia and Pain Medicine Evidence-Based Guidelines (Third Edition). *Reg Anesth Pain Med.* 2010;35(1):64-101.

47. Mood GR, Tang WHW, Perioperative DVT Prophylaxis: eMedicine. *http://emedicine.medscape.com/article/284371-overview.* Accessed February 14, 2011.

48. Huntington S, Acomb C. Reducing the risk of thromboembolic events with warfarin. *Br J Card Nurs.* 2008;3(6):248-263.

49. AORN guidance statement: safe medication practices in perioperative settings across the life span. in: *Perioperative Standards and Recommended Practices.* Denver, CO: AORN, Inc; 2010: 665-672.

50. Stewart D, Zalamea N, Waxman K, Schuster R, Bozuk M. A prospective study of nurse and patient education on compliance with sequential compression devices. *Am Surg.* 2006;72(10):921-923.

51. Pruitt B, Lawson R. What you need to know about venous thromboembolism. *Nurs*. 2009;39(4):22- 28.

52. Goldhaber SZ, Tapson VF, DVT FREE Steering Committee. A prospective registry of 5,451 patients with ultrasound-confirmed deep vein thrombosis. *Am J Cardiol*. 2004;93(2):259-262.

53. Arcelus JI, Kudrna JC, Caprini JA. Venous thromboembolism following major orthopedic surgery: what is the risk after discharge? *Orthop*. 2006;29(6):506-516.

54. Medical device reporting: manufacturer reporting, importer reporting, user facility reporting, distributor reporting. Food and Drug Administration, HHS. Final rule. *Fed Regist*. 2000;65(17):4112-4121.

Acknowledgements

LEAD AUTHOR
Byron Burlingame, MS, RN, CNOR
Perioperative Nursing Specialist
AORN Center for Nursing Practice
Denver, CO

CONTRIBUTING AUTHORS
Sharon Van Wicklin, MSN, RN, CNOR, CRNFA, CPSN, PLNC
Perioperative Nursing Specialist
AORN Center for Nursing Practice
Denver, CO

David L. Feldman, MD, MBA, CPE, FACS
American College of Surgeons

Patricia Graybill-D'Ercole, MSN, RN, CNOR, CRCST
Nurse Manager
Wellspan Health/York Hospital
York, Pennsylvania

PUBLICATION HISTORY
Originally published March 2011 online in *Perioperative Standards and Recommended Practices*.

AORN Perioperative Standards and Recommended Practices, 2012 Edition

Recommended Practices for the
Prevention of Unplanned Perioperative Hypothermia

The following recommendations for protecting patients from unplanned perioperative hypothermia were developed by the AORN Recommended Practices Committee and have been approved by the AORN Board of Directors. They were presented as proposed recommendations for comments by members and others. They are effective January 1, 2008.

These recommended practices are intended as achievable recommendations representing what is believed to be an optimal level of practice. Policies and procedures will reflect variations in practice settings and/or clinical situations that determine the degree to which the recommended practices can be implemented.

AORN recognizes the various settings in which perioperative registered nurses practice. These recommended practices are intended as guidelines adaptable to various practice settings. Practice settings include traditional operating rooms, ambulatory surgery centers, physicians' offices, cardiac catheterization suites, endoscopy suites, radiology departments, and all other areas where operative and other invasive procedures may be performed.

Purpose

These recommended practices are intended to guide perioperative registered nurses in optimizing patient care practices to maintain normothermia and prevent unplanned hypothermia. Hypothermia, defined as a core body temperature less than 36° C (96.8° F), presents a constant challenge for perioperative registered nurses because many surgical patients are at risk for unplanned hypothermia during surgery. There are three phases of unplanned hypothermia: the redistribution phase, the linear decrease phase, and the thermal plateau phase. These recommended practices focus on the prevention of the redistribution phase of unplanned hypothermia. Planned or therapeutic hypothermia is outside the scope of this document.

In the redistribution phase of unplanned hypothermia, a rapid shift of body heat from the body's core to its periphery occurs, resulting in a core temperature drop of approximately 1.6° C (2.7° F) during the first hour after induction of anesthesia.[1,2] The initial temperature drop of the redistribution phase is followed by a slow linear decrease phase during the second and subsequent hours of anesthesia, in which heat loss exceeds the body's abil-ity to metabolically produce heat. In this second phase, warming the patient can effectively limit further heat loss. After approximately three to five hours of anesthesia, the patient's core temperature often plateaus and is characterized by a core body temperature that remains constant, even during prolonged surgery.[3,4]

Unplanned hypothermia is among the most common complications of surgery. It results from anesthesia-induced thermoregulation impairment and the heat loss inherent to surgery and the surgical environment.[5] The risk of hypothermia is greater in some patients (eg, neonates,[6,7] trauma patients,[8] patients with extensive burns[9]). All patients, however, are at risk of hypothermia as the duration of anesthesia time increases.[1,2,10,11]

Randomized clinical trials have demonstrated that mild hypothermia increases the incidence of serious adverse consequences including surgical site infections[12] and adverse cardiac events including ventricular tachycardia.[13,14] In trauma patients, hypothermia is associated with increased mortality.[15] Mild hypothermia inhibits platelet activation, resulting in increased blood loss.[16,17] A 2° C (3.6° F) drop in temperature increases blood loss by approximately 500 mL.[18] Mild hypothermia also alters medication metabolism and increases the duration of muscle relaxant action.[19,20] Hypothermia extends postanesthesia recovery time[21,22] and prolongs hospitalization.[12,23] The risk of these complications is considered greater for frail, elderly patients undergoing extensive surgery than it is for young, generally healthy patients undergoing comparatively minor procedures.[24]

Recommendation I

The perioperative registered nurse should assess the patient for risk of unplanned perioperative hypothermia.

I.a   Perioperative registered nurses should evaluate the patient's risk for unplanned hypothermia. Sources of data include chart review, physical assessment and patient interview, and review of the anesthesia planned and proposed surgical procedure.

I.b.   Infancy or neonatal status should be considered. Neonates and infants are more susceptible to hypothermia than adults because they have a high ratio of body surface area to weight, which leads to more heat loss through their skin.[6,7] Studies show that greater temperature decreases occurred in infants and neonates when undergoing major surgery involving an open procedure.[7]

I.c. The extent and severity of a patient's traumatic injuries should be considered.

Patients with severe traumatic injuries are more likely to be hypothermic upon hospital admission and are at high risk of development of unplanned perioperative hypothermia. Between 21% and 50% of severely injured trauma patients become hypothermic.[8] Predisposing factors include exposure in the field, blood loss and shock, rapid infusions of cool fluids, removal of clothing, and impaired heat production. Hypothermia triggers a cascade of coagulopathy and acidosis. Studies have consistently found that hypothermia increases the risk of death in trauma patients.[15,25,26] In one large study more than half of the hypothermic trauma patients died.[27]

I.d. The extent and severity of any patient burns should be considered.

Patients with extensive burns lose body heat readily by radiation from burned tissue and convection when tissue is exposed to air currents. Burned patients are at high risk for unplanned hypothermia. The threshold for physiologic response to external temperature is set higher in these patients, triggering a metabolic response to cold at higher ambient temperatures than in unburned patients. The set point is estimated to be 0.03° C higher for each percent of total body surface area burned (eg, 50% burn = 1.5° C higher set point).[9] The natural insulating effect of skin is also impaired. The higher set point, combined with the lack of insulation, places patients with severe burns at high risk for hypothermia.

I.e. The type and duration of planned anesthesia should be reviewed.

Hypothermia in the operating room results from impaired thermoregulation induced by anesthetic agents and exposure to the relatively cool environment. General or major regional anesthesia (eg, epidural, spinal) for periods longer than one hour induces hypothermia. General anesthetics inhibit tonic vasoconstriction and cause vasodilatation. This results in a shift of heat from the body's core to its periphery and a drop in core temperature of approximately 1.6° C over the first hour after induction. During the subsequent two hours of anesthesia time, core temperature continues to decrease an additional 1.1° C.[1] Epidural and spinal anesthesia decrease the vasoconstriction and shivering to a slightly lesser degree, depending on the level of the block.[28,29]

I.f. Perioperative registered nurses should be aware of factors influencing the severity of potential hypothermia in patients under general or major regional anesthesia. These factors include, but are not limited to, the following:

I.f.1. **Older adults.** In a case control study of adult general surgery patients, increased age was found to be a predictive risk factor for perioperative hypothermia.[30] This has been found in patients receiving either general or epidural anesthesia,[31] or spinal anesthesia.[32] Older patients lose heat more rapidly than younger adults due to decreased fat or muscle mass and changes in vascular tone that inhibit vasoconstriction and decrease heat production.[32] Older patients' thermoregulatory defenses are also impaired more than younger patients by general[11] and neuraxial[33] anesthesia.

I.f.2. **Body weight.** Low body weight has been identified as a risk factor for perioperative hypothermia in general surgery patients.[30] Thin patients have a large body-surface-area-to-weight ratio and limited insulation to prevent heat loss. Obese patients have a high weight-to-body-surface ratio and maintain peripheral tissues at high temperatures due to high body fat and a consistent vasodilated state in the time before induction of anesthesia. These patients generally have low core-to-peripheral temperature gradients and little redistribution hypothermia.[34]

I.f.3. **Metabolic disorders.** Some metabolic disorders inhibit thermoregulation by impeding heat production or physiologic responses to changes in external temperatures. Central nervous system dysfunctions may cause insufficient thermoregulation. Cardiovascular diseases may cause peripheral vasoconstriction. Hypothyroidism and hypopituitarism may inhibit heat production. Patients with diabetic neuropathies have been found to have lower core body temperature after two hours of anesthesia than generally healthy adults undergoing similar surgery.[35]

I.f.4. **Chronic treatment with antipsychotics or antidepressants.** Antipsychotics impair the central thermoregulatory effect of the hypothalamus, resulting in decreased heat production and increased heat loss.[36] The cause of thermoregulation impairment during anesthesia in chronically depressed patients remains unclear.[37]

I.f.5. **Use of a pneumatic tourniquet.** Pneumatic tourniquets help prevent hypothermia while inflated; however, they cause abrupt hypothermia when released. Pneumatic tourniquets reduce hypothermia by preventing blood and heat exchange between the isolated extremity and the remainder of the body. More metabolic heat is thus conserved in the core thermal compartment. Upon release of the tourniquet, a redistribution of heat from the core to the extremity results in a rapid decrease in core temperature.[38-41]

I.f.6. **Cold surgical environment.** Environmental temperature determines the rate at which metabolic heat is lost through radiation and convection from the skin, and by evaporation of skin-preparation solutions.[4,42]

I.f.7. **Open-cavity surgery.** There is substantial heat loss into the relatively cool environment of the operating room from surgical incisions. This decrease in core temperature is more pronounced during large open-cavity procedures than small-cavity procedures.[4,43]

I.f.8. **Infusions of cool fluids, blood, and blood products.** A unit of refrigerated blood or one liter of crystalloid solution administered at ambient temperature decreases mean body temperature approximately 0.25° C in a 70-kg patient.[44]

I.f.9. **Cool irrigation solutions in body cavities.** Irrigation solutions placed into the abdomen, pelvis, or thorax enhance heat transfer from the body core to the solution and increase heat loss.

I.g. Patients' preoperative baseline temperature should be assessed. When preoperative hypothermia is identified, interventions should be undertaken to normalize patients' core temperature before surgery when possible. Preexisting hypothermia is considered one of the most significant contributing factors to intraoperative hypothermia.[6]

Recommendation II

The perioperative registered nurse should develop a plan of care to minimize the risk of unplanned perioperative hypothermia in patients identified at risk.

II.a. The perioperative registered nurse should establish expected outcomes and collaborate with anesthesia care providers in the selection of appropriate temperature monitoring technology and interventions to reduce the risk of unplanned hypothermia.

II.b. The perioperative registered nurse should identify and assure the availability of temperature monitoring technology and patient warming equipment and supplies, as needed, and adjust environmental conditions according to individualized patient needs.[45]

Recommendation III

Equipment to monitor core temperature should be selected based upon reliability and access to the route.

III.a. The perioperative registered nurse should ensure that equipment to monitor the patient's temperature is readily available. Temperature monitoring devices that provide the most accurate and consistent readings during each phase of perioperative care should be selected. The selection of the best monitoring device should depend upon the accuracy of measuring core body temperature, reliability of the device, accessibility of the monitoring site, patient safety, and ease of use. The ideal thermometer should be accurate within +/– 0.1° C and not sensitive to outside temperature influences.[46] The device should accurately identify temperatures that are above and below normal.

III.a.1.   There are four reliable sites for measurement of core temperature:

- **Tympanic membrane.** The tympanic membrane temperature, measured by a thermocouple, is the preferred method in many preoperative and postoperative areas.[47,48] This method is noninvasive, and the monitoring site receives blood supply from the carotid artery, which supplies the thermoregulatory center of the hypothalamus.

- **Distal esophagus.** The distal esophagus is considered a desirable site to measure temperature, particularly in the operating room, and is less prone to artifact than most others. It is an alternative to the pulmonary artery and is widely used intraoperatively. Placement of the probe in the lower fourth of the esophagus prevents artifactual cooling of the probe by respiratory gases.[48]

- **Nasopharynx.** The nasopharynx is another reliable monitoring site for intraoperative measurement because it approximates core temperature.[48] A thermistor probe is inserted through the nares to the nasopharynx. Measurements may be influenced by the temperature of inspired gases and often are 0.5° C lower than pulmonary artery temperatures.[49,50]

- **Pulmonary artery.** The most accurate measurement of core body temperature is through the pulmonary artery, which is bathed in blood from the core.[48] This invasive form of monitoring, however, is not justified solely for temperature assessment.

III.a.2.   Less reliable sites for estimating core temperature include the following:

- **Axillary.** Temperatures can be measured through a thermocouple or an infrared axillary reading. Axillary temperatures are not accurate.[51-58] Read-

ings have been found to be significantly lower than pulmonary artery measurements.[52] Accuracy of readings in pediatric patients has been shown to decrease as temperature increases.[55]

- **Bladder.** Temperatures can be measured using urinary catheters containing temperature transducers. Bladder temperatures are close to core temperature, but the accuracy of the measurement decreases during cardiopulmonary bypass,[59] when the patient is hypothermic and urinary output is lower,[50] and during lower abdominal surgery. This method is a better approximation of core temperature than rectal or axillary methods.[59]

- **Oral.** A systematic review of research studies comparing oral temperatures taken at the posterior sublingual site found that in the absence of a pulmonary catheter, this method provides a reliable estimate of core temperature, even in intubated patients.[48] This method does not detect malignant hyperthermia, however, and is not recommended for intraoperative use.

- **Rectal.** Temperatures taken by the rectal route are directly related to the area's blood flow, and measurements seriously lag behind core temperatures.[50,60] This method of measurement does not appropriately detect malignant hyperthermia and is not a good alternative for general use.[61,62]

- **Skin.** Skin temperature may be measured using a crystal skin-surface thermometer. Studies have demonstrated that peripheral skin temperature correlates poorly with core temperature.[58,63] A recent study found that redistribution of body heat has little effect on the core-to-forehead temperature difference.[64]

- **Temporal artery.** Temporal artery temperature may be measured noninvasively with a scanner probe attached to the forehead. The temporal artery is a branch of the carotid artery and provides a measurement of core temperature; however, this method has been found to be unreliable.[65-67]

III.b. Equipment selected for measuring temperature should be free of mercury. Mercury is a heavy metal that can cause serious adverse health consequences, including chromosomal abnormalities. Environmental contamination can cause harmful effects on wildlife. Mercury thermometers are identifiable by the liquid mercury bubble used for reading the thermometer. Disposal of mercury is regulated by the Resource Conservation and Recovery Act.[68,69]

III.c. Temperature monitoring devices should be used according to the manufacturers' written instructions. Manufacturers' instructions provide details that may enhance the reliability of measurements.

Recommendation IV

The core temperature of patients at risk for unplanned hypothermia should be monitored preoperatively, intraoperatively, and postoperatively.

Monitoring patient temperature alerts the provider to the need for preventive or corrective action. Changes can be a decrease in core temperature or an increase in temperature associated with application of a heating device or inflation of a pneumatic tourniquet. It is important to measure core temperature because peripheral temperature is often significantly different from core temperature. The perception of cold is an inadequate measure. For example, hypothermia during regional anesthesia may not trigger a perception of cold by the patient.[62]

IV.a. The patient's temperature should be assessed preoperatively. Assessment of the patient's temperature preoperatively provides a baseline for planning patient care. This assessment alerts care providers of the need to treat pre-existing hypothermia or to avoid overheating the patient with an elevated temperature.

IV.b. The patient's core body temperature should be monitored intraoperatively. Intraoperative temperature monitoring is used to provide information to prevent or mitigate hypothermia and to avoid overheating.

IV.c. The temperature of patients should be monitored when undergoing general anesthesia that exceeds 30 minutes and during regional anesthesia when changes are anticipated or suspected.[62]

IV.c.1. The American Society of Anesthesiologists (ASA) recommends that temperature be continually evaluated and monitored "when clinically significant changes in body temperature are intended, anticipated, or suspected."[70]

IV.c.2. The American Association of Nurse Anesthetists recommends monitoring body temperature continuously in pediatric patients receiving general anesthesia and, when indicated, on all patients.[71]

IV.d. The patient's core body temperature should be evaluated postoperatively. The patient's postoperative core temperature provides a basis for evaluation of the effectiveness of intraoperative measures to prevent unplanned hypothermia and provides data to guide the postoperative plan of care.

IV.e. Abnormal patient temperatures should be communicated to the appropriate patient care providers. Managing the patient's temperature requires a coordinated effort among members of the entire perioperative team.

Recommendation V

Interventions should be implemented to prevent unplanned hypothermia.

V.a. Prewarming the patient for a minimum of 15 minutes immediately prior to induction of anesthesia should be considered for patients at risk of unplanned hypothermia. Warming the patient's skin and peripheral tissues before induction of general or major regional anesthesia prevents redistribution hypothermia. The temperature of the peripheral tissues is increased and vasodilatation triggered. This results in a smaller core to periphery temperature gradient and minimizes the effect of anesthesia-induced vasodilatation.

In a randomized clinical trial of patients undergoing cesarean section, 15 minutes of prewarming and intraoperative forced-air warming resulted in a higher core body temperature in both patients and their infants.[72] In outpatients, 15 minutes of forced-air prewarming resulted in higher core body temperatures upon arrival in the postanesthesia care unit, when compared to prewarming with warm cotton blankets.[73] In a study of volunteers, 30 minutes of forced-air warming resulted in an increase in peripheral temperature determined to be more than the amount typically redistributed from core to periphery under anesthesia.[74]

V.b.   Patients should be kept normothermic intraoperatively. Patients who remain normothermic intraoperatively experience fewer adverse outcomes. Insulating blankets (eg, cotton, reflective) reduce heat loss by 30%,[75,76] but this is usually insufficient to prevent hypothermia in anesthetized patients.[77] Circulating fluid mattresses under the patient are nearly ineffective at minimizing the risk of hypothermia.[62,78-81] The patient's body weight, in combination with the heat of the fluid mattress, increases the risk of pressure ulcer or necrosis.[62]

V.c.   Effective methods of preventing unplanned hypothermia should be used. These methods involve skin surface warming including, but not limited to, the following:

–   **Forced-air warming** is safe and the most widely used skin surface warming method. The efficacy of forced-air warming in preventing unplanned hypothermia has been proven in many clinical trials.[11,81-86] The method is effective in neonates,[87] pediatric patients,[85] and morbidly obese patients.[88] Forced-air warming has also been found to be effective in rewarming patients after cardiopulmonary bypass.[89-91] Forced-air warming does not increase the risk of wound contamination.[83,92]

–   **Circulating-water garments** circulate warm water through a special, segmented, conductive-heating garment wrapped around the patient. This method has been found to effectively transfer heat to the patient and maintains normothermia in adult[93-97] and pediatric patients.[98] Circulating-water garments maintained normothermia better than a combination of water blanket and fluid warmer in patients undergoing on-pump[96] or off-pump[94,95] cardiopulmonary bypass. Studies have shown that more heat is transferred to the patient by a circulating water garment than forced-air warming.[97] Compared to an upper body forced-air blanket, normothermia was maintained better using the circulating-

water garments in patients undergoing abdominal surgery.[99] Circulating-water garments have also been found to effectively rewarm patients after cardiopulmonary bypass[94,100,101] and to rewarm hypothermic patients better than a full-body forced-air blanket.[97]

–   **Energy transfer pads** circulate water through a set of heat-exchange pads that adhere to the patient's skin. Energy transfer pads have been found to be an effective tool to reduce intraoperative hypothermia during off-pump cardiac surgery.[102]

V.d.   Warming intravenous (IV) fluids should be considered only if large volumes (ie, more than 2 liters/hour for adults) are being administered. Warming IV fluids to near 37° C (98.6° F) prevents heat loss from the administration of cold IV fluids and should be considered as an adjunct to skin surface warming. When less than 2 liters of volume is given, fluid warming is of limited value because fluid-induced cooling is minimal. In studies of patients undergoing major surgery, the combination of forced-air warming and fluid warming decreased the risk of hypothermia more than forced-air warming alone.[103,104] In one study, however, the average temperature in patients in both groups was normothermic.[104] Fluid warming is not a substitute for forced-air warming, which usually transfers far more heat, and warmed fluids alone will not usually keep patients normothermic.[60,104,105] When fluids are being warmed, technology designed for this purpose should be used according to the manufacturers' written instructions.

V.e.   Warming irrigation solutions to be used inside the abdomen, pelvis, or thorax should be considered. Warmed irrigation fluid [near 37° C (98.6° F)] should be used as an adjunct therapy to decrease heat loss, but it is insufficient alone to prevent hypothermia. In a study of patients undergoing laparoscopy without forced-air warming, patients receiving warmed irrigation solutions maintained higher core body temperatures than those receiving room temperature solutions;[24,106] however, warmed irrigation fluids alone did not prevent hypothermia.[106] No improvement in body temperature was found when using warmed irrigation during arthroscopic surgery.[107] When using warmed irrigation solutions, the temperature of the solution should be measured with a thermometer at the point of use and verified before instillation. Irrigating with hot solutions has resulted in patient injuries.

V.f.   Increasing the room temperature should be considered when active skin warming is not feasible, or in addition to active skin warming in cases where active skin warming alone is insufficient. When a large surface area must be exposed for the surgical procedure, forced-air warming may not be sufficient. For these patients, the severity of hypothermia may be reduced by raising the room temperature to more than 23° C (73.4° F).[62,108] In orthopedic procedures, normothermia was successfully maintained without forced-air warming when the room temperature remained above 26° C (78.8° F).[109]

V.g.   Equipment to humidify warm anesthetic gases should be available for pediatric patients. Less than 10% of metabolic heat is lost through the respiratory tract, and heating and humidification of the airway have little effect on core temperature.[62] This intervention is more effective in infants and children.[110] This method transfers much less heat than forced air and should not be used in lieu of forced-air warming.

V.h.   Skin preparation solutions should be used at a temperature recommended by the solution manufacturer. Heating some skin preparation agents may increase the risk of a chemical or thermal burn. Heating flammable antimicrobial skin preparation agents creates a fire hazard. Manufacturers' written instructions provide guidance for the appropriate storage temperature.

V.i.   Additional precautions should be taken to prevent unplanned hypothermia in infants and neonates.

V.i.1.   The room should be prewarmed and maintained higher than 26° C (78.8° F).[62] In a study of anesthetized neonates and infants, operating room temperatures less than 23° C (73.4° F) increased the risk of hypothermia by 1.96 times.[7]

V.i.2.   Skin exposure should be minimized and limited in time as much as possible.

V.i.3.   Equipment should be available to humidify and warm the airway. Active humidification and heating of inspired gases has been found to result in a 0.25° to 0.5° C higher core temperature in infants.[110,111]

V.i.4.   Equipment should be available to warm IV fluids.[112]

V.i.5.   Irrigation fluids should be warmed to normal body temperature (37° C [98.6° F]) and the fluid temperature verified before use. Instillation of warmed irrigation fluids minimizes heat lost through radiation.

V.i.6.   Patient temperature should be monitored continuously intraoperatively. An infant's temperature decreases within 10 minutes after induction of anesthesia.[7] Vigorous warming may cause hyperthermia. Continuous monitoring provides early identification of temperature changes, including hyperthermia caused by overheating.

V.j.   Additional precautions should be taken to prevent unplanned hypothermia in patients with severe trauma.

V.j.1.   Patients with severe trauma are at risk of hypothermia. In this patient population, hypothermia is associated with increased risk of death.[113] The patient may be hypothermic upon arrival in the perioperative area. Forced-air warming may not be appropriate because of the amount of tissue exposed for the surgical procedure. Extra measures are required to minimize heat loss if forced-air warming is contraindicated and may be necessary in addition to forced-air warming.

V.j.2.   The room temperature should be prewarmed higher than 29.4° C (85° F).[45,114]

V.j.3.   The room temperature should be maintained higher than 29.4° C (85° F) until active warming devices achieve normothermia.[45,114]

V.j.4.   Equipment should be available to warm IV fluids. Large volumes of fluids may be given rapidly to stabilize the patient. Warming these fluids minimizes heat lost through radiation.

V.j.5. Irrigation fluids should be warmed to normal body temperature (ie, 37° C [98.6° F]).

V.j.6. Equipment should be available to humidify and warm the airway.

V.j.7. Patient temperature should be monitored continuously intraoperatively.

V.k. Additional precautions should be taken to prevent unplanned hypothermia in patients with extensive burns.

V.k.1. Forced-air warming should be used when feasible. It may not be feasible for patients with extensive burns, however, when a large amount of tissue must be exposed for the surgical procedure. Extra measures are required for extensive burns to minimize heat loss.

V.k.2. The room temperature should be prewarmed and maintained higher than 29.4° C (85° F). High ambient temperatures minimize heat loss through radiation and convection.

V.k.3. Body surfaces not involved in the surgical procedure should be covered. Covering these surfaces minimizes heat lost through convection.

V.k.4. Equipment should be available to warm IV fluids.

V.k.5. Irrigation fluids should be warmed to near 37° C (98.6° F).

V.k.6. Equipment should be available to warm and humidify anesthetic gases.

V.k.7. Intraoperative patient temperature should be monitored continuously.

Recommendation VI

Warming devices should be used in a manner that minimizes the potential for patient injuries.

IV.a. Prewarming and continued normothermia management must be provided using only US Food and Drug Administration (FDA)-cleared devices.

IV.b. Intravenous fluid bags or irrigation bottles of heated fluid should not be used to warm patients' skin. In 1994, the ASA Closed Claims Project reported that 52% of burn injuries in the operating room were associated with the use of unapproved devices. Sixty-four percent of these injuries resulted from using heated IV fluid bags to warm patients' skin.[115]

IV.c. Warming devices should be used in accordance with manufacturers' written instructions and in a manner that minimizes the potential for injury. Forced-air warming technology should be used only with the appropriate blanket attached to the hose. The hose end has a dangerously high air temperature, and the blanket serves to disperse this heat. Using the air unit without a blanket has resulted in serious burns.[116,117] Intravenous fluid should be warmed only by technology designed for this purpose, at temperatures recommended by the fluid manufacturer.

IV.d. Ischemic tissue should never be heated. Heat is inadequately distributed in ischemic tissue, and application of heat increases the risk of thermal injury.

Recommendation VII

Competency
Personnel should receive initial education and competency validation and updates on the prevention of unplanned hypothermia and the use of warming equipment.

VII.a. Personnel providing perioperative patient care should be knowledgeable about principles of thermoregulation, risks and consequences of hypothermia, correct use of temperature measurement technology, and measures to minimize the risk of unplanned hypothermia. Personnel should be instructed in the proper operation, care, and handling of warming devices and accessories before use. Initial education of the underlying principles of unplanned hypothermia provides direction for personnel in providing safe care. Additional, periodic educational programs provide reinforcement of these principles and new information on changes in technology, its application, compatibility of equipment and accessories, and potential hazards.

VII.b. Administrative personnel should assess and document annual competency of personnel in prevention of unplanned hypothermia and safe use of warming devices and accessories according to hospital and department policy. Incorrect use of warming devices can result in serious injury to patients. Competency assurance verifies that personnel have a basic understanding of thermoregulation, risks of unplanned hypothermia, and safe use of warming equipment. This knowledge is essential to minimizing the risks of misuse of the equipment and to providing safe care.

Recommendation VIII

Documentation

Patient assessments, the plan of care, interventions implemented, and evaluation of care to prevent unplanned perioperative hypothermia should be documented.

VIII.a. Documentation should include a patient assessment, a plan of care, nursing diagnoses, identification of desired outcomes, interventions, and an evaluation of the patient's response to care provided. The Perioperative Nursing Data Set (PNDS), the uniform perioperative nursing vocabulary, should be used to document patient care and to develop policies and procedures related to prevention of unplanned perioperative hypothermia.

VIII.a.1. Potential diagnoses include:
- Risk for imbalanced body temperature (X57),
- Ineffective thermoregulation (X58), and
- Hypothermia (X26).[15]

VIII.a.2. An expected outcome of primary importance to these recommended practices is "The patient is at or returning to normothermia at the conclusion of the immediate postoperative period." (O12) This outcome falls within the physiologic domain (D2).[45]

VIII.a.3. Interventions that may lead to the desired outcome include the following: assesses risks for unplanned hypothermia (I131); implements thermoregulation measures (I78); monitors body temperature (I86); and evaluates response to thermoregulation measures (I55).[45]

VIII.b. The patient's temperature and the interventions taken to protect him or her from unplanned hypothermia should be documented in the perioperative record. Documentation should include, but not be limited to,
- preoperative assessment with baseline temperature measure;
- plan of care for prevention of hypothermia;
- patient temperature measurements taken throughout perioperative care;
- use of temperature-regulating devices, including identification of the unit and temperature settings used;
- other thermoregulation interventions; and
- postoperative outcome evaluation.

Recommendation IX

Policies and Procedures

Policies and procedures for prevention of unplanned hypothermia should be developed in collaboration with anesthesia care providers, reviewed periodically, revised as necessary, and readily available in the practice setting.

IX.a. These recommended practices should be used as guidelines for the development of policies and procedures in the perioperative practice setting. Policies and procedures establish authority, responsibility, and accountability within the facility. They also serve as operational guidelines.

IX.b. Policies and procedures for prevention of unplanned hypothermia should be developed and include, but not be limited to,
- preoperative, intraoperative, and postoperative patient assessments;
- interventions to be employed;
- documentation of care provided;
- use, care, and cleaning of equipment;
- maintenance of equipment;
- reporting and removal from service of malfunctioning equipment;
- reporting of incidence of hypothermia or injuries; and
- competency verification.

IX.c. Policies and procedures should be reviewed and revised at regularly scheduled intervals and be readily available in the practice setting.

Recommendation X

Quality

A quality improvement/management program should be in place to evaluate the structure, process, and outcomes of interventions used to protect patients from unplanned perioperative hypothermia.

X.a.   Unplanned hypothermia should be evaluated as part of the perioperative quality management program. The patient outcomes of preventive measures should be evaluated. Outcomes in high-risk populations should be included (eg, neonates, infants, severe trauma, burn patients). The Surgical Care Improvement Project includes "colorectal surgery patients with immediate postoperative normothermia" as an evidence-based indicator of quality.[118]

X.b.   Measures should be implemented as necessary to minimize the incidence of unplanned hypothermia. Corrective measures may include increasing the availability of warming equipment and educational programs, and providing clinicians with feedback about outcomes.

X.c.   Adverse events related to warming devices should be reported through the facility's incident reporting system and investigated in compliance with the Safe Medical Devices Act of 1990, amended in March 2000.[119]

X.d.   Adverse events should be investigated and analyzed to minimize the risk of recurrence. An injury related to the use of a warming device must be reported to the FDA. Serious injuries and deaths must be reported to the FDA and manufacturer within 10 days. Device identification, maintenance and service information, and adverse event information should be included in the report from the practice setting. Retaining the equipment and accessories allows for a complete evaluation and facilitates determination of the cause of the injury. Semiannual reports must be submitted to the FDA as follow-up to any adverse event report submitted during the previous six-month period.

Glossary

Active skin warming: The application of conductive, convective, or radiative warming to the skin.

Ambient temperature: The temperature of the immediate environment, usually ranging from 20° C to 25° C (68° F to 77° F).

Circulating-fluid garment: A microprocessor-controlled heating and cooling device with temperature sensors; skin thermistor; and a specially designed, segmented garment that wraps around the patient.

Core temperature: The temperature of the thermal compartment of the body containing highly perfused tissues and major organs.

Energy transfer pads: A servo-regulated system circulating temperature-controlled water through energy transfer pads adhered to the patient's skin and used to cool or warm the patient.

Forced-air warming: Convection warming technology dispersing a blanket of warm air over the patient's skin in a controlled manner.

Infant: A child one month after birth to approximately 12 months of age.

Mild hypothermia: A core temperature between 34° C to 36° C (93.2° F to 96.8° F).[24]

Neonate: An infant from birth to 28 days of age.

Neuraxia anesthesia: Spinal or epidural regional nerve blocks.

Normothermia: A core temperature between 36° C to 38° C (96.8° F to 100.4° F).

Passive insulation: Method of containing body heat and insulate the body from heat loss through radiation (eg, blankets, clothing).

Redistribution hypothermia: A decrease in body temperature occurring as heat is exchanged from the body's core compartment to the peripheral tissues.

Thermistor: An electrical resistor using a semiconductor whose resistance varies sharply in a known manner with the temperature.

Thermocouple: A device for measuring temperature in which a pair of wires of dissimilar metals is joined and the free ends connected to an instrument that measures the difference in potential created at the junction of the two metals.

Thermometer: An instrument for measuring temperature.

Thermostat: A device that automatically establishes and mains a desired temperature.

REFERENCES

1. Matsukawa T, Sessler DI, Christensen R, Ozaki M, Schroeder M. Heat flow and distribution during epidural anesthesia. *Anesthesiology.* 1995;83:961-967.

2. Matsukawa T, Sessler DI, Sessler AM, Schroeder M, Ozaki M, Kurz A, Cheng C. Heat flow and distribution during induction of general anesthesia. *Anesthesiology.* 1995;82:662-673.

3. Buggy DJ, Crossley AW. Thermoregulation, mild perioperative hypothermia and postanaesthetic shivering. *Br J Anaesth.* 2000;84:615-628.

4. Sessler DI. Perioperative heat balance. *Anesthesiology.* 2000;92:578-596.

5. Sessler DI. Perioperative thermoregulation and heat balance. *Ann N Y Acad Sci.* 1997;813:757-777.

6. Macario A, Dexter F. What are the most important risk factors for a patient's developing intraoperative hypothermia? *Anesth Analg.* 2002;94:215-220.

7. Tander B, Baris S, Karakaya D, Ariturk E, Rizalar R, Bernay F. Risk factors influencing inadvertent hypothermia in infants and neonates during anesthesia. *Paediatr Anaesth.* 2005;15:574-579.

8. Tisherman S. Hypothermia, cold injury, and drowning. In: Peitzman A, Rhodes M, Schwab C, Yealy D, Fabian T, eds. *The Trauma Manual,* 2nd ed. Philadelphia: Lippincott, Williams, & Wilkins; 2002:404-410.

9. Caldwell FT, Jr., Wallace BH, Cone JB. The effect of wound management on the interaction of burn size, heat production, and rectal temperature. *J Burn Care Rehabil.* 1994;15:121-129.

10. Sessler DI, Moayeri A, Stoen R, Glosten B, Hynson J, McGuire J. Thermoregulatory vasoconstriction decreases cutaneous heat loss. *Anesthesiology.* 1990;73:656-660.

11. Kurz A, Plattner O, Sessler DI, Huemer G, Redl G, Lackner F. The threshold for thermoregulatory vasoconstriction during nitrous oxide/isoflurane anesthesia is lower in elderly than in young patients. *Anesthesiology.* 1993; 79:465-469.

12. Kurz A, Sessler DI, Lenhardt R. Perioperative normothermia to reduce the incidence of surgical-wound infection and shorten hospitalization. Study of Wound Infection and Temperature Group. *N Engl J Med.* 1996; 334:1209-1215.

13. Flores-Maldonado A, Guzman-Llanez Y, Castaneda-Zarate S, Pech-Colli J, Alvarez-Nemegyei J, Cervera-Saenz M, Canto-Rubio A, Terrazas-Olguin MA. Risk factors for mild intraoperative hypothermia. *Arch Med Res.* 1997; 28:587-590.

14. Frank SM, Beattie C, Christopherson R, Norris EJ, Perler BA, Williams GM, Gottlieb SO. Unintentional hypothermia is associated with postoperative myocardial ischemia. The Perioperative Ischemia Randomized Anesthesia Trial Study Group. *Anesthesiology.* 1993;78:468-476.

15. Gentilello LM, Jurkovich GJ, Stark MS, Hassantash SA, O'Keefe GE. Is hypothermia in the victim of major trauma protective or harmful? A randomized, prospective study. *Ann Surg.* 1997;226:439-447; discussion 447-439.

16. Michelson AD, MacGregor H, Barnard MR, Kestin AS, Rohrer MJ, Valeri CR. Reversible inhibition of human platelet activation by hypothermia in vivo and in vitro. *Thromb Haemost.* 1994;71:633-640.

17. Reed RL, 2nd, Johnson TD, Hudson JD, Fischer RP. The disparity between hypothermic coagulopathy and clotting studies. *J Trauma.* 1992;33:465-470.

18. Schmied H, Kurz A, Sessler DI, Kozek S, Reiter A. Mild hypothermia increases blood loss and transfusion requirements during total hip arthroplasty. *Lancet.* 1996;347:289-292.

19. Heier T, Caldwell JE. Impact of hypothermia on the response to neuromuscular blocking drugs. *Anesthesiology.* 2006;104:1070-1080.

20. Leslie K, Sessler DI, Bjorksten AR, Moayeri A. Mild hypothermia alters propofol pharmacokinetics and increases the duration of action of atracurium. *Anesth Analg.* 1995;80:1007-1014.

21. Kurz A, Sessler DI, Narzt E, Bekar A, Lenhardt R, Huemer G, Lackner F. Postoperative hemodynamic and thermoregulatory consequences of intraoperative core hypothermia. *J Clin Anesth.* 1995;7:359-366.

22. Lenhardt R, Marker E, Goll V, Tschernich H, Kurz A, Sessler DI, Narzt E, Lackner F. Mild intraoperative hypothermia prolongs postanesthetic recovery. *Anesthesiology.* 1997;87:1318-1323.

23. Frank SM, Fleisher LA, Breslow MJ, Higgins MS, Olson KF, Kelly S, Beattie C. Perioperative maintenance of normothermia reduces the incidence of morbid cardiac events. A randomized clinical trial. *JAMA.* 1997;277:1127-1134.

24. Sessler DI. Complications and treatment of mild hypothermia. *Anesthesiology.* 2001;95:531-543.

25. Jurkovich GJ, Greiser WB, Luterman A, Curreri PW. Hypothermia in trauma victims: an ominous predictor of survival. *J Trauma.* 1987;27:1019-1024.

26. Luna GK, Maier RV, Pavlin EG, Anardi D, Copass MK, Oreskovich MR. Incidence and effect of hypothermia in seriously injured patients. *J Trauma.* 1987;27:1014-1018.

27. Rutherford EJ, Fusco MA, Nunn CR, Bass JG, Eddy VA, Morris JA, Jr. Hypothermia in critically ill trauma patients. *Injury.* 1998;29:605-608.

28. Sessler DI, Moayeri A. Skin-surface warming: heat flux and central temperature. *Anesthesiology.* 1990;73:218-224.

29. Kurz A, Sessler DI, Schroeder M, Kurz M. Thermoregulatory response thresholds during spinal anesthesia. *Anesth Analg.* 1993;77:721-726.

30. Kasai T, Hirose M, Yaegashi K, Matsukawa T, Takamata A, Tanaka Y. Preoperative risk factors of intraoperative hypothermia in major surgery under general anesthesia. *Anesth Analg.* 2002;95:1381-1383.

31. Frank SM, Shir Y, Raja SN, Fleisher LA, Beattie C. Core hypothermia and skin-surface temperature gradients. Epidural versus general anesthesia and the effects of age. *Anesthesiology.* 1994;80:502-508.

32. Frank SM, Raja SN, Bulcao C, Goldstein DS. Age-related thermoregulatory differences during core cooling in humans. *Am J Physiol Regul Integr Comp Physiol.* 2000; 279:R349-354.

33. Vassilieff N, Rosencher N, Sessler DI, Conseiller C. Shivering threshold during spinal anesthesia is reduced in elderly patients. *Anesthesiology.* 1995;83:1162-1166.

34. Kurz A, Sessler DI, Narzt E, Lenhardt R, Lackner F. Morphometric influences on intraoperative core temperature changes. *Anesth Analg.* 1995;80:562-567.

35. Kitamura A, Hoshino T, Kon T, Ogawa R. Patients with diabetic neuropathy are at risk of a greater intraoperative reduction in core temperature. *Anesthesiology.* 2000;92:1311-1318.

36. Kudoh A, Takase H, Takazawa T. Chronic treatment with antipsychotics enhances intraoperative core hypothermia. *Anesth Analg.* 2004;98:111-115.

37. Kudoh A, Takase H, Takazawa T. Chronic treatment with antidepressants decreases intraoperative core hypothermia. *Anesth Analg.* 2003;97:275-279.

38. Estebe JP, Le Naoures A, Malledant Y, Ecoffey C. Use of a pneumatic tourniquet induces changes in central temperature. *Br J Anaesth.* 1996;77:786-788.

39. Sanders BJ, D'Alessio JG, Jernigan JR. Intraoperative hypothermia associated with lower extremity tourniquet deflation. *J Clin Anesth.* 1996;8:504-507.

40. Akata T, Kanna T, Izumi K, Kodama K, Takahashi S. Changes in body temperature following deflation of limb pneumatic tourniquet. *J Clin Anesth.* 1998;10:17-22.

41. Bloch EC, Ginsberg B, Binner RA, Jr., Sessler DI. Limb tourniquets and central temperature in anesthetized children. *Anesth Analg.* 1992;74:486-489.

42. Sessler DI, Sessler AM, Hudson S, Moayeri A. Heat loss during surgical skin preparation. *Anesthesiology.* 1993;78:1055-1064.

43. Roe CF. Effect of bowel exposure on body temperature during surgical operations. *Am J Surg.* 1971; 122:13-15.

44. Sessler DI. Consequences and treatment of perioperative hypothermia. *Anesthesiology Clinics of North America.* 1994;23:425-456.

45. Felciano D. Abdominal vascular injury. In: Moore E, Feliciano D, Mattox K, eds. *Trauma.* 5th ed. New York, NY: McGraw-Hill; 2002:755-880.

46. Moran DS, Mendal L. Core temperature measurement: methods and current insights. *Sports Med.* 2002; 32:879-885.

47. American Society of PeriAnesthesia Nurses. Clinical guideline for the prevention of unplanned perioperative hypothermia. *J Perianesth Nurs.* 2001;16:305-314.

48. Hooper VD, Andrews JO. Accuracy of noninvasive core temperature measurement in acutely ill adults: the state of the science. *Biol Res Nurs.* 2006;8:24-34.

49. Ilsley AH, Rutten AJ, Runciman WB. An evaluation of body temperature measurement. *Anaesth Intensive Care.* 1983;11:31-39.

50. Holtzclaw BJ. Monitoring body temperature. *AACN Clin Issues Crit Care Nurs.* 1993;4:44-55.

51. Bailey J, Rose P. Axillary and tympanic membrane temperature recording in the preterm neonate: a comparative study. *J Adv Nurs.* 2001;34:465-474.

52. Erickson RS, Kirklin SK. Comparison of ear-based, bladder, oral, and axillary methods for core temperature measurement. *Crit Care Med.* 1993;21:1528-1534.

53. Giuffre M, Heidenreich T, Carney-Gersten P, Dorsch JA, Heidenreich E. The relationship between axillary and core body temperature measurements. *Appl Nurs Res.* 1990;3:52-55.

54. Hicks MA. A comparison of the tympanic and axillary temperatures of the preterm and term infant. *J Perinatol.* 1996;16:261-267.

55. Jean-Mary MB, Dicanzio J, Shaw J, Bernstein HH. Limited accuracy and reliability of infrared axillary and aural thermometers in a pediatric outpatient population. *J Pediatr.* 2002;141:671-676.

56. Jensen BN, Jensen FS, Madsen SN, Lossl K. Accuracy of digital tympanic, oral, axillary, and rectal thermometers compared with standard rectal mercury thermometers. *Eur J Surg.* 2000;166:848-851.

57. Weiss ME, Richards MT. Accuracy of electronic axillary temperature measurement in term and preterm neonates. *Neonatal Netw.* 1994;13:35-40.

58. Cork RC, Vaughan RW, Humphrey LS. Precision and accuracy of intraoperative temperature monitoring. *Anesth Analg.* 1983;62:211-214.

59. Lefrant JY, Muller L, de La Coussaye JE, Benbabaali M, Lebris C, Zeitoun N, Mari C, Saissi G, Ripart J, Eledjam JJ. Temperature measurement in intensive care patients: comparison of urinary bladder, oesophageal, rectal, axillary, and inguinal methods versus pulmonary artery core method. *Intensive Care Med.* 2003;29:414-418.

60. Lenhardt R. Monitoring and thermal management. *Best Pract Res Clin Anaesthesiol.* 2003;17:569-581.

61. Iaizzo PA, Kehler CH, Zink RS, Belani KG, Sessler DI. Thermal response in acute porcine malignant hyperthermia. *Anesth Analg.* 1996;82:782-789.

62. Sessler DI. Temperature Monitoring. In: Miller RD, ed. *Miller's Anesthesia.* 6th ed. Philadelphia, PA: Elsevier; 2005:1571-1597.

63. Bissonnette B, Sessler DI, LaFlamme P. Intraoperative temperature monitoring sites in infants and children and the effect of inspired gas warming on esophageal temperature. *Anesth Analg.* 1989;69:192-196.

64. Ikeda T, Sessler DI, Marder D, Xiong J. Influence of thermoregulatory vasomotion and ambient temperature variation on the accuracy of core-temperature estimates by cutaneous liquid-crystal thermometers. *Anesthesiology.* 1997;86:603-612.

65. Hebbar K, Fortenberry JD, Rogers K, Merritt R, Easley K. Comparison of temporal artery thermometer to standard temperature measurements in pediatric intensive care unit patients. *Pediatr Crit Care Med.* 2005; 6:557-561.

66. Suleman MI, Doufas AG, Akca O, Ducharme M, Sessler DI. Insufficiency in a new temporal-artery thermometer for adult and pediatric patients. *Anesth Analg.* 2002;95:67-71.

67. Greenes DS, Fleisher GR. Accuracy of a noninvasive temporal artery thermometer for use in infants. *Arch Pediatr Adolesc Med.* 2001;155:376-381.

68. AORN guidance statement: environmental responsibility. In: *Standards, Recommended Practices, and Guidelines.* 2006 ed. Denver: AORN, Inc; 2006:243-250.

69. U.S. Environmental Protection Agency. Mercury. Available at: *http://www.epa.gov/mercury/index.htm.* Accessed August 26, 2006.

70. American Society of Anesthesiologists. Standards for basic anesthetic monitoring. Available at: *http://www.asahq.org/publicationsAndServices/standards/02.pdf.* Accessed August 26, 2006.

71. Scope and standards for nurse anesthesia practice. *Professional Practice Manual for the Certified Registered Nurse Anesthetist.* Park Ridge, IL: American Association of Nurse Anesthetists; 1996:1-4.

72. Horn EP, Schroeder F, Gottschalk A, Sessler DI, Hiltmeyer N, Standl T, Schulte am Esch J. Active warming during cesarean delivery. *Anesth Analg.* 2002;94:409-414.

73. Fossum S, Hays J, Henson MM. A comparison study on the effects of prewarming patients in the outpatient surgery setting. *J Perianesth Nurs.* 2001;16:187-194.

74. Sessler DI, Schroeder M, Merrifield B, Matsukawa T, Cheng C. Optimal duration and temperature of prewarming. *Anesthesiology.* 1995;82:674-681.

75. Sessler DI, Schroeder M. Heat loss in humans covered with cotton hospital blankets. *Anesth Analg.* 1993;77:73-77.

76. Sessler DI, McGuire J, Sessler AM. Perioperative thermal insulation. *Anesthesiology.* 1991;74:875-879.

77. Ng SF, Oo CS, Loh KH, Lim PY, Chan YH, Ong BC. A comparative study of three warming interventions to determine the most effective in maintaining perioperative normothermia. *Anesth Analg.* 2003;96:171-176.

78. Matsuzaki Y, Matsukawa T, Ohki K, Yamamoto Y, Nakamura M, Oshibuchi T. Warming by resistive heating maintains perioperative normothermia as well as forced air heating. *Br J Anaesth.* 2003;90:689-691.

79. Morris RH, Kumar A. The effect of warming blankets on maintenance of body temperature of the anesthetized, paralyzed adult patient. *Anesthesiology.* 1972;36:408-411.

80. Negishi C, Hasegawa K, Mukai S, Nakagawa F, Ozaki M, Sessler DI. Resistive-heating and forced-air warming are comparably effective. *Anesth Analg.* 2003;96:1683-1687.

81. Hynson JM, Sessler DI. Intraoperative warming therapies: a comparison of three devices. *J Clin Anesth.* 1992;4:194-199.

82. Borms SF, Engelen SL, Himpe DG, Suy MR, Theunissen WJ. Bair hugger forced-air warming maintains normothermia more effectively than thermo-lite insulation. *J Clin Anesth.* 1994;6:303-307.

83. Huang JK, Shah EF, Vinodkumar N, Hegarty MA, Greatorex RA. The Bair Hugger patient warming system in prolonged vascular surgery: an infection risk? *Crit Care.* 2003;7:R13-16.

84. Lamb FJ, Rogers R. Forced-air warming maintains normothermia during orthotopic liver transplantation. *Anaesthesia.* 1995;50:745.

85. Murat I, Berniere J, Constant I. Evaluation of the efficacy of a forced-air warmer (Bair Hugger) during spinal surgery in children. *J Clin Anesth.* 1994;6:425-429.

86. Russell SH, Freeman JW. Prevention of hypothermia during orthotopic liver transplantation: comparison of three different intraoperative warming methods. *Br J Anaesth.* 1995;74:415-418.

87. Komatsu H, Chujo K, Ogli K. Forced-air warming system for perioperative use in neonates. *Paediatr Anaesth.* 1996;6:427-428.

88. Mason DS, Sapala JA, Wood MH, Sapala MA. Influence of a forced air warming system on morbidly obese patients undergoing Roux-en-Y gastric bypass. *Obes Surg.* 1998;8:453-460.

89. Janke EL, Pilkington SN, Smith DC. Evaluation of two warming systems after cardiopulmonary bypass. *Br J Anaesth.* 1996;77:268-270.

90. Rajek A, Lenhardt R, Sessler DI, Brunner G, Haisjackl M, Kastner J, Laufer G. Efficacy of two methods for reducing postbypass afterdrop. *Anesthesiology.* 2000;92:447-456.

91. Mort TC, Rintel TD, Altman F. The effects of forced-air warming on postbypass central and skin temperatures and shivering activity. *J Clin Anesth.* 1996;8:361-370.

92. Zink RS, Iaizzo PA. Convective warming therapy does not increase the risk of wound contamination in the operating room. *Anesth Analg.* 1993;76:50-53.

93. Hofer CK, Worn M, Tavakoli R, Sander L, Maloigne M, Klaghofer R, Zollinger A. Influence of body core temperature on blood loss and transfusion requirements during off-pump coronary artery bypass grafting: a comparison of 3 warming systems. *J Thorac Cardiovasc Surg.* 2005;129:838-843.

94. Nesher N, Insler SR, Sheinberg N, Bolotin G, Kramer A, Sharony R, Paz Y, Pevni D, Loberman D, Uretzky G. A new thermoregulation system for maintaining perioperative normothermia and attenuating myocardial injury in off-pump coronary artery bypass surgery. *Heart Surg Forum.* 2002;5:373-380.

95. Nesher N, Uretzky G, Insler S, Nataf P, Frolkis I, Pineau E, Cantoni E, Bolotin G, Vardi M, Pevni D, Lev-Ran O, Sharony R, Weinbroum AA. Thermo-wrap technology preserves normothermia better than routine thermal care in patients undergoing off-pump coronary artery bypass and is associated with lower immune response and lesser myocardial damage. *J Thorac Cardiovasc Surg.* 2005;129:1371-1378.

96. Nesher N, Wolf T, Kushnir I, David M, Bolotin G, Sharony R, Pizov R, Uretzky G. Novel thermoregulation system for enhancing cardiac function and hemodynamics during coronary artery bypass graft surgery. *Ann Thorac Surg.* 2001;72:S1069-1076.

97. Taguchi A, Ratnaraj J, Kabon B, Sharma N, Lenhardt R, Sessler DI, Kurz A. Effects of a circulating-water garment and forced-air warming on body heat content and core temperature. *Anesthesiology.* 2004;100:1058-1064.

98. Nesher N, Wolf T, Uretzky G, Oppenheim-Eden A, Yussim E, Kushnir I, Shoshany G, Rosenberg B, Berant M. A novel thermoregulatory system maintains perioperative normothermia in children undergoing elective surgery. *Paediatr Anaesth.* 2001;11:555-560.

99. Janicki PK, Higgins MS, Janssen J, Johnson RF, Beattie C. Comparison of two different temperature maintenance strategies during open abdominal surgery: upper body forced-air warming versus whole body water garment. *Anesthesiology.* 2001;95:868-874.

100. Motta P, Mossad E, Toscana D, Lozano S, Insler S. Effectiveness of a circulating-water warming garment in rewarming after pediatric cardiac surgery using hypothermic cardiopulmonary bypass. *J Cardiothorac Vasc Anesth.* 2004;18:148-151.

101. Nesher N, Zisman E, Wolf T, Sharony R, Bolotin G, David M, Uretzky G, Pizov R. Strict thermoregulation attenuates myocardial injury during coronary artery bypass graft surgery as reflected by reduced levels of cardiac-specific troponin I. *Anesth Analg.* 2003;96:328-335.

102. Grocott HP, Mathew JP, Carver EH, Phillips-Bute B, Landolfo KP, Newman MF. A randomized controlled trial of the Arctic Sun Temperature Management System versus conventional methods for preventing hypothermia during off-pump cardiac surgery. *Anesth Analg.* 2004;98:298-302.

103. Camus Y, Delva E, Cohen S, Lienhart A. The effects of warming intravenous fluids on intraoperative hypothermia and postoperative shivering during prolonged abdominal surgery. *Acta Anaesthesiol Scand.* 1996;40:779-782.

104. Smith CE, Desai R, Glorioso V, Cooper A, Pinchak AC, Hagen KF. Preventing hypothermia: convective and intravenous fluid warming versus convective warming alone. *J Clin Anesth.* 1998;10:380-385.

105. Sessler DI. Mild perioperative hypothermia. *N Engl J Med.* 12 1997;336:1730-1737.

106. Moore SS, Green CR, Wang FL, Pandit SK, Hurd WW. The role of irrigation in the development of hypothermia during laparoscopic surgery. *Am J Obstet Gynecol.* 1997;176:598-602.

107. Kelly JA, Doughty JK, Hasselbeck AN, Vacchiano CA. The effect of arthroscopic irrigation fluid warming on body temperature. *J Perianesth Nurs.* 2000;15:245-252.

108. Morris RH. Influence of ambient temperature on patient temperature during intraabdominal surgery. *Ann Surg.* 1971;173:230-233.

109. El-Gamal N, El-Kassabany N, Frank SM, Amar R, Khabar HA, El-Rahmany HK, Okasha AS. Age-related thermoregulatory differences in a warm operating room environment (approximately 26° C). *Anesth Analg.* 2000; 90:694-698.

110. Bissonnette B, Sessler DI. Passive or active inspired gas humidification increases thermal steady-state temperatures in anesthetized infants. *Anesth Analg.* 1989;69:783-787.

111. Bissonnette B, Sessler DI, LaFlamme P. Passive and active inspired gas humidification in infants and children. *Anesthesiology.* 1989;71:350-354.

112. Bissonnette B. Temperature monitoring in pediatric anesthesia. *Int Anesthesiol Clin.* Summer 1992;30:63-76.

113. Hildebrand F, Giannoudis PV, van Griensven M, Chawda M, Pape HC. Pathophysiologic changes and effects of hypothermia on outcome in elective surgery and trauma patients. *Am J Surg.* 2004;187:363-371.

114. Rodrick M, Krugh J, Hanson W. Anesthesia for the trauma patient. In: Peitzman A, Rhodes M, Schwab C, Yealy D, Fabian T, eds. *The Trauma Manual.* 2nd ed. Philadelphia, PA: Lippincott, Williams & Wilkins; 2002: 386-395.

115. Cheney FW, Posner KL, Caplan RA, Gild WM. Burns from warming devices in anesthesia. A closed claims analysis. *Anesthesiology.* 1994;80:806-810.

116. Misusing forced-air hyperthemia units can burn patients. *Health Devices.* (17-950).

117. U.S. Food and Drug Administration. Burns from misuse of forced-air warming devices. Available at: *http://www .fda.gov/cdrh/psn/show9.html.* Accessed August 26, 2006.

118. Surgical Care Improvement Project. Available at: *http://www.medqic.org/dcs/ContentServer?cid=112290 4930422&pagename=Medqic%2FContent%2FParent ShellTemplate&parentName=Topic&c=MQParents.* Accessed August 27, 2006.

119. Medical device reporting: Manufacturer reporting, importer reporting, user facility reporting, distributor reporting. *Federal Register.* Jan 26, 2000;65:4112-4121.

PUBLICATION HISTORY

Originally published in *Perioperative Standards and Recommended Practices,* 2008 edition.

Recommended Practices for
Perioperative Health Care Information Management

The following Recommended Practices for Perioperative Health Care Information Management have been approved by the AORN Recommended Practices Advisory Board. They were presented as proposed recommendations for comments by members and others. They are effective December 1, 2011. These recommended practices are intended as achievable recommendations representing what is believed to be an optimal level of practice. Policies and procedures will reflect variations in practice settings and/or clinical situations that determine the degree to which the recommended practices can be implemented. AORN recognizes the various settings in which perioperative nurses practice. These recommended practices are intended as guidelines adaptable to various practice settings. These practice settings include traditional operating rooms (ORs), ambulatory surgery centers, physicians' offices, cardiac catheterization laboratories, endoscopy suites, radiology departments, and all other areas where surgery and other invasive procedures may be performed.

Purpose

These recommended practices provide guidance to assist perioperative nurses in documenting and managing patient care information within the perioperative practice setting. Highly reliable data collection is not only necessary to chronicle the patient response to nursing interventions, but also to demonstrate the health care organization's progress toward quality care outcomes. Health care data collection and retention is rapidly transitioning from traditional paper formats to standardized electronic applications that incorporate criteria from statutes and regulations, accreditation requirements, and standards setting bodies. Whether patient data are captured using paper or electronic formats, the nursing process should be completed for each surgical or procedural intervention performed.[1,2] The nursing process is a formalized systematic approach to providing and documenting patient care and is embedded within perioperative patient care workflow (ie, clinical workflow). Comprehensive perioperative documentation accurately reflects the patient experience and is essential for the continuity of goal-directed nursing care and for effective comparison of realized versus anticipated patient outcomes.[3,4]

This document should be viewed as a conceptual outline that can be used to create a comprehensive documentation platform. It is not inclusive of all documentation elements, nor should it be seen as the only guideline that may be used when developing or revising a clinical documentation system.

Recommendation I

The patient's health care record should reflect the perioperative patient's plan of care, including assessment, nursing diagnosis, outcome identification, planning, implementation, and evaluation of progress toward the outcome.[1,3-5]

The nursing process provides the guiding framework for documenting perioperative nursing care. When the nursing process is used in perioperative practice settings, it demonstrates the critical-thinking skills practiced by the registered nurse (RN) in caring for the patient undergoing surgical and other procedural interventions.[1,3,6-8] Documentation includes related information about the patient's current and past health status, nursing diagnoses and interventions, expected patient outcomes, and evaluation of the patient's response to perioperative nursing care.[5,9,10]

I.a. The perioperative RN conducts a patient assessment (eg, physical, psychosocial, cultural, spiritual) and should record the findings in the patient health care record before the surgical or other invasive procedure.[1,4]

The patient assessment forms a baseline for identifying the patient's health status, developing nursing diagnoses, and establishing an individualized plan of care. Concurrent reassessment throughout the patient's perioperative experience contributes to continuity in the delivery of care.[1,3,5,10]

Intraoperative nursing interventions for inpatient and ambulatory settings are embedded within the delivery of care but are not consistently reflected in clinical documentation.[7] In a systematic review of nursing documentation literature, inadequacies in the use of nursing process structure within clinical documentation resulted in one or more deficiencies in the application of the assessment process.[11] Using the structured data elements (eg, Perioperative Nursing Data Set [PNDS]) that include nursing diagnoses, interventions, and outcomes in clinical documentation demonstrates nursing contributions to patient outcomes and represents professional nursing practice.[7,8]

I.b.	The health care record should include the nursing interventions performed and the time performed, the location of care, and the person performing the care.[4,5,12,13]

Clinical judgments are based on actual or potential patient problems (eg, nursing diagnoses), which determine the nursing interventions to be implemented to achieve expected perioperative patient outcomes.[1,10,14] Documenting nursing interventions promotes continuity of patient care and improves the exchange of patient care information between health care team members.[4,5]

I.c.	Expected and interim patient outcomes that are identified by the perioperative RN should be recorded in the patient health care record.[10]

The goals for nursing interventions are to prevent potential patient injury or complications and treat actual patient problems (eg, nursing diagnoses). Identified nursing diagnoses contribute to interim and expected patient outcomes for the planned operative or procedural intervention. Research also indicates that nurses who associate the patient diagnoses with planned interventions are more outcome focused than task oriented.[15]

I.d.	The patient health care record should reflect continuous reassessment and evaluation of perioperative nursing care and the response to implemented nursing interventions.[1,3,5,16]

The nursing process directs perioperative nurses to evaluate the effectiveness of nursing interventions toward attaining desired patient outcomes. The evaluation process provides information for continuity of care, performance improvement activities, perioperative nursing research, and management of risk. Documentation provides a mechanism for comparing actual versus expected outcomes.[1,3,5]

I.d.1.	Patient data must be collected concurrently with each assessment, reassessment, or evaluation and recorded in the patient health care record.[17,18]

Continuous evaluation of the patient's condition establishes a baseline to determine fluctuations in the patient's status.[1,3,12,13,19] Appropriately captured patient data contribute to a centralized repository that members of the health care team can use to monitor the patient's status, coordinate prescribed treatments, and evaluate the effectiveness of care rendered.[4,16,20]

Recommendation II

Perioperative nursing documentation should be synchronized with the nursing work flow.[21-23]

Nursing work flow represents the cognitive process of nursing care activities and establishes the process for patient care data collection. Documentation of nursing activities is dictated by health care organization policy and regulatory and accrediting agency requirements and is necessary to inform other health care professionals involved in the patient's care. To accurately represent the patient experience and promote quality delivery of care, data aggregation should be coordinated with clinical work flow.[8,21-25] Incorporating nursing process work flow into the framework of clinical documentation platforms has been shown to improve documentation completeness and compliance with regulatory requirements.[26]

II.a.	Clinical documentation should facilitate data capture using a format designed to support clinical work flow activities while eliminating redundancy in data entry.[2,22,25,27]

The burden of clinical documentation has been associated with decreased nursing attention to patient care activities and has been shown to affect patient safety.[28] Work inefficiencies, such as how or where clinical data are captured within perioperative documentation systems, have a negative correlation on clinical reasoning and decision making.[14,23,24,29,30] Interruption of established clinical processes competes for cognitive resources and may contribute to an adverse event or patient harm by reducing situational awareness.[31-34] Redundancy in the design of documentation activities further reduces the nurse's ability to focus on the clinical environment and may pose a risk for error.[27] When processes are simplified and data capture is standardized and organized, there is a reduction in the reliance on memory to complete tasks, thereby eliminating potential harmful events.[23,25,29]

An observational study on nursing work flow examined the percentage of time nurses dedicated to patient care and documentation activities.[35] The study identified that nursing time is focused primarily on patient care (eg, assessment, interventions) with documentation being completed in intervals and not concurrently with patient care. This, with the frequency of switching between nursing activities (ie, patient care, documentation), was correlated with nursing cognitive disruption, which resulted in slower performance and raised the potential for error.

A follow-up observational and randomized investigation examined the effect of new electronic documentation implementation on nursing activities and work flow. Findings indicated that the repeated clustering of patient care and documentation activities, though evenly distributed, affected nursing work flow by increasing the amount of time dedicated to electronic documentation without negatively affecting direct patient care time.[36]

II.a.1. Clinical documentation should reflect patient-focused care.[37-40]

Perioperative RNs provide patient-focused interventions that should be incorporated into the patient health care record.[41] Clinical (eg, nursing) documentation systems often do not support health care personnel in accommodating the specific needs of the individual (eg, teaching needs, age-specific criteria, self-care requirements).[37,42,43] Two research studies highlight the discrepancy between quality of care delivered and what is captured in documentation.[44,45] Health care currently relies on the technology centered medical model of care, which often does not replicate patient-centric,

evidence-based care within documentation platforms.

II.a.2. Perioperative RNs should evaluate perioperative electronic documentation systems for their effect on clinical work flow and patient safety, and their ability to accommodate the objectives of the implementation site.[11,21,22,30,46] Clinical information systems should address

- clinical work flow,[21,22,24-26,47-49]
- information needs of the patient care environment,[38]
- patient population characteristics,[37,39,42] and
- clinician and provider usability requirements.[26,34,48,50]

Effective information systems collect, store, and organize patient information to allow real-time updates, support clinical decision making, and be accessible to health care professionals when needed.[51-55] Research on the effect of health information technology implementation has shown that changes in contextual clinical work processes made to accommodate clinical information systems have both positive and negative influence on clinical work flow and patient safety.[23,34,35,43,50] Technology implementation with the most positive effects on clinical work flow, data availability, patient outcomes, and health care provider satisfaction occurs when clinicians are involved in the selection and implementation of the information system.[44,46,56]

Recommendation III

Electronic perioperative nursing documentation should use structured vocabulary (eg, PNDS) inclusive of the nursing process work flow with discrete representation of each phase of the perioperative patient care continuum (ie, preadmission, preoperative, intraoperative, postoperative).[26,57]

The use of structured vocabulary facilitates the capture of expressed observations, treatments, and patient responses within the clinical domain of care. Structured vocabulary describes patient care using controlled (ie, standardized) and unambiguous terms that are interpreted with consistent meaning between health care clinicians.[26,58] Patient information gathered from the collection of standardized data creates the knowledge perioperative RNs use to provide individualized patient care. The synthesis of knowledge for patient care interventions is in turn documented, resulting in the wisdom of perioperative nursing practice.[59,60]

III.a.   The PNDS should be incorporated into the documentation platform.[7,61,62]

The PNDS is a controlled, structured, and coded nursing language that describes perioperative nursing influence on the effectiveness and safety of patient care delivery, and the contributions of perioperative nursing toward patient outcomes. Clinical documentation systems incorporating standardized language provide patient care data that can be aggregated and analyzed to determine clinical efficiencies, examine operational metrics, and facilitate new evidence for sustainable improvements in health care quality.[21,61,63]

III.a.1.   Each phase of perioperative nursing documentation should incorporate nursing process work flow and require unambiguous representation of the patient experience.[64-68]

The phases of perioperative patient care collectively represent the unique domain of perioperative nursing. Standardization of patient care information improves the quality of the data[69] and can be used to support the extraction and interpretation of data for
- clinical decision support,[70,71]
- improved quality metrics,[26,71,72]
- information exchange,[71,72]
- research,[72,73]
- policy making,[26,72] and
- nursing visibility.[7,8,26,57,58,61,64,74-76]

III.b.   The health care organization should implement a documentation system that includes a standardized perioperative electronic framework.

Standardization in documentation platforms promotes uniformity in comprehensive patient care data capture between health care organizations and creates a foundation for sharing health care data. The

burgeoning cost of health care and the drive for improved quality have created urgency for implementation of electronic medical records (EMRs) and interoperable electronic health record (EHR) systems.[77-79] Adoption of EHR systems is a component of the American Recovery and Reinvestment Act (ARRA) of 2009 to facilitate access to quality care and improved patient safety[80] through high-reliability processes using data analysis to evaluate performance and outcomes.[81] Data quality facilitated by the adoption of an EHR and established by compliance with laws, clinical practice standards, and national quality measures adds to the relevance in efficiency benchmarks. The adoption of EHR technology also will lead to quantifiable improvements in reducing the time required for patient care data capture by nurses.[47,72,78,82]

Inpatient and ambulatory EHR implementation has been stimulated by the ARRA incentives for EHR adoption and subsequent analysis and dissemination of performance metrics.[71] Achieving success with the national Health Information Technology for Economic and Clinical Health (HITECH) agenda for comparative analysis between health care organizations may be accomplished by implementing an electronic documentation framework embedded with standardized sets of documentation values that are applicable across multiple perioperative settings to increase the confidence in data quality and research validity.[69,72,83]

Recommendation IV

Perioperative nursing documentation should be structured to meet professional and regulatory compliance requirements for a comprehensive representation of patient care.[66,84-87]

Patient care information collected and entered into the health care record is a tool for monitoring and evaluating the patient's health status and response to care, a resource to evaluate compliance with regulatory requirements, and a method to equate provision of services for reimbursement.[4,5,8]

IV.a.   Perioperative nursing documentation should correspond to the elements of regulatory statutes, health care accreditation measures, national practice standards, and mandatory quality and reimbursement for quality performance criteria.

Clinical documentation serves as the legal record of care delivery and assists with cross-disciplinary patient care coordination.[5,84,88]

IV.a.1. The components for clinical documentation should include the following:
- "assessments;
- clinical problems;
- communications with other health care professionals regarding the patient;
- communication with and education of the patient, the patient's family members, the patient's designated support person, and other third parties;
- medication records (MAR);
- order acknowledgement, implementation, and management;
- [patient care interventions];
- patient clinical parameters;
- patient responses and outcomes, including changes in the patient's status; and
- plans of care that reflect the social and cultural framework of the patient."[8]

IV.a.2. Perioperative nursing documentation should correspond to professional guidelines and standards. The following organizations' guidelines and standards should be incorporated into the clinical documentation platform:
- AORN,
- American Association of Blood Banks (AABB),
- Agency for Healthcare Research and Quality (AHRQ),
- American National Standards Institute (ANSI),
- American Society of Anesthesiologists (ASA),
- Association for the Advancement of Medical Instrumentation (AAMI),
- American Association of Anesthesia Clinical Directors (AACD),

- Association of PeriAnesthesia Nurses (ASPAN),
- Institute for Safe Medication Practices (ISMP),
- Malignant Hyperthermia Association of the United States (MHAUS),
- National Fire Protection Agency (NFPA),
- National Institute for Occupational Safety and Health (NIOSH),
- National Quality Forum (NQF),
- US Pharmacopeia (USP), and
- United Network for Organ Sharing (UNOS).

Examples of guidance from professional standards setting agencies that may be considered for incorporation into perioperative documentation include:
- AACD Glossary of Times,
- national patient safety guidelines,
- organ and tissues tracking guidelines,
- perioperative recommendations for safe patient care, and
- safe medication administration guidelines.

As licensed health care professionals, perioperative RNs have a responsibility to maintain the established standards of perioperative nursing care. The standards of nursing practice require documentation to be based on the patient's condition or needs and the relationship to the proposed intervention, and have relevance to the period of patient care (eg, preadmission testing, preoperative, intraoperative, and postoperative care).[1,3,5,8] National practice standards cross all disciplines of nursing care and are applicable to perioperative nursing.

IV.a.3. Perioperative nursing documentation should correspond to established recommended practices for perioperative nursing care.[89] Elements of perioperative recommended practices that should be incorporated into clinical documentation include
- aseptic technique maintenance;[65,90-93]
- local anesthesia administration;[85,94-104]
- medication administration practices (eg, use of abbreviations);[20,94-96,101,105-111]

- moderate sedation/analgesia administration;[85,95-104,112,113]
- patient care considerations (eg, latex allergy, implanted electronic device, dentures);[19,65,66,87,95,101,114-119]
- patient positioning;[65,85,97,101,116,120,121]
- patient information exchange;[19,66,85,86,97,101,103,104,119,122-128]
- safety precautions including
  - electrical,[101,119,129-133]
  - environment of care preparation (eg, device alarms, blanket warmer temperatures),[65,98,131,134-137]
  - equipment use (eg, laser, MRI),[41,120,138,139]
  - fire prevention,[65,101,108,124,129,134,139-142]
  - human tissue procurement, processing, and preservation,[65,101,103,104,124,143-148]
  - infection prevention,[65,97,101,108,109,111,112,137,149-155]
  - tissue protection,[97,101,108,124,139,141,156-158]
  - radiation exposure prevention,[156]
  - retained surgical items prevention,[101,159,160]
  - correct site, side, person surgery processes,[19,65,66,78,87,99,103,104,108,118,119,121,124,161-167] and
  - skin preparation and antisepsis;[65,85,95,97,98,100-102,108,110,113,140,150,154,168-171]
- specimens and tissues;[65,87,97,101-103,124,144-147,160,166]
- sterilization/disinfection practices;[65,97,101,102,113,114,126,129,131,134,140,142,152,166,172-178] and
- traffic control measures.[65,102,134,140,149,152,176]

The AORN recommended practices for perioperative nursing care are nationally recognized as the standard of care for all operative or invasive procedure patient care settings. Perioperative recommended practices are not mandatory nursing care criteria but have been incorporated into regulatory and other standards setting agencies' guidelines and have been used to support judicial decisions.[179-185]

IV.a.4. Perioperative nursing documentation should correspond to local, state, and national regulatory requirements.

State and federal regulations are a collection of general and permanent rules (ie, laws) established to protect the welfare of the public and fortify the guiding principles of the nation. Many statutes or laws are established at the national level and may be amplified at the state level. The amplified statute would become the mandatory authority for the state. An example of this would be document retention requirements that vary between states. Failure to comply with the final law-making authority could result in monetary penalties or incarceration of the offending body. Agencies with regulatory authority include

- Centers for Medicare & Medicaid Services (CMS),
- Department of Health and Human Services (HHS),
- Occupational Safety and Health Administration (OSHA), and
- US Food and Drug Administration (FDA).

Criteria identified by national regulatory agencies for patient care documentation include

- allergies,[65,66,84,87,88,168,186]
- cultural variables,[66,84,88,99,118,187]
- equipment used for patient care (eg, type, model number),[65,66,85,86,98,117,118,129,130,160,168,186,188]
- names of legal guardian(s) and patient support person(s),[65,86,99,118,186]
- nutritional considerations,[66,86,87,186]
- ordered tests and services provided,[65,66,117,189]
- patient and family education,[66,84,88,118,151,186]
- patient identifiers and demographics,[65,66,87,117,160,163]
- patient attributes and status,[65,66,84,85,87,88,118,162,163,186,190]
- safety precautions,[65,84,88,129,155,189]
- surgical consent(s),[65,66,118,163] and
- surgical implants and explants.[65,66,84,88,117,146,188,191,192]

IV.a.5. Perioperative nursing documentation should correspond to health care accreditation organization requirements.

Compliance with state or national health care accreditation agency criteria is mandatory for organizations seeking CMS reimbursement or striving to meet established patient safety goals. Accrediting bodies review documentation for compliance to the minimum standards on an element of performance. The following accreditation agencies have deemed status:

- American Association for Accreditation of Ambulatory Surgery Facilities, Inc (AAAASF),[132]
- Accreditation Association for Ambulatory Health Care, Inc (AAAHC),[111]
- State CMS,[193]
- DNV Healthcare, Inc (DNV),[194]
- Healthcare Facilities Accreditation Program (HFAP),[195] and
- The Joint Commission.[196,197]

Elements of performance identified by accreditation agencies may include evidence of

- blood and tissue tracking;
- compliance with The Joint Commission's National Patient Safety Goals;
- elimination of nationally identified unacceptable abbreviations, acronyms, and symbols;
- hand off communications;
- identification of implantable objects;
- identification of designated support person(s);
- infection control practices;
- medication reconciliation;
- patient care elements (eg, care plans, tests, services provided);
- pain management interventions;
- patient and family member education;
- patient demographics; and
- presence of current history and physical.

IV.a.6. Perioperative nursing documentation should incorporate mandatory reporting and reimbursement for quality performance criteria.

To improve population health, the US government is coordinating evidence-based standards development to be incorporated into the national agenda on health care reform. These efforts are incentivized through inclusion within CMS reimbursement programs and made public through national reporting forums (eg, Hospital Compare[198]). Agencies responsible for national standards development or reimbursement for quality performance criteria include, but are not limited to, the following:

- Centers for Disease Control (CDC),
- NQF, and
- AHRQ.

Measurement criteria for quality performance reimbursement are included in the following regulations and criteria:

- Ambulatory Surgical Center Payment System (ASCPS),[199]
- Deficit Reduction Act of 2005,[160]
- Hospital Inpatient Prospective Payment System (IPPS),[199]
- Hospital Outpatient Prospective Payment System (OPPS),[199]
- Surgical Care Improvement Project (SCIP),[200] and
- Value-based Purchasing (VBP).[201,202]

IV.a.7. Perioperative documentation should include all patient care orders occurring in the perioperative patient care setting.[66] Patient care orders are to be entered into the clinical documentation system as close to the time when the order is communicated or intervention is initiated. All orders, including verbal orders, standing orders, orders included on surgeon preference cards, and order sets must be dated, timed, and authenticated by the ordering health care practitioner with prescriptive authority.[66,196,203-205] Verbal orders must be documented when they are communicated and verified using a read-back process that involves the ordering health care practitioner.[206-209]

Using standing orders and preprinted order sets has been shown to reduce medication errors and improve documentation compliance.[210] To prevent patient harm from outdated, incomplete, or erroneous entries, well-constructed standing orders and pre-printed order sets should

- avoid the use of unacceptable abbreviations,
- eliminate trailing zeros in medication dosages,
- use standardized names and terms to describe treatments and interventions (eg, brand vs generic medications, device instructions), and
- be reviewed frequently by the attending surgeon for accuracy of information for the intended procedure.[206-208,211]

IV.a.8. The patient care record must include a complete and accurate informed patient consent for each surgical or invasive procedure to be performed.[66,99,163] The informed consent process must be documented for procedures and treatments that are identified in the health care facility's medical staff policies as requiring informed consent.[66,84,163] Unless designated as an emergency situation in the health care facility's informed consent policy, a "properly executed informed consent"[99] must include

- the name of the health care facility providing the surgery or invasive procedure;
- the specific name of the intervention to be performed;
- indications for the proposed intervention;
- the name of the responsible health care provider performing the intervention;
- a statement identifying the risks and benefits associated with the proposed intervention and indication of discussion with the patient or patient's legal representative;
- the signature of the patient or the patient's legal representative;
- the date and time the patient or the patient's legal representative signed the informed consent document;
- the date and time, and signature of the person who witnessed the patient or the patient's legal representative

signing the informed consent document; and

- the signature of the responsible health care provider who executed the informed consent discussion with the patient or the patient's legal representative.[84,87,88]

Additional content that may be identified on the informed consent document and may be regulated by state statutes and administrative rules includes

- identification of assisting physicians including, but not limited to, medical residents who will be contributing significantly to the proposed intervention and
- identification of assisting health care personnel who are not physicians but who are performing within their scope of practice (eg, registered nurse first assistant [RNFA], nurse practitioner) and who will be contributing significantly to the proposed intervention.[84,87,88]

The patient or the patient's legal representative is entitled to participate in the informed decision-making process for planning care and treatment, including the right to request or refuse treatment.[99,204]

IV.a.9. Individuals participating in the patient's perioperative care, as well as those not directly involved in the scheduled surgical or procedural intervention (eg, x-ray technicians, industry representatives, approved observers), must be recorded in the patient health care record.[66,99,204] Documentation must include the names, roles, and credentials of individuals participating in the patient's perioperative care experience and may include[84,88]

- surgical or procedural patient care team members,
- identified legal representatives,
- identified patient support person(s),
- recipients of patient care information on behalf of the patient,
- health care professionals contributing to the patient's care (eg,

pathologist, approved health care student), and

- law enforcement officers (eg, prison guards).

A comprehensive patient-centric record of care reflects interactions between the patient's health care team and those individuals legally representing or providing physical, spiritual, or other support services to the patient.[84,88] Documentation of interactions provides the groundwork for transparency in care planning through effective representation of the patient's involvement in the plan of care and contributions made toward the treatment plan.

IV.b. Clinical documentation platforms (ie, paper, electronic) should support the collection of tailored health care information using a format that accommodates and is customized to the clinical environment.[42,43] Formats selected for the collection of tailored patient care information should be established based on nationally recognized standards of practice that outline the nurse's responsibilities to the patient.[12]

Tailoring patient health information allows the collection of unique patient care data (eg, communicable diseases, responses to medications, psychosocial considerations) that may affect the planned operative or other invasive procedure. The collection of tailored health care information is standardized to the clinical setting (eg, surgical versus interventional radiology) but may vary by the requirements of the environment where perioperative care is delivered (eg, pediatric hospital, cancer treatment center, ambulatory surgery center).[42,43]

IV.b.1. Charting by exception processes should be well constructed and reviewed by the health care organization's risk management and legal representatives.[80]

Charting by exception, also known as variance charting,[212] has been successfully implemented using a well-researched and -designed documentation system.[213] A well-designed documentation system corresponds to the health care organization's policy for charting by exception and allows for an undisputable description of the patient condition. Charting by exception may lead to litigious situations when organizational policy has not been well formulated or updated for changes in statutory requirements or when the nurse has not followed the established guidance for charting by exception.[12,16,184,214]

The minimum criteria for charting by exception include

- identifying objective physical assessment criteria for the patient population being served (eg, endoscopy population, orthopedic population);
- identifying and defining what constitutes normal findings;
- describing the process for documenting normal findings (eg, "within normal limits");
- describing the process for identifying, describing, and documenting objective abnormal or key findings;
- listing the practice standards, care guidelines, and clinical pathways used to guide patient care;
- listing a rationale, including decisions and interventions, for deviations from established guidance for patient care;
- setting the frequency of documentation entries; and
- adhering to state or national statutory requirements (eg, record authentication).

IV.c. Cognitive processes used in patient care should be supported by clinical support technologies that are embedded within electronic clinical documentation systems.[23,218,219]

The processes within perioperative patient care are classified as cognitive performance or the intellectual processing of information to complete a finite task.[218] Multitasking, environmental stimulation, and availability of information contribute to the nurse's ability, or inability, to accommodate needed adjustments in patient care activities. Poorly designed clinical information systems, those not conforming to national data standards, and those without consideration of clinical work flow and work process requirements may contribute to patient harm.[23,24,30, 218-220] Conversely, clinical information systems that incorporate technology innovations (eg, order entry, decision support, clinical alerts) and support the cognitive processes of patient care are believed to enhance health care worker performance and result in improved patient safety and quality patient outcomes.[23,24,52,218-220]

Recommendation V

Patient care information must be secure, held confidential, and protected from unauthorized disclosure.[221]

The Health Insurance Portability and Accountability Act (HIPAA) of 1996 guarantees the privacy of individuals receiving health services and the confidentiality of "individually identifiable health information."[222] Updated to correspond with the HITECH Act, HIPAA now includes security standards for protecting electronic health information (ie, Security Rule) and regulations that specify compliance, investigation, payments, and penalties (ie, Enforcement Rule) that were established in 1996.[221]

V.a.   Access to patient health information should be limited to authorized individuals based on the health care role (eg, surgeon, RN, perfusionist), responsibility, and function (eg, postanesthesia care unit RN assisting in the endoscopy unit).[223-225] Risk-reduction strategies to proactively mitigate potential access violations should include[225-228]

- establishing perioperative information management policies that include remote access protocols, on/off site information storage practices, and employee exit strategies that are reviewed frequently and updated as the environment changes (eg, new regulations, transitions from paper to electronic documentation platforms);
- identifying procedures for the use of mobile devices (eg, cell phone, tablet technologies, video imaging) within the perioperative care environment;
- establishing awareness and sensitivity to data security and privacy by reinforcing

the existing health care organization's information security policy for monitoring and auditing access to patient health information;

- restricting access to electronic health information to users with individualized, unique authorization credentials that are associated with time-sensitive passwords using alpha-numeric-symbol combinations; and
- holding annual, competency-based education programs on information access and sharing for all employees within the perioperative care environment.

Controlling access to the patient's health information prevents privacy and security breaches for HIPAA covered entities.[221,223,224] The health care organization has a legal responsibility to create procedures to circumvent unauthorized access to sensitive patient health information and to execute a plan for data breach notification practices should a breach occur.[221,222,229,230]

V.b.   Perioperative health care workers should be familiar with the health care organization's information policies before sharing electronic patient information. Considerations for recipients of electronic health information that should be incorporated into the organization's information policies include[228,229,231] ensuring that

- electronic patient health information, either to or from outside organizations or with the patient, meets current requirements for information exchange and security (eg, malware protection),
- validation occurs for original source authenticity and the accuracy of transmitted information, and
- electronically transmitted content is evaluated for potential corruption.

Electronic transmissions of patient health information is held to the same privacy and security criteria as facility-based EHRs. Sensitive patient information in paper, electronic text, or image formatting can be exposed to unintended or unauthorized disclosure without proper sharing safeguards in place.[80,221,222,224,231] Electronic transmission of patient health information by fax, e-mail, mobile storage media, or other formats may introduce malicious software into the health care information system.

V.b.1. Recipients of electronic patient health information should validate original source authenticity and accuracy of information and evaluate content for potential corruption.[228,229,231]

V.b.2. The patient must have a signed consent for release of information in the health care record before graphic imaging takes place and before the release of patient specific information, including remote access to and relocation of health information from the treating organization.[163,221,222,228,232-237] Non-consented disclosure of sensitive patient health information requires execution of the data breach notification process by the health care organization.[221,222,238,230] To complete full disclosure and reporting, the organization's information technology and risk management personnel should collaborate to discover all patient care records that were involved in the non-consented disclosure.[238]

V.c. Documentation entries made into the patient health care record must include an authentication process at the completion of the documentation process or according to the organization's established policies.[66,85,227,239,240,241] Health care records must accurately reflect the patient care experience, be promptly completed, and be associated with an author identification procedure to ensure the integrity of the content.[66,87,242] The authentication process may include, but is not limited to, the following:[227,243,244]

- using an electronic or digital signature or a code key in the format designated by the health care organization as the legal representation of an individual's written signature for the EHR.
- completing a pen-to-paper signature, using initials with a signature legend on the same document, or a rubber signature stamp for paper-based documentation platforms (eg, faxed, scanned documents) and as permitted by the health care organization's policy.

- Initials with a signature legend should be avoided on narrative documentation (eg, comments, patient quotes, consultation), assessment data collection, or when a signature is required by law (eg, patient informed consent).
- Digitized inked signatures (ie, signature image) should only be used when deemed acceptable by the health care organization and allowed by state or federal reimbursement regulations.
- using a countersignature demonstrating accuracy of content entered into a patient health care record; once countersigned, the content is legally considered the cosigner's entry (eg, nursing student entry).

Authentication identifies the author of the documentation entry and indicates responsibility for the interventions performed and patient information collected. Authentication legally binds the owner of the signature with the responsibility for accuracy of the content within the document.[227]

V.c.1. Authentication of verbal orders must occur within the time frame specified by state statutory guidelines. If state law does not specify a time frame, the federal mandate applies for verbal orders to be authenticated by the responsible physician within 48 hours of entering the order.[66]

V.d. The patient care record must be retained in the original or a legally reproducible format for the minimum allocation of time dictated by federal regulations and state statutes of limitations. Organizational policies may address other time frames for record retention based on the patient population served (eg, pediatrics, cancer treatment), facility demographics (eg, research, trauma, academic), media used to store patient data (eg, paper, microfilm, optical disc), or operational requirements (eg, regulatory compliance).[66,87,227,242,245-247]

The American Health Information Management Association (AHIMA) recommends retaining operative indexes for a minimum

Table 1

US FEDERAL MINIMUM RETENTION GUIDELINES		
Documentation type	**Retention period**	**Source**
Ambulatory surgical services	Not specified	42 CFR §416.47 Condition of participation: Medical records[1]
Hospitals	Five years from the date of discharge	42 CFR §482.24(b)(1) Condition of participation: Medical record services[2]
Hospitals, critical access	Six years from date of last entry or longer as mandated by state statutory guidelines or as necessary for legal proceedings	42 CFR §485.638 Condition of participation: Clinical records[3]
Department of Veterans Affairs operation log file (including type of operation, date, patient's name, surgeon, assistant scrub nurse [scrub person], sponge count, anesthetist, agent, method, preoperative and postoperative diagnoses, complications, and other information)	Destroy after 20 years	National Archives Job No. N1-015-94-2, Item 1[4]
Department of Veterans Affairs (date the surgery was performed, members of the surgical and nursing teams, and other information pertaining to the surgery of a patient)	Destroy after 3 years	National Archives Job No. N1-015-94-2, Item 2[5]

REFERENCES:

1. *Centers for Medicare & Medicaid Services. 42 CFR §416.47: Condition of participation: Medical records. 2010.*
2. *Centers for Medicare & Medicaid Services. 42 CFR §482.24: Condition of participation: Medical record services. 2010.*
3. *Centers for Medicare & Medicaid Services. 42 CFR §485.638: Conditions of participation: Clinical records. 2010.*
4. *Veterans Health Administration Records Control Schedule 10-1. Washington, DC. Veterans Health Administration; 2011. http://www1.va.gov/vhapublications/RCS10/rcs10-1.pdf. Accessed October 20, 2011.*
5. *Veterans Health Administration Records Control Schedule 10-1. Washington, DC. Veterans Health Administration; 2011. http://www1.va.gov/vhapublications/RCS10/rcs10-1.pdf. Accessed October 20, 2011.*

of 10 years and the register of surgical procedures permanently.[245] The minimum retention guidelines for perioperative information according to US Federal regulations are detailed in Table 1.

V.e. Electronic documentation platforms should have an alternate data entry and backup process.[248] Perioperative services should formalize a thorough downtime process addressing hardware, operating system, and network disruptions to preserve data accuracy and uninterrupted health care processes. Downtime planning should incorporate strategies to
- facilitate an uninterrupted patient care schedule (eg, paper forms, documentation backup media),
- identify changes to existing work flows (eg, how new orders are communicated, clinical resources),
- recover potential loss of patient care data, and

- incorporate patient care data that are captured using alternate documentation platforms (eg, paper forms) into the electronic information system.[31,248,249]

Perioperative personnel with system access responsibilities should receive ongoing education on the policies, procedures, and alternate work flows associated with the downtime or technology performance issues.[31,248,249]

Backup processes will mitigate interruptions in patient care caused by technology failures. Dependance on technology can significantly influence the effectiveness and efficiency of patient care delivery.

Recommendation VI

Modifications to existing content in the patient health care record must comply with relevant federal and state regulations, health care accreditation requirements, and national practice guidelines.[8,227] **Amendments, corrections, or addendums**

to the patient care record should only occur to present an accurate description of the care provided or to protect the patient's interest.[4,250]

The patient care record is a legal representation of services provided by the health care organization. Perioperative nurses are obligated to accurately represent the patient's care within the health care record.[66,87,242] Using inappropriate methods to correct, clarify, or change existing entries in the patient health care record may expose the health care organization or clinicians to liability for falsification of patient care information.[8,12,16]

VI.a. The health care organization's information management policy should outline the processes to make legally acceptable modifications to the patient care record.

Corrections, amendments, and addendums that are completed are limited by the functionality of the documentation platform used.[227,250]

VI.a.1. Amendments or addendums to the patient care record should follow established organizational policies and procedures. Corrections, amendments, and addendums in paper records should be performed by[4,227]

- placing a single line through the incorrect entry, being careful not to obliterate the inaccurate information;
- writing "error," "mistaken entry," or "omit" next to the incorrect text as determined by organizational policy;
- providing the rationale for the correction above the inaccurate entry if room is available or adding it to the margin of the document;
- signing and dating the entry; and
- entering the correct information in the next available space or adjacent to the acknowledged inaccurate information.

VI.a.2. Corrections, amendments, and addendums in EHRs should[80,227,250]

- have versioning or "track corrections" function (eg, electronic strike-through with time stamp) to identify the alterations made to an entry that has been authenticated;

- automatically date-, time-, and author-stamp each entry;
- generate a symbol or other notation to identify when an alteration has been made to existing content by creating a new version of the document;
- retain and link the original document version to the newly created version; and
- reflect corrections made to the EHR on the paper copy.

Additionally,

- corrections completed after a final signature or authentication process has occurred will comply with the functionality of the information system and established organizational policies and procedures,
- corrections completed before the final signature or authentication process may not be classified as a "correction" according to organizational policy and the information system that is in place,
- addendums should be completed where the original document was created using the source information system when available and should be reflected in the permanent patient care record or data repository system, and
- deletions and retractions of content from a closed EHR system should be made according to organizational policies and procedures and the functionality of the information system that is in place.

Recommendation VII

Perioperative personnel should receive initial and ongoing education related to accurately documenting patient care and should demonstrate competency in documentation processes and best practices to maintain security and privacy of patient care information.[8,80,251,252]

Initial and periodic competency-based education programs made available to maintain proficiency in the application of knowledge and use of the documentation platform improve the effectiveness of documentation practices and reinforce strategies to avert unintentional disclosure of patient care information.

VII.a. A review of the health care organization's policies for information management and the procedures for documentation processes and activities should be incorporated into orientation and ongoing education for personnel within the perioperative care environment.

Perioperative personnel receiving ongoing education and periodic review of policies and procedures develop the knowledge, skills, and attitudes that affect patient outcomes.

VII.a.1. Perioperative nurses should have knowledge of the significance and use of structured vocabularies for clinical documentation. Minimum education criteria on structured terminologies include
- the value structured terminology brings to clinical documentation;
- an overview of the PNDS;
- the contributions of the PNDS to perioperative nursing practice and patient outcomes; and
- how standardized documentation facilitates benchmarks, comparative analysis, and efficiency reporting.

VII.a.2. Minimum education and competency activities for perioperative RNs should include reviewing
- national and organizational documentation standards, guidelines, and requirements;
- procedures for completing amendments, addendums, and corrections;
- procedures for sharing patient information securely while maintaining patient privacy;
- procedures for initiating breach notification;
- compliance requirements for health care data capture; and
- legal implications for failure to comply with documentation standards.

Additional education and competency considerations for users of perioperative information systems, a

component of the EHR, should also incorporate the following minimum skills by demonstrating
- accessing and closing the patient care record;
- information system's functionality (eg, data entry, order acknowledgment);
- authentication processes;
- downtime procedures including alternate work flows to accommodate patient care; and
- compliance requirements for health care data capture.

Recommendation VIII

Policies and procedures related to perioperative information management should be developed, reviewed annually, revised as needed to accommodate changes in practice and documentation standards, and be readily available in the practice setting.

Policies and procedures establish authority, responsibility, and accountability and serve as operational guidelines that are used to minimize patient risk factors, standardize practice, direct health care personnel, and establish guidelines for continuous performance improvement activities. As new evidence emerges, policies and procedures will evolve to accommodate best practices and technology developments.

VIII.a. The perioperative services information management policy should complement and reinforce existing organization-wide policies (ie, risk management, quality improvement, health information privacy and security) and include the unique considerations of the perioperative care environment.

A collaborative approach to policy development and the provision of access to policies for all health care personnel will result in improved communications and compliance to established practices within the health care organization.

VIII.a.1. Information management policies and documentation procedures for EHR systems should include guidance on[250]

- forwarding addendums to each destination where patient information is retained,
- editing content before a final signature or authentication process occurs,
- using cut-copy-paste and "carry forward" functionality to populate the patient care record,
- completing corrections in an active or locked patient care record,
- rectifying a misidentification of patient health information (ie, wrong name association),
- amending clinical content in an active or locked patient care record,
- completing a delayed entry and updating the long-term record or data repository,
- deleting or retracting information from a locked patient care record while maintaining the integrity of the record, and
- defining components that are required for record completion.

VIII.a.2. Policies and procedures must include information on data privacy and security and identify risk-reduction strategies to proactively mitigate potential violations of patient health information access.[221] Risk-reduction strategies should include[225-228]

- establishing remote access protocols, on/off site information storage practices, and employee exit strategies to protect patient health information;
- frequently reviewing and updating policies as the health care information environment changes (eg, new regulations, transitions from paper to electronic documentation platforms);
- identifying procedures for using mobile devices (eg, cell phone, tablet technologies, video imaging) within the perioperative care environment;
- reinforcing the existing health care organization's information security policy for monitoring and auditing access to patient health informa-

tion within the perioperative care environment;
- restricting access to electronic health information by user type with individualized unique authorization credentials associated with time-sensitive passwords using alpha-numeric-symbol combinations; and
- holding annual competency-based education programs on information access and sharing for all employees within the perioperative care environment.

Recommendation IX

A quality management program should be established to ensure the integrity of the data within the patient health care record.

A fundamental precept for the professional perioperative nurse is the responsibility to provide safe, high-quality nursing care to patients undergoing operative and other invasive procedures.[3] Regularly monitoring and validating documentation processes is necessary for variance reporting, which supports process and performance measurement to quantify organizational effectiveness and nursing influence on patient outcomes.[8]

IX.a. Perioperative personnel should participate in the organization-wide clinical documentation improvement (CDI) program.

Participation in a CDI program facilitates data and documentation analysis while providing a structured framework to achieve consistency in quality processes that affect patient satisfaction, accreditation standing, and reimbursement status.[253] Representation in the CDI program ensures concerns specific to perioperative practice parameters are addressed and that areas for improvement are identified.

IX.a.1. Minimum criteria that should be reviewed for a perioperative CDI program should include[227,252]
- use of unacceptable abbreviations,
- timeliness and chronology of patient information,
- legibility,
- use of vague or generalized language,

- blank spaces or data fields,
- content omissions (eg, missing informed consent),
- delayed entries (eg, next day entry),
- inconsistencies (eg, conflicting assessment findings, procedure start times),
- inappropriate information (eg, communications with attorneys),
- authentication of verbal orders,
- absence of signatures or countersignature,
- appropriate documentation practices (eg, charting by exception/variance charting), and
- alterations to clinical content.

IX.b. Validation procedures for the perioperative information system should be incorporated into the quality management program. Data quality may be ensured by periodically evaluating the information system for the integrity of
  - collected patient care information,
  - report generation,
  - file storage and retrieval,
  - data security, and
  - control for document versioning.[227,250,251]
Validation procedures for the perioperative information system should be incorporated into the health care organization's comprehensive strategies for EHR system security and maintenance.

Perioperative information systems are complex systems that contribute to improved care or may add to error-prone documentation processes.[32,251,254] Validation procedures help to maintain the integrity of patient health information.

IX.b.1. Routine audits should be performed as a part of a quality-driven information management program. Audit trails should be retained and placed on a retention schedule following the state statute of limitations and needs of the health care organization.[227,255] Audit trails may include[227,255]
  - paper-based sign-out processes,
  - logbook activities,
  - EHR access and operations performed,

- electronic tracking system, and
- data mining activities.

Auditing procedures help to establish user and organizational accountability for the legal integrity of the patient health care record.

IX.b.2. Perioperative information systems should be included in the organizational information technology risk mitigation plan.[251] Collaborating with the organization's risk manger, information services department, and engineering department, perioperative nursing leaders should coordinate efforts to plan for
  - perioperative information system upgrades and maintenance;
  - system redundancies (eg, remote patient care record access, backup generators);
  - unanticipated access to and theft of patient health care information; and
  - organizational information technology network infrastructure maintenance, upgrades, and conversions on the perioperative information system.[251]

Proactive contingency planning for information system failures and disaster response procedures will help maintain continuity in patient care activities.

Glossary

Addendum: New documentation used to add information to an original documentation entry of patient health information.

American Recovery and Reinvestment Act (ARRA): An economic stimulus package enacted by the US Congress in 2009 with a defined purpose to stimulate jobs, investments, and consumer spending. ARRA contains provisions for improved health care quality through the use of health information technology. (Source: American Recovery and Reinvestment Act – H.R.1. *http://frwebgate. access.gpo.gov/cgi-bin/getdoc.cgi?dbname=111_ cong_bills&docid=f:h1enr.pdf.* Accessed October 20, 2011.)

Amendments: Additional documentation completed to clarify a preexisting entry of patient health information.

Authentication: A security measure to establish the validity of an electronic transmission, message, or original source (eg, author) or to verify the authorization of an individual to receive specific information. Authentication is used to confirm that an individual or system is who or what it claims to be.

Clinical information systems: Computer technology used in the patient care environment for collecting patient health care information.

Clinical support technologies: Assorted technologies used in the patient care environment to facilitate the clinician's ability to provide safe, comprehensive interventions for delivery of quality health care.

Code key: A computer code used to authenticate entries in an electronic health record as permitted by state, federal, and reimbursement regulations.

Controlled terminology: Terminology developed according to specific characteristics so that each data element is expressed as a single, clear, and unambiguous concept. Controlled terminology concepts maintain their meaning permanently.

Corrections: A change made to the documented patient health information meant to clarify the entry after the document has been authenticated.

Customize: To specifically select or set preferences or options for health care information.

Data mining: The process of extracting and analyzing data for usable information from relationships, patterns, information clusters, and data trends. The new information may be used for predictive modeling in decision support processes for clinical, operational, and research utilization.

Data quality: Data remaining unchanged from its original meaning; it is complete, correct, comprehensive, and consistent for the intended use.

Data repository: A central location where health care data (eg, clinical, financial, operational) and files are stored and maintained for later retrieval and use.

Deemed status: The "deeming" authority granted to national accreditation organizations (eg, The Joint Commission, DNV-Hospital Accreditation) by the Centers for Medicare & Medicaid Services (CMS) to determine, on CMS's behalf, whether a health care provider organization is in compliance with the regulations to provide and receive payment for Medicare services. Six areas are deemable: quality assurance, antidiscrimination, access to services, confidentiality and accuracy of enrollee records, information on advance directives, and provider participation rules.

Digital signature: A cryptographic signature (ie, digital key) used to authenticate the user, provide legal ownership, and ensure integrity of the unit of information.

Digitized inked signatures: A handwritten signature using a pen pad to create an electronic representation of the actual signature.

Downtime: Periods of time when the clinical information system (ie, electronic health record) is unavailable because of scheduled maintenance or upgrade, technology failure, power outage, or other unscheduled event.

Electronic health record: An electronic record of health-related information for an individual that conforms to nationally recognized interoperability standards and that can be created, managed, and consulted by authorized clinicians and staff members across more than one health care organization.

Electronic medical records: Electronic records of health-related information for individuals that can be created, gathered, managed, and consulted by authorized clinicians and staff members within one health care organization.

Electronic signature: The technology-neutral electronic process used to sign (ie, attest) content for authorship and legal responsibility for a section of information. The electronic signature format is determined by the technology used to collect or create the signature.

Health Information Technology for Economic and Clinical Health (HITECH): A component of the American Recovery and Reinvestment Act of 2009 addressing the use of electronic health information technology to improve health care quality, coordination of care, and health information privacy and security.

Integrity: The accuracy, consistency, and reliability of information content, processes, and systems.

Interoperable: The ability for health information systems to exchange or share health information within and across organizational boundaries.

Malware: Software considered harmful to a computer system including, but not limited to, the following: viruses, worms, trojan horses, spyware, and unauthorized adware.

Signature legend: A document that identifies an author's full signature and title when initials are used to authenticate entries in the health care record.

Tailored health care information: The unique patient characteristics based on multiple factors influencing health status and health behaviors and collected to inform individualized nursing interventions.

Versioning: The process of assigning a unique version name or number to an electronic heath record and used to identify revisions occurring to previously documented content.

REFERENCES

1. *Nursing: Scope and Standards of Practice.* Silver Spring, MD: American Nurses Association; 2010.

2. Gugerty B, Maranda MJ, Beachley M, et al. *Challenges and Opportunities in Documentation of the Nursing Care of Patients.* Baltimore, MD: Maryland Nursing Workforce Commission, Documentation Work Group; 2007.

3. Standards of perioperative nursing. In: *Perioperative Standards and Recommended Practices.* Denver, CO: AORN, Inc; 2010: 9-27.

4. Iyer PW, Koob SL. Nursing documentation. In: Iyer PW, Levin BB, Agosto M, eds. *Nursing Malpractice.* Tucson, AZ: Lawyers and Judges Pub Co; 2007: 181-227.

5. *Complete Guide to Documentation.* Philadelphia, PA: Wolters Kluwer Health/Lippincott Williams & Wilkins; 2008.

6. *Nursing's Social Policy Statement: The Essence of the Profession.* Silver Spring, MD: American Nurses Association; 2010.

7. Beyea SC. Describing professional nursing through a universal record in perioperative settings. *Int J Nurs Terminol Classif.* 2003;14(4):23.

8. *ANA Principles for Documentation.* Silver Spring, MD: American Nurses Association; 2010.

9. Kuc JA. Perioperative records. In: Iyer PW, Levin BL, Shea MA, eds. *Medical Legal Aspects of Medical Records.* Tucson, AZ: Lawyers & Judges Publishing Company; 2006: 657-677.

10. Junttila K, Hupli M, Salanterä S. The use of nursing diagnoses in perioperative documentation. *Int J Nurs Terminol Classif.* 2010;21(2):57-68.

11. Wang N, Hailey D, Yu P. Quality of nursing documentation and approaches to its evaluation: a mixed-method systematic review. *J Adv Nurs.* 2011;67(9):1858-1875. doi:10.1111/j.1365-2648.2011.05634.x; 10.1111/j.1365-2648.2011.05634.x.

12. Ferrell KG. Documentation, part 2: the best evidence of care. Complete and accurate charting can be crucial to exonerating nurses in civil lawsuits. *Am J Nurs.* 2007;107(7):61-64. doi:10.1097/01.NAJ.0000279271.41357.fa.

13. McGeehan R. Best practice in record-keeping. *Nurs Stand.* 2007;21(17):51.

14. Potter P, Wolf L, Boxerman S, et al. Understanding the cognitive work of nursing in the acute care environment. *J Nurs Adm.* 2005;35(7-8):327-335.

15. Micek WT, Berry L, Gilski D, Kallenbach A, Link D, Scharer K. Patient outcomes: the link between nursing diagnoses and interventions. *J Nurs Adm.* 1996;26(11):29-35.

16. Monarch K. Documentation, part 1: principles for self-protection. Preserve the medical record—and defend yourself. *Am J Nurs.* 2007;107(7):58-60. doi:10.1097/01.NAJ.0000279270.41357.b3.

17. Provision of care, treatment, and services. PC.02.02.01. In: *2011 Comprehensive Accreditation Manual for Hospitals.* Oakbrook Terrace, IL: Joint Commission Resources; 2011.

18. Provision of care, treatment, and services. PC.02.02.01. In: *2011 Comprehensive Accreditation Manual for Ambulatory Care.* Oakbrook Terrace, IL: Joint Commission Resources; 2011.

19. AORN guidance statement: Preoperative patient care in the ambulatory surgery setting. In: *Perioperative Standards and Recommended Practices.* Denver, CO: AORN, Inc; 2011: 227-232.

20. AORN guidance statement: Postoperative patient care in the ambulatory surgery setting. In: *Perioperative Standards and Recommended Practices.* Denver, CO: AORN, Inc; 2011: 219-226.

21. Whittenburg L. Workflow viewpoints: analysis of nursing workflow documentation in the electronic health record. *J Healthc Inf Manag.* 2010;24(3):71-75.

22. Lee S, McElmurry B. Capturing nursing care workflow disruptions: comparison between nursing and physician workflows. *Comput Inform Nurs.* 2010;28(3):151-159. doi:10.1097/NCN.0b013e3181d77d3e.

23. Karsh BT, Holden RJ, Alper SJ, Or CK. A human factors engineering paradigm for patient safety: designing to support the performance of the healthcare professional. *Qual Saf Health Care.* 2006;15 Suppl 1:i59-65. doi:10.1136/qshc.2005.015974.

24. Institute of Medicine; Page A, eds. *Keeping Patients Safe: Transforming the Work Environment of Nurses.* Washington, DC: National Academies Press; 2004.

25. Keohane CA, Bane AD, Featherstone E, et al. Quantifying nursing workflow in medication administration. *J Nurs Adm.* 2008;38(1):19-26.

26. Häyrinen K, Lammintakanen J, Saranto K. Evaluation of electronic nursing documentation—nursing process model and standardized terminologies as keys to visible and transparent nursing. *Int J Med Inform.* 2010;79(8):554-564.

27. Capuano T, Bokovoy J, Halkins D, Hitchings K. Work flow analysis: eliminating non-value-added work. *J Nurs Adm.* 2004;34(5):246-256.

28. Hendrich A, Chow M, Skierczynski B, Lu Z. A 36-hospital time and motion study: how do medical-surgical nurses spend their time? *Permanente J.* 2008;12(3):25-34.

29. Benner P, Sheets V, Uris P, Malloch K, Schwed K, Jamison D. Individual, practice, and system causes of errors in nursing: a taxonomy. *J Nurs Adm.* 2002;32(10):509-523.

30. Ammenwerth E, Eichstadter R, Haux R, Pohl U, Rebel S, Ziegler S. A randomized evaluation of a computer-based nursing documentation system. *Methods Inf Med.* 2001;40(2):61-68.

31. Bloomrosen M, Starren J, Lorenzi NM, Ash JS, Patel VL, Shortliffe EH. Anticipating and addressing the unintended consequences of health IT and policy: a report from the AMIA 2009 Health Policy Meeting. *J Am Med Inform Assoc.* 2011;18(1):82-90. doi:10.1136/jamia.2010.007567.

32. Clancy CM. Nursing, system design, and health care quality. *AORN J.* 2009;90(4):581-583. doi:10.1016/j.aorn.2009.09.008.

33. Ash JS, Berg M, Coiera E. Some unintended consequences of information technology in health care: the nature of patient care information system-related errors. *J Am Med Inform Assoc.* 2004;11(2):104-112. doi:10.1197/jamia.M1471.

34. Harrison MI, Koppel R, Bar-Lev S. Unintended consequences of information technologies in health care—an interactive sociotechnical analysis. *J Am Med Inform Assoc.* 2007;14(5):542-549. doi:10.1197/jamia.M2384.

35. Cornell P, Herrin-Griffith D, Keim C, et al. Transforming nursing workflow, part 1: the chaotic nature of nurse activities. *J Nurs Adm.* 2010;40(9):366-373. doi:10.1097/NNA.0b013e3181ee4261.

36. Cornell P, Riordan M, Herrin-Griffith D. Transforming nursing workflow, part 2: the impact of technology on nurse activities. *J Nurs Adm.* 2010;40(10):432-439. doi:10.1097/NNA.0b013e3181f2eb3f.

37. Irwin RS, Richardson ND. Patient-focused care: using the right tools. *Chest.* 2006;130(1 Suppl):73S-82S. doi:10.1378/chest.130.1_suppl.73S.

38. Allan J, Englebright J. Patient-centered documentation: an effective and efficient use of clinical information systems. *J Nurs Adm.* 2000;30(2):90-95.

39. Nailon RE. The assessment and documentation of language and communication needs in healthcare systems: current practices and future directions for coordinating safe, patient-centered care. *Nurs Outlook.* 2007;55(6):311-317. doi:10.1016/j.outlook.2007.04.005.

40. Institute of Medicine. *Crossing the Quality Chasm: A New Health System for the 21st Century.* Washington, DC: National Academies Press; 2001. http://www.nap.edu/openbook.php?record_id=10027. Accessed October 6, 2011.

41. Recommended practices for the use of the pneumatic tourniquet in the perioperative practice setting. In: *Perioperative Standards and Recommended Practices.* Denver, CO: AORN, Inc; 2011: 177-190.

42. Spooner SA; Council on Clinical Information Technology. Special requirements of electronic health record systems in pediatrics. *Pediatrics.* 2007;119(3):631-637. doi:10.1542/peds.2006-3527.

43. Park EJ, McDaniel A, Jung MS. Computerized tailoring of health information. *Comput Inform Nurs.* 2009;27(1):34-43. doi:10.1097/NCN.0b013e31818dd396.

44. Payne TH, tenBroek AE, Fletcher GS, Labuguen MC. Transition from paper to electronic inpatient physician notes. *J Am Med Inform Assoc.* 2010;17(1):108-111. doi:10.1197/jamia.M3173.

45. Korst LM, Eusebio-Angeja AC, Chamorro T, Aydin CE, Gregory KD. Nursing documentation time during implementation of an electronic medical record. *J Nurs Adm.* 2003;33(1):24-30.

46. Urquhart C, Currell R, Grant MJ, Hardiker NR. Nursing record systems: effects on nursing practice and healthcare outcomes. *Cochrane Database Syst Rev.* 2009;(1). doi:10.1002/14651858.CD002099.pub2.

47. Mahler C, Ammenwerth E, Wagner A, et al. Effects of a computer-based nursing documentation system on the quality of nursing documentation. *J Med Syst.* 2007;31(4):274-282.

48. Poissant L, Pereira J, Tamblyn R, Kawasumi Y. The impact of electronic health records on time efficiency of physicians and nurses: a systematic review. *J Am Med Inform Assoc.* 2005;12(5):505-516. doi:10.1197/jamia.M1700.

49. Stead WW, Lin HS, eds. *Computational Technology for Effective Health Care: Immediate Steps and Strategic Directions.* Washington, DC: National Academies Press; 2009. http://www.nap.edu/openbook.php?record_id=12572&page=R1. Accessed October 6, 2011.

50. Asaro PV, Boxerman SB. Effects of computerized provider order entry and nursing documentation on workflow. *Acad Emerg Med.* 2008;15(10):908-915. doi:10.1111/j.1553-2712.2008.00235.x.

51. Manasse HR Jr. Not too perfect: hard lessons and small victories in patient safety. *Am J Health Syst Pharm.* 2003;60(8):780-787.

52. Amarasingham R, Plantinga L, Diener-West M, Gaskin DJ, Powe NR. Clinical information technologies and inpatient outcomes: a multiple hospital study. *Arch Intern Med.* 2009;169(2):108-114. doi:10.1001/archinternmed.2008.520.

53. Shojania KG, Jennings A, Mayhew A, Ramsay CR, Eccles MP, Grimshaw J. The effects of on-screen, point of care computer reminders on processes and outcomes of care. *Cochrane Database Syst Rev.* 2009;3(3):CD001096. doi:10.1002/14651858.CD001096.pub2.

54. Institute of Medicine. *The Future of Nursing: Leading Change, Advancing Health.* Washington, DC: National Academies Press; 2011. http://books.nap.edu/openbook.php?record_id=12956. Accessed October 6, 2011.

55. Previte JP. Information and communication system implementation in anesthesia. *Int Anesthesiol Clin.* 2006;44(1):179-197.

56. American Academy of Nursing. Position statement: use of electronic information for health and health care. 2008. http://www.aannet.org/files/public/EMR%20Position%20Statement%20Recommendation%20Post%20NIEP.doc. Accessed October 10, 2011.

57. Kim H, Dykes P, Mar P, Goldsmith D, Choi J, Goldberg H. Towards a standardized representation to support data reuse: representing the ICNP semantics using the HL7 RIM. *Stud Health Technol Inform.* 2009;146:308-313.

58. Zielstorff RD. Characteristics of a good nursing nomenclature from an informatics perspective. *Online J Issues Nurs.* 1998;3(2).

59. *Nursing Informatics: Scope and Standards of Practice.* Silver Spring, MD: American Nurses Association; 2008.

60. Graves JR, Corcoran S. The study of nursing informatics. *Image J Nurs Sch.* 1989;21(4):227-231.

61. Petersen C, ed. *Perioperative Nursing Data Set.* 3rd ed. Denver, CO: AORN, Inc; 2011.

62. Beyea SC. Standardized language—making nursing practice count. *AORN J.* 1999;70(5):831-838.

63. Lundberg C, Warren J, Brokel J, et al. Selecting a standardized terminology for the electronic health record that reveals the impact of nursing on patient care. *Online J Nurs Inform.* 2008;12(2). *http://www.ojni .org/12_2/lundberg.pdf.* Accessed October 6, 2011.

64. Saba VK, Taylor SL. Moving past theory: use of a standardized, coded nursing terminology to enhance nursing visibility. *Comput Inform Nurs.* 2007;25(6):324-333. doi:10.1097/01.NCN.0000299654.13777.9f.

65. Centers for Medicare & Medicaid Services. Department of Health and Human Services. Condition of participation: Surgical services. 42 CFR §482.51. *http://edocket.access.gpo.gov/cfr_2004/octqtr/ pdf/42cfr482.51.pdf.* Revised November 27, 2007. Accessed October 6, 2011.

66. Centers for Medicare & Medicaid Services. Department of Health and Human Services. Condition of participation: Medical record services. 42 CFR §482.24. *http://edocket.access.gpo.gov/cfr_2004/ octqtr/pdf/42cfr482.24.pdf.* Revised November 27, 2007. Accessed October 6, 2011.

67. Record of care, treatment, and services. RC.01.01.01. The hospital maintains complete and accurate medical records for each individual patient. In: *Comprehensive Accreditation Manual for Hospitals.* Oakbrook Terrace, IL: Joint Commission Resources; 2011.

68. Record of care, treatment, and services. RC.02.01.01. The medical record contains information that reflects the patient's care, treatment, and services. In: *Comprehensive Accreditation Manual for Hospitals.* 2011 ed. Oakbrook Terrace, IL: Joint Commission Resources; 2011.

69. Westra BL, Subramanian A, Hart CM, et al. Achieving "meaningful use" of electronic health records through the integration of the Nursing Management Minimum Data Set. *J Nurs Adm.* 2010;40(7-8):336-343. doi:10.1097/NNA.0b013e3181e93994.

70. Mangalmurti SS, Murtagh L, Mello MM. Medical malpractice liability in the age of electronic health records. *N Engl J Med.* 2010;363(21):2060-2067. doi:10.1056/NEJMhle1005210.

71. Electronic health record incentive program. Final rule. *Fed Regist.* 2010;75(144):44314-44588. 42 CFR §412, 413, 422, et al. *http://edocket.access.gpo .gov/2010/pdf/2010-17207.pdf.* Accessed October 18, 2011.

72. Häyrinen K, Saranto K, Nykanen P. Definition, structure, content, use and impacts of electronic health records: a review of the research literature. *Int J Med Inform.* 2008;77(5):291-304. doi:10.1016/j .ijmedinf.2007.09.001.

73. Hyun S, Bakken S. Toward the creation of an ontology for nursing document sections: mapping section names to the LOINC semantic model. *AMIA Annu Symp Proc.* 2006:364-368.

74. Executive summary. In: *Health Information Technology Automation of Quality Measure: Quality Data Set and Data Flow.* Washington, DC: National Quality Forum; 2009:iii-vi.

75. Kahn MG, Ranade D. The impact of electronic medical records data sources on an adverse drug event quality measure. *J Am Med Inform Assoc.* 2010;17(2):185-191. doi:10.1136/jamia.2009.002451.

76. Goossen WT, Ozbolt JG, Coenen A, et al. Development of a provisional domain model for the nursing process for use within the Health Level 7 reference information model. *J Am Med Inform Assoc.* 2004;11(3):186-194. doi:10.1197/jamia.M1085.

77. Jha AK, DesRoches CM, Campbell EG, et al. Use of electronic health records in U.S. hospitals. *N Engl J Med.* 2009;360(16):1628-1638. doi:10.1056/ NEJMsa0900592.

78. Brown DS, Donaldson N, Burnes Bolton L, Aydin CE. Nursing-sensitive benchmarks for hospitals to gauge high-reliability performance. *J Healthc Qual.* 2010;32(6):9-17. doi:10.1111/j.1945-1474.2010.00083.x.

79. US Department of Health and Human Services. *Report to Congress: Medicare Ambulatory Surgical Center Value-Based Purchasing Implementation Plan.* Washington, DC: Centers for Medicare & Medicaid Services; 2011. *http://www.cms.gov/ASCPayment/downloads/C_ ASC_RTC%202011.pdf.* Accessed October 7, 2011.

80. ECRI. Electronic health records. *Healthcare Risk Control.* 2011;2(Medical Records 1.1).

81. Hines S, Luna K, Lofthus J, et al. *Becoming a High Reliability Organization: Operational Advice for Hospital Leaders.* Rockville, MD: Agency for Healthcare Research and Quality; 2008.

82. Thompson D, Johnston P, Spurr C. The impact of electronic medical records on nursing efficiency. *J Nurs Adm.* 2009;39(10):444-451. doi:10.1097/ NNA.0b013e3181b9209c.

83. Shekelle PG, Morton SC, Keeler EB, et al. *Costs and Benefits of Health Information Technology.* Rockville, MD: Agency for Healthcare Research and Quality; April 2006.

84. Centers for Medicare & Medicaid Services. Department of Health and Human Services. Conditions for participation for hospitals. 42 CFR §482. *http://www .access.gpo.gov/nara/cfr/waisidx_10/42cfr482_10.html.* Accessed October 7, 2011.

85. Centers for Medicare & Medicaid Services. Department of Health and Human Services. Condition of participation: nursing services. 42 CFR §482.23. Revised November 27, 2007. *http://edocket.access.gpo.gov/cfr_2010/ octqtr/pdf/42cfr482.23.pdf.* Accessed October 7, 2011.

86. Centers for Medicare & Medicaid Services. Department of Health and Human Services. Condition for coverage—nursing services. 42 CFR §416.46. *http://edocket.access.gpo.gov/cfr_2010/octqtr/ pdf/42cfr416.46.pdf.* Accessed October 7, 2011.

87. Centers for Medicare & Medicaid Services. Department of Health and Human Services. Condition of participation: medical records. 42 CFR §416.47. *http://edocket.access.gpo.gov/cfr_2010/octqtr/ pdf/42cfr416.47.pdf.* Accessed October 7. 2011.

88. Centers for Medicare & Medicaid Services. Department of Health and Human Services. Ambulatory

surgical services. 42 CFR §416. *http://www.access.gpo .gov/nara/cfr/waisidx_10/42cfr416_10.html*. Accessed October 7. 2011.

89. *Perioperative Standards and Recommended Practices*. Denver, CO: AORN, Inc; 2011.

90. Centers for Medicare & Medicaid Services. Department of Health and Human Services. Conditions for coverage—infection control. 42 CFR §416.51. *http://edocket.access.gpo.gov/cfr_2010/octqtr/ pdf/42cfr416.51.pdf*. Accessed October 7, 2011.

91. National Patient Safety Goal. NPSG.07.05.01. Implement evidence-based practices for preventing surgical site infections. In: *Comprehensive Accreditation Manual for Hospitals*. Oakbrook Terrace, IL: Joint Commission Resources; 2011.

92. Infection prevention and control. Standard IC.01.05.01. The hospital has an infection prevention and control plan. In: *Comprehensive Accreditation Manual for Hospitals*. Oakbrook Terrace, IL: Joint Commission Resources; 2011.

93. Infection prevention and control. Standard IC.02.01.01. Hospital leaders allocate needed resources for the infection prevention and control program. In: *Comprehensive Accreditation Manual for Hospitals*. Oakbrook Terrace, IL: Joint Commission Resources; 2011.

94. Recommended practices for managing the patient receiving local anesthesia. In: *Perioperative Standards and Recommended Practices*. Denver, CO: AORN, Inc; 2011: 321-326.

95. Recommended practices for medication safety. In: *Perioperative Standards and Recommended Practices*. Denver, CO: AORN, Inc. In press.

96. Krenzischek DA, Wilson L; ASPAN. ASPAN pain and comfort clinical guideline. *J Perianesth Nurs.* 2003;18(4).232-236.

97. Practice recommendation 2: components of initial, ongoing, and discharge assessment and management. In: *Perianesthesia Nursing Standards and Practice Recommendations 2010-2012*. Cherry Hill, NJ: American Society of PeriAnesthesia Nurses; 2010: 73-78.

98. Centers for Medicare & Medicaid Services. Department of Health and Human Services. Condition for coverage— pharmaceutical services. 42 CFR §416.48. *http://edocket.access.gpo.gov/cfr_2010/ octqtr/pdf/42cfr416.48.pdf*. Accessed October 7, 2011.

99. Centers for Medicare & Medicaid Services. Department of Health and Human Services. Condition of participation: patient's rights. 42 CFR §482.13. *http://edocket.access.gpo.gov/cfr_2010/octqtr/ pdf/42cfr482.13.pdf*. Accessed October 7, 2011.

100. Medication management. In: *Comprehensive Accreditation Manual for Hospitals*. Oakbrook Terrace, IL: Joint Commission Resources; 2011: MM-1 MM-23.

101. Provision of care, treatment, and services. In: *Comprehensive Accreditation Manual for Hospitals*. Oakbrook Terrace, IL: Joint Commission Resources; 2011: PC-1–PC-66.

102. Standard 5.001: Facility safety manual. In: *Medicare Standards and Checklist for Accreditation of Ambulatory Surgery Facilities*. Gurnee, IL: American Association for Accreditation of Ambulatory Surgery Facilities; 2005: 24-29.

103. Standard 04: Quality of care provided. In: *Accreditation Handbook for Ambulatory Health Care*. Skokie, IL: Accreditation Association for Ambulatory Health Care; 2009: 32-33.

104. Standard 06: Clinical records and health information. In: *Accreditation Handbook for Ambulatory Health Care*. Skokie, IL: Accreditation Association for Ambulatory Health Care; 2009:38-39.

105. AORN guidance statement: "do-not-use" abbreviations, acronyms, dosage designations, and symbols. In: *Perioperative Standards and Recommended Practices*. Denver, CO: AORN, Inc; 2011: 487-490.

106. AORN position statement on preventing wrong-patient, wrong-site, wrong-procedure events. AORN. *http:// www.aorn.org/PracticeResources/AORNPositionStatements/ PositionCorrectSiteSurgery*. Accessed October 7, 2011.

107. AORN position statement on pediatric medication safety. In: *Perioperative Standards and Recommended Practices*. Denver, CO: AORN, Inc; 2010: 737-738.

108. Recommended practices for preoperative patient skin antisepsis. In: *Perioperative Standards and Recommended Practices*. Denver, CO: AORN, Inc; 2011: 361-380.

109. Rights and responsibilities of the individual. In: *Comprehensive Accreditation Manual for Hospitals*. Oakbrook Terrace, IL: Joint Commission Resources; 2011:RI-1–RI-18.

110. National Patient Safety Goal. NPSG Goal 8: accurately and completely reconcile medications across the continuum of care. In: *Comprehensive Accreditation Manual for Hospitals*. Oakbrook Terrace, IL: Joint Commission Resources; 2011.

111. Accreditation Association for Ambulatory Health Care. *http://www.aaahc.org/eweb/StartPage.aspx*. Accessed October 11, 2011.

112. Recommended practices for prevention of transmissible infections in the perioperative practice settings. In: *Perioperative Standards and Recommended Practices*. Denver, CO: AORN, Inc; 2011: 291-302.

113. Standard 310: PACU rooms. In: *Regular Standards and Checklist for Accreditation of Ambulatory Surgery Facilities*. Gurnee, IL: American Association for Accreditation of Ambulatory Surgery Facilities; 2007: 22-23.

114. AORN malignant hyperthermia guideline. In: *Perioperative Standards and Recommended Practices*. Denver, CO: AORN, Inc; 2011: 541-576.

115. AORN guidance statement: Care of the perioperative patient with an implanted electronic device. In: *Perioperative Standards and Recommended Practices*. Denver, CO: AORN, Inc; 2011: 503-524.

116. Recommended practices for prevention of deep vein thrombosis. In: *Perioperative Standards and Recommended Practices*. Denver, CO: AORN, Inc; 2011: e1-e11.

117. Centers for Medicare & Medicaid Services. Department of Health and Human Services. Condition of participation: laboratory services. 42 CFR §482.27. *http://edocket.access.gpo.gov/cfr_2010/octqtr/ pdf/42cfr482.27.pdf*. Accessed October 7, 2011.

118. Centers for Medicare & Medicaid Services. Department of Health and Human Services. Condition of participation: patient admission, assessment and discharge. 42

CFR §416.52. *http://edocket.access.gpo.gov/cfr_2010/ octqtr/pdf/42cfr416.52.pdf.* Accessed October 7, 2011.

119. Record of care, treatment, and services. In: *Comprehensive Accreditation Manual for Hospitals.* Oakbrook Terrace, IL: Joint Commission Resources; 2011:RC-1–RC-14.

120. Recommended practices for positioning the patient in the perioperative practice setting. In: *Perioperative Standards and Recommended Practices.* Denver, CO: AORN, Inc; 2011: 337-360.

121. Universal Protocol for Preventing Wrong Site, Wrong Procedure, and Wrong Person Surgery. In: *Comprehensive Accreditation Manual for Hospitals.* Oakbrook Terrace, IL: Joint Commission Resources; 2011:NPSG-12–NPSG-24.

122. Recommended practices for transfer of patient care information. In: *Perioperative Standards and Recommended Practices.* Denver, CO: AORN, Inc; 2011: 381-388.

123. Standards of perioperative nursing. In: *Perioperative Standards and Recommended Practices.* Denver, CO: AORN, Inc; 2011: 3-52.

124. Standard 10: Surgical and related services. In: *Accreditation Handbook for Ambulatory Health Care.* Skokie, IL: Accreditation Association for Ambulatory Health Care; 2009: 50-54.

125. Standard 17: Behavioral health services. In: *Accreditation Handbook for Ambulatory Health Care.* Skokie, IL: Accreditation Association for Ambulatory Health Care; 2009: 64.

126. Standard 8.000: Operating room suite operations & management. In: *Medicare Standards and Checklist for Accreditation of Ambulatory Surgery Facilities.* Gurnee, IL: American Association for Accreditation of Ambulatory Surgery Facilities; 2005: 35-41.

127. Standard 630: Laboratory, pathology, x-ray, consultation and treating physician reports. In: *Regular Standards and Checklist for Accreditation of Ambulatory Surgery Facilities.* Gurnee, IL: American Association for Accreditation of Ambulatory Surgery Facilities; 2007: 33-34.

128. Standard 4.007: X-ray reports. In: *Medicare Standards and Checklist for Accreditation of Ambulatory Surgery Facilities.* Gurnee, IL: American Association for Accreditation of Ambulatory Surgery Facilities; 2005:20.

129. Centers for Medicare & Medicaid Services. Department of Health and Human Services. Condition of participation: Physical environment. 42 CFR §482.41. *http://edocket.access.gpo.gov/cfr_2010/ octqtr/pdf/42cfr482.41.pdf.* Accessed October 7, 2011.

130. Centers for Medicare & Medicaid Services. Department of Health and Human Services. Condition for coverage—Environment. 42 CFR §416.44. *http://edocket.access.gpo.gov/cfr_2010/octqtr/ pdf/42cfr416.44.pdf.* Accessed October 6, 2011.

131. Environment of care. In: 2011 *Comprehensive Accreditation Manual for Hospitals.* Oakbrook Terrace, IL: Joint Commission Resources; 2011.

132. American Association for Accreditation of Ambulatory Surgery Facilities. *http://www.aaaasf.org/.* Accessed October 6, 2011.

133. Standard 10.Q: Surgical and related services. In: *Accreditation Handbook for Ambulatory Health Care.* Skokie, IL: Accreditation Association for Ambulatory Health Care, Inc; 2009: 51.

134. Recommended practices for a safe environment of care. In: *Perioperative Standards and Recommended Practices.* Denver, CO: AORN, Inc; 2011: 215-236.

135. Recommended practices for electrosurgery. In: *Perioperative Standards and Recommended Practices.* Denver, CO: AORN, Inc; 2011: 99-118.

136. AORN latex guideline. In: *Perioperative Standards and Recommended Practices.* Denver, CO: AORN, Inc; 2011: 525-540.

137. Quality Indicators. Agency for Healthcare Research and Quality. *http://www.qualityindicators .ahrq.gov/.* Published November 2000. Updated August 2011. Accessed October 6, 2011.

138. Recommended practices for minimally invasive surgery. In: *Perioperative Standards and Recommended Practices.* Denver, CO: AORN, Inc; 2011: 143-176.

139. Recommended practices for laser safety in perioperative practice settings. In: *Perioperative Standards and Recommended Practices.* Denver, CO: AORN, Inc; 2011: 125-142.

140. Infection prevention and control. In: 2011 *Comprehensive Accreditation Manual for Hospitals.* Oakbrook Terrace, IL: Joint Commission Resources; 2011.

141. Standard 410: General Safety in the Facility. General. In: *Regular Standards and Checklist for Accreditation of Ambulatory Surgery Facilities.* Gurnee, IL: American Association for Accreditation of Ambulatory Surgery Facilities; 2007:25.

142. *ANSI/AAMI ST79:2006 and A1:2008, A2:2009: Comprehensive Guide to Steam Sterilization and Sterility Assurance in Health Care Facilities.* Arlington, VA: Association for the Advancement of Medical Instrumentation; 2009.

143. Recommended practices for surgical tissue banking. In: *Perioperative Standards and Recommended Practices.* Denver, CO: AORN, Inc; 2011: 201-214.

144. Recommended practices for the care and handling of specimens in the perioperative environment. In: *Perioperative Standards and Recommended Practices.* Denver, CO: AORN, Inc; 2011: 283-290.

145. Standardized packaging, labeling and transporting of organs, vessels, and tissue typing materials. Organ Procurement and Transplantation Network. *http://optn.transplant. hrsa.gov/PoliciesandBylaws2/policies/pdfs/policy_17.pdf.* Updated June 29, 2011. Accessed October 6, 2011.

146. Centers for Medicare & Medicaid Services. Department of Health and Human Services. Condition of participation: organ, tissue, and eye procurement. 24 CFR §482.45. *http://ecfr.gpoaccess.gov/cgi/t/text/text-idx?c=e cfr&sid=161a6bff7c036b1836ab37d4d1604d53&rgn=di v8&view=text&node=42:5.0.1.1.1.3.4.13&idno=42.* Published June 22, 1998. Accessed October 6, 2011.

147. US Department of Labor, Occupational Safety and Health Standards. Bloodborne pathogens. 29 CFR §1910.1030. *http://www.osha.gov/pls/oshaweb/owa disp.show_document?p_table=standards&p_id=10051.* Accessed October 6, 2011.

148. Transplant safety. In: 2011 *Comprehensive Accreditation Manual for Hospitals.* Oakbrook Terrace, IL: Joint Commission Resources; 2011.

149. Recommended practices for traffic patterns in the perioperative practice setting. In: *Perioperative Standards and Recommended Practices*. Denver, CO: AORN, Inc; 2011: 95-98.

150. Mangram AJ, Horan TC, Pearson ML, Silver LC, Jarvis WR. Guideline for prevention of surgical site infection, 1999. *Infect Control Hosp Epidemiol*. 1999;20(4):247-278. doi:10.1086/501620.

151. Centers for Medicare & Medicaid Services. Department of Health and Human Services. Condition of participation: discharge planning. 42 CFR §482.43. *http://edocket.access.gpo.gov/cfr_2010/octqtr/pdf/42cfr482.43.pdf*. Accessed October 6, 2011.

152. National Patient Safety Goal 7: reduce the risk of health care–associated infections. In: *2011 Comprehensive Accreditation Manual for Hospitals*. Oakbrook Terrace, IL: Joint Commission Resources; 2011.

153. SCIP-Inf-4: Cardiac surgery patients with controlled 6 a.m. postoperative blood glucose. In: *The Specifications Manual for National Hospital Inpatient Quality Measures*. Version 3.3. Centers for Medicare & Medicaid Services and Joint Commission; 2011.

154. SCIP-Inf-6: Surgery patients with appropriate hair removal. In: *The Specifications Manual for National Hospital Inpatient Quality Measures*. Version 3.3. Centers for Medicare & Medicaid Services and Joint Commission; 2011.

155. *Guide to Patient Safety Indicators*. Version 3.1. Rockville, MD: Department of Health and Human Services Agency for Healthcare Research and Quality; 2007.

156. Recommended practices for reducing radiological exposure in the perioperative practice setting. In: *Perioperative Standards and Recommended Practices*. Denver, CO: AORN, Inc; 2011: 251-262.

157. ANSI Z136.4-2010: American National Standard Recommended Practice for Laser Safety Measurements for Hazard Evaluation. Orlando, FL: Laser Institute of America; 2010.

158. ANSI Z136.7-2008: American National Standard for Testing and Labeling of Laser Protective Equipment. Orlando, FL: Laser Institute of America; 2008.

159. Recommended practices for prevention of retained surgical items. In: *Perioperative Standards and Recommended Practices*. Denver, CO: AORN, Inc; 2011: 263-282.

160. 109th US Congress. Deficit Reduction Act of 2005. Pub L 109-171. February 8, 2006. *http://frwebgate.access.gpo.gov/cgi-bin/getdoc.cgi?dbname=109_cong_public_laws&docid=f:publ171.109.pdf*. Accessed October 6, 2011.

161. AORN guidance statement: creating a patient safety culture. In: *Perioperative Standards and Recommended Practices*. Denver, CO: AORN, Inc; 2011: 577-582.

162. Centers for Medicare & Medicaid Services. Department of Health and Human Services. Condition of participation: medical staff. 42 CFR §482.22. *http://edocket.access.gpo.gov/cfr_2004/octqtr/pdf/42cfr482.23.pdf*. Accessed October 6, 2011.

163. Centers for Medicare & Medicaid Services. Department of Health and Human Services. Condition for coverage—surgical services. 42 CFR §416.42. *http://www.gpo.gov/fdsys/pkg/CFR-2010-title42-vol3/pdf/CFR-2010-title42-vol3-sec416-42.pdf*. Published 2010. Accessed October 7, 2011.

164. Centers for Medicare & Medicaid Services. Department of Health and Human Services. Condition for coverage—laboratory and radiologic services. 42 CFR §416.49. *http://edocket.access.gpo.gov/cfr_2010/octqtr/pdf/42cfr416.49.pdf*. Published 2010. Accessed October 7, 2011.

165. Standard 1010: Anesthesia. Pre-anesthesia care. In: *Regular Standards and Checklist for Accreditation of Ambulatory Surgery Facilities*. 11th ed. Gurnee, IL: American Association for Accreditation of Ambulatory Surgery Facilities; 2007: 50-51.

166. Standard 4.020: Additional Medicare standards. In: *Medicare Standards and Checklist for Accreditation of Ambulatory Surgery Facilities*. 3rd ed. Gurnee, IL: American Association for Accreditation of Ambulatory Surgery Facilities; 2005: 22-24.

167. Standard 4.003: Patient charts. Medical history. In: *Medicare Standards and Checklist for Accreditation of Ambulatory Surgery Facilities*. 3rd ed. Gurnee, IL: American Association for Accreditation of Ambulatory Surgery Facilities; 2005: 19.

168. Centers for Medicare & Medicaid Services. Department of Health and Human Services. Condition of participation: pharmaceutical services. 42 CFR §482.25. *http://edocket.access.gpo.gov/cfr_2010/octqtr/pdf/42cfr482.25.pdf*. Published 2010. Accessed October 7, 2011.

169. National Patient Safety Goal. NPSG 2: Improve the effectiveness of communication among caregivers. In: *2011 Comprehensive Accreditation Manual for Hospitals*. Oakbrook Terrace, IL: Joint Commission Resources; 2011.

170. Standard 04.E. Quality of care provided. In: *Accreditation Handbook for Ambulatory Health Care*. 2009 ed. Skokie, IL: Accreditation Association for Ambulatory Health Care, Inc; 2009: 32.

171. Standard 06K. Clinical records and health information. In: *Accreditation Handbook for Ambulatory Health Care*. Skokie, IL: Accreditation Association for Ambulatory Health Care, Inc; 2009:38-39.

172. Recommended practices for high-level disinfection. In: *Perioperative Standards and Recommended Practices*. Denver, CO: AORN, Inc; 2011: 399-414.

173. Recommended practices for sterilization in the perioperative practice setting. In: *Perioperative Standards and Recommended Practices*. Denver, CO: AORN, Inc; 2011: 463-486.

174. Standard 230. Operating room policy, environment and procedures. Procedures—sterilization. In: *Regular Standards and Checklist for Accreditation of Ambulatory Surgery Facilities*. 11th ed. Gurnee, IL: American Association for Accreditation of Ambulatory Surgery Facilities; 2007: 14.

175. Standard 9.001. Requirements for facility classification. In: *Medicare Standards and Checklist for Accreditation of Ambulatory Surgery Facilities*. 3rd ed. Gurnee, IL: American Association for Accreditation of Ambulatory Surgery Facilities; 2005: 42-45.

176. Standard 10M. In: *2009 Accreditation Handbook for Ambulatory Health Care*. Skokie, IL: Accreditation Association for Ambulatory Health Care, Inc; 2009: 51.

177. Recommended practices for the prevention of unplanned perioperative hypothermia. In: *Perioperative Standards and Recommended Practices*. Denver, CO: AORN, Inc; 2011: 307-320.

178. Clinical practice guideline 1: ASPAN's evidence-based clinical practice guideline for the promotion of perioperative normothermia. In: *Perianesthesia Nursing Standards and Practice Recommendations 2010-2012*. Cherry Hill, NJ: American Society of PeriAnesthesia Nurses; 2010: 24-45.

179. Preventing the retention of foreign objects during interventional radiology procedures. *Pa Patient Saf Advis*. 2008;5(1):24-27.

180. Sales representatives and other outsiders in the OR. *Oper Room Risk Manag*. 2007; 2(Quality Assurance/Risk Management 7):1-9.

181. Use of blunt-tip suture needles to decrease percutaneous injuries to surgical personnel: safety and health information bulletin. Atlanta, GA. National Institute for Occupational Safety and Health; 2007: *http://www.cdc.gov/niosh/docs/2008-101/*. Accessed October 20, 2011.

182. Rutala WA, Weber DJ; Healthcare Infection Control Practices Advisory Committee (HICPAC). *Guideline for Disinfection and Sterilization in Healthcare Facilities, 2008*. Atlanta, GA: Centers for Disease Control and Prevention; 2008.

183. *Pommier v ABC Insurance Company*, 715 So2d 1270, 1297-1342 (La.App.3dCir. 1998).

184. *Lama v Borras*, 1994 16 F3d 473 (United States Court of Appeals, First Circuit, February 25, 1994). *http://law.justia.com/cases/federal/appellate-courts/F3/16/473/491880/*. Accessed October 20, 2011.

185. *Ledesma v Shashoua*, 2007 WL 2214650 (Tex App, August 3, 2007). *http://www.nalnc.org/lnc_court_cases/Ledesma%20v.%20Shashoua.htm*. Accessed October 20, 2011.

186. Centers for Medicare & Medicaid Services. Department of Health and Human Services. Condition of participation: Anesthesia services. 42 CFR §482.52. Published 2009.

187. Centers for Medicare & Medicaid Services. Department of Health and Human Services. Condition of participation: food and dietetic services. 42 CFR §482.28.

188. US Food and Drug Administration. Department of Health and Human Services. Medical device tracking requirements. 21 CFR §821. Updated April 2010. Accessed May 20, 2010.

189. Centers for Medicare & Medicaid Services. Department of Health and Human Services. Condition of participation: radiologic services. 42 CFR §482.26. Published 2010.

190. Social Security Act, 42 USC 1396d §1905, Pub L No. 74-271.

191. Medical device tracking; guidance for industry and FDA staff. US Food and Drug Administration. 2010. *http://www.fda.gov/MedicalDevices/DeviceRegulationandGuidance/GuidanceDocuments/ucm071756.htm*. Accessed October 20, 2011.

192. Food and Drug Administration Modernization Act of 1997, S 830, 105th Cong, 1st Sess (1997), Pub L No 105-115.

193. Overview certification & compliance. Centers for Medicare & Medicaid Services. Updated December 14, 2005. *http://www.cms.gov/certificationandcomplianc/01_overview.asp?*. Accessed October 20, 2011.

194. About DNV accreditation. DNV. *http://www.dnvaccreditation.com/pr/dnv/about.aspx*. Accessed October 20, 2011.

195. Overview. Healthcare Facilities Accreditation Program. *http://www.hfap.org/about/overview.aspx*. Accessed October 20, 2011.

196. *2011 Comprehensive Accreditation Manual for Hospitals*. Oakbrook Terrace, IL: Joint Commission Resources; 2011.

197. *2011 Comprehensive Accreditation Manual for Ambulatory Care*. Oakbrook Terrace, IL: Joint Commission Resources; 2011.

198. Hospital compare. US Department of Health and Human Services. *http://www.hospitalcompare.hhs.gov/*. Accessed October 20, 2011.

199. US Department of Health and Human Services. Ambulatory surgical center payment system and CY 2011 payment rates. *Fed Regist*. 2010;75(226):71799-72580. *http://edocket.access.gpo.gov/2010/pdf/2010-27926.pdf*. Accessed October 20, 2011.

200. Surgical Care Improvement Project. *http://www.qualitynet.org/dcs/ContentServer?c=Page&pagename=QnetPublic%2FPage%2FQnetTier2&cid=1141662756099*. Accessed October 20, 2011.

201. US Department of Health and Human Services. Medicare program: hospital inpatient value-based purchasing program. *Fed Regist*. 2011;76(9):2454-2491. *http://www.gpo.gov/fdsys/pkg/FR-2011-01-13/pdf/2011-454.pdf*. Accessed October 20, 2011.

202. 2010 ORYX Performance Measure Reporting Requirements for Hospitals and Guidelines for Measure Selections. 2010. *http://www.jointcommission.org/assets/1/18/2010_ORYX_Performance_Measure_Reporting_Requirements.pdf*. Accessed October 20, 2011.

203. Straube BM. Letter to David T. Tayloe Jr. [written communication]. Baltimore, MD: Department of Health & Human Services; 2010. *http://practice.aap.org/public/Straube%20Letter%20to%20Tayloe.PDF*. Accessed September 30, 2011.

204. Centers for Medicare & Medicaid Services. US Department of Health and Human Services. Condition for coverage—patient rights. 42 CFR §416.50. Published 2010.

205. Record of care, treatment, and services. RC.02.03.07. Qualified staff receive and record verbal orders. In: *2011 Comprehensive Accreditation Manual for Ambulatory Care*. Oakbrook Terrace, IL: Joint Commission Resources; 2011.

206. Dawson A, Orsini MJ, Cooper MR, Wollenburg K. Medication safety—reliability of preference cards. *AORN J*. 2005;82(3):399.

207. Cole LM. Med report. Documenting to reduce medication errors. *OR Nurse*. 2008;2(7):17-19.

208. Medication management. MM.04.01.0. Medication orders are clear and accuarate. In: *2011 Comprehensive Accreditation Manual for Hospitals*. Oakbrook Terrace, IL: Joint Commission Resources; 2011.

209. Medication management. MM.04.01.01. Medication orders are clear and accurate. In: *2011 Comprehensive Accreditation Manual for Ambulatory Care*. Oakbrook Terrace, IL: Joint Commission Resources; 2011.

210. Broussard M, Bass PF 3rd, Arnold CL, McLarty JW, Bocchini JA Jr. *J Pediatr.* 2009;154(6):865-868. doi:10.1016/j.jpeds.2008.12.022.

211. Stevenson JG, Brunetti L, Santell JP, Hicks RW. USP medication safety forum. The impact of abbreviations on patient safety. *Joint Comm J Qual Patient Saf.* 2007;33(9):576-583.

212. Smith L. How to chart by exception. *Nursing.* 2002;32(9):30.

213. Noone JM. How to chart by exception. *J Nurs Adm.* 2000;30(7-8):342-343.

214. Murphy EK. Charting by exception. *AORN J.* 2003;78(5):821-823.

215. Anderson LA, Schramm CA. Adapting charting by exception to the perianesthesia setting. *J Perianesth Nurs.* 1999;14(5):260-269.

216. Short MS. Charting by exception on a clinical pathway. *Nurs Manage.* 1997;28(8):45-46.

217. Samuels JG. Abstracting pain management documentation from the electronic medical record: comparison of three hospitals. *Appl Nurs Res.* In press. doi:10.1016/j.apnr.2010.05.001.

218. Holden RJ. Cognitive performance-altering effects of electronic medical records: an application of the human factors paradigm for patient safety. *Cogn Technol Work.* 2011;13(1):11-29.

219. *Driving Quality and Performance Measurement—A Foundation for Clinical Decision Support: A Consensus Report.* Washington, DC: National Quality Forum; 2010.

220. Committee on Data Standards for Patient Safety, Board on Health Care Services, Institute of Medicine of the National Academies. *Key Capabilities of an Electronic Health Record System: Letter Report.* Washington, DC: National Academies Press; 2003.

221. Modifications to the HIPAA Privacy, Security, and Enforcement Rules Under the Health Information Technology for Economic and Clinical Health Act: Proposed Rule. *Fed Regist.* 2010;75(134):40868-40924. Codified at 45 CFR §160 and §164. *http://edocket.access.gpo.gov/2010/pdf/2010-16718.pdf.* Accessed October 11, 2011.

222. Health Insurance Portability and Accountability Act of 1996, 42 USC §201 (1996), Pub L No. 104-191, 110 Stat 1936.

223. Nelson ML. HIE provider verification: the privacy and security elephant in the room. *JHIM.* 2011;25(1):44-47.

224. Walsh D, Passerini K, Varshney U, Fjermestad J. Safeguarding patient privacy in electronic healthcare in the USA: the legal view. *Int J Electron Healthc.* 2008;4(3-4):311-326.

225. Malin B, Airoldi E. Confidentiality preserving audits of electronic medical record access. *Stud Health Technol Inform.* 2007;129(Pt 1):320-324.

226. *2010 HIMSS Analytics Report: Security of Patient Data Commissioned by Kroll's Fraud Solutions.* Chicago, IL: HIMSS Analytics; 2010.

227. AHIMA e-HIM Work Group on Maintaining the Legal EHR. Maintaining a legally sound health record: paper and electronic. *J AHIMA.* 2005;76(10):64A-L.

228. Kane B, Sands DZ. Guidelines for the clinical use of electronic mail with patients. The AMIA Internet Working Group, Task Force on Guidelines for the Use of Clinic-Patient Electronic Mail. *J Am Med Inform Assoc.* 1998;5(1):104-111.

229. US Department of Health and Human Services. *Nationwide Privacy and Security Framework for Electronic Exchange of Individually Identifiable Health Information.* Washington, DC: Office of the National Coordinator for Health Information Technology; 2008. *http://healthit.hhs.gov/portal/server.pt/gateway/PTARGS_0_10731_848088_0_0_18/NationwidePS_Framework-5.pdf.* Accessed October 11, 2011.

230. US Federal Trade Commission. Health breach notification rule. 16 CFR §318 (2009). *http://ecfr.gpoaccess.gov/cgi/t/text/text-idx?c=ecfr&tpl=/ecfrbrowse/Title16/16cfr318_main_02.tpl.* Accessed October 11, 2011.

231. Connecting for Health Work Group on Consumer Access Policies for Networked Personal Health Information. *Security and Systems Requirements.* New York, NY: Markle Foundation; 2008.

232. Centers for Medicare & Medicaid Services. Department of Health and Human Services. Condition of participation: surgical services. Standard: delivery of service. 42 CFR §482.51(b) (2004). *http://edocket.access.gpo.gov/cfr_2010/octqtr/pdf/42cfr482.51.pdf.* Accessed October 11, 2011.

233. Condition for Coverage—Medical Records. Standard: Form and Content of Record. 42 CFR §416.47(b). In: *State Operations Manual Appendix L - Guidance for Surveyors: Ambulatory Surgical Centers.* Rev.56, issued December 30, 2009. Baltimore, MD: Centers for Medicare & Medicaid Services; 2009. *http://cms.gov/manuals/Downloads/som107ap_l_ambulatory.pdf.* Accessed October 11, 2011.

234. Rights and responsibilities of the individual. RI.01.03.01. The hospital honors the patient's right to give or withhold informed consent. In: *2011 Comprehensive Accreditation Manual for Ambulatory Care.* Oakbrook Terrace, IL: Joint Commission Resources; 2011.

235. Rights and responsibilities of the individual. RI.01.03.03. The hospital honors the patient's right to give or withhold informed consent to produce or use recordings, films, or other images of the patient for purposes other than his or her care. In: *2011 Comprehensive Accreditation Manual for Ambulatory Care.* Oakbrook Terrace, IL: Joint Commission Resources; 2011.

236. Rights and responsibilities of the individual. RI.01.03.01. The hospital honors the patient's right to give or withhold informed consent. In: *2011 Comprehensive Accreditation Manual for Hospitals.* Oakbrook Terrace, IL: Joint Commission Resources; 2011.

237. Rights and responsibilities of the individual. RI.01.03.03. The hospital honors the patient's right to give or withhold informed consent to produce or use recordings, films, or other images of the patient for purposes other than his or her care. In: *2011 Comprehensive Accreditation Manual for Hospitals.* Oakbrook Terrace, IL: Joint Commission Resources; 2011.

238. The AMA Code of Medical Ethics' opinion on computerized medical records. *AMA J Ethics.* 2011;13(3):161-162.

239. Record of care, treatment, and services. RC.01.02.01. Entries in the medical record are authenticated. In: *2011 Comprehensive Accreditation*

Manual for Ambulatory Care. Oakbrook Terrace, IL: Joint Commission Resources; 2011.

240. Record of care, treatment, and services. RC.01.04.01. The hospital audits its medical records. In: *2011 Comprehensive Accreditation Manual for Hospitals*. Oakbrook Terrace, IL: Joint Commission Resources; 2011.

241. Electronic health record incentive program: final rule. *Fed Regist*. 2010;75(144):44314-44588. Codified at 42 CFR §412, 413, 422, et al. *http://edocket.access .gpo.gov/2010/pdf/2010-17207.pdf*. Accessed October 21, 2011.

242. Centers for Medicare & Medicaid Services. Department of Health and Human Services. Conditions of participation: clinical records. 42 CFR §485.638. *http://www.gpo.gov/fdsys/pkg/CFR-2010-title42-vol5/ pdf/CFR-2010-title42-vol5-sec485-638.pdf*. Accessed October 11, 2011.

243. Electronic Signatures in Global and National Commerce Act. Pub L No. 106-229, 114 Stat 464.

244. US Food and Drug Administration. Department of Health and Human Services. Electronic records; electronic signatures. 21 CFR §11. Revised 2010.

245. *Practice Brief: Retention of Health Information (Updated)*. Chicago, IL: American Health Information Management Association; 2002.

246. Record of care, treatment, and services. RC.01.05.01. The hospital retains its medical records. In: *2011 Comprehensive Accreditation Manual for Hospitals*. Oakbrook Terrace, IL: Joint Commission Resources; 2011.

247. Record of care, treatment, and services. RC.01.05.01. The hospital retains its medical records. In: *2011 Comprehensive Accreditation Manual for Ambulatory Care*. Oakbrook Terrace, IL: Joint Commission Resources; 2011.

248. Campbell EM, Sittig DF, Guappone KP, Dykstra RH, Ash JS. Overdependence on technology: an unintended adverse consequence of computerized provider order entry. *AMIA Annu Symp Proc*. 2007:94-98.

249. Agrawal A, Glasser AR. Barcode medication. Administration implementation in an acute care hospital and lessons learned. *J Healthc Inf Manag*. 2009;23(4):24-29.

250. *Amendments, Corrections, and Deletions in the Electronic Health Record Toolkit*. Chicago, IL: American Health Information Management Association; 2009.

251. ECRI. Electronic health records. *Oper Room Risk Manag*. 2007;1A(Medical Records 7):1-23.

252. ECRI. Medical records. *Oper Room Risk Manag*. 2008;1(Medical Records 3):1-16.

253. Russo R, American Health Information Management Association. *Clinical Documentation Improvement*. Chicago, IL: American Health Information Management Association; 2010.

254. Magrabi F, Ong M, Runciman W, Coiera E. An analysis of computer-related patient safety incidents to inform the development of a classification. *J Am Med Inform Assoc*. 2010;17(6):663-670. doi:10.1136/ jamia.2009.002444.

255. Nunn S. Managing audit trails. *J AHIMA*. 2009;80(9):44-45.

Acknowledgements

LEAD AUTHOR
Sharon Giarrizzo-Wilson, MS, RN-BC, CNOR
Informatics Nurse Specialist
AORN, Inc
Denver, Colorado

CONTRIBUTING AUTHORS
Christine A. Anderson, PhD, RN
Educator/Staff Development
University of Michigan School of Nursing
Ypsilanti, Michigan

Antonia B. Hughes, MA, BSN, RN, CNOR
Perioperative Education Specialist
Baltimore Washington Medical Center
Edgewater, Maryland

Cathy A. Klein, JD, MSN, MSEd, RN-C
Attorney and Counselor at Law
Greenwood Village, CO

PUBLICATION HISTORY
Originally published March 1982, *AORN Journal*, as "Recommended practices for documentation of perioperative nursing care."

Format revision July 1982.

Revised March 1987; revised September 1991; revised November 1995; published June 1996.

Revised; published January 2000, *AORN Journal*. Reformatted July 2000.

Revised November 2011; published online as "Recommended practices for perioperative health care information management" in *Perioperative Standards and Recommended Practices*.

Recommended Practices for Managing the Patient Receiving Local Anesthesia

The following recommended practices were developed by the AORN Recommended Practices Committee and have been approved by the AORN Board of Directors. They were presented as proposed recommended practices for comments by members and others. They are effective January 1, 2007.

These recommended practices are intended as achievable recommendations representing what is believed to be an optimal level of practice. Policies and procedures will reflect variations in practice settings and/or clinical situations that determine the degree to which the recommended practices can be implemented.

AORN recognizes the numerous types of settings in which perioperative registered nurses practice. These recommended practices are intended as guidelines adaptable to various practice settings. These practice settings include traditional operating rooms, ambulatory surgery centers, physicians' offices, cardiac catheterization suites, endoscopy suites, radiology and interventional radiology departments, and all other areas where operative and other invasive procedures may be performed.

Purpose

These recommended practices provide guidelines for perioperative registered nurses managing patients receiving local infiltration or topical anesthesia, without the use of sedation or regional anesthesia. If any sedation is used, AORN's "Recommended practices for managing the patient receiving moderate sedation/analgesia" should be followed.[1] It is not the intent of these recommended practices to address situations that require the services of anesthesia care providers or to substitute the services of perioperative registered nurses in those situations that require the services of anesthesia care providers, regardless of the complexity of the surgical procedure.

Recommendation I

Patients should be assessed preoperatively by a perioperative registered nurse and an individualized plan of care developed.[2]

1. The criteria for the selection of patients to receive local anesthesia should be established through consensus and collaboration of the perioperative registered nurse, physicians, and other health care professionals within the organization where care is provided.[2-4] Although it has been shown that a variety of patients can be successfully managed with a local anesthetic, local anesthesia is not appropriate for every patient or all types of surgical procedures.[4,5] Highly nervous, apprehensive, or excitable patients, or those who are unable to cooperate because of their mental state or age may not be appropriate candidates for local anesthesia.[6]

2. A perioperative registered nurse should perform a preoperative nursing assessment for all patients undergoing local anesthesia.[3] The perioperative registered nurse should review the patient's history, physical examination findings, laboratory results, and other diagnostic test results as indicated. At a minimum, the perioperative registered nurse should assess the patient for
   - pulse, blood pressure, arterial oxygen percent saturation, skin integrity, level of consciousness, temperature, and respiration;[2]
   - allergies and sensitivities (eg, food, medications, tape, latex, prep solutions);[2]
   - age;
   - current medications and use of alternative/complementary therapies;
   - NPO status (ie, when the patient last consumed solids and/or liquids by mouth);
   - any chronic conditions such as coughs or tremors that may impede the ability of the surgeon to perform the procedure;[5]
   - ability to tolerate the required operative position for the duration of the procedure, as well as draping that may cover the face;[5,6]
   - past or present substance abuse (these conditions may require dosage adjustments for the anesthetics used);[2,7]
   - weight, particularly in children;[8]
   - the need for IV access and/or fluids based upon patient assessment data and plan of care;[9]
   - understanding of the plan of care;
   - ability to understand expectations for participation and ability to cooperate;[6]
   - preoperative pain level and expectation of intraoperative and postoperative pain control; and
   - signs and symptoms of anxiety and fear.[2]

Significant assessment findings allow the surgical team to make adjustments in patient care to provide the safest approach to the procedure and anesthesia.[3]

Each patient has a variety of unique physical characteristics that can influence his or her response to medications. Considerations include, but are not limited to, the patient's weight, age, presence of co-morbidities, medication tolerance.[3,4]

3. The appropriate staffing for the care of the patient should be based on the competency of the staff member and individualized patient assessment. The patient's clinical assessment or behavior may require the presence of a perioperative registered nurse whose sole responsibility is to monitor the patient.

Recommendation II

The perioperative registered nurse should provide information to the patient regarding expected outcomes, benefits, risks, surgical experience, and recovery process related to the operative or invasive procedure.

1. Information should include
   ♦ the expected sequence of events before, during, and immediately after the procedure;
   ♦ performance of pain assessment and administration of pain relief measures during and after the procedure; and
   ♦ postoperative signs and symptoms that should be reported to a designated health care provider.[2]

Recommendation III

The perioperative registered nurse should be knowledgeable about medication administration and be able to recognize both desired responses and adverse reactions to anesthetic medications.

1. Perioperative registered nurses should be familiar with potential adverse medication reactions, especially those associated with local anesthetics. Although rare, local anesthetic agents may cause cardiovascular, respiratory, or central nervous system depression. Adverse reactions stemming from hypersensitivity to the amide group of local anesthetics, the most common local agents (eg, lidocaine, bupivicaine, mepivicaine), are extremely rare and are usually reactions to the preservatives

used. Toxicity may occur if large amounts of local anesthetics are absorbed rapidly.[8-10]

Symptoms of toxicity include, but are not limited to,
♦ metallic taste,
♦ tinnitus,
♦ light-headedness,
♦ syncope,
♦ visual disturbances,
♦ numbness of tongue and lips,
♦ confusion,
♦ tremors,
♦ shivering,
♦ generalized seizures,
♦ tachycardia/hypertension (initially),
♦ bradycardia/hypotension (with increased toxicity),
♦ ventricular arrhythmias or cardiac arrest, and
♦ respiratory arrest.[8-11]

2. Emergency medications, a source of supplemental oxygen, suction apparatus, resuscitative equipment, and qualified personnel should be readily available.[9-11] At a minimum, personnel should be competent in basic life support. Serious cardiac or respiratory complications can occur abruptly after the administration of local anesthetic medications. If the medication enters the bloodstream directly, seizures, circulatory and respiratory distress, cardiovascular collapse, or even death can result.[9-11]

3. Techniques should be considered to aid in minimizing the amount of discomfort associated with administration of local anesthetic. These include, but are not limited to:
   ♦ reassurance and distraction (eg, deep breathing, music, conversing with patient),
   ♦ prior application of a topical anesthetic (eg, a cream mixture of lidocaine 2.5% and prilocaine 2.5% in an emulsion base);
   ♦ warming the anesthetic to 37°–42° C;
   ♦ buffering of the local anesthetic agent;
   ♦ use of fine gauge needles (ie, 27–29 gauge);
   ♦ slow, incremental injections; and
   ♦ using smallest volume of solution necessary.[10-13]

Recommendation IV

The perioperative registered nurse managing the nursing care of the patient receiving local anesthesia should monitor and interpret the patient's physiological and psychological responses throughout the procedure.

1. The parameters monitored and the frequency of observation should be individualized to the patient and the surgical procedure.

2. Minimum patient monitoring throughout the procedure should include the patient's
   ♦ heart rate and regularity,
   ♦ respiratory rate,
   ♦ level of consciousness,[9]
   ♦ amount of local anesthetic administered,[13]
   ♦ pain level,[2] and
   ♦ response to medications.[2]

   Additional monitoring parameters may include, but are not limited to,
   ♦ blood pressure,[14]
   ♦ oxygen saturation by pulse oximetry,[14] and
   ♦ skin temperature and color[9,14,]

3. The perioperative registered nurse should monitor the amount of local anesthetic given. Toxic effects are dose-related, especially in children, because the dose-to-weight ratio can easily be overestimated.[8,10] The patient should be monitored not only for physiological changes but for any behavioral changes that may occur due to medications and/or other factors related to the surgical encounter. Monitoring the patient's physiological and psychological status facilitates early detection of potential complications.[10,11,13,14]

4. The perioperative registered nurse should recognize and report to the physician significant changes in the patient's status and should be prepared to initiate appropriate interventions. Immediate intervention at the earliest signs of toxicity can prevent serious complications.[11]

5. The perioperative registered nurse should reassess the patient postprocedure and before discharge to identify any potential latent reactions that may put the patient at risk.[15] If indicated by the postoperative assessment, the patient should be discharged in the company of a responsible adult who is given the appropriate postoperative care instructions.

Recommendation V

Holistic care interventions should be considered and offered to the local anesthetic patient to promote an atmosphere of comfort throughout the procedural experience.

1. Holistic comfort interventions should be considered as they have been shown to positively affect physical and psychological patient outcomes. The use of holistic interventions should be coordinated between the patient and procedural team members. While giving the patient a sense of control, the use of one or more interventions may reduce patient stress and anxiety, decrease pain and narcotic use, decrease side effects, and length of stay.[16-19]

2. Interventions may include, but are not limited to,
   ♦ therapeutic communication,
   ♦ guided imagery,
   ♦ music, and
   ♦ touch.[17-19]

3. Therapeutic communication should begin with the preoperative encounter. The perioperative registered nurse should ask the patient about concerns he or she may have. It is important for the perioperative registered nurse to listen actively to the patient's responses and react with kindness and caring concern for the patient's well-being.

   Additional forms of therapeutic communication, such as guided imagery, may be considered for enhancing patient comfort. Guided imagery is a technique used to divert and focus the patient's thoughts into a state in which the mind is calm, thus leading to relaxation.[16] Patients experience less preoperative and postoperative anxiety, report less pain, and require nearly 50% less narcotic medication when guided imagery is used.[19] Although the actual guided imagery techniques may vary, many organizations supply patients with scripted tapes or CDs to listen to up to several weeks before and, in many cases, during and after their surgery.[16,18,20,21]

4. Music may be used either with guided imagery or alone to enhance relaxation and divert the patient's attention away from frightening or unfamiliar noises. Music can aid in decreasing pain by stimulating the release of endorphins.[16] Patients also experience a decrease in epinephrine levels resulting in lower respiratory rate, heart rate, blood pressure, and anxiety scores when listening to music.[22]

   Research has shown that offering a choice of music to patients or allowing them to bring their own (ie, giving them a sense of situational control) has a particularly beneficial effect.[23-25]

Patients wearing headphones report positive experiences because surrounding noises and conversations within the perioperative care areas were filtered out.[17,24,26-29]

5. Touch may be used to convey a sense of reassurance, comfort, and caring. Whether it is simply holding an anxious patient's hand or performing therapeutic touch or massage, the effect conveys compassion and caring on the nurse's part. This promotes a more positive nurse-patient relationship.[17,29]

Recommendation VI

The perioperative nurse should document information to facilitate continuity of care and provide retrievable information for evaluating the care given.

1. Documentation of patient care should reflect the perioperative plan of care which includes assessment, diagnosis, outcome identification, planning, implementation, and evaluation.[30] Documentation of all nursing care is legally and professionally important for clear communication, collaboration among health care providers, and continuity of patient care.

2. Documentation should include, but not be limited to,
   - preoperative assessment;
   - vital signs;
   - level of consciousness;
   - dosage, route, time, and effect of local anesthetics;
   - significant untoward patient reactions and their resolutions; and
   - postoperative evaluation based on preoperative assessment data.

3. The Perioperative Nursing Data Set, the uniform perioperative nursing vocabulary, should be used to document patient care and to develop policies and procedures related to managing the patient receiving local anesthesia. The outcomes of primary importance to this recommended practice include the following.
   - The patient demonstrates and/or reports adequate pain control throughout the perioperative period (O29).
   - The patient receives appropriate medication(s) safely administered during the perioperative period (O9).

   - The patient demonstrates knowledge of the expected responses to the operative or invasive procedure (O31).

   These outcomes fall within the domains of Safety (D1), Physiologic Responses (D2), and Behavioral Responses (D3). The associated interventions that may lead to the desired outcomes include, but are not limited to, the following.
   - Administers prescribed medications (I8).
   - Assesses pain control (I16).
   - Develops individualized plan of care (I30).
   - Elicits perceptions of surgery (I32).
   - Evaluates response to medications (I51).
   - Evaluates response to pain management interventions (I54).[2]

Recommendation VII

The health care facility's quality management program should include investigation of adverse events and near misses associated with administration of local anesthesia.

1. Adverse patient outcomes and near misses associated with administration of local anesthesia should be collected, analyzed, and used for performance improvement as part of the institution-wide performance improvement program. To evaluate the quality of patient care and formulate plans for corrective action, it is necessary to maintain a system of evaluation. When an adverse event occurs, the surgical team is responsible for reporting the event as soon as possible following the discovery.[31]

2. Following organizational policy, documentation of an event should include what happened, the date and time of incident, its location, and witnesses. Measures taken to reverse the situation and communications made regarding the outcome should also be included. This is considered a sound professional practice and demonstrates that all reasonable efforts were made to protect the patient's safety.[31]

3. A critical investigation should be conducted of any adverse patient safety process or outcome. Error and near miss reporting are the first steps to addressing error reduction.[32]

4. Elements of the root cause analysis tool should be considered in addressing the contributing

causes of an incident or adverse event (eg, human, process, system), identification of risks, and preventive measures.[33,34] Multidisciplinary teams should be involved in the process of review and address any changes in practice that can improve patient safety.

5. Action plans should be developed, approved, and implemented to provide solutions and improve care. Action plans should be based on the understanding of the processes in question, supporting policies/procedures, and relevant knowledge-based information.[35]

6. Action plans should be nonpunitive. Attention should be given to correct knowledge deficits, defects in the system, and deficient behavioral performances.[35]

Recommendation VIII

Education, competency assessment, and validation should be conducted prior to the perioperative registered nurse managing the care of a patient undergoing a procedure with local anesthesia.

1. Perioperative registered nurses should complete initial education and competency validation, to include
   - ♦ roles and responsibilities of personnel involved in a procedure with local anesthesia,
   - ♦ local anesthetics and safe medication administration,
   - ♦ care of the patient receiving local anesthesia,
   - ♦ patient safety,
   - ♦ guidelines and techniques for holistic comfort interventions,
   - ♦ processes for reporting adverse events, and
   - ♦ documentation.

2. Continuing education and competency assessment should occur at regular intervals, as designated by the organization's policy and the identified learning needs of the individual.

Recommendation IX

Policies and procedures for managing the patient receiving local anesthesia should be developed, reviewed, and revised at regularly scheduled intervals by a multidisciplinary team and be readily available in the practice setting.

1. These recommended practices should be used as guidelines for developing policies and pro-

cedures in the practice setting. Policies and procedures establish authority, responsibility, and accountability. They also serve as operational guidelines and assist in the development of patient safety, quality assessment, and quality improvement activities.[35]

2. Policies and procedures for managing patients receiving local anesthesia should include, but are not limited to,
   - ♦ patient selection criteria,
   - ♦ type and frequency of monitoring,
   - ♦ method and frequency of documentation,
   - ♦ medications that may be administered by the perioperative registered nurse and the level of monitoring skills required,
   - ♦ interventions that may be implemented based on preapproved protocol and that are within the scope of nursing practice,
   - ♦ discharge criteria,[15]
   - ♦ staffing requirements based upon the individualized needs of the patient, and
   - ♦ management of medical emergencies.

3. Ambulatory surgery facilities should develop policies and procedures for immediately transferring patients that require emergency care beyond the ambulatory surgical center's capability to an acute care facility.[36,37]

4. A review of policies and procedures should be included in orientation and ongoing staff member education.

REFERENCES
1. "Recommended practices for managing the patient receiving moderate sedation/analgesia," in *Standards, Recommended Practices, and Guidelines* (Denver: AORN, Inc, 2006) 433-440.
2. S C Beyea, ed, *Perioperative Nursing Data Set: The Perioperative Nursing Vocabulary*, second ed (Denver: AORN, Inc, 2002).
3. J Cassidy, R A Marley, "Preoperative assessment of the ambulatory patient," (Ambulatory Surgery) *Journal of PeriAnesthesia Nursing* 11 (October 1996) 334-343.
4. E N George et al, "Re-evaluating selection criteria for local anesthesia in day surgery," *The British Journal of Plastic Surgery* 57 (July 2004) 446-449.
5. R MacPherson, "Structured assessment tool to evaluate patient suitability for cataract surgery under local anesthesia," *British Journal of Anesthesia* 93 (August 2004) 521-524.
6. B Hutchisson, C B Nicoladis, "Topical anesthesia—A new approach to cataract surgery," *AORN Journal* 74 (September 2001) 339-360.
7. C F Iocolano, "Perioperative pain management in the chemically dependent patient," *Journal of PeriAnesthesia Nursing* 51 (October 2000) 329-347.

8. M J Donald, S Derbyshire, "Lignocaine toxicity; A complication of local anesthesia administered in the community," *Emergency Medicine Journal* 21 (2004) 249-250. Also available at *http://www.emjonline.com* (accessed 6 Sept 2006).

9. D Fogg, "Expiration dates; alcohol disinfection; OR consents; local anesthesia; marking surgical sites; moderate sedation," (Clinical Issues) *AORN Journal* 78 (August 2003) 295-302.

10. S Achar, S Kundu, "Principles of office anesthesia: Part I. Infiltrative anesthesia," *American Family Physician* 66 (July 2002) 91-94.

11. G L Weinberg, "Current concepts in resuscitation of patients with local anesthesia cardiac toxicity," *Regional Anesthesia and Pain Medicine* 27 (November/ December 2002) 568-575.

12. O Quaba et al, "A users guide for reducing pain of local anesthetic," *Emergency Medicine Journal* (Short Report) 22 (2005) 188-189. Also available at *http://www.emjonline.com* (accessed 6 Sept 2006).

13. D W Smith et al, "Local anesthesia: Topical application, local infiltration, and field block," *Postgraduate Medicine Online, http://www.postgradmed.com /issues/1999/08_99/smith.htm* (accessed 6 Sept 2006).

14. R H Stein, "The perioperative nurse's role in anesthesia management," *AORN Journal* 62 (November 1995) 794-804.

15. "Failure to monitor local anesthesia patient before discharge," (Nursing Law Case of the Month) *Nursing Law's Regan Report* 45 (1) 2 (June 2004).

16. D L Tusek, R E Cwynar, "Strategies for implementing a guided imagery program to enhance patient experience," (Clinical Issues Advanced Practice Acute Critical Care) *American Association of Critical-care Nurses* 11 (February 2000) 68-76.

17. C L Norred, "Minimizing preoperative anxiety with alternative caring-healing therapies," *AORN Journal* 72 (November 2000) 840-843.

18. C D Knight, "Alternative medicine calms perioperative patients," (Career Management) *Nursing Spectrum* (21 August 2000). Also available at *http://community .nursingspectrum.com/MagazineArticles/article.cfm?2060* (accessed 6 Sept 2006).

19. D Tusek et al, "Guided imagery as a coping strategy for perioperative patients," *AORN Journal* 66 (October 1997) 644-649.

20. L S Halpin et al, "Guided imagery in cardiac surgery," *Outcomes Management* 6 no 3 (2002) 132-137.

21. "Guided imagery: Its use in heart surgery and other procedures," (2005) Cleveland Clinic Heart and Vascular Institute, *http://www.clevelandclinic.org/heart center/pub/guide/prevention/stress/guided_imagery.htm* (accessed 6 Sept 2006).

22. M Brunges, G Avigne, "Music therapy for reducing surgical anxiety," *AORN Journal* 78 (November 2003) 816-818.

23. K Stevens, "Patients' perceptions of music during surgery," *Journal of Advanced Nursing* 15 (September 1990) 1045-1051.

24. E Mok, K Wong, "Effects of music on patient anxiety," *AORN Journal* 77 (February 2003) 396-410.

25. M Reilly, "Incorporating music into the surgical environment," *Plastic Surgical Nursing* 19 no 1 (Spring 1999) 35-38.

26. M F Cunningham et al, "Introducing a music program in the perioperative area," *AORN Journal* 66 (October 1997) 674-682.

27. P Augustin, A Hains, "Effect of music on ambulatory surgery patients' preoperative anxiety," *AORN Journal* 63 (April 1996) 750-758.

28. V Steelman, "Intraoperative music therapy: Effects on anxiety, blood pressure," *AORN Journal* 52 (November 1990) 1026-1034.

29. L D McRee et al, "Using massage and music therapy to improve postoperative outcomes," *AORN Journal* 78 (September 2003) 433-447.

30. "Recommended practices for documentation of perioperative nursing care," in *Standards, Recommended Practices, and Guidelines* (Denver: AORN, Inc, 2006) 477-479.

31. D Dunn, "Incident reports—Their purpose and scope," *AORN Journal* 74 (July 2003) 45-68.

32. B A Liang, "The adverse event of unaddressed medical error: Identifying and filling holes in the healthcare and legal systems," (Symposium: Patient Injury, Medical Errors, Liability and Reform) *The Journal of Law, Medicine & Ethics* 29 (2001) 346-368.

33. H Wald, K G Shojania, "Chapter 5: Root cause analysis," Agency for Healthcare Research and Quality, *http://www.ahrq.gov/clinic/ptsafety/chap5.htm* (accessed 6 Sept 2006).

34. "Root cause analysis", VA National Center for Patient Safety, *http://www.patientsafety.gov/rca.html* (accessed 6 Sept 2006).

35. "Quality and performance improvement standards for perioperative nursing," in *Standards, Recommended Practices, and Guidelines* (Denver: AORN, Inc, 2006) 405-414.

36. Joint Commission on Accreditation of Healthcare Organizations, *Comprehensive Accreditation Manual for Ambulatory Care* (Oakbrook Terrace, Ill: Joint Commission on Accreditation of Healthcare Organizations, 2006) PC-25.

37. Accreditation Association for Ambulatory Health Care, *Accreditation Handbook for Ambulatory Health Care, 2004* (Wilmette, IL: Accreditation Association for Ambulatory Health Care, 2004) 49.

RESOURCES

Stoelting, R K, Miller R D, "Chapter 7: Local anesthetics," in *Basics of Anesthesia*, fourth ed (Philadelphia: Churchill Livingstone, 2000) 80-88.

Guidelines of Care for Local and Regional Anesthesia, American Academy of Dermatology Practice Management, *http://www.aadassociation.org/Guidelines/anesthesia .html* (accessed 6 Sept 2006).

PUBLICATION HISTORY

Originally published May 1984, *AORN Journal.* Revised September 1989. Revised August 1993.

Revised November 1997; published February 1998. Reformatted July 2000.

Revised November 2001; published April 2002, *AORN Journal.*

Revised 2006; published in *Standards, Recommended Practices, and Guidelines,* 2007 edition.

Recommended Practices for Managing the Patient Receiving Moderate Sedation/Analgesia

The following recommended practices for managing the patient receiving moderate sedation/analgesia were developed by the AORN Recommended Practices Committee and have been approved by the AORN Board of Directors. They were presented as proposed recommendations for comments by members and others. They are effective January 1, 2008.

These recommended practices are intended as achievable recommendations representing what is believed to be an optimal level of practice. Policies and procedures will reflect variations in practice settings and/or clinical situations that determine the degree to which the recommended practices can be implemented.

AORN recognizes the various settings in which perioperative nurses practice. These recommended practices are intended as guidelines adaptable to various practice settings. These practice settings include traditional operating rooms, ambulatory surgery centers, physician's offices, cardiac catheterization laboratories, endoscopy suites, radiology departments, and all other areas where surgery may be performed.

References to nursing interventions (I) used in the Perioperative Nursing Data Set, second edition, (PNDS) are noted in parentheses when a recommended practice corresponds to a PNDS intervention.[1] The reader is referred to the PNDS for further explanation of perioperative nursing diagnoses, interventions, and outcomes.

Purpose

Moderate sedation/analgesia is a drug-induced, mild depression of consciousness achieved by the administration of sedatives or the combination of sedatives and analgesic medications, most often administered intravenously, and titrated to achieve a desired effect. The primary goal of moderate sedation/analgesia is to reduce the patient's anxiety and discomfort. Moderate sedation/analgesia also can facilitate cooperation between the patient and caregivers.[2] Moderate sedation/analgesia produces a condition in which the patient exhibits a mildly depressed level of consciousness and an altered perception of pain, but retains the ability to respond appropriately to verbal and/or tactile stimulation. The patient maintains protective reflexes, may experience some degree of amnesia, and has a rapid return to activities of daily living.[3]

The desired effect is a level of sedation with or without analgesia whereby the patient is able to tolerate diagnostic, therapeutic, and invasive procedures through relief of anxiety and pain. The four distinct characteristics of moderate sedation/analgesia are:

- The patient is able to respond purposefully to verbal commands or light tactile stimulation.
- The patient is able to maintain his or her protective reflexes and communicate verbally.
- The patient can maintain adequate, spontaneous ventilation.
- There are minimal variations in vital signs.[2]

Recommendation I

The perioperative registered nurse administering moderate sedation/analgesia must practice within the scope of nursing practice as defined by his or her state and should be compliant with state advisory opinions, declaratory rules, and other regulations that direct the practice of the registered nurse.[4]

The methods of monitoring used with patients who receive moderate sedation/analgesia, the medications selected and administered, and the interventions taken must be within the legal definitions of the scope of practice of the registered nurse.[5]

I.a. In accordance with state and local laws and regulations, a licensed independent practitioner qualified by education, training, and licensure to administer moderate sedation should supervise the administration of moderate sedation.

I.b. The perioperative registered nurse should consult with his or her state board of nursing for any changes or revisions to declaratory rulings and other guidelines that relate to the perioperative registered nurse's role as a provider of moderate sedation/analgesia.[5] (PNDS: I1)

The professional obligation of the perioperative registered nurse to safeguard clients is grounded in the ethical obligation to the patient, the profession, society, the American Nurses Association's (ANA) *Standards of Clinical Nursing Practice*, AORN's "Explications for perioperative nursing," and state nurse practice acts.[4,6]

Table 1

PHYSICAL STATUS CLASSIFICATION		
Status	**Definition of patient status**	**Example**
P1	A normal healthy patient	No physiologic, psychological, bio-chemical, or organic disturbance.
P2	A patient with mild systemic disease	Cardiovascular disease, asthma, chronic bronchitis, obesity, or diabetes mellitus.
P3	A patient with severe systemic disease	Cardiovascular or pulmonary disease that limits activity; severe diabetes with systemic complications; history of myocardial infarction, angina pectoris, or poorly controlled hypertension.
P4	A patient with severe systemic disease that is a constant threat to life	Severe cardiac, pulmonary, renal, hepatic, or endocrine dysfunction.
P5	A moribund patient who is not expected to survive without the operation	Surgery is done as a last recourse or resuscitative effort; major multi-system or cerebral trauma, ruptured aneurysm, or large pulmonary embolus.
P6	A declared brain-dead patient whose organs are being removed for donor purposes	

Reproduced with permission from the American Society of Anesthesiologists, Park Ridge, IL.

Recommendation II

Patient selection for moderate sedation/analgesia should be based on established criteria developed through interdisciplinary collaboration by health care professionals.

Certain patients may not be candidates for moderate sedation/analgesia administered by perioperative registered nurses. Such patients may require care provided by an anesthesia provider qualified to administer monitored anesthesia care and to rescue the patient from a deeper level of sedation, or qualified to convert to general anesthesia if needed.[5,7,8]

II.a. The perioperative registered nurse should assess the patient to determine the appropriateness of registered nurse-administered sedation/analgesia based on selection criteria defined by the health care organization. (PNDS: I59, I144, I60, I66, I68)

The American Society of Anesthesiologists (ASA) Physical Status Classification (**Table 1**) may be used as a means of determining patient appropriateness for registered nurse-administered sedation/analgesia. Patients classified as P1, P2, and a medically stable P3 are normally considered appropriate for registered nurse-administered moderate sedation/analgesia.[5,6]

II.b. Consultation with an anesthesia provider should be obtained if a patient presents with any one of the following:
- known history of respiratory or hemodynamic instability;
- previous difficulties with anesthesia or sedation;[2]
- severe sleep apnea or other airway related issues;[2]
- one or more significant co-morbidities;[2] (I58)
- pregnancy;[2]
- inability to communicate (eg, aphasic);
- inability to cooperate (eg, mentally incapacitated);[2]
- multiple drug allergies;
- multiple medications with potential for drug interaction with sedative analgesics;[2,3]
- current substance use (eg, street drugs, herbal supplements, nonprescribed prescription drugs);[5]
- ASA physical classification of an unstable P3;[3,5] and
- ASA physical classification of P4 or above.[3,5] (PNDS: I92, I111)

Recommendation III

The perioperative registered nurse should complete a patient assessment before administering moderate sedation/analgesia.

A presedation assessment determines a patient's suitability for registered nurse-administered moderate sedation/analgesia by identifying the potential for adverse events.

III.a. The presedation assessment should include, but is not limited to,[2,5,7]

– verification of consent explaining the risks, benefits, and alternatives to sedation;[2,5] (PNDS: I124)

– review of medical history; (PNDS: I111)

– review of physical examination of the cardiac and pulmonary systems, including vital signs;[1] (PNDS: I66, I58)

– review of height and weight;[3,5] (PNDS: I66)

– verification of pregnancy test results, when applicable; (PNDS: I66)

– review of present medication regimen (eg, prescribed, over-the-counter, herbals, supplements), medication taken within the last 48 hours including any as needed medications, especially opioids or other narcotics;[5] (PNDS: I17)

– review of substance use;[1,2,5] (PNDS: I66, I114)

– review of tobacco and alcohol use;[1,2,5] (PNDS: I66, I114)

– verification of allergies and sensitivities to medications, latex, chemical agents, foods, and adhesives;[1,2,5] (PNDS: I123)

– confirmation of NPO status;[2,5] (PNDS: I56, I66)

– determination of patient's ability to tolerate and maintain the required position for the duration of the planned procedure; and (PNDS: I64, I127)

– verification of a responsible adult caregiver to escort the patient home.[5,9] (PNDS: I80)

The fasting guidelines developed by the ASA may be used.[2]

III.b. The perioperative registered nurse should perform an assessment of the patient's airway before administering moderate sedation/analgesia. (PNDS: I66, I60, I15)

Support of the airway and positive-pressure bag-mask ventilation may be necessary if respirations are compromised by the respiratory depressive effects of moderate sedation medications.[2,5]

III.b.1. The presedation airway assessment should include, but is not limited to, the following risk factors for difficult mask ventilation:

- age > 55 years;[10]
- significant obesity (especially of the face, neck, and tongue);[2]
- missing teeth or edentulous;[10]
- presence of a beard;[10]

- history of snoring or sleep apnea;[10] and
- presence of stridor.[2]

III.c. The perioperative registered nurse should consult with an anesthesia provider if the patient presents with a history of severe obstructive sleep apnea.[2] (PNDS: I92, I64, I15, I111)

Administration of sedatives to the patient with central sleep apnea may inhibit the brain's signal to wake up and breathe.[11]

III.d. Additional precautions should be taken for patients with sleep apnea. (PNDS: I64, I92, I87, I121)

Moderate sedation medications may cause relaxation of the oropharyngeal structures resulting in partial or total airway obstruction.[2,11]

III.d.1. Care of the patient with sleep apnea should include, but is not limited to,

- management by an anesthesia provider if the patient has severe central sleep apnea;[2]
- positioning in the lateral or semi-Fowlers position, if at all possible;
- use of continuous positive airway pressure (CPAP) machines during the procedure and recovery periods for patients who routinely use CPAP machines when they sleep;[11] and
- continuous monitoring and positioning to facilitate an open airway.[11]

III.e. The perioperative registered nurse should collaborate with the licensed independent practitioner in developing and documenting the sedation/analgesia plan.[7]

Recommendation IV

The perioperative registered nurse monitoring the patient receiving moderate sedation/analgesia should have no other responsibilities that would require leaving the patient unattended or would compromise continuous monitoring during the procedure.[12]

Continuous monitoring of the patient's physiological and psychological status by the perioperative registered nurse leads to early detection of potential complications.[12]

IV.a. A designated perioperative registered nurse should continually monitor the patient during administration of moderate sedation/analgesia.[1,2,7] (PNDS: I30, I27, I128)

IV.b.   An additional perioperative registered nurse should be assigned to the circulating role during the administration of moderate sedation.[7]

IV.c.   When moderate sedation is administered, the supervising licensed independent practitioner should remain immediately available during the procedure and recovery period.

Recommendation V

The perioperative registered nurse should know the recommended dose, recommended dilution, onset, duration, effects, potential adverse reactions, drug compatibility, and contraindications for each medication used during moderate sedation/analgesia.

Safe administration of medications for moderate sedation and analgesia requires knowledge of the intended purpose and potential adverse effects of each medication and continuous monitoring of the patient responses to the medications.[2,5]

V.a.   When medications are administered by the oral, rectal, intramuscular, or transmucosal routes, sufficient time should be allowed for drug absorption and onset before considering additional medication.[2] (PNDS: I8, I51)

       The absorption rate of nonintravenous medications is unpredictable.[2]

V.b.   The need for IV access should be assessed and will vary depending on the level of sedation intended; the route of sedative administration (eg, oral); and organizational policy, procedure, and protocol. (PNDS: I34)

      – Maintaining IV access throughout the procedure allows for additional sedation as well as resuscitative medications.[2]

      – Intravenous administration of both a sedative and an analgesic provides effective moderate sedation/analgesia.[2]

      – Sedatives (eg, benzodiazepines) may be prescribed to reduce anxiety.[2,3,5]

      – Analgesics (eg, opioid agonists) may be prescribed to manage pain.[2,3,5]

V.c.   Each IV agent should be administered separately in incremental doses and titrated to desired effect (ie, moderate sedation/analgesia that enables the patient to maintain his or her protective reflexes, airway patency, spontaneous ventilation).[2,5] (PNDS: I51, I89)

The incremental administration of agents decreases the risk for overdose and respiratory or circulatory depression because the person administrating the agents may better observe the patient's response to the medications given.[2,3,5]

V.d.   Opioid antagonists (ie, naloxone) and benzodiazepine antagonists (ie, flumazenil) should be readily available whenever opioids and benzodiazepines are administered.[2,3] (PNDS: I51, I89)

V.e.   Only persons trained in administering general anesthesia should administer propofol for moderate sedation/analgesia. (PNDS: I1)

      On April 14, 2004, the American Association of Nurse Anesthetists (AANA) and the ASA in a joint statement said:

> *"Because sedation is a continuum, it is not always possible to predict how an individual patient will respond. Due to the potential for rapid, profound changes in sedative/analgesia depth and the lack of antagonistic medications, agents such as propofol require special attention.*
>
> *Whenever propofol is used for sedation/anesthesia, it should be administered only by persons trained in the administration of general anesthesia, who are not simultaneously involved in these surgical or diagnostic procedures. This restriction is concordant with specific language in the propofol insert, and failure to follow these recommendations could put patients at increased risk of significant injury or death.*
>
> *Similar concerns apply when other intravenous induction agents are used for sedation, such as thiopental, methohexital or etomidate."*[2,7,13]

The AORN Board of Directors endorsed this statement on January 14, 2005.

Recommendation VI

The perioperative registered nurse should continuously monitor the patient throughout the procedure.[1,5,7]

Continuous monitoring throughout the procedure enables the perioperative registered nurse to use clinical data to implement or modify the plan of care.[5]

VI.a. The perioperative registered nurse, at a minimum, should continuously monitor the patient's heart rate and function via electrocardiogram (ECG); oxygenation using pulse oximetry; respiratory rate and adequacy of ventilation; blood pressure; level of consciousness (LOC); comfort level; and skin condition at regular intervals.[2,7] (PNDS: I89, I87, I59, I128)

VI.b. The method and the flow rate of administering oxygen should be determined based upon achieving the patient's optimal level of oxygen saturation level as measured with pulse oximetry. (PNDS: I87)

A patient's restlessness resulting from hypercapnia and hypoxia may be misinterpreted as discomfort.

The administration of oxygen does not prevent apnea. Patients manifesting restlessness in the absence of a change in pulse oximetry readings may be overmedicated.[14]

VI.c. Monitoring end-tidal carbon dioxide by capnography should be considered for those patients whose ventilation cannot be directly observed during the procedure.[2] (PNDS: I87, I89, I128)

VI.d. Vital signs should be monitored before the start of the procedure, after administration of sedative or analgesic medications, and at least every five minutes during the procedure based on the patient's condition, type and amount of medication administered, and length of procedure.[2] (PNDS: I89, I128)

VI.e. The patient's LOC and ability to respond to verbal commands should be a routine assessment indicator, except in patients unable to respond (eg, young children, mentally impaired, dental surgery).[2,3] (PNDS: I144, I145, I128)

Assessing the patient's LOC by his or her verbal responses at regular intervals during the procedure can quickly determine if the patient is also breathing well. In addition, verbally reassuring the patient can divert his or her attention and assist in reducing anxiety.[2]

VI.f. Equipment should be present, working properly, and and immediately available in the room where the procedure is performed.[7] (PNDS: I122, I138, I120, I87)

VI.f.1. The following age- and size-appropriate equipment and supplies should be present:
- suction;
- airway management devices (eg, oral, nasal airways; mask ventilation devices);
- noninvasive blood pressure monitoring device;
- pulse oximetry;
- electrocardiograph; and
- sedative and analgesic antagonists.[2,15]

VI.g. An emergency resuscitation cart should be immediately available in every location in which moderate sedation/analgesia is administered. (PNDS: I121, I120, I87)

While careful titration of sedation and analgesics to obtain the desired effect can be very safe when using short-acting agents; respiratory depression, hypotension, or impaired cardiovascular function are common sequelae of sedation and analgesia.[2,5]

VI.g.1. An emergency cart should include
- resuscitation medications;
- intravenous access equipment;
- intravenous fluids; and
- life-support equipment (eg, defibrillator, endotracheal intubation equipment, mechanical positive bag-value mask device).

Recommendation VII

The perioperative registered nurse should monitor the patient who receives moderate sedation/analgesia postoperatively.

Recovery time will depend on the type and amount of sedation/analgesia given, procedure performed, and organizational policy.

VII.a. The same monitoring parameters used during the procedure should be used during the recovery phase. (PNDS: I45, I44, I87, I120, I121)

VII.a.1. Postoperative patient care and monitoring should be consistent for all patients.

VII.a.2. Postoperative monitoring should include, but is not limited to,
- heart rate and rhythm;[5,9]
- LOC;[5,7,9]
- blood pressure;[5,9]
- cardiac monitoring;[5]

- oxygenation monitored by pulse oximetry with an audible pulse rate and alarms;[9] and
- ventilation monitored by direct observation and/or auscultation.[9]

VII.b. All patients should be assessed postoperatively. (PNDS: I4, I3, I16, I130, I153, I54)

VII.b.1. Postoperative patient care assessments should include, but are not limited to:
- wound condition;[5,9]
- dressing condition;[5,9]
- line patency,[5]
- amount of drainage in drains;[5] and
- level of pain.[5,7,9]

Recommendation VIII

The perioperative registered nurse should evaluate the patient for discharge readiness based on specific discharge criteria.[5,7]

Recovery time will depend on the type and amount of sedation/analgesia given, procedure performed, and organizational policy.

VIII.a. Discharge criteria should be developed collaboratively and agreed upon by nursing, surgery, medicine, and anesthesia services. (PNDS: I92)

Establishing discharge criteria may minimize the risk of cardiorespiratory depression after the patient has been released.[16-18]

VIII.b. Patients should remain awake for at least 20 minutes without stimulation before they are considered ready for discharge.[9] (PNDS: I146)

The incorporation of a sedation scale in combination with a modified wakefulness test has been reported as ensuring a more objective criterion as compared to using the caregiver's judgment alone.[9]

VIII.c. Children receiving medication with a long half-life should be monitored post-procedure until able to meet discharge criteria and remain awake for at least 20 minutes without stimulation.[15]

There are numerous reports of deaths of prematurely discharged children that have died in the back seats of cars on the ride home from airway obstruction related to the administration of long-acting agents (eg, chloral hydrate).[9,17]

VIII.d. Discharge criteria should be consistently applied to all patients. (PNDS: I89, I27, I146, I44, I45, I51, I143)

VII.d.1. Criteria for discharge may include, but are not limited to:
- return to preoperative, baseline LOC;
- stability of vital signs;
- sufficient time interval (eg, two hours) since the last administration of an antagonist (eg, naloxone, flumazenil) to prevent resedation of the patient;[2,19]
- use of an objective patient assessment scoring system (eg, Aldrete Recovery Score);[2,20]
- absence of protracted nausea;
- intact protective reflexes;
- adequate pain control; and
- return of motor/sensory control.

VIII.e. Patients and/or their caregivers should receive verbal and written discharge instructions.[5] (PNDS: I50, I80)

Medications used for moderate sedation/analgesia cause retrograde amnesia reducing patient's ability to recall events during the immediate postoperative period.

VIII.e.1. A copy of the written discharge instructions should be given to the patient and a copy should be placed in the patient's medical record.[20]

VIII.e.2. The patient and/or caregiver should be able to verbalize an understanding of the discharge instructions.

Recommendation IX

Competency
The perioperative registered nurse should be clinically competent, possessing the skills necessary to manage the nursing care of the patient receiving moderate sedation/analgesia.

Competency assurance verifies that personnel have an understanding of moderate sedation; the risks of unplanned, deeper sedation; and the safe use of monitoring equipment. This knowledge is essential to minimize the risks of moderate sedation and to provide safe care.[21]

IX.a. The competency of the perioperative registered nurse to administer moderate sedation/analgesia should be assessed, demonstrated, documented, and maintained.[21] (PNDS: I1, I128, I138, I15, I89, I51, I8, I121, I120, I111)

IX.a.1.   Competencies related to administration of moderate sedation/analgesia should include, but are not limited to,
- patient selection and assessment criteria;
- selection, function, and proficiency in use of physiological monitoring equipment;[1]
- pharmacology of the medications used;
- airway management;
- CPAP use;
- basic dysrhythmia recognition and management;
- emergency response and management;
- advanced cardiac life support (ACLS) and pediatric advanced life support (PALS) according to patients served;[18]
- recognition of complications associated with sedation/analgesia; and
- knowledge of anatomy and physiology.[12]

IX.b.   The perioperative registered nurse administering moderate sedation/analgesia should be able to rescue patients whose level of sedation progresses to deep sedation. (PNDS: I1, I89, I92)

Sedation occurs on a continuum from fully conscious to deep sedation[2,7] (**Table 2**).

XI.c.   The perioperative registered nurse should, at a minimum, have the ability to manage a compromised airway and to provide adequate oxygenation and ventilation. (PNDS: I1)

Patients receiving moderate sedation/analgesia may unexpectedly slip to the next level (ie, deep sedation or general anesthesia). A provider with bag-, valve-, mask-ventilation; advance life support; and resuscitation skills should be immediately available (eg, within one to five minutes).[2,7]

IX.d.   Administrators should ensure that initial and ongoing educational opportunities are provided to meet the needs of personnel who perform moderate sedation/analgesia. (PNDS: I1)

Initial education provides a baseline to support a beginning level of competency to assist in the development of knowledge, skills, and attitudes that positively affect patient outcomes. Ongoing education offers personnel an opportunity to enhance skills and learn about changes in practice, regulations, and standards.[21]

IX.d.1.   An introduction and review of moderate sedation/analgesia policies and procedures should be included in the orientation and ongoing education of personnel.

Table 2

CONTINUUM OF DEPTH OF SEDATION				
Levels of sedation/ analgesia	Minimal sedation (ie, anxiolysis)	Moderate sedation/ analgesia (ie, conscious sedation)	Deep sedation/ analgesia	General anesthesia
Responsiveness	Normal response to verbal stimulation	Purposeful response to verbal or tactile stimulation	Purposeful response following repeated or painful stimulation	Unarousable even with painful stimulation
Airway	Unaffected	No intervention required	Intervention may be required	Intervention often required
Ventilations	Unaffected	Adequate	May be adequate	Frequently inadequate
Cardiovascular function	Unaffected	Usually maintained	Usually maintained	May be impaired
Reproduced with permission from the American Society of Anesthesiologists, Park Ridge, IL.				

IX.e. Administrators should ensure that perioperative registered nurses who administer moderate sedation/analgesia for procedures are competent to perform these skills.[21] (PNDS: I1)

IX.f. Competencies should reflect current regulations, nurse practice acts, standards, recommended practices, and guidelines affecting the administration of moderate sedation/analgesia. (PNDS: I1)

Regulations, nurse practice acts, standards, recommended practices, and guidelines affecting the administration of moderate sedation/analgesia are evolving and may change over time.

IX.g. The perioperative registered nurse should have the additional knowledge and skills necessary to provide care to the pediatric patient populations they serve.[15]

Recommendation X

Documentation

The perioperative registered nurse should document the care of the patient and their physiological responses throughout the continuum of care.[7]

Documentation of all nursing activities performed is legally and professionally important for clear communication and collaboration between health care team members, and for continuity of patient care.

X.a. Documentation using the PNDS, should include a patient assessment, a plan of care, nursing diagnoses, identification of desired outcomes, interventions, and an evaluation of the patient's response to the care provided.

X.b. Documentation should be recorded in a manner consistent with health care organization policies and procedures and should include, but is not limited to,
   - name, dose, route, time, and effects of all medications;
   - patient's LOC;
   - ventilation and oxygenation status;
   - vital signs documented at intervals dependent on the type and quantity of medication administered;
   - procedure start and end times; and
   - condition of the patient.[1]

Recommendation XI

Policies and Procedures

Policies and procedures for managing patients who receive moderate sedation/analgesia should be written, reviewed periodically, and readily available within the practice setting.

Policies and procedures are operational guidelines that are used to minimize patient risk factors, standardize practice, direct staff members, and establish guidelines for continuous performance improvement activities.

XI.a. Policies and procedures should establish authority, responsibility, and accountability.

XI.b. Policies and procedures for managing patients receiving moderate sedation/analgesia should include, but are not limited to,
   - patient selection criteria;
   - personnel requirements;
   - staffing requirements;
   - monitoring;
   - risk assessment and criteria for consultation (eg, anesthesia);
   - moderate sedation/analgesia medication administration and dosage guidelines;
   - recovery and discharge criteria;
   - documentation;
   - emergency procedures;[3,7] and
   - alternative care arrangements when the patient's acuity and or level of care required is outside the capabilities and scope of practice of the perioperative registered nurse.[22]

Recommendation XII

Quality

A quality assurance/performance improvement process should be in place that measures patient, process, and structural (eg, system) outcome indicators.

A fundamental precept of AORN is that it is the responsibility of professional perioperative registered nurses to ensure safe, high-quality nursing care to patients undergoing operative and invasive procedures.[24]

XII.a. Structure, process, and clinical outcomes performance measures should be identified that can be used to improve patient care and that also monitor compliance with facility policy and procedure, national standards and regulatory requirements.[23,25]

XII.a.1. The measures should have universality across the continuum and relevance to all providers of sedation for procedures.[25]

XII.a.2. Process indicators may include, but are not limited to,
- consent for sedation and procedure;
- NPO status confirmed;
- history and physical completed;
- airway assessment conducted;
- factors requiring anesthesia consultation are noted;
- ASA classification;
- anesthesia intervention required (eg, loss of protective reflexes, bag mask ventilation required);
- reversal agents used;
- providers credentialed for procedure/sedation and practice in compliance with facility policy and procedure; and
- adherence to required physiological monitoring.

XII.b. Adverse events should be reported and investigated through the health care organization's quality review process (eg, root cause analysis).[25]

XII.b.1. Any of the following adverse events should be reviewed, and some may require reporting to the appropriate regulatory agency or accrediting organization:[25]
- death;
- aspiration;
- use of antagonists (eg, reversal agents);
- unplanned transfer to a higher level of care;
- cardiac or respiratory arrest;
- sedation using nonapproved agents (eg, anesthetic agent by nonanesthesia provider); and
- emergency procedure without a licensed, independent practitioner in attendance.

Glossary

Anxiolytic: Pharmacologic agent used to treat anxiety. Synonym for anti-anxiety agent.[21]

Benzodiazepine: Pharmacological agent that has sedative, anxiolytic, amnesic, muscle relaxant, and anticonvulsant properties.[24]

Deep sedation/analgesia: A medication-induced depression of consciousness that allows patients to respond purposefully only after repeated or painful stimulation. The patient cannot be aroused easily, and the ability to independently maintain a patent airway may be impaired with spontaneous ventilation possibly inadequate. Cardiovascular function usually is adequate and maintained.[21]

General anesthesia: Patients cannot be aroused, even by painful stimulation, during this medication-induced loss of consciousness. Patients usually require assistance in airway maintenance and often require positive pressure ventilation due to depressed spontaneous ventilation or depression of neuromuscular function. Cardiovascular function also may be impaired.

Immediately available: Defined by the ASA practice guidelines as having a health care provider trained in ACLS and resuscitation skills available to assist with patient care within one to five minutes.[2]

Licensed independent practitioner: Any individual who is permitted by law and the health care organization to provide care and services, without supervision or direction. The care and services should be within the scope of the individual's license and granted clinical privileges.

Moderate sedation/analgesia: A minimally depressed level of consciousness that allows a surgical patient to retain the ability to independently and continuously maintain a patent airway and respond appropriately to verbal commands and physical stimulation. Often referred to as *conscious sedation.*

Opioid: Pharmacologic agent that produces varying degrees of analgesia and sedation, and relieves pain. Fentanyl, morphine, and hydromorphone are opiod analgesic medications that may be used for moderate sedation/analgesia.[3]

Sedative: Pharmacologic agent that reduces anxiety and may induce some degree of short-term amnesia. Diazapam and midazolam are two benzodiazepines commonly used for sedation.

REFERENCES
1. Beyea SC, ed. *Perioperative Nursing Data Set.* Rev 2nd ed. Denver CO: AORN, Inc; 2007.
2. American Society of Anesthesiologists Task Force on Sedation and Analgesia by Non-Anesthesiologists. Practice guidelines for sedation and analgesia by non-anesthesiologists. *Anesthesiology.* 2002; 96:1004-1017.

3. King CA. *Moderate Sedation/Analgesia Competency Assessment Module.* 2nd ed. Denver CO: Competency & Credentialing Institute; 2005:9, 13-16, 19-21, 23, 25-26, 29, 37-38.

4. AORN explications for perioperative nursing. In: *Standards, Recommended Practices, and Guidelines.* Denver CO: AORN, Inc; 2007:171-201.

5. Odom-Forren J, Watson D. *Practical Guide to Moderate Sedation/Analgesia.* St. Louis MO: Elsevier Mosby; 2005:4-5;242-257.

6. American Nurses Association. *Nursing: Scope and Standards of Practice.* Washington DC: Nursebooks.org; American Nurses Association; 2004:36;39;42.

7. Operative and other high-risk procedures and/or the administration of moderate or deep sedation or anesthesia. In: *Comprehensive Accreditation Manual for Hospitals: The Official Handbook.* Oakbrook Terrace IL: Joint Commission on Accreditation of Healthcare Organizations; 2007 PC-41 to PC-43.

8. American Society of Anesthesiologists. Distinguishing monitored anesthesia care ("MAC") from moderate sedation/analgesia (conscious sedation) (Oct 27, 2004). *http://www.asahq.org/publicationsAndServices/standards/35.pdf.* Accessed July 23, 2007.

9. Malviya S, Voepel-Lewis T, Ludomirsky A, Marshall J, Tait AR. Can we improve the assessment of discharge readiness? a comparative study of observational and objective measures of depth of sedation in children. [Comment]. *Anesthesiology.* 2004; 100:218-224.

10. Langeron O, Masso E, Huraux C, et al. Prediction of difficult mask ventilation. *Anesthesiology.* 2000; 92:1229-1236.

11. Gross JB, Bachenberg KL, Benumof JL, et al. Practice guidelines for the perioperative management of patients with obstructive sleep apnea: a report by the American Society of Anesthesiologists task force on perioperative management of patients with obstructive sleep apnea. *Anesthesiology.* 2006; 104:1081-1093.

12. American Nurses Association. The role of the registered nurse (RN) in the management of patients receiving IV conscious sedation for short-term therapeutic, diagnostic, or surgical procedures. In: *Compendium of American Nurses Association Position Statements.* Washington, DC: American Nurses Pub; 1996; 148-150.

13. American Association of Nurse Anesthetists, American Society of Anesthesiologists. *AANA-ASA Joint Statement Regarding Propofol Administration.* Available at: *http://www.asahq.org/news/propofolstatement.htm.* Accessed September13, 2007.

14. Harkness GA, Dincher JR. *Medical-Surgical Nursing: Total Patient Care.* 10th ed. St Louis, MO: Mosby; 1999:502.

15. Committee on Drugs American Academy of Pediatrics. Guidelines for monitoring and management of pediatric patients during and after sedation for diagnostic and therapeutic procedures: addendum. *Pediatrics.* 2002; 110:836-838.

16. Newman DH, Azer MM, Pitetti RD, Singh S. When is a patient safe for discharge after procedural sedation? The timing of adverse effects events in 1367 pediatric procedural sedations. *Ann Emerg Med.* 2003; 42:627-635.

17. Cote CJ, Karl HW, Notterman DA, Weinberg JA, McCloskey C. Adverse sedation events in pediatrics: analysis of medications used for sedation. *Pediatrics.* 2000; 106:633-644.

18. Cote CJ, Notterman DA, Karl HW, Weinberg JA, McCloskey C. Adverse sedation events in pediatrics: a critical incident analysis of contributing factors. *Pediatrics.* 2000; 105:805-814.

19. *Drug Information Handbook for Perioperative Nursing.* Hudson OH: Lexi-Comp; 2006: 739, 1220.

20. American Society of PeriAnesthesia Nurses. *Standards of Perianesthesia Nursing Practice.* Thorofare NJ: American Society of Perianesthesia Nurses; 2004:63-67.

21. Management of human resources. In: *Comprehensive Accreditation Manual for Hospitals: The Official Handbook.* Oakbrook Terrace IL: Joint Commission on Accreditation of Healthcare Organizations; 2007: HR-2.

22. America Nurses Association. The right to accept or reject an assignment. Available at: *http://nursingworld.org/MainMenuCategories/HealthcareandPolicyIssues/ANAPositionStatements/workplac/wkassign14540.aspx.* Accessed September 18, 2007.

23. AORN. Quality and performance improvement standards for perioperative nursing. In: *Standards, Recommended Practices, and Guidelines.* Denver, CO: AORN, Inc; 2007:437-446.

24. Lee A, Fan LT, Gin T, Karmakar MK, Ngan Kee WD. A systemic review (meta-analysis) of the accuracy of the Mallampati tests to predict the difficult airway. *Anesth & Analg.* 2006;102:1867-1878.

25. Improving organization performance. In: *Comprehensive Accreditation Manual for Hospitals: The Official Handbook.* Oakbrook Terrace IL: Joint Commission on Accreditation of Healthcare Organizations; 2007:PI-8 to PI-9.

PUBLICATION HISTORY

Originally published April 1993, *AORN Journal,* as "Recommended practices for monitoring the patient receiving intravenous conscious sedation."

Revised; published in January 1997, *AORN Journal,* as "Recommended practices for managing the patient receiving conscious sedation/analgesia." Reformatted July 2000.

Revised November 2001; published March 2002, *AORN Journal,* as "Recommended practices for managing the patient receiving moderate sedation/analgesia."

Revised 2007; published in *Perioperative Standards and Recommended Practices,* 2008 edition.

Recommended Practices for Positioning the Patient in the Perioperative Practice Setting

The following recommended practices for positioning the patient in the perioperative practice setting were developed by the AORN Recommended Practices Committee and have been approved by the AORN Board of Directors. They were presented as proposed recommendations for comments by members and others. They are effective January 1, 2008.

These recommended practices are intended as achievable recommendations representing what is believed to be an optimal level of practice. Policies and procedures will reflect variations in practice settings and/or clinical situations that determine the degree to which the recommended practices can be implemented.

AORN recognizes the various settings in which perioperative registered nurses practice. These recommended practices are intended as guidelines adaptable to various practice settings. These practice settings include traditional operating rooms, ambulatory surgery centers, physicians' offices, cardiac catheterization laboratories, endoscopy suites, radiology departments, and all other areas where surgery may be performed.

References to nursing interventions (I) used in the Perioperative Nursing Data Set (PNDS) are noted in parentheses when a recommended practice corresponds to a PNDS intervention.[1] The reader is referred to the PNDS for further explanation of nursing diagnoses, interventions, and outcomes.

Purpose

These recommended practices provide guidelines for positioning the patient in the perioperative setting. They are not intended to cover aspects of perioperative patient care addressed in other recommended practices. Prevention of positioning injury requires anticipation of the positioning equipment necessary based on the patient's identified needs and the planned operative or invasive procedure, application of the principles of body mechanics and ergonomics, ongoing assessment throughout the perioperative period, and coordination with the entire perioperative team.[1] Attention should be given to patient comfort and safety, as well as to assessing circulatory, respiratory, integumentary, musculoskeletal, and neurological structures. Working as a member of the team, the perioperative registered nurse can minimize the risk of perioperative complications related to positioning.

Recommendation I

Personnel who purchase positioning equipment should make decisions based on the health care organization's patient population, current research findings, and the equipment design safety features required to minimize risks to patients and personnel.

The technology used to create mattresses, padding, and other positioning equipment continues to evolve, and it is important for perioperative registered nurses to be aware of products and current research to support their product selection.

The primary safety feature consideration for positioning equipment is that it redistribute pressure, especially at bony prominences on the patient's body. The National Pressure Ulcer Advisory Panel Support Surface Standards Initiative defines a support surface as "a specialized device for pressure redistribution designed for management of tissue loads, micro-climate, and/or other therapeutic functions (ie, any mattresses, integrated bed system, mattress replacement, overlay, or seat cushion, or seat cushion overlay)."[2]

Although physiologic blood and lymphatic flow rates vary among individuals, capillary pressures may increase to as much as 150 mm Hg during prolonged, unrelieved pressure without position change.[3]

The traditional procedure bed mattress usually is constructed of one to two inches of foam covered with a vinyl or nylon fabric. Research studies have found that foam overlays or replacement pads, which represent most OR and procedure bed mattresses, do not have effective pressure-reduction capabilities.[4] Studies comparing the pressure-reducing abilities of standard foam procedure bed mattresses to gel mattresses (ie, visco-elastic polymer) have found gel mattresses to be more effective.[4,5] One research study reported that polyether mattresses generate a lower capillary interface pressure when the patient was in the supine position than gel mattresses or foam mattresses.[6] Another study found that foam and gel mattresses are effective for preventing skin changes, but visco-elastic overlays are effective for preventing both skin changes and pressure sore formation.[7]

Clinical support surfaces (ie, padding) function differently for persons of different height and weight.[8] A performance improvement study reported that supplemental padding on the procedure bed mattress or the use of other positioning devices may not

RP: Positioning the Patient

reduce capillary interface pressure for all body types or for all areas of bony prominences even in patients with the same body type.[9]

Postoperative use of alternating pressure mattresses has been found to minimize the incidence of pressure ulcers. Intraoperative use of this technology may be limited due to concerns about patient movement, electrical safety, and asepsis.[3]

There are studies reporting a reduction in the postoperative incidence of pressure ulcers when pressure-relieving overlays are used on procedure bed mattresses and in the postoperative period; however, use of mattress overlays intraoperatively may not minimize this risk.[10] It is difficult, therefore, to draw firm conclusions about the most effective means of intraoperative pressure relief. Future studies of pressure-relieving surfaces are needed and must address methodological deficiencies associated with many of the available studies. Examples of current study limitations include the following:

♦ Trials that do not clearly reflect whether a reduction in risk for skin changes is due to intraoperative or postoperative pressure relief or whether application of the trial is necessary in both settings to achieve a risk reduction.[10]

♦ Studies that do not include information gathered on the postoperative skin care of the patient make it difficult to assess the clinical significance of the studies' findings.[10]

♦ Cross comparisons of study results often are not effective because of variations of selection criteria. In addition, limited sample sizes, interrater reliability, and contradictory findings further contribute to weak scientific support for recommendations on how to predict and prevent pressure ulcers resulting from intraoperative procedure bed mattresses.[11]

♦ Studies that measure only interface pressure (ie, the pressure on different parts of the patient's body that are in contact with the support surface) have serious limitations. The process that leads to the development of a pressure ulcer involves the complex interplay of several factors.[10]

The most frequent predictors of perioperative pressure ulcers have been found to be

♦ increasing age of the patient,
♦ a patient diagnosed with diabetes or vascular disease, and
♦ vascular procedures.[11]

I.a.   Personnel selecting procedure bed mattresses and positioning equipment for purchase and use should make decisions based on criteria that include, but are not limited to,
– ability to hold the patient in the desired position;
– available in a variety of sizes and shapes;
– suitable for the patient population and anticipated position requirements;
– ability to support maximum weight requirements;
– durable material and design (eg, maintains resilience under constant use);
– evidence that it is able to disperse skin interface pressure;
– resistance to moisture;
– low risk for moisture retention;
– radiolucent, if necessary;
– fire retardant;
– nonallergenic;
– promotes air circulation;
– low risk of harboring bacteria (eg, replacements may be needed when soiled);
– easy to use and store; and
– cost effective.[3,4,7,12]

One study found the viscoelastic mattress overlay appears to offer the most benefit for older patient populations; patients who have more serious or chronic health problems, where there is a prevalence of vascular disease; or in situations where surgical procedures extend beyond two-and-one-half hours.[7]

I.a.1.   Positioning equipment for obese patients should include, but is not limited to,
• lateral transfer devices or patient lifts to move obese patients from stretcher procedure bed to the OR procedure bed;[13] and
• stretchers and beds in the postanesthesia care unit (PACU) that are able to accommodate at least a 30-degree elevation of the patient's upper body and head to avoid respiratory distress.

Whether or not a facility has a bariatric surgery program, it is necessary to accommodate the unique needs of the obese patient population. Patient demographics, baseline utilization requirements, and peek census requirements may help to determine whether caseloads justify purchasing rather than leasing special bariatric equipment. Upgrading existing equipment with bariatric accessories may be a viable option rather than replacing equipment in its entirety.[14]

I.a.2. The manufacturer should be consulted for both weight capacity and articulation abilities of the procedure bed.

Many procedure beds are designed to safely support a 500-pound patient, but maximum weight for special functioning capabilities is an important consideration. Heavy-duty procedure beds are available that lift, articulate, and support patients weighing 800 to 1,000 lbs.[15]

I.b. Procedure bed mattresses and positioning equipment should be evaluated according AORN's "Recommended practices for product selection in the perioperative practice setting."[16]

Recommendation II

During the planning phase of patient care, the perioperative registered nurse should anticipate the positioning equipment needed for the specific operative or invasive procedure.

The patient's position should provide optimum exposure for the procedure while providing access to IV lines and monitoring devices. The nurse determines the equipment to be used based on the planned procedure, surgeon's preference, and patient condition. Assessment of surgical case characteristics (eg, procedure length, surgical approach, use of radiological equipment) helps determine positioning equipment and modifications in positioning needed to safely accommodate a patient's physical needs.

II.a. The perioperative registered nurse should review the surgery schedule before the patient's arrival, preferably before the day of surgery, to identify potential conflicts in availability of positioning equipment. (PNDS: I85, I30, I138)

Compromises in patient safety may result when proper equipment is not available.

II.a.1. When a procedure is scheduled, the availability of special equipment should be verified.

II.b. The perioperative registered nurse should confirm that the room is set up appropriately for the planned procedure before the patient arrives. (PNDS: I85, I30, I138)

Compromises in patient safety may result when the room arrangement is not specific to the planned procedure and its laterality.[17]

II.b.1. The correct patient position and related equipment should be verified during the time out period.[18]

Recommendation III

Positioning and transporting equipment should be periodically inspected and maintained in properly functioning condition.

Properly functioning equipment contributes to patient safety and assists in providing adequate exposure of the surgical site. Patients and health care workers are at risk for injury if equipment is not used according to manufacturers' specifications.

III.a. Scheduled preventive maintenance and repair should be performed on all equipment used for patient transport. (PNDS: I138)

Preventive maintenance and repair promote proper functioning and decrease the risk for injury to patients and personnel.

III.b. Surfaces of positioning and transporting equipment should be smooth and intact. (PNDS: I122, I138)

Loss of equipment surface integrity can result in bacterial growth. Surfaces that hold moisture or wrinkle contribute to skin breakdown.

III.c. Proper working condition of positioning and transporting equipment should be verified before use. (PNDS: I122, I138)

Creating a culture of safety includes designing a work environment that minimizes factors that contribute to errors or injuries.[19]

III.d. Potential hazards associated with the use of positioning and transporting equipment should be identified, and safe practices should be established in accordance with AORN's "Recommended practices for a safe environment of care."[20] (PNDS: I122, I138)

Recommendation IV

During the preoperative assessment, the perioperative registered nurse should identify unique patient considerations that require additional precautions for procedure-specific positioning.

Assessing patients for pressure ulcer development risk factors serves as a key step to preventing them. Patients who are immobile, as is required during operative procedures, are at increased risk.[3]

Additional precautions may be necessary when positioning special patient populations (eg, neonatal, elderly, malnourished, morbidly obese patients; patients with chronic diseases; patients with existing pressure ulcers) to reduce the risk for integumentary, respiratory, or cardiovascular compromises, and nerve impairment.[12,21] For example:

♦ Obesity adversely affects most body systems.[22] Routine skin condition assessments may be difficult because of the patient's size, lack of landmarks, and chronic conditions.[23] Traditional foam positioning products may prove ineffective, due to compression resulting from the patient's weight.[15,23]

♦ Patients with vascular disease may have existing tissue ischemia and often have additional risk factors (eg, age, nutritional deficits, obesity, diabetes). Patients with vascular disease who are hypertensive may react unexpectedly to a reduction in blood pressure that is considered normotensive for many patients, but which results in loss of blood flow through stenotic vessels.[24]

♦ Patients who smoke often experience vasoconstriction, another mechanism that contributes to pressure ulcer formation.[24]

IV.a. Patient needs should be assessed by a registered nurse before transport to determine the required equipment and the skill level and number of transport personnel needed. (PNDS: I64)

Advance preparation for transport may be required for obese patients or other patients with special needs.[21]

IV.b. The preoperative nursing assessment should include questions to determine patient tolerance to the planned operative position. (PNDS: I15, I60, I64, I66, I127, I144, I148)

IV.b.1. The perioperative registered nurse should take additional precautions to decrease the risk for pressure ulcers in patients who

• are more than 70 years of age;
• require vascular procedures or any procedure lasting longer than four hours;

• are thin, small in stature, or who have poor preoperative nutritional status;
• are diabetic or have vascular disease; and
• have a preoperative Braden Scale score that is less than 20.[11]

Studies report that the duration of a procedure is a significant predictor of pressure ulcer development. One study reported that intraoperative pressure ulcers increased when the procedure time extended beyond three hours. Cardiac, general, thoracic, orthopedic, and vascular procedures were reported to be the most common types of procedures associated with pressure ulcer formation.[25]

IV.b.2. Preoperative assessment should include evaluation of both patient and intraoperative factors.

• Patient assessment should include, but is not limited to,
  ▪ age;
  ▪ height;
  ▪ weight;
  ▪ body mass index (BMI);
  ▪ skin condition;
  ▪ presence of jewelry;
  ▪ nutritional status;
  ▪ allergies (eg, latex);
  ▪ preexisting conditions (eg, vascular, respiratory, circulatory, neurological, immune system suppression);
  ▪ laboratory results;
  ▪ physical or mobility limitation (eg, range of motion);
  ▪ presence of prosthetics or corrective devices;
  ▪ presence of implanted devices (eg, pacemakers, orthopedic implants);
  ▪ presence of external devices (eg, catheters, drains, orthopedic immobilizers);
  ▪ presence of peripheral pulses;
  ▪ perception of pain;
  ▪ level of consciousness; and
  ▪ psychosocial and cultural considerations.[1,12]
• Intraoperative assessment factors should include, but are not limited to,

- anesthesia care provider's access to patient;
- estimated length of procedure; and
- desired procedural position.

IV.c. Special procedure beds and accessories designed to meet unique patient needs should be used. (PNDS: I30, I64, I122)

When assessing a patient's body weight and condition it is important to assess more than just their BMI. Patients of the same BMI (a relative ratio of height and weight) can have significantly different body composition that affects positioning needs and their risk for pressure ulcer development; therefore, procedure bed and positioning device requirements may be quite different.

The perioperative nursing assessment should include the length and weight capacity of the procedure bed.

IV.d. Perioperative registered nurses should participate in their health care organization's fall-reduction program by including an assessment of the patient's risk for falling. (PNDS: I64)

Patients may be prone to falls before they enter the operating room, during transfer to the procedure bed, and when attempting to sit up or transfer to a recliner in the PACU.[26] Patients may be at a higher risk for falling if the following conditions are present:

- history of a fall during the past three months;
- use of certain medications (eg, psychotropics, antidepressants, benzodiazepines, cardiovascular agents, antihypertensives, diuretics, anticoagulants, antihistamines, bowel preparation medications, medications related to treating nocturia);[27]
- confusion or depression;
- function or mobility problems (ie, gait),
- age, and
- dizziness.[27,28]

The top three risk factors for predicting falls include a previous fall, medications used, and gait.[27] Age ranks fourth as a risk factor, however, it is not a good predictor of falls because studies show a wide range of age groups experience falls. One study reported a high percentage of injuries due to falls occurring in the 20- to24-year-old age group.[28]

IV.d.1. Regardless of age, patients who have poor vision, postural hypotension, or an altered mental status should be considered to be at a high risk for falling.[27]

Recommendation V

Perioperative personnel should use proper body mechanics when transporting, moving, lifting, or positioning patients.

The incidence of work-related back injuries in nursing is among the highest of any profession worldwide.[29] Manual lifting and other patient-handling tasks are high-risk activities that can result in musculoskeletal disorders.[13] Most injuries are due to overexertion when lifting patients; tasks that require staff members to twist or bend forward; and high-risk tasks performed on a horizontal plane (eg, lateral transfer from bed to stretcher, repositioning patient in bed).[29,30]

Biomechanical studies have demonstrated that health care personnel are at risk for injury, despite the use of proper body mechanics, if patient-handling tasks are beyond reasonable limits and the caregiver's capabilities.[29] The combination of frequency, duration, and the stress of performing high-risk tasks that push the limits of human capabilities (eg, heavy loads; sustained, awkward positions; bending and twisting; reaching fatigue or stress; force; standing for long periods of time) predisposes nurses to musculoskeletal disorders.[13]

V.a. An adequate number of personnel should be available to ensure patient and personnel safety when transporting the patient. (PNDS: I30, I77)

Procedure beds can be very heavy and difficult to move, even without the presence of a patient. When a procedure bed is moved with a patient on it, the risk of injury is increased for both the worker and the patient.[13]

V.b. The perioperative registered nurse should identify high risk tasks and implement ergonomic solutions to eliminate or reduce occupational risks for injury.

Transferring, lifting, and handling patients have been identified as the most frequent precipitating trigger of back and shoulder problems for nurses.[13] Nurses are often required to use the weaker muscles of the arms and shoulders as the primary lifting muscles, rather than the stronger muscles of the legs, because lifting, turning, or repositioning patients is often performed on a horizontal plane, such as a bed or stretcher.[29]

Experts do not always agree on the safest methods for lifting or assisting dependent patients. One research center recommends the use of a roller or mechanical lifting equipment to reduce the risk of strain when moving a patient who is unable to move independently. The same center studied nurses' behaviors regarding use of lifting equipment and identified the following reasons for continued manual lifting:

- devices were purchased in insufficient quantities,
- lifts were stored in inconvenient locations, and
- equipment was not maintained adequately.[29]

V.c. All perioperative personnel should be educated in the principles of body mechanics and ergonomics.

The majority of musculoskeletal disorders reported by nurses working in the private sector are back injuries that require time away from work. Several studies report that nurses complain of chronic back pain, are unable to do their work because of injuries to shoulder and neck, or are planning to leave the profession because of their concern for personal safety in the health care environment.[13]

Recommendation VI

Potential hazards associated with patient transport and transfer activities should be identified, and safe practices should be established.

Preoperative patient observation and assessment by a perioperative registered nurse allows for identification of potential problems during transport and transfer activities that can be prevented by the implementation of appropriate precautions.

VI.a. When selecting the appropriate transport vehicle, design features to be considered should include, but are not limited to,
- locking devices on wheels;
- protective devices (eg, safety straps, side rails, cribs rails high enough to prevent a standing child from falling out);
- stable, adjustable IV poles or stands;
- holding devices for oxygen tanks;
- positioning capabilities;
- controls that are easy to operate and within reach of the operator;
- maneuverability;
- sufficient size;
- removable head and foot boards;
- mattress-stabilizing devices;
- easily cleanable surfaces; and
- a rack or shelf to hold monitoring equipment. (PNDS: I138)

Equipment safety design features help reduce the risk of injury to patients and personnel during transport.

VI.b. The patient should be attended during transport and transfer by personnel deemed appropriate by the perioperative registered nurse or as determined by the anesthesia care provider or surgeon. (PNDS: I138)

VI.c. Safety measures to be implemented during transport and transfer activities should include, but are not limited to,
- presence of locking wheels on the transport vehicle and the patient's bed during transfer activities;
- side rails that can be elevated;
- use of safety straps;
- hanging and securing IV containers away from the patient's head;
- ensuring that the patient's head, arms, and legs are protected;
- ensuring that one staff member remains at the head of the patient transport vehicle;
- pushing the transport vehicle with the patient's feet first and avoiding rapid movement through hallways or when turning corners;
- maintaining the integrity and function of IV infusions, indwelling catheters, tubes, drainage systems, and monitoring equipment; and
- obtaining appropriately skilled assistance personnel and specific instructions for the patient with special needs. (PNDS: I138)

Locking wheels, raising side rails, and securing safety straps reduce the risk of patient falls. Maintaining proximity to the patient's head provides access to the patient's airway in the event of respiratory distress or vomiting. Rapid movements can cause patient disorientation, nausea and vomiting, and dizziness.

Recommendation VII

Positioning equipment should be used in a safe manner and according to manufacturers' written instructions.

To reduce the risk of injury, it is important to follow manufacturers' written instructions regarding weight limits in flat, articulated, and reverse orientation positions for each type of procedure bed. One researcher reviewed 16 perioperative incident reports and found that 63% involved patients who were above the specified weight limit for the positioning equipment used for back surgery. In all of the reports, it was noted that a staff member notified the surgeon of the problem before the beginning of the surgery, but the equipment was used anyway because alternative equipment was not available.[31]

VII.a. The perioperative registered nurse should verify that the positioning equipment to be used has been designed specifically for surgical procedure positioning. (PNDS: I122)

The goal of using positioning equipment is to use equipment that is designed to redistribute pressure and that decreases the risk for positioning injuries.

The number of pads, blankets, and warming blankets beneath the patient has been implicated as a risk factor for pressure ulcer development.[4,11,26,32,33]

- Foam pads may not be effective as padding devices because they quickly compress under heavy body areas.[33-35] In some situations, however, foam can be an effective pressure-reducing material equal to that of gel or visco-elastic.
- Convoluted foam mattress overlays (eg, egg crate mattresses) may be more effective in redistributing pressure if they are made of thick, dense foam that resists compression. The effectiveness of this type of mattress overlay depends on the weight of the patient and may not provide adequate pressure reduction in obese patients.
- Pillows, blankets, and molded-foam devices may produce only a minimum amount of pressure redistribution and are less effective during long procedures.
- Towels and sheet rolls do not reduce pressure and may contribute to friction injuries.[3]

VII.b. The perioperative registered nurse should select a surface that is able to reduce excessive pressure on the patient's bony prominences. (PNDS: I11, I122)

Pressure against the skin above 32 mm Hg interferes with tissue perfusion.[36,37] Firm, stable devices may help hold the patient in position but may not help redistribute pressure. If care is not taken to minimize pressure points caused by positioning equipment, the positioning equipment may not adequately decrease the potential for injury and may actually increase the potential for pressure injury.

VII.b.1. Rolled sheets and towels should not be used beneath the procedure bed mattress or an overlay. When using positioning equipment such as a uterine displacing wedge or chest rolls, the positioning devices should be placed underneath the patient and not beneath the mattress or overlay.

When rolled towels, sheets, or other positioning equipment are placed beneath the mattress or the overlay, they may negate the pressure-reducing effect of the mattress or overlay.[11]

VII.c. Patients should not be transported in procedure beds unless the manufacturer's written instructions state that the bed is safe to use as a transportation device. (PNDS: I122)

Procedure bed designs vary. Unlocking the bed may make it unstable. Moving an occupied procedure bed is not recommended because the risk of injury increases for both the worker and the patient.[13] There are some procedure beds, however, that are designed for patient transport. It is important to consult the manufacturers' written instructions to determine if unlocking and moving a patient-occupied procedure bed is recommended.

Recommendation VIII

The perioperative registered nurse should actively participate in safely positioning the patient under the direction of and in collaboration with the surgeon and anesthesia provider.

The physiologic effects of anesthesia increase the patient's vulnerability to the effects of pressure. Patients may have preexisting conditions that limit the positions they can assume and may influence the positions they can tolerate.[37]

VIII.a. The perioperative registered nurse should provide for patient dignity and privacy during transport, transfer, and positioning. (PNDS: I100, I102, I150)

Maintaining patient privacy is essential to preserving the trust developed in the nurse-patient relationship. The perioperative registered nurse is responsible for developing a caring environment that promotes the well-being of patients. Perioperative registered nurses should provide care that recognizes the importance of each patient's values, beliefs, and health practices and is culturally relevant to a diverse patient population.[38]

VIII.a.1. The perioperative registered nurse should implement actions that include, but are not limited to, the following:
- Restrict OR patient care area access to designated authorized personnel only.
- Keep doors to patient care areas closed.
- Limit traffic coming into OR procedure rooms.
- Expose only the areas of the patient's body needed to provide care or access to the surgical site during the planned procedure.
- Provide auditory privacy for patient and staff member conversations during transport and transfer.
- Provide care without prejudicial behavior.[38]

VIII.b. Patient jewelry and body piercing accessories should be removed before positioning or transferring to the procedure bed if it will cause potential injury or interfere with the surgical site. (PNDS: I138)

Patients positioned on jewelry may be subject to pressure injuries.[39] Patient jewelry can become entangled in bedding or caught on equipment while moving the patient and cause injuries due to accidental removal.

VIII.c. Movement or positioning of the patient should be coordinated with the surgical team. (PNDS: I96, I77)

Sliding or pulling the patient can result in shearing forces and/or friction on the patient's skin. Shearing can occur when the patient's skin remains stationary and underlying tissues shift or move, as might occur when the patient is pulled or dragged without support to the skeletal system or while using a draw sheet. Friction occurs when skin surfaces rub over a rough stationary surface.[3,40]

VIII.c.1. Specific patient needs should be communicated to the perioperative team before initiating transfer or positioning the patient.

VIII.c.2. Attention should be given to protecting the patient's airway at all times during patient transfer and positioning.

VIII.c.3. Before and during transfer or positioning, perioperative team members should communicate with each other regarding securing tubes, drains, and catheters; take actions to support these devices and prevent dislodging; and confirm that the devices have maintained patency after transfer, positioning, or repositioning.

Indwelling catheters, tubes, or cannulas may be dislodged without proper support.

VIII.c.4. The perioperative registered nurse should actively participate in monitoring the patient's body alignment and confirming that the patient's legs are not crossed during transfer and positioning.

Maintaining the patient's correct body alignment and supporting his or her extremities and joints decreases the potential for injury during transfer and positioning.[12]

VIII.c.5. When on the procedure bed, the patient should be attended by surgical team members at all times.

A lack of clear communication about who should be watching the patient after the safety straps are removed or before the patient is transferred has been reported as a contributing factor for patient falls in the operating room.[28]

VIII.d. The number of personnel and required equipment should be adequate to safely position the patient. (PNDS: I64, I138)

Inadequate numbers of personnel and/or equipment can result in patient or personnel injury.

VIII.e. The perioperative registered nurse should actively participate in monitoring the patient's tissue integrity based on sound physiologic principles. (PNDS: I15, I42, I64, I96, I145)

VIII.f. The perioperative registered nurse should implement general positioning safety measures including, but not limited to, the following:

- Positioning equipment should be used to protect, support, and maintain the patient's position.
- Padding should be used to protect the patient's bony prominences.
- The patient's arms should be positioned to protect them from nerve injury.[37,41]
- The location of the patient's fingers should be confirmed to ensure they are in a position that is clear of procedure bed breaks or other hazards.
- Safety restraints should be applied carefully to avoid nerve compression injury and compromised blood flow.[42]
- The patient's body should be protected from coming in contact with metal portions of the procedure bed.
- The patient's heels should be elevated off the underlying surface when possible.[43]
- The patient's head and upper body should be in alignment with the hips. The patient's legs should be parallel and the ankles uncrossed to reduce pressure to occiput, scapulae, thoracic vertebrae, olecranon processes (ie, elbows), sacrum/coccyx, calcaneae (ie, heel),[12,44] and ischial tuberosities.[9,45]
- The patient's head should be in a neutral position and placed on a headrest.
- A pillow may be placed under the back of the patient's knees to relieve pressure on the lower back.[12]
- If the patient is pregnant, a wedge should be inserted under the patient's right side to displace the uterus to the left and prevent supine hypotensive syndrome, caused by the gravid uterus compressing the aorta and vena cava.[46]
- If patient is attached to a robot, caution should be used before moving either the patient or the robot. (PNDS: I77, I92, I96, I139)

VIII.f.1. Unless necessary for surgical reasons, the patient's arms should not be tucked at his or her sides when in the supine position. If there are surgical reasons to secure the patient's arms at his or her side with the use of a draw sheet, the draw sheet should extend above the elbows and should be tucked between the patient and the procedure bed's mattress.[37,44]

When a patient's arms are tucked tightly at his or her side with sheets, it may add unnecessary pressure on the tucked arms and may lead to tissue injury and ischemia. It may also cause interference with physiologic monitoring (eg, blood pressure monitoring, arterial catheter monitoring) and result in an inability to resuscitate during an emergency due to unrecognized IV infiltration in the tucked arm. There is also an increased risk for the patient to develop compartment syndrome in the upper extremity.[47]

VIII.f.2. Direct pressure on the eye should be avoided to reduce the risk of central retinal artery occlusion and other ocular damage, including corneal abrasion.

Patients who are at increased risk for development of postoperative visual loss are those that are undergoing procedures that are prolonged (ie, > 6.5 hrs), have substantial blood loss (ie, > 44.7% of estimated blood volume), or who are in a prone position.[48]

- Patients at risk for ocular injury should be positioned so that their heads are level with or higher than their hearts, when possible. In addition, their heads should be maintained in a neutral forward position without significant neck flexion, extension, lateral flexion, or rotation, when possible. The use of a horseshoe headrest may increase the risk of ocular compression.
- The eyes of patients in the prone position should be assessed regularly.
- The surgeon may consider using a series of staged spine procedures for high-risk patients.

VIII.g. Perioperative team members should implement measures to reduce the risk of nerve injuries when positioning the patient's extremities. (PNDS: I38, I144)

– Patients who undergo general anesthesia are at an increased risk for nerve injury resulting from patient positioning.[42]

– Trauma may result from compression or stretching of nerves, with the most frequent injuries involving the ulnar nerve and brachial plexus. Why some of these injuries occur is unknown.[12,41,42,49,50,51]

– The saphenous, sciatic, and peroneal nerves are vulnerable when the patient is in the lithotomy position. The peroneal nerve is also at risk with the patient in the lateral position.[50]

– Injury to the pudendal nerve may result from inadequate padding or incorrect placement of the positioning post, when using a fracture table.[37,52,53]

VIII.g.1. To minimize the risk of nerve injury, safety measures should include, but are not limited to, the following:

• Padded arm boards should be attached to the procedure bed at less than a 90-degree angle for supine patients.[37,41,44,50]

• The patient's palms should be facing up and the fingers should be extended when his or her arms are placed on arm boards.[37,41,50]

• When the patient's arms are placed at the side of the body, they should be in a neutral position (ie, elbows slightly flexed, wrist in neutral position, palms facing inward).[37,41,50]

• Patient shoulder abduction and lateral rotation should kept be to a minimum.[42]

• Patient extremities should be prevented from dropping below procedure bed level.

• The patient's head should be placed in a neutral position, if not contraindicated by the surgical procedure or the patient's physical limitations.[50]

• Adequate padding is required for the saphenous, sciatic, and peroneal nerves, especially when the patient is in a lithotomy or lateral position.[50]

• A well-padded perineal post should be placed against the perineum between the genitalia and the uninjured leg when a patient is positioned on a fracture table.[37,52,53]

VIII.h. Perioperative team members should implement measures to reduce the risk of injuries when positioning the patient in the supine position. (PNDS: I3, I11, I77, I96, I122)

The supine position may be modified into a sitting or semi-sitting position for access to the shoulder, posterior cervical spine, or posterior or lateral head. While there is better lung excursion and diaphragmatic activity in these positions, there is increased risk for poor venous return from the lower extremities and pooling of blood in the patient's pelvis.[12]

– When using only a draw sheet without a lateral transfer device for a lateral patient transfer in the supine position, the care provider exerts a pull force up to 72.6% of the patient's weight.[54]

– When one care provider (eg, anesthesia care provider) supports the patient's head and neck, the remaining mass of the patient's body equals 91.6% of his or her total body mass.[55] To accommodate this body mass, each caregiver can safely contribute a pull force required to transfer up to 48 lbs.[13]

– When moving the patient into and out of a sitting or modified sitting position, the mass of a patient's body from the waist up, including the head, neck, and upper extremities, equals almost 69% of the patient's total body weight.[55]

VIII.h.1. A lateral transfer device (eg, friction-reducing sheets, slider board, air-assisted transfer device) should be used for supine-to-supine patient transfer. One caregiver and one anesthesia care provider (who is managing the airway, head, and neck) should be assigned to safely transfer a patient who weighs 52 lbs. Two caregivers plus the anesthesia care provider should be assigned to safely transfer a patient up to 104 lbs. Three caregivers plus the anesthesia care provider should be assigned to safely transfer a patient up to 157 lbs. For patients who weigh more than 157 lbs, an appropriate mechanical lifting device (ie, mechanical lift with supine sling, mechanical lateral transfer device, or air-assisted lateral transfer device) should be used and a minimum of three to four caregivers should be assigned.[13]

VIII.h.2.   When moving the patient into and out of a sitting or modified sitting position, three caregivers should be assigned to work together to lift up to 67 lb (30 kg). It is preferable to use mechanical devices and a minimum of three caregivers if the patient weighs more than 68 lbs.[13]

VIII.i.   The perioperative team should implement measures to reduce the risk of injuries when positioning the patient in the prone position. (PNDS: I3, I11, I77, I96, I122)

The prone position may be modified into the jackknife position to provide exposure to sacral, rectal, and perineal areas, or modified into the knee-chest position to provide exposure for spinal procedures.[11,36]

Respiratory function may be affected by the ultimate positioning of the patient and is mitigated by many factors, including the angle of incline, external pressure on the rib cage, and whether the diaphragm is free to move.

Respiratory function may be decreased as a result of mechanical restriction of the rib cage and diaphragm when the patient is in a prone position.[12,37]

Ophthalmic complications, including vision loss, have been reported in association with patients undergoing spinal surgery in a prone position.[56] There is an increased risk for direct compression to the orbit and corneal abrasion when the patient is in a prone position. During spinal surgeries, the patient may be turned to a prone position using a frame that causes the head to be lower than the rest of the body. This cerebral-dependent position may lead to a decreased venous return from the head, which can lead to capillary bed stasis and decreased perfusion to the optic nerve and result in blindness[57]

When transferring a patient from a supine position to a prone position, the most common physiologic changes are related to hypotension.[37]

VIII.i.1.   General safety considerations for the prone position should include, but are not limited to, the following.

- The patient's cervical neck alignment should be maintained.
- Protection for the patient's forehead, eyes, and chin should be provided.
- A padded headrest should be used to provide airway access.
- Chest rolls (ie, from clavicle to iliac crest) should be used to allow chest movement and decrease abdominal pressure.
- Breasts and male genitalia should be positioned in a way that frees them from torsion or pressure.
- The patient's toes should be positioned to allow them to hang over the end of the bed or to be elevated off the bed by placing padding under the patient's shins so the shins are high enough to avoid pressure on the tips of the toes.[11]

VIII.i.2.   When in the prone position, direct pressure on the patient's eyes and face should be avoided.[58]

Although ocular injuries have been reported with and without the use of a headrest (eg, the head held with pins), the use of a horseshoe headrest may increase the risk of ocular compression and perioperative central retinal artery occlusion.[57]

VIII.i.3.   Ideally, the patient's arms should be placed down by his or her sides in the prone position. If this is not possible, each arm should be placed on an arm board with the arms abducted to less than 90 degrees, the elbows flexed, and the palms facing downwards. To safely secure the patient's arms at his or her sides, the palms of the hands should be facing in toward the thighs, the elbows and hands should be protected with padding, and the hands and wrists should be kept in anatomical alignment.[37]

Positioning the arms above the patient's head can cause a stretch injury to the lower trunks of the brachial plexus.[50]

VIII.i.4.   Four caregivers should be available for a supine-to-prone patient transfer. One anesthesia care provider should maintain the airway and support the patient's head, while other members of the team are responsible for the patient's trunk and extremities.

Two caregivers, plus the anesthesia care provider, can safely transfer a patient weighing up to 48.5 lb (22.0 kg) from the supine to the prone position. Three caregivers, plus an anesthesia care provider, can safely transfer a patient weighing up to 72.7 lb (33.0 kg). If the patient's weight is greater than 73 lbs, it is necessary to use assistive technology and a minimum of three to four caregivers.[13]

VIII.j. The perioperative team should implement measures to reduce the risk of injuries when positioning the patient in the Trendelenburg's and reverse Trendelenburg's positions. (PNDS: I3, I11, I77, I96, I122)

When the patient is in Trendelenburg's position, excessive pressure on the clavicle can compress the brachial plexus as it exits the thorax between the clavicle and the first rib. Morrell closed claims files revealed that brachial plexus injuries were related to the use of shoulder braces and the head-down position.[51]

Positioning a patient with a history of heart failure secondary to increased venous return and increased pulmonary blood flow in a steep, head-down tilt may adversely affect heart function. Trendelenburg's position causes redistribution of the blood supply due to increased venous return from the lower extremities. To ventilate the patient's lungs while in this position, the diaphragm must push against the displaced abdominal contents, which increases the risk for the alveoli to collapse resulting in atelectasis.[12,44]

Circulatory response changes can be rapid and dramatic when moving the patient into or out of Trendelenburg's position. During surgery, there is gravitational flow of blood away from the surgical field, which can mask significant blood loss. The patient may be hypotensive as a result of hypovolemia when returned from Trendelenburg's position to the supine position. Cerebral blood flow may fall as venous and intracranial pressure rises; therefore, patients with known or suspected intracranial pathology should not be placed in Trendelenburg's position if it can be avoided.[12,44] Trendelenburg's position can lead to visual loss related to decreased venous return from the head.[57]

VIII.j.1. Measures should be taken to prevent patient from sliding on the procedure bed.

Risk for shear injuries increase when changing the patient's position from supine to Trendelenburg's or reverse Trendelenburg's.[59]

VIII.j.2. To prevent injury to the shoulders, brachial plexus, or feet in Trendelenberg's or reverse Trendelenberg's positions,[41,42,49,60]

- shoulder braces should be avoided, and
- a padded footboard should be used for reverse Trendelenburg's position.

VIII.k. The perioperative team should implement measures to reduce the risk of injury to patients and caregivers associated with the lithotomy position. (PNDS: I3, I11, I77, I96, I122)

- Some type of leg holder is used in all lithotomy positions. Modifications of the position include low, standard, high, and exaggerated positions depending on how high the legs and pelvis need to be elevated for the procedure.[37,61]
- The length of time that a patient may remain in the lithotomy position without risk of injury is unknown and is related to patient condition.
- In the lithotomy position the patient's heels are at risk for pressure ulcers at the heel support sites, particularly when the legs are supported by the heel in the standard, high, or exaggerated lithotomy position for prolonged procedures.[61]
- Injury to the peroneal nerve on the lateral aspect of the knee is common and results from the fibular neck resting against the vertical post of the stirrup when the patient is in the lithotomy position. This injury can result in foot drop and lateral, lower-extremity paresthesia.[12,37,50,60]
- Compartment syndrome, although infrequent, has been reported as a complication of surgical positioning, especially the lithotomy position.[37,62-64]

There is increased risk for poor venous return from the lower extremities and pooling of blood in the patient's pelvis when the patient is in a lithotomy position. At the end of the procedure, the patient's overall circulating blood volume may be depleted when the patient's legs are lowered to the procedure bed due to the blood returning quickly into the patient's peripheral circulation. Respiratory compromises may occur due to pulmonary congestion. There is increased risk for deep vein thrombus formation due to the increased risk of blood pooling in the calf muscles.[12]

When positioning the patient into and out of the lithotomy position, the maximum load for a two-handed lift is 22.2 lb (10.1kg). Each complete lower patient extremity (including thigh, calf, and foot) weighs almost 16% of the patient's total body mass.[13]

VIII.k.1. General positioning considerations for patients in the lithotomy position include, but are not limited to, the following:
- Stirrups should be placed at an even height.
- The patient's buttocks should be even with the lower break of the procedure bed and positioned in a manner that securely supports the sacrum on the bed surface. Confirm proper positioning of the patient buttocks before surgery is initiated.[12]
- The patient's legs should be moved slowly and simultaneously into the leg holders to prevent lumbosacral strain.
- The patient's legs should be removed from stirrups slowly and brought together simultaneously before lowering the legs to the bed surface when removing the patient from leg holders, to prevent lumbosacral strain. To maintain the patient's hemodynamic status, his or her legs should be slowly returned to the bed, one at a time if possible.[37]
- The patient's arms should be placed on padded arm boards, extended less than 90 degrees from the long axis of the procedure bed, with the patient's palms up and gently secured.[37,60] The arms should be tucked at the patient's

sides only if surgically necessary. When it is necessary to tuck the arms at the patient's side, the elbows should be padded and the palms should be facing in toward the patient's body. The hands should be enclosed and secured within a foam protector.[37]
- The patient's fingers should be protected from injury when the foot of the procedure bed is repositioned.[37]
- The patient's heels should be placed in the lowest position possible.[61]
- Support should be provided over the largest surface area of the leg possible.[61]
- The patient's legs should not rest against the stirrup posts.[60]
- Scrubbed personnel should not lean against the patient's thighs.[60,62]
- The patient should be in the lithotomy position for the shortest time possible.[61]
- Care should be exercised to avoid shearing when moving the patient to the break in the procedure bed during repositioning.

VIII.k.2. In prolonged procedures (ie, longer than four hours), the perioperative team should consider repositioning the patient in the lithotomy position as a strategy to reduce the risk of pressure injury (eg, skin damage, nerve injury, compartment syndrome).[60,62]

One research review suggests that perioperative team members remove the patient's legs from support structures every two hours, if the procedure is anticipated to last four hours or more.[63] Research does not identify how long the patient's legs should be out of the stirrups before repositioning.

VIII.k.3. The perioperative registered nurse should monitor the patient at all times, especially when the safety strap is removed.

Proper placement of the safety strap is difficult in the lithotomy position. The perioperative registered nurse may not be able to place the safety strap low across the patient's pelvis without restricting access to the surgical site. Use of a safety strap that is placed high or too tight across the abdomen increases the risk of restricting respiration or causing pressure injuries. The patient's legs may seem to be secure in leg holders with his or her arms tucked at the side. It is important to remember that there is still a risk for the patient to shift on the procedure bed, especially when moving into or out of Trendelenburg's position, which is often used in conjunction with the lithotomy position.

VIII.k.4. When positioning the patient into and out of the lithotomy position, a minimum of two caregivers is needed to lift the legs. Mechanical devices such as support slings can be used to lift the legs to and from the lithotomy position.[13]

VIII.l. The perioperative team should implement measures to reduce the risk of injury to patient and caregivers associated with the lateral position. (PNDS: I3, I11, I77, I96, I122)

The patient in the lateral position is at risk of injury due to spinal misalignment and vulnerable pressure points on the dependent side, specifically the ear, acromion process, iliac crest, greater trochanter, lateral knee, and malleolus.[9]

In a lateral position, the patient is positioned on the nonoperative side. This dependent side is the reference point for documentation. For example, when documenting a right lateral position, the patient is lying on his or her right side. This position provides exposure for a left-sided procedure (eg, upper chest or kidney procedure). When documenting the left lateral position, the patient is lying on the left side. The left lateral position provides exposure for a surgical or invasive procedure on the patient's right side.

One research study on interface pressures found that the highest pressures occurred in the lateral position and that there was an increased risk for the procedure bed mattress to become fully compressed under the weight of the patient's body and cause a "bottoming out" effect.[6] Another study found an increased risk for ulceration when a solid object or positioning device (eg, "bean bag" product) is used to maintain patients in a specific position. The firm pressure of the positioning device may compromise the circulatory system due to the tight restraint and because of

the overall effect of gravity on the horizontal body posture.[25]

The lateral position increases the risk of damage to the common peroneal nerve if there is not padding to protect the nerve on the dependent leg from being compressed between the fibula and the procedure bed.[50]

VIII.l.1. Safety considerations for the lateral position should include, but are not limited to, the following:
- The patient's spinal alignment should be maintained during turning.
- The patient's dependent leg should be flexed for support.[37]
- The patient's straight upper leg should be padded and supported with pillows between the legs.
- Padding should be used under the patient's dependent knee, ankle, and foot.
- A headrest or pillow should be placed under the patient's head to keep the cervical and thoracic vertebrae aligned.
- The patient's dependent ear should assessed to ensure that it is not folded, and the ear should be well padded.[37]
- The patient's arm should be secured to prevent movement during the procedure.

VIII.l.2. To safely position a patient weighing up to 76 lb (ie, 34.5 kg) into and out of the lateral position, three caregivers should be assigned; one caregiver (eg, the anesthesia care provider) should be assigned specifically to support the patient's head and neck and maintain the patient's airway during the lateral transfer.

When positioning or repositioning the anesthetized patient into and out of the lateral position, pushing and pulling forces can occur rather than lifting forces. Three caregivers plus an anesthesia care provider can safely position a patient weighing up to 115 lb (ie, 52.2 kg). If the patient's weight exceeds 115 lb (ie, 52.2 kg), it is important to use lateral positioning devices.[13]

VIII.m. The perioperative team members should implement measures to reduce the risk of injury to patient and caregivers associated with the morbidly obese patient. (PNDS: I3, III, I64, I77, I96, I122)

Morbid obesity is associated with patients who have a BMI of greater than 40 or who weigh 100 lb or more over their recommended weight. Patients who are morbidly obese tend to have other health conditions, such as type II diabetes, hypertension, atherosclerosis, arthritis of weight bearing joints, sleep apnea, alveolar hypoventilation, urinary stress incontinence, and gastroesophageal reflux disease. Morbidly obese patients are at increased risk for stroke and sudden death.[65]

It is essential for perioperative team members to understand the pathophysiology of obesity and the effects that various positions have on the obese patient's cardiopulmonary function.[66]

- Respiratory issues include
  - airway compromise due to a patient's short, thick neck;
  - risk of difficult intubation;
  - increased risk for hypoxia;
  - increased risk for intra-abdominal pressure on diaphragm; and
  - increased risk of aspiration.
- Circulatory issues include
  - increased cardiac output,
  - increased pulmonary artery pressure, and
  - risk of inferior vena cava compression.

VIII.m.1. Safety considerations for positioning the morbidly obese patient should include, but are not limited to, the following:
- The procedure bed should be capable of articulating and supporting patients weighing 800 to 1000 lb (363.2 kg to 454 kg.[15] Specialized hydraulics should be capable of lifting patients weighing 800 to 1000 lb (363.2 kg to 454 kg).[67]
- Mattresses should provide sufficient support and padding and should not "bottom out."[23]
- The width of the patient's legs determines whether the lower legs will remain on the procedure bed or must be supported by stirrups. Side attachments may be available on more recent procedure bed models.

- The patient's size may cause difficulty in determining if arms are positioned at less than a 90-degree angle. Padded sleds/toboggans may be used to contain the patient's arms at the side of the body if necessary, provided they can be used without causing excessive pressure on the arms.
- An extra wide, extra long safety strap should be used for patients who exceed the length limits for a regular size safety strap. Sheets should not be substituted for inadequately sized safety straps. Two separate safety straps may be necessary to decrease the risk for the patient falling off the procedure bed due to instability and weight load shifts. One safety strap should be placed across the patient's thighs and one over the patient's lower legs.[22]
- When in the supine position, a roll or wedge should be placed under the patient's right flank to relieve compression of vena cava.
- Patients may not be able to tolerate the supine position due to respiratory or circulatory compromises; it may be necessary to reposition the patient into a sitting or lateral position.[66]
- When in the prone position, the patient's upper chest and pelvis should be adequately supported to free the abdominal viscera to reduce pressure on the diaphragm and inferior vena cava.[66]
- Trendelenburg's position should be avoided because the added weight of the abdominal contents press against the diaphragm causing respiratory compromise, and the increased blood flowing from the lower extremities into central and pulmonary circulation causes vascular congestion.
- In reverse Trendelenburg's position, care should be taken when placing the patient's feet against a padded footboard to ensure that his or her feet are aligned and flat against the board. This prevents rotation and increased pressure on the ankle.
- The lithotomy position should be avoided, if possible, due to the weight

of the patient's thighs pressing on his or her abdomen and raising intra-abdominal pressure, thus increasing the risk of circulatory complications.

- If the patient is placed in the lithotomy position, heavy-duty stirrups should be used, and the perioperative nurse should be aware of and institute measures to reduce risks for respiratory, circulatory, and neurological complications.

- The lateral position may be preferred over the prone position as the bulk of the patient's panniculus can be displaced off the abdomen. The perioperative nurse should be aware, however, that a shift of the patient's panniculus may increase the risk of falling or other injury due to unintentional change in position.[15]

Recommendation IX

After positioning the patient, the perioperative registered nurse should assess the patient's body alignment, tissue perfusion, and skin integrity.

Respiratory function may be compromised after positioning the surgical patient depending on individual factors and patient position.[12,37]

Circulatory function is influenced by anesthetic agents and surgical techniques that may result in vasodilatation, hypertension, decreased cardiac output, and inhibition of normal compensatory mechanisms.[37]

Intraoperative skin injury occurs because of a combination of events:

- ♦ unrelieved pressure,
- ♦ duration of the pressure, and
- ♦ the individual patient's ability to withstand the insult.

Several studies indicate that procedures over two-and-one-half to three hours significantly increase the patient's risk for pressure ulcer formation.[37,68] External skin pressure exceeding normal capillary interface pressure (ie, 23 to 32 mm Hg) can cause capillary occlusion that will restrict or block blood flow. The resulting tissue ischemia leads to tissue breakdown. Both high pressure for a short duration and low pressure for extended duration are pressure injury risk factors. Other extrinsic factors for skin injury include shear forces and friction.[3,4,7,34,64,68]

IX.a.   After the desired patient position is attained, the perioperative registered nurse should reassess the patient to include, but not be limited to, the following systems:
- respiratory,
- circulatory,
- neurological, and
- musculoskeletal/integumentary.[1,11] (PNDS: I38, I87, I96, I128)

Positions such as lithotomy and Trendelenburg's can cause redistribution and congestion of the patient's blood supply.[12,43]

Circulatory responses to certain positions or position changes can be rapid and dramatic.[12,43]

IX.b.   The perioperative registered nurse should monitor the patient for external pressure from surgical team members leaning against the patient's body. (PNDS: I77, I128)

Retractors, equipment, or instruments resting on the patient and members of the perioperative team resting or leaning on the patient add to the risk of pressure injuries that cause nerve or tissue damage.[37,60]

IX.b.1.   The perioperative registered nurse should communicate with the surgical team about the position of surgical instruments, retractor frames, Mayo stands, or other items placed on or over the patient throughout the procedure.[12,60]

IX.c.   The perioperative registered nurse should reassess the patient's body alignment, placement of the safety strap, and the placement of all padding after repositioning or any movement of the patient, procedure bed, or any equipment that attaches to the procedure bed.[12] (PNDS: I11; I128)

Changing the patient's position may expose or damage otherwise protected body tissue. The safety strap may shift and apply increased pressure when repositioning the patient or adding extra padding.

Patient repositioning may increase the risk of pressure ulcer development due to shearing of tissue.[24,40]

An injury may result from adding or deleting positioning equipment, adjusting the procedure bed, or moving the patient on the procedure bed.[12]

In nonsurgical settings, patients who are identified as being at risk for developing pressure injuries are turned or repositioned at least once every two hours. If a patient is chair-bound preoperatively, it is optimal to reposition the patient once every hour.[3] When patients receive anesthesia, they are even more vulnerable to the effects of pressure due to physiological changes.[67] One study found that the incidence of occipital alopecia was significantly reduced when the patient's head was repositioned at regular intervals during prolonged procedures (ie, longer than four hours).[69]

When a prolonged surgical procedure is expected, a patient who is in the lithotomy position may need to be repositioned every two hours to reduce the risk of pressure injury and compartment syndrome.[60,62,63]

Patients who have a radial intra-arterial catheter in place throughout the procedure may have their wrists in a hyperextended position for the duration of the surgical procedure. One study suggests that patients' wrists should be returned to the neutral position following arterial catheter placement as a strategy to decrease the risk of injury to the median nerve.[70]

Literature searches demonstrate that it is difficult to determine the effect of patient repositioning during a surgical procedure because, while position changes are documented, these changes are not normally identified as a strategy to prevent pressure injuries.[71,72]

IX.c.1. The perioperative registered nurse should communicate with anesthesia personnel and the surgeon when assessing the need for repositioning the patient every two hours for prolonged procedures.

IX.c.2. The perioperative registered nurse should place his or her hand between the safety strap and the patient to ensure the strap is not applying excessive pressure to the patient's tissue.[12]

IX.c.3. The perioperative registered nurse should assess the patient for adequate padding by positioning a hand, palm up, below the part of the body at risk to be sure there is more than an inch of support material between the body part and any hard surface.[3]

IX.c.4. The perioperative registered nurse should confirm that prep solutions have not pooled beneath the patient and check for excessive moisture (eg, urine from incontinence) between the patient and positioning devices before the start of the surgical procedure.

A patient's skin may be more susceptible to pressure and friction due to prep solutions that change the pH of the skin and remove protective oils. When prep solutions pool beneath a patient, there is increased risk for skin maceration.[1,24]

Recommendation X

The perioperative registered nurse should collaborate with the postoperative patient caregiver to identify patient injury due to intraoperative positioning.

The incidence of pressure ulcers occurring as a result of surgery may be as high as 66%. Pressure ulcers that originate in surgery may be assessed and documented as burns and may not appear until one to four days postoperatively. Operating room-acquired pressure injuries have a unique purple appearance initially. They tend to progress outwardly with origination at the muscle overlying bony prominences, which explains why they may not be detected when the initial skin assessment is done in the operating room. Pressure injuries in nonsurgical patients progress inward, getting deeper as the tissue injury advances[3] (**Table 1**).

Epithelialization may be delayed in patients who are obese, which may cause poor postoperative wound healing and increased risk of infection.[21]

X.a. Perioperative registered nurses should evaluate the patient for signs and symptoms of physical injury related to intraoperative positioning. (PNDS: I44, I45, I46, I146; I152)

Pressure ulcers are staged according to the degree of tissue damage.[4,73,74] Refer to **Table 1** for assessment descriptors.

X.a.1. Perioperative registered nurses should identify patients who are high risk for postoperative injuries due to positioning and communicate areas of concern with postoperative care provider. (PNDS: I64)

X.a.2. When the patient has been in the lateral position for an extended amount of time in the OR, the perioperative nurse

Policies and procedures establish authority, responsibility, and accountability. Policies also assist in the development of performance improvement activities. These recommended practices should be used to guide the development of policies and procedures within the individual perioperative practice setting.

XIII.a. Policies and procedures for positioning should include, but not be limited to,
- assessment and evaluation criteria,
- required documentation,
- safety interventions,
- positioning equipment care and maintenance, and
- ergonomic safety.

XIII.b. Perioperative policies on positioning should be consistent with the health care organization's risk-control plan for pressure ulcer prevention and management.

Recommendation XIV

Quality
A quality management program should be in place to evaluate the outcomes of patient positioning practices and to improve patient safety.

To evaluate the quality of patient care and formulate plans for corrective action, it is necessary to maintain a system of evaluation.[77,78]

XIV.a. Perioperative administration members should participate in developing and monitoring an organization-wide risk control plan for pressure ulcer prevention and management.

XIV.a.1. Pressure ulcer prevention and management risk-control plans should include, but not be limited to, the following:
- a method for identifying patients at risk for pressure ulcers;
- a documentation system to follow the progress of a wound;
- prevention protocols that protect the patient's skin integrity; and
- education programs for caregivers, patients, and family members.[3,79]

XIV.b. Information about adverse patient outcomes and "near-miss incidents" associated with positioning should be collected, analyzed, and used for performance improvement as part of the institution-wide performance improvement program.

To demonstrate that all reasonable efforts were made to protect the patient's safety, it is considered a sound professional practice to document information according to organizational policy when an event occurs.[80]

XIV.b.1. Following organizational policy, documentation of an event related to positioning should include, but not be limited to,
- a description of what happened,
- the date and time of the incident,
- location of the incident,
- witnesses,
- corrective action to be implemented, and
- communications made regarding the outcome.

XIV.b.2. Data on health care personnel injuries related to positioning activities should be collected, analyzed, and used for performance improvement.

Glossary

Body mass index (BMI): The measure of a person's body fat based on height and weight that applies to both adult men and women.

Braden scale: A widely used assessment tool for predicting the development of pressure sores.

Capillary interface pressure: The amount of pressure placed on the skin's resting surface over a bony prominence.

Compartment syndrome: A pathologic condition caused by the progressive development of arterial compression and consequent reduction of blood supply. Clinical manifestations include swelling, restriction of movement, vascular compromise, and severe pain or lack of sensation.

Ergonomics: The science of fitting the demands of work to the anatomical, physiological, and psychological capabilities of the worker to enhance efficiency and well-being.

Friction: The act of rubbing one object (or tissue surface) against another.

Morbid obesity: A person whose body mass index (BMI) is more than 40.

Procedure bed: A type of bed used in ORs or procedure rooms that allow the surgical team access to the patient and the ability to position the patient for a surgical procedure through the use of the bed, its positions, and its attachments.

Positioning equipment/devices: Any device or piece of equipment used for positioning the patient and/or providing maximum anatomic exposure. Devices include, but are not limited to,

- support devices for head, arms, chest, iliac crests, and lumbar areas;
- pads in a variety of sizes and shapes for pressure points (eg, head, elbows, knees, ankles, heels, sacral areas);
- securing devices (eg, safety belts, tapes, kidney rests, vacuum-pack positioning devices);
- procedure beds equipment (eg, headrest/ holders, overhead arm supports, stirrups, footboard); and
- specialty surgical beds (eg, fracture table, ophthalmology carts/stretchers, chairs).[16]

Shearing: A sliding movement of skin and subcutaneous tissue that leaves the underlying muscle stationary.

REFERENCES

1. Petersen C, ed. *Perioperative Nursing Data Set.* Rev 2nd ed. Denver, CO: AORN, Inc; 2007:43-44, 64-66.
2. National Pressure Ulcer Advisory Panel Support Surface Standards Initiative. Terms and definitions related to support surfaces. Ver. 01/29/07. *http://invisiblecaregiver.com/docs/NPUAP_Standards.pdf.* Accessed December 7, 2007.
3. ECRI. Pressure ulcers. *HRC Risk Analysis.* 2006;3(Nursing 4):1-37.
4. Armstrong D, Bortz P. An integrative review of pressure relief in surgical patients. *AORN J.* 2001;73:645, 647-648, 650-653.
5. Nixon J, McElvenny D, Mason S, Brown J, Bond S. A sequential randomised controlled trial comparing a dry visco-elastic polymer pad and standard operating procedure bed mattress in the prevention of postoperative pressure sores. *Int J Nurs Stud.* 1998;35:193-203.
6. Defloor T, De Schuijmer JD. Preventing pressure ulcers: an evaluation of four operating table bed mattresses. *Applied Nursing Research.* 2000;13:134-141.
7. Hoshowsky VM, Schramm CA. Intraoperative pressure sore prevention: an analysis of bedding materials. *Res Nurs Health.* 1994;17:333-339.
8. Shelton F, Lott JW. Conducting and interpreting interface pressure evaluations of clinical support surfaces. *Geriatr Nurs.* 2003;24:222-227.
9. King CA. Comparison of pressure relief properties of operating room surfaces. *Perioperative Nursing Clinics.* 2006;1.261-265.
10. Cullum N, McInnes E, BellSyer SEM, Legood R. Support surfaces for pressure ulcer prevention. *Cochrane Database Syst Rev.* 2007;(1):ID1030007532000000-01074.
11. Schultz A. Predicting and preventing pressure ulcers in surgical patients. *AORN J.* 2005;81:986-1006.
12. McEwen DR. Intraoperative positioning of surgical patients. *AORN J.* 1996;63:1058-1063, 1066-1075, 1077-1082.
13. Petersen C, ed. *AORN Guidance Statement: Safe Patient Handling and Movement in the Perioperative Setting.* Denver, CO: AORN, Inc; 2007:1-32.
14. Facility design, equipment, and supplies. In: *Bariatric Services: Safety, Quality, and Technology Guide.* Plymouth Meeting, PA: ECRI; 2004:77-110.
15. Dybec RB. Intraoperative positioning and care of the obese patient. *Plastic Surgical Nursing.* 2004;24:118-122.
16. Recommended practices for product selection in perioperative practice settings. In: *Standards, Recommended Practices, and Guidelines.* Denver, CO: AORN, Inc; 2007:637-640.
17. AORN position statement on correct site surgery. In: *Standards, Recommended Practices, and Guidelines.* Denver, CO: AORN, Inc; 2007:371-374.
18. Joint Commission. Implementation expectations for the universal protocol for preventing wrong site, wrong procedure, and wrong person surgery, 2003. *http://www.jointcommission.org/NR/rdonlyres/DEC4A816-ED52-4C04-AF8C-FEBA74A732EA/0/up_guidelines.pdf.* Accessed May 3, 2007.
19. AORN guidance statement: creating a patient safety culture. In: *Standards, Recommended Practices, and Guidelines.* Denver, CO: AORN, Inc; 2007:305-310.
20. Recommended practices for a safe environment of care. In: *Standards, Recommended Practices, and Guidelines.* Denver, CO: AORN, Inc; 2008:351-373.
21. Keller C. The obese patient as a surgical risk. *Semin Perioper Nurs.* 1999;8:109-117.
22. Graling P, Elariny, H. Perioperative care of the patient with morbid obesity. *AORN J.* 2003;77:801-819.
23. Bushard S. Trauma in patients who are morbidly obese. *AORN J.* 2002;76:585-589.
24. Sieggreen M. OR-acquired pressure ulcers in vascular surgery patients. *Adv Wound Care.* 1998;11:12.
25. Aronovitch SA. Intraoperatively acquired pressure ulcer prevalence: a national study. *Journal of WOCN.* 1999/5;26:130-136.
26. Catalano, K. Update on the national patient safety goals—changes for 2005. *AORN J.* 2005;81:336-341.
27. Robey-Williams C, Rush KL, Bendyk H, Patton LM, Chamberlain D, Sparks T. Spartanburg Fall Risk Assessment Tool: a simple three-step process. *Applied Nursing Research.* 2007;20:86-93.
28. Beyea S. Preventing patient falls in perioperative settings. [Patient Safety First]. *AORN J.* 2005; 81:393-395.
29. Nelson A, Fragala G, Menzel N. Myths and facts about back injuries in nursing. *Am J Nurs.* 2003;103:32-40.
30. Stetler CB, Burns M, Sander-Buscemi K, Morsi D, Grunwald E. Use of evidence for prevention of work-related musculoskeletal injuries. *Orthop Nurs.* 2003; 22:32-41.
31. Chappy, S. Perioperative patient safety: a multi-site qualitative analysis. *AORN J.* 2006; 83:871-897.
32. Sewchuk D, Padula C, Osborne E. Prevention and early detection of pressure ulcers in patients undergoing cardiac surgery. *AORN J.* 2006; 84:75-96.
33. Feuchtinger J, de Bie R, Dassen T, Halfens R. A 4-cm thermoactive viscoelastic foam pad on the operating room procedure bed to prevent pressure ulcer during cardiac surgery. *J Clin Nurs.* 2006;15:162-167.

34. Ramsay J. Pressure ulcer risk factors in the operating room. *Advances in Wound Care*. 1998;11:5-6.

35. Reddy M, Gill SS, Rochon PA. Preventing pressure ulcers: a systematic review. *JAMA*. 2006; 296: 974-984.

36. Landis EM. Micro-injection studies of capillary blood pressure in human skin. *Heart*. 1930;15:209-228.

37. O'Connell MP. Positioning impact on the surgical patient. *Nurs Clin North Am*. 2006;41:173-192.

38. AORN explications for perioperative nursing. In: *Standards, Recommended Practices, and Guidelines*. Denver, CO: AORN, Inc; 2007;171-201.

39. Larkin BG. The ins and outs of body piercing. *AORN J*. 2004;79:333-342.

40. Aronovitch SA, Wilber M, Slezak S, Martin T, Utter D. A comparative study of an alternating air mattress for the prevention of pressure ulcers in surgical patients. *Ostomy Wound Management*. 1999;45:34-40.

41. Practice advisory for the prevention of perioperative peripheral neuropathies: a report by the American Society of Anesthesiologists Task Force on Prevention of Perioperative Peripheral Neuropathies. *Anesthesiology*. 2000;92:1168-1182.

42. Fritzlen T, Kremer M, Biddle C. The AANA Foundation Closed Malpractice Claims Study on nerve injuries during anesthesia care. *AANA J*. 2003;71:347-352.

43. Ayello EA. Preventing pressure ulcers and skin tears. In: Mezey M, Fulmer T, Abraham I, Zwicker DA, eds. *Geriatric Nursing Protocols for Best Practice*. 2nd. ed. New York, NY: Springer Publishing Company, Inc; 2003:165-184.

44. Walsh J. *AANA Journal* course: update for nurse anesthetists—patient positioning. *AANA J*. 1994;62:289-298.

45. Lindgren M, Unosson M, Krantz AM, Ek AC. Pressure ulcer risk factors in patients undergoing surgery. *J Adv Nurs*. 2005;50:605-612.

46. Birnbach DJ, Browne IM. Anesthesia for obstetrics. In: *Miller's Anesthesia, Volume Two*. Miller RD, ed. 6th ed. Philadelphia, PA: Elsevier; 2006: 2309.

47. Liau, DW. Injuries and liability related to peripheral catheters: a closed claims analysis. *ASA Newsletter*. June 2006. *http://www.asahq.org/newsletter/2006/06/liau06_06.html*. Accessed December 12, 2007.

48. Faust RJ, Cucchiara RF, Bechtel PS. Patient positioning. In: *Miller's Anesthesia, Volume One*. Miller RD, ed. 6th ed. Philadelphia, PA: Elsevier; 2006:1155-1158.

49. Coppieters MW, Van de Velde M, Stappaerts KH. Positioning in anesthesiology: toward a better understanding of stretch-induced perioperative neuropathies. [Comment]. *Anesthesiology*. 2002;97:75-81.

50. Sawyer RJ, Richmond MN, Hickey JD, Jarrratt JA. Peripheral nerve injuries associated with anaesthesia. [Comment]. *Anaesthesia*. 2000;55:980-991.

51. Cheney FW, Domino KB, Caplan RA, Posner KL. Nerve injury associated with anesthesia: a closed claims analysis. *Anesthesiology*. 1999;90:1062-1069.

52. France MP, Aurori BF. Pudendal nerve palsy following fracture procedure bed traction. *Clinical Orthopaedics & Related Research*. 1992;276:272-276.

53. Toolan BC, Koval KJ, Kummer FJ, Goldsmith ME, Zuckerman JD. Effects of supine positioning and fracture post placement on the perineal countertraction force in awake volunteers. *J Orthop Trauma*. 1995;9:164-170.

54. Lloyd JD, Baptiste A. Friction-reducing devices for lateral patient transfers: a biomechanical evaluation. *American Association of Occupational Health Nurses*. 2006;54:113-119.

55. Chaffin DB, Andersson G, Martin BJ. *Occupational Biomechanics*. 3rd ed. New York: J Wiley & Sons; 1999:73.

56. American Society of Anesthesiologists Task Force on Perioperative Blindness. Practice advisory for perioperative visual loss associated with spine surgery: a report by the American Society of Anesthesiologists Task Force on Perioperative Blindness. *Anesthesiology*. 2006; 104:1319-1328.

57. Rupp-Montpetit K, Moody, ML. Visual loss as a complication of non-ophthalmologic surgery: a review of the literature. *AANA Journal*. 2004;72:285-292.

58. Giarrizzo-Wilson S. Postoperative vision loss; cellular telephones; medical gas handling; roller latches. [Clinical Issues]. *AORN J*. 2006;84:107-108, 111-114.

59. Biddle C, Cannaday MJ. Surgical positions. their effects on cardiovascular, respiratory systems. *AORN J*. 1990;52:350-359.

60. Irvin W, Andersen W, Taylor P, Rice L. Minimizing the risk of neurologic injury in gynecologic surgery. *Obstet Gynecol*. 2004;103:374-382.

61. Roeder RA, Geddes LA, Corson N, Pell C, Otlewski M, Kemeny A. Heel and calf capillary-support: pressure in lithotomy positions. *AORN J*. 2005;81:821-830.

62. Wilde S. Compartment syndrome. the silent danger related to patient positioning and surgery. *Br J Perioper Nurs*. 2004;14:546-550.

63. Raza A, Byrne D, Townell N. Lower limb (well leg) compartment syndrome after urological pelvic surgery. *J Urol*. 2004;171:5-11.

64. Pfeffer SD, Halliwill JR, Warner MA. Effects of lithotomy position and external compression on lower leg muscle compartment pressure. [Comment]. *Anesthesiology*. 2001;95:632-636.

65. Recommendations for facilities performing bariatric surgery. *Bull Am Coll Surg*. 2000;85:20-23.

66. Brodsky JB. Positioning the morbidly obese patient for anesthesia. *Obesity Surg*. 2002;12:751-758.

67. ECRI. Bariatric surgery. *Operating Room Risk Management*. May 2005:14-17.

68. Schouchoff B. Pressure ulcer development in the operating room. *Crit Care Nurs Q*. 2002;25:76-82.

69. Lawson N, Mills NL, Oschner JL. Occipital alopecia following cardiopulmonary bypass. *J Thorac Cardiovasc Surg*. 1976;71:342-347.

70. Chowet AL, Lopez JR, Brock-Utne JG, Jaffe RA. Wrist hyperextension leads to median nerve conduction block: Implications for intra-arterial catheter placement. *Anesthesiology*. 2004;100:287-291.

71. Stotts, NA. Risk assessment of pressure ulcer development in surgical patients. *Adv Skin Wound Care*. 1998;11(suppl 3):7.

72. Price MC, Whitney JD, King CA. Wound care. development of a risk assessment tool for intraoperative pressure ulcers. *J WOCN*. 2005;32:19-32.

73. Schoonhoven L, Defloor T, Grypdonck MH. Incidence of pressure ulcers due to surgery. *J Clin Nurs*. 2002;11:479-487.

74. National Pressure Ulcer Advisory Panel. Pressure ulcer definition and stages. February 2007. *http://www.npuap.org/pr2.htm*. Accessed November 6, 2007.

75. Roth S, Thisted RA, Erickson JP, Black S, Schreider BD. Eye injuries after nonocular surgery. A study of 60,965 anesthetics from 1988 to 1992. *Anesthesiology*. 1996;85:1020-1027.

76. Recommended practices for documentation of perioperative nursing care. In: *Standards, Recommended Practices, and Guidelines*. Denver, CO: AORN, Inc; 2007:511-514.

77. Dunn D. Incident reports: their purpose and scope. First in a two-part series. [Home Study Program]. *AORN J*. 2003;78:45-46, 49-61, 65-70.

78. Quality and performance improvement standards for perioperative nursing. In: *Standards, Recommended Practices, and Guidelines*. Denver, CO: AORN, Inc; 2007:437-446.

79. Agency for Healthcare Research and Quality. Pressure Ulcers in Adults: Prediction and Prevention. *Clinical Practice Guideline Number 3*. Pub No 92-0047 (May 1992). *http://www.ncbi.nlm.nih.gov/books/bv.fcgi?rid=hstat2.chapter.4409*. Accessed November 6, 2007.

80. Liang BA. The adverse event of unaddressed medical error: Identifying and filling the holes in the health-care and legal systems. *J Law Med Ethics*. 2001;29:346-368.

PUBLICATION HISTORY

Originally published November 1990, *AORN Journal*. Revised November 1995; published August 1996, *AORN Journal*.

Revised and reformatted; published January 2001, *AORN Journal*.

Revised 2007; published in *Perioperative Standards and Recommended Practices*, 2008 edition.

Recommended Practices for Preoperative Patient Skin Antisepsis

The following recommended practices for preoperative patient skin antisepsis were developed by the AORN Recommended Practices Committee and have been approved by the AORN Board of Directors. They were presented as proposed recommendations for comments by members and others. They are effective January 1, 2008.

These recommended practices are intended as achievable recommendations representing what is believed to be an optimal level of practice. Policies and procedures will reflect variations in practice settings and/or clinical situations that determine the degree to which the recommended practices can be implemented.

AORN recognizes the various settings in which perioperative nurses practice. These recommended practices are intended as guidelines adaptable to various practice settings. These practice settings include traditional operating rooms, ambulatory surgery centers, physician's offices, cardiac catheterization laboratories, endoscopy suites, radiology departments, and all other areas where surgery may be performed.

References to nursing interventions (I) used in the Perioperative Nursing Data Set, second edition, (PNDS) are noted in parentheses when a recommended practice corresponds to a PNDS intervention.[1] The reader is referred to the PNDS for further explanation of perioperative nursing diagnoses, interventions, and outcomes.

Purpose

These recommended practices provide a guideline for achieving skin preparation of the surgical site. The goal of preoperative preparation of the patient's skin is to reduce the risk of postoperative surgical site infection by removing soil and transient microorganisms from the skin; reduce the resident microbial count to subpathogenic levels in a short period of time and with the least amount of tissue irritation; and inhibit rapid, rebound growth of microorganisms. The following recommended practices are considered established guidelines for perioperative practice.

Recommendation I

Patients undergoing open Class I surgical procedures below the chin should have two preoperative showers with chlorhexidine gluconate (CHG) before surgery, when appropriate.[2]

The act of washing and rinsing removes microorganisms from the skin. Some organisms may be difficult or impossible to kill with the application of CHG alone.

Staphylococcus aureus is the most common organism causing surgical site infections.[2,3] In 2003, 64.4% of health care-associated *Staphylococcus aureus* infections were from methicillin-resistant *Staphylococcus aureus* (MRSA).[4,5] Many surgical site infections result from colonization of the surgical site with the patient's own flora; and colonization with *Staphylococcus aureus* is a known risk factor for surgical site infection.[2,6,7] Clinical trials support the use of preoperative antiseptic showers to reduce the number of microorganisms on the skin, including *Staphylococcus aureus*.[8-11] In 1999, the Centers for Disease Control and Prevention recommend requiring patients to "shower or bathe with an antiseptic agent at least the night before the operative day" (Category IB).[2]

I.a.   Unless contraindicated, patients should be instructed or assisted to perform two preoperative baths or showers with CHG before surgery to reduce the number of microorganisms on the skin and reduce the risk of subsequent contamination of the surgical wound. (PNDS: I48, I123, I104, I50, I36, I106)

I.a.1.   Four percent CHG is more effective than povidone-iodine or soap, and more than one shower is necessary to achieve maximum antiseptic effectiveness.[8,9] One preoperative shower with 4% CHG was found to be twice as effective in reducing skin bacterial flora as showering with nonmedicated soap.[3] Two showers with 4% CHG were found to result in lower microbial counts than showers with bar soap, medicated soap, or povidone-iodine.[8,9] This greater reduction in microbial counts persisted for more than 11 hours.[8] One randomized clinical trial found two consecutive showers or baths with 4% CHG resulted in lower surgical site infection rates than bar soap (ie, 9% versus 12.8%).[9] Showering three times with 4% CHG was found to reduce skin flora 20-fold preoperatively and to lower bacterial counts of the incision taken at the end of the procedure.[10]

Researchers studied the effects of preoperative showering with 4% CHG and povidone-iodine on skin microbial counts of patients colonized with *Staphylococcus aureus*. Two consecutive showers with 4% CHG the evening before surgery reduced microbial counts in the subclavian and groin areas; however, povidone-iodine had little effect on colonization of the groin. Showering both the evening before and the morning of surgery with 4% CHG reduced the bacterial count further at both sites; povidone-iodine provided inconsistent results; and showering with lotion soap increased the colony counts in both the subclavian site and groin.[11]

A sequential process of two applications of CHG with a minimum of two minutes contact time for intraoperative skin preps is suggested by manufacturers' recommendations and supported by one efficacy study for surgical scrub agents.[12-15]

I.a.2. The reduction of the patient's own flora is more important with regard to surgical wounds that are classified as clean or surgical wound Class I.[2] For wounds that are partially or heavily contaminated, other organisms are more likely to contribute to surgical site infection, and showering with CHG may not be as advantageous. Research has not addressed the value of decolonizing patients before surgery on the eyes, ears, face, or before laparoscopic procedures.

I.a.3. Although there is sufficient evidence of the effectiveness of two CHG showers to reduce microbial counts, there is insufficient research to definitively link this decrease in microbial count to a reduction in surgical site infection rates.

I.a.4. Following each preoperative shower, the skin should be
- thoroughly rinsed;
- dried with a fresh, clean, dry towel; and
- the patient should don clean clothing.

Rinsing the skin removes residual CHG that may cause skin irritation. After use, towels contain microorganisms that can grow in the presence of moisture. Using a fresh towel after each shower and donning clean clothing minimizes the risk of reintroducing microorganisms to clean skin.

I.b. Chlorhexidine gluconate preparation products used for preoperative showers should be US Food and Drug Administration (FDA)-approved or cleared for use as a general cleansing agent. (PNDS: I22, I75)

The FDA determines the appropriate uses for all approved or cleared products.[16,17]

I.c. Patients undergoing surgery on the head should be instructed or assisted to perform two preoperative shampoos with 4% CHG before surgery to reduce the number of microorganisms and subsequent contamination of the surgical site. (PNDS: I48, I123, I104, I51, I36, I106, I50)

Two shampoos with 4% CHG reduce the emergence of resident skin flora and contamination of the surgical wound.[18] Researchers found that patients receiving two 4% CHG-shampoos and an intraoperative skin prep with 4% CHG had fewer bacteria on the scalp, both preoperatively and postoperatively, and had significantly fewer positive postoperative scalp cultures than patients receiving either shampoos with povidone-iodine or no shampoos.[18]

Conditioners and other hair care products should not be used after performing preoperative shampoos because a chemical reaction between CHG and the hair care product may impede the antiseptic effectiveness of the CHG.[19]

I.c.1. Hair spray and other alcohol-based hair products should not be used during head and neck surgery.

Alcohol-based hair products are flammable and should not be left on the hair during head and neck surgery because they pose a fire hazard.[19,20]

I.d. Caution should be exercised to avoid CHG contact with the eyes, the inside of the ears, the meninges, or other mucous membranes. (PNDS: I75, I104, I36, I51)

Chlorhexidine gluconate is irritating to the eye and can cause corneal damage.[19] Exposure of CHG to the inner ear can result in permanent deafness.[13,19,22]

I.d.1.   If CHG solution gets into the eye, immediately rinse the area with copious amounts of running water for at least 15 minutes and seek medical attention.[23]

I.d.2.   Chlorhexidine gluconate should not be used on the head if the patient's tympanic membrane is not intact.

I.e.   Chlorhexidine gluconate should not be used on patients for whom it is contraindicated, including patients with a known hypersensitivity to CHG or any other ingredient in the product.[19,22] (PNDS: I123, I75)

Isolated incidents of hypersensitivity to CHG have been reported. Relatively minor symptoms upon exposure have preceded more serious reactions in some patients.[19]

Recommendation II

Preoperative skin antiseptic agents that have been FDA-approved or -cleared and approved by the health care organization's infection control personnel should be used for all preoperative skin preparation. (PNDS: I122)

The FDA determines the appropriate uses for products which the agency has approved or cleared.[16]

II.a.   Current research, recommendations from the Association for Professionals in Infection Control and Epidemiology, FDA information, manufacturers' literature, and material safety data sheets (MSDSs) should be consulted when selecting antiseptic agents for skin preparation within health care organizations. (PNDS: I122, I75)

Decisions about which skin antiseptics should be used in the practice setting are complex. A variety of products may be necessary to meet the needs of various patient populations. Input from an infection control professional knowledgeable about antiseptics is helpful when reviewing the current research and documentation provided by manufacturers.

II.b.   The preoperative skin antiseptic agent should:
- significantly reduce microorganisms on intact skin,
- contain a nonirritating antimicrobial preparation,

- be broad spectrum,
- be fast acting, and
- have a persistent effect.[17]

An antimicrobial ingredient is intended to kill microorganisms. A characteristic of certain antiseptic agents that sets them apart from plain soap is their ability to bind with the stratum corneum of the skin, resulting in persistent chemical activity. Alcohols provide the most rapid and greatest reduction in initial microbial counts on skin, but have no persistent activity.[8]

Persistent antimicrobial activity (ie, measured in hours) helps decrease rebound microbial growth after skin preparation. **Table 1** provides a summary of the characteristics of commonly used skin antiseptic agents.

II.c.   Products selected for preoperative skin preparation should meet FDA requirements, as outlined in the Tentative Final Monograph (TFM) for Health-Care Antiseptic Drug Products, or be the subject of a "New Drug Approval" or an "Abbreviated New Drug Approval" process.[16,17,24] (PNDS: I75, I122)

The FDA requires products for preoperative skin preparation to be
- fast acting (ie, a two-log bacterial reduction on the abdomen and three-log reduction on the groin within 10 minutes), and
- persistent (ie, no return to baseline flora count at six hours post application).[16]

II.c.1.   Persistence of the antimicrobial effect suppresses the regrowth of residual skin flora not removed by preoperative prepping, as well as suppressing transient microorganisms contacting the prepped site.

II.c.2.   Infection control professionals and committees should review the data provided by manufacturers to ensure that surgical antisepsis agents comply with current FDA testing and labeling criteria. The testing should be performed at an independent testing laboratory complying with current FDA requirements and subject to FDA inspection.

The laboratory should employ either ASTM International (formerly known as the American Society for Testing and Materials) standard methods, or methods

Table 1

ACTIVITY AND CONSIDERATIONS FOR PREOPERATIVE SKIN PREPARATION ANTISEPTICS						
Antiseptic agent	Mechanism of action	Gram + bacteria	Gram – bacteria	Viruses	Rapidity of action	(continues on next page)
Alcohol	Denatures proteins.[1]	Excellent[1]	Excellent[1]	Good[1]	Excellent[1]	
Chlorhexidine gluconate	Disrupts cell membrane.[1]	Excellent[1]	Good[1]	Good[1]	Moderate[1]	
Povidone-iodine	Oxidation/substitution with free iodine.[1]	Excellent[1]	Good[1]	Good[1]	Moderate[1]	
Chlorhexidine gluconate with alcohol	Disrupts cell membrane and denatures proteins.[1,2]	Excellent	Excellent	Good	Excellent	
Iodine-based with alcohol	Oxidation/substitution by free iodine denatures proteins.[1,3,4]	Excellent [1,3,4]	Excellent	Good	Excellent	
Parachoroxylenol (PCMX)	Disrupts cell membrane.[1]	Good[1]	Fair[1]	Fair[1]	Moderate[1]	

REFERENCES

1. Mangram AJ, Horan TC, Pearson ML, Silver LC, Jarvis WR. Guideline for prevention of surgical site infection, 1999. *Infect Control Hosp Epidemiol.* 1999;20:250-278.

2. Denton GW. Chlorhexidine. In: *Disinfection, Sterilization and Preservation.* 5th ed. Block SS, ed. Philadelphia, PA: Lippincott Williams & Wilkins; 2001: 321-36.

3. Bryant WP, Zimmerman D. Iodine-induced hyperthyroidism in a newborn. *Pediatrics.* 1995;95:434-436.

4. Smerdely P, Lim A, Boyages SC, et al. Topical iodine-containing antiseptics and neonatal hypothyroidism in very-low-birthweight infants. *Lancet.* 1989;2:661-664.

5. EnviroSystems, Incorporated. Technical Overview, Biocides. *http://www.envirosi.com/TechInfo/technical overview.html.* Accessed November 6, 2007.

(continued on following page)

Table 1 *(continued)*

	ACTIVITY AND CONSIDERATIONS FOR PREOPERATIVE SKIN PREPARATION ANTISEPTICS					
(continued from previous page)	Antiseptic agent	Persistent/ residual activity	Use on eye or ear	Use on mucous membranes	Contraindi- cations	Cautions
	Alcohol	None[1]	No. Can cause corneal damage or nerve damage.[1]	No		Flammable. Does not penetrate organic material. Optimum concentration is 60% to 90%.[1]
	Chlorhexidine gluconate	Excellent[1]	No. Can cause corneal damage. Can cause deafness if in contact with inner ear.[1]	Use with caution.[2]	Known hypersensitivity to drug or any ingredient.[2] Lumbar puncture and use on meninges.[2]	Prolonged skin contact may cause irritation in sensitive individuals. Rare severe hypersensitivity reactions have been reported.[2] Use with caution on mucous membranes.
	Povidone-iodine	Minimal[1]	Yes. Moderate ocular irritant.	Yes	Sensitivity to povidone-iodine. (Shellfish allergies are not a contraindication).[6]	Prolonged skin contact may cause irritation. May cause iodism in susceptible individuals; avoid use in neonates.[3,4] Inactivated by blood.[7,8]
	Chlorhexidine gluconate with alcohol	Excellent	No. Can cause corneal damage. Can cause deafness if in contact with inner ear.	No	Known hypersensitivity to drug or any ingredient. Lumbar puncture and use on meninges.	Flammable.
	Iodine-based with alcohol	Moderate	No. Can cause corneal damage or nerve damage.	No	Sensitivity to povidone-iodine. (Shellfish allergies are not a contraindication.)	Flammable.
	Parachoroxylenol (PCMX)	Moderate[1]	Yes[5]	Yes[5]	Known hypersensitivity to PCMX or any ingredient.[5]	Minimally effective in the presence of organic matter. The FDA has classified PCMX as a Category III (data are insufficient to classify it as safe and effective). The FDA continues to evaluate PCMX.[5]

(continued from previous page)

6. American Academy of Allergy Asthma and Immunology. Academy Position Statement: *The Risk of Severe Allergic Reactions from the Use of Potassium Iodide for Radiation Emergencies.* http://www.aaaai.org/media /resources/academy_statements/position_statements /potassium_iodide.asp. Accessed August 28, 2007.

7. Zamora JL, Price MF, Chuang P, Gentry LO. Inhibition of povidone iodine's bactericidal activity by common organic substances: an experimental study. *Surgery.* 1985;98:25-9.

8. Gottardi W. Iodine and iodine compounds. In: *Disinfection, Sterilization and Preservation.* 5th ed. Block SS, ed. Philadelphia, PA: Lippincott Williams & Wilkins; 2001:159-83.

specifically approved by the FDA for use in conjunction with a particular New Drug Application subject product.

II.c.3. Consult scientific data when selecting new products for use.[25]

Recommendation III

The antiseptic agent used should be selected based on the patient assessment. (PNDS: I94)

The patient should be assessed for considerations affecting skin preparation.

III.a. The patient should be assessed for allergy or sensitivity to skin preparation agents. (PNDS: I123)

II.a.1. Povidone-iodine can cause contact dermatitis or irritant reactions and does not indicate an allergy to iodine. Anaphylaxis to povidone-iodine is extremely rare and has not been proven to be from the iodine.[26] There is no correlation between reactions to povidone-iodine and allergy to seafood or contrast media.[27,28]

II.a.2. Chlorhexidine gluconate has triggered allergic reactions in sensitized individuals ranging from mild local symptoms to severe anaphylaxis. Mild symptoms may precede severe attacks.[29]

III.b. The patient should be assessed for contraindications to specific skin preparation agents. (PNDS: I75, I122)
- Alcohol can cause tissue trauma (ie, necrosis, burns) in neonates with underdeveloped stratum corneum.[30-32]
- Transcutaneous absorption of iodine in neonates can result in iodism.[33-36]
- Safe use of CHG on neonates with underdeveloped stratum corneum has not been established.
- Chlorhexidine gluconate is neurotoxic and can cause permanent injury if the inner ear is exposed to CHG through a nonintact tympanic membrane. Chlorhexidine gluconate can cause corneal irritation if allowed to contact the eye.[19]
- Use of any agent is contraindicated if the patient has a known sensitivity.

III.b.1. The manufacturer's written instructions should be reviewed for additional information about their product's use.

III.c. The surgical site should be identified before skin preparation. (PNDS: I143, I124, I26)

The surgical site should be confirmed before initiating the skin prep. This verification minimizes the risk of prepping the wrong area, which could contribute to wrong-site surgery.

III.c.1. Verification should be done in advance of the "time out" period, which occurs immediately before the surgeon makes the incision.

III.d. The marker used to make the surgical site mark should
- not facilitate microbial growth, and
- provide a mark that remains visible after the surgical prep.[25,37] (PNDS: I138, I122, I98, I77, I75)

Marking the skin with an alcohol-based surgical site marker before skin preparation does not increase the amount of microorganisms on the skin.[38] Water-based skin markers may wash off during skin preparation and have been found to transmit MRSA in laboratory tests.[39]

III.d.1. Ballpoint pens should not be used for surgical skin marking because they may cause trauma to the skin during use.

III.e. The patient's skin condition should be assessed for the presence of lesions or other tissue conditions at the surgical site before skin preparation begins. (PNDS: I94, I77, I15, I21)

Unintentional removal of lesions (eg, nevi) traumatizes the skin at the surgical site and provides an opportunity for wound colonization by microorganisms.

III.e.1. The presence of excessive hair that may interfere with the surgical procedure should be identified.

III.f. The antiseptic product used for an individual patient should be selected based on
- patient allergies;
- a patient's report of significant skin irritation from specific antiseptic agents;
- contraindications to specific antiseptic agents;

– the surgical site to be prepped;
– the presence of organic matter, including blood;
– neonatal status;
– large, open wounds;
– a review of written manufacturer's information; and
– surgeon preference. (PNDS: I123, I94, I21, I75, I85)

Antiseptic agents used on the skin of patients with known hypersensitivity reactions (ie, allergies) may cause adverse outcomes (eg, blisters, rashes). Some antiseptic agents are affected by organic matter and/or saline and are rendered less effective (see **Table 1**). Some antiseptic agents may be absorbed by the skin or mucous membranes and become neurotoxic or ototoxic. Certain antiseptic agents are believed to be potentially harmful to neonates. Products made specifically for use on mucous membranes should be used following manufacturers' recommendations.

Recommendation IV

Hair at the surgical site should be left in place (ie, not removed) whenever possible. (PNDS: I94)

Research studies have found that preoperative shaving of the surgical site increases the risk of surgical site infection[40-42] and results in higher surgical site infection rates than using a depilatory cream or clipping.[42] Hair has successfully been left in place for neurosurgery without increasing the risk of surgical site infection.[43,44]

IV.a.   The patient should be instructed not to shave or use a depilatory on the surgical site before surgery. (PNDS: I136, I77, I106)

Removing hair at the surgical site abrades the skin surface and enhances microbial growth. Shaving has been found to increase the risk of surgical site infection.[40-42] Depilatory creams may cause skin reactions in some individuals, which could result in cancellation of surgery.[42]

IV.b.   Hair at the surgical site should not be removed with a razor. (PNDS: I77, I94)

Shaving increases the risk of surgical site infection.[39-41]

IV.b.1.   Alternatives to hair removal for head and neck surgery include:

• braiding hair instead of shaving; and
• using a nonflammable gel to keep the hair away from the incision.[44]

IV.b.2.   If the presence of hair will interfere with the surgical procedure and removal is in the best interest of the patient, the following precautions should be taken:

• Hair removal should be performed the day of surgery, in a location outside of the operating or procedure room.
• Only hair interfering with the surgical procedure should be removed.
• Hair should be clipped using a single-use electric or battery-operated clipper, or a clipper with a reusable head that can be disinfected between patients.

Clipping hair the morning of surgery has resulted in fewer surgical site infections than shaving or clipping the day before surgery.[45] Limiting the amount of clipping minimizes the risk of microscopic nicks. Clipping the hair outside of the operating room minimizes the dispersal of loose hair and the potential for contamination of the sterile field and surgical wound. During use, the clipper handle is contaminated with the patient's skin flora. The clipper head may become contaminated with microscopic blood or body fluids; therefore, decontamination for bloodborne pathogens is necessary to prevent transmission.

IV.b.3.   Depilatories may be used for hair removal if skin testing has been performed without tissue irritation.

Depilatories may be used when hair is to be removed from the operative site. The use of depilatories, however, does increase the risk of hypersensitivity reactions. The written manufacturers' instructions regarding skin testing and the use of chemical depilatories should be followed.

Recommendation V

The skin around the surgical site should be free of soil, debris, exudates, and transient microorganisms to minimize contamination of the surgical wound before application of the antiseptic skin preparation. (PNDS: I94)

The efficacy of antiseptic agents is dependent on the cleanliness of the skin. Removal of superficial soil, debris, and transient microbes before applying antiseptic agents reduces the risk of wound contamination by decreasing the organic debris on the skin.

♦ No skin antiseptic alone is effective in killing spores (eg, *clostridium*).

♦ Some anatomic areas contain more debris than others (eg, umbilicus, under fingernails, under foreskin). Cleaning these areas separately from the surgical prep prevents distribution of microorganisms from these areas to the surgical site.

♦ Cleaning the foot before antiseptic skin preparation for surgery was found more effective in reducing bacterial counts between the toes than application of the antiseptic alone.[46]

V.a.   If preoperative showers have not been performed, perioperative personnel should wash the surgical site either in the preoperative area or immediately before applying the antiseptic agent in the practice setting. (PNDS: I94, I85)

Preoperative washing removes gross contaminants and oils that may block penetration of the antiseptic agent and removes spores and other organisms that are not killed by the antiseptic agent.

V.b.   Cosmetics should be removed before the preoperative skin prep. (PNDS: I94, I85)

Cosmetics may contribute to increased soil and contamination and impede the effectiveness of the antiseptic agent. The removal of facial cosmetics also may be indicated to prevent debris from irritating the eyes, to facilitate securing the endotracheal tube, or for other reasons identified by the surgical team.

V.b.1.   To remove facial cosmetics, the face should be gently cleansed with a non-irritating agent.

Initial cleansing of the eyes, before application of the antiseptic agent, is not necessary because tears naturally rinse most contaminants from the eye.

V.c.   For abdominal surgery, the umbilicus should be cleaned before the antiseptic skin preparation. (PNDS: I94, I98)

The organic and inorganic material in the umbilicus is a contaminant and cannot be adequately disinfected.

V.c.1.   To soften umbilical detritus, antiseptic solution may be instilled into the umbilicus before cleaning.

V.c.2.   Cotton applicators may be used to remove the detritus.

V.d.   Jewelry (eg, body piercing ornaments) at the surgical site should be removed before cleansing the skin. (PNDS: I94, I98, I102, I77, I72, I75, I57)

Jewelry harbors microorganisms and traps these organisms in adjacent skin. Wearing of rings has been associated with up to a 10-fold increase in median skin microorganism count (ie, bioload).[47] Removal of jewelry before skin cleansing provides an opportunity to more effectively remove these microorganisms from the area that will be prepped.

V.d.1.   Jewelry should be removed to reduce the risk of injury related to
• positioning,[48] and
• proximity to the incision site or active electrosurgical unit (ESU) electrode.[49]

V.e.   An intestinal or urinary stoma within the surgical field should be cleansed gently and separately from the rest of the prepped area. (PNDS: I94, I98, I85)
– Some antiseptics are ineffective in the presence of organic material.
– Cleansing of the stoma removes mucin and organic material that impedes the effectiveness of the antiseptic agent.

V.f.   Surgical fields that include the penis require the foreskin (ie, prepuce), if present, to be retracted before the glans is gently cleansed. (PNDS: I94, I98, I85, I75, I150, I152)

Organic material (ie, smegma) and microorganisms accumulate under the foreskin.

V.f.1.   After cleaning, the foreskin should be pulled back over the glans to prevent circulatory compromise.

V.g.   For surgery on the hand or wrist, the patient's nails should be short and natural without artificial nail surfaces (eg, extensions, overlays, acrylic, silk wraps, enhancements) in the prepped area. (PNDS: I94, I98, I85, I138)

The subungual region harbors the majority of microorganisms found on the hand. The variety and amount of potentially pathogenic bacteria cultured from fingertips of persons wearing artificial nails is greater than from those with natural nails, both before and after handwashing.[50-52]

There is insufficient evidence to determine whether fresh or chipped nail polish in the surgical field increases the risk of surgical site infection.[53] There is, however, a theoretical risk of chipped nail polish fragments entering the wound.

V.h. Cleansing traumatic orthopedic injuries with exposed bone may be facilitated by pulse lavage, high-pressure parallel water-jet, or brush-suction irrigation. (PNDS: I94, I98, I85, I138, I152, I122, I77, I128, I38)

In a randomized clinical trial, low-pressure pulse lavage decreased wound contamination by 86.9% and high-pressure parallel water-jet decreased contamination by 90.8%.[54] In a laboratory study, high-pressure lavage removed less inorganic contaminants and caused more tissue damage than a brush-suction method.[55]

When irrigating traumatic wounds:
- sterile 0.9% saline solution should be used for the irrigation;
- caution should be exercised to avoid aerosolization of wound contaminants onto the sterile field during irrigation; and
- the use of a pulse lavage protective shield may be beneficial.

Recommendation VI

Protective measures should be implemented to prevent skin and tissue injury due to prolonged contact with skin prep agents. (PNDS: I94, I98, I85, I138, I75, I70)

Chemical burns and skin irritations are more likely when antiseptic solutions are not allowed to dry and remain in contact with the skin for prolonged periods of time.[22,31,56]

The iodine in povidone-iodine prep solutions remains free until it has dried and can chemically irritate the skin. When the skin is occluded, the solution is unable to dry, the chemical contact is sustained, and the skin is macerated. The use of forced-air warming under the surgical drapes adds heat to antiseptic solutions, which may increase the likelihood of a chemical or thermal injury. In a series of povidone-iodine burns, authors reported burns resulting from
- soaked linen,
- soaked adhesive tape,
- drips on padding under tourniquet cuffs,
- solution running off surgical sites and onto the patients' backs, and
- a povidone-iodine-soaked gauze being used to cover an epidural site during surgery.[56]

VI.a. Sheets, padding, positioning equipment, and adhesive tape should be protected from the dripping or pooling of prep agents beneath and around the patient. (PNDS: I94, I75, I138)

If antiseptic solutions drip onto fabrics and positioning equipment, the surgical drapes may prevent the solution from evaporating, thus prolonging skin contact with the wet solution.

VI.a.1. Special attention should be paid when the patient is in lithotomy position because antiseptic solution running down the gluteal cleft may not be apparent.

VI.a.2. For vaginal procedures, using a fluid-resistant towel or drape with an adhesive strip below the patient's buttocks may be beneficial.

VI.b. Electrodes, including the ESU dispersive electrode, should be protected from dripping or pooling of antiseptic agents. (PNDS: I122, I75, I72)

Antiseptic solutions contacting these electrical devices may cause chemical or thermal burns. The adhesive material holds the solution next to the skin, and the solution is unable to dry. Solution between the skin and the electrode increases impedance and increases the risk of a pad-site injury or equipment malfunction.

VI.b.1. If antiseptic solution contacts the ESU dispersive electrode,
- the dispersive electrode should be removed,
- the antiseptic solution cleaned from the patient's skin, and
- a new dispersive electrode applied.

VI.c. If a tourniquet is used, the cuff, padding, and skin under the cuff should be protected from contact with prep solutions. (PNDS: I75, I77, I122)

Antiseptic solutions contacting tourniquet cuffs are compressed against and occlude the skin, increasing the likelihood of a chemical burn.

VI.c.1. Use of an impervious tourniquet cuff protector or towelette drape with an adhesive strip may prevent prep solution contact with the skin under the tourniquet.

VI.c.2. If contact occurs, the cuff and/or padding should be replaced before draping.

Recommendation VII

The antiseptic agent should be applied to the skin over the surgical site and surrounding area in a manner to minimize contamination, preserve skin integrity, and prevent tissue damage. (PNDS: I10, I77, I75, I94, I98, I122, I152, I150)

VII.a. Nonscrubbed personnel should apply the skin antiseptic. (PNDS: I10, I94, I98)

The risk of contamination to sterile gown and gloves is high, in most circumstances, when scrubbed personnel perform the prep.

VII.b. Hand hygiene should be performed before initiating the surgical prep.[57,58] (PNDS: I98, I138, I122) Hand hygiene prevents contamination of the prepped area in the event of a glove failure.

VII.c. Antiseptic agents used for skin preparation should be applied using sterile supplies. (PNDS: I70, I94)

There is insufficient evidence to determine if using only clean supplies is a safe practice. In one study, using a combination povidone-iodine scrub and paint, researchers found that using clean prep kits with reusable sponge sticks for the paint, assembled in a central sterilizing area, did not result in higher microbial counts on the skin than when similar trays were sterilized first.[59]

VII.c.1. Sterile gloves should be worn unless the antiseptic prep applicator is of sufficient length to prevent the antiseptic and patient's skin from contact with the nonsterile glove.

VII.c.2. Any supplies touching the prepped area after the prep has been completed should be sterile to prevent introduction of microorganisms.

VII.d. When not part of the surgical procedure, a highly contaminated site (eg, anus, colostomy) should be isolated from the area to be prepped. (PNDS: I21, I94, I98)

Isolating the contaminated area confines and contains microorganisms away from the surgical site.

VII.d.1. An adhesive, fluid-resistant or plastic drape may be beneficial in sealing the contaminated area.[60,61]

VII.e. Application of the skin antiseptic should progress from the incision site to the periphery of the surgical site. (PNDS: I94, I98)

In most surgical procedures, the incision site is in close proximity to anatomic areas with high microbial counts (eg, laparotomy incision/umbilicus/groin; neck/mouth/nares; ankle/toes; shoulder/axilla; hand/fingernails). Progressing from the incision site to the periphery prevents reintroducing microorganisms from these areas into the incision site.

VII.e.1. The prep sponge or applicator should be used for a single application and discarded.

VII.e.2. Subsequent applications should be applied with a fresh sponge or applicator to prevent contamination of the incision site.

VII.e.3. When using a commercially available applicator, refer to the manufacturer's instructions to ensure uniform distribution of the antiseptic.

VII.f. Special consideration on skin prep implementation is necessary when the incision site is more highly contaminated than the surrounding skin. (PNDS: I21, I94, I98, I150)

VII.f.1. If a highly contaminated area is part of the procedure, the area with a lower bacterial count is prepped first, followed by the area of higher contamination, as opposed to working from the incision site toward the periphery.

VII.f.2. When prepping the anus or vagina or a stoma, sinus, ulcer, or open wound, the sponge should be applied once to that area and then discarded.

VII.f.3. An antiseptic-soaked sponge may be applied to the contaminated area during prepping of the surrounding skin.

VII.f.4. Vaginal preps for procedures that include the abdomen should be performed in a manner to prevent splashing of antiseptic agent expelled from the vagina onto the prepped abdomen.

VII.f.5. Urinary catheter insertion should be performed using sterile supplies and aseptic technique. Using sterile supplies for the urinary catheter insertion prevents the risk of cross-contamination of the genitourinary tract.

VII.g. Special precautions and consideration for skin prep implementation is necessary for burns, open wounds, and fragile skin. (PNDS: I21, I94, I98, I36, I75, I77, I152, I131, I138, I122, I128, I51)

VII.g.1. When prepping fragile tissues, gentle friction should be used to prevent tissue damage.

VII.h. The prepared area of skin should extend to an area large enough to accommodate potential shifting of the drape fenestration, extension of the incision, the potential for additional incisions, and all potential drain sites. (PNDS: I21, I94, I98, I138)

An unprepared area may be exposed when enlarging the drape fenestration or if shifting of the drapes occurs, resulting in contamination of the surgical site.

VII.h.1. Consideration of the potential need to convert a minimally invasive procedure to an open procedure will determine the extent of the area to be included in the prep.

VII.i. The antiseptic agent should remain in place for the full time suggested by the manufacturer's written recommendations. (PNDS: I94, I122)

Testing of antiseptic agents has demonstrated effectiveness under specific conditions and contact times. Complying with recommended exposure times facilitates the occurrence of the best antiseptic conditions.

For example, povidone-iodine reaches maximum effectiveness only after it has dried.

VII.i.1. To prevent surgical fires, flammable prep agents must have thoroughly dried and vapors dissipated before applying drapes.[62-64]

VII.j. Adhesive incision drapes may be used to minimize the gaping and shifting of surgical drapes and to contain residual microorganisms on the skin. (PNDS: I70, I98)

Adhesive incision drapes may be advantageous in sealing the surgical field; however, the utility of the iodine-impregnation of these drapes has not been demonstrated.[65] One randomized clinical trial investigating the utility of these drapes after povidone-iodine prep reported no reduction in surgical site infection risk when using iodine-impregnated incision drapes.[66]

Recommendation VIII

If a flammable prep agent is used, additional precautions should be taken to minimize the risk of a surgical fire and patient burn injury. (PNDS: I76, I75, I122)

Using flammable skin prep agents in the operating room or procedural area poses a serious risk of fire because of the common use of ignition and heat sources (eg, electrosurgery, lasers, drills, fiberoptic cables). Special precautions have been developed by the National Fire Protection Association (NFPA), and have been incorporated in the National Patient Safety Goals by the Joint Commission.[63,67]

VIII.a. Perioperative personnel should be familiar with the flammability characteristics of all prep agents stored or used in the patient care area. (PNDS: I122)

Fires have resulted when personnel did not know or remember that a prep agent was flammable and used a heat source during the procedure.[68]

VIII.b. When flammable prep agents are used, they should be packaged in small quantities appropriate for a single application or be prepackaged in a unit dose.[63,67] (PNDS: I122)

Packaging in small quantities may minimize the risk of soaking materials adjacent to the prepped area and limits the amount left over for disposal.

VIII.c. The prep agent should not contact fabric or be allowed to pool on or under body parts (eg, umbilicus, groin). (PNDS: I75, I76, I122)

Solution in contact with fabric may not dry adequately. Pooled prep agents require longer periods of time for evaporation.

VIII.d. If pooling occurs, the excess solution should be wicked away. Any solution-soaked materials should be removed from the procedure room before draping or using electrosurgery, laser, or other heat source.[63,64,67] (PNDS: I75, I76, I122)

Wicking solution away from pooled areas allows the remaining solution to dry adequately. Solution-soaked materials are easily ignitable, and removal from the operating room minimizes the risk of fire.

VIII.e. The prep agent should be allowed to dry and vapors to dissipate before application of an incise drape or surgical drape, or use of electrosurgery, laser, or other heat source.[62-64] (PNDS: I75, I76, I122)

The prep agent remains flammable until completely dry. Vapors occurring during evaporation are also flammable. Trapping of solution or vapors under drapes increases the risk of fire or burn injury.

VIII.f. The use of a flammable prep agent should be discussed during the "time out" period used to verify the surgical procedure and site. (PNDS: I75, I76, I122)

Active communication about the use of flammable prep agents alerts all personnel to the inherent risks and verifies that appropriate precautions have been taken. At times, the person operating the heat (ie, ignition) source may be unaware that a flammable prep agent was used. Active communication prevents this misunderstanding.

VIII.f.1. Active communication between the surgical team members should include that
- a flammable prep agent was used;
- the application site was dry before draping;
- pooling of the prep solution did not occur or has been corrected; and
- any materials soaked with the prepping agent have been removed from the procedure room.[63,67]

VIII.g. Disposal of unused flammable prep agents must be handled in a manner to decrease the risk of fire and in accordance with federal, state, and local regulations. (PNDS: I138, I122)

Disposal of residual flammable prep agents is regulated by the Environmental Protection Agency.[69] Fires can occur when these agents are discarded in nonhazardous trash. Incineration or autoclaving of biohazardous waste can rapidly ignite flammable prep agents.

VIII.g.1. Residual flammable prep agents may be safely discarded in a chemical hazardous waste receptacle outside of the operating or procedure room or immersed in water in a soiled utility room to render the agents nonhazardous.

VIII.h. Flammable skin preparation agents should not be heated. (PNDS: I122)

Heating flammable preparation agents poses a serious risk of fire. When the temperature of these agents increases, they become more unstable and may ignite easily.

Recommendation IX

Manufacturers' written recommendations and MSDSs for handling, storing, and heating of all skin preparation agents should be readily available, reviewed, and followed. (PNDS: I122)

Testing antimicrobial agents is a complex process and not practical in the patient care setting. Data from current research, manufacturers' literature, and the FDA provide direction for storage, safe use, and product efficacy.

IX.a. Skin antiseptic agents should be stored in their original containers; these containers should not be refilled. (PNDS: I138, I122)

Prolonged use of a multi-use container, transferring solutions to secondary containers, and refilling containers of povidone-iodine has resulted in contamination of the antiseptic with *Pseudomonas aeruginosa*.[70-74] These microorganisms can survive more than one year in povidone-iodine;[71] and contaminated povidone-iodine has resulted in transmission of the contaminating organism and subsequent infections.[71,72,74-76] Use of single-dose containers eliminates this risk.

IX.b. If the skin preparation solution is poured into a secondary container, it should be labeled and the label verified before use of the prep agent. (PNDS: I138)

A label placed on the secondary container communicates to anyone using the agent the contents of the container. A patient death resulted when a skin preparation agent was erroneously mistaken for another drug and injected.[77] Health care accreditation agencies require labeling to identify the skin preparation name and strength.[78-80]

IX.c. Heating of nonflammable skin preparation solutions should only be performed in accordance with the manufacturer's written instructions. (PNDS: I122)

Heating these solutions may cause thermal or chemical burns. Heating may alter the chemical composition of the prepping agent and may alter the effectiveness of the antiseptic. Heating povidone-iodine alters the equilibrium of the iodine content.[81] Manufacturers may have a time limit that an antiseptic agent may be warmed slightly, after which it should be discarded.

IX.d. Skin preparation agents should never be warmed in a microwave oven or autoclave. (PNDS: I122)

The temperature of the skin preparation agent is uncontrolled when heated in a microwave or autoclave, and temperature extremes may result in a patient injury.

IX.e. Material safety data sheets for all antiseptic agents and other chemicals used must be available in the practice area.[82] (PNDS: I122, I138)

Material safety data sheets provide information about the flammability of skin antiseptic agents and the maximum safe storage temperature. The Occupational Safety and Health Administration (OSHA) requires that MSDSs be available for all chemicals used in the practice setting. These documents outline the hazards related to the chemicals and appropriate action to be taken in the event of an exposure (eg, splash to the eyes).[82]

IX.f. Storage of flammable preparation agents must be in compliance with local, state, and federal regulations. (PNDS: I138, I122)

Alcohol-based antiseptics are flammable and should be stored away from high temperatures, sparking devices, or flames.[62-64,67]

IX.f.1. Alcohols are extremely volatile, and their containers should be sealed to prevent spilling, leaking, and evaporation.

IX.f.2. Flammable antiseptic agents should not be stored in egress hallways.

IX.f.3. Large quantities of flammable preparation agents should not be stored in an operating room or procedure area.

The NFPA recommends solutions are to be stored in a flammable solutions cabinet designed to minimize the risk of ignition when the amount of alcohol stored in one location is 10 gallons or more.[83]

IX.f.4. Perioperative personnel should refer to their facility's policies and procedures and individual state regulations for additional information.

Recommendation X

At the end of the surgical procedure, the skin preparation agent should be thoroughly removed from the skin unless otherwise indicated by the manufacturer's written instructions. (PNDS: I75, I122, I51, I36)

Active and inactive ingredients in the solution may cause skin irritation and contact dermatitis in sensitive individuals.[19,22,56]

X.a. Residual antiseptic agent should be removed before application of an occlusive dressing or tape.

Removing the solution as soon possible after completion of the procedure minimizes the risk of ongoing irritation. Trapping antiseptic solutions under occlusive dressings has resulted in chemical burns.

X.a.1. All visible antiseptic agent should be removed from the skin.

Residual antiseptics can cause irritation.[22,56] Some manufacturers recommend that specific preparation agents be left on the skin and allowed to wear off naturally.

X.a.2. As soon as feasible, the patient should be rolled to the side and posterior skin surfaces examined to identify any residual antiseptic that should be removed.

A thorough evaluation of the patient's skin may need to be postponed until after the patient is transferred to the postoperative area.

Recommendation XI

Competency
Personnel should receive initial education, training, and competency validation on skin preparation agent selection, application procedures, and patient assessments.

Initial competency validation, in addition to the annual review and evaluation of individual competency skills, should be performed to maintain proficiency in application of knowledge and use of critical thinking concerning performance of skin preparation.

XI.a. Personnel who could be potentially exposed to antiseptic preparation agents must be made aware of the exposure risk associated with these chemicals.[82]

Workers have the right to know about workplace hazards and OSHA requires employers to provide this information. Information about chemical hazards should be offered during initial orientation.[82]

XI.b. Personnel should receive education and training on selection of skin preparation agents.

Personnel should be knowledgeable about skin preparation agents, indications, contraindications, and special precautions to be used when handling flammable antiseptic agents.

XI.c. Personnel providing preoperative patient instructions should receive education on the evidence base for preoperative patient showers.

Patient compliance is enhanced by appropriate education about the importance of preoperative showers, strategies for facilitating the shower, and preventing recontamination of the skin.

XI.d. Personnel removing hair should receive instruction on the risks associated with shaving, shaving alternatives, and proper hair-removal techniques.

Understanding risks and alternatives to hair removal reinforces discernment to avoid hair removal. Appropriate hair-removal techniques minimize the risk of skin injury and surgical site infection.

XI.e. Personnel should receive education and guidance on skin preparation for the types of procedures performed and precautions to be taken.

Skin preparation techniques vary by surgical procedure and patient condition. Educating personnel about these variations and providing didactic instruction enhances required skills.

XI.f. Administrative personnel should validate the competence of personnel participating in skin preparation activities. (PNDS: I1)

Validation of competence provides an indication that personnel are able to appropriately perform skin preparation.

Recommendation XII

Documentation
Patient skin preparation should be documented in the medical record. (PNDS: I27;I30;I116)

Documentation provides communication among all care providers involved in planning and implementing the patient's care. Documentation of surgical skin preparation may assist in the investigation of infections or adverse reactions and identify opportunities for performance improvement. Accountability is established by recording names of personnel who perform procedures. Predetermined documentation fields or indicators also may prompt compliance with policies and procedures.

XII.a. Documentation should include, but not be limited to,
- preoperative instructions;
- patient report of compliance with preoperative showering instructions;
- removal and disposition of any jewelry;
- condition of the skin at the surgical site (eg, presence of rashes, skin eruptions, abrasions, redness, irritation, burns);
- hair removal, if performed, including method, time of removal, and area;
- antiseptic agent used;
- area prepped;
- name(s) of person(s) performing skin preparation;
- precautions taken when flammable agents are used (eg, agent allowed to completely dry);
- removal of prepping agent; and

– postoperative skin condition, including any skin irritation or hypersensitivity (allergic) response to preparation solutions.

Recommendation XIII

Policies and Procedures
Policies and procedures on the skin preparation of patients should be written, reviewed annually, and readily available within the practice setting.

Policies and procedures assist in the development of patient safety, and quality assessment and improvement activities. Policies and procedures establish authority, responsibility, and accountability and serve as operational guidelines. Policies and procedures establish guidelines for performance improvement activities to be used when monitoring and evaluating skin preparation in the operating room.

XIII.a. Policies about preoperative skin preparation should be developed in collaboration with surgeons and an infection control professional.

XIII.a.1. Policies should include, but not be limited to,

- patient education or assistance in performing two CHG-showers;
- appropriate restrictions on and alternatives to hair removal;
- removal of jewelry at the surgical site;
- assessments to be performed before skin preparation;
- approved skin antiseptic agents;
- if flammable skin preparation agents are permitted or not;
- precautions to be taken if flammable skin preparation agents are used;
- removal of preparation agents and evaluation of the skin condition at the end of the procedure;
- documentation;
- storage of flammable skin preparation agents;
- maintenance of MSDS sheets; and
- reporting adverse events.

XIII.b. An introduction and review of policies and procedures should be included in the initial orientation and ongoing education of health care personnel.

Review of policies and procedures assist health care professionals in the development of knowledge, skills, and attitudes that affect patient outcomes.

Recommendation XIV

Quality
A quality management program should be in place to evaluate skin preparation procedures and identify and respond to opportunities for improvement.

A fundamental precept of AORN is that it is the responsibility of professional perioperative registered nurses to ensure safe, high-quality nursing care to patients undergoing operative and invasive procedures.

XIV.a. A quality management program should be in place to evaluate skin preparation procedures and to identify and respond to opportunities for improvement.

"Surgery patients with appropriate hair removal" is a Surgical Care Improvement Project and National Hospital Quality Measures evidence-based practice indicator used by the Centers for Medicare and Medicaid Services and the Joint Commission.[84-86] The abstraction criterion indicating compliance is: "Surgical patients with surgical site hair removal by clippers or depilatory or no surgical site hair removal."[84] Public reporting of the percent of compliance with this indicator is required for Medicare or Medicaid reimbursement.[86,87]

XIV.b. Adverse reactions to skin antiseptic agents should be reported in the health care organization's adverse event reporting system and reviewed for potential opportunities for improvement. (PNDS: I92)

XIV.b.1. Surgical fires resulting from skin preparation agents should be reported and investigated as serious adverse events through a root cause analysis and corrective action taken to prevent recurrence.

XIV.b.2. Near misses should be investigated and corrective action taken to prevent serious adverse events.

Glossary

Antisepsis: The prevention of sepsis by preventing or inhibiting the growth of resident and transient microbes.

Antiseptic: A product with antimicrobial activity that formerly may have been referred to as an *antimicrobial agent.*

Antiseptic agent: Antimicrobial substance applied to the skin to reduce the log number of microbial flora. Examples include alcohols, chlorhexidine gluconate, chlorine, hexachlorophene, iodine, parachloroxylenol, quaternary ammonium compounds, and triclosan.

Denature: To alter the chemical structure of a protein so that biological activity is diminished or eliminated. Made unnatural or changed from the normal in any of a substance's characteristics.

Detritus: Accumulated debris resulting from the wearing away or deterioration of tissue or other deposited material. Any broken-down material.

Flammable: Capable of being easily ignited and burning rapidly.

Gluteal cleft: Cleft of the buttocks.

Iodism: Poisoning by iodine, manifested by severe rhinitis, frontal headache, emaciation, weakness, and skin eruptions. Caused by the administration of iodine or one of the iodides.

Log reduction: The logarithmic death progression of microorganisms after exposure to a sterilant or antiseptic agent. The reduction difference between average surviving microbes for control and test carriers used as an efficacy parameter.

Neurotoxic: Poisonous or destructive to nerves, nerve tissue, or nervous system.

Ototoxic: Having a toxic or injurious effect on the ear, especially the nerve supply, affecting hearing and balance.

Oxidation: The combination of a substance with oxygen, altering cell biologic activity.

Subungual: Under the nail (eg, fingernail).

Toxicity: The degree to which a substance can harm humans or animals.

References

1. Peterson, C, ed. *Perioperative Nursing Data Set.* Rev 2nd ed. Denver, CO: AORN, Inc; 2007.

2. Mangram AJ, Horan TC, Pearson ML, Silver LC, Jarvis WR. Guideline for prevention of surgical site infection, 1999. *Infect Control Hosp Epidemiol.* 1999;20:250-278.

3. Centers for Disease Control and Prevention. Management of multidrug-resistant organisms in healthcare settings, 2006. *Clin Infect Dis.* 2006; 42, 389-391.2. Also available at *http://www.cdc.gov/ncidod/dhqp/pdf /ar/mdroGuideline2006.pdf.* Accessed October 5, 2007.

4. Centers for Disease Control and Prevention. MRSA in Healthcare Settings, 2007. *http://www.cdc.gov/ncidod /dhqp/ar_MRSA_spotlight_2006.html.* Accessed November 5, 2007.

5. Klevens RM, Edwards JR, Tenover FC, McDonald LC, Horan T, Gaynes R. Changes in the epidemiology of methicillin-resistant *Staphylococcus aureus* in intensive care units in US hospitals, 2992-2003. *Clin Infect Dis.* 2006:42:389-91.

6. Kluytmans JA, Mouton JW, Ijzerman EP, et al. Nasal carriage of *Staphylococcus aureus* as a major risk factor for wound infections after cardiac surgery. *J Infectious Disease.* 1995;171:216-219.

7. Leigh DA, Stronge JL, Marriner J, Sedgwick J. Total body bathing with 'hibiscrub' (chlorhexidine) in surgical patients: a controlled trial. *J Hosp Infect.* 1983;4: 229-235.

8. Garibaldi RA. Prevention of intraoperative wound contamination with chlorhexidine shower and scrub. *J Hosp Infect.* 1988;11(Suppl B):5-9.

9. Hayek L, Emerson JM, Gardner AMN. A placebo-controlled trial of the effect of two preoperative baths or showers with chlorhexidine detergent on postoperative wound infection rates. *J Hosp Infect.* 1987;10:165-72.

10. Byrne DJ, Napier A, Phillips G, Cuschieri A. Effects of whole body disinfection on skin flora in patients undergoing elective surgery. *J Hosp Infect.* 1991;17:217-222.

11. Kaiser AB, Kernodle DS, Barg NL, Petracek MR. Influence of preoperative showers on staphylococcal skin colonization: a comparative trial of antiseptic skin cleansers. *Ann Thorac Surg.* 1988;45:35-38.

12. Aly R, Maibach HI. Comparative antibacterial efficacy of a 2-minute surgical scrub with chlorhexidine gluconate, povidone-iodine, and chloroxylenol sponge-brushes. *Am J Infect Control.* 1988;16:173-177.

13. Molnlycke Health Care. Product information Hibiclens® Antiseptic/Antimicrobial Skin Cleanser. *http:// www.molnlycke.com/item.asp?id=23793&lang=2&si=182.* Accessed September 10, 2007.

14. Steris Corporation. Product information Bactosheild CHG 2% and 4% (Chlorhexidine Gluconate) Handwash/ preoperative/surgical scrub technical data. Mentor, IL: Steris Corporation; 1999.

15. Cardinal Health. Exidene® CHG (Chlorhexidene Gluconate) Directions for Use. McGaw Park, IL: Cardinal Health; 2003.

16. US Department of Health and Human Services, Food and Drug Administration. Tentative final monograph for health care antiseptic drug products proposed rule. CFR.21.333, CFR.21.369. *Federal Register.* June 17, 1994: 31402-31452.

17. US Department of Health and Human Services, Food and Drug Administration, Food and Drug Administration Center. Tentative final monograph for health-care antiseptic drug products; proposed rule. 21 CFR Parts 33 and 369. *Federal Register.* June 17, 1994.

18. Leclair JM, Winston KR, Sullivan BF, O'Connell JM, Harrington SM, Goldmann DA. Effect of preoperative shampoos on resident scalp flora. *Today's OR Nurse.* 1988;10:15-21.

19. Denton GW. Chlorhexidine. In: *Disinfection, Sterilization and Preservation.* 5th ed. Block SS, ed. Philadelphia, PA: Lippincott Williams & Wilkins; 2001: 321-36.

20. National Fire Protection Association. Germicide. In: NFPA 99, *Standard for Health Care Facilities.* Quincy, MA: National Fire Protection Association; 2005:99-109.

21. ECRI. Surgical fire safety. In: *Health Devices.* Plymouth Meeting, PA: ECRI; 2006:45-66.

22. LexiComp, AORN. *Drug Information Handbook for Perioperative Nursing.* Hudson, OH: Lexi-Comp, Inc; 2006:373-375.

23. Chlorhexidine gulconate solution materials safety data sheet. ScienceLab.com. *http://www.sciencelab.com/xMSDS-Chlorhexidine_Gluconate_Solution-9923401.* Accessed August 28, 2007.

24. US Department of Health and Human Services, Food and Drug Administration Center for Drug Evaluation and Research (CDER). Guidance for Insustry: Changes to an Approved NDA or ANDA. *http://www.fda.gov/cder/guidance/2766fnl.htm.* Accessed July 25, 2007.

25. Recommended practices for product section in perioperative practice settings. In: *Standards, Recommended Practices, and Guidelines.* Denver, CO: AORN, Inc; 2007:637-40.

26. Adachi A, Fukunaga A, Hayashi K, Kunisada M, Horikawa T. Anaphylaxis to polyvinalpyrrolidone after vaginal application of povidone iodine. *Contact Dermatitis.* 2003;48:133-36.

27. American Academy of Allergy Asthma and Immunology. Academy Position Statement: The Risk of Severe Allergic Reactions from the Use of Potassium Iodide for Radiation Emergencies. *http://www.aaaai.org/media/resources/academy statements/position_statements/potassium_iodide.asp.* Accessed August 28, 2007.

28. Sampson AH. Food allergy. *J Allergy Clin Immunol.* 2003; 111[2 Suppl]:S540-547.

29. Aalto-Korte K, Makinen-Kiljunen S. Symptoms of immediate chlorhexidine hypersensitivity in patients with a positive prick test. *Contact Dermatitis.* 2006;55:173-177.

30. Harpin V, Rutter N. Percutaneous alcohol absorption and skin necrosis in a preterm infant. *Arch Dis Child.* 1982;57:477-479.

31. Reynolds PR, Banerjee S, Meek JH. Alcohol burns in extremely low birthweight infants: still occurring. *Arch Dis Child Fetal Neonatal Ed.* 2005;90:F10.

32. Schick JB, Milstein JM. Burn hazard of isopropyl alcohol in the neonate. *Pediatrics.* 1981;68:587-588.

33. Bryant WP, Zimmerman D. Iodine-induced hyperthyroidism in a newborn. *Pediatrics.* 1995;95:434-436.

34. Pyati SP, Ramamurthy RS, Krauss MT, Pildes RS. Absorption of iodine in the neonate following topical use of povidone iodine. *J Pediatr.* 1977;91:825-828.

35. Smerdely P, Lim A, Boyages SC, et al. Topical iodine-containing antiseptics and neonatal hypothyroidism in very-low-birthweight infants. *Lancet.* 1989;2:661-664.

36. Linder N, Davidovic N, Reichman B, et al. Topical iodine-containing antiseptics and subclinical hypothyroidism in preterm infants. *J Pediatr* 1997;131:434-39.

37. Joint Commission. Frequently Asked Questions about the Universal Protocol for Preventing Wrong Site, Wrong Procedure, Wrong Person Surgery. *http://www.jointcommission.org/PatientSafety/UniversalProtocol/up_faqs.htm.* Accessed August 28, 2007.

38. Cronen G, Ringus V, Sigle G, Ryu J. Sterility of surgical site marking. *J Bone Joint Surg Am.* 2005;87:2193-2195.

39. Wilson J, Tate D. Can preoperative skin marking transfer methicillin-resistant *Staphylococcus aureus* between patients? a laboratory experiment. *J Bone Joint Surg Br.* 2006;88:541-542.

40. Mishriki SF, Law DJ, Jeffery PJ. Factors affecting the incidence of postoperative wound infection. *J Hosp Infect.* 1990;16:223-230.

41. Moro ML, Carrieri MP, Tozzi AE, Lana S, Greco D. Risk factors for surgical wound infections in clean surgery: a multicenter study. Italian PRINOS study group. *Ann Ital Chir.* 1996;67:13-19.

42. Tanner J, Moncaster K, Woodings D. Preoperative hair removal: a systematic review. *J Perioper Pract.* 2007;17:118-21, 124-32.

43. Bekar A, Korfali E, Dogan S, Yilmazlar S, Baskan Z, Aksoy K. The effect of hair on infection after cranial surgery. *Acta Neurochir* (Wien). 2001;143:533-6; [discussion] 537.

44. Kretschmer T, Braun V, Richter HP. Neurosurgery without shaving: indications and results. *Br J Neurosurg.* 2000;14:341-344.

45. Alexander JW, Fischer JE, Boyajian M, Palmquist J, Morris MJ. The influence of hair-removal methods on wound infections. *Arch Surg.* 1983;118:347-352.

46. Brooks RA, Hollinghurst D, Ribbans WJ, Severn M. Bacterial recolonization during foot surgery: a prospective randomized study of toe preparation techniques. *Foot Ankle Int.* 2001;22:347-350.

47. Trick WE, Vernon MO, Hayes RA, et al. Impact of ring wearing on hand contamination and comparison of hand hygiene agents in a hospital. *Clin Infect Dis.* 2003; 36:1383-1390.

48. Recommended practices for positioning the patient in the perioperative practice setting. In: *Standards, Recommended Practices, and Guidelines.* Denver, CO: AORN, Inc; 2007:631-36.

49. Recommended practices for electrosurgery. In: *Standards, Recommended Practices, and Guidelines.* Denver, CO: AORN, Inc; 2007:515-29.

50. Hedderwick SA, McNeil SA, Lyons MJ, Kauffman CA. Pathogenic organisms associated with artificial fingernails worn by health care workers. *Infect Control Hosp Epidemiol.* 2000;21:505-509.

51. McNeil SA, Foster CL, Hedderwick SA, Kauffman CA. Effect of hand cleansing with antimicrobial soap or alcohol-based gel on microbial colonization of artificial fingernails worn by health care workers. *Clin Infect Dis.* 2001;32:367-372.

52. Moolenaar RL, Crutcher JM, San Joaquin VH, et al. A prolonged outbreak of *Pseudomonas aeruginosa* in a neonatal intensive care unit: did staff fingernails play a role in disease transmission? *Infect Control Hosp Epidemiol.* 2000;21:80-85.

53. Arrowsmith VA, Maunder JA, Sargent RJ, Taylor R. Removal of nail polish and finger rings to prevent surgical infection. *Cochrane Database Syst Rev.* 2007; (2): CD003325.

54. Granick MS, Tenenhaus M, Knox KR, Ulm JP. Comparison of wound irrigation and tangential hydrodissection in bacterial clearance of contaminated wounds: results of a randomized controlled clinical study. *Ostomy Wound Manage.* 2007;53:64-6, 68-70, 72.

55. Draeger RW, Dahners LE. Traumatic wound debridement: a comparison of irrigation methods. *J Orthop Trauma.* 2006;20:83-88.

56. Lowe DO, Knowles SR, Weber EA, Railton CJ, Shear NH. Povidone iodine-induced burn: case report

and review of the literature. *Pharmacotherapy.* 2006;26:1641-1645.

57. Boyce JM, Pittet D, Health care Infection Control Practices Advisory Committee. Society for Health Care Epidemiology of America. Association for Professionals in Infection Control. Infectious Diseases Society of America. Hand Hygiene Task Force. Guideline for hand hygiene in health-care settings: recommendations of the health care infection control practices advisory committee and the HICPAC/SHEA/ APIC/IDSA hand hygiene task force. *Infect Control Hosp Epidemiol.* 2002;23[12 suppl]:S3-40.

58. Recommended practices for surgical hand antisepsis/ hand scrubs. In: *Standards, Recommended Practices, and Guidelines.* Denver, CO: AORN, Inc; 2007:565-73.

59. Pearce BA, Miller LH, Martin MA, Roush DL. Efficacy of clean vs sterile surgical prep kits. *AORN J.* 1997;66:464-470.

60. Association for the Advancement of Medical Instrumentation. Selection and use of protective apparel and surgical drapes in health care facilities. In: *Technical Information Report:TIR11:2005.* Arlington, VA: Association for the Advancement of Medical Instrumentation, 2005.

61. Recommended practices for selection and use of surgical gowns and drapes. In: *Standards, Recommended Practices, and Guidelines.* Denver, CO: AORN, Inc; 2007:559-564.

62. ECRI. A clinician's guide to surgical fires: How they occur, how to prevent them, how to put them out. *Health Devices.* January 2003;32:5-24.

63. National Fire Protection Association. Tentative interim amendment. In: NFPA 99 *Standard for Healthcare Facilities.* Quincy, MA: NFPA; 2005:13.4.1.2.2-A-13.4.1.2.2.3.

64. AORN guidance statement: Fire prevention in the operating room. In: *Standards, Recommended Practices, and Guidelines.* Denver, CO: AORN Inc; 2007:259-267.

65. Pottinger JM, Starks SE, Steelman VM. Skin preparation. *Periop Nurs Clin.* 2006;1:203-210.

66. Dewan PA, Van Rij AM, Robinson RG, Skeggs GB, Fergus M. The use of an iodophor-impregnated plastic incise drape in abdominal surgery—a controlled clinical trial. *Aust N Z J Surg.* 1987;57:859-863.

67. Joint Commission. FAQs for the Joint Commission's 2007 National Patient Safety Goals Questions about Goal 11 (Reduce surgical fires). *http://www.jointcommission.org /NR/rdonlyres/61AEFEC2-3970-4856-B518-C9CCDB7B 5779/0/07_NPSG_FAQs_11.pdf.* Accessed August 28, 2007.

68. Best practices for fire prevention in perioperative settings. *AORN Journal.* 2006;84 [Suppl 1]:S37-S44. 2007.

69. Environmental Protection Agency. RCRA Online. *http://www.epa.gov/rcraonline.* Accessed August 28, 2007.

70. Anderson RL, Vess RW, Panlilio AL, Favero MS. Prolonged survival of Pseudomonas cepacia in commercially manufactured povidone iodine. *Appl Environ Microbiol.* 1990;56:3598-3600.

71. Berkelman RL, Lewin S, Allen JR, et al. Pseudobacteremia attributed to contamination of povidone iodine with *Pseudomonas cepacia. Ann Intern Med.* 1981;95:32-36.

72. Craven DE, Moody B, Connolly MG, Kollisch NR, Stottmeier KD, McCabe WR. Pseudobacteremia caused by povidone iodine solution contaminated with *Pseudomonas cepacia. N Engl J Med.* 1981;305:621-623.

73. Oie S, Kamiya A. Microbial contamination of antiseptics and disinfectants. *Am J Infect Control.* 1996; 24:389-395.

74. Parrott PL, Terry PM, Whitworth EN, et al. *Pseudomonas aeruginosa* peritonitis associated with contaminated poloxamer-iodine solution. *Lancet.* 1982;2:683-685.

75. O'Rourke E, Runyan D, O'Leary J, Stern J. Contaminated iodophor in the operating room. *Am J Infect Control.* 2003;31:255-256.

76. Panlilio AL, Beck-Sague CM, Siegel JD, et al. Infections and pseudoinfections due to povidone iodine solution contaminated with *Pseudomonas cepacia. Clin Infect Dis.* 1992;14:1078-1083.

77. Institute for Safe Medication Practices. Loud wake-up call: unlabeled containers lead to patient's death. *http://www.ismp.org/Newsletters/acutecare/articles /20041202.asp.* Accessed August 28, 2007.

78. Joint Commission. National Patient Safety Goals: Goal 3 (Improve the Safety of Using Medications). *http:// www.jointcommission.org/PatientSafety/National PatientSafetyGoals.* Accessed August 28, 2007.

79. Accreditation Association for Ambulatory Health Care. *Accreditation Handbook for Ambulatory Health Care: 2006.* Wilmette, IL: Accreditation Association for Ambulatory Health Care, Inc; 2006:63.

80. Accreditation Association for Ambulatory Health Care. *Accreditation Guidebook for Office Based Surgery: 2006.* Wilmette, IL: Accreditation Association for Ambulatory Health Care, Inc; 2006:63.

81. Gottardi WJ. The influence of the chemical behaviour of iodine on the germicidal action of disinfectant solutions containing iodine. *Hosp Infection.* 1985; 6 [suppl]:1-11.

82. Occupational Safety and Health Administration. Hazard Communication Standard. *http://osha.gov/SLTC /hazardcommunications/standards.html.* Accessed August 28, 2007.

83. National Fire Protection Association. NFPA 30: Flammable and Combustible Liquids Code. Quincy MA: National Fire Protection Association; 2003.

84. Joint Commission. National Hospital Quality Measures/The Joint Commission Core Measures. *http://www .jointcommission.org/NR/rdonlyres/A929F4B9-4F77-4983 -9D9A-8661FDE01F1B/0/oryx_hap_cm_list.pdf.* Accessed October 10, 2007.

85. Centers for Medicare and Medicaid Services. SCIP Process and Outcome Measures. *http://www.medqic.org /dcs/BlobServer?blobcol=urldata&blobheader=multi part%2Foctet-stream&blobheadername1=Content-Dis position&blobheadervalue1=attachment%3Bfilename% 3DNumbered+Measures+for+SCIP+21006.pdf&blobkey =id&blobtable=MungoBlobs&blobwhere=114297 4279114.* Accessed October 10, 2007.

86. CMS plans changes in guidelines for consent, alcohol-based preps. *OR Manager.* 2007;23:1, 7.

87. Centers for Medicare and Medicaid Services. Details for: FY 2008 Inpatient prospective payment system proposed rule improving the quality of hospital cares. *http://www.cms.hhs.gov/apps/media/press/fact sheet.asp?Counter=2119&intNumPerPage=10&check Date=&checkKey=&srchType=1&numDays=3500&srch Opt=0&srchData=&keywordType=All&chkNewsType= 6&intPage=&showAll=&pYear=&year=&desc=& cboOrder=date.* Accessed August 28, 2007.

RESOURCES

AORN guidance statement: Fire prevention in the operating room In: *Standards, Recommended Practices, and Guidelines.* Denver, CO: AORN, Inc; 2007:259-267.

Association for Professionals in Infection Control and Epidemiology. *http://www.apic.org.* Accessed August 28, 2001.

Centers for Disease Control and Prevention. *http://www.cdc.gov/ncidod/dhqp/index.html.* Accessed August 28, 2007.

Environmental Protection Agency. Treatment, storage, and disposal of hazardous waste. *http://www.epa.gov/epaoswer/osw/tsds.htm#dispose.* Accessed August 28, 2007.

US Food and Drug Administration. *http://www.fda.gov.* Accessed August 28, 2007.

PUBLICATION HISTORY

Originally published May 1976, *AORN Journal,* as "Standards for preoperative skin preparation of patients." Format revision March 1978, July 1982.

Revised February 1983, November 1988, November 1992, June 1996. Published November 1996, *AORN Journal;* reformatted July 2000.

Revised November 2001; published January 2002, *AORN Journal.*

Revised 2007; published as "Recommended practices for preoperative patient skin antisepsis" in *Perioperative Standards and Recommended Practices,* 2008 edition.

clinical categories, 27% of adverse events were rule-based errors that could possibly have been prevented by the implementation of some type of standardized documentation format such as a checklist.[4] Additional study results indicated that data loss was minimal when nurses used both verbal communication and a pre-printed form during the process to transfer patient information.[5] Aside from the written portion, an effective communication exchange between the giver and receiver of patient information provides time for the opportunity to dialogue and ask questions.[6] Direct communication reduces the number of assumptions made by the practitioners regarding patient status, allows for a more effective exchange of information, and provides an opportunity to ask questions. In face-to-face exchanges, all communication channels are available including body language, facial expression, and eye contact.[7] Results from an observational study of hand-off strategies showed that a face-to-face exchange of information improved the effectiveness of the hand off.[8]

I.b.1. Only individuals involved with the patient's care should be allowed to view or hear protected information. Examples include, but are not limited to,

- appropriate members of the health care team,
- family members, and
- designated support person(s).

Confidentiality ensures compliance with Health Insurance Portability and Accountability Act (HIPAA) regulations[9] and protects the patient's right to privacy.[10,11]

I.c. All phases of patient care should be addressed in the process for transferring patient information. Phases of care should include, but not be limited to, the

- surgeon's office;
- scheduling department;
- preanesthesia testing unit;
- preoperative holding unit;
- OR;
- postanesthesia care unit (PACU); and
- other areas where postoperative care is provided (eg, intensive care unit, ambulatory care discharge unit).

Research results have indicated that information loss and degradation has occurred across the major phases of patient care.[12,13]

I.d. Contents of the transfer-of-patient-information process for each perioperative phase should include, but not be limited to, the following:

Preoperative phase:
- verification of correct patient (ie, two identifiers), site, and procedure;
- evidence of site marking, if applicable;
- diagnosis, surgeon, anesthesia type;
- required legal documents (eg, complete and signed consent form, durable power of attorney);
- required clinical documentation (eg, complete and signed history and physical by attending physician, informed consent statement);
- laboratory/diagnostic/radiologic test results;
- required blood products, implants, devices, and/or special equipment or instrumentation;
- precautions (eg, isolation, respiratory);
- presence of prostheses and implants (eg, sensory aids, hardware, pacemaker, implanted electronic device [IED]);
- NPO status, allergies, vital signs (eg, temperature, pulse, respiration, blood pressure, pain assessment), as well as pulse oximetry, height, and weight);
- advanced directives documents;
- medication profile including preoperative medications;
- relevant cultural, generational, spiritual, and/or educational patient needs;
- primary language;
- family/significant other information;
- risk for hypothermia, deep vein thrombosis (DVT), difficult airway, and surgical site infection;
- performance measures (eg, antibiotic prophylaxis, beta-blocker administration);
- patient seen by surgeon and anesthesia care provider; and
- patient ready for transfer.

Intraoperative phase:
- verification of correct patient (ie, two identifiers), site, position, and procedure;
- allergies;

- diagnosis, surgeon, and anesthesia type;
- current or pending laboratory or other test results;
- precautions (eg, isolation, respiratory);
- advanced directives;
- special equipment, instrumentation, and implants;
- surgical count status;
- family communication;
- available blood products and blood loss;
- catheter and/or invasive lines present;
- medications (including dose and time);
- IV and irrigation fluids;
- specimens;
- thermal interventions;
- DVT prophylaxis; and
- patient family and/or significant other information.

Postoperative phase:
- verification of correct patient (ie, two identifiers), site, position, and procedure;
- anesthesia type;
- anesthesia care provider's orders related to oxygenation/ventilation, and IV medications;
- surgeon's orders for drains, diet, and medications;
- administered medications including dose and time;
- administered IV fluids and irrigation;
- advanced directives;
- estimated blood loss;
- related information about the surgical site (eg, dressings, tubes, drains, packing);
- vital signs;
- hemodynamic status;
- airway and oxygenation status;
- thermal status;
- urine output;
- presence or absence of surgical complications;
- precautions (eg, isolation, respiratory);
- any significant events; and
- patient family and/or significant other information.

Patient needs vary among phases of perioperative care. Key elements for inclusion may depend on different circumstances (eg, clinical environment, health care provider involved in the transfer process, patient acuity, identified safety risks).[14,15]

I.e. The timing of the transfer of patient information during a change in personnel (eg, breaks, permanent shift relief) or during periods of high activity (eg, conducting counts) should be addressed.

Communicating case status and critical information in the transfer of patient information during a change in personnel (eg, breaks, permanent shift relief) or during periods of high activity (eg, counting protocol) has been identified as a point of vulnerability to information loss, which may have a negative effect on patient safety.[12,13,16]

I.f. Standardized documentation formats (eg, checklists, electronic records, scripts, briefings) should be adopted in processes for the transfer of patient information. Practitioners should ensure that the format for the safe transfer of patient information allows for a smooth and efficient exchange of information.

Standardized documentation formats provide adequate and purposeful information to ensure safe patient care transitions.[17] Standardized transfers and hand-off protocols have the potential to reduce communication breakdowns.[2] Examples of standardized documentation formats include
- SBAR: situation, background, assessment, recommendation;[18]
- I PASS the BATON: introduction, patient, assessment, situation, safety concerns, (the) background, actions, timing, ownership, next;[19]
- SURgical PAtient Safety System (SUR-PASS);[15] and
- SHARED: situation, history, assessment, request, evaluate, document.[20]

I.g. Interruptions and distractions (eg, cellular telephones, pagers, music) during the transfer of patient information should be minimized and eliminated, if possible.

Interruptions and distractions during verbal and/or written patient information exchanges can lead to errors, forgetfulness on the part of the practitioner, and decreased attention. An interruption-driven environment can cause failures in a person's working memory, which is described as the memory that actively processes information.[21] In an analysis of observational data for evidence of use of 21 hand-off strategies in non-health care formats, limiting interruptions was found to be a useful strategy for improving the effectiveness of the hand-off process.[8]

I.h. Transfer of patient information should be delayed until members of the patient care team have had an opportunity to ask and respond to patient care questions or concerns. Questions may include but not be limited to
   - the process,
   - the readiness of the incoming provider, and
   - staffing or bed availability.[22,23]

I.i. Health care organization leaders should support the implementation of a process for the transfer of patient information.

Support at all levels of the organization, including clinical, is needed to implement safe patient practices.[24-26] Encouragement on the part of health care organization leaders creates a familiar environment in which all team members feel safe to speak and participate.[24] It was found in a prospective study that OR leaders and managers were supportive if shown how the use of a preoperative checklist could improve communication and promote safer teamwork.[27]

Recommendation II

Patients, families, and significant others should have an active role in transfer of patient information processes whenever possible.

It was found that a structured, individualized method of transfer that engaged the patient and family members reduced family members' anxiety. The intervention provided family members with details regarding what to expect after the patient and relevant information were transferred.[28]

II.a. Patients, families, and significant others should be informed as soon as possible if the patient's transfer plan changes (eg, patient is transferred directly to a unit instead of the PACU).

It was concluded from an extensive review of the literature that patients' families incur transfer anxiety that can be reduced through nursing interventions.[29] Patient and family anxiety, related to changes in care providers and the physical environment, was reduced after they received written information. Anxiety was decreased in patients and

their relatives when they received individualized education on transfers.[30,31]

Recommendation III

Personnel should receive education, training, and competency validation on effective communication skills and processes for the transfer of patient information.

Communication is central in maintaining the continuity of patient care.[32] Communication was cited as the root cause of the nearly 3,000 sentinel events, such as unexpected deaths and catastrophic injuries, reported to the Joint Commission between 1995 and 2005.[33] A relationship exists between effective communication skills and positive patient outcomes.[34,35]

III.a. The health care organization leaders should determine the type and frequency of competency assessment (eg, upon hire and periodically thereafter) for processes for the transfer of patient information. Team members accompanying the patient should be selected according to their training and validated competency and the patient's ongoing or anticipated needs during transport.[36]

Competency assessment validates the clinician's knowledge acquisition to implement processes for the transfer of patient information.

III.b. Training sessions, using different teaching modalities (eg, simulation, role-playing, case studies), should be conducted to educate personnel.

Simulation is a valuable tool in aiding effective communication and teamwork during the transfer of patient information.[24] Data has shown that simulation improves communication and teamwork skills.[37-39]

Recommendation IV

The perioperative registered nurse should document the process for the transfer of patient information using a standardized documentation format, and the document should be recorded and retained in a manner consistent with the health care organization's policies and procedures.

Documentation of the process for the transfer of patient information provides a record of patient care. A standardized documentation format allows clear and timely communication of patient information affecting patient safety. The Perioperative Nursing Data Set (PNDS) contains specific data elements related to the continuity of care and communication of patient information.[40]

Recommendation V

Policies and procedures for standardized transfer of patient information processes should be developed, reviewed periodically, readily available in the practice setting, and reflect the rules and recommendations from regulatory and accreditation bodies.

Policies and procedures are operational guidelines that are used to minimize patient risk factors, standardize practice, direct staff members, and establish guidelines for continuous performance improvement activities.

V.a. The policy and procedure for the transfer of patient information should be developed by a multidisciplinary team and written according to the established guidelines and format of the health care organization. Components of the policy should include the documentation and communication methods as well as tools and what information and equipment (eg, electrocardiogram monitor, portable oxygen, lifting devices) are needed in various patient information transfer situations.

V.b. The policy and procedure should outline a contingency plan should a patient's status change.

A contingency plan has been shown to improve the effectiveness of the transfer of information in settings with high consequences for failure.[8]

Recommendation VI

A quality management program should be implemented to evaluate and monitor the processes for the transfer of patient information. Components should include patient; process; and structural (eg, format) outcome indicators. A fundamental precept of AORN is that it is the responsibility of professional perioperative registered nurses to provide safe, high-quality nursing care to patients undergoing operative and invasive procedures.[11]

Feedback should be solicited from practitioners to validate the implementation of the standardized documentation format, its ease of use, and the required

training process.[20] Regularly evaluating and monitoring processes for the transfer of patient information may assist in identifying areas for improvement.[22]

VI.a. Barriers to effective communication that interfere with processes for the transfer of patient information should be identified and corrected through quality review activities. The areas that should be evaluated include but are not limited to
- physical setting;
- social setting (eg, status, hierarchy);
- language; and
- communication.[7]

Barriers to effective communication resulting in poorly executed patient care processes can result in delays in surgical intervention, delays in obtaining consents, and delays and/or duplications of tests or treatments thereby placing the patient at risk.[41] Methods to reduce information loss include confirming and repeating verbal orders; using standardized and accepted abbreviations, symbols, acronyms, and dose designations; and avoiding colloquialisms.[6,42] A combination of verbal and written communication provides multiple pathways for the exchange of information.[7]

VI.b. An evaluation period should occur to assess the efficacy of the standardized documentation format. Data on past transfer of patient information processes that were deemed deficient and compromised patient safety should be reviewed. Ongoing evaluation efforts may include focus groups, surveys, and direct observations.

During the evaluation period following the implementation of a preoperative team checklist, team members indicated that the most valuable functions of the checklist were providing detailed case-related information and team-building.[43] Results from a follow-up study using the same checklist showed that communication failures were reduced after the checklist was implemented.[27] Improved accuracy and completeness of transfer-of-patient information may result from evaluation efforts by team members.[44]

VI.c. An evaluation tool for measuring the effectiveness of the standardized documentation process should be considered, and if desired, completed anonymously by health care personnel.[45]

Through the use of an evaluation tool, particular transfer of patient information situations can be evaluated for efficiency, including determining risks that could cause miscommunication. Areas to assess include adequate time, likelihood of interruptions, accessible information, and how many personnel are required.[16] Data results should be shared with the team members to solicit suggestions or comments on identified deficiencies.[1] Review of data may provide insight into the success of the transfer of patient information process.[46]

REFERENCES

1. Arora V, Johnson J. A model for building a standardized hand-off protocol. *Jt Comm J Qual Patient Saf.* 2006;32(11):646-655.
2. Greenberg CC, Regenbogen SE, Studdert DM, et al. Patterns of communication breakdowns resulting in injury to surgical patients. *J Am Coll Surg.* 2007; 204(4):533-540.
3. Manning ML. Improving clinical communication through structured conversation. *Nurs Econ.* 2006;24(5): 268-271.
4. Wilson RM, Runciman WB, Gibberd RW, Harrison BT, Newby L, Hamilton JD. The Quality in Australian Health Care Study. *Med J Aust.* 1995;163(9):458-471.
5. Pothier D, Monteiro P, Mooktiar M, Shaw A. Pilot study to show the loss of important data in nursing handover. *Br J Nurs.* 2005;14(20):1090-1093.
6. National Patient Safety Goals. In: *Comprehensive Accreditation Manual for Hospitals: The Official Handbook.* Oakbrook Terrace, IL: The Joint Commission; 2009: NPSG-1–NPSG-24.
7. Solet DJ, Norvell JM, Rutan GH, Frankel RM. Lost in translation: challenges and opportunities in physician-to-physician communication during patient handoffs. *Acad Med.* 2005;80(12):1094-1099.
8. Patterson ES, Roth EM, Woods DD, Chow R, Gomes JO. Handoff strategies in settings with high consequences for failure: lessons for health care operations. *Int J Qual Health Care.* 2004;16(2):125-132.
9. *Summary of the HIPAA Privacy Rule.* Washington, DC: US Department of Health and Human Services; 2003.
10. Code of Ethics for Nurses With Interpretive Statements. American Nurses Association. *http://nursing world.org/ethics/code/protected_nwcoe813.htm.* Accessed October 6, 2009.
11. Standards of perioperative nursing. In: *Perioperative Standards and Recommended Practices.* Denver, CO: AORN, Inc; 2010. In press.
12. Christian CK, Gustafson ML, Roth EM, et al. A prospective study of patient safety in the operating room. *Surgery.* 2006;139(2):159-173.
13. Roth EM, Christian CK, Gustafson M, et al. Using field observations as a tool for discovery: analysing

cognitive and collaborative demands in the operating room. *Cogn Tech Work.* 2004;6(3):148-157.
14. Committee on Patient Safety and Quality Improvement. Communication strategies for patient handoffs [ACOG committee opinion, Number 367]. *Obstet Gynecol.* 2007;109(6):1503-1505.
15. de Vries EN, Hollmann MW, Smorenburg SM, Gouma DJ, Boermeester MA. Development and validation of the SURgical PAtient Safety System (SURPASS) checklist. *Qual Saf Health Care.* 2009;18(2):121-126.
16. Gregory BS. Patient safety first. Standardizing hand-off processes. *AORN J.* 2006;84(6):1059-1061.
17. Vidyarthi AR, Arora V, Schnipper JL, Wall SD, Wachter RM. Managing discontinuity in academic medical centers: strategies for a safe and effective resident sign-out. *J Hosp Med.* 2006;1(4):257-266.
18. SBAR checklist can cut risk at patient handoff. *Healthc Risk Manage.* 2006;28(9):102-104.
19. *Strategies and Tools to Improve Healthcare Handoffs and Transitions.* Washington, DC: US Department of Defense; 2005.
20. Sharing information at transfers: proven technique to aid handoff communications. *Joint Comm Perspect Patient Saf.* 2005;5(12):9-10.
21. Parker J, Coiera E. Improving clinical communication: a view from psychology. *J Am Med Inform Assoc.* 2000;7(5):453-461.
22. Simpson KR. Handling handoffs safely. *MCN Am J Matern Child Nurs.* 2005;30(2):152.
23. 2010 National Patient Safety Goals. The Joint Commission. *http://www.jointcommission.org/PatientSafety /NationalPatientSafetyGoals.* Accessed October 6, 2009.
24. Leonard M, Graham S, Bonacum D. The human factor: the critical importance of effective teamwork and communication in providing safe care. *Qual Saf Health Care.* 2004;13(Suppl 1):85-90.
25. Pronovost PJ, Goeschel CA, Marsteller JA, Sexton JB, Pham JC, Berenholtz SM. Framework for patient safety research and improvement. *Circulation.* 2009;119(2):330-337.
26. Pronovost PJ, Rosenstein BJ, Paine L, et al. Paying the piper: investing in infrastructure for patient safety. *Jt Comm J Qual Patient Saf.* 2008;34(6):342-348.
27. Lingard L, Regehr G, Orser B, et al. Evaluation of a preoperative checklist and team briefing among surgeons, nurses, and anesthesiologists to reduce failures in communication. *Arch Surg.* 2008;143(1):12-17.
28. Mitchell ML, Courtney M. Reducing family members' anxiety and uncertainty in illness around transfer from intensive care: an intervention study. *Int J Qual Health Care.* 2004;20(4):223-231.
29. Mitchell ML, Courtney M, Coyer F. Understanding uncertainty and minimizing families' anxiety at the time of transfer from intensive care. *Nurs Health Sci.* 2003; 5(3):207-217.
30. Paul F, Hendry C, Cabrelli L. Meeting patient and relatives' information needs upon transfer from an intensive care unit: the development and evaluation of an information booklet. *J Clin Nurs.* 2004;13(3):396-405.
31. Tel H, Tel H. The effect of individualized education on the transfer anxiety of patients with myocardial infarction and their families. *Heart Lung.* 2006;35(2):101-107.

32. Kerr MP. A qualitative study of shift handover practice and function from a socio-technical perspective. *J Adv Nurs*. 2002;37(2):125-134.

33. *Front Line of Defense: the Role of Nurses in Preventing Sentinel Events*. Oakbrook Terrace, IL: Joint Commission Resources; 2007.

34. Mazzocco K, Petitti DB, Fong KT, et al. Surgical team behaviors and patient outcomes. *Am J Surg*. 2009;197(5):678-685.

35. McKeon LM, Cunningham PD, Oswaks JS. Improving patient safety: patient-focused, high-reliability team training. *J Nurs Care Qual*. 2009;24(1):76-82.

36. Warren J, Fromm RE Jr, Orr RA, Rotello LC, Horst HM; American College of Critical Care Medicine. Guidelines for the inter- and intrahospital transport of critically ill patients. *Crit Care Med*. 2004;32(1):256-262.

37. Gettman MT, Pereira CW, Lipsky K, et al. Use of high fidelity operating room simulation to assess and teach communication, teamwork and laparoscopic skills: initial experience. *J Urol*. 2009;181(3):1289-1296.

38. Paige JT, Kozmenko V, Yang T, et al. High-fidelity, simulation-based, interdisciplinary operating room team training at the point of care. *Surgery*. 2009;145(2):138-146.

39. Powers KA, Rehrig ST, Irias N, et al. Simulated laparoscopic operating room crisis: an approach to enhance the surgical team performance. *Surg Endosc*. 2008;22(4):885-900.

40. Petersen C, ed. *Perioperative Nursing Data Set*. 2nd ed Rev. Denver, CO: AORN, Inc; 2007.

41. Carr DD. Case managers optimize patient safety by facilitating effective care transitions. *Prof Case Manag*. 2007;12(2):70-80.

42. Sutcliffe KM, Lewton E, Rosenthal MM. Communication failures: an insidious contributor to medical mishaps. *Acad Med*. 2004;79(2):186-194.

43. Lingard L, Espin S, Rubin B, et al. Getting teams to talk: development and pilot implementation of a checklist to promote interprofessional communication in the OR. *Qual Saf Health Care*. 2005;14(5):340-346.

44. Wayne JD, Tyagi R, Reinhardt G, et al. Simple standardized patient handoff system that increases accuracy and completeness. *J Surg Educ*. 2008;65(6):476-485.

45. Measure understanding during handoffs: a naval hospital uses an evaluation tool to determine whether information is understood. *Brief Patient Saf*. 2006;7(7):4-5.

46. SBAR initiative to improve staff communication. *Healthcare Benchmarks Qual Improv*. 2005;12(4):40-41.

Acknowledgements

LEAD AUTHOR
Robin Chard, RN, PhD, CNOR
Perioperative Nursing Specialist
AORN Center for Nursing Practice
Denver, Colorado

CONTRIBUTING AUTHORS
Jane Kuhn, RN, MSN, CNOR, CNAA
Health Care Consultant
Carson, California

Maria C. Arcilla, RN, BSN, CNOR
Education Coordinator
Texas Children's Hospital
Houston, Texas

Terri Goodman, PhD, RN
Health Care Consultant
Dallas, Texas

Thomas Hilbert, CRNA, MS
American Association of Nurse Anesthetists Liaison
Marshfield Clinic Ambulatory Surgery Center
Marshfield, Wisconsin

PUBLICATION HISTORY
Originally published December 2009 online in *Perioperative Standards and Recommended Practices*.

Minor editing revisions made in November 2010 for publication in *Perioperative Standards and Recommended Practices*, 2011 edition.

AORN Perioperative Standards and Recommended Practices, 2012 Edition

Recommended Practices for Cleaning, Handling, and Processing Anesthesia Equipment

The following recommended practices were developed by the AORN Recommended Practices Committee and have been approved by the AORN Board of Directors. They were presented as proposed recommended practices for comment to members and others. These recommended practices are effective January 1, 2005.

These recommended practices are intended as achievable recommendations representing what is believed to be an optimal level of practice. Policies and procedures will reflect variations in practice settings or clinical situations that determine the degree to which the recommended practices can be implemented.

AORN recognizes the numerous types of settings in which perioperative nurses practice. These recommended practices are intended as guidelines adaptable to various practice settings. These practice settings include traditional operating rooms, ambulatory surgery units, physicians' offices, cardiac catheterization suites, endoscopy suites, radiology departments, and all other areas where operative and other invasive procedures may be performed.

Purpose

Anesthesia equipment is a potential vector in the transmission of microorganisms. Proper handling and processing of medications, supplies, and equipment can reduce the risk of infection to the patient. These recommended practices provide guidelines for the handling, cleaning, disposal, and reprocessing of anesthesia equipment and instrumentation.

Recommendation I

Anesthesia equipment that comes in contact with the vascular system or sterile body tissue should be sterile at the time of use.

1. Items such as IV catheters, tubing, and stopcocks; syringes and needles; and medication vials and ampules are considered critical items. The Centers for Disease Control and Prevention (CDC) uses Spaulding's criteria to determine the potential for transmission of infectious agents. In this classification, items contacting the vascular system or sterile tissues pose the greatest risk of infection and are classified as critical.[1] Using sterile items when contacting the vascular system or sterile tissues minimizes the risk of infection.

2. Aseptic technique should be used when preparing medications. Breaks in aseptic technique have contaminated IV anesthetic agents and medications, resulting in clusters of infections.[2-9] Good practices include
   ◆ performing hand hygiene before preparing medications,
   ◆ cleaning vial stoppers before puncturing them,
   ◆ using multiple needles to withdraw medication into multiple syringes,
   ◆ not transferring syringes of unused medication between patients, and
   ◆ not storing syringes of propofol at room temperature for the day.

   Medications should be stored in a clean area. Personnel should perform basic hand hygiene according to the CDC's "Guideline for hand hygiene in health-care settings,"[10] before preparing medication. Vial stoppers should be cleaned with alcohol before they are punctured. Single-dose vials should be used for only one patient. Syringes of unused medication should be discarded at the end of the procedure. Propofol should be withdrawn immediately before administration.

3. Aseptic technique should be used when administering medications. Bacteria from hands can contaminate syringes and their contents.[11-16] Multidose vials have been found to be contaminated.[17] Syringe contents have been found to contain blood or bloodborne pathogens after one injection or entry into IV tubing.[13,18-23] Using a common syringe in the IV tubing ports of more than one patient has transmitted infectious diseases.[9,24] Syringes and needles should be used for only one application (eg, one syringe and one needle per entry into a multidose vial). Intravenous tubing ports should be cleaned with alcohol before they are punctured with a needle.

Recommendation II

Anesthesia equipment that comes in contact with mucous membranes should be sterilized or undergo high-level disinfection before use.

1. Reusable items (eg, airways, breathing circuits, connectors, fiberoptic endoscopes, forceps, laryngoscope blades, masks, self-inflating bags,

some laryngeal mask airways [LMAs], transducer tubing, transesophageal probes) are considered semicritical. The CDC has determined that their potential for transmitting infectious agents is significant and has classified these items as semicritical.[1]

2. Reusable semicritical items should be cleaned as the first step in reprocessing. Removal of organic material provides optimal conditions for proper exposure of equipment to disinfectants and sterilants.[1,25,26] Rigid laryngoscopes should be disassembled and all components cleaned, including handles. Some automated pasteurization equipment has a cleaning step within the pasteurizing cycle.

3. Clean, semicritical reusable items should be processed by high-level disinfection, pasteurization, or sterilization with a US Food and Drug Administration (FDA)-approved agent, according to AORN's "Recommended practices for high-level disinfection" or "Recommended practices for sterilization in the practice setting."[27,28] Written instructions from the manufacturers of reprocessing equipment, chemicals, and instruments should be followed. High-level disinfection kills vegetative bacteria, tubercle bacilli, some spores, fungi, and viruses.[1] The CDC recommends that reusable semicritical items be high-level disinfected, pasteurized, or sterilized to minimize the risk of transmission of infectious agents.[1] This recommendation is supported by professional organizations, including the Association for Professionals in Infection Control and Epidemiology, Inc (APIC), the American Society of Anesthesiologists (ASA), and the American Association of Nurse Anesthetists (AANA).[1,29,30] Inadequately disinfected laryngoscope blades have been implicated in clusters of infections.[31-33] Laryngoscopes should be disassembled and all parts thoroughly cleaned and the blades high-level disinfected before they are reassembled. Some LMAs are designed for limited reuse. Manufacturers' instructions should be followed.

4. Flexible endoscopes should be processed according to AORN's "Recommended practices for cleaning and processing endoscopes and endoscope accessories,"[34] and the manufacturer's written instructions. Infections have been transmitted when flexible endoscopes have been reprocessed in an automated endoscope reprocessor with the biopsy port caps off or adapters that were incompatible with the equipment.[35,36] Users of this equipment should verify compatibility of the reprocessor with the endoscope and that adapters are approved by the manufacturer of the reprocessing equipment for use with the particular endoscope being processed. Manufacturers' written instructions should be followed.

5. Residual chemicals should be removed and the reprocessed item thoroughly dried before storage or use on a patient. Residual chemicals on items have led to allergic reactions and tissue burns.[37] Chemical stains have occurred when orthophthalaldehyde was not rinsed off adequately before use.[38] Users of chemical disinfectants should verify the appropriateness of the chemical's use on items being disinfected and thoroughly rinse the items according to the manufacturer's written instructions. These recommendations may include a triple rinse. Disinfected items should be dried thoroughly and stored in manner that prevents recontamination or damage. Use of contaminated tap water to rinse semicritical items has resulted in transmission of *Pseudomonas aeruginosa*.[39-43] This agent proliferates in the channels of endoscopes.[39,40,43] Items should be rinsed with sterile water after the chemical disinfection process. If sterile water is not used, the item should be rinsed first with water and then with 70% alcohol, and it should be thoroughly dried, along with its lumens and channels.[43]

6. Disinfected semicritical items should be stored in a clean location in a manner that prevents recontamination or damage. Storing semicritical items in a clean location minimizes the risk of contamination with pathogens before use. Endoscopes should be stored vertically with control valves, caps, and hoods removed.[43]

7. Personnel should be trained in the reprocessing procedures and equipment. Training personnel regarding the complexities of the equipment, chemicals, and processes used minimizes the risk of human error.

8. Quality control of reprocessing procedures should be performed and documentation maintained in accordance with

- AORN's "Recommended practices for high-level disinfection,"[27]
- AORN's "Recommended practices for sterilization in the practice setting,"[28] and
- manufacturers' written instructions.

Quality control measures provide assurance that mechanical and chemical conditions are optimal for high-level disinfection. Documentation provides a mechanism for process improvement and investigation of adverse events.

Recommendation III

Anesthesia equipment contacting intact skin should be clean at the time of use.

1. Items such as blood pressure cuffs, electrocardiogram (ECG) leads, and oximeter probes that contact only intact skin are considered noncritical. The CDC
   - has determined that the potential for transmission of infectious agents is lower when items contact only intact skin,
   - has classified these items as noncritical, and
   - recommends low-level disinfection.[1]

2. Reusable items and surfaces contacting intact skin (eg, blood pressure cuffs, ECG leads, skin temperature probes) should be cleaned between use on patients. Cleaning removes organic and inorganic material, which allows the disinfectant to contact all surfaces.[1,25,26]

3. Reusable laryngoscope handles should be cleaned and low-level disinfected between patients. Laryngoscope handles become contaminated during airway management. In studies, 40% to 50% of handles tested positive for blood.[44,45] Cleaning and disinfecting these handles minimizes the risk of transmission of bloodborne pathogens. The disinfectant selected should be registered with the Environmental Protection Agency (EPA) for use as a hospital disinfectant and used according to the manufacturer's written instructions.[46]

4. Reusable noncritical items should be low-level disinfected between patients. Low-level disinfection with an EPA-registered hospital disinfectant kills most bacteria and some viruses and fungi but may not kill tubercle bacilli or bacterial spores.[1] After subjection to low-level disinfection, the device is considered safe to come in contact with intact skin.

5. Surfaces of anesthesia equipment that are touched by personnel while they are providing patient care or handling contaminated items should be cleaned and low-level disinfected between use on patients, according to manufacturers' written instructions. Surfaces of anesthesia equipment become contaminated with oral secretions and blood during surgical procedures.[47-50] Researchers have found occult or visible blood on 29.5% to 35.5% of anesthesia machines, carts, and monitors.[47,48] Blood also has been found on ventilator controls, flow meter knobs, vapor controls, ECG leads, oximeter probes, and blood pressure cuffs (ie, 25% to 64.3%).[48] Surfaces of anesthesia carts, drawer handles, touch screens, flow meter knobs, ventilator controls, ECG leads, oximeter probes, and blood pressure cuffs should be cleaned and disinfected between use on patients. Other surfaces known to have been touched during patient care also should be cleaned and disinfected between patients.

6. Exterior surfaces of anesthesia equipment (eg, anesthesia cart, machine, monitors) that are not knowingly contaminated during patient care should be terminally low-level disinfected at the end of the day according to manufacturers' written instructions. Contact with blood and body fluids is routinely associated with tasks performed by anesthesia care providers.[50] These surfaces may become contaminated during use, without the knowledge of the provider.[51] Low-level disinfection with an EPA-registered hospital disinfectant renders the surfaces safe to contact intact skin.[1] Manufacturers recommend specific agents to clean complex electronic equipment. These instructions should be followed.

Recommendation IV

Single-use items (eg, breathing circuits, endotracheal tubes, filters, needles, some LMAs, stylets, suction catheters, syringes) should be used once and discarded in accordance with local, state, and federal regulations.

1. Single-use items should be used for a single patient and not reused on subsequent patients. Patient care equipment and supplies are potential vectors of microorganisms and can transmit infectious agents. Safe cleaning and reuse of single-use items has not been established.

These items should be discarded after use on a single patient.

2. Single-use items should not be reprocessed unless requirements for validation testing can be met. Reuse of items designed for single use creates the potential for injury related to mechanical failure, residual bioburden, and chemical residue from the reprocessing agent. For these reasons, reprocessing of items designed for single use is regulated by the FDA. Under the Federal Food, Drug, and Cosmetic Act, facilities reprocessing single-use devices must meet all regulatory requirements of a device manufacturer, including

♦ facility registration and device listing,
♦ premarket clearance or approval,
♦ labeling,
♦ corrections and removals,
♦ medical device tracking,
♦ medical device reporting, and
♦ quality system regulation.[52]

These requirements exceed the capabilities of most perioperative settings.

Recommendation V

Anesthesia equipment should meet performance and safety criteria established by the practice setting and that is consistent with the manufacturer's written instructions.

1. Written information regarding safety and testing methods, warranties, and a manual for maintenance and inspections should be obtained from the manufacturer for all anesthesia equipment. These manuals help in developing operational, safety, and maintenance guidelines. Recommendations vary by manufacturer and equipment model. Manuals should be maintained for each.

2. Anesthesia equipment should be assigned an identification number. Identification numbers allow for documentation of inspections, safety checks, preventive maintenance, repairs, and tracking in the event of a patient or equipment problem.

3. Before placing anesthesia equipment into service, the safety features of the equipment should be tested by qualified, trained personnel, according to manufacturers' written instructions. These tests should be specific to the type and model of equipment involved and include, but not be limited to, calibrations and alarms. Testing the equipment before initial use minimizes the risk of patient injury resulting from faulty equipment.

4. Before use, anesthesia equipment should be tested according to manufacturers' written instructions and the safety standards of the facility. This check provides assurance that basic safety features of the equipment are operational. The FDA's "Anesthesia apparatus checkout recommendations" can be adapted for this purpose.[53]

5. Routine maintenance of anesthesia machines should be conducted on a regular schedule by qualified, trained personnel, according to manufacturers' written instructions. Regular preventive maintenance minimizes the risk of mechanical failure of anesthesia equipment.

6. Any equipment not meeting safety standards should be removed from service. Equipment failing safety checks poses a risk to patients and/or personnel. Removal of the equipment minimizes these risks. The ASA has published guidelines for determining when anesthesia machines should be considered obsolete.[54] Obsolete machines and equipment should be replaced.

7. Before use on a patient susceptible to malignant hyperthermia (MH), the anesthesia machine should be prepared in a manner that minimizes trace anesthetic agents. Halogenated anesthetic agents may trigger MH in susceptible patients.[55] Removing traces of these agents minimizes this risk. The Malignant Hyperthermia Association of the United States recommends changing the soda lime and breathing circuit, draining and inactivating vaporizers, and flushing the machine with 10 L of air or oxygen for 10 minutes before using the machine for an MH-susceptible patient.[56]

8. Equipment containing mercury should be replaced with alternatives that are mercury-free. Mercury poses a risk to patients and personnel as well as the environment. Removing mercury from the health care environment minimizes these risks.[57]

Recommendation VI

Internal components of the anesthesia machine breathing circuit should be cleaned regularly.

1. Reusable absorbers and valves should be cleaned on a regular basis according to manufacturers' written instructions. Particular attention should be given to the valves. An appropriate and cost-effective schedule for reprocessing has not been established.[58] Single-use absorbers are available and should be used for only one patient. Routine sterilization or high-level disinfection of the internal components of anesthesia machines is unnecessary.[29,30,58]

2. Anesthesia ventilator bellows should be cleaned regularly according to manufacturers' written instructions.

3. Soda lime should be changed according to the manufacturer's written instructions. Soda lime canisters do not filter bacteria adequately.[59-61] In one study, 40% of bacteria passed through the soda lime.[61] The bactericidal activity of soda lime also is unreliable.[61,62] Mycobacterium tuberculosis has been found to survive three hours in soda lime.[61] Soda lime, therefore, should not be used as the only method of filtration. Canisters and contents should be replaced according to the manufacturer's written instructions.

4. Routine use of single-use breathing circuits with bacterial filters should be considered. Bacteria circulate through the anesthesia circuit and proliferate inside the absorber and accessories.[63-65] Filters prevent microorganisms from contaminating the ventilator and escaping into the OR through the positive pressure relief valve of the waste gas scavenging system.[62,66-73] Research findings indicate that the absence of bacterial filters does not lead to an increased rate of nosocomial pneumonias.[58,74] In one investigation, however, contamination of the anesthetic circuit was identified as the likely cause of transmission of hepatitis C virus.[75] Currently, there is no consensus about the routine use of bacterial filters.[29,30,58,76,77] For patients with known or suspected tuberculosis, the CDC, ASA, and AANA recommend using a bacterial filter between the patient and breathing circuit.[29,30,58] The Canadian Society of Anesthesiologists also recommends use of bacterial filters for patients with severe acute respiratory syndrome (SARS).[78] With the increased prevalence of tuberculosis, increased numbers of immunocompromised patients, and the advent of SARS, it is prudent to consider the routine use of bacterial filters on the inspiratory and expiratory limbs of the anesthesia circuit. Some single-use circuits have a heat and moisture exchanger equipped with these filters. Reusable circuits should be cleaned and undergo high level disinfection, pasteurization, or sterilization between use on patients.

5. Humidifiers should be used and cleaned according to manufacturers' written instructions. The water in humidifiers is heated to temperatures that reduce or eliminate microbial growth.[79] Tap water may contain stationary-phase forms of Legionella pneumophila, which are heat resistant.[66] Sterile water should be used in humidifiers.[58,79-81] Reusable humidifying chambers should undergo sterilization or high-level disinfection between patient uses.[58,79] Single-use chambers should be discarded after use on one patient.

Recommendation VII

Waste must be disposed of in a manner consistent with local, state, and federal regulations.

1. Biohazardous waste should be placed in a biohazardous waste bag. Some anesthetic waste poses a risk of transmission of bloodborne pathogens. Placing it in designated biohazardous containers alerts handlers to this risk. Management of biohazardous waste within the health care facility is regulated by the Occupational Safety and Health Administration (OSHA).[82] State and local laws also apply. Perioperative professionals should be aware of and act in accordance with these laws.

2. Sharps should be handled in a manner that minimizes the risk of percutaneous injury. To minimize the risk of injury from contaminated sharps, OSHA requires that puncture-resistant sharps containers be located at the point of use.[82] Placing the container next to or on the anesthesia equipment meets this expectation. Sharps should be placed directly into the container.

3. Waste that is hazardous upon disposal must be managed in a way that minimizes environmental impact. Some waste poses a risk to the environment (eg, alcohol, benzoin, epinephrine, mercury). This waste is classified by the EPA as hazardous upon disposal and is regulated

under the Resource Conservation and Recovery Act.[83] The EPA requires that this waste be placed in hazardous waste containers at the point of use to alert handlers to the need to take precautions upon its disposal.[84] State and local laws also may apply.

Recommendation VIII

Potential hazards to perioperative personnel that are associated with handling and processing clean and contaminated anesthesia equipment (eg, exposure to infectious organisms, chemicals) should be identified, and practices should be established to reduce the risk of injury.

1. Contaminated sharps must be discarded in a puncture-resistant container at the point of use. Immediate disposal of sharps prevents injuries to people unaware of the location of the sharp and is required by OSHA.[82]

2. All personnel involved with cleaning and processing anesthesia equipment should practice according to AORN's "Recommended practices for standard and transmission-based precautions."[85] These precautions define general measures for infection control.

3. Anesthesia equipment should be processed using methods that reduce the risk of exposure to pathogens and injury. Manual cleaning methods that minimize splashing, spraying, spattering, and generation of droplets protect personnel from exposure to blood, body fluids, and cleaning agents.

4. Personnel must be apprised of the hazards in the workplace, including chemicals used for reprocessing anesthesia equipment. Knowledge of the hazards in the workplace, preventive measures, and exposure management minimize the risk of injury to employees and are required by OSHA.[86]

5. Personal protective equipment (PPE) must be provided to minimize the risk of exposure to bloodborne pathogens and chemicals used in the workplace. Use of barrier protection minimizes the risk of exposure to bloodborne pathogens by personnel performing tasks likely to generate contact with blood. According to OSHA regulations, employers are required to provide PPE (eg, gloves, gown, mask, protective eyewear, face shield) for their employees.[82]

6. Personnel should actively participate in the evaluation of engineering devices and work practice controls to minimize the risk of exposure to bloodborne pathogens. Active participation in the selection of PPE and practices provides the best opportunity for designing a safer workplace. According to OSHA regulations, employers are required to solicit nonmanagerial employee input during evaluation of engineering devices and work practice controls to minimize exposures to bloodborne pathogens.[87]

Recommendation IX

Anesthesia equipment should be handled, cleaned, processed, or discarded in the same manner in all areas of the practice setting.

1. Guidelines should be developed and approved by appropriate mechanisms and governing bodies in the practice setting. Equipment may be located in satellite areas (eg, labor and delivery). Guidelines should be consistent throughout the practice setting because all patients are entitled to the same standard of care.[88]

Recommendation X

Policies and procedures on cleaning and processing anesthesia equipment should be developed, reviewed periodically, and readily available in the practice setting.

1. These recommended practices should be used as guidelines for developing policies and procedures in the practice setting. Policies and procedures establish authority, responsibility, and accountability for cleaning, handling, and processing anesthesia equipment and serve as operational guidelines. Policies and procedures also help in developing performance improvement activities.

2. Policies and procedures for cleaning and processing anesthesia equipment should include, but not be limited to,
   ◆ disposal of single-use items,
   ◆ equipment maintenance programs,
   ◆ equipment quality checks,
   ◆ personal protection,
   ◆ personnel education,
   ◆ processing reusable equipment, and
   ◆ waste disposal.

Glossary

Anesthesia equipment: Equipment used to provide anesthesia and/or monitor the patient under sedation or anesthesia.

Cleaning: A process using friction, detergent, and water to remove organic debris.

Critical item: An item that contacts the vascular system or enters sterile tissue, posing the highest risk of transmission of infection.

High-level disinfection: A process that uses a government-registered agent that kills vegetative bacteria, tubercle bacilli, some spores, fungi, and lipid and nonlipid viruses, given appropriate concentration, submersion, and contact time.

Low-level disinfection: A process by which most bacteria, some viruses, and some fungi are killed. This process may not kill resistant organisms, such as mycobacterium tubercle or bacterial spores.

Noncritical item: An item that comes in contact with intact skin but not with mucous membranes, sterile tissue, or the vascular system.

Pasteurization: A process that employs time and hot water (ie, 160° to 170° F [71.1° C to 76.7° C] for 30 minutes) for high-level disinfection. The intensity of heat and duration of exposure must be determined by the manufacturer of the pasteurization unit and the manufacturer of the product or device to be cleaned.

Semicritical item: An item that comes in contact with mucous membranes or with skin that is not intact.

REFERENCES

1. W A Rutala, APIC Guidelines Committee, "APIC guideline for selection and use of disinfectants," *American Journal of Infection Control* 24 (August 1996) 313-342.

2. Centers for Disease Control and Prevention, "Postsurgical infections associated with an extrinsically contaminated intravenous anesthetic agent—California, Illinois, Maine, and Michigan, 1990," *Morbidity and Mortality Weekly Report* 39 (June 29, 1990) 426-427, 433.

3. M J Daily, J B Dickey, K H Packo, "Endogenous Candida endophthalmitis after intravenous anesthesia with propofol," *Archives of Ophthalmology* 109 (August 1991) 1081-1084.

4. M E Villarino et al, "Postsurgical infectious associated with an extrinsically contaminated intravenous anesthetic agent," program and abstracts of the 31st Interscience Conference on Antimicrobial Agents and Chemotherapy, Chicago, 29 Sept-2 Oct 1991.

5. B Veber et al, "Severe sepsis after intravenous injection of contaminated Propofol," *Anesthesiology* 80 (March 1994) 712-713.

6. K Kidd-Ljunggren et al, "Nosocomial transmission of hepatitis B virus infection through multiple-dose vials," *Journal of Hospital Infection* 43 (September 1999) 57-62.

7. M J Kuehnert et al, "*Staphylococcus aureus* bloodstream infections among patients undergoing electroconvulsive therapy traced to breaks in infection control and possible extrinsic contamination by Propofol," *Anesthesia and Analgesia* 85 (August 1997) 420-425.

8. M Massari et al, "Transmission of hepatitis C virus in a gynecological surgery setting," *Journal of Clinical Microbiology* 39 (August 2001) 2860-2863.

9. Centers for Disease Control and Prevention, "Transmission of hepatitis B and C viruses in outpatient settings—New York, Oklahoma, and Nebraska, 2000-2002," *Morbidity and Mortality Weekly Report* 52 (Sept 26, 2003) 901-906.

10. J M Boyce, D Pittet, "Guideline for hand hygiene in health-care settings: Recommendations of the Healthcare Infection Control Practices Advisory Committee and the HICPAC/SHEA/APIC/ISAD Hand Hygiene Taskforce," *Morbidity and Mortality Weekly Report* 51 (Oct 25, 2002) (RR16) 1-44.

11. C F Blogg, M A Ramsey, J D Jarvis, "Infection hazard from syringes," *British Journal of Anaesthesia* 46 (April 1974) 260-262.

12. M R Lessard et al, "A microbiological study of the contamination of the syringes used in anaesthesia practice," *Canadian Journal of Anaesthesia* 35 (November 1988) 567-569.

13. C T Lutz et al, "Allergy testing of multiple patients should no longer be performed with a common syringe," *The New England Journal of Medicine* 310 (May 17, 1984) 1335-1337.

14. J W Koepke, J C Selner, "Allergy testing of multiple patients with a common syringe," *The New England Journal Medicine* 311 (Nov 1, 1984) 1188-1189.

15. D J Shulan et al, "Contamination of intradermal skin test syringes," *Journal of Allergy and Clinical Immunology* 76 (August 1985) 226-227.

16. J W Koepke et al, "Viral contamination of intradermal skin test syringes," *Annals of Allergy* 55 (December 1985) 776-778.

17. A Carbonne et al, "Patient to patient transmission of hepatitis C in surgery clinic through multi-dose vials," abstract presented at the 13th annual meeting of the Society for Healthcare Epidemiology of America, Arlington, VA, 5-8 April 2003.

18. A Fleming, A C Ogilvie, "Syringe needles and mass inoculation technique," *British Medical Journal* 1 (March 17, 1951) 543-546.

19. R R Hughes, "Post-penicillin jaundice," *British Medical Journal* 2 (Nov 9, 1946) 685-688.

20. R Uren, C Commens, R Howman-Giles, "Intradermal injections: A potential health hazard?" *Medical Journal of Australia* 161 (August 994) 226.

21. H A Hein et al, "Recapping needles in anesthesia—Is it safe?" *Anesthesiology* 67 (September 1987) A161.

22. C A Trepanier et al, "Risk of cross-infection related to the multiple use of disposable syringes," *Canadian Journal of Anaesthesia* 37 (March 1990) 156-159.

23. J L Parlow, "Blood contamination of drug syringes used in anaesthesia," *Canadian Journal of Anaesthesia* 36 suppl (1989) S61-S62.

24. B Meier, "Reuse of needle at hospital infects 50 with hepatitis C," *New York Times,* Oct 10, 2002.

25. Association for the Advancement of Medical Instrumentation, "Safe handling and biological decontamination of reusable medical devices in health care facilities and in nonclinical settings; ANSI/AAMI ST35" (Arlington, Va: Association of the Advancement of Medical Instrumentation, 2003) 16.

26. "Sterilization or disinfection of medical devices: General principles," Centers for Disease Control and Prevention, *http://www.cdc.gov/ncidod/hip/sterile/sterilgp.htm* (accessed 24 Sept 2004).

27. "Recommended practices for high-level disinfection," in *Standards, Recommended Practices, and Guidelines* (Denver: AORN, Inc, 2004) 235-240.

28. "Recommended practices for sterilization in the practice setting," in *Standards, Recommended Practices, and Guidelines* (Denver: AORN, Inc, 2004) 373-384.

29. American Society of Anesthesiologists Committee on Occupational Health of Operating Room Personnel, *Recommendations for Infection Control for the Practice of Anesthesiology,* second ed (American Society of Anesthesiologists: Park Ridge, Ill, 1998). Also available at *http://www.asahq.org/publicationsAndServices/infection control.pdf* (accessed 24 May 2004).

30. American Association of Nurse Anesthetists, *Infection Control Guide* (Park Ridge, Ill: American Association of Nurse Anesthetists, 1997) 13-23.

31. J E Foweraker, "The laryngoscope as a potential source of cross-infection," *Journal of Hospital Infections* 29 (April 1995) 315-316.

32. T J Neal et al, "The neonatal laryngoscope as a potential source of cross-infection," *Journal of Hospital Infections* 30 (August 1995) 315-317.

33. K E Nelson et al, "Transmission of neonatal listerosis in a delivery room," *American Journal of Diseases of Children* 139 (September 1985) 903-905.

34. "Recommended practices for cleaning and processing endoscopes and endoscope accessories," in *Standards, Recommended Practices, and Guidelines* (Denver: AORN, Inc, 2004) 261-266.

35. Centers for Disease Control and Prevention, "Bronchoscopy-related infections and pseudoinfections—New York, 1996 and 1998," *Morbidity and Mortality Weekly Report* 48 (July 9, 1999) 557-560.

36. US Department of Health and Human Services, "Infections from inadequately processed endoscopes," *User Facility Reporting* 28 (Fall 1999) 1-5.

37. "Manufacturer and User Facility Device Experience Database. Report Numbers 2084725-2002-00033; 2084725-2003-00084; 2084725-2004-00010; 2084725-2004-00003; 2084725-2004-00011; 2084725-2004-00012; 3003723454-2004-0001," US Food and Drug Administration, *http://www.accessdata.fda.gov /scripts/cdrh/cfdocs/cfMAUDE/Search.cfm* (accessed 30 Sept 2004).

38. "Manufacturer and User Facility Device Experience Database. Report Numbers 2084725-2003-00008; 3003723454-2004-0001," US Food and Drug Adminis-

tration, *http://www.accessdata.fda.gov/scripts/cdrh /cfdocs/cfMAUDE/Search.cfm* (accessed 30 Sept 2004).

39. H J O'Conner, J R Babb, G A Ayliffe, "*Pseudomonas aeruginosa* infection in endoscopy," *Gastroenterology* 93 (December 1987) 1451.

40. J I Allen et al, "*Pseudomonas* infection of the biliary system resulting from use of contaminated endoscope," *Gastroenterology* 92 (March 1987) 759-763.

41. D E Low et al, "Infectious complications of endoscopic retrograde cholangio-pancreatography. A prospective assessment," *Archives of Internal Medicine* 140 (August 1980) 1076-1077.

42. M J Arfa, D L Sitter, "In-hospital evaluation of contamination of duodenoscopes: A quantitative assessment of the effect of drying," *Journal of Hospital Infections* 19 (October 1991) 89-98.

43. C J Alvarado, M Reichelderfer, "APIC guideline for infection prevention and control in flexible endoscopy," *American Journal of Infection Control* 18 (April 2000) 138-155.

44. R C Morell et al, "A survey of laryngoscope contamination at a university and a community hospital," *Anesthesiology* 80 (April 1994) 960.

45. R A Phillips, W P Monaghan, "Incidence of visible and occult blood on laryngoscope blades and handles," *AANA Journal* 65 (June 1997) 241-246.

46. Centers for Disease Control and Prevention, "Guidelines for environmental infection control in healthcare facilities: Recommendations of CDC and the Healthcare Infection Control Practices Advisory Committee (HICPAC)," *Morbidity and Mortality Weekly Report* 52 (June 6, 2003) No RR-10 22.

47. J R Hall, "Blood contamination of anesthesia equipment and monitoring equipment," *Anesthesia and Analgesia* 78 (June 1994) 1136-1139.

48. S M Perry, W P Monghan, "The prevalence of visible and/or occult blood on anesthesia and monitoring equipment," *Journal of the American Association of Nurse Anesthetists* 69 (February 2001) 44-48.

49. H Arkoff, R A Ortega, "Touchscreen technology: Potential source of cross-infections," *Anesthesia and Analgesia* 75 (December 1992) 1073.

50. M S Kristensen, E Sloth, T K Jensen, "Relationship between anesthetic procedure and contact of anesthesia personnel with patient body fluids," *Anesthesiology* 73 (October 1990) 619-624.

51. L A Herwaldt, J M Pottinger, S A Coffin, "Nosocomial infections associated with anesthesia," in *Hospital Epidemiology and Infection Control,* third ed, C G Mayhall ed (Philadelphia: Lippincott Williams & Wilkins, 2004).

52. US Food and Drug Administration, "Important enforcement date for reprocessing single-use devices," *User Facility Reporting* 39 (Summer 2002). Also available at *http://www.fda.gov/cdrh/fusenews/ufb39.html#1* (accessed 24 Sept 2004).

53. "Anesthesia apparatus checkout recommendations, 1993," US Food and Drug Administration, *http://www.fda.gov/cdrh/humfac/anesckot.html* (accessed 24 Sept 2004).

54. "Guidelines for determining anesthesia machine obsolescence," American Society of Anesthesiologists,

http://www.asahq.org/PublicationsAndServices/machine obsolescense.pdf (accessed 24 Sept 2004).

55. B Abraham et al, "Malignant hyperthermia susceptibility: Anaesthetic implications and risk stratification," *Quarterly Journal of Medicine* 90 (January 997) 13-18.

56. "Medical FAQs," Malignant Hyperthermia Association of the United States, *http://www.mhaus.org/index.cfm/fuseaction/Content.Display/PagePK/Medical FAQs.cfm* (accessed 24 Sept 2004).

57. "Reducing mercury use in healthcare: Promoting a healthier environment: A how-to manual," US Environmental Protection Agency, *http://www.epa.gov/glnpo/bnsdocs/merchealth* (accessed 24 Sept 2004).

58. Centers for Disease Control and Prevention, "Guidelines for prevention of nosocomial pneumonia, 2003," *Morbidity and Mortality Weekly Report* 53 (March 26, 2004) (RR03) 1-36.

59. G E Dryden, "Risk of contamination from the anesthesia circle absorber: An evaluation," *Anesthesia and Analgesia* 48 (November/December 1969) 939-943.

60. J R Jenkins, W M Edgar, "Sterilization of anaesthetic equipment," *Anaesthesia* 19 (April 1964) 177-190.

61. P M Murphy, R B Fitzgeorge, F Barrett, "Viability and distribution of bacteria after passage through a circle anaesthetic system," *British Journal of Anaesthesia* 66 (March 1991) 300-304.

62. D T Leijten, V S Rejger, R P Mouton, "Bacterial contamination and the effect of filters in anaesthetic circuits in a simulated patient model," *Journal of Hospital Infections* 21 (May 1992) 51-60.

63. G E Dryden, "Uncleaned anesthesia equipment," *JAMA* 233 (September 1975) 1297-1298.

64. B C Stratford, R R Clark, S Dixson, "The disinfection of anaesthetic apparatus," *British Journal of Anaesthesia* 36 (August 1964) 471-476.

65. "Bacterial contamination of anesthesia machines revealed," *Excerpta Medica* (Lawrenceville, NJ: Convention Reporter, 1991) 12-14.

66. H Aranha-Creado et al, "Removal of *Mycobacterium* species by breathing circuit filters," *Infection Control and Hospital Epidemiology* 18 (April 1997) 252-254.

67. A J Berry, F S Nolte, "An alternative strategy for infection control of anesthesia breathing circuits: A laboratory assessment of the Pall HME filter," *Anesthesia and Analgesia* 72 (May 1991) 651-655.

68. I Hogbarth, "Anaesthetic machine and breathing system contamination and the efficacy of bacterial/viral filters," *Anaesthesia and Intensive Care* 25 (April 1996) 154-163.

69. G Lloyd et al, "Barriers to hepatitis C transmission within breathing systems: Efficacy of a pleated hydrophobic filter," *Anaesthesia and Intensive Care* 25 (June 1997) 235-238.

70. H H Luttropp, L Berntman, "Bacterial filters protect anaesthetic equipment in a low-flow system," *Anaesthesia* 48 (June 1993) 520-523.

71. J Rathgeber et al, "Prevention of patient bacterial contamination of anaesthesia-circle-systems: A clinical study of the contamination risk and performance of different heat and moisture exchanges with electret filter (HMEF)," *European Journal of Anaesthesia* 14 (July 1997) 368-373.

72. G M Shiotani et al, "Prevention of contamination of the circle system and ventilators with a new disposable filter," *Anesthesia and Analgesia* 50 (September/October 1971) 844-845.

73. C Smith et al, "An evaluation of one and two airflow filters preventing the movement of bacterial through the anesthesia circle system," *Journal of the American Association of Nurse Anesthetists* 64 (April 1996) 153-156.

74. S Van Hassel et al, "Bacterial filters in anesthesia: Results of nine years of surveillance," *Infection Control and Hospital Epidemiology* 20 (January 1999) 58-60.

75. K Chant et al, "Investigation of possible patient-to-patient transmission of hepatitis C in a hospital," *New South Wales Public Health Bulletin* 5 (May 1994) 47-51.

76. Association of Anaesthetists of Great Britain and Ireland, *Infection Control in Anaesthesia* (London: The Association of Anaesthetists of Great Britain and Ireland, 2002) 4.

77. "Policy on infection control in anaesthesia, 1995," Australian and New Zealand College of Anaesthetists, *http://www.medeserv.com.au/anzca/pdfdocs/P28_1995.PDF* (accessed 25 Sept 2004).

78. "Anesthetic management of a SARS-Infected patient," Canadian Society of Anesthesiologists, *http://www.asahq.org/clinical/pracadvsars.htm* (accessed 25 Sept 2004).

79. Centers for Disease Control and Prevention, "Guidelines for prevention of nosocomial pneumonia," *Morbidity and Mortality Weekly Report* 46 (Jan 3, 1997) (RR-1) 1-77.

80. P M Anrow et al, "Nosocomial Legionnaire's disease caused by aerosolized tap water from respiratory devices," *Journal of Infectious Diseases* 146 (October 1982) 460-467.

81. D E Craven, T A Goularte, B J Make, "Contaminated condensate in mechanical ventilator circuits: A risk factor for nosocomial pneumonia?" *American Review of Respiratory Disease* 129 (April 1984) 625-628.

82. "Bloodborne pathogens—1910.1030," US Department of Labor Occupational Safety and Health Administration, *http://www.oshaslc.gov/pls/oshaweb/owadisp.show_document?p_table=STANDARDS&p_id=10051* (accessed 25 Sept 2004).

83. "RCA online," US Environmental Protection Agency, *http://www.epa.gov/rcraonline* (accessed 25 Sept 2004).

84. "Identification and listing of hazardous waste," in *Electronic Code of Federal Regulations (e-CFR)* 40: Protection of Environment, Part 261, *http://www.epa.gov/epahome/cfr40.htm* (accessed 25 Sept 2004).

85. "Recommended practices for standard and transmission-based precautions," in *Standards, Recommended Practices, and Guidelines* (Denver: AORN, Inc, 2004) 361-366.

86. "Hazard communication in the 21st century workplace," US Department of Labor, Occupational Safety and Health Administration, *http://www.osha.gov/dsg/hazcom/finalmsdsreport.html* (accessed 25 Sept 2004).

87. "Bloodborne pathogens and needlestick prevention," US Occupational Safety and Health Administration, *http://www.osha.gov/SLTC/bloodbornepathogens/index.html* (accessed 25 Sept 2004).

88. Joint Commission on Accreditation of Healthcare Organizations, "Crosswalk of 2003 standards for hospitals to 2004 leadership standards for hospitals," in *2004 Comprehensive Accreditation Manual for Hospitals: The Official Handbook* (Oakbrook Terrace, Ill: Joint Commission on Accreditation of Healthcare Organizations, 2003) LD.3.20.

PUBLICATION HISTORY

Originally published June 1977, *AORN Journal, as* AORN "Recommended practices for cleaning and processing anesthesia equipment."

Revised March 1978; July 1982; March 1991. Published as proposed recommended practices September 1994.

Revised; published November 1999, *AORN Journal.* Reformatted July 2000.

Revised November 2004; published in *Standards, Recommended Practices, and Guidelines,* 2005 edition. Reprinted April 2005, *AORN Journal.*

Minor editing revisions made in June 2011 for publication in *Perioperative Standards and Recommended Practices,* 2012 edition.

Recommended Practices for High-Level Disinfection

The following recommended practices were developed by the AORN Recommended Practices Committee and have been approved by the AORN Board of Directors. They were presented as proposed recommendations for comments by members and others. They are effective January 1, 2009.

These recommended practices are intended as achievable recommendations representing what is believed to be an optimal level of practice. Policies and procedures will reflect variations in practice settings and/or clinical situations that determine the degree to which the recommended practices can be implemented. AORN recognizes the various settings in which perioperative nurses practice. These recommended practices are intended as guidelines adaptable to various practice settings. These practice settings include traditional operating rooms, ambulatory surgery centers, physician's offices, cardiac catheterization laboratories, endoscopy suites, radiology departments, and all other areas where surgery may be performed.

Purpose

These recommended practices provide guidance for achieving safe and effective high-level disinfection (HLD) of reusable instruments and equipment. Care and cleaning of flexible endoscopes is outside the scope of these recommended practices. Refer to the AORN "Recommended practices for cleaning and processing endoscopes and endoscope accessories."

Recommendation I

Items to be reprocessed should be categorized as critical, semicritical, and noncritical.

The Spaulding classification system, developed by Earle Spaulding in 1968, has withstood the passage of time and continues to be used today by infection preventionists and others to determine the correct processing methods for preparing instruments and other items for patient use. According to the Spaulding system, the level of processing required is based on the nature of the item requiring processing and the manner in which it is to be used (**Table 1**).[1-5]

I.a.   Items that enter sterile tissue or the vascular system are categorized as critical and should be sterile when used. Sterility may be achieved by physical or chemical processes.[1,5-9]

When critical items are contaminated with microorganisms, including bacterial spores, the risk of infection is substantial.[2,10-12] Examples of critical items include, but are not limited to,

- surgical instruments;
- cutting endoscopic accessories that break the mucosal barrier;
- endoscopes used in sterile body cavities;
- cardiac, vascular, and urinary catheters;
- implants;
- needles; and
- ultrasound probes used in sterile body cavities.

I.b.   Items that come in contact with nonintact skin or mucous membranes are considered semicritical and should receive a minimum of high-level disinfection.[1,5-9,13]

Intact mucous membranes generally provide a barrier to common bacterial spores but not to organisms such as tubercle bacilli and viruses.[2,11] Examples of semicritical items include, but are not limited to,

- vaginal and rectal probes, even when sheaths are used;
- respiratory therapy equipment;
- anesthesia equipment;
- bronchoscopes; and
- gastrointestinal endoscopes and accessories.

I.b.1.   Semicritical devices contaminated or potentially contaminated with hepatitis B virus (HBV), hepatitis C virus (HCV), HIV, multi-drug resistant bacteria, or *Mycobacterium tuberculosis* (TB) should receive a minimum of high-level disinfection.[2]

Literature has supported and research has demonstrated that high-level disinfectants inactivate these and other pathogens that may contaminate semicritical devices.[3,6,10,14-22] The practice of using HLD is consistent with standard precautions, which presume that all patients potentially are infected.[2]

I.c.   Items that contact only intact skin are categorized as noncritical items and should receive intermediate-level disinfection, low-level disinfection, or cleaning.[1,5-9]

Table 1

SPAULDING CLASSIFICATION SYSTEM[1-7]			
Device category/ Classification	**Level of Disinfection**	**Effectiveness of Method**	**Examples**
Critical Items that come in contact with the blood-stream or sterile body tissues	**Sterilization** *Examples:* saturated steam, ethylene oxide, dry heat, ozone, low-temperature hydrogen peroxide gas plasma, glutaraldehyde-based formulations, peracetic acid, stabilized hydrogen peroxide 6% **Chemical sterilants** *Examples:* glutaraldehyde-based formulations, peracetic acid, stabilized hydrogen peroxide 6%, wet pasteurization, sodium hypochlorite	Sterilization kills all microbial life, including pathogenic and nonpathogenic micro-organisms and spores.	• surgical instruments • acupuncture needles • foot care instruments • implants • cardiac and urinary catheters • endoscope accessories that penetrate the mucosal barrier
Semicritical Items that come in contact with mucous membranes or non-intact skin	**High-level disinfection** Use when sterilization is not possible. *Examples:* glutaraldehyde-based formulations, peracetic acid, stabilized hydrogen peroxide 6%, wet pasteurization, sodium hypochlorite	High-level disinfection kills all microorganisms but not necessarily a large number of bacterial spores.	• scopes (eg, bronchoscopes, colonoscopes, and similar scopes) • laryngoscope handles and blades, • reusable peak flow meters • vaginal and rectal probes • cryosurgical instruments • thermometers
Noncritical Items that come in contact with intact skin and those exposed to blood or other potentially infectious material	**Intermediate-level disinfection** Use an EPA-registered hospital disinfectant with label claim for tuberculocidal activity. *Examples:* chlorine-based products, phenolics	Intermediate-level disinfection kills viruses, mycobacteria, fungi, and vegetative bacteria but not bacterial spores.	• skin probes • blood pressure cuffs • pneumatic tourniquet cuffs • hydrotherapy tanks • examination tables
Items that do not come in contact with the patient's skin and have not been exposed to blood or other potentially infectious material	**Low-level disinfection** Use an EPA-registered hospital disinfectant without label claim for tuberculocidal activity. *Examples:* chlorine-based products, phenolics, quaternary ammonium compounds, hydrogen peroxide (approximately 3%), iodophors, 70% to 90% alcohol	Low-level disinfection kills vegetative forms of bacteria, some fungi, and lipid viruses but cannot be relied on to destroy mycobacteria, bacterial endospores, or nonlipid viruses.	• stethoscopes • dishes • scales • furniture • bed pans

REFERENCES

1. Spaulding EH. Clinical disinfection and antisepsis in the hospital. *J Hosp Res.* 1972:95.

2. Appendix B: Decontamination and disinfection. In: *Biosafety in Microbiological and Biomedical Laboratories (BMBL).* 5th ed. Centers for Disease Control and Prevention; National Institutes of Health, eds. Washington, DC: US Government Printing Office; 2007:328-336. Available at http://www.cdc.gov/od/ohs/biosfty/bmbl5/bmbl5toc.htm. Accessed December 5, 2008.

3. Alvarado CJ, Reichelderfer M. APIC guideline for infection prevention and control in flexible endoscopy. Association for Professionals in Infection Control. *Am J Infect Control* 2000;28(2):138.

4. *AAMI TIR12:2004—Designing, Testing and Labeling Reusable Medical Devices for Reprocessing in Health Care Facilities: A Guide for Medical Device Manufacturers.* Arlington, VA: Association for the Advancement of Medical Instrumentation; 2005.

5. Rutala WA, Weber DJ. How to assess risk of disease transmission to patients when there is a failure to follow recommended disinfection and sterilization guidelines. *Infect Control Hosp Epidemiol.* 2007;28(2):146.

6. Multi-society guideline for reprocessing flexible gastrointestinal endoscopes. *Am J Infect Control.* 2003; 31(5):309.

7. Rutala WA, Weber DJ. Cleaning, disinfection, and sterilization in healthcare facilities. In: *APIC Text of Infection Control and Epidemiology.* Washington, DC: Association for Professionals in Infection Control and Epidemiology; 2005:21-31.

Intact skin acts as an effective barrier to most organisms.[2] Examples of noncritical items include, but are not limited to,
- tourniquets and blood pressure cuffs,
- linens,
- Mayo stands, and
- other OR furnishings.

Recommendation II

Items should be thoroughly cleaned and decontaminated before high-level disinfection.[10]

Cleaning and decontamination are the initial and most critical steps in breaking the chain of disease transmission. Debris, blood, mucous, fat, tissue, and organic matter will interfere with the action of the disinfectant. Microbial biofilms (ie, collections of bacteria and fungi existing in a multicellular matrix) adhere to each other or to medical devices, particularly those with lumens, where they affect tissues adjacent to virtually any medical device. Biofilms are difficult to remove and may serve as sources of bacterial toxin that can affect remote locations in the body. Friction and oxidizing chemicals must be used to remove biofilms. Initiating cleaning immediately after use reduces or eliminates the growth of biofilm-forming microorganisms.[10,23-43]

II.a. Appropriate personal protective equipment (PPE) should be worn during cleaning and decontamination.[6,22,44]

Personal protective equipment protects the worker from hazardous chemicals and exposure to blood and other potentially infectious materials.

II.a.1. Personnel should wear PPE that may include, but is not limited to,
- 100% nitrile rubber or 100% butyl rubber gloves when handling glutaraldehyde (polyvinyl chloride [PVC] gloves are not recommended because they absorb glutaraldehyde);[18]
- less than 100% nitrile or butyl rubber gloves for handling all other HLD solutions except glutaraldehyde;
- protective eyewear (eg, goggles, face shields);
- masks (ie, to prevent contact with skin and not inhalation of fumes); and
- moisture-repellent or splash-proof skin protection (eg, gowns, jumpsuits, aprons).[45]

Chemical disinfectants can irritate or stain skin and mucous membranes.[46,47] Use of protective apparel decreases the potential for exposure to the chemical agent.[48]

II.b. Soiled instruments and devices should be handled using PPE and transported in a contained, covered, and secure manner to the point of decontamination and processing.[22]

These practices prevent environmental contamination and protect employees from bloodborne pathogen exposure.

II.c. Meticulous cleaning and decontamination should precede high-level disinfection.

Adherence to a written cleaning protocol results in consistency of practice and facilitates the disinfection process.[6,12,22,44,49,50] According to the US Food and Drug Administration (FDA), manufacturers are obliged to provide users with adequate instructions for the safe and effective use of an instrument or device, including methods to clean and disinfect or sterilize the item if it is marked as reusable.[51,52]

II.c.1. Particular attention should be given to complex medical devices with multiple pieces (eg, endoscopes, robotic devices) that have crevices, joints, lumens, ports, and channels because they are difficult to clean.[12]

II.d. Instruments to be disinfected should be cleaned according to AORN's "Recommended practices for cleaning and care of surgical instruments and powered equipment"[49] and "Recommended practices for cleaning and processing flexible endoscopes and endoscope accessories."[53]

Adherence to a written cleaning protocol results in consistency of practice and facilitates the disinfection process.[12,22,49]

II.e. High-level disinfection should not be used for items exposed to prions. Refer to the AORN "Recommended practices for sterilization in the perioperative practice setting."[15,49,53-55]

Prions present unique infection prevention and control challenges. Prions are proteinaceous, infectious agents containing no DNA or RNA and may be transmitted iatrogenically by direct inoculation. Prions cause transmissible spongiform encephalopathies (TSE), including Creutzfeldt-Jakob disease (CJD) and variant Creutzfeldt-Jakob disease (vCJD). Prions are resistant to traditional chemical and physical decontamination methods. High-level disinfection does not inactivate prions. Critical and semicritical items or surfaces contaminated with the CJD agent require unique decontamination procedures because of an extremely resistant subpopulation of prions.[36,49] Although some discrepancies exist between studies, all studies show that these prions resist normal inactivation methods.[33,54,56]

II.e.1. Critical and semicritical devices that come into contact with internal tissues of patients with known or suspected TSE should be processed using the highest level and method of decontamination that can be tolerated by the instrument.[54]

Many complex and expensive instruments such as intracardiac monitoring devices, fiber-optic endoscopes, and microscopes cannot be decontaminated by the harsh procedures recommended for the decontamination of critical items exposed to high-infectivity tissue.

II.e.2. Extended steam sterilization cycles are the preferred method of inactivating resistant prions on critical and semicritical devices. Effective exposure inactivation parameters for gravity displacement is 30 minutes at 131° C (268° F) and 18 minutes at 134° C to 138° C (273° F to 280° F) for dynamic-air removal.[2] Critical and noncritical items used in low-infectivity tissue (eg, intestines) do not have to be incinerated.[54]

II.e.3. Disposable endoscopic accessories should be used whenever possible when there is a patient with known or suspected TSE infectivity.

Prions are highly resistant to chemical and physical processes that normally inactivate microorganisms. The risk of transferring prion protein is greatest in cases that manipulate high- risk tissue (ie, brain, dura matter, cornea). Few reports have revealed transmission of spongiform encephalopathy from endoscopic procedures; however, iatrogenic transmission of the disease has catastrophic consequences that warrants conservative treatment of accessories.[39,57]

II.e.4. Disposable cover sheets should be used whenever possible to avoid environmental contamination of noncritical items.[54]

Transmissible spongiform encephalopathy infectivity persists for long periods on work surfaces, although they have not been implicated in iatrogenic transmission.

II.e.5. Noncritical patient care items and surfaces should be disinfected with double-strength sodium hydroxide solution (2N NaOH) or undiluted sodium hypochlorite for one hour and rinsed with water. Sodium hypochlorite may be corrosive to some surfaces.[57]

Noncritical patient care items and surfaces have not been implicated in disease transmission.[2]

Recommendation III

Pasteurization may be used to achieve thermal high-level disinfection.

Pasteurization is a heat-automated high-level disinfection process that employs time and heat (ie, 160° F to 170° F [21.7° C to 25° C] for 30 minutes) for HLD of heat-sensitive semicritical patient care items. Pasteurization destroys all microorganisms except high numbers of bacterial spores.[15] The process originally developed by Louis Pasteur consists of heating milk, wine, or other liquids to between 140° F and 212° F (60° C to 100° C) for approximately 30 minutes to kill or significantly reduce the number of pathogenic and spoilage organisms.

III.a. Items to be high-level disinfected using pasteurization should be placed inside the washer/pasteurizer chamber according to the manufacturer's written instructions.

Medical washer/pasteurizers have wash, rinse, and pasteurization cycles. The wash cycle is accomplished either through a horizontal agitation method or a vertical rotational method, depending on the manufacturer's specifications, using warm water and detergent cleaning solution. The length of this cycle is determined by the manufacturer's written instructions. At the conclusion of the wash and rinse cycles, the tank automatically drains in preparation for the pasteurization cycle. Pasteurization is achieved by immersing all devices in a hot water bath heated to 140° F to 212° F (60° C to 100° C) and held for 30 minutes.[58] Medical washer/pasteurizers may offer quality assurance data recorders that document the temperature of the pasteurizing bath and cycle time.

Recommendation IV

An FDA-cleared agent should be used to achieve chemical high-level disinfection of medical devices.

The FDA has primary responsibility for premarket review of safety and efficacy requirements for liquid chemical germicides intended for use on critical and semicritical devices.[59] A list of products that have been cleared for marketing by the FDA can be found on the web site of the FDA Center for Devices and Radiological Health (CDRH).[17]

IV.a.   Products selected for chemical disinfection should be efficacious and compatible with the materials or items to be disinfected. Many disinfectants are used in the practice setting (eg, glutaraldehyde, stabilized hydrogen peroxide, peracetic acid, orthophthalaldehyde [OPA]). These agents are not interchangeable.[48]

Devices may be damaged by these chemicals. The use of incompatible chemicals can damage the surfaces of the instrument, causing corrosion, scratches, and other surface irregularities. This damage can create a challenge for cleaning and high-level disinfection, interfere with the proper function, and reduce the life and cosmetic appearance of the device.

IV.a.1.   Factors that influence the efficacy of a chemical agent include, but may not be limited to,
- organic load present on the items to be disinfected;
- type and level of microbial contamination;
- precleaning, rinsing, and drying of the items;
- active ingredients of the chemical agent;
- concentration of the chemical agent;
- exposure time to the chemical agent;
- physical configuration of the item;
- temperature and pH of the chemical agent;
- inorganic matter present;
- water hardness; and
- presence of surfactants.

IV.a.2.   An ideal high-level disinfectant should
- possess a broad spectrum of antimicrobial effectiveness,
- demonstrate rapid activity,
- possess material compatibility,
- be nontoxic,
- be odorless,
- have no disposal restrictions,
- possess prolonged reuse and shelf life,
- be easy to use,
- demonstrate resistance to organic material,
- be able to be monitored for concentration, and
- be cost effective.[17]

Emerging pathogens such as *Cryptosporidium parvum,* human papilloma virus, rotavirus, Norwalk virus, *Helicobacter pylori, Escherichia coli 0157:H7,* multidrug-resistant bacteria, nontuberculous mycobacteria *(M chelonae),* and prions are a growing concern for members of the public and infection preventionists. The susceptibility of each of these pathogens has been studied, and with the exception of *C parvum* and prions, all are susceptible to available chemical disinfectants and chemical sterilants.[21,46] Glutaraldehyde-resistant strains of *M chelonae* have been isolated in some automated endoscope reprocessors but have been found to be sensitive to other high-level disinfectants such as ortho-phthalaldehyde.[38,47]

IV.a.3.   FDA-approved high-level disinfectant liquid chemical agents should be used according to workload requirements, instrumentation characteristics, and workplace design (**Table 2**). *Note:* A full and comprehensive list of high-level disinfectant solutions and contact conditions is available from the FDA.

IV.a.4.   High-level disinfection should occur at appropriate temperature, contact time,

Table 2

USE OF FDA-APPROVED CHEMICAL AGENTS FOR HIGH-LEVEL DISINFECTION (HDL)[1-5]

NOTE: This is not intended to be a comprehensive list of all HLD products. Manufacturers' directions for use should be followed.

HLD chemical	Advantages	Disadvantages	Concentration	Contact time/Conditions
Peracetic acid (PA) and hydrogen peroxide solutions	No activation required. Odor or irritation not significant.	Concerns regarding compatibility with materials (eg, lead, brass, copper, zinc) and both cosmetic and functional damage. Limited clinical use. Potential for eye and skin damage.	0.08% PA and 1.0% hydrogen peroxide 0.23% PA and 7.35% hydrogen peroxide	25 min contact time at 20° C (68° F); 14 days maximum reuse 15 min contact time at 20° C (68° F); 14 days maximum reuse
Glutaraldehyde solutions	Numerous published studies of use. Relatively inexpensive. Excellent compatibility with materials.	Respiratory irritation from glutaraldehyde vapor. Pungent and irritating odor. Relatively slow mycobactericidal activity. Coagulates blood and fixes tissue to surfaces. Allergic contact dermatitis.	2.5% glutaraldehyde automated endoscopic reprocessor (AER) 1.12% glutaraldehyde and 1.93% phenol	5.0 min at 35° C (95° F); 28 days maximum reuse 20 min contact time at 25° C (77° F); 14 days maximum reuse
Hydrogen peroxide	No activation required. May enhance removal of organic material and organisms. No disposal issues. No odor or irritation issues. Does not coagulate blood or fix tissues to surfaces. Inactivates *Cryptosporidium*. Published studies of use.	Concerns regarding compatibility with materials (eg, brass, zinc, copper, nickel/silver plating) and both cosmetic and functional damage. Serious eye damage with contact.	7.5% hydrogen peroxide	30 min contact time at 20° C (68° F); 21 days maximum reuse
Ortho-phthalaldehyde	Fast-acting high-level disinfectant. No activation required. Odor not significant. Claim of excellent compatibility with materials. Claim of not coagulating blood or fixing tissues to surfaces.	Stains protein gray (eg, skin, mucous membranes, clothing, environmental surfaces). More expensive than glutaraldehyde. Eye irritation with contact. Slow sporicidal activity. Repeated exposure may result in hypersensitivity in some patients with bladder cancer.	5.75% ortho-phthalaldehyde 0.55% ortho-phthalaldehyde manual processing AER	5 min at 50° C (122° F); single use 12 min at 20° C (68° F); 14 days maximum reuse 5 min at 25° C (77° F); 14 days maximum reuse
Peracetic acid *Indication for sterilization only*	Environmentally friendly byproducts (ie, acetic acid, oxygen, and water). Fully automated. Single-use system eliminates need for concentration testing. Standardized cycle. May enhance removal of organic material and endotoxins. No adverse health effects to operators under normal operating conditions.	Potential incompatibility with materials (eg, aluminum anodized coating becomes dull). Used for immersible instruments only. Biological indicator may not be suitable for routine monitoring. Only one endoscope or a small number of instruments can be processed in a cycle. More expensive (eg, endoscope repairs, operating costs, purchase costs) than high-level disinfection. Serious eye and skin damage after contact with concentrated solution. Point-of-use system; cannot save sterilized items for later use or storage.	0.2% peracetic acid	rapid sterilization cycle time (30–45 min) low-temperature (50°–55°C/122°–131° F) liquid-immersion sterilization; single use

REFERENCES

1. Appendix B: Decontamination and disinfection. In: *Biosafety in Microbiological and Biomedical Laboratories (BMBL)*. 5th ed. Centers for Disease Control and Prevention; National Institutes of Health, eds. Washington, DC: US Government Printing Office; 2007:328-336. Available at *http://www.cdc.gov/od/ohs/biosfty/bmbl5/bmbl5toc.htm*. Accessed December 5, 2008.

2. Alvarado C J, Reichelderfer M. APIC guideline for infection prevention and control in flexible endoscopy. Association for Professionals in Infection Control. *Am J Infect Control* 2000;28(2):138.

3. Favero MS, Bond WW. Chemical disinfection of medical and surgical materials. In: Block SS, ed. *Disinfection, Sterilization, and Preservation*. 5th ed. Philadelphia, PA: Lippincott Williams & Wilkins; 2001:881.

4. FDA-cleared sterilants and high-level disinfectants with general claims for processing reusable medical and dental devices; September 28, 2006. US Food and Drug Administration. *http://www.fda.gov/cdrh/ode/germlab.html*. Accessed December 5, 2008.

5. Association for the Advancement of Medical Instrumentation. *ANSI/AAMI ST58:2005—Chemical Sterilization and High-Level Disinfection in Health Care Facilities*. Arlington, VA: Association for the Advancement of Medical Instrumentation; 2005.

and length of use following solution activation. **Table 2** provides FDA-approved chemicals for HLD with recommended conditions for use.[2,16,17,27,46,51,56,60,61]

Improper use of cleaners and disinfectants can cause contamination and lead to outbreaks.[62]

IV.b. Chemical high-level disinfection should be achieved by immersing an item for specified contact conditions (ie, period of time, temperature, concentration) in a chemical agent (also called a chemical germicide) that has been cleared by the FDA as a high-level disinfectant.

Disease transmission can result from improper selection and/or use of disinfecting agents.

IV.c. Manufacturers' written instructions should be followed when preparing disinfectant solutions, calculating expiration dates, and labeling solution soaking containers.

The appropriate conditions for use are provided on solution container labels. Labels indicate clearly the appropriate time for discarding solutions that may no longer be effective. Most chemical disinfectants are effective for only a specific period of time.[36]

IV.c.1. Manufacturers' written instructions about the type of container used should be followed.

The correct container ensures that no interaction occurs between the container and the active ingredients of the disinfectant.[36]

IV.c.2. A test strip or other FDA-cleared testing device specific for the disinfectant and minimum effective concentration of the active ingredient should be used for monitoring solution potency prior to each use.[36,51]

The test strip expiration date should be checked before use.

IV.c.3. If a solution falls below its minimum effective concentration, it should be discarded, even if the designated expiration date has not been reached.

High-level disinfection solution potency cannot be guaranteed when the solution falls below the minimum effective concentration.

IV.d. Items to be chemically disinfected should be cleaned and completely immersed in the disinfectant solution according to device and HLD solution manufacturers' written instructions and consistent with established infection control practice.

Total immersion permits contact of all surfaces. Perfusion of the disinfectant into all channels eliminates air pockets and ensures contact with internal channels.

IV.e. Lumens and ports should be flushed and filled with the disinfectant and the entire item completely immersed for the designated exposure time.

Disinfection of all surfaces can be achieved only if all surfaces of the items are clean and in constant contact with the disinfecting solution. Flushing lumens and ports eliminates air pockets and facilitates contact of the disinfectant with internal channels.[2,12,21]

IV.f. The automated endoscopic reprocessor (AER) manufacturer's written instructions should be congruent with the endoscope manufacturer's written instructions when an AER is used for high-level disinfection, or the endoscope should not be processed in the AER.

Device-specific instructions ensure adequate function of the reprocessing equipment and prevent damage to the scope.[6]

IV.g. After being exposed to the disinfectant solution for the required exposure time, critical and semicritical items should be thoroughly rinsed with water according to the manufacturer's written instructions.

Rinsing removes toxic and irritating residues that can result in tissue damage or staining.[7,63] Rinsing critical and semicritical items with sterile water prevents potential recontamination that could result from tap water.[2,6,9,15,25]

Recommendation V

HLD items should be protected from contamination until the item is delivered to the point of use.

Use of aseptic technique will protect the items from being contaminated before patient use.[2,6,36,59]

V.a. High-level disinfected items should be transported to the point of use using a technique that does not result in recontamination of the instrument (eg, aseptic technique).

Performance of hand hygiene, donning gloves to handle HLD items, and transferring immediately to point of use following processing are examples of practices that minimize recontamination.

V.b. High-level disinfected items should be processed immediately before use. Flexible endoscopes should be cleaned, high-level disinfected, and stored according to the "Recommended practices for cleaning and processing flexible endoscopes and endoscope accessories.[36,53]

HLD devices that cannot be placed in appropriate barrier materials are prone to recontamination when stored.

Recommendation VI

Health care organizations should provide a safe environment for personnel who are using chemical disinfectants.

Health care organizations are responsible for providing a safe work and patient care environment. Patients, visitors, and health care workers should be protected from injuries and illnesses caused by hazardous chemicals used in the facility.

VI.a. When handling chemical disinfectants, personnel should wear protective apparel that may include, but is not limited to,
  – 100% nitrile rubber or 100% butyl rubber gloves when handling glutaraldehyde (polyvinyl chloride [PVC] gloves are not recommended because they absorb glutaraldehyde);[18]
  – less than 100% nitrile or butyl rubber gloves for handling all other HLD solutions except glutaraldehyde;
  – protective eyewear (eg, goggles, face shields);
  – masks (ie, to prevent contact with skin and not inhalation of fumes); and
  – moisture-repellent or splash-proof skin protection (eg, gowns, jumpsuits, aprons).[45]
  Chemical disinfectants can irritate or stain skin and mucous membranes, cause allergic reactions, and may pose other health risks.[46,47] Use of protective apparel decreases the potential for exposure to the chemical agent.[36]

VI.b. Chemical disinfectants should be contained and used in well-ventilated areas.

Vapor generated from glutaraldehyde can be irritating to the respiratory tract and may aggravate preexisting respiratory conditions. Glutaraldehyde should be used in well-ventilated areas or in freestanding or vented chemical fume hoods. The American Conference of Governmental Industrial Hygienists (ACGIH) recommends a ceiling limit of 0.05 parts per million (ppm) for occupational exposure to glutaraldehyde vapors. The Occupational Safety and Health Administration (OSHA) has established occupational exposure limits for several agents. No exposure limits have been established by OSHA for glutaraldehyde; however, OSHA can regulate exposure to glutaraldehyde and has recommended that the ACGIH limits be followed.[22]

VI.b.1. Chemical disinfectants should be kept in covered containers with tight-fitting lids and clearly labeled with contents and expiration date.

VI.b.2. Methods (eg, transfer pumps) should be used to limit worker exposure during loading of chemical disinfectants into automated endoscopic reprocessors.

VI.b.3. Chemical disinfectants should be used according to manufacturers' written instructions and federal, state, and local regulations.

Recommendation VII

Chemical disinfectants should be disposed of according to federal, state, and local regulations.[64,65]

The most stringent regulations should be followed. State and local regulations may be more stringent than those imposed at the federal level.[36,66]

VII.a. Personnel should know their obligations under state laws and local ordinances and use appropriate PPE when disposing of high-level disinfectants.

Recommendation VIII

Personnel should receive initial education and competency validation on procedures, chemicals used, and personal protection and should receive additional training when new equipment, instruments, supplies, or procedures are introduced.

Ongoing education and competency validation of perioperative personnel facilitates the development of knowledge, skills, and attitudes that affect patient and worker safety.[8,67]

VIII.a. Personnel should receive initial education on
- decontamination methods;
- preparation of instruments and equipment for high-level disinfection;
- selection of cleaning agents and methods;
- proper use of cleaning agents, including an understanding of specific applications, appropriate dilution, and special precautions;
- decontamination of specific instruments and equipment used within the practice setting;
- procedures for decontamination of instruments contaminated with prions and the effectiveness of various methods of deactivation;
- personal protection required during instrument processing; and
- exposure risk associated with chemical cleaning agents.[22]

Workers have the right to know the about the safe use of disinfectants and about the hazards in the workplace. The OSHA requires that employers provide hazardous material safety information to employees.[22]

VIII.b. Personnel should receive education on new instruments and equipment, new cleaning agents and methods, and new procedures.[9,67-69]

VIII.c. Personnel responsible for HLD should maintain the technical skills needed to establish and maintain a safe practice environment for patients and other staff members.

Adverse effects resulting from the exposure to HLD is well documented in patients and health care workers.[70-74] Adverse effects include, but are not limited to,
- OPA-related anaphylaxis in patients with carcinoma of the urinary bladder,[32,56]
- OPA-related bronchial asthma in health care workers,[75]
- glutaraldehyde-related asthma and contact dermatitis,[76]
- glutaraldehyde-induced bowel injury after laparoscopy,[77] and,
- toxic anterior segment syndrome with glutaraldehyde.[78]

VIII.d. Administrative personnel should ensure competency validation of personnel participating in decontamination and high-level disinfection of invasive instruments.[67,79]

Competency validation is an essential component to providing safe and effective patient care.

VIII.e. The validation of competencies should include all types of instruments that the individual is authorized to reprocess.

Validation of competency supports demonstration of mastery level knowledge and skill required to correctly perform decontamination procedures.

VIII.f. Employers must provide employees with the information and training needed to protect themselves from chemical hazards in the workplace according to federal standards.[22]

Employers must provide a written hazard communication program, hazard evaluation, hazardous materials inventory, materials safety data sheets (MSDS), labels on all containers of hazardous chemicals, and employee training.

VIII.f.1. Employee training includes an explanation of the standard, identification of hazards and health effects, location of the written hazard communication program and MSDS, procedures to detect and measure contaminants, safe work practices, appropriate PPE, an explanation of labeling, and locations of spill kits and eyewash stations in accordance with employees' right to know about hazards in the workplace.[6,22]

VIII.f.2 The latest version of the MSDS must be maintained on site and be readily accessible to personnel when they are in their work areas. Material may be available in hard copy and/or electronic format.[22]

The MSDS provides users with valuable information about toxicity, reactivity, required protective equipment and apparel, storage, and disposal of the material.[36]

Recommendation IX

Documentation should be completed to enable the identification of trends and demonstrate compliance with regulatory and accrediting agency requirements.

Documentation policies and procedures establish authority, responsibility, and accountability and serve as operational guidelines.[80]

IX.a. HLD processing records should be kept and include, but not be limited to,
- the patient identifier, when applicable;
- the procedure and physician;
- load contents (item description, serial number if applicable);
- name of the individual performing cleaning, disinfection, rinsing, and transport;
- method of cleaning;
- number or identifier of the mechanical decontaminator;
- date and time disinfection was performed;
- type of disinfectant used and lot number;
- test results before each load indicating the solution used was at the proper concentration (ie, MEC) and within the expiration date;
- temperature of the disinfectant;
- submersion time;
- verification of rinsing of the disinfected item;
- use of device-specific biological and chemical indicators (BI, CI) for automated peracetic acid processors;
- testing results of insulated electrical instruments, and;
- disposition of defective equipment.[2,36,81]

Some washer decontaminators have digital readouts or printers that facilitate recordkeeping. Records of washer testing provide a source of evidence for review when investigating clinical issues, including surgical site infections.

IX.b. Records should be maintained for a time period specified by the health care organization and in compliance with local, state, and federal regulations.[22]

Employers are required to maintain hazardous communication training to ensure that employees are aware and knowledgeable of hazardous chemical exposure and exposure consequences.[22]

Recommendation X

Policies and procedures for high-level disinfection should be developed using the validated instructions provided by the medical device manufacturers, reviewed at regular intervals, revised as necessary, and readily available in the practice setting.

Policies and procedures establish authority, responsibility, and accountability and serve as operational guidelines. Policies and procedures also assist in the development of patient safety, quality assessment, and improvement activities. Policies and procedures are subject to change with the advent of new technologies.

X.a. Policies regarding high-level disinfection should be developed by a multidisciplinary team to include perioperative nurses, sterile processing personnel, surgeons, and infection preventionists.

Using a multidisciplinary team provides varied input and improved ownership of policies and procedures. Involving surgeons in review of policies educates them on the expectations for high-level disinfection and facilitates planning for instrument use. The expertise of infection preventionists facilitates establishment of minimum standards of infection control.

X.b. Policies should include, but not be limited to
- review of validated manufacturers' written instructions before purchase or consignment,
- cleaning of instruments before initial use,
- precautions to be taken when handling contaminated items,
- precautions to be taken when handling chemical agents,
- frequency of AER checks,
- frequency and method of evaluation of manual cleaning,
- criteria for identification and precautions taken for instruments used on patients with known or suspected prion disease,
- documentation of high-level disinfection,
- initial education and annual competency,
- maintenance of material safety data sheets,
- reporting exposures to bloodborne pathogens, and
- reporting adverse events.

X.c. Introduction to and review of policies and procedures should be included in the orientation and ongoing education of personnel to help develop knowledge, skills, and attitudes that affect patient care and occupational safety.

Policies and procedures may guide performance improvement activities.

X.d. Written policies and procedures should be in place to designate how critical and semicritical items are transported from the area where disinfection takes place to the point of use in patient areas.[44,48,82]

Recommendation XI

A quality-control program should be established for the health care organization in all areas where high-level disinfection is used.

The health care organization's quality management program should evaluate high-level disinfection to improve patient and worker safety.[52,67,79,83-85]

XI.a. Quality-control programs should be documented and should include, but not be limited to,
- orientation programs;
- competency assurance;
- continuing education;
- quality-control checks;
- investigation of adverse events, including outbreaks and exposures; and
- monitoring of solution replacement intervals.

Quality and performance improvement functions ensure that organizations design processes well and systematically monitor, analyze, and improve their outcomes.

XI.a.1. The HLD solution should be tested prior to each use.[9,86]

XI.a.2. The solution should be discarded even if it is within its use life if the test strip indicates the solution is below the minimum effective concentration.[36]

The test strip is the only indicator that the solution is effective.

XI.a.3. In the event of test strip failure, items processed with HLD solution below the minimum effective concentration should be considered inadequately processed and should not be used until reprocessed in an acceptable minimum effective concentration of high-level disinfection solution.[36]

XI.b. A comprehensive quality management program should include ongoing monitoring including scheduled testing of mechanical cleaning and AER equipment with supportive documentation.

Adequate cleaning and processing of endoscopes is essential to remove or destroy microorganisms and eliminate endotoxins.

XI.b.1. Mechanical instrument washers and AERs should be tested for proper functioning according to AORN "Recommended practices for cleaning and processing flexible endoscopes and endoscope accessories."[53]

Testing washer decontaminators and AERs on a regular basis verifies that the equipment is functioning properly or identifies an opportunity for corrective action. Washer-testing products are commercially available.

XI.b.2. Manual cleaning processes and skills should be evaluated when new types of instruments are reprocessed and periodically, at intervals determined by the health care organization.

Periodic testing provides an opportunity to evaluate the health care worker's understanding of principles and validate performance. Manual cleaning is a learned skill and subject to human error. New instruments can pose unique challenges when cleaning.

XI.b.3. Personnel should identify and respond to opportunities for improvement.

XI.c. Reporting mechanisms for adverse events and near misses related to HLD should be in place.

Systematic performance measures (ie, indicators) and/or priority areas are identified as opportunities for improvement based on the functions and processes of the perioperative episode.[87]

XI.c.1. Adverse events should be reported in the adverse event reporting system and reviewed for potential opportunities for improvement.[36]

Continuous quality improvement opportunities arise from documented and structured quality processes and measures that can define and resolve problems.

XI.c.2. Near misses should be investigated and corrective action taken to prevent serious adverse events.

XI.d. When investigating surgical infections, documentation of the decontamination and HLD processes should be reviewed.[6,8,9,32,39]

Pathogen transmission from endoscopy has been associated with failure to follow cleaning and disinfection protocols.[6,9,15]

Glossary

Automated endoscope reprocessor: A unit for mechanical cleaning, disinfecting, and rinsing of flexible endoscopes.

Bioburden: The degree of microbial load; the number of viable organisms contaminating an object.

Biofilms: "A thin coating containing biologically active organisms, that have the ability to grow in water, water solutions, or in vivo, which coat the surface of structures (eg, teeth, inner surfaces of catheters, tubes, implanted or indwelling devices, instruments, other medical devices). Biofilms contain viable and nonviable microorganisms that adhere to surfaces and become trapped within a matrix of organic matter (eg, proteins, glycoproteins, carbohydrates), which prevents antimicrobial agents from reaching the cells." *(Source: Favero MS, Bond WW. Chemical disinfection of medical and surgical materials. In: Disinfection, Sterilization, and Preservation. 5th ed. Block SS, ed. Philadelphia, PA: Lippincott Williams & Wilkins; 2001:910-911.)*

Cavitation: "A process by which high-frequency sound wave energy is produced in an ultrasonic cleaner causing microscopic bubbles to form, become unstable, and implode, thus creating minute vacuum areas that draw particles of debris off of instrument surfaces and from crevices in instruments." *(Source: Topical antimicrobial drug products for over-the-counter human use; tentative final monograph for health-care antiseptic drug products. In: Code of Federal Regulations (CFR) 21: Food and Drugs, Parts 333 and 369. Washington, DC: US Government Printing Office; 1994:31402-31453.)*

Chemical disinfectant/germicide: A generic term for a government-registered agent that destroys microorganisms. Germicides are classified as sporicides, general disinfectants, sanitizers, and others.

Critical item: An item that has contact with the vascular system or enters sterile tissue, or body cavities and thus poses the highest risk of transmission of infection.

Decontamination: A process that removes contaminating infectious agents and renders reusable medical products safe for handling.

Disinfection: A process that kills most forms of microorganisms on inanimate surfaces. Disinfection destroys pathogenic organisms (excluding bacterial spores) or their toxins or vectors by direct exposure to chemical or physical means.

Free-rinsing: Ability to be removed without leaving residue.

High-level disinfection: A process that kills all microorganisms with the exception of high numbers of bacterial spores and prions. High-level disinfectants have the capability to inactivate the hepatitis B and C viruses, HIV, and *Mycobacterium tuberculosis,* but do not inactivate the virus-like prion that causes Creutzfeld-Jakob disease. Government-registered high-level disinfection agents kill vegetative bacteria, tubercle bacilli, some spores and fungi, and lipid and nonlipid viruses, given appropriate concentration, submersion, and contact time.

Hospital disinfectant: A chemical germicide with label claims for effectiveness against *Salmonella, Staphylococcus,* and *Pseudomonas.* Hospital disinfectants may be low-, intermediate-, or high-level disinfectants.

Iatrogenic: A response to a medical or surgical treatment, usually denoting an unfavorable response.

In vitro: Outside the living body and in an artificial environment.

Intermediate-level disinfection: A process that kills *Mycobacterium tuberculosis,* vegetative bacteria, most viruses, and most fungi, but does not necessarily kill bacterial spores.

Low-level disinfection: A process by which most bacteria, some viruses, and some fungi are killed. This process cannot be relied on to kill resistant microorganisms such as *Mycobacterium tuberculosis* or bacterial spores.

Minimum effective concentration: The minimum concentration of a liquid chemical germicide that achieves the claimed microbicidal activity as determined by dose-response testing.

Nidus; (pl) nidi: A focus of infection; or the coalescence of small particles that is the beginning of a solid deposit.

Pasteurization: "A process originally developed by Louis Pasteur of heating milk, wine, or other liquids to between 140° F and 212° F (60° C to 100° C) for approximately 30 minutes to kill or significantly reduce the number of pathogenic and spoilage organisms" *(Source: Block SS. Definition of terms. In: Disinfection, Sterilization, and Preservation. 5th ed. Block SS, ed. Philadelphia, PA: Lippincott Williams & Wilkins; 2001:19-28.)* A process that employs time and heat (ie, 160° F to 170° F [71.1° C to 76.7° C] for 30 minutes) for high-level disinfection. The intensity of heat and duration of exposure must be determined by the manufacturer of the pasteurization unit and the manufacturer of the product or device to be cleaned.

Personal protective equipment (PPE): Specialized equipment or clothing for eyes, face, head, body, and extremities; protective clothing; respiratory devices; and protective shields and barriers designed to protect the worker from injury or exposure to a patient's blood, tissue, or body fluids. Used by health care workers and others whenever necessary to protect themselves from the hazards of processes or environments, chemical hazards, or mechanical irritants encountered in a manner capable of causing injury or impairment in the function of any part of the body through absorption, inhalation, or physical contact.

Sterilization: Processes by which all microbial life, including pathogenic and nonpathogenic microorganisms, and spores, are killed.

REFERENCES

1. Spaulding EH. Clinical disinfection and antisepsis in the hospital. *J Hosp Res* 1972;95.

2. Rutala WA. APIC guideline for selection and use of disinfectants. 1994, 1995, and 1996 APIC Guidelines Committee. Association for Professionals in Infection Control and Epidemiology, Inc. *Am J Infect Control* 1996; 24(4):313.

3. Tablan OC, Anderson LJ, Besser R, Bridges C, Hajjeh R, et al. Guidelines for preventing health care-associated pneumonia, 2003: Recommendations of CDC and the Healthcare Infection Control Practices Advisory Committee. *MMWR Recomm Rep* 2004;53(RR-3):1.

4. Class II special controls guidance document: Medical washers and medical washer-disinfectors; guidance for the medical device industry and FDA review staff. US Food and Drug Administration. *http://www.fda.gov/cdrh/ode/guidance/1252.html.* Accessed December 5, 2008.

5. Appendix B: Decontamination and disinfection. In: *Biosafety in Microbiological and Biomedical Laboratories (BMBL).* 5th ed. Centers for Disease Control and Prevention; National Institutes of Health, eds. Washington, DC: US Government Printing Office; 2007:328-336. Available at *http://www.cdc.gov/od/ohs/biosfty/bmbl5/bmbl5toc.htm.* Accessed December 5, 2008.

6. Alvarado CJ, Reichelderfer M. APIC guideline for infection prevention and control in flexible endoscopy. Association for Professionals in Infection Control. *Am J Infect Control* 2000;28(2):138.

7. *AAMI TIR12:2004—Designing, Testing and Labeling Reusable Medical Devices for Reprocessing in Health Care Facilities: A Guide for Medical Device Manufacturers.* Arlington, VA: Association for the Advancement of Medical Instrumentation; 2005.

8. Rutala WA, Weber DJ. How to assess risk of disease transmission to patients when there is a failure to follow recommended disinfection and sterilization guidelines. *Infect Control Hosp Epidemiol* 2007;28(2):146.

9. Multi-society guideline for reprocessing flexible gastrointestinal endoscopes. *Am J Infect Control* 2003;31(5):309.

10. Rutala WA, Gergen MF, Weber DJ. Disinfection of a probe used in ultrasound-guided prostate biopsy. *Infect Control Hosp Epidemiol* 2007;28(8):916.

11. Perkins JJ. *Principles and methods of sterilization in health sciences.* 2nd ed. Springfield, Ill.: Thomas; 1969.

12. Favero MS, Bond WW. Chemical disinfection of medical and surgical materials. In: Block SS, ed. *Disinfection, Sterilization, and Preservation.* 5th ed. Philadelphia, PA: Lippincott Williams & Wilkins; 2001:881.

13. Thomas LA. Essentials for endoscopic equipment. High-level disinfection. *Gastroenterol Nurs* 2006;29(2):179.

14. Camp S, Dawson C. Best practice forum: Standard high-level disinfection protocol development. *ORL Head Neck Nurs* 2003; 21(2):18-21.

15. Rutala WA, Weber DJ. Disinfection and sterilization in health care facilities: what clinicians need to know. *Clin Infect Dis.* 2004;39(5):702-709.

16. Bolding B. Choosing a reprocessing method. *Can Oper Room Nurs J.* 2004;22(2):24.

17. FDA-cleared sterilants and high-level disinfectants with general claims for processing reusable medical and dental devices; September 28, 2006. US Food and Drug Administration. *http://www.fda.gov/cdrh/ode/germlab.html.* Accessed December 5, 2008.

18. Society of Gastroenterology Nurses and Associates Inc. Guidelines for the use of high-level disinfectants and sterilants for reprocessing of flexible gastrointestinal endoscopes. *Gastroenterol Nurs* 2004;27(4):198.

19. Lee J H, Rhee P L, Kim J H, Kim J J, Paik S W, Rhee J C, Song J H, Yeom J S, Lee N Y. Efficacy of electrolyzed acid water in reprocessing patient-used flexible upper endoscopes: Comparison with 2% alkaline glutaraldehyde. *J Gastroenterol Hepatol* 2004;19(8):897-903.

20. Bhattacharyya N, Kepnes L J. The effectiveness of immersion disinfection for flexible fiberoptic laryngoscopes. *Otolaryngol Head Neck Surg* 2004;130(6):681.

21. Rutala WA, Weber DJ. Disinfection of endoscopes: Review of new chemical sterilants used for high-level disinfection. *Infect Control Hosp Epidemiol* 1999; 20(1):69.

22. *Hazard Communication.* (29 CFR §1910.) Occupational Safety and Health Administration. Washington, DC: US Government Printing Office; 2007. Available at *http://www.osha.gov/SLTC/hazardcommunications/standards.html.* Accessed December 5, 2008.

23. Rutala WA, Weber DJ. Cleaning, disinfection, and sterilization in healthcare facilities. In: *APIC Text of Infection Control and Epidemiology.* Washington, DC: Association for Professionals in Infection Control and Epidemiology; 2005:21-31.

24. Cantrell S. High-level disinfection vs sterilization: Six of one, half dozen of the other? *Healthc Purchasing News* 2005;29(4):38, 40, 42.

25. Rutala WA, Weber DJ. Reprocessing endoscopes: United States perspective. In: Proceedings of the 7th International BODE Hygiene Days, May 2003. *J Hosp Infect* 2004 (April); 56 Supplement 2:S27-S39.

26. Alfa MJ. Can biofilm prevent high-level disinfection? *J Genca* 2006;16(1):23.

27. Raffo P, Salliez AC, Collignon C, Clementi M. Antimicrobial activity of a formulation for the low temperature disinfection of critical and semicritical medical equipment and surfaces. *New Microbiol* 2007;30(4):463.

28. Marion K, Freney J, James G, Bergeron E, Renaud FN, Costerton JW. Using an efficient biofilm detaching agent: An essential step for the improvement of endoscope reprocessing protocols. *J Hosp Infect* 2006;64(2):136.

29. Murdoch H, Taylor D, Dickinson J, Walker JT, Perrett D, Raven ND, Sutton JM. Surface decontamination of surgical instruments: An ongoing dilemma. *J Hosp Infect* 2006;63(4):432.

30. Rerknimitr R, Eakthunyasakul S, Nunthapisud P, Kongkam P. Results of gastroscope bacterial decontamination by enzymatic detergent compared to chlorhexidine. *World J Gastroenterol* 2006;12(26):4199.

31. Thomas LA. Manual cleaning. *Gastroenterol Nurs* 2005;28(6):512.

32. Dettenkofer M, Block C. Hospital disinfection: Efficacy and safety issues. *Curr Opin Infect Dis* 2005; 18(4):320.

33. Kampf G, Bloss R, Martiny H. Surface fixation of dried blood by glutaraldehyde and peracetic acid. *J Hosp Infect* 2004;57(2):139.

34. Vickery K, Pajkos A, Cossart Y. Removal of biofilm from endoscopes: Evaluation of detergent efficiency. *Am J Infect Control* 2004;32(3):170.

35. Cowen AE. The clinical risks of infection associated with endoscopy. *Can J Gastroenterol* 2001;15(5):321.

36. Association for the Advancement of Medical Instrumentation. *ANSI/AAMI ST58:2005—Chemical Sterilization and High-Level Disinfection in Health Care Facilities.* Arlington, VA: Association for the Advancement of Medical Instrumentation; 2005.

37. Morck DW, Olson ME, Ceri H. Microbial biofilms: Prevention, control, and removal. In: Block SS, ed. *Disinfection, Sterilization, and Preservation.* 5th ed. Philadelphia, PA: Lippincott Williams & Wilkins; 2001:675.

38. McDonnell G, Pretzer D. New and developing antimicrobials. In: Block SS, ed. *Disinfection, Sterilization, and Preservation.* 5th ed. Philadelphia, PA: Lippincott Williams & Wilkins; 2001:431.

39. Cowen A, Jones D, Wardle E. *Guidelines: Infection Control in Endoscopy.* 2nd ed. Sydney, Australia: Gastroenterological Society of Australia; 2003.

40. Spach DH, Silverstein FE, Stamm WE. Transmission of infection by gastrointestinal endoscopy and bronchoscopy. *Ann Intern Med* 1993;118(2):117.

41. Weber DJ, Rutala WA, DiMarino AJ. The prevention of infection following gastrointestinal endoscopy: The importance of prophylaxis and reprocessing. In: DiMarino AJ, Benjamin SB, eds. *Gastrointestinal Disease: An Endoscopic Approach.* Thorofare, NJ: Slack; 2002:87.

42. Miner N, Harris V, Ebron T, Cao T. Sporicidal activity of disinfectants as one possible cause for bacteria in patient-ready endoscopes. *Gastroenterol Nurs* 2007; 30(4):285.

43. Cheetham NWH. Comparative efficacy of medical instrument cleaning products in digesting some blood proteins [corrected]. *Aust Infect Control* 2005;10(3):103; erratum *Aust Infect Control* 2005;10(4):142.

44. Nelson DB, Jarvis WR, Rutala WA, et al; Society for Healthcare Epidemiology of America. Multi-society guideline for reprocessing flexible gastrointestinal endoscopes. *Infect Control Hosp Epidemiol* 2003;24(7):532.

45. Hospital eTool: Healthcare-wide hazards module—Glutaraldehyde. Occupational Safety and Health Administration. *http://www.osha.gov/SLTC/etools/hospital /hazards/glutaraldehyde/glut.html.* Accessed December 5, 2008.

46. Fraud S, Maillard J Y, Russell AD. Comparison of the mycobactericidal activity of ortho-phthalaldehyde, glutaraldehyde, and other dialdehydes by a quantitative suspension test. *J Hosp Infect* 2001;48(3):214.

47. Rutala W A, Weber D J. New disinfection and sterilization methods. *Emerg Infect Dis* 2001;7(2):348.

48. *ANSI/AAMI ST58:2005—Chemical Sterilization and High-Level Disinfection in Health Care Facilities.* Arlington, VA: Association for the Advancement of Medical Instrumentation; 2005.

49. Recommended practices for cleaning and care of surgical instruments and powered equipment. In: *Perioperative Standards and Recommended Practices.* Denver, CO: AORN; 2008:421-446.

50. Banerjee S, Nelson DB, Dominitz JA, et al. Reprocessing failure. *Gastrointest Endosc* 2007; 66(5):869.

51. Lin CS, Fuller J, Mayhall ES. Federal regulation of liquid chemical germicides by the US Food and Drug Administration. In: Block SS, ed. *Disinfection, Sterilization, and Preservation.* 5th ed. Philadelphia, PA: Lippincott Williams & Wilkins; 2001:1293.

52. Procedures for performance standards development. (21 CFR §861.) US Food and Drug Administration. Washington, DC: US Government Printing Office; 2008. Available at *http://www.accessdata.fda.gov/scripts/cdrh/cfdocs/cfcfr/ CFRSearch.cfm?CFRPart=861.* Accessed December 5, 2008.

53. Recommended practices for cleaning and processing flexible endoscopes and endoscope accessories. In: *Perioperative Standards and Recommended Practices.* Denver, CO: AORN; 2009:595-610.

54. WHO infection control guidelines for transmissible spongiform encephalopathies. Report of a WHO consultation, Geneva, Switzerland, 23-26 March 1999. World Health Organization. *http://www.who.int/csr/resources /publications/bse/WHO_CDS_CSR_APH_2000_3/en.* Accessed December 5, 2008.

55. Rutala WA, Weber DJ. Creutzfeldt-Jakob disease: Recommendations for disinfection and sterilization. *Clin Infect Dis* 2001;32(9):1348.

56. Gray J. How safe is your endoscope disinfectant? *Br J Perioper Nurs* 2005;15(3):134.

57. NINDS Creutzfeldt-Jakob disease information page. National Institute of Neurological Disorders and Stroke. *http://www.ninds.nih.gov/disorders/cjd/cjd.htm.* Accessed December 5, 2008.

58. Definition of terms. In: Block SS, ed. *Disinfection, Sterilization, and Preservation.* 5th ed. Philadelphia, PA: Lippincott Williams & Wilkins; 2001:19.

59. Nelson DB, Jarvis WR, Rutala WA, et al. Multi-society guideline for reprocessing flexible gastrointestinal endoscopes. *Dis Colon Rectum* 2004;47(4):413.

60. Acosta-Gío AE, Rueda-Patiño JL, Sánchez-Pérez L. Sporicidal activity in liquid chemical products to sterilize

or high-level disinfect medical and dental instruments. *Am J Infect Control* 2005;33(5):307-309.

61. Omidbakhsh N. A new peroxide-based flexible endoscope-compatible high-level disinfectant. *Am J Infect Control* 2006;34(9):571.

62. Weber DJ, Rutala WA, Sickbert-Bennett EE. Outbreaks associated with contaminated antiseptics and disinfectants. *Antimicrob Agents Chemother* 2007; 51(12):4217.

63. *AAMI TIR34:2007—Water for the Reprocessing of Medical Devices*. Arlington, VA: Association for the Advancement of Medical Instrumentation; 2007.

64. Guidelines for protecting the safety and health of health care workers, chapter 6: Hazardous waste disposal. National Institute for Occupational Safety and Health. *http://www.cdc.gov/niosh/hcwold6.html*. Accessed December 5, 2008.

65. *Code of Federal Regulations*. Title 40: Protection of Environment. *http://ecfr.gpoaccess.gov/cgi/t/text/text-idx?c=ecfr;sid=4990e762d7b81851bef18f82dc851826;rgn=div5;view=text;node=40:25.0.1.1.2;idno=40;cc=ecfr #40:25.0.1.1.2.3.1.4*. Accessed December 5, 2008.

66. Public health notification from FDA, CDC, FPA and OSHA: Avoiding hazards with using cleaners and disinfectants on electronic medical equipment. US Food and Drug Administration. *http://www.fda.gov/cdrh/safety/103107-cleaners.html*. Accessed December 5, 2008.

67. AORN explications for perioperative nursing. In: *Perioperative Standards and Recommended Practices*. Denver, CO: AORN; 2008:633-660.

68. Newsome C. Education in product safety: glutaraldehyde in high-level disinfection applications. *Occup Health Rev* 2005;118:18-20.

69. Rideout K, Teschke K, DimichWard H, Kennedy S M. Considering risks to healthcare workers from glutaraldehyde alternatives in high-level disinfection. *J Hosp Infect* 2005;59(1):4-11.

70. Suzukawa M, Yamaguchi M, Komiya A, Kimura M, Nito T, Yamamoto K. Ortho-phthalaldehyde-induced anaphylaxis after laryngoscopy. *J Allergy Clin Immunol* 2006; 117(6):1500.

71. Cohen NL, Patton CM. Worker safety and glutaraldehyde in the gastrointestinal lab environment. *Gastroenterol Nurs* 2006;29(2):100.

72. Ghasemkhani M, Jahanpeyma F, Azam K. Formaldehyde exposure in some educational hospitals of Tehran. *Ind Health* 2005;43(4):703.

73. Cogliano V, Grosse Y, Baan R, Straif K, Secretan B, El Ghissassi F; WHO International Agency for Research on Cancer. Advice on formaldehyde and glycol ethers. *Lancet Oncol* 2004; 5(9):528.

74. Sokol WN. Nine episodes of anaphylaxis following cystoscopy caused by Cidex OPA (ortho-phthalaldehyde) high-level disinfectant in 4 patients after cytoscopy. *J Allergy Clin Immunol* 2004; 114(2):392.

75. Fujita H, Ogawa M, Endo Y. A case of occupational bronchial asthma and contact dermatitis caused by ortho-phthalaldehyde exposure in a medical worker. *J Occup Health* 2006; 48(6):413.

76. Best practices for the safe use of glutaraldehyde in health care. OSHA document number 3258-08N-2006. Occupational Safety and Health Administration. *http://www.osha.gov/Publications/3258-08N-2006-English .html*. Accessed December 5, 2008.

77. Karpelowsky JS, Maske CP, Sinclair-Smith C, Rode H. Glutaraldehyde-induced bowel injury after laparoscopy. *J Pediatr Surg* 2006; 41(6):e23.

78. Unal M, Yücel I, Akar Y, Oner A, Altin M. Outbreak of toxic anterior segment syndrome associated with glutaraldehyde after cataract surgery. *J Cataract Refract Surg* 2006 Oct;32(10):1696-1701.

79. Standards of perioperative administrative practice. In: *Perioperative Standards and Recommended Practices*. Denver, CO: AORN; 2008:15.

80. Recommended practices for documentation of perioperative nursing care. In: *Perioperative Standards and Recommended Practices*. Denver, CO: AORN; 2008:311-314.

81. American Society for Healthcare Central Service Professionals. *Training Manual for Health Care Central Service Technicians*. 5th ed. San Francisco, CA: Jossey-Bass; 2006.

82. Thomas LA. Essentials for endoscopic equipment. Recommended care and handling of flexible endoscopes: Endoscope storage. *Gastroenterol Nurs* 2005; 28(1):45.

83. Perioperative patient care quality. In: *Perioperative Standards and Recommended Practices*. Denver, CO: AORN; 2008:11-12.

84. Standards of perioperative professional practice. In: *Perioperative Standards and Recommended Practices*. Denver, CO: AORN; 2008:23-26.

85. Sciortino CV Jr, Xia EL, Mozee A. Assessment of a novel approach to evaluate the outcome of endoscope reprocessing. *Infect Control Hosp Epidemiol* 2004; 25(4):284.

86. Standards of infection control in reprocessing of flexible gastrointestinal endoscopes. Society of Gastroenterology Nurses and Associates. *http://www.sgna.org/Resources/standards.cfm*. Accessed December 5, 2008.

87. Quality and performance improvement standards for perioperative nursing. In: *Perioperative Standards and Recommended Practices*. Denver, CO: AORN; 2008:27-36.

Acknowledgments

LEAD AUTHORS

Sheila Mitchell, RN, BSN, MS, CNOR
Perioperative Nursing Specialist
AORN Center for Nursing Practice
Denver, Colorado

Judith Goldberg, RN, MSN, CNOR
Clinical Director
Backus Hospital
Norwich, Connecticut

CONTRIBUTING AUTHOR

Ardene Nichols, RN, MSN, CNS, CNOR, PAHM
Health Care Consultant
Conroe, Texas

RP: High-Level Disinfection

PUBLICATION HISTORY

Originally published August 1980, *AORN Journal,* as AORN "Recommended practices for sterilization and disinfection."

Format revision July 1982; revised February 1987.

Revised October 1992 as "Recommended practices for disinfection"; published as proposed recommended practices September 1994 as "Recommended practices for chemical disinfection."

Revised November 1998 as "Recommended practices for high-level disinfection"; published March 1999, *AORN Journal.*

Revised November 2004; published in *Standards, Recommended Practices, and Guidelines,* 2005 edition. Reprinted February 2005, *AORN Journal.*

Revised November 2008; published in *Perioperative Standards and Recommended Practices,* 2009 edition.

Minor editing revisions made in November 2009 for publication in *Perioperative Standards and Recommended Practices,* 2010 edition.

Recommended Practices for Cleaning and Processing Flexible Endoscopes and Endoscope Accessories

The following recommended practices were developed by the AORN Recommended Practices Committee and have been approved by the AORN Board of Directors. They were presented as proposed recommendations for comments by members and others. They are effective January 1, 2009.

These recommended practices are intended as achievable recommendations representing what is believed to be an optimal level of practice. Policies and procedures will reflect variations in practice settings and/or clinical situations that determine the degree to which the recommended practices can be implemented. AORN recognizes the various settings in which perioperative nurses practice. These recommended practices are intended as guidelines adaptable to various practice settings. These practice settings include traditional operating rooms, ambulatory surgery centers, physician's offices, cardiac catheterization laboratories, endoscopy suites, radiology departments, and all other areas where surgery may be performed.

Purpose

These recommended practices provide guidelines to assist personnel in the care, cleaning, decontamination, maintenance, handling, storage, sterilization, and/or disinfection of flexible endoscopes and related accessories. Use of these recommended practices will assist personnel in providing a safe environment for patients and health care workers.

These recommended practices are based on the most current evidence available at the time of development. They should be used to develop policies and procedures for care of flexible endoscopes and accessories in the practice setting. As new information becomes available, perioperative nurses should consult with infection preventionists and epidemiologists to review and revise procedures as appropriate. These recommended practices pertain only to flexible endoscopes and are divided into the following sections:

- following manufacturer's instructions,
- precleaning,
- transport to decontamination,
- leak testing,
- cleaning,
- high-level disinfection
- alcohol treatment,
- drying,
- storage,

- handling damaged flexible endoscopes,
- care of accessories, and
- personal protective equipment (PPE).

Competencies, documentation, policies and procedures, and quality management suggestions also are discussed. For more information on the care and cleaning of rigid endoscopes and related equipment, refer to the AORN "Recommended practices for care and cleaning of instruments and powered surgical equipment."[1]

Recommendation I

Flexible endoscopes should be cleaned and stored in accordance with the manufacturer's written instructions.

Failure to follow the manufacturer's written instructions could result in ineffective cleaning that interferes with high-level disinfection or sterilization, creating a risk of infection for the patient. The manufacturer's warranty may be void if the written instructions for care and use of the device are not followed.

I.a. The manufacturer's written instructions for flexible endoscopes and all accessories should be followed regarding
   - cleaning processes,
   - selection of cleaning product,
   - selection of disinfectant/sterilization products,
   - use of alcohol, and
   - compatibility with automatic endoscope reprocessors.

   Flexible endoscopes manufactured by different companies require different cleaning processes as described in the manufacturer's written instructions. The flexible endoscope manufacturer is required to demonstrate to the US Food and Drug Administration in the premarket clearance application that the cleaning/disinfecting instructions are adequate and that the results are reproducible.[2] All flexible endoscopes and accessories cannot be processed successfully in all automatic endoscopic reprocessors.[3]

I.b. High-level disinfectant and chemical cleaner manufacturers' written instructions should be followed regarding

- compatibility with the flexible endoscope and accessories,
- water quality,
- dilution,
- temperature of solution,
- testing for minimum effective concentration,
- time of exposure, and
- rinsing.[4]

Following the manufacturer's written instructions will deliver the recommended concentration of cleaning solution, disinfectant, or sterilant required for adequate cleaning and to create effective high-level disinfection or sterilization.[5,6] Improper dilution may result in ineffective high-level disinfection or sterilization if the solution is too weak. If the solution is too strong, it may become abrasive or corrosive, possibly contributing to corrosion and degradation of the surfaces of the flexible endoscope.[7] The high-level disinfectant and chemical cleaner may remain on the scope if the manufacturer's written instructions for rinsing are not followed. For more information on high-level disinfection, refer to the AORN "Recommended practices for high-level disinfection."[8]

I.c. New, repaired, or refurbished flexible endoscopes and accessories should be leak tested, cleaned, and high-level disinfected or sterilized before use in a health care organization.

Cleaning and high-level disinfection of newly acquired or repaired flexible endoscopes removes any soil related to manufacturing, repairing, refurbishing, or shipping. Leak tests determine if perforations in either the outer covering or the lining of the internal channels may have occurred during manufacturing, shipping, repairing, or refurbishing.[9]

Recommendation II

Precleaning of flexible endoscopes and accessories should occur at the point of use, before organic material has dried on the surface or in the channels of the endoscope, and before transport to the decontamination area.

Flexible endoscopes, by virtue of the body cavities in which they are used, acquire high levels of microbial contamination during each use. Failure to completely follow the defined cleaning process, beginning with precleaning, has been shown to cause inadequate decontamination leading to patients being exposed to infectious agents.[10] Precleaning of endoscopes and related equipment at the point of use before transport to the decontamination area helps prevent drying of the organic material on the flexible endoscope surfaces.

The presence of dried organic material makes decontamination/disinfection more difficult. Organic materials (eg, blood and body fluids) that have dried on the flexible endoscope surfaces are difficult to remove and can inhibit sterilization and high-level disinfection.[11] Precleaning reduces the likelihood of the formation of biofilms, which contain viable and nonviable microorganisms that become trapped within a matrix of organic matter (eg, proteins, glycoproteins, carbohydrates) and adhere to the surfaces of flexible endoscopes. Biofilms are difficult to remove, and it is difficult for sterilizing/disinfecting agents to penetrate and kill the microorganisms within the biofilms. The biofilm formation process can begin within minutes after completion of a procedure.[7,12]

II.a. Precleaning measures include the following:

(1) External surfaces of the flexible endoscope insertion tube should be washed with an enzymatic detergent solution using a soft cloth or sponge.

(2) Internal suction/biopsy channels should be cleaned by suctioning copious amounts of enzymatic solution (ie, enzymatic detergent mixed with tap water) and air.

(3) Air and water channels should be flushed with an enzymatic solution, then flushed using low-pressure compressed air (ie, pressure should not exceed maximum channel pressure specified by manufacturer), if available. If low-pressure compressed air is not available, a syringe may be used for flushing with air.

(4) Additional complex design components or channels (eg, forward water jet channel, exposed elevator wire channels, balloon channels) should be flushed or purged with water and/or enzymatic detergent solution as described in the manufacturer's written instructions.

(5) The tip of the endoscope should be visually inspected for damage to any surface and any working part and for cleanliness.

(6) The video protective cap, if available, should be attached after removing the

flexible endoscope from the light source and suction.

(7) All detachable parts (eg, hoods, valves, water bottle) should be removed and immersed in an enzymatic detergent solution until transport to the decontamination room. When flexible endoscopes and accessories are used on a sterile field,

- the external surfaces should be wiped with a lint-free cloth saturated with sterile water;
- sterile water and air should be alternately suctioned through the channels; and
- the endoscope and accessories should be handed to the circulator as soon as possible, enabling steps 1–7 to be accomplished.

(8) The enzymatic detergent solution should be discarded after a single use.

Washing the external surfaces of the endoscope and flushing the internal channels with enzymatic solution helps to soften, moisten, dilute, and remove organic soils (eg, blood, feces, respiratory secretions).[13]

Alternating cleaning solution with air may help to soften, moisten, dilute, and remove organic soils (eg, blood, feces, respiratory secretions). It is more effective to alternate the use of air and water when cleaning rather than prolonged use of either.[13]

Flushing with low-pressure compressed air helps to dry the channel. Low-pressure compressed air should be used because it is possible to damage the channel linings with uncontrolled or high-flow air.[7]

Depending upon design and intended use, endoscopes vary in complexity. Certain flexible endoscopes may have more channels than the standard air, water, and suction. Therefore, whenever scopes have additional channels or complex components, each should also be flushed or purged by following the original scope manufacturer's recommendations.

A visual inspection after precleaning should be done to verify that no obvious organic debris remains.

The video protective cap protects video connections from moisture during decontamination and disinfection.[13]

Soaking the detachable parts of the endoscope in enzymatic detergent solution assists in degrading and preventing biofilms.[7] Wiping the flexible endoscope and accessories with lint-free cloth saturated with sterile water and alternately suctioning sterile water and air while the endoscope remains on the sterile field will prevent drying of proteins on the endoscope surfaces until the cleaning process may be accomplished.

The enzymatic detergent cleaning solution should be discarded after each use because it does not possess bactericidal activity and may support growth of organisms if stored. There are no tests to verify the strength of the solution prior to use.

Recommendation III

After precleaning, contaminated flexible endoscopes and accessories should be transported to the decontamination area before remaining organic material dries on the surface or in the channels of the endoscope.

Transport to the decontamination area before remaining organic material is able to dry on the surface or in the channels of the flexible endoscope facilitates cleaning which helps to reduce the formation of biofilms.[7,12]

III.a.   During transport to the decontamination area, soiled flexible endoscopes must be contained (eg, enclosed by a plastic bag, container with a lid) in a manner to prevent exposure of environmental surfaces, patients, and personnel to bloodborne pathogens and other potentially infectious organisms. If the decontamination area is adjacent to the procedure room, the contaminated items may be transported in an open container by personnel wearing appropriate PPE.[14]

Contaminated flexible endoscopes and accessories present a risk of contaminating the environment and can expose health care workers to blood and other potentially infectious materials during transport to the decontamination area.[14]

III.b.   The transport container must be labeled to indicate biohazardous contents. The types of label may include, but are not limited to, magnetic signs, stickers, or plastic placards.[14]

Labeling the transport container communicates to others that the items are potentially infectious.[14]

Recommendation IV

In the decontamination area and before cleaning, pressure (ie, leak) tests should be performed on flexible endoscopes with leak testing capabilities.[9]

Leak tests determine if there are any openings in the external surfaces and internal channels that would permit fluid to enter the internal body of the endoscope.[9]

IV.a. During leak testing, the flexible endoscope control knobs should be manipulated in all directions.

Manipulating the flexible endoscope control knobs in all directions exposes the surfaces to the maximum extension, thereby revealing small perforations if present.[9]

IV.b. When using a leak test system requiring water, the leak test system should be attached to the flexible endoscope, followed by submersion of the entire endoscope in water that does not contain cleaning agents, to check for the presence of bubbling.[9]

Leakage in either the covering or one or more of the internal channels can be determined by the presence of air bubbles when air pressure is applied to the inside of the insertion tube. Discoloration and foam caused by the detergent agent may prevent small bubbles from being visible.[9]

IV.b.1. When a leak is detected, the leak testing device should remain attached to the flexible endoscope and under pressure until the endoscope is removed from the water.[9]

Continuous air pressure helps to prevent water from entering the internal (ie, working) portions of the flexible endoscope which may cause more extensive damage to the internal parts.[15]

IV.c. When using a leak test system that does not require water, the leak test should be completed before submersion in water or cleaning solution.[9]

Leaks in either the covering or one or more of the inside channels can be determined by a drop in pressure after inflation or by the inability to inflate the inside of the insertion tube.[9]

Recommendation V

Following leak testing and before high-level disinfection using a manual process or an automatic endoscope reprocessor, flexible endoscopes and their accessories should be manually cleaned before any remaining organic material dries on the surface or in the channels of the endoscope.[16]

Immediate cleaning reduces the amount of microbial contamination and the formation of biofilms. For the high-level disinfectant to be effective, the solution must reach all surfaces of the flexible endoscope. If the microbial contamination and biofilm are not removed, the surface under the bioburden will not be disinfected.[7]

V.a. When manually cleaning flexible endoscopes:
(1) The flexible endoscope should be submerged in an enzymatic detergent solution.
(2) The insertion tube of the flexible endoscope should be washed using a soft, lint-free cloth or sponge.[17]
(3) All internal channels should be flushed thoroughly with an enzymatic detergent using manufacturer-provided channel cleaning adapters.
(4) All endoscope components (eg, shroud, valves) should be flushed thoroughly with an enzymatic detergent.
(5) Brushes should be inspected prior to insertion to confirm that they are sized appropriately to the channel(s), not kinked, not missing bristles, and that a protective tip is present to prevent damage to the channel.[17]
(6) The brush should be inserted through the channel with the entire endoscope submerged to prevent aerosolization. The bristles should be wiped to remove excess moisture prior to retracting the brush back through the channel.[17] All channels should be flushed thoroughly and all exterior surfaces of the flexible endoscope and accessories rinsed with potable tap water.[4]
(7) The flexible endoscope should be dried using low-pressure forced air through the internal channels and the exterior surfaces wiped with a soft cloth before placing the endoscope in high-level disinfecting solution or an automatic endoscope reprocessor.

Submersion of the flexible endoscope in enzymatic detergent solution helps ensure contact between the solution and all surfaces of the endoscope and decreases the potential for the cleaning solution to splash.[17]

Washing the exterior of the insertion tube with an enzymatic detergent and a soft cloth removes organic material remaining after precleaning.

Flushing all internal channels with detergent solution exposes these surfaces to the enzymatic detergent solution. Using the manufacturer-provided channel cleaning adapters facilitates opening of the ports.

Brushing accessible channels removes particulate matter. Using the appropriate size brush will maximize the amount of soil removed without damaging the inside of the channel. Using a brush that is kinked or missing bristles or without its protective tip may cause damage to the flexible endoscope.[12,17]

The tip of the flexible endoscope and the lens may be abraded by vigorous brushing and wiping. Brushing and wiping the tip of the flexible endoscope removes any debris or tissue that might be lodged around the air-water outlet.[17] Thorough flushing of the channels and rinsing of the flexible endoscope and accessories with potable tap water removes residual debris and cleaning agents. Potable tap water may be used at this point if it does not cause corrosion or tarnishing or leave salt deposits on the flexible endoscope or its accessories. If corrosion, tarnishing, or salt deposits are found on the flexible endoscope, the water filtration process should be examined.[4]

Moisture remaining on the surface and in the flexible endoscope's lumens may dilute the high-level disinfecting solution, potentially reducing its effectiveness.

Recommendation VI

After cleaning, flexible endoscopes and accessories should be high-level disinfected or sterilized.[9,10]

Flexible endoscopes and accessories contact mucous membranes and/or nonintact skin during use and require a minimum of high-level disinfection. Some flexible endoscopes are heat-labile and cannot be steam sterilized. Sterilization is only required if the flexible endoscope is to be used on a sterile field.[11]

VI.a. When using a manual process for high-level disinfection:
  (1) The flexible endoscope and its accessories should be manually cleaned, as described in Recommendation V, before beginning the manual high-level disinfection process.
  (2) The flexible endoscope and its accessories should be completely immersed in the disinfecting solution.
  (3) All channels should be flushed with disinfecting solution after immersion.[19]

For the high-level disinfectant to be effective, the solution must reach all surfaces of the item. If the microbial contamination and biofilm are not removed, the surface under the bioburden will not be disinfected.[7,16] Complete immersion is required to ensure complete coverage of all surfaces of the flexible endoscope.[20] Flushing helps to ensure that the high-level disinfectant has contact with all surfaces, including internal channels, which is necessary for complete disinfection.[19,20]

VI.b. When using an automatic endoscope reprocessor for high-level disinfection:
  (1) Manual cleaning should be accomplished as described in Recommendation V.
  (2) The flexible endoscope and components should be inserted into the automatic endoscope reprocessor.
  (3) All the flexible endoscope channels should be attached to the unit using compatible connectors.[19]

For the high-level disinfectant to be effective, the solution must reach all surfaces of the flexible endoscope. If the microbial contamination and biofilm are not removed, the surface under the bioburden will not be disinfected.[7,16] Failure to use approved connectors may result in disinfection failure because the disinfectant/sterilant may not reach all surfaces of the flexible endoscope. The use of incompatible connectors have lead to the transmission of infections.[7,21]

VI.b.1. When the compatible connectors of the automatic endoscope reprocessor cannot be connected to a specific channel (ie, the wire elevator channel of a duodenoscope), the steps for manual high-level disinfection should be followed for this channel or for the entire flexible endoscope.[7,22]

Manual high-level disinfection is the only method by which the high-level disinfectant will reach the entire inner surface of the channel.[3,7,21,22]

Recommendation VII

After high-level disinfection, flexible endoscopes should be rinsed and the internal channels flushed with water (eg, sterile water, filtered or unfiltered tap water) followed by a 70% to 90% ethyl or isopropyl alcohol rinse and flush, unless contraindicated by the manufacturer's written instructions.[4,19]

The water rinse and flush removes the residual disinfecting solution. Use of filtered tap water or sterile water reduces the potential for recontamination by waterborne microorganisms. Filtered tap water is created at the point of use, using a filter with 0.2 or 0.1 micron pores.[4,7,19] Rinsing with alcohol assists with removing the water because the alcohol binds with the water remaining in the channel, facilitating the drying process and killing any microorganisms contained in the water.[7,19,23]

VII.a. After rinsing with 70% to 90% ethyl or isopropyl alcohol, the channels should be dried using low pressure forced air.

Using forced air assists with removal of moisture remaining in the channels. Dry air channels do not support microbial growth.[7]

Recommendation VIII

Flexible endoscopes, accessories, and associated equipment should be inspected for integrity, function, and cleanliness:
- before use,
- during the procedure,
- after the procedure,
- immediately after decontamination, and
- before disinfection or sterilization.[24]

Visual inspection helps to identify structural damage, when and where the damage occurred, what caused the damage, and how to prevent further damage. Loss of function and gross soil that may affect further processing and patient outcomes can also be identified during visual inspection.[16]

VIII.a. Damaged flexible endoscopes and accessories should be removed from use, and the manufacturer should be consulted for directions regarding actions to be taken prior to shipping for repair, such as reprocessing or not reprocessing the damaged flexible endoscope.

Immediate removal from use will prevent further damage to the internal mechanisms of the flexible endoscope that may be caused by water entering the mechanism and will prevent the damaged endoscope from being inadvertently used. The manufacturer will determine the correct method of shipping and whether the endoscope should be cleaned before shipping based on the nature of the damage.[9]

VIII.a.1. Unless otherwise specified in the manufacturer's instructions, a damaged flexible endoscope should not be submerged.[9]

Submersion may lead to additional damage related to water entering the interior of the flexible endoscope.[9]

VIII.a.2. Before shipping a contaminated flexible endoscope or its accessories, the item must be packaged in impervious material in compliance with Department of Transportation shipping regulations.[14]

Flexible endoscopes and accessories returned to the manufacturer for repair are considered a biohazard and precautions must be taken to protect anyone who may come in contact with the device.[14]

VIII.a.3. Flexible endoscopes and accessories returned to the manufacturer for repair must be labeled with a biohazardous label visible during shipping.

Contaminated flexible endoscopes and accessories returned to the manufacturer for repair are considered a biohazard. The biohazard label will act as a warning of potentially infectious material for anyone who handles the package.[14]

Recommendation IX

Flexible endoscopes should be stored in a manner that protects the device from damage and minimizes microbial contamination.

IX.a. Flexible endoscopes should be stored
- in a closed cabinet with
  - venting that allows air circulation around the flexible endoscopes,
  - internal surfaces composed of cleanable materials,

- adequate height to allow flexible endoscopes to hang without touching the bottom of the cabinet, and
- sufficient space for storage of multiple endoscopes without touching;
- hanging in a secure vertical position;
- with all removable endoscope components (eg, valve mechanisms, biopsy valve covers, irrigation tubes) detached;
- with all accessories removed; and
- with scope protectors applied if the protector does not interfere with the flexible endoscope hanging straight or restrict the air movement around channel openings.[25-28]

When flexible endoscopes are hung in the vertical position, coiling or kinking is prevented, allowing any remaining moisture to drain out of the endoscope and decreasing the potential development of an environment conducive to microbial growth in the endoscope. Proper storage facilitates drying and decreases potential for contamination. Opening all valves and removing all accessories facilitates drying. The scope protector may create an environment favorable for microbial growth if the flexible endoscope is not dry and cannot hang straight.[28-30]

IX.a.1.   Flexible endoscopes should not be stored in the original shipment cases.

The cases are difficult to clean, may be contaminated, and are designed for shipping only.

IX.b.   Flexible endoscopes should be reprocessed before use if unused for more than five days.[25-27,31]

In research studies, flexible endoscopes cleaned and processed as recommended and stored by hanging in closed cabinets have been shown to grow organisms after five days of no use. In a prospective observational study, flexible endoscopes in active service during the three-week study period were microbiologically sampled prior to reprocessing before the first case of the day. The contamination rate was 15.5%, with a pathogenic contamination rate of 0.5%. Mean shelf life (ie, time between the last reprocessing one day and reprocessing before the first case on the following day) was 37.62 hours (SD 36.47). Median shelf life was 18.8 hours (range 5.27 to 165.35 hours). The most fre-

quently identified organism was coagulase-negative *Staphylococcus*, an environmental nonpathogenic organism.[31]

One study evaluated the contamination of high-level disinfection of upper endoscopes, duodenoscopes, and colonoscopes endoscopes stored in a dust-proof cabinet for five days. After completion of the endoscopic procedure, the endoscopes were subjected to an initial decontamination, followed by manual cleaning with the endoscope immersed in detergent. The endoscopes then were placed in an automatic reprocessor that provides high-level disinfection. They then were stored by hanging in a dust-proof cabinet. Bacteriologic samples were obtained from the surface of the endoscopes, the openings for the piston valves, and the accessory channels daily for five days and by flush-through (combined with brushing) from the accessory channels after five days of storage. Samples were cultured for all types of aerobic and anaerobic bacteria, including bacterial spores, and for *Candida* species. For all assays, all endoscopes were bacteria-free immediately after high-level disinfection. Only four assays (of 135) were positive (for skin bacteria cultured from endoscope surfaces) during the subsequent five-day assessment. All flush-through samples were sterile. The study concluded that when endoscope reprocessing guidelines are strictly observed and endoscopes are stored in appropriate cabinets for up to five days, reprocessing before use may not be necessary.[25]

In a multiphase study, four endoscopic retrograde cholangiopancreatography (ERCP) scopes and three colonoscopes were evaluated. In phase 1, endoscopes were assayed after initial high-level disinfection and daily for a period of two weeks. In phase 2, this procedure was repeated to confirm phase 1 results. In phase 3, endoscopes were assayed after high-level disinfection and again following a seven-day storage period. In phase 1, 6 of 70 (8.6%) assays were positive. This involved two colonoscopes and two ERCP scopes out of the seven total scopes (57%) and was limited to the first five days of the study. No cultures were positive in phase 2. In phase 3, one endoscope had a positive culture.

Positive cultures grew only *Staphylococcus epidermidis,* a low-virulence skin organism.[27]

One study conducted in the clinical environment to determine shelf life for flexible colonoscopes, which were processed using peracetic acid, suggests that colonoscopes with all channels thoroughly reprocessed and dried may be stored for up to one week before needing to be reprocessed. This study was limited by the small sample size, completion at a single site with a single processing method, and artificial contamination of a single colonoscope without a control measure to measure the level of contamination following inoculation.[26]

IX.c.   Flexible endoscopes should be reprocessed before use if evidence of improper drying exists (eg, evidence of discoloration, wet spots, or stains, or soil in the storage cabinet) when the scope is removed from storage.[25-27,31]

Evidence of improper drying may include wet spots or stains on the bottom of the cabinet where the flexible endoscopes have been hanging. Improper drying creates an environment conducive to growth of microorganisms.[31]

IX.d.   Storage cabinets should be cleaned and disinfected with an Environmental Protection Agency (EPA)-registered disinfectant when visibly soiled and on a weekly or monthly schedule.[32]

Cleaning and disinfecting storage cabinets periodically will decrease dust and soil build up.[32]

Recommendation X

Flexible endoscope accessories (eg, water bottle, cap, water tubing, biopsy forceps, cytology brushes, cleaning brushes) should be decontaminated after use and inspected for damage.

Flexible endoscope accessories have been found to be a source of contamination.[30,33]

X.a.   Endoscopic accessories (eg, biopsy forceps, cytology brushes) that enter sterile tissue or the vascular system should be cleaned and sterilized between use as described in the AORN "Recommended practices for care and cleaning of surgical instruments and powered equipment" and the AORN "Recommended

practices for sterilization in the perioperative practice setting."[1]

These devices enter sterile tissue and, if contaminated, increase the risk of patient infection.[11]

X.b.1.   All surfaces of accessories should be brushed using brushes of the appropriate size and style.

Brushing all surfaces of accessories, some of which may be irregular, assists with removing all organic debris.[17]

X.b.2.   Insulated electrosurgical instruments should be handled as described in the AORN "Recommended practices for care and cleaning of surgical instruments and powered equipment" and the AORN "Recommended practices for electrosurgery."[1,34]

X.b.3.   Reusable cleaning brushes should be thoroughly cleaned using an ultrasonic cleaner, inspected for integrity, and sterilized or high-level disinfected after each use.[17]

Damaged reusable brushes can cause perforations in any flexible endoscope surface. Reusable brushes may be a cause for cross contamination. Ultrasonic cleaning of reusable endoscopic accessories removes soil and organic material from hard to clean places. Disposable cleaning brushes are available commercially and may be safer, more efficient, and more economic to use.[17]

Recommendation XI

Flexible endoscopes should be decontaminated in an area physically separated from locations where clean items are handled and patient care activities are performed.[35]

Physical separation of decontamination areas from areas where clean items are handled minimizes the risk of cross-contamination. Cross-contamination can result when soiled items are placed in close proximity to clean items or placed on surfaces upon which clean items are later placed. Aerosols created during cleaning can also cause cross-contamination.[7]

XI.a.   The decontamination area should be physically separated from clean patient care areas and include a door.[35] This area should contain, but not be limited to,

- sinks to manually clean flexible endoscopes,
- hand-washing facilities,[14]
- eyewash station,[36]
- automated equipment consistent with the types of flexible endoscopes to be decontaminated,
- adapters and accessories to connect the flexible endoscopes with cleaning equipment and utilities,
- leak testing equipment,
- low-pressure air,
- closed storage facilities, and
- proper ventilation.

The design of the decontamination area facilitates the safe and effective decontamination of flexible endoscopes and accessories. Appropriate equipment and utilities facilitate desired infection control practices. Keeping the door closed supports the functioning of the building ventilation system which is designed to vent potentially contaminated room air out of the building, minimizing contamination of adjacent areas.

Sinks are required to manually clean or remove gross bioburden from flexible endoscopes before high-level disinfection via manual or automatic endoscope reprocessor methods.

Hand washing facilities are required to decontaminate hands after removal of PPE.[14]

An eyewash station is required to flush eyes when cleaning and disinfecting chemicals are accidentally splashed into the health care worker's face.[37]

Automated cleaning and decontamination of flexible endoscopes and accessories provides a high level of cleaning that is difficult to consistently replicate using manual methods.

Compressed air is needed to dry lumens after cleaning.[7]

Closed storage facilities help to prevent contamination of stored supplies.[1]

Adequate ventilation is required to protect personnel from the high-level disinfecting fumes.[35]

XI.b. The decontamination area should be supplied at a minimum with

- enzymatic detergent,
- soft-bristle brushes,
- cleaning cloths,
- alcohol, and
- personal protective equipment (PPE).

Enzymatic cleaner is used for manual and automated cleaning of flexible endoscopes. Soft-bristle brushes, designed for flexible endoscope cleaning, can effectively clean scopes and accessories without damaging surfaces. Cleaning cloths are used for external surfaces. Alcohol is used to irrigate after the final rinse to assist with drying. When cleaning flexible endoscopes with water, it can be reasonably anticipated that there is a potential for exposure to chemicals and bloodborne pathogens.[14]

XI.c. Flexible endoscopes and accessories should not be decontaminated in scrub or hand sinks.

Cleaning soiled instruments in a scrub or hand sink can contaminate the sink and faucet, which also may be used for clean activities (eg, hand washing, surgical hand antisepsis).

Recommendation XII

Personnel handling contaminated endoscopic equipment must wear appropriate PPE.[14]

Personal protective equipment (PPE) helps to protect the employee from exposure to bloodborne pathogens and other potentially infectious materials.

XII.a. Personal protective equipment consistent with the anticipated exposure must be worn.[14,37] The appropriate PPE for these types of exposures include, but is not limited to,

- a fluid-resistant gown,
- disposable chemical resistant glove,
- a mask, and
- face protection.

Splashes, splatters, and skin contact can be reasonably anticipated when handling contaminated flexible endoscopes. Glutaraldehyde may be absorbed through neoprene and PVC gloves; use gloves made of butyl rubber, nitrile, and Viton®. Latex surgical exam or polyethylene gloves may be used for short-term, or incidental contact only.[8,38]

XII.a.1. Hands must be washed after removing PPE.[14]

Perforations can occur in gloves, and hands can become contaminated when removing PPE.[14]

XII.a.2. Reusable protective attire must be decontaminated and the integrity of the attire confirmed between uses.[14]

Reusable gloves, gowns, aprons, and face shields become contaminated and their integrity can be compromised during use. Decontamination and confirmation of integrity helps to protect the wearer from exposure.[37]

Recommendation XIII

Personnel should demonstrate competency in the use, care, and processing of flexible endoscopes and related equipment periodically and before new endoscopic equipment and/or accessories are introduced into the practice setting.[11]

Ongoing competency validation and education of personnel facilitates the development of knowledge, skills, and attitudes that affect patient and health care worker safety.

XIII.a. Personnel working with flexible endoscopes and accessories should demonstrate competency commensurate with their responsibilities, including but not limited to,
- cleaning/decontamination methods;
- preparation of flexible endoscopes and related accessories for sterilization/high-level disinfection;
- selection of cleaning agents and methods;
- proper use of cleaning agents, including an understanding of specific applications, appropriate dilution, and special precautions;
- decontamination of specialized flexible endoscopes and related accessories used within the practice setting;
- personal protection required during instrument processing;
- exposure risk associated with chemical cleaning agents; and
- location of material safety data sheets.[11,37]
Workers have the right to know the hazards that exist in the workplace.[37] An understanding of procedures involved in cleaning each type of flexible endoscope is necessary to provide the foundation for compliance with procedures. Failure to follow decontamination practices has been shown to be the leading cause of flexible endoscope contamination.[10] Knowing the location of the material safety data sheets assists in obtaining information in the event of an emergency.

XIII.a.1. Education programs should be specific to the type and design of flexible endoscopes used and the procedures performed in the facility.[11]

XIII.a.2. Orientation and ongoing education activities for personnel should include an introduction to and/or review of policies and procedures to be applied in the practice setting.

XIII.b. Personnel should receive education before new flexible endoscopes, accessories, cleaning agents, cleaning methods, and procedures are introduced.

XIII.c. Designated administrative personnel should validate the competencies of personnel participating in decontamination of flexible endoscopes and accessories. The validation of competencies should include all types of flexible endoscopes and accessories the individual is authorized to reprocess.

Validation of competencies provides an indication that personnel are able to appropriately perform inspection, decontamination, cleaning, and sterilization or high-level disinfection procedures.

Recommendation XIV

Cleaning and processing of flexible endoscopes, accessories, and related equipment should be documented to enable the identification of trends and demonstrate compliance with regulatory and accrediting agency requirements.

Documentation provides a source of data to review processes and evaluate corrective actions.

XIV.a. Records of flexible endoscope cleaning and processing should include, but not be limited to,
- date,
- time,
- flexible endoscope identification,
- method of cleaning,

- number or identifier of automatic endoscope reprocessor,
- name of person performing the cleaning,
- dilution testing results on high-level disinfectants if used multiple times,
- routine and unscheduled maintenance or repairs, and
- disposition of defective equipment.

Most high-level disinfection and sterilization failures result from inadequate cleaning. Some automatic endoscope reprocessors have digital readouts or printers that facilitate recordkeeping. Records of testing of the dilution of the high-level disinfectant provide a source of evidence for review when investigating clinical issues.[7]

XIV.b. High-level disinfection and sterilization records should be maintained for a time period specified by the health care organization and in compliance with local, state, and federal regulations.

Recommendation XV

Policies and procedures for cleaning and processing flexible endoscopes, accessories, and related equipment should be developed, reviewed regularly, revised as necessary, and readily available in the practice setting.

Policies and procedures serve as operational guidelines to develop/reinforce knowledge, skills, and attitudes and establish authority, responsibility, and accountability within the organization. Policies and procedures also assist in the development of patient safety guidelines and quality assessment and improvement activities.

XV.a. Policies and procedures should establish authority, responsibility, and accountability for flexible endoscope care, cleaning, and processing; should be developed by a multidisciplinary team; and should be based on current literature and manufacturer's written instructions.

Multidisciplinary team participation in policy and procedure development and review provides varied input and improves compliance. Involving surgeons, infection preventionists, and health care workers in review of policies educates them on the requirements of flexible endoscope reprocessing and facilitates safe patient care.

XV.b. Policies should include, but not be limited to,
- review of manufacturers' written instructions before purchase,
- cleaning of flexible endoscopes and accessories before initial use,
- precautions to be taken when handling contaminated items,
- precautions to be taken when handling chemical agents,
- frequency and method of evaluation of mechanical washers,
- frequency and method of evaluation of manual cleaning,
- frequency of checking insulated electrosurgery instruments for leakage current,
- documentation of cleaning,
- initial education and annual competency,
- maintenance of material safety data sheets,
- reporting exposures to bloodborne pathogens, and
- reporting adverse events.

XV.c. A procedure should be developed in the event of a potential disinfection or sterilization failure and should include, but not be limited to,
- assessment to confirm failure;
- assessment of patient risk;
- removal of all improperly disinfected equipment;
- removal of defective cleaning equipment from use;
- notification of departments and physicians involved;
- root cause analysis;
- corrective action plan;
- identification of potentially involved patients;
- determination if patients require notification;
- identification of regulatory, accrediting, and governing agencies requiring notification;
- notification of all medical device manufacturers potentially related to the disinfection or sterilization failure, and
- development of an action plan for disinfection/sterilization failure prevention.[11]

A procedure provides an outline of the steps to follow after a potential disinfection or sterilization failure has occurred.

Recommendation XVI

The health care organization's quality management program should evaluate the cleaning and processing of flexible endoscopes and accessories.

Evaluation of cleaning and processing of flexible endoscopes and accessories improves patient safety.

XVI.a. A quality management program should be in place to test mechanical and manual cleaning processes when new types of flexible endoscopes and accessories are purchased and at intervals determined by the health care organization.[39]

Testing of mechanical cleaners assures proper functioning to the equipment because malfunctioning automatic endoscope reprocessors have been shown to cause contamination of flexible endoscopes.[10] Periodic testing of cleaning methods provides an opportunity to evaluate the performance of personnel and equipment. Manual cleaning is a learned skill and subject to human error.[23,39] New instruments can pose unique challenges when cleaning.

XVI.a.1. Automatic endoscope reprocessors should be tested for proper functioning before initial use, annually during service, and after major repair.[40]

Testing automatic endoscope reprocessors on a regular basis verifies that the equipment is functioning properly or identifies an opportunity for corrective action. Washer testing products (eg, protein indicators) are commercially available to assist with this evaluation.[39]

XVI.a.2. Adverse events and near misses related to flexible endoscope and accessory cleaning should be reported in the health care organization's adverse event reporting system and reviewed for potential opportunities for improvement.

Reporting mechanisms assist in the discovery of opportunities for improvement and prevention of repeat adverse events.

XVI.b. Water quality should be tested periodically for bacterial contamination and purity (eg, hardness, mineral content, pH).[4]

Contaminated water has been shown to cause contamination of flexible endoscopes after the decontamination process has been completed.[4,10]

XVI.c. Perioperative nurses should collaborate with infection preventionists to monitor and validate flexible endoscope cleaning, disinfection, and storage processes.

XVI.d. A program should be developed to monitor appropriate storage conditions, including but not limited to,
- length of storage time, and
- lack of evidence of the presence of moisture in or on the flexible endoscope after hanging.

Improper storage conditions may cause bacterial growth.

XVI.d.1. The length of storage time after high-level disinfection and before next use should be measured and monitored using a system to determine the date for removal of the flexible endoscope from use for reprocessing (eg, expiration date label on endoscope, log of serial numbers and the date of processing).

Recording the date the flexible endoscope was last processed will reduce the risk of a flexible endoscope being used more than five days after processing.

Glossary

Automated endoscope reprocessor: A unit for mechanical cleaning, disinfecting, and rinsing of flexible endoscopes.

Bioburden: The degree of microbial load; the number of viable organisms contaminating an object.

Biofilms: "A thin coating containing biologically active organisms, that have the ability to grow in water, water solutions, or in vivo, which coat the surface of structures (eg, teeth, inner surfaces of catheters, tubes, implanted or indwelling devices, instruments, other medical devices). Biofilms contain viable and nonviable microorganisms that adhere to surfaces and become trapped within a matrix of organic matter (eg, proteins, glycoproteins, carbohydrates), which prevents antimicrobial agents from reaching the cells." *(Source: Favero MS, Bond WW. Chemical disinfection of medical and surgical materials. In: Disinfection, Sterilization, and Preservation. 5th ed. Block SS, ed. Philadelphia, PA: Lippincott Williams & Wilkins; 2001:910-911.)*

Chemical disinfectant/germicide: A generic term for a government-registered agent that destroys microorganisms. Germicides are classified as sporicides, general disinfectants, sanitizers, and others.

Cleaning. A process using friction, detergent, and water to remove organic debris; the process by which any type of soil, including organic debris, is removed. Cleaning removes rather than kills microorganisms.

Contaminated: The presence of potentially infectious, pathogenic organisms (eg, blood, other potentially infectious material) on or in animate or inanimate objects.

Critical item: An item that has contact with the vascular system or enters sterile tissue, or body cavities and thus poses the highest risk of transmission of infection.

Decontamination: A process that removes contaminating infectious agents and renders reusable medical products safe for handling.

Disinfection: A process that kills most forms of microorganisms on inanimate surfaces. Disinfection destroys pathogenic organisms (excluding bacterial spores) or their toxins or vectors by direct exposure to chemical or physical means.

Electrosurgical accessories: Electrosurgical accessories are defined as the active electrode with tip(s), dispersive electrode, adapters, and connectors to attach these devices to the generator.

Enzymatic cleaner: A cleaner that uses enzymes to remove protein from surgical instruments.

High-level disinfection: A process that kills all microorganisms with the exception of high numbers of bacterial spores and prions. High-level disinfectants have the capability to inactivate the hepatitis B and C viruses, HIV, and *Mycobacterium tuberculosis,* but do not inactivate the virus-like prion that causes Creutzfeld-Jakob disease. Government-registered high-level disinfection agents kill vegetative bacteria, tubercle bacilli, some spores and fungi, and lipid and nonlipid viruses, given appropriate concentration, submersion, and contact time.

Minimum effective concentration: The minimum concentration of a liquid chemical germicide that achieves the claimed microbicidal activity as determined by dose-response testing.

Personal protective equipment (PPE): Specialized equipment or clothing for eyes, face, head, body, and extremities; protective clothing; respiratory devices; and protective shields and barriers designed to protect the worker from injury or exposure to a patient's blood, tissue, or body fluids. Used by health care workers and others whenever necessary to protect themselves from the hazards of processes or environments, chemical hazards, or mechanical irritants encountered in a manner capable of causing injury or impairment in the function of any part of the body through absorption, inhalation, or physical contact.

Potable water: Water that is of sufficient quality to be considered appropriate for drinking.

Semicritical item: An item that comes in contact with mucous membranes or with skin that is not intact.

Sterile: The absence of all living microorganisms.

Sterilization: Processes by which all microbial life, including pathogenic and nonpathogenic microorganisms, and spores, are killed.

Tap water: High-quality potable water that meets federal clean water standards at the point of use.

REFERENCES:

1. Recommended practices for cleaning and care of surgical instruments and powered equipment. In: *Perioperative Standards and Recommended Practices.* Denver, CO: AORN; 2008:421-446.

2. *ANSI/AAMI ST81:2004—Sterilization of Medical Devices: Information to Be Provided by the Manufacturer for the Processing of Resterilizable Medical Devices.* Arlington, VA: Association for the Advancement of Medical Instrumentation; 2004.

3. The Steris Reliance EPS endoscope processing system: A new automated endoscope reprocessing technology. *Health Devices* 2007;36(1):22.

4. *AAMI TIR34:2007—Water for the Reprocessing of Medical Devices.* Arlington, VA: Association for the Advancement of Medical Instrumentation; 2007.

5. Zuhlsdorf B, Emmrich M, Floss H, Martiny H. Cleaning efficacy of nine different cleaners in a washer-disinfector designed for flexible endoscopes. *J Hosp Infect* 2002;52(3):206.

6. Zuhlsdorf B, Winkler A, Dietze B, Floss H, Martiny H. Gastroscope processing in washer-disinfectors at three different temperatures. *J Hosp Infect* 2003;55(4):276.

7. Rutala WA, Weber DJ. Reprocessing endoscopes. United States perspective. In: Proceedings of the 7th International BODE Hygiene Days, May 2003. *J Hosp Infect* 2004 (April); 56 Supplement 2:S27-S39.

8. Recommended practices for high-level disinfection. In: *Perioperative Standards and Recommended Practices.* Denver, CO: AORN; 2008:303-310.

9. Thomas L A. Essentials for endoscopic equipment: Leak testing. *Gastroenterol Nurs* 2005;28(5):430.

10. Seoane-Vazquez E, Rodriguez-Monguio R, Visaria J, Carlson A. Endoscopy-related infections and toxic reactions: An international comparison. *Endoscopy* 2007;39(8):742.

11 Rutala WA, Weber DJ. How to assess risk of disease transmission to patients when there is a failure to follow recommended disinfection and sterilization guidelines. *Infect Control Hosp Epidemiol* 2007;28(2):146.

12. Martiny H, Floss H, Zuhlsdorf B. The importance of cleaning for the overall results of processing endoscopes. In: Proceedings of the 7th International BODE Hygiene Days, May 2003. *J Hosp Infect* 2004 (April); 56 Supplement 2:S16.

13. Standards of infection control in reprocessing of flexible gastrointestinal endoscopes. *Gastroenterol Nurs* 2006;29(2):142.

14. *Bloodborne Pathogens.* (29 CFR §1910.1030.) Occupational Safety and Health Administration. *http://www.osha.gov/pls/oshaweb/owadisp.show_document?p_table=STANDARDS&p_id=10051.* Accessed December 15, 2008.

15. Thomas LA. Essentials for endoscopic equipment: Endoscope staging. *Gastroenterol Nurs* 2005;28(3):243.

16. Garces E. Endoscope repair prevention: It takes a team. *Healthc Purchasing News* 2006;30(11):50, 55.

17. Thomas L A. Essentials for endoscopic equipment: Manual cleaning. *Gastroenterol Nurs* 2005;28(6):512.

18. Recommended practices for sterilization in the perioperative practice setting. In: *Perioperative Standards and Recommended Practices.* Denver, CO: AORN; 2008:575.

19. Pang J, Perry P, Ross A, Forbes GM. Bacteria-free rinse water for endoscope disinfection. *Gastrointest Endosc* 2002;56(3):402.

20. *ANSI/AAMI ST58:2005—Chemical Sterilization and High-Level Disinfection in Health Care Facilities.* Arlington, VA: Association for the Advancement of Medical Instrumentation; 2005.

21. Thomas LA. Essentials for endoscopic equipment: Care of the specialty scope. *Gastroenterol Nurs* 2006;29(1):68.

22. Nelson DB, Jarvis WR, Rutala WA, et al; Society for Healthcare Epidemiology of America. Multi-society guideline for reprocessing flexible gastrointestinal endoscopes. *Infect Control Hosp Epidemiol* 2003;24(7):532.

23. Alfa MJ, Olson N, Degagne P, Jackson M. A survey of reprocessing methods, residual viable bioburden, and soil levels in patient-ready endoscopic retrograde choliangiopancreatography duodenoscopes used in Canadian centers. *Infect Control Hosp Epidemiol* 2002;23(4):198.

24. Fisher C. The blame game: Don't play it. *Surg Technol* 2007;39(3):121.

25. Rejchrt S, Cermak P, Pavlatova L, McKova E, Bures J. Bacteriologic testing of endoscopes after high-level disinfection. *Gastrointest Endosc* 2004;60(1):76.

26. Riley R, Beanland C, Bos H. Establishing the shelf life of flexible colonoscopes. *Gastroenterol Nurs* 2002; 25(3):114.

27. Vergis AS, Thomson D, Pieroni P, Dhalla S. Reprocessing flexible gastrointestinal endoscopes after a period of disuse: Is it necessary? *Endoscopy* 2007; 39(8):737.

28. Thomas L A. Essentials for endoscopic equipment. Recommended care and handling of flexible endoscopes: Endoscope storage. *Gastroenterol Nurs* 2005; 28(1):45.

29. Goldstine S. Endoscopy storage: Preventing distal tip protector contamination. *Gastroenterol Nurs* 28(1), 45-46.

30. Bisset L, Cossart YE, Selby W, West R, Catterson D, O'Hara K, Vickery K. A prospective study of the efficacy of routine decontamination for gastrointestinal endoscopes and the risk factors for failure. *Am J Infect Control* 2006; 34(5):274.

31. Osborne S, Reynolds S, George N, Lindemayer F, Gill A, Chalmers M. Challenging endoscopy reprocessing guidelines: a prospective study investigating the safe shelf life of flexible endoscopes in a tertiary gastroenterology unit. *Endoscopy* 2007; 39(9):825.

32. Recommended practices for environmental cleaning in the perioperative setting. In: *Perioperative Standards and Recommended Practices.* Denver, CO: AORN; 2008:375-382.

33. Reprocessing of endoscopic accessories and valves. *Gastroenterol Nurs* 2006; 29(5):394.

34. Recommended practices for electrosurgery. In: *Perioperative Standards and Recommended Practices.* Denver, CO: AORN; 2008:315-330.

35. AIA Health Facilities Guidelines Institute. *Guidelines for Design and Construction of Health Care Facilities.* Washington, DC: American Institute of Architects; 2006.

36. *OSH Act of 1970.* Public Law 91-596 84; STAT. 1590; 91st Congress, S.2193 (December 29, 1970). *http://www.osha.gov/pls/oshaweb/owadisp.show_document?p_id=2743&p_table=OSHACT.* Accessed December 15, 2008.

37. *Hazard Communication.* (29 CFR §1910.) Occupational Safety and Health Administration. Washington, DC: US Government Printing Office; 2007. Available at *http://www.osha.gov/SLTC/hazardcommunications/standards.html.* Accessed December 5, 2008.

38. Hospital eTool: Healthcare wide hazards module—Glutaraldehyde. Occupational Safety and Health Administration. *http://www.osha.gov/SLTC/etools/hospital/hazards/glutaraldehyde/glut.html.* Accessed December 5, 2008.

39. *ANSI/AAMI ST79:2006—Comprehensive Guide to Steam Sterilization and Sterility Assurance in Health Care Facilities.* Arlington, VA: Association for the Advancement of Medical Instrumentation; 2008.

40. Gillespie EE, Kotsanas D, Stuart RL. Microbiological monitoring of endoscopes: 5-year review. *J Gastroenterol Hepatol* 2008 (July); 23(7 Pt 1):1069-1074.

Acknowledgments

LEAD AUTHORS
Byron Burlingame, RN, BSN, MS, CNOR
Perioperative Nursing Specialist
AORN Center for Nursing Practice
Denver, Colorado

Maria Arcilla, RN, BSN, CNOR
Perioperative Coordinator
Texas Children's Hospital
Houston, Texas

CONTRIBUTING AUTHOR
Carla McDermott, RN, CNOR
Educator, Staff Development
South Florida Baptist Hospital
Plant City, Florida

PUBLICATION HISTORY
Originally published February 1993, *AORN Journal.* Revised November 1997; published January 1998. Reformatted July 2000.

Revised November 2002; published in *Standards, Recommended Practices, and Guidelines,* 2003 edition. Reprinted February 2003, *AORN Journal.*

Revised November 2008; published in *Perioperative Standards and Recommended Practices,* 2009 edition.

Recommended Practices for Cleaning and Care of Surgical Instruments and Powered Equipment

The following recommended practices for the cleaning and care of surgical instruments and powered equipment were developed by the AORN Recommended Practices Committee and have been approved by the AORN Board of Directors. They were presented as proposed recommendations for comments by members and others. They are effective January 1, 2008.

These recommended practices are intended as achievable recommendations representing what is believed to be an optimal level of practice. Policies and procedures will reflect variations in practice settings and/or clinical situations that determine the degree to which the recommended practices can be implemented.

AORN recognizes the various settings in which perioperative nurses practice. These recommended practices are intended as guidelines adaptable to various practice settings. These practice settings include traditional operating rooms, ambulatory surgery centers, physicians' offices, cardiac catheterization laboratories, endoscopy suites, radiology departments, and all other areas where surgery may be performed.

References to nursing interventions (I) used in the Perioperative Nursing Data Set, second edition, (PNDS) are noted in parentheses when a recommended practice corresponds to a PNDS intervention.[1] The reader is referred to the PNDS for further explanation of nursing diagnoses, interventions, and outcomes.

Purpose

These recommended practices provide guidelines to assist perioperative nurses in decontaminating and preparing surgical instruments and powered equipment for terminal sterilization and disinfection. These recommended practices are general recommendations, as it is impossible to make a separate recommendation for every instrument used. These recommended practices complement AORN's "Recommended practices for sterilization in perioperative practice settings"[2] and "Recommended practices for high-level disinfection in perioperative practice settings."[3]

Perioperative nurses should consult these documents to assist them in providing a safe environment for the patient. Perioperative nurses are advised to review the Association for the Advancement of Medical Instrumentation (AAMI)

standards for additional practice details. Information about flexible endoscope cleaning can be found in the AORN "Recommended practices for cleaning and processing endoscopes and endoscopic accessories."[4]

Recommendation I

The manufacturer's written, validated instructions for handling and reprocessing should be obtained and evaluated to determine the ability to adequately clean and reprocess the equipment within the health care facility before purchasing surgical instruments and powered equipment. (PNDS: I122)

Cleaning and handling instructions recommended by the device manufacturer vary widely. Specific types of equipment, pneumatically powered instruments, and specialty instruments can require special cleaning and maintenance procedures.[5]

I.a. The manufacturer's written instructions should be used to determine how to replicate the validated cleaning and processing methods.[6] (PNDS: I122)

I.a.1. The manufacturer's written instructions should identify requirements related to
- utilities (eg, type of water, compressed air);
- cleaning equipment;
- accessories (eg, adaptors) for creating a proper connection between the instruments and equipment, utilities, and cleaning equipment;
- accessories for cleaning lumens, ports, and internal parts;
- cleaning agents;[6]
- lubricants; and
- processing methods.

I.b. The accessories necessary to reprocess the instrument according to the manufacturer's validated instructions should be obtained at the time of purchase. (PNDS: I122)

Using the proper accessories that fit the instruments and equipment and that were used during testing provides the best opportunity to replicate validated cleaning methods.

Recommendation II

New, repaired, and refurbished instruments should be examined, cleaned, and sterilized according to manufacturers' written instructions before use in a health care organization.

II.a. When new, repaired, or refurbished instruments are received into a facility all moving parts, tips, box locks, ratchets, screws, and cutting edges should be examined for defects and to ensure proper working order. (PNDS: I98, I138)

Inspecting the instrument verifies that the instrument has no obvious defects and has not sustained damage during shipping.

II.b. When indicated, new instruments should be pretreated according to the instrument manufacturer's written instructions. (PNDS: I122)

Some manufacturers recommend a series of treatments in a steam sterilizer to harden the coating on the instruments before initial cleaning. When this is indicated, details are provided in the manufacturer's written instructions.

II.c. New, repaired, or refurbished instruments should be decontaminated according to the manufacturer's written instruction before use. (PNDS: I70, I122, I138)

Decontamination of newly acquired or repaired instruments removes any soil related to manufacturing, repair, refurbishing, or shipping.

Recommendation III

Borrowed or consigned (ie, loaner) instruments should be examined, cleaned, and sterilized by the receiving health care organization before use, according to manufacturers' written instructions. (PNDS: I38, I70, I85, I98, I122)

Parameters of in-house sterilization can be verified. If an instrument has been sterilized by another health care organization, the user will have no record of the sterilization process in the event of a recall. There is a high probability of an event occurring during transport that could compromise sterility.

III.a. Before receiving loaner instruments, the instrument manufacturer's instructions for handling and reprocessing should be obtained and evaluated to determine the ability to adequately clean and reprocess the equipment. (PNDS: I122, I138)

When instructions are received in advance, proper conditions can be created for cleaning and sterilization before the arrival of the instruments. This can prevent a potential delay in the scheduled case and help ensure adequate sterilization. Requests that cleaning instructions arrive before receiving the instrument tray improves the efficiency of reprocessing.[7]

III.b. The accessories necessary to reprocess loaner instruments according to the manufacturer's validated instructions should be received at the same time as the instruments. (PNDS: I85, I122, I138)

The best opportunity to replicate valid cleaning methods is to use the proper accessories that fit the instruments and equipment and that have been used during testing.

III.c. When a loaner instrument is received, all moving parts, tips, box locks, ratchets, screws, and cutting edges should be examined for defects and to ensure proper working order. (PNDS: I85, I128, I138)

Inspecting the instrument verifies the absence of obvious defects and damage during shipping.

III.d. Loaner instruments should be decontaminated and sterilized in the borrowing facility according to the manufacturer's written instructions before use. (PNDS: I70, I98, I122)

Instruments consigned or borrowed from other facilities may not have been adequately decontaminated. Conditions during storage and transport are not known. The quality of any previous processing has not been verified, and sterile storage conditions have not been maintained during transport.[7]

III.e. Loaner instruments should be requested when the surgery is scheduled and delivered to the health care organization with sufficient time available before the surgical procedure to allow inspection and inventory of the instruments and to perform reprocessing in the same manner as a facility-owned instrument. (PNDS: I85)

Managing loaner instruments requires planning. Requesting the instruments when the surgery is scheduled allows the vendor to deliver the instruments far enough in advance for proper cleaning, decontamination, inspection, and sterilization to occur. Vendor collaboration is more likely when delivery and other expectations are communicated in advance.

III.f.   Loaner instruments should be logged in and inventoried within the receiving facility before use.

Keeping logs and inventory lists of instruments helps to provide verification that the instrument set is complete and available for the intended surgical procedure upon their arrival. Requesting that an inventory list accompany the instrument tray improves the efficiency of reprocessing.[7] Digital images may be used for documentation.

III.g.   Loaner instruments should be disassembled and decontaminated after use. (PNDS: I98)

III.g.1.   Loaner instruments should be inventoried and documentation created regarding the disposition of the items after completion of decontamination.

Recommendation IV

Instruments should be kept free of gross soil during surgical procedures. (PNDS: I70, I98)

Blood and body fluids can cause pitting of instruments and, if left to dry, can be difficult to remove. If blood and body fluids are not removed, they can prevent adequate sterilization, which could be an avenue for transmission of other potentially infectious materials.

IV.a.   Instruments should be wiped as needed with sterile surgical sponges moistened with sterile water during the procedure to remove gross soil. (PNDS: I70, I98)

Blood and body fluids, as well as saline, are highly corrosive. Corrosion, rusting, and pitting occur when saline, blood, and debris are allowed to dry in or on surgical instruments. Dried blood and debris can be difficult, if not impossible, to remove from all surfaces during the decontamination process; therefore, subsequent disinfection or sterilization may not be achieved.

IV.b.   Instruments with lumens should be irrigated with sterile water as needed throughout the surgical procedure. (PNDS: I70, I98)

Cannulated instruments or instruments with lumens can become obstructed with organic material. Irrigating these instruments with sterile water helps remove residue. Instruments should be rinsed with water because of the corrosive nature of saline.

IV.c.   Electrosurgical unit (ESU) active electrode tips should be cleaned frequently, away from the surgical site, to remove eschar. (PNDS: I72)

Eschar on the ESU electrode tip impedes the current flow, causing the equipment to work less efficiently. Eschar also serves as a fuel source that can lead to surgical fires.[8] Debris on the tip can cause tissues to tear and lead to bleeding.[9]

Recommendation V

Cleaning and decontamination should occur as soon as possible after instruments and equipment are used. (PNDS: I70, I98)

Cleaning and decontamination should occur as soon as possible after instruments and equipment are used to prevent the formation of biofilm. Cleaning and decontamination must be thoroughly accomplished or disinfection and sterilization may not be effective.

V.a.   Preparation for decontamination of instruments should begin at the point of use. (PNDS: I70, I98)

Removing gross soil and moistening soil at the point of use improves the efficiency and effectiveness of decontamination.

V.b.   All instruments opened in the operating or procedure room should be decontaminated whether or not they have been used. (PNDS: I70, I98)

All instruments opened during a surgical procedure are considered contaminated. Scrubbed persons may touch instruments without being aware of it. Used instruments also may come in contact with other instruments.

V.c.   Sharp instruments should be segregated from other instruments.

Segregation of sharp instruments minimizes the risk of injury to personnel handling the instruments during decontamination. The Occupational Safety and Health Administration (OSHA) prohibits processes that require employees to place their hands into basins of sharp instruments submerged in water because of the risk of a percutaneous exposure to bloodborne pathogens.[10]

V.c.1. Disposable sharps (eg, scalpel blades, suture needles) should be removed and discarded into the proper receptacles.

V.c.2. Reusable sharp instruments, including scissors, should be placed in a separate receptacle.

V.c.3. Reusable scalpel handles should be considered sharp and placed in a receptacle designated for sharp instruments.

Considering a reusable scalpel handle to be sharp minimizes the risk of injury if a blade has been left on the handle.

V.c.4. Reusable sharps must be placed in a puncture-proof container for transport.[10]

V.d. When instruments are composed of more than one piece, they should be opened, disassembled, and arranged in an orderly fashion within the original set configuration. (PNDS: I70, I98)

Disassembling and opening of instruments followed by their placement into original set configuration minimizes the risk of instrument displacement and improves the efficiency of reprocessing.

V.d.1. Instruments should be placed in a perforated or mesh-bottom instrument tray before mechanical decontamination.

Using perforated trays allows all surfaces to be exposed when processed in an automated cleaner.

V.d.2. Instrument box locks should be fully open and the instrument secured to prevent closing by using stringers, racks, or instrument pegs designed to contain instruments.

V.e. Delicate instruments should be protected from damage.

Instruments may shift during transport. The weight of heavy instruments can easily damage delicate instruments, unless preventive measures are taken.

V.e.1. Lightweight instruments should be placed on top of heavier instruments or segregated into separate containers.

V.e.2. Microsurgical instruments should be segregated into separate containers.

V.e.3. Heavy instruments should be placed on the bottom of storage containers or in a separate tray.

V.f. Instruments should be treated with an instrument cleaner according to the instrument or device manufacturer's recommendation before transport. (PNDS: I70, I98)

When decontamination will not occur immediately, or the decontamination area is remote from the surgical suite, treating instruments with an instrument cleaner at the point of use can facilitate the efficiency and effectiveness of cleaning. Corrosion, rusting, and pitting occur when blood and debris are allowed to dry in or on surgical instruments. Cannulas or lumens can become obstructed with organic material.

V.f.1. If items are soaked in water or an instrument cleaning solution at the point of use, the liquid should be contained or discarded before transport.

Disposal of cleaning solution before transport of instruments minimizes the risk of a spill and limits the weight of the container, which makes transportation easier and less likely to result in injury to personnel. When disposal at the point of use is not feasible, containing the solution will prevent spills and subsequent exposures.

V.f.2. A towel soaked with water, not saline, may be used to cover instruments to keep them moist.

Recommendation VI

Contaminated instruments must be contained during transport and should be transported in a timely manner to a location designed for decontamination.[10]

Proper containment of instruments decreases the potential for injury to personnel or their exposure to infectious organisms and prevents damage to the instruments during transport.

VI.a. During transport to a decontamination area, soiled instruments must be contained in a manner to prevent exposure of patients or personnel to bloodborne pathogens and other potentially infectious organisms.[10] (PNDS: I98)

The OSHA requires that contaminated instruments be contained in a leak-proof container to minimize the risk of exposing personnel to contaminants during transport.[10]

VI.a.1. Hand-carried items must be contained (eg, enclosed by a plastic bag, container with a lid).[10]

VI.a.2. Large quantities of items may be contained within a larger transport container (eg, transport cart with doors or plastic cover).

VI.a.3. Items placed on top of a transport cart must be contained (eg, plastic bag).[10]

VI.a.4. Items with sharp or pointed edges must be contained in a puncture-resistant container.[10]

VI.a.5. Liquids must be contained in a spill-proof container.[10]

VI.a.6. Transport carts should be designed to prevent items from falling over or off the cart during transport to the decontamination area.

VI.b. The transport container must be labeled to indicate biohazardous contents.[10] The type of label may include, but is not limited to, magnetic signs, stickers, or plastic placards.

Labeling the transport container communicates to others that the items are potentially infectious. This labeling is required by OSHA.[10]

VI.c. Care should be taken to avoid contaminating the outside of the transport containment method. If the outside container has been contaminated, it must be either cleaned at the point of use or enclosed during transport.[10]

Contact with contaminated surfaces can transmit infectious agents during transport.

VI.d. Transport of soiled instruments should be separated from the delivery of clean and sterile supplies to the operating or procedure room.[11] (PNDS: I98)

Separation of soiled instruments from clean supplies minimizes the risk of cross-contamination.[11]

VI.e. Contaminated surgical instruments should be transported to the decontamination area as soon as possible after completion of the surgical procedure.

Removal of organic material from instruments becomes more difficult after the debris has dried. Blood and body fluids that have dried on the instruments are hard to remove, can cause continuing surface corrosion damage (ie, pitting) over time, and can inhibit sterilization.

Recommendation VII

Instruments should be decontaminated in an area separated from locations where clean activities are performed.[12] (PNDS: I70, I98)

Physical separation of decontamination areas from areas where clean items are handled minimizes the risk of cross-contamination. Cross-contamination can result when soiled items are placed in close proximity to clean items or placed on surfaces upon which clean items are later placed. Aerosols created during cleaning can also cause cross-contamination.

VII.a. Instruments should not be decontaminated in scrub or hand sinks. (PNDS: I98)

Cleaning soiled instruments in a scrub or hand sink can contaminate the sink and faucet, which also may be used for clean activities (eg, hand washing, surgical hand antisepsis).

VII.b. The decontamination area should be physically separate from clean areas and include a door.[12] This area should contain, but not be limited to, the following equipment:
- sinks to manually clean instruments,
- hand-washing facilities,[10]
- eye wash station,[13]
- automated equipment consistent with the types of instruments to be decontaminated,
- adaptors and accessories to connect instruments with cleaning equipment and utilities, and
- a compressed air supply. (PNDS: I70, I98)

The design of the decontamination area facilitates the appropriate decontamination of instruments. Having equipment and utilities in place facilitates desired infection control practices. Keeping the door closed exhausts aerosols out of the building, minimizing contamination of adjacent rooms.

Sinks are required to provide a place to manually clean or remove gross bioburden from instruments before using a washer decontaminator and are required for single instruments.

Hand-washing facilities are required by OSHA for use after removal of personal protective equipment (PPE).[10]

An eye wash station is required by OSHA when chemicals such as those used to clean instruments are used.[13]

Automated cleaning and decontamination of equipment is recommended because it provides a high level of cleaning that is difficult to consistently replicate using manual methods. Compressed air is needed to clear lumens after cleaning.

VII.c. The decontamination area heating, ventilation, and air conditioning (HVAC) system should be controlled and monitored according to local requirements. (PNDS: I98)

Proper HVAC controls facilitate desired infection control practices. Local requirements vary depending upon the location.

VII.c.1. At a minimum, the following HVAC settings should be maintained in the decontamination area:
- negative air pressure,[12]
- at least six air exchanges per hour,[12]
- temperature of 68° F to 73° F (20° to 23° C),[12] and
- 30% to 60% humidity.[5]

VII.c.2. Doors to the decontamination area should be kept closed, except when moving personnel and equipment.

Keeping the door closed exhausts aerosols out of the building, minimizing contamination of adjacent areas. Negative pressure within the decontamination room cannot be maintained, if the door is held open.

VII.d. The decontamination area should be stocked, at a minimum, with the following supplies:
- soft-bristle brushes,
- cleaning cloths,
- alcohol, and
- appropriate PPE.

Enzymatic cleaner is used for manual and automated cleaning of instruments. Soft-bristle brushes, designed for surgical instrument cleaning can effectively clean instruments without damaging surfaces. Cleaning cloths are used for external surfaces. Alcohol is used to render instruments safe to handle after cleaning, if not rendered safe by another means. When cleaning instruments with water, it can be reasonably anticipated that there will be some splatter or splash of potentially infectious material. In these situations OSHA requires that personnel wear skin and mucous membrane protection (ie, fluid-resistant or impervious gown, gloves, face protection).[10]

Recommendation VIII

The type of water available for cleaning should be consistent with the manufacturer's written instructions and intended use of the equipment and cleaning agent. (PNDS: I122)

Water quality is affected by conductivity; the presence of dissolved mineral solids, chlorides, and other impurities; and its acidity or alkalinity. Water quality also fluctuates over time. The optimum combination of chemicals used in a washer decontaminator is based on the hardness of the available water.

VIII.a. Potable water should be used for manual or mechanical (ie, automated) decontamination methods unless contraindicated by instrument manufacturers' instructions.[5]

VIII.b. Softened or deionized water should be used for the final rinse.

Softened or deionized water removes soil and detergent residues more efficiently. Water with a high chloride or chlorine content can damage surgical instruments and equipment. Water softeners remove the calcium and magnesium ions that cause spots on instruments. Deionizing water removes ionized salts and particles that could harm instruments.[5]

VIII.c. A water quality assessment should be performed periodically and after major maintenance to the water source.

Water quality varies seasonally and after water source maintenance. Periodic testing can indicate if the chemical combination used to condition the cleaning and decontamination water should be adjusted. Water quality checks determine the hardness of the water and if any impurities are present.

Impurities present in the water also can be a reflection of insufficient filtration. Repairs or modifications in the filtration system should be made based upon this testing.

Recommendation IX

Surgical instrument, medical device, and equipment manufacturers' validated instructions should be followed regarding the types of cleaning agents (eg, enzyme preparations, detergents) to be used for decontamination. (PNDS: I122)

Following manufacturers' instructions decreases the possibility of selecting cleaning agents that can be harmful to instruments (eg, abrasives can damage the protective surfaces of instruments, contribute to corrosion, impede sterilization). Use of inappropriate cleaning agents can result in damage to surgical instruments and equipment, and possibly limit their warranties.

IX.a. Manufacturers' written instructions and AORN's "Recommended practices for product selection in perioperative practice settings" should be followed for cleaning agent selection and proper use.[14] (PNDS: I122, I138)

IX.a.1. Neutral detergents with a pH of seven that are low-foaming and free-rinsing should be used for manual or mechanical cleaning of surgical instruments and equipment unless contraindicated by instrument or equipment manufacturers' instructions.

Neutral pH detergents work well when enzymatic solutions are used as a part of the cleaning regimen. Low-foaming detergents are more easily removed during rinsing and are generally recommended for use by mechanical washer manufacturers.

IX.b. Highly acidic or highly alkaline pH detergents should be handled carefully and used only if recommended by instrument or equipment manufacturers.

Highly acidic or highly alkaline detergents can cause injuries to the skin or mucous membranes. Careful handling minimizes the risk of exposure.

IX.c. Cleaning agent manufacturers' written instructions should be followed
– during dilution,
– when selecting water temperature, and
– during use. (PNDS: I75, I122)

IX.c.1. A titration unit may be used to efficiently dilute chemicals at a consistent ratio.

IX.d. Abrasive cleaning devices and agents (eg, metal scouring pads, metal brushes, cleaning agents containing chlorides, abrasive cleaners, scouring powders) should not be used.

Abrasive cleaning devices and agents can cause permanent damage to the instruments and equipment.

Recommendation X

All surgical instrument and medical device or equipment manufacturers' validated instructions should be followed regarding the types of cleaning methods (eg, manual, automated) to be used for decontamination. (PNDS: I70, I75, I98, I122)

Use of inappropriate cleaning methods could result in damage and can limit the warranty of the surgical instruments or equipment.

X.a. Before beginning the cleaning process, instruments received into the decontamination area should be rinsed with cold running water.

A rinse with cold running water will remove gross debris and help prevent coagulation of the blood present on instruments.[5]

X.b. When manually cleaning, instruments should be washed in a manner that provides proper decontamination.[5] (PNDS: I70, I98)

Although automated methods are preferred, some delicate instruments (eg, microsurgery, eye), powered equipment, and other instruments that cannot be submerged can require manual cleaning.

X.b.1. Manual cleaning should be accomplished by submerging the instrument in warm water with an appropriate detergent followed by complete submersion of the instrument in rinse solution to minimize aerosolization of contaminants.[5]

Aerosolization of contaminants, splashing of infectious material, and injury from sharp objects are possible when manual cleaning is performed under a stream of running tap water.

X.c. Mechanical cleaning of surgical instruments should be accomplished by ultrasonic cleaners, washer decontaminators/disinfectors, or washer sterilizers.[5]

Mechanical cleaning is preferred because it removes soil efficiently and provides consistent washing and rinsing parameters during the process. Mechanical equipment specifically designed to decontaminate (ie, clean, disinfect) special types of medical devices also is available.

X.c.1. Ultrasonic cleaners should be used according to the manufacturer's operating instructions.

Ultrasonic cleaners use a process called *cavitation* that facilitates removal of small particles and debris from instrument joints, crevices, and hard to reach places (eg, lumens).[5] Ultrasonic energy is passed through a water bath, creating bubbles that implode. This process of implosion creates a suction action that pulls debris away from instrument surfaces.[15]

X.c.2. Ultrasonic cleaners should be used only after gross soil has been removed.

X.c.3. Manufacturers' instructions should be followed regarding detergent selection for use in ultrasonic cleaning devices.

Low-foaming detergents are commonly used in ultrasonic cleaning devices.

X.c.4. Ultrasonic cleaning device manufacturers' written instructions should be followed regarding "degassing" the cleaning solution before processing instruments.

Degassing conditions the solution by removing some air to improve cavitation and soil removal.

X.c.5. Only instruments made of similar metals should be combined in the ultrasonic cleaner unless specified otherwise in the instrument manufacturer's written instructions.[15]

Placing only instruments made of similar metals in the ultrasonic cleaner will prevent instrument etching and pitting from occurring because of the transfer of ions from one instrument surface to another.

X.c.6. Some instruments should not be placed in an ultrasonic cleaner; these include
- chrome-plated instruments;
- power instruments;
- rubber, silicone, or plastic instruments; and
- endoscopic lenses.

The mechanical vibrations of the ultrasonic cleaner can cause chrome plating to flake.[15]

Power instruments can be damaged by fluid contacting internal parts. Rubber materials, plastics, and endoscopic lenses can be damaged by the vibration.[6]

X.c.7. Instruments with lumens should be fully submerged and filled with cleaning solution to remove air from within the channel.

The presence of air prevents the solution from contacting the inner lumen of instruments and affects the cavitation process.[5]

X.c.8. Instruments should be thoroughly rinsed after ultrasonic cleaning.[5]

X.c.9. A lid should be in place when the ultrasonic cleaner is in use.

The presence of the lid prevents aerosolization of contaminants.[5]

X.c.10. Cleaning solution should be checked between cycles and changed if visibly soiled.

The presence of gross soil in the water impedes the effectiveness of cavitation on the instruments surface.[5]

X.c.11. Ultrasonic cleaners should be emptied, cleaned, rinsed with sterile water, and the chamber wiped with alcohol or other disinfectant, as recommended by the equipment manufacturer, when visibly soiled and at least daily.

The fluid in the ultrasonic cleaner can harbor gram-negative bacteria. Growth of these bacteria results in the production of endotoxins, which are heat-resistant, can survive steam sterilization, and can have serious patient consequences. Endotoxins from contaminated eye instruments have been shown to cause toxic anterior segment syndrome (TASS), an acute inflammation of the anterior segment of the eye.[16] Alcohol disinfects the ultrasonic cleaner and prevents microbial growth.

X.c.12. Automated washer decontaminators or disinfectors and washer sterilizers should be used according to the manufacturer's written instructions.

Washer decontaminator cycles are intended to process instruments and equipment to a level that renders them safe to handle by persons who will inspect and prepare them for terminal sterilization. This type of decontamination equipment can use a single chamber for rinsing, cleaning, and drying or can use multiple chambers and is usually referred to as a *tunnel washer* (ie, one chamber for each phase of the cycle). These phases can include

- an initial cool-water rinse to remove protein debris,
- an enzymatic rinse,
- a detergent wash,
- an ultrasonic cleaning,
- a sustained hot-water rinse,
- a deionized water final rinse,
- a lubrication rinse,
- a liquid chemical germicide rinse, and
- a drying cycle.[15]

The sequencing and number of stages can vary among manufacturers.

Washer decontaminators or disinfectors can accomplish the microbicidal part of the process by thermal or chemical means, once the items have been thoroughly cleaned and rinsed.

The washer sterilizer first cleans instruments through several phases of a cycle that can include a cold water pre-rinse, a high-temperature wash with final rinse, and then sterilization. This process can be accomplished in a small or large chamber.

X.c.13. The instrument manufacturer's instructions should be used to determine the amount of time necessary to efficiently clean and rinse the instruments.

X.c.14. The operator should ensure that the proper cycle is being used.

Many mechanical washers have pre-programmed cycles, and the wash and rinse phases of the cycles are often adjustable. The manufacturer of the mechanical washer should be consulted to determine

- what level of decontamination is achieved with the washer decontaminator (ie, low-level, intermediate, high-level disinfection); and
- how the user can verify that a cycle was sufficient to render the processed items safe to handle.

Recommendation XI

Surgical instruments should be inspected for cleanliness and proper working order after decontamination. (PNDS: I70, I98, I138)

Inspecting instruments for sterilization before assembly of trays provides an opportunity to identify those instruments that require additional cleaning or repair before use.

XI.a. Instruments should be inspected for
- cleanliness;
- alignment;
- corrosion, pitting, burrs, nicks, and cracks;
- sharpness of cutting edges;
- loose set pins;
- wear and chipping of inserts and plated surfaces;
- missing parts;
- any other defects;
- removal of moisture; and
- proper functioning. (PNDS: I70, I98)

Instruments can become damaged during use or decontamination. Sterilization may not occur in the presence of soil or water.

XI.b. Instruments should be thoroughly dried. (PNDS: I70, I98)

Elimination of moisture helps prevent rust formation during instrument storage. The presence of moisture can impede the sterilization process.

Moisture on instrument surfaces alters the moisture content of steam and can pose a challenge for effective heating of the instrument.

Ethylene oxide (EO) combines with water and creates ethylene glycol (ie, antifreeze), which is toxic and is not removed during aeration.

Excess moisture inhibits the hydrogen peroxide plasma sterilization process and can result in an aborted cycle.[2]

XI.c. The instrument manufacturer's written instructions should be followed for selection and appropriate use of lubricants. (PNDS: I122)

Lubricants decrease friction between working surfaces. Some instruments do not require lubrication. Cleaning, particularly ultrasonic cleaning, removes lubricants from instruments.

XI.c.1. Instruments should be clean before lubricant is applied.

Applying lubricants to soiled instruments can compound the problem of stiff joints and inhibit smooth movement.

XI.c.2. Lubricants should be compatible with the method of sterilization to be used.

Water soluble lubricants allow steam penetration during sterilization; oil-based products, however, cannot be penetrated and prevent the sterilant from contacting the instrument's surface.

XI.d. Instruments in disrepair should be tagged or labeled and removed from service until repaired. (PNDS: I70, I77, I138)

Identification of defective instruments facilitates segregation of these instruments from those to be used when assembling sets and prevents defective instruments from being used on patients.

XI.e. Instruments to be sterilized should be packaged according to AORN's "Recommended practices for selection and use of packaging systems for sterilization."[17] (PNDS: I70, I98)

XI.f. The AORN "Recommended practices for sterilization in the perioperative practice setting"[2] should be referred to for recommendations regarding instrument sterilization. (PNDS: I70, I98)

Recommendation XII

Cleaned surgical instruments should be organized for packaging in a manner to allow the sterilant to contact all exposed surfaces. (PNDS: I70)

Proper organization will facilitate sterilant contact on all surfaces and adequate drying.

XII.a. Instruments should be placed in a container tray or basket that is large enough to evenly distribute the metal mass in a single layer. (PNDS: I70)

Instruments should be contained within the tray or basket in a manner that protects the instruments from damage and prevents puncturing of the sterilization wraps. Overloading trays can cause wet packs because an increase in metal mass in the tray results in more condensate, which requires additional drying at the end of the cycle.

XII.b. Broad-surfaced instruments and those with concave surfaces (eg, malleable retractors, hip skids) should be placed on edge. (PNDS: I70)

Instruments placed on edge facilitate drying because in this position, steam condensate will drain off the instrument rather than pool on it.

XII.c. Instruments with hinges should be opened and those with removable parts should be disassembled when placed in trays designed for sterilization, unless the manufacturer has provided validated instructions to the contrary. (PNDS: I70)

Sterilization occurs only on surfaces that have direct contact with the sterilant. Disassembly of multiple-part instruments and those with sliding parts (eg, retractors) enables the sterilant to contact all surfaces.

XII.c.1. Instruments should be kept in the open and unlocked position using instrument stringers, racks, or instrument pegs designed to contain instruments.

XII.d. Delicate and sharp instruments should be protected using a device such as a tip protector. The tip protector should be used according to the manufacturer's instructions. (PNDS: I70)

Damage to delicate and sharp instruments can render them ineffective.

XII.d.1. Tip protectors should be
- used for sharp or delicate instruments,
- validated for use with the chosen method of sterilization,
- used according to manufacturers' instructions, and
- loose-fitting so that the sterilant can contact the surface to be sterilized.

XII.d.2. Heavy instruments should be positioned on the bottom of trays.

Positioning heavy instruments on the bottom of trays helps prevent damage to delicate items that may be present.

XII.e. Only validated containment devices should be used to organize or segregate instruments within sets. (PNDS: I70)

Many devices used to organize or segregate instruments within sets have not been validated as safe and effective by container or wrap/pouch manufacturers. The presence of these devices inside of a packaged instrument set can prohibit
- air removal,
- sterilant contact with instruments in close proximity to the containment device,
- sterilant evacuation, and
- condensate drainage and drying.

XII.e.1. Rubber bands should not be used to keep several instruments together.

Sterilant cannot contact surfaces beneath rubber bands and instruments may not be sterilized.

XII.e.2. Paper-plastic peel pouches should not be used to organize or segregate instruments within sets unless their use is validated by the containment device manufacturer.

XII.e.3. Small accessory baskets or boxes with lids or covers to contain instruments, parts, or accessories should not be incorporated into sets unless their use is validated by the containment device manufacturer.

XII.e.4. Nonabsorbent, nonwoven disposable wrap material (eg, polyolefin spunbound) should not be used as a tray liner or to organize or segregate a small group of instruments to be placed into the instrument set.

This type of material is not intended for use within an instrument set that is to be steam-sterilized because it does not absorb moisture. Moisture can pool on this material, causing a wet pack.

XII.f. Suction lumens and other devices with similar channels should be flushed with distilled, demineralized, or sterile water before steam sterilization.[5] (PNDS: I70)

When the moisture within the lumen is heated it will produce steam, which moves air out of the lumen resulting in lumen sterilization. The steam in the compartment does not move into the lumen because the lumen acts as a diffusion restrictor. Tap water might contain pyrogens.

XII.g. Stylets should be removed from lumens.

Removal of stylets enables sterilant contact with the inside of lumens.

XII.h. The instrument tray or basket should be lined with an absorbent, lint-free surgical towel if indicated.

The towel will absorb and disperse moisture to assist in drying the set.[5]

XII.i. Nonabsorbent plastic or silicone fingered mats should be used according to the mat manufacturer's validated instructions for the various sterilization cycles in which they will be used. (PNDS: I122)

Improper use of nonabsorbent plastic or silicone mats may cause condensate to pool and inhibit drying.

XII.j. Information provided by the container manufacturer describing how instruments should be placed within the container or tray should be followed for each sterilization method used. (PNDS: I70, I122)

Recommendation XIII

Powered surgical instruments and all attachments should be decontaminated, lubricated, assembled, sterilized, and tested before use according to the manufacturer's written instructions. (PNDS: I122, I138)

Proper care and handling of powered surgical instruments minimizes the risk of injury to patients and personnel. Manufacturers' instructions are validated for specific instruments only and are not transferable to other devices because the design of powered surgical instruments and equipment varies.

XIII.a. Powered equipment and attachments should be cleaned and maintained according to manufacturers' written instructions. (PNDS: I70, I122)

Improper care and cleaning of powered equipment lead to patient and personnel exposure to pathogens and potential injury.

XIII.b. Attachments should be properly affixed to the units and tested before use. (PNDS: I77, I138)

Improperly seated attachments can be ejected from the equipment with great force and cause injury to patients and personnel. Testing the equipment or device before use can decrease the risk of injury.

XIII.b.1. Trigger handles should be placed in the safety position when changing attachments.

Accidental activation of powered equipment can cause injury.

XIII.c. Medical-grade compressed air or compressed dry nitrogen (ie, 99% pure) should be used to operate air-powered equipment according to the manufacturer's written instructions.

Use of contaminated gases to run powered equipment can result in equipment damage and injury to patients or personnel.

XIII.d. Manufacturers' written instructions should be used to determine the correct pressure settings required to operate equipment. The setting should be measured with the equipment operating. (PNDS: I77, I122)

Using excessive pressure can damage equipment and exert great stress on air hoses. Unless pressure is set with the equipment operating, incorrect pressures can result. Pneumatic equipment may not perform in the designated manner, if the pressure is set above or below recommended limits.

XIII.d.1. When an extension hose is used, the manufacturer should be consulted for appropriate pressure setting.

Pressure at the hand piece decreases when an extension hose is used.

XIII.e. Only grounded outlets should be used for electrical powered equipment.

XIII.f. Powered equipment should be cleaned and decontaminated thoroughly after use, following manufacturers' written, validated cleaning instructions. (PNDS: I98, I122)

Organic debris left on powered equipment hinders the sterilization process and can interfere with proper functioning. Powered instruments contain complex lumens, movable parts, and intricate internal components and may not be immersible in cleaning solutions. Permanent damage can result if fluid enters the internal mechanisms of powered equipment. Special attention is required to ensure that blood and contaminated tissue are adequately removed from the instrument before sterilization. Following manufacturers' instructions reduces the possibility of damaging or inadequately cleaning the instrument.

XIII.f.1. Blades and drill bits should be removed from powered equipment in the OR by the scrub person after the procedure has ended.

XIII.f.2. Instrument manufacturers' written recommendations for detergent or germicide use should be followed.

Abrasive detergents can damage protective surfaces, contribute to corrosion, and impede sterilization.

XIII.f.3. Powered equipment should not be immersed or placed under running water, in ultrasonic cleaners, washer disinfectors, or washer sterilizers, unless indicated in the equipment manufacturers' instructions.

XIII.f.4. When pneumatic hand pieces are cleaned, air hoses should be attached.

Attaching the air hose to the pneumatic hand piece during cleaning facilitates keeping the internal parts of the hand piece dry.

XIII.f.5. All traces of detergent or germicide and excess fluids should be wiped from the equipment and attachments.

XIII.f.6. The outer surfaces of the powered equipment and attachments should be dried with lint-free towels.

XIII.f.7. Powered equipment, batteries, attachments, and power cords should be inspected for damage or wear after decontamination and before use.

XIII.g. Air hoses should not be immersed or placed in ultrasonic cleaners, washer disinfectors, or washer sterilizers, unless indicated in the air hose manufacturer's instructions. (PNDS: I122)

Ultrasonic cleaners, washer sterilizers, and washer decontaminators force fluids into internal parts. Fluid in air hoses is not evacuated during these cycles, possibly leading to evacuation of this contaminated fluid during the surgical procedure.

XIII.g.1. Air hoses should be inspected for damage or wear before and after decontamination and before use.

XIII.g.2. Air hoses should be wiped with a clean, damp cloth using detergent or germicidal solution.

XIII.g.3. All traces of detergent or germicide and excess fluids should be wiped from the surface of the air hose.

XIII.h. Powered equipment and attachments should be lubricated with a product specifically recommended by the manufacturer and applied according to manufacturers' instructions. (PNDS: I122)

Lubricants decrease friction between working surfaces, which is essential for optimal functioning of the instrument and helps to prolong equipment life. Some instruments are sealed and do not require lubrication. Manufacturers may recommend oil-based or non-oil based lubricant for powered equipment.

XIII.i. Manufacturers' written instructions for packaging powered equipment and attachments should be followed. Packaging instructions should include methods to
– disassemble powered equipment before sterilization,
– protect delicate parts of the equipment, and
– loosely coil air hoses when packaged for sterilization. (PNDS: I70, I122)

Manufacturers' validated sterilization parameters should be followed for powered equipment, batteries, and attachments.

Recommendation XIV

Special precautions should be taken for reprocessing ophthalmic surgical instruments.[18] **(PNDS: I70, I98)**

Toxic anterior segment syndrome (TASS) can result from contaminants introduced into the eye during ophthalmic surgery.[16,19,20,21] An incidence of TASS can cause serious damage to a patient's intraocular tissue and result in vision loss.[16] More than 300 cases of TASS associated with balanced salt solution contaminated with endotoxins were reported to the US Food and Drug Administration (FDA), leading to the contaminated product being recalled by the FDA.[22] Other potential etiologies of TASS include
♦ antiseptics,[23,24]
♦ antibiotic ointment,[19]

♦ medications,[25] and
♦ powder from surgical gloves.[26,27]

Most cases of TASS appear to result from inadequate instrument cleaning and sterilization.[16] Other reported TASS cases were associated with gluteraldehyde and detergent residue on instruments,[28,29] endotoxins from gram-negative bacteria in ultrasonic cleaners,[30,31] impurities in steam from improperly maintained sterilizers,[20] and degradation of brass surgical instruments sterilized by hydrogen peroxide gas plasma.[32] Prevention of TASS requires thorough cleaning and rinsing of surgical instruments.[18]

XIV.a. Instruments should be wiped clean with sterile water and a lint-free sponge during the surgical procedure. (PNDS: I70, I75, I98)

Viscoelastic solution can harden on instruments within minutes.

XIV.b. Instruments should be immersed in sterile water immediately at the end of the procedure. (PNDS: I70, I98)

Biofilm adheres to the surfaces of instruments and is very difficult to remove. Keeping the organic material moist prevents the formation of biofilm.

XIV.c. Single-use cannulae should be used whenever possible. If reusable cannulae are used, the lumens should be flushed with sterile water immediately at the end of the procedure. (PNDS: I70, I75, I98)

Lumens are difficult to clean and can harbor contaminants.

XIV.d. Manufacturers' written instructions for cleaning each instrument should be reviewed and followed. (PNDS: I122)

The method of cleaning and the compatibilities of cleaning agents are unique to each instrument. Instructions for cannulated instruments indicate the type and volume of solution to be used for rinsing and cleaning, the frequency of flushing, and the number of times the cannula should be flushed.

XIV.e. The irrigation and aspiration ports of phacoemulsification handpieces, tips, and tubing should be flushed before disconnecting the handpiece from the unit. (PNDS: I70, I98)

Several centers have reported occluded tips as a potential cause of TASS.[16] Flushing the handpiece prevents build-up of material inside the handpiece, which is difficult to remove during cleaning.

XIV.f. Intraocular lens injectors/inserters should be carefully cleaned. (PNDS: I70, I98)

Residue in the injector can be inserted into the eye chamber and cause TASS.[16]

XIV.g. Single-use items must be used only once and discarded or reprocessed using validated methods in accordance with FDA regulations.[33]

XIV.h. Detergents and enzymatic detergents should be used and diluted according to cleaning agent manufacturers' written instructions. (PNDS: I70, I75, I122)

Some cleaning agent manufacturers' instructions require the use of deionized or distilled water for diluting the detergent.

XIV.i. Enzymatic detergents should be used only if recommended by the surgical instrument manufacturer. (PNDS: I75, I122)

Following instrument manufacturers' instructions assures compatibility of the detergent with the instrument.

XIV.j. After cleaning or decontamination, instruments should be thoroughly rinsed with distilled or deionized sterile water and dried. (PNDS: I70, I75)

Residual enzymes and detergents not rinsed from the instruments can cause TASS.[16,18]

XIV.k. After cleaning, lumens should be thoroughly flushed with sterile water (expelling the liquid into a drain not the rinse water) and dried with filtered, oil-free compressed air. (PNDS: I70, I75)

Sterile water removes detergent residue. Expelling the lumen rinse into a drain prevents recontamination of the instrument with lumen contents. Compressed air forced through the lumen eliminates moisture that can serve as a medium for microbial growth.

XIV.l. Syringes and brushes used to clean ophthalmic instruments and cleaning solutions should be discarded after each use (if designed for single use) or sterilized following all recommended precautions.

Cleaning tools can harbor contaminants that can be reintroduced during cleaning of the next instrument.

XIV.m. After manual or ultrasonic cleaning, instruments should be wiped with alcohol before preparation for sterilization.

Wiping with alcohol disinfects the instruments and renders them safe to handle.

XIV.n. After cleaning and disinfection, instruments contacting viscoelastic material should be inspected for residue under magnification.

Viscoelastic material is difficult to remove during cleaning, and inspection with magnification can enhance detection of residual material.

XIV.o. Records should be maintained of all cleaning methods, detergent solutions used, and lot numbers of cleaning solutions.

These records can be used to facilitate investigation of any suspected or confirmed cases of TASS.

XIV.p. An adequate inventory of instruments should be provided to allow for thorough instrument cleaning and sterilization.

An adequate inventory of instruments facilitates compliance with proper decontamination and sterilization processes.

XIV.q. Adequate time should be provided for thorough instrument cleaning and sterilization.

Time constraints may create a disincentive for personnel to adhere to decontamination procedures and may result in noncompliance.

Recommendation XV

Insulated electrosurgery instruments should be decontaminated after use according to manufacturers' validated, written instructions and inspected for damage. (PNDS: I70, I98, I122)

Breaks in the insulation of electrosurgery instruments can occur during use and handling. These insulation failures can result in current leakage and subsequent burns. Inspection of the instruments provides a screening mechanism to identify visible insulation breaks.[34] Additional information about electrosurgery can be found in AORN's "Recommended practices for electrosurgery."[9]

XV.a. Insulated electrosurgical instruments should be inspected for small breaks in the insulation before initial use. (PNDS: I72)

Breaks in insulation can occur during manufacturing and transportation.

XV.b. Insulated instruments should be handled in a manner to prevent sharp instruments from contacting the insulation, and they should be segregated from sharp objects during use, transport, and decontamination.

Sharp objects and rough handling can damage the insulation during use, transport, and decontamination.

XV.c. Electrosurgical instruments should be decontaminated according to manufacturers' written instructions using care to avoid damaging the insulation on the device. (PNDS: I72, I122) Abrasive cleaning may damage insulation.

XV.d. The insulation on electrosurgical instruments should be inspected for impairment using a magnifying lens after decontamination. (PNDS: I72)

Visual inspection identifies obvious breaks in insulation, but will not identify all insulation failures. Using a magnifying lens can assist with identifying small imperfections.[34]

XV.e. Technology should be used to conduct stray current leakage tests at the end of each decontamination cycle.

Current can leak through insulation, even when breaks are not clearly visible. Performing a visual inspection and performing any recommended technological evaluation before preparation for sterilization minimizes the risk of using defective instruments that could lead to patient injury. Detecting insulation failures well in advance of a surgical procedure provides time for equipment replacement.

XV.f. Equipment found to have insulation damage should be immediately removed from service and repaired or replaced.

Instruments with impaired insulation are unsafe for use.

XV.g. Manufacturers' written recommendations limiting the use of insulated instruments to a specific time frame or number of reprocessings should be followed. (PNDS: I122)

Manufacturers validate the life span of the equipment insulation, and use after that period of time can result in injury to the patient. If injury occurs in this situation, the health care organization may have to assume the liability.

Recommendation XVI

Special precautions should be taken when cleaning robotic instruments.(PNDS: I70)

Robotic instruments and equipment have lumens with complex, difficult to clean internal and external components that require special attention to adequately decontaminate the instruments.

XVI.a. Gross soil should be removed from the external surfaces using a soft-bristled brush. (PNDS: I70, I98)

Robotic "wrists" and electrosurgical tips can become soiled during use.

XVI.b. The ports of robotic instruments and equipment should be flushed
- with a water line,
in the sequence and for the duration identified by the manufacturer's written instructions,
- while moving the robotic wrist through a full range of motion, and
- until the fluid exiting the ports is clear.
Moving the robotic wrist through a full range of motion exposes all of its surfaces to the cleaning solution.

XVI.b.1. The fluid expelled from the ports during flushing should be directed into a drain and not allowed to run into the receptacle of clean solution.

XVI.c. Ports should be primed with clean enzymatic cleaner and the device cleaned in an ultrasonic cleaner according the manufacturer's written instructions. (PNDS: I70, I122)

Ultrasonic cleaning facilitates removal of debris that has adhered to components.

XVI.c.1. After ultrasonic cleaning, ports should be flushed
- with deionized water, under pressure; and
- in the sequence and for the duration identified by the manufacturer's written instructions.
Flushing of ports removes residual cleaning solution.

XVI.d. Ports should be cleared with compressed air in the sequence and duration identified by the manufacturer's written instructions. (PNDS: I70, I98, I122)

Clearing lumens and internal components with compressed air removes residual water that can serve as a medium for microbial growth.

XVI.e. Movable parts of the robotic instruments and equipment should be lubricated according to the manufacturer's written instructions. (PNDS: I122)

Lubrication facilitates the functioning of the hinges and joints of robotic instruments and equipment which coordinate fine dissection and manipulation of tissue.

XVI.f. The outside of the instruments should be wiped with alcohol or an instrument disinfectant, before preparation for steam sterilization. (PNDS: I70, I98)

Wiping with alcohol or another disinfectant renders the instrument safe to handle.

Recommendation XVII

Special precautions should be taken to minimize the risk of transmission of prion diseases. (PNDS: I98, I145)

Prions are a unique classification of infectious agents with a genetic component that are thought to be transmitted through direct inoculation, rather than the traditional routes (ie, bloodborne, skin contact, droplet, airborne). The resulting human prion diseases (ie, Creutzfeldt-Jakob disease [CJD], variant CJD, fatal familial insomnia, Gertsmann-Straussler syndrome) are fatal, degenerative neurological disorders.[35]

Prions have been transmitted experimentally through direct inoculation (eg, oral ingestion, inoculation of scratched skin, injection, implantation) and have been transmitted iatrogenically through transplanted contaminated tissue (eg, cornea, dura mater) and injections of human pituitary hormones (eg, growth hormone, gonadotropin).[36] Six cases of transmission via neurosurgical instruments occurred before 1980 in Europe.[36] No other cases have been reported resulting from transmission via instruments in other types of surgery or since that time.

Prions are resistant to chemical disinfection (eg, alcohol, gluteraldehyde) and routine sterilization (ie, steam, ethylene oxide, gas plasma, peracetic acid).[37] These agents remain infective for years, and special precautions are required to eliminate their infectivity.[38]

XVII.a. An interdisciplinary team should develop processes to minimize the risk of prion disease transmission. These processes should be based upon the probability or possibility of
- a patient having a prion disease,
- the level of infectivity of the tissue involved, and
- the characteristics of the surgical instruments involved. (PNDS: I98, I145)

Use of a defined protocol helps protect patients and health care workers from pathogen transmission. Including personnel with different types of expertise (eg, anesthesia providers, central sterilizing employees, housekeeping personnel, infection control team members, neurosurgeons, perioperative services personnel) in the protocol development maximizes the likelihood of developing effective strategies and enhances compliance with the procedures that are developed.

Diagnostic criteria for CJD have been developed by the World Health Organization (WHO). Diagnosis can be confirmed, but cannot be ruled out, by brain biopsy.[35] Prion diseases can be genetically acquired or acquired through contact with infectious material; however, all prion diseases are infectious regardless of mode of acquisition.

Patients at high risk of having or developing prion diseases include
- patients with rapidly progressive dementia consistent with CJD in whom a diagnosis has not been confirmed or ruled out;
- members of families in which prion disease has occurred (eg, two or more family members with a confirmed diagnosis); and
- recipients of cadaveric dura mater grafts or human pituitary gland hormones (eg, growth hormone, gonadotropin).

Cadaveric dura mater has been replaced with fascia grafts, and synthetic pituitary hormones have replaced those derived from human pituitary glands to reduce the risk of prion transmission.[36]

While all prion diseases are infectious, infectivity is based primarily on laboratory studies of different prion diseases in humans and animals.[36,39] Central nervous system tissue (eg, brain, spinal cord, dura mater, pituitary) has been shown to be highly infectious as has tissue from the posterior eye (eg, optic nerve, retina). Other tissues and fluids that have shown to have a lower level of infectivity include

- corneal tissue;
- lymphoid tissue, the spleen, thymus, appendix, tonsils, and lymph nodes;
- the kidneys, liver, lungs, and placenta;
- skeletal muscle;
- olfactory cilia and pathways;
- cerebral spinal fluid; and
- blood.

Other areas of the body demonstrate no infectivity, such as

- the heart muscle, intestine, peripheral nerves, prostate, testis, thyroid;
- adipose tissue, bone marrow, skin; and
- feces, milk, nasal mucus, saliva, semen, serous fluid, sweat, tears, urine, and vaginal secretions.

XVII.a.1. Considerations regarding instruments used on patients suspected of having prion disease should include, but not be limited to,
- the use of single-use versus reusable instruments if possible;
- the ability of the instrument to tolerate heat;
- the complexity of cleaning required (eg, lumens); and
- the intended use of the instrument (eg, in internal tissues).

XVII.b. Patients should be screened for the risk of prion disease and any information discovered should be conveyed to the OR during scheduling of the surgical procedure. (PNDS: I98, I145)

Screening patients provides a mechanism to identify which patients are at high risk of having a prion disease. Conveying this information during scheduling provides adequate time to plan instrument use and decontamination and to discuss alternatives to the use of complex instruments and implant sets requiring reprocessing.

XVII.c. When treating patients at high risk for a prion diseases, instruments used on highly infective tissue should be minimized, limited to those that are easily cleaned, and replaced with single-use devices, when possible. (PNDS: I98, I145)

Minimizing the number of instruments limits the number of items that need to be decontaminated and reduces the risk of an error that can result in exposure of subsequent patients or personnel.

XVII.c.1. Single-use brain biopsy sets should be used. Creutzfeld-Jacob disease is often definitively diagnosed by brain biopsy. Single-use brain biopsy sets are commercially available or can be assembled using older instruments.

XVII.c.2. Instruments with lumens (eg, suction tips, needles) should be single use when possible.

Lumens are difficult to effectively decontaminate.

XVII.c.3. Flexible neuroendoscopes should be replaced with rigid alternatives.

Flexible endoscopes are difficult to clean and will be damaged during the cleaning and sterilization methods known to deactivate prions infectivity.

XVII.c.4. Power drills should not be used.

Power drills may splatter potentially infective material and are difficult to clean, and the cleaning and sterilization methods known to eliminate prion infectivity damage these instruments.

XVII.c.5. Surgical drapes, gowns, and single-use supplies should be used whenever possible and incinerated after use.

Drapes and gowns are in contact with highly infectious tissue during these procedures. Routine hospital laundry does not deactivate prions.

XVII.c.6. Work surfaces should be covered with disposable, impervious material that can be removed and incinerated after the procedure.

Minimizing contamination of the room minimizes the need for special precautions during environmental cleaning.

XVII.c.7. Trays of implants (eg, burr hole covers, screws) should be limited to those implants essential for the specific patient. Implants opened and handled by scrubbed personnel after the surgery has started should be discarded and not reprocessed for subsequent patient use.

The determination of the need for and size of implant rests with the surgeon. Collaboration between the perioperative nurse and surgeon can result in elimination of implants that the surgeon determines are nonessential. If implants normally delivered to the sterile field in sets (eg, plates and screws) are required, removing implants that are not needed for the patient before sterilizing the tray decreases the amount of implant inventory needing to be discarded.

XVII.d. Single-use instruments that have come in contact with tissue considered to be highly infective from patients at high risk for a prion disease should be incinerated.

XVII.e. Work surfaces contaminated with prions should be cleaned with sodium hydroxide (NaOH) or sodium hypochlorite (ie, bleach).[40]

No transmissions of prion diseases from environmental surfaces have been reported; however, it remains prudent to eliminate highly infectious material from operating room surfaces that patients and personnel will be in contact with during subsequent surgeries.

For more information on cleaning of contaminated work surfaces consult AORN's "Recommended practice for environmental cleaning in the surgical practice setting."[41]

XVII.f. Reusable instruments that have come in contact with highly infective tissue of patients at high risk for a prion disease should be treated to reduce infectivity using the following steps listed below. (PNDS: I70)

When a potentially contaminated device can be cleaned and prion or tissue load decreased or physically removed, the probability of infection transmission is reduced significantly. There is currently no consensus on the best method of managing instruments that are likely contaminated with prions. Peracetic acid is ineffective and hydrogen peroxide gas plasma alone is only partially effective against prions.[42]

XVII.f.1. Instruments that cannot be adequately cleaned or require low-temperature sterilization (ie, ethylene oxide, hydrogen peroxide gas plasma) should be discarded.

XVII.f.2. Instruments should be kept moist until they are cleaned and decontaminated.

Drying renders prions more resistant to steam sterilization. Keeping instruments moist and cleaning them immediately after use minimizes drying.

XVII.f.3. Personnel should wear impervious gowns, heavy-duty gloves, and face shields while decontaminating instruments.

XVII.f.4. Instruments should be cleaned with an instrument cleaner as soon as possible after use.

Instrument cleaners reduce the amount of contamination and challenge to subsequent sterilization.[43] If allowed to dry, prion-contaminated material adheres to the surface of instruments, which can make subsequent terminal sterilization ineffective.[44]

XVII.f.5. After thorough cleaning, one of the following methods should be used to steam sterilize the instruments.

- Eighteen minutes in a prevacuum sterilizer with a cycle temperature of 134° C (272° F).
- Sixty minutes in a gravity-displacement sterilizer with a cycle temperature of 132° C (272° F).
- Immersion of instruments in 1N sodium hydroxide (NaOH) (ie, 1 Normal or 1 Molar concentration of NaOH) for one hour, followed by removal and a water rinse, followed by a steam sterilization cycle as noted above.

The WHO has recommended instruments exposed to prions be immersed in 1N sodium hydroxide for one hour followed by steam sterilization of the immersed instruments in the container at 121° C (250° F) for 30 minutes. Sterilizing instruments in a bath of sodium hydroxide creates dangerous vapors that can injure the airway and eyes of health care workers and can cause burns.[45] This practice also damages sterilizers, invalidates the sterilizer warranty, and corrodes some surgical instruments.[46,47] Using a polypropylene containment pan with a lid when sterilizing the instruments in the 1N sodium hydroxide bath has been found to contain the vapors within the pan.[45]

XVII.f.6. After initial cleaning, instruments should be processed in a washer decontaminator and sterilized in the usual fashion.

XVII.f.7. Solidify and incinerate any liquids used for cleaning.

XVII.g. Devices that have been contaminated with medium-, low-, or no-infectivity tissue can be cleaned and disinfected or sterilized using conventional protocols of heat, chemical sterilization, or high-level disinfection.

When a device is contaminated with tissue or body fluids that are not deemed to be of high-infectivity and the device can be cleaned effectively, the probability of infection transmission appears to be so low that it would not be measurable. During surgery on patients at high risk for prion disease, most surfaces in the operating room are not contaminated with highly infectious material and routine cleaning will limit contamination to what is considered a safe level.[40]

XVII.h. If a patient is identified postoperatively as having had a prion disease at the time of surgery, special precautions should be taken. Devices determined to be potentially contaminated with highly infectious tissue of this patient should be pulled from service and decontaminated as described above after the device has been reprocessed.

Prions can survive for years.[38] Inadequately decontaminated instruments pose a risk to subsequent patients who have had contact with the instruments.

XVII.i. Perioperative nurses should review current research on methods of detecting prion infectivity and decontamination methods.

Knowledge about detection of prion contamination on instruments and the effectiveness of various methods of deactivation is evolving as new research is published.

Recommendation XVIII

Personnel handling contaminated instruments and equipment must wear appropriate personal protective equipment (PPE)[10] and should be vaccinated against the hepatitis B virus.

Personal protective equipment helps to protect the employee from exposure to bloodborne pathogens and other potentially infectious materials.

XVIII.a. Personal protective equipment consistent with the anticipated exposure must be worn.[10,48]

Splashes, splatters, and skin contact can be reasonably anticipated when handling contaminated instruments.

XVIII.a.1. The appropriate PPE for these types of exposures include, but are not limited to,
- a fluid-resistant gown,
- heavy-duty gloves,
- a mask, and
- face protection.

XVIII.b. Hands must be washed after removing PPE.[10]

Perforations can occur in gloves, and hands can become contaminated when removing PPE. The OSHA requires hand washing after removal of PPE.[10]

XVIII.c. Reusable protective attire must be decontaminated and the integrity of the attire confirmed between uses.[10]

Reusable gloves, gowns, aprons, and face shields become contaminated and their integrity can be compromised during use. Decontamination and confirmation of integrity helps to protect the wearer from exposure.[48]

XVIII.d. Two pairs of gloves should be worn when cleaning instruments and equipment, if there is a risk for perforation of the outer glove.

XVIII.e. Personnel working with contaminated instruments should be vaccinated against hepatitis B virus.

Hepatitis B vaccination provides protection against one of the most common bloodborne pathogens. The OSHA requires the vaccination be offered to employees at risk of exposure at no charge.[10]

XVIII.f. Exposures to bloodborne pathogens should be reported immediately through the approved health care organization channels.

Antiviral medication is most effective if given as soon as possible after an exposure.

Recommendation XIX

Competency
Personnel should receive initial education and competency validation on procedures, chemicals used, and personal protection and should receive additional training when new equipment, instruments, supplies, or procedures are introduced.

Ongoing education and competency validation of perioperative personnel facilitates the development of knowledge, skills, and attitudes that affect patient and worker safety.

XIX.a. Personnel should receive initial education on
- decontamination methods;
- preparation of instruments and equipment for sterilization;
- selection of cleaning agents and methods;
- proper use of cleaning agents, including an understanding of specific applications, appropriate dilution, and special precautions;
- decontamination of specific instruments and equipment used within the practice setting;
- procedures for decontamination of instruments contaminated with prions and the effectiveness of various methods of deactivation;
- personal protection required during instrument processing; and
- exposure risk associated with chemical cleaning agents.[48]

Workers have the right to know the hazards that exist in the workplace and OSHA requires that employers provide this information.[48] An understanding of procedures involved in cleaning each type of instrument is necessary to provide the foundation for compliance with procedures.

XIX.b. Personnel should receive education on
- new instruments and equipment,
- new cleaning agents and methods, and
- new procedures.

XIX.c. Administrative personnel should validate the competencies of personnel participating in decontamination of surgical instruments. The validation of competencies should include all types of instruments that the individual is authorized to reprocess.

Validation of competencies provides an indication that personnel are able to appropriately perform decontamination procedures.

Recommendation XX

Documentation
Documentation should be completed to enable the identification of trends and demonstrate compliance with regulatory and accrediting agency requirements.

Documentation provides a source of data to review processes and evaluate corrective actions.

XX.a. Documentation should include maintaining records of the cleaning of instruments including, but not limited to,

- date,
- time,
- instruments,
- method of cleaning,
- number or identifier of mechanical decontaminator,
- name of person performing the cleaning,
- lot numbers of chemicals used,
- testing results on mechanical instrument washers,
- testing results on insulated electrical instruments, and
- disposition of defective equipment.

Most sterilization failures result from inadequate cleaning of the instruments before sterilization. Toxic anterior segment syndrome has been associated with inadequate cleaning processes. Some washer decontaminators have digital readouts or printers that facilitate recordkeeping. Bar code scanning technology also is available making this process more efficient. Records of washer testing provide a source of evidence for review when investigating clinical issues including surgical site infections.

XX.b. Records should be maintained for a time period specified by the health care organization and in compliance with local, state, and federal regulations.

Recommendation XXI

Policies and Procedures
Policies and procedures regarding the care and cleaning of surgical instruments and powered equipment should be developed using the validated instructions provided by the medical device manufacturers, reviewed at regular intervals, revised as necessary, and be readily available in the practice setting.

Policies and procedures serve as operational guidelines and establish authority, responsibility, and accountability within the organization. Policies and procedures also assist in the development of patient safety guidelines and quality assessment and improvement activities.

XXI.a. Policies regarding instrument cleaning should be developed by a multidisciplinary team to include perioperative nurses, sterile processing personnel, surgeons, and an infection control professional.

Using a multidisciplinary team provides varied input and improved ownership of policies and procedures. Involving surgeons in review of policies educates them on the expectations for instrument cleaning and facilitates planning for instrument use. The expertise of infection control professionals facilitates establishment of minimum standards of infection control.

XXI.b. Policies should include, but not be limited to,
- review of validated manufacturers' written instructions before purchase or consignment;
- cleaning of instruments before initial use;
- management of loaner instruments, to include advanced notification of vendors, required time frame for advance delivery, a process for cleaning and sterilization before use, and a process for cleaning and return after use;
- precautions to be taken when handling contaminated items;
- precautions to be taken when handling chemical agents;
- reprocessing powered surgical equipment;
- reprocessing ophthalmic surgical instruments;
- reprocessing robotic instruments and equipment;
- frequency of mechanical washer checks;
- frequency and method of evaluation of manual cleaning;
- frequency of checking insulated electrosurgery instruments for leakage current;
- criteria for identification and precautions taken for instruments used on patients with known or suspected prion disease;
- documentation of cleaning;
- initial education and annual competency;
- maintenance of material safety data sheets;
- reporting exposures to bloodborne pathogens; and
- reporting adverse events.

Recommendation XXII

Quality
The health care organization's quality management program should evaluate the care of instruments to improve patient safety.

XXII.a. A quality management program should be in place to test mechanical cleaning equipment.
- Mechanical instrument washers should be tested for proper functioning before initial use, weekly during service, and after major maintenance.
- Manual cleaning should be evaluated when new types of instruments are reprocessed and periodically, at intervals determined by the health care organization.
- Insulated electrical instruments should be tested for leakage current before initial use and after decontamination. Testing after decontamination allows a defective device to be replaced before sterilization.
- Personnel should identify and respond to opportunities for improvement.
- Reporting mechanisms for adverse events and near misses related to instrument cleaning should be in place.

XXII.a.1. Adequate cleaning of surgical instruments is essential to remove or destroy microorganisms and eliminate endotoxins. Testing washer decontaminators on a regular basis verifies that the equipment is functioning properly or identifies an opportunity for corrective action. Washer testing products are commercially available.

XXII.a.2. Periodic testing provides an opportunity to evaluate the performance of personnel. Manual cleaning is a learned skill and subject to human error. New instruments can pose unique challenges when cleaning. Protein indicators are commercially available to assist with this evaluation.

XXII.a.3. Visual inspection of insulation on electrosurgery instruments provides a screening mechanism to identify obvious breaks. Electrical testing can identify very small insulation failures that may not be apparent visually. Doing this testing after decontamination provides an opportunity to take corrective action well in advance of the surgical procedure.

XXII.a.4. Adverse events should be reported in the adverse event reporting system and reviewed for potential opportunities for improvement. When investigating surgical infections, documentation of the cleaning process of instruments should be reviewed. Near misses should be investigated and corrective action taken to prevent serious adverse events.

Glossary

Biofilm: A thin coating containing biologically active organisms that have the ability to grow in water, water solutions, or in vivo and which coat the surface of structures (eg, teeth, inner surfaces of catheters, tubes, implanted or indwelling devices, instruments and other medical devices). Biofilms contain viable and nonviable microorganisms that adhere to the surface and are trapped within a matrix of organic matter (eg, proteins, glycoprotein's, carbohydrates), which prevents antimicrobial agents from reaching the cells.

Decontamination: Any physical or chemical process that removes or reduces the number of microorganisms or infectious agents and renders reusable medical products or equipment safe for handling or disposal; the process by which contaminants are removed, either by hand cleaning or mechanical means, using specific solutions capable of rendering blood and debris harmless and removing them from the surface of an object or instrument.

Endotoxin: A toxin produced by certain bacteria and released upon destruction of the bacterial cell.

Enzymatic cleaner: A cleaner that uses enzymes to remove protein from surgical instruments.

Eschar: Charred tissue residue.

Ethylene oxide: An alkylating agent that, under the right conditions of time, temperature, concentration, and humidity, can result in microbial death.

Free-rinsing: Ability to be removed without leaving residue.

Iatrogenic: A response to medical or surgical treatment, usually denoting an unfavorable response.

Normal: Denotes a solution containing 1 equivalent of replaceable hydrogen ion per liter or a solution containing 1 gram of a substance or its equivalent in hydrogen ions.

Personal protective equipment (PPE): Specialized equipment or clothing for eyes, face, head, body, and extremities; protective clothing; respiratory devices; and protective shields and barriers designed to protect the worker from injury or exposure to a patient's blood, tissue, or body fluids. Used by health care workers and others whenever necessary to protect themselves from the hazards of processes or environments, chemical hazards, or mechanical irritants encountered in a manner capable of causing injury or impairment in the function of any part of the body through absorption, inhalation, or physical contact.

Potable water: Water that is of sufficient quality to be considered appropriate for drinking.

Prion: A proteinaceous and infectious agent containing no DNA or RNA.

Robotic surgical instruments: A remote-controlled surgical instrument system, including scalpels, scissors, forceps, and needle holders, used to perform minimally invasive surgery.

Toxic anterior segment syndrome (TASS): A complication of ophthalmic surgery involving a severe, noninfectious inflammation of the anterior segment of the eye, caused by various contaminants in solutions, medications, steam, and residue on surgical instruments and supplies.

Ultrasonic cleaner: A processing unit that transmits ultrasonic waves through the cleaning solution in a mechanical process known as cavitation. Ultrasonic cleaning is particularly effective in removing soil deposits from hard-to-reach areas.

Viscoelastic: A gel injected into the anterior chamber during ophthalmic surgery to maintain the depth of the chamber, protect the corneal endothelium, and stabilize the vitreous.

Washer/decontaminator: A processing unit that cleans by a spray-force action known as impingement. This machine combines a vigorous agitation bath with jet-stream air to create underwater turbulence. A sterilization cycle follows the washing cycle.

REFERENCES

1. Peterson C, ed. *Perioperative Nursing Data Set: Rev 2nd ed.* Denver, CO: AORN, Inc; 2007.

2. Recommended practices for sterilization in the perioperative practice setting. In: *Standards, Recommended Practices, and Guidelines.* Denver, CO: AORN, Inc; 2007:673-688.

3. Recommended practices for high-level disinfection. In: *Standards, Recommended Practices, and Guidelines.* Denver, CO: AORN, Inc; 2007:503-510.

4. Recommended practices for cleaning and processing endoscopes and endoscope accessories. In: *Standards, Recommended Practices, and Guidelines.* Denver, CO: AORN, Inc; 2007:531-536.

5. Association for the Advancement of Medical Instrumentation. *ANSI/AAMI ST79: 2006 Comprehensive Guide to Steam Sterilization and Sterility Assurance in Health Care Facilities.* Arlington, VA: Association for the Advancement of Medical Instrumentation, 2006.

6. Association for the Advancement of Medical Instrumentation. *ANSI/AAMI ST81: 2004 Sterilization of Medical Devices: Information to Be Provided by the Manufacturer for the Processing of Resterilizable Medical*

Devices. Arlington, VA: Association for the Advancement of Medical Instrumentation; 2004.

7. American Society of Healthcare Central Service Professionals, International Association of Healthcare Central Service Materiel Management. ASHCSP/IAHCSMM position paper on loaner instrumentation. *http://www.iahcsmm.org/current_issues_Joint_paper_loaner_instrumentation.htm.* Accessed October 27, 2007.

8. Ignition of debris on active electrosurgical electrodes. *Health Devices.* 1998;27:367-370.

9. Recommended practices for electrosurgery. In: *Standards, Recommended Practices, and Guidelines.* Denver, CO: AORN, Inc; 2007:515-530.

10. Occupational Safety and Health Administration. Bloodborne pathogens. 29CFR 1910.1030. *http://www.osha.gov/pls/oshaweb/owadisp.show_document?p_table=STANDARDS&p id=10051.* Accessed October 27, 2007.

11. Recommended practices for traffic patterns in the perioperative practice setting. In: *Standards, Recommended Practices, and Guidelines.* Denver, CO: AORN, Inc; 2007:703-706.

12. American Institute of Architects Academy of Architecture for Health. Facilities Guidelines Institute. *Guidelines for Design and Construction of Health Care Facilities.* Washington, DC: American Institute of Architects; 2006.

13. Occupational Safety and Health Administration. OSHA Act of 1970. *http://www.osha.gov/pls/oshaweb/owasrch.search_form?p_doc_type=OSHACT&p_toc_level=0&p_keyvalue=&p_status=CURRENT.* Accessed October 27, 2007.

14. Recommended practices for product selection in the perioperative practice setting. In: *Standards, Recommended Practices, and Guidelines.* Denver, CO: AORN, Inc; 2007:637-640.

15. American Society for Healthcare Central Service Professionals. *Training Manual for Health Care Central Service Technicians.* San Francisco, CA: Jossey-Bass; Health Forum; 2006.

16. Mamalis N, Edelhauser HF, Dawson DG, Chew J, LeBoyer RM, Werner L. Toxic anterior segment syndrome. *J Cataract Refract Surg.* 2006;32:324-333.

17. AORN. Recommended practices for selection and use of packaging systems for sterilization. In: *Standards, Recommended Practices, and Guidelines.* Denver, CO: AORN, Inc; 2007:607-616.

18. American Society of Cataract and Refractive Surgery, American Society of Ophthalmic Registered Nurses. Recommended practices for cleaning and sterilizing intraocular surgical instruments. *J Cataract Refract Surg.* 2007;33:1095-1100.

19. Werner L, Sher JH, Taylor JR, et al. Toxic anterior segment syndrome and possible association with ointment in the anterior chamber following cataract surgery. *J Cataract Refract Surg.* 2006;32:227-235.

20. Hellinger WC, Hasan SA, Bacalis LP, et al. Outbreak of toxic anterior segment syndrome following cataract surgery associated with impurities in autoclave steam moisture. *Infect Control Hosp Epidemiol.* 2006; 27:294-298.

21. American Society of Cataract and Refractive Surgery. Final TASS Report. *http://www.ascrs.org/press_releases/Final-TASS-Report.cfm.* Accessed October 27, 2007.

22. US Food and Drug Administration. FDA-Requested Recall:Cytosol Laboratories, Inc. Product Contains Dangerous Levels of Endotoxin. *http://www.fda.gov/bbs/topics/news/2006/NEW01315.html.* Accessed October 27, 2007.

23. Mac Rae SM, Brown B, Edelhauser HF. The corneal toxicity of presurgical skin antiseptics. *Am J Ophthalmol.* 1984;97:221-232.

24. Phinney RB, Mondino BJ, Hofbauer JD, et al. Corneal edema related to accidental Hibiclens exposure. *Am J Ophthalmol.* 1988;106:210-215.

25. Anderson NJ, Nath R, Anderson CJ, Edelhauser HF. Comparison of preservative-free bupivacaine vs. lidocaine for intracameral anesthesia: a randomized clinical trial and *in vitro* analysis. *Am J Ophthalmol.* 1999; 127:393-402.

26. Cox MJ, Woods JA, Newman S, Edlich RF. Toxic effects of surgical glove powders on the eye. *J Long Term Eff Med Implants.* 1996;6:219-226.

27. Bene C, Kranias G. Possible intraocular lens contamination by surgical glove powder. *Ophthalmic Surg.* 1986;17:290-291.

28. Unal M, Yucel I, Akar Y, Oner A, Altin M. Outbreak of toxic anterior segment syndrome associated with glutaraldehyde after cataract surgery. *J Cataract Refract Surg.* 2006;32:1696-1701.

29. Breebaart AC, Nuyts RM, Pels E, Edelhauser HF, Verbraak FD. Toxic endothelial cell destruction of the cornea after routine extracapsular cataract surgery. *Arch Ophthalmol.* 1990;108:1121-1125.

30. Kreisler KR, Martin SS, Young CW, Anderson CW, Mamalis N. Postoperative inflammation following cataract extraction caused by bacterial contamination of the cleaning bath detergent. *J Cataract Refract Surg.* 1992;18:106-110.

31. Richburg FA, Reidy JJ, Apple DJ, Olson RJ. Sterile hypopyon secondary to ultrasonic cleaning solution. *J Cataract Refract Surg.* 1986;12:248-251.

32. Duffy RE, Brown SE, Caldwell KL, et al. An epidemic of corneal destruction caused by plasma gas sterilization. The toxic cell destruction syndrome investigative team. *Arch Ophthalmol.* 2000;118:1167-1176.

33. US Food and Drug Administration. Medical devices; reprocessed single-use devices; requirement for submission of validation data. *Fed Reg.* 2006;71: 55729-55737.

34. ECRI Institute. Safety technologies for laparoscopic monopolar electrosurgery: devices for managing burn risks. *Health Devices.* 2005;34:259-271.

35. Blattler T. Implications of prion diseases for neurosurgery. *Neurosurg Rev.* 2002;25:195-203.

36. Pana A, Jung M. Prion diseases and iatrogenic infections I. A review. *Ig Sanita Pubbl.* 2005;61:325-377.

37. Jung M, Pistolesi D, Pana A. Prion diseases and iatrogenic infections II. decontamination. *Ig Sanita Pubbl.* 2005;61:379-410.

38. Brown P. Survival of scrapie after 3 years' intement. *Lancet* [- 8736]. 1991;337:269-270.

39. Peden AH, Ritchie DL, Head MW, Ironside JW. Detection and localization of PrPSc in the skeletal muscle of patients with variant, iatrogenic, and sporadic forms of Creutzfeldt-Jakob disease. *Am J Pathol.* 2006;168:927-935.

40. Rutala W.A, Weber DJ. Creutzfeldt-Jakob disease: Recommendations for disinfection and sterilization. *Clin Dis Inf.* 2001;32:1348-1356.

41. Recommended practices for environmental cleaning in the surgical practice setting. In: *Standards, Recommended Practices, and Guidelines.* Denver, CO: AORN, Inc; 2008:475-482.

42. Fichet G, Comoy E, Duval C, et al. Novel methods for disinfection of prion-contaminated medical devices. *Lancet.* 2004;364:521-526.

43. Yan ZX, Stitz L, Heeg P, Pfaff E, Roth K. Infectivity of prion protein bound to stainless steel wires: a model for testing decontamination procedures for transmissible spongiform encephalopathies. *Infect Control Hosp Epidemiol.* 2004;25:280-283.

44. Lipscomb IP, Pinchin H, Collin R, Keevil CW. Effect of drying time, ambient temperature and pre-soaks on prion-infected tissue contamination levels on surgical stainless steel: concerns over prolonged transportation of instruments from theatre to central sterile service departments. *J Hosp Infect.* 2007;65:72-77.

45. Brown SA, Merritt K. Use of containment pans and lids for autoclaving caustic solutions. *Am J Infect Control.* 2003;31:257-260.

46. STERIS. Overview of current CJD decontamination and sterilization methods and possible effects on product warranty. Document M236OEN. *http://www.steris.com/search/search2.cfm#.* Accessed December 24, 2007.

47. Brown SA, Merritt K, Woods TO, Busick DN. Effects on instruments of the World Health Organization recommended protocols for decontamination after possible exposure to transmissible spongiform encephalopathy-contaminated tissue. *J Biomed Mater Res B Appl Biomater.* 2005;72:186-190.

48. Occupational Safety and Health Administration. Hazard Communication: OSHA Standards. *http://osha.gov/SLTC/hazardcommunications/standards.html.* Accessed October 27, 2007.

PUBLICATION HISTORY

Originally published February 1988, *AORN Journal.* Revised March1992.

Revised November 1996; published January 1997, *AORN Journal.* Reformatted July 2000.

Revised November 2001; published March 2002, *AORN Journal.*

Revised 2007; published in *Perioperative Standards and Recommended Practices,* 2008 edition.

Recommended Practices for Selection and Use of Packaging Systems for Sterilization

The following recommended practices were developed by the AORN Recommended Practices Committee and have been approved by the AORN Board of Directors. They were presented as proposed recommended practices for comments by members and others. They are effective January 1, 2007.

These recommended practices are intended as achievable recommendations representing what is believed to be an optimal level of practice. Policies and procedures will reflect variations in practice settings and/or clinical situations that determine the degree to which the recommended practices can be implemented.

AORN recognizes the numerous settings in which perioperative nurses practice. These recommended practices are intended as guidelines adaptable to various practice settings. These practice settings include traditional operating rooms, ambulatory surgery centers, physicians' offices, cardiac catheterization suites, endoscopy suites, radiology departments, and all other areas where operative and other invasive procedures may be performed.

Purpose

These recommended practices provide guidelines for the evaluation, selection, and use of packaging systems for items to be sterilized. Packaging systems should ensure the integrity of the sterilized contents until opened for use and should permit aseptic delivery of the contents to the sterile field. These packaging systems include woven fabrics, nonwoven materials, paper-plastic pouches, plastic-plastic pouches, and containment devices (eg, rigid sterilization containers, instrument cases and cassettes, and organizing trays). These recommended practices do not include recommendations for loading the sterilizer or sterilization processes.

Recommendation I

Packaging systems should be evaluated before purchase and use to ensure that items to be packaged can be sterilized by the specific sterilizers and or sterilization methods to be used.[1]

1. Packaging systems should be appropriate for items being sterilized. The package system should
   - provide an adequate barrier to microorganisms, particulates, and fluids;

- maintain sterility of package contents until opened;
- allow sterilant penetration and direct contact with the item and surfaces, and removal of the sterilant;
- be free of toxic ingredients and nonfast dyes;
- permit aseptic delivery of contents to the sterile field (eg, minimal wrap memory, removal of lids from containers);
- permit complete and secure enclosure of item(s);
- protect package contents from physical damage (eg, compression, stacking);
- provide adequate seal integrity;
- resist tears, punctures, abrasions, and prevent the transfer of microorganisms;
- be tamper-proof and able to seal only once;
- permit adequate air removal;
- be low-linting;
- permit identification of contents;
- be large enough to evenly distribute the mass;[2]
- allow ease of use by personnel preparing and/or opening the package or container;
- have a favorable cost/benefit ratio; and
- include manufacturer's instructions for use.

2. Packaging systems should be appropriate to the method of sterilization. The packaging system should be compatible with, and designed and approved for use with, the specific technology employed, and able to withstand physical conditions of the sterilization process. Purchasers should request, review, and be familiar with the manufacturer's written sterilization validation studies.[2]

3. Purchasers should evaluate and test the performance of each packaging system before selection and use this information to determine that conditions for sterilization, shelf life, transport, storage, and handling can be met. The packaging system compatibility with the intended sterilization process(es) and equipment should be verified before purchase. If the packaging represents a major change in product type (eg, change from woven textiles to nonwoven materials, increased weight of trays) product testing should be performed. Product testing should include
   - placing biological indicators (BIs) inside a variety of items to be processed (eg, basin sets, instrument sets). The BI should be

located in the most challenging location inside the package (eg, geometric center of the pack, in between folds of gowns in linen packs, between nested basins in basin sets);

♦ packages containing the test BIs should be placed in the most challenging locations inside the sterilizer (eg, over the drain) in a full chamber;

♦ sterilization of the test packages and removal and incubation of the BIs. Test package contents should be reprocessed before use; and

♦ documentation of the test results should be maintained with the sterilization records.[2]

4. The total weight of instrument containment devices should not exceed 25 pounds including the contents and containment method (eg, wrappers, rigid container systems, cassettes, organizing trays).[2] Excessively heavy instrument sets may compromise sterilization and drying. The focus should be on the set configuration (ie, how the instruments are distributed in the set) and the overall weight of the set. Lifting and moving heavy instrument sets may cause health care worker injury.[2]

Recommendation II

Packaging systems should be compatible with the specific sterilization process for which it is designed.

1. Packaging systems for steam sterilization should permit adequate drying.[2]

    The efficacy of steam sterilization can be affected by humidity; altitude; packaging material; package contents; load; position of items within the sterilizer; size, weight, and density of the pack or container; and the parameters of the sterilization cycle. Practice settings should follow manufacturers' written instructions for each packaging system for steam sterilization.[2]

2. Packaging systems for ethylene oxide (EO) should
    ♦ be permeable to EO, moisture, and air;
    ♦ permit aeration;
    ♦ be constructed of a material recommended by the sterilizer and sterilant manufacturer; and
    ♦ maintain material compatibility (ie, nondegradable) with the sterilization process.[3]

    Woven, nonwoven, peel-pouch packages, and some rigid container materials are permeable to EO and do not impede rapid aeration of

contents. Woven materials, however, may absorb a large amount of the relative humidity that is needed for EO sterilization. This may prevent adequate hydration of microorganisms for penetration of EO gas to all surfaces of the package contents.[3]

3. Packaging systems for low-temperature gas plasma sterilization should
    ♦ allow sterilizing plasmas to penetrate packaging materials;
    ♦ be compatible (ie, nondegradable, nonabsorbable) with the sterilization process;
    ♦ be constructed of a material recommended by the sterilizer manufacturer; and
    ♦ be used according to the packaging manufacturer's written instructions.

    Low-temperature gas plasma sterilization is affected by absorbable packaging materials (eg, cellulose-based packaging material, textile wrappers, paper-plastic pouches, or porous wrap); both the packaging and sterilizer manufacturer's written instructions should be followed.[4] The absorption of the plasma sterilant (ie, hydrogen peroxide) by paper-plastic pouches or porous wrap could have an adverse effect on the effectiveness of the sterilization process. Pouches used in low-temperature gas plasma sterilizers should be made of all plastic (eg, polypropylene).[4,5] Not all containment systems are compatible with low-temperature gas plasma; the user should obtain the manufacturer's technical data verifying the containment device has been validated for use in low-temperature gas plasma. If the containment device requires a filter, the filter should be made of noncellulose material.

4. Packaging systems for ozone sterilization should comply with the sterilizer manufacturer's written recommendations. Packaging not intended for use in ozone sterilizers may compromise the sterilization process. Packaging materials suitable for ozone sterilization include uncoated non-woven material, polyethylene pouches and commercially available anodized aluminum containers using noncellulose disposable filters.[5]

Recommendation III

Packaging materials should be stored and processed to maintain the qualities required for sterilization.

1. Reusable woven textile materials should be laundered between every use for rehydration. Re-sterilization without relaundering may lead to superheating and could be a deterrent to achieving sterilization.[2] Over-drying, heat-pressing, and storage in areas of low humidity also may lead to superheating and sterilization failure. When woven textiles are not rehydrated after sterilization, and/or if repeated sterilization is attempted, the textiles may absorb the available moisture present in the steam, thereby creating a dry or superheated steam effect.[2]

2. Packaging materials should be stored at 20° C to 23° C (68° F to 73° F) and at a relative humidity of 30% to 60% for least two hours before use. Maintaining room temperature and moisture content of packaging materials facilitates steam penetration and prevents superheating during the sterilization process. Room temperature and humidity levels in the packaging area should be monitored.[2]

3. Single-use packaging material should be used for one sterilization cycle. Disposable packaging material should be discarded after opening.

Recommendation IV

Package contents should be assembled, handled, and wrapped in a manner that provides for an aseptic presentation of package contents.

1. The appropriate size wrapping material should be selected to achieve adequate coverage of the item being packaged. The item should be wrapped securely to prevent gapping, billowing, or air pockets from forming, which may lead to compromised sterilization.

2. The method of packaging should be performed in a manner that facilitates the aseptic presentation of the contents.

   Sequential wrapping using two barrier-type wrappers provides a tortuous pathway to impede microbial migration and permits ease of presentation to the sterile field without compromising sterility. A fused or bonded, double-layer, disposable, nonwoven wrapper used according to manufacturers' written recommendations may provide a bacterial barrier comparable to the sequential double wrap, allowing safe and easy presentation to the sterile field. Correct use of a single disposable, nonwoven, double-bonded wrapper may eliminate the need to double-wrap sequentially.[6]

3. Count sheets should not be placed inside wrapped sets or rigid containers. Although there are no known reports of adverse events related to sterilized count sheets, there is no available research regarding the safety of toners and/or various papers subjected to any sterilization method. Chemicals used in the manufacture of paper and toner ink pose a theoretical risk of reaction in some sensitized individuals.[7]

Recommendation V

Paper-plastic pouch packages should be used according to manufacturers' written instructions.

1. Paper-plastic pouch packages should be used only for small, lightweight, low-profile items (eg, one or two clamps, scissors). Heavy metal instruments (eg, drills, retractors, weighted vaginal speculums) should not be sterilized in peel pouches because problems (eg, wet packages following sterilization) and sterility maintenance problems (eg, package seal break) may occur.[2]

2. Paper-plastic pouch packages should have as much air removed as possible before sealing. Air acts as a barrier to heat and moisture. Expansion of air may cause rupturing of packages during the sterilization process.[8]

3. Paper-plastic pouch packages should provide a seal of proven integrity and not allow resealing. A break in the seal may allow microorganisms to enter and contaminate package contents.[8]

4. Paper-plastic pouch packages should be sealed airtight. Air-tight sealing can be accomplished by applying heat to the open end of the peel pouch or pressure to the mating surfaces of self-sealing pouches to cure and make the seal permanent.[5]

5. Paper-plastic pouch packages should be inspected for intact seals and barrier integrity before and after sterilization and before use.

6. Double paper-plastic pouch packaging is not routinely required for sterilization; however, double packaging may be used to facilitate containment of multiple small items to be sterilized and facilitate aseptic presentation to the sterile field.[5]

   ◆ Double paper-plastic pouch packages should be used in such a manner as to avoid folding the inner package to fit into the outer package. Folding the edges of inner peel packages may entrap air and inhibit the sterilization process.[2,5]

♦ During sterilization of double paper-plastic pouch packages, the paper portions should be placed together to ensure penetration and removal of the sterilant, air, and moisture. Sterilizing agents penetrate paper portions of peel-pouch packages; plastic portions allow items to be viewed.[2]

7. Paper-plastic pouches should not be used within wrapped sets or containment devices because the pouches cannot be positioned to ensure adequate air removal, sterilant contact, and drying. The practice of confining instruments in paper-plastic pouches and then including them in wrapped or containerized sets has not been validated as appropriate and efficacious by packaging and container manufacturers.[2]

8. Paper-plastic pouch packages should open without tearing, linting, shredding, or delaminating. Contamination of sterile contents can occur due to functional failure of plastic-paper pouch packages.[9]

Recommendation VI

Design, material, and construction of the containment device (eg, rigid containers, instrument cases/cassettes, organizing trays) should be considered before selection, purchase, and use.

1. Purchasers should verify that the containment device has been tested and validated for the sterilization method and cycles to be used. Purchasers should request, review, and be familiar with the manufacturer's sterilization validation studies.[2]

2. Pre-purchase evaluation and biological testing of the containment device should be performed.[2]

♦ Pre-purchase evaluation should determine
   - whether the facility can verify the manufacturer's test results;
   - if the container device has been cleared by the US Food and Drug Administration (FDA) for use in a sterilization process;
   - if the container device is compatible with the design of the sterilizer(s) in which it will be used;

   - if the container device will allow complete air removal, adequate sterilant penetration, and drying; and
   - requirements for disassembly and cleaning.[2]

♦ Pre-purchase biological testing should be performed according to the Association for the Advancement of Medical Instrumentation standards. Each size container should be tested under the sterilization methods and cycles to be used.[2]

♦ Sealed flash sterilization containers should be biologically tested during the pre-purchase evaluation and routinely thereafter. The container manufacturer should provide technical data regarding the best method for biologically testing the container.[2]

3. The recommended sterilization method and cycle exposure times for each rigid container system should be provided in the manufacturers' data and instructions. Construction materials and container design may affect compatibility with the sterilization process (eg, penetration of sterilant [gas plasma], release of moisture or sterilant [EO]). Recommendations related to the type of sterilization method vary by the container manufacturer. Prevacuum sterilizers may be preferred because air removal is difficult in gravity displacement sterilizers.[2]

4. Rigid containers with single-use or reusable filters and valve systems should be secured and in proper working order before sterilization.
   ♦ Filter plates should be examined for integrity both before installation and after the sterilization process. If the filter is damp; dislodged; or has holes, tears, or punctures, the contents should be considered unsterile.[2]
   ♦ Only components of the rigid container system specified by the manufacturer and compatible with the system should be used.
   ♦ The integrity of the rigid container should be inspected and damaged items repaired or replaced after each use. Inspection should ensure that
      - sealing and mating surfaces and edges of the container and lid are free of dents or chips;
      - filter retention mechanisms and fasteners (eg, screws, rivets) are secure and not distorted or burred;
      - securing mechanisms are functioning;

- integrity of the filter media is not compromised;
- gaskets are pliable, securely fastened, and without breaks or cuts; and
- valves work freely.[2]

Loosened rivets, improperly maintained valves, worn gaskets, dents, or other damage compromises the integrity of the container and will compromise the sterilization process.[2]

5. Rigid container systems should be cleaned after each use. All components (eg, filter retention plates) should be disassembled for proper cleaning.[2]

6. The manufacturer's written instructions for cleaning, inspection, repair, and preventive maintenance should be followed.[2]

7. The manufacturer's written instructions for loading rigid containers should be followed. Instructions should include instrument set configuration requirements.[2]

8. The manufacturer's instructions for recommended filter material, security locks, and external chemical indicators should be followed.[2]

9. Additional materials placed inside rigid containers (eg, silicone mats, surgical towels) should not be used unless the container manufacturer has provided validation for their use.

10. The manufacturer's technical data for types of devices validated for use inside the container (eg, power equipment, items with lumens) should be obtained and special instructions for sterilization followed.

Recommendation VII

Packages to be sterilized should be labeled.

1. Packaging systems should be labeled before sterilization. The label information should include, but not be limited to,
   - a description of the package contents,
   - a method to identify the package assembler, and
   - lot control number.

2. Package labels should be visible and remain securely fixed to the package throughout processing, storage, and distribution to the point of use. If tape or a computer-generated label is used, it may be placed on either side of the peel-pouch package.

3. Label information should be written on indicator tape and not on the packing material. Markers used to label packages should be indelible, nonbleeding, and nontoxic. If a marking pen is used to label peel-pouch packages, the information should be written only on the plastic side of the pouch. If a marking pen is used to label wrapped packages, the information should be written on the indicator tape or affixed labels.[2]

Recommendation VIII

Sterilized packages should be considered sterile until an event occurs to compromise the package barrier integrity.[2]

1. Health care organizations should determine the best methods and materials for packaging sterile items, based upon the anticipated storage, handling, and environmental events that may be encountered. Loss of sterility of a packaged sterile item is event related. An event must occur to compromise package content sterility. Events that may affect the sterility of a package include, but are not limited to,
   - multiple handling that leads to seal breakage or loss of package integrity;
   - compression during storage;
   - moisture penetration;
   - exposure to airborne and other environmental contaminants;
   - storage conditions (eg, type of shelving, cleanliness, temperature, humidity, traffic control);
   - type and configuration of packaging materials used; and
   - use of sterility maintenance covers and method of sealing.

2. Sterile packages should be stored under environmentally controlled conditions. Sterile storage area temperature should be controlled and should not exceed 75° F (24° C). The humidity should not exceed 70%. There should be a minimum of four air exchanges per hour, and the air flow should be under positive pressure in relation to adjacent areas.[2]

3. The end user should visually inspect the package or container before opening for package integrity (eg, free of holes in fabric/paper, effective seal in containers).

Recommendation IX

A chemical indicator/integrator should be placed inside each package and an external chemical indicator affixed outside each package to be processed.[2]

1. External chemical indicators, classified as Class I chemical indicators, should be specific to the sterilization process selected.

2. Internal chemical indicators should be specific to the sterilization process. Class III (single parameter indicators), Class IV (multi-parameter indicators), or Class V (chemical integrators) may be used.

3. End users should obtain and follow the chemical indicator manufacturer's instructions for storage, use, and expiration.

4. The internal chemical indicator/integrator should be placed in the geometric center of the package, not on top, to verify that air has been removed and that the sterilant has penetrated into the center of the pack or set. The indicator should be visible to the user when the package is opened so the user can see that the indicator has changed before touching the contents.

5. Two chemical indicators/integrators should be placed inside rigid containers, one in each of two opposite corners of the inside basket.[2])

    Multi-level containers should have a chemical indicator/integrator placed in two opposite corners (eg, one in each of two corners) of each level.

6. A chemical indicator/integrator should be placed on each level of multi-level wrapped sets.[2]

Recommendation X

The health care organization's quality management program should include sterile packaging selection and use.

1. Product testing should be performed whenever there is a major change in packaging systems, materials, tray configuration, or content density[2] Two types of testing should be performed.
    - **Biological testing.** The biological indicator should be placed inside the tray, set, or pack being tested, usually in each corner and in the center of the set.
    - **Verification of the ability to dry the set under user conditions.** The set should be observed for any condensate on the instruments or package contents, wet or moist towels or silicone mats, or visible water inside the container. Evidence of retained moisture will require additional steps to determine the necessary cycle parameters and sterilizer load configuration required to ensure adequate drying.

2. Wet packs should be investigated and resolved.[10] Internal or external moisture has the potential to provide a pathway for microorganisms to enter and contaminate a sterilized item.[2]
    - Measures to resolve wet packs should include, but are not limited to,
        - determine the set/tray configuration and weight,
        - evaluate the packaging materials and methods used,
        - evaluate the pan/tray used to contain the set,
        - determine the placement (ie, location) of the tray/set on the sterilizer cart,
        - determine the entire contents of the sterilizer load in question (eg, the number and various types of items) including placement on the sterilizer cart,
        - determine if the chamber drain line basket is clogged,
        - investigate the steam quality with the engineering department, and
        - determine if the steam sterilizer is functioning properly (eg, insufficient vacuum during the drying cycle).[2]
    - One method that may be used to minimize wet pack issues is to "precondition" the load. Instruments should be placed inside the steam sterilizer before starting the cycle for 10 to 15 minutes with the door closed. The heat in the chamber, from steam stored in the jacket, will heat the instruments. The heating of the instruments before injection of steam may resolve wet pack issues that are not associated with steam quality or packaging/loading errors.[2]

3. A quality control program should be developed and implemented when woven textile packaging is used.
    - All woven textiles should be de-linted after washing and before packaging. Textiles should be inspected on a light table for defects (eg, holes, tears) each time they are processed. Any defects should be repaired using a vulcanized patch applied with a heat patch machine. Vulcanized patches

do not permit penetration of most sterilants; therefore, the quantity as well as the
location of the patches should be evaluated. The defect should be patched on
both sides. If there are multiple patches in
the same general area, the item should be
removed from service even if the overall
quality of the material is acceptable.

♦ Tears should not be sewn. Sewing increases
the number of holes in the textile where
microbes can enter. Cross stitching of textiles is not recommended due to the number
of holes created in the woven material.

♦ A system of inspection for the overall integrity of the material should be developed,
implemented, and monitored for quality. If
the material appears very thin, even though
there are no patches on the item, the item
should be removed from use.

♦ Reusable textiles should maintain a protective
barrier throughout the life of the product.
Multiple processing will eventually diminish
the protective barrier of the material. Manufacturers' instructions should be followed for
the suggested number of re-processings.[11] A
method should be established to monitor,
control, and determine useful life when reprocessing woven materials. This should include,
but not be limited to, the number of sterilization processes and washing cycles that may
occur while maintaining the acceptable barrier quality of the material.[11] If a printed area
(eg, grid system) for marking the number of
uses is available on the woven textile, the
printed area should be marked each time the
item is processed. When the grid is full, the
item should be removed from service.[11]

4. Evaluation and biological testing of rigid containers should be performed periodically in
each specific sterilizer and with each cycle
type used.[2] Various sterilizers having the same
sterilization cycles may have different air-
removal efficiencies.

Recommendation XI

**Personnel should demonstrate competence in the use
of sterilization packaging systems and accessories.**

1. Personnel selecting and using packaging systems should be knowledgeable about the principles of sterilization, manufacturers' instruc-

tions, risks, measures to minimize these risks,
and corrective actions to employ in the event
of a failure of the packaging system.

2. Personnel should be competent in the proper
selection and use of packaging systems before
use. Education should be provided during the
orientation period. Additional periodic educational programs should be provided to reinforce safe use; new information on changes in
technology, its application, and compatibility
of sterilization equipment and processes; and
potential hazards.

3. Administrative personnel should periodically
assess and document the competency of personnel in the use of packaging systems, according
to hospital and department policy. Incorrect use
can result in serious injury to patients. Competency assurance verifies that personnel have a
basic understanding of packaging systems, risks,
and appropriate corrective action to take in the
event of a product or process failure. This knowledge is essential to minimizing the risks of misuse and providing a safe environment of care.

4. An introduction to related policies and procedures should be included in the orientation
and ongoing education of personnel to assist in
the development of knowledge, skills, and
behaviors that affect patient outcomes.

Recommendation XII

**Policies and procedures for the selection and use
of packaging systems should be written, reviewed
periodically, and readily available within the practice setting.**

1. These recommended practices should be used
as guidelines for the development of policies
and procedures for packaging. The AORN recommended practices that deal with sterilization and protective barrier materials also
should be consulted when developing policies
and procedures. Policies and procedures establish authority, responsibility, and accountability
for the selection and use of packaging systems
within the practice setting.

2. Maximum weight and tray configurations
should be identified in the policy.

3. Policies and procedures establish guidelines for performance improvement activities to be used in monitoring packaging system efficacy.

4. The Perioperative Nursing Data Set, the uniform perioperative nursing vocabulary, should be used to develop policies and procedures related to sterilization and sterile packaging. The expected outcome of primary import to this recommended practice is, "The patient is free from signs and symptoms of infection" (O10). This outcome falls within the domain of Physiologic Responses (D2). The associated nursing diagnosis is "Risk for infection" (X28). The associated interventions that may lead to the desired outcome may include "Protects from cross-contamination" (I98).[12]

Glossary

Chemical indicators: Devices used to monitor exposure to one or more sterilization parameters.

Class I: Process indicator that demonstrates that the package has been exposed to the sterilization process to distinguish between processed and unprocessed packages.

Class II: Process indicators that are used for a specific purpose such as the dynamic air removal test (formerly called the Bowie-Dick test).

Class III: A single-parameter indicator that reacts to one of the critical parameters of sterilization.

Class IV: A multi-parameter indicator that reacts to two or more of the critical parameters of sterilization.

Class V *(integrating indicator):* An indicator that reacts to all critical parameters of sterilization.

Containment device: Reusable rigid sterilization container, instrument case, cassette, or organizing tray intended for the purpose of containing reusable medical devices for sterilization.

Flash sterilization container: A container specifically designed for steam flash sterilization. The container is used to contain a device before, during, and after the sterilization process. It is sealed and may require special extended sterilization exposure times.

Instrument case/cassette: A device with a lid and a base to sterilize devices that permits air removal and sterilant penetration/removal. These devices require wrapping in packaging material if sterility of the contents is to be maintained.

Low-temperature gas plasma sterilization: This type of sterilization process involves an ionizing hydrogen peroxide gas or cloud or low-temperature plasma produced by exciting a strong electrical field over a contained precursor vapor that serves as a sterilizing agent.

Nonwoven materials: A fabric made by bonding fibers together as opposed to weaving threads.

Organizing tray: A reusable metal or plastic tray that permits organization of the contents and provides protection for the contents. Some organizing trays have diagrams of the respective instruments etched onto the surface of the tray to facilitate their location inside. These trays must be wrapped with an approved packaging material.

Package integrity: Unimpaired physical condition of a final package.

Packaging material: Any material used in the fabrication or sealing of a packaging system or primary package.

Packaging systems: One or more packaging materials assembled into a single unit intended as part or all of a primary package.

Paper-plastic pouch: A type of packaging suitable for steam and EO sterilization usually made of Mylar® (a polyester film manufactured by DuPont) and paper. The plastic (Mylar®) side is clear, permitting viewing of the contents. Paper-plastic pouches are available in various size pouches or on rolls and can be self-sealed or heat-sealed. They should not be confused with all-plastic (eg, Tyvek®, a polyethylene material manufactured by DuPont) pouches, which are not compatible with steam sterilization.

Rigid sterilization container system: Specifically designed heat-resistant, metal, plastic, or anodized aluminum receptacles used to package items, usually surgical instruments, for sterilization. The lids and/or bottom surfaces contain steam- or gas-permeable, high-efficiency microbial filters.

Sequential wrapping: A double-wrapping procedure that creates a package within a package.

Sterilization validation studies: Tests performed by the device manufacturer that demonstrate that a sterilization process will consistently yield sterile container contents under defined parameters.

Superheating: A condition in which dehydrated textiles are subjected to steam sterilization. The superheated package or product becomes too dry, which causes destructive effects on the strength of the cloth fibers. When woven textiles are not rehydrated after sterilization, and/or if repeated sterilization is attempted, the textiles could absorb the available moisture present in the steam, thereby creating a dry or superheated steam effect and adversely affecting the steam sterilization process.[2]

Shelf life: When this term is used in conjunction with a sterile device, shelf life is considered the length of time a device is considered safe to use.

Sterility maintenance cover (synonym: dust cover): A plastic bag, usually 2 to 3 thousandths of an inch (ie, mils) in thickness, applied to a cooled, sterilized item to provide extra protection from dust, moisture, and other environmental contaminates. These covers can be heat-sealed or self-sealed closed.

Useful life: Length of time, as determined by the manufacturer, for which a product maintains acceptable safety and performance characteristics. The manufacturer should provide data to support useful life of the material.

Wet packs: Packs are considered wet when there is moisture in the form of dampness, droplets, or puddles of water found on or within a textile pack, instrument, basin set, rigid container or containment device after a completed sterilization cycle and at least one hour after cooling. Wet packs generally are associated with steam sterilization; however, they also can occur with EO sterilization.

Woven textile: A reusable fabric constructed from yarns made of natural and/or synthetic fibers or filaments that are woven or knitted together to form a web in a repeated interlocking pattern.

REFERENCES

1. "Recommended practices for product selection in perioperative practice settings," in *Standards, Recommended Practices, and Guidelines* (Denver: AORN, Inc, 2006) 593-596.

2. Association for the Advancement of Medical Instrumentation, "Comprehensive guide to steam sterilization and sterility assurance in health care facilities," ANSI/AAMI ST79:2006 (Arlington, Va: Association for the Advancement of Medical Instrumentation, 2006) 54-111.

3. Association for the Advancement of Medical Instrumentation, "Ethylene oxide sterilization in health care facilities: Safety and effectiveness," ANSI/AAMI ST41-1999 (Arlington, Va: Association for the Advancement of Medical Instrumentation, 1990) Section 6.7.1.

4. Association for the Advancement of Medical Instrumentation, "Chemical sterilization and high level disinfection in health care facilities," ANSI/AAMI ST-58 (Arlington, Va: Association for the Advancement of Medical Instrumentation, 2005) Annex "H", H.3.

5. American Society for Healthcare Central Service Professionals, *Training Manual for Central Service Technicians,* fifth ed (San Francisco: Jossey-Bass, 2006) 175.

6. N Gorman-Annis, "Non-wovens," in *Sterilization Technology for the Health Care Facility,* second ed, M Reichert, J H Young, eds (Gaithersburg, Md: Aspen Publishers, Inc, 1997) 60.

7. N Chobin, personal communication with Consumer Response Center, Georgia Pacific Paper and J Kerns, Xerox Corporation, November17, 2005.

8. D Alexander, "Packaging: Pouches," in *Sterilization Technology for the Health Care Facility,* second ed, M. Reichert, J H Young, eds (Gaithersburg, Md: Aspen Publishers, Inc, 1997) 69.

9. L Nicolette, "Sterilization and disinfection," in *Perioperative Nursing,* third ed, L K Groah, ed (Stamford, Conn: Appleton & Lang, 1996) 169.

10. D Karle, "Solving wet pack problems," *Journal of Hospital Supply, Processing & Distribution* 2 (January/February 1984) 22-27.

11. Association for the Advancement of Medical Instrumentation, "Processing of reusable surgical textiles for use in health care facilities," ANSI/AAMI ST65:2000 (Arlington, Va: Association for the Advancement of Medical Instrumentation, 2000) Section 7.1.

12. S C Beyea, ed, *Perioperative Nursing Data Set: The Perioperative Nursing Vocabulary,* second ed (Denver: AORN, Inc, 2002).

PUBLICATION HISTORY

Originally published February 1983, *AORN Journal.* Revised November 1988, February 1992.

Revised November 1995; published May 1996, *AORN Journal.*

Revised and reformatted; published December 2000, *AORN Journal.*

Revised 2006; published in *Standards, Recommended Practices, and Guidelines,* 2007 edition.

AORN Perioperative Standards and Recommended Practices, 2012 Edition

Recommended Practices for Sterilization in the Perioperative Practice Setting

T he following recommended practices for sterilization were developed by the AORN Recommended Practices Committee and have been approved by the AORN Board of Directors. They were presented as proposed recommended practices for comments by members and others. They are effective January 1, 2008.

These recommended practices are intended as achievable recommendations representing what is believed to be an optimal level of practice. Policies and procedures will reflect variations in practice settings and/or clinical situations that determine the degree to which the recommended practices can be implemented.

AORN recognizes the various settings in which perioperative nurses practice. These recommended practices are intended as guidelines adaptable to various practice settings. These practice settings include traditional operating rooms, ambulatory surgery centers, physician's offices, cardiac catheterization laboratories, endoscopy suites, radiology departments, and all other areas where surgery may be performed.

References to nursing interventions (I) used in the Perioperative Nursing Data Set, second edition, (PNDS) are noted in parentheses when a recommended practice corresponds to a PNDS intervention.[1] The reader is referred to the PNDS for further explanation of nursing diagnoses, interventions, and outcomes.

Purpose

These recommended practices provide guidance for sterilizing items to be used in the surgical environment. The creation and maintenance of an aseptic environment has a direct influence on patient outcomes. A major responsibility of the perioperative registered nurse is to minimize patient risk for surgical site infection. One of the measures for preventing surgical site infections is to provide surgical items that are free of contamination at the time of use. This can be accomplished by subjecting them to cleaning and decontamination, followed by a sterilization process.[2] Steam, ethylene oxide (EO), low-temperature hydrogen peroxide gas plasma, peracetic acid, ozone, and dry heat are sterilization methods that are used in the health care environment. Sterilization provides the highest level of assurance that surgical items are free of viable microbes.

Recommendation I

Items to be sterilized should be cleaned, decontaminated, sterilized, and stored in a controlled environment and in accordance with AORN's "Recommended practices for cleaning and caring of instruments and powered equipment"[2] and the device manufacturer's written instructions.

Effective sterilization cannot take place without effective cleaning. The process of sterilization is negatively affected by the amount of bioburden and the number, type, and inherent resistance of microorganisms, including biofilms, on the items to be sterilized. Soils, oils, and other materials may shield microorganisms on items from contact with the sterilant or combine with, and inactivate, the sterilant.[3,4]

I.a.   Functional workflow patterns should be established to create and maintain physical separation between the decontamination and sterilization areas. (PNDS: I81, I98)

Physical separation aids in environmental and microbial control. During manual cleaning of instruments, particulates, aerosolized matter, dust, and microbial counts are elevated. Physical separation and vented airflow to the outside minimizes contamination of processed items.

I.a.1.   Attire, use of personal protective equipment (PPE), and limitations in personnel access and movement should be based on expected contamination levels (**Table 1**).

I.a.2.   Functional workflow patterns should be established in the following order from potentially high contamination areas to clean areas:
• decontamination,
• preparation and packaging,
• sterilization processing,
• sterile storage, and
• clean distribution.

I.a.3.   Traffic patterns should be established that define access restrictions, movement of personnel, and appropriate attire according to AORN's "Recommended practices for traffic patterns in the perioperative practice setting" to

Table 1

ATTIRE AND PERSONAL PROTECTIVE EQUIPMENT REQUIREMENTS[1]						
Work area	Scrubs	Head cover	Gloves*	Gown or apron#	Eye protection+	Masks or face shields±
Decontamination	X	X	X	X	X	X
Preparation and packaging	X	X				
Sterilization processing	X	X				
Sterile storage	X	X				

*Gloves should be waterproof, general-purpose utility, or heavy duty.
#Gowns must be liquid-resistant with sleeves. Aprons may be liquid-resistant but do not need to have sleeves.
+Eye protection includes goggles/eye glasses with side shields or chin-length face shields.
± Masks should be fluid-resistant.

REFERENCE
1. US Department of Labor, Occupational Safety and Health Administration. 29 CFR Bloodborne pathogens—1910.1030, Occupational safety and standards, Appendix A. Federal Register. 1991;56:64004.

protect personnel, equipment, supplies, and instrumentation from sources of potential contamination.[5]

I.b. Room temperature, humidity, and ventilation should be controlled in accordance with local, state, and federal policy and regulation. **Table 2** provides parameters for the controlled environment.[3] (PNDS: I81, I98)

Bacteria and fungi thrive at warm temperatures; cooler temperatures may impede bacterial and fungal growth in the decontamination area. Regulated environmental controls in work areas are essential for the comfort of personnel wearing appropriate attire and PPE.[3]

I.c. Room temperature, humidity, and ventilation for each work area should be monitored and recorded daily.[3] (PNDS: I98)

I.c.1. Organizations should monitor and record environmental controls in each area to ensure that, at minimum, recommended parameters are met and maintained.

I.d. Health care personnel should refer to the "Recommended practices for cleaning and care of surgical instruments and powered

equipment" and must use standard precautions when performing decontamination activities.[2] (PNDS: I70, I98)

Standard precautions are designed to protect patients and health care workers from contact with recognized and unrecognized sources of infectious diseases.

Recommendation II

Items to be sterilized should be packaged in accordance with AORN's "Recommended practices for selection and use of packaging systems for sterilization."[6]

Appropriate packaging ensures that sterility can be achieved and maintained to the point of use.

II.a. Manufacturers of packaging systems should be consulted for package preparation, configuration, and sterilization.[6,7] (PNDS: I70: I98)

II.b. The total weight of an instrument set should not exceed 25 lbs. (PNDS: I122)

Instrument sets weighing more than 25 lbs are known to be difficult to dry without lengthy drying times and present an increased risk of ergonomic injury.[3,8]

Table 2

PARAMETERS FOR CONTROLLED ENVIRONMENTS DURING STERILIZATION[1]					
Functional area	Airflow	Minimum number of air exchanges per hour	All air exhausted directly to the outdoors	Temperature	Relative humidity
Soiled/ decontaminated	Negative (in)	10	Yes	60° F to 65° F (16° C to 18° C)	30% to 60%
Sterilizer equipment access	Negative (in)	10	Yes	75° F to 85° F (24° C to 29° C)	30% to 60%
Sterilizer loading/ unloading	Positive (out)	10	Yes	68° F to 73° F (20° C to 23° C)	30% to 60%
Restrooms/ housekeeping	Negative (in)	10	Yes	≤ 75° F (≤ 24° C)	30% to 60%
Preparation and packaging	Positive (out)	10 (downdraft type)	No	68° F to 73° F (20° C to 23° C)	30% to 60%
Textile packaging room	Positive (out)	10 (downdraft type)	No	68° C to 73° F (20° C to 23° C)	30% to 60%
Clean/sterile storage	Positive (out)	4 (downdraft type)	No	≤ 75° F (≤ 24° C)	≤ 70%

REFERENCE

1. Association for the Advancement of Medical Instrumentation. ANSI/AAMI ST79: 2006 Comprehensive Guide to Steam Sterilization and Sterility Assurance in Health Care Facilities. Arlington, VA: Association for the Advancement of Medical Instrumentation; 2006:24-25. Adapted with permission.

II.c. Combination paper/plastic peel pouches should not be placed in a container or wrapped set.[3,6] (PNDS: I70, I122)

It may not be possible to position pouches to ensure adequate air removal, steam contact, or drying. The practice of using wraps or pouches inside container systems has not been validated by pouch or container manufacturers. Medical-grade, all-paper pouches may be used for this purpose.[3]

Recommendation III

Saturated steam under pressure should be used to sterilize heat- and moisture-stable items unless otherwise indicated by the device manufacturer.

Saturated steam under pressure is the preferred sterilization method. It is an effective, inexpensive, and relatively rapid sterilization method for most porous and nonporous materials.[9]

III.a. Manufacturers' written instructions for operating steam sterilizers should be followed. (PNDS: I98, I122).

Steam sterilizers vary in design and performance characteristics. A variety of steam sterilization cycles are used in health care organizations. Some examples are gravity-displacement cycles, dynamic air-removal (ie, prevacuum), steam-flush pressure-pulse cycles, flash cycles, and express cycles (ie, abbreviated steam sterilization cycles used for flash sterilization).[2] In addition, some sterilizers may be designed to permit only one type of cycle. For example, some sterilizers are identified as gravity-displacement sterilizers because that is the only type of cycle this type of sterilizer permits.

Table 3 and **Table 4** provide typical minimum sterilization times for gravity-displacement and dynamic air-removal steam sterilization cycles.[3]

Table 3

TYPICAL MINIMUM CYCLE TIMES FOR GRAVITY-DISPLACEMENT STEAM STERILIZATION[1]					
Item	Exposure time at 250° F (121° C)	Minimum drying time	Exposure time at 270° F (132° C)	Minimum drying time	Exposure time at 275° F (135° C)	Minimum drying time
Wrapped instruments	30 min	15 to 30 min	15 min	15 to 30 min	10 min	30 min
Textile packs	30 min	15 min	25 min	15 min	10 min	30 min
Wrapped utensils	30 min	15 to 30 min	15 min	15 to 30 min	10 min	30 min

1. *Association for the Advancement of Medical Instrumentation. ANSI/AAMI ST79:2006 Comprehensive Guide to Steam Sterilization and Sterility Assuring in Health Care Facilities. Arlington, VA: Association for the Advancement of Medical Instrumentation; 2006. Reprinted with permission.*

III.b.   Cycle parameters recommended by the device manufacturer should be reconciled with the sterilizer manufacturer's written instructions for the specific sterilization cycle and load configuration.[3,10] Certain types of equipment and implants (eg, some pneumatically powered instruments; specialty orthopedic, neurosurgery, trauma instruments) may require prolonged exposure times or drying times.[3,10] (PNDS: I98, I122)

III.c.   Following steam sterilization, the contents of the sterilizer should be removed from the chamber and left untouched for a period of 30 minutes to two hours depending on the load contents.[3] (PNDS: I70, I98, I122)

The potential for the formation of condensation is decreased by allowing the contents of the sterilizer to remain untouched until the equalization of the temperature differential between the chamber and outside environment has occurred.[3]

III.c.1.   Steam sterilizer doors should not be left ajar to cool loads following a cycle.[11]

Removing the sterilizer load from the sterilizer as soon as possible after steam sterilization allows the cooling process to begin earlier.

Cracking the sterilizer door may hinder the drying process.

Wet packs may be a result of excessively wet steam, poor loading techniques, or a true sterilizer malfunction.

III.d.   Warm or hot items should not be placed on cool or cold surfaces. (PNDS: I70, I98, I122)

When hot and cold surfaces are brought together, moisture condenses from both inside and outside the package. At the end of the steam sterilization cycle and after an appropriate drying time, items still may contain some steam vapor. Touching packages at this vulnerable stage could compromise the barrier properties of the packaging material by causing moisture and/or contaminants to wick through the package. Droplets inside or outside of the container can form because rigid container materials are nonabsorbent. Condensate can drip onto surrounding containers, compromising the sterility of other packages.[3]

III.e.   Sterilized packages or containers that have formed condensate should be considered unsterile and none of the contents used.[3] (PNDS: I70, I98, I122)

Moisture can compromise the integrity of barrier material and the sterility of the contents. Moisture may indicate problems with the packaging and sterilization process.[3]

Recommendation IV

Use of flash sterilization should be kept to a minimum. Flash sterilization should be used only in selected clinical situations and in a controlled manner.

Flash sterilization may be associated with increased risk of infection to patients because of

Table 4

TYPICAL MINIMUM CYCLE TIMES FOR DYNAMIC AIR-REMOVAL STEAM STERILIZATION[1]				
Item	Exposure time at 270° F (132° C)	Minimum drying time	Exposure time at 275° F (135° C)	Minimum drying time
Wrapped instruments	4 min	20 to 30 min	3 min	16 min
Textile packs	4 min	5 to 20 min	3 min	3 min
Wrapped utensils	4 min	20 min	3 min	16 min

1. *Association for the Advancement of Medical Instrumentation. ANSI/AAMI ST79:2006 Comprehensive Guide to Steam Sterilization and Sterility Assurance in Health Care Facilities. Arlington, VA: Association for the Advancement of Medical Instrumentation; 2006. Reprinted with permission.*

pressure on personnel to eliminate one or more steps in the cleaning and sterilization process.

IV.a. Flash sterilization should be used only when there is insufficient time to process by the preferred wrapped or container method. Flash sterilization should not be used as a substitute for sufficient instrument inventory.[12] (PNDS: I70, I98)

Proper decontamination is essential in removing bioburden and preparing an item for sterilization by any method. Failures in instrument cleaning have resulted in transmission of infectious agents.[3]

IV.a.1. Items to be flash sterilized should be subjected to the same decontamination processes as described in AORN's "Recommended practices for cleaning and care of surgical instruments and powered equipment."[2]

IV.a.2. Flash sterilization should be performed only if all of the following conditions are met:
- The device manufacturer's written instructions on cycle type, exposure times, temperature settings, and drying times (if recommended) are available and followed.
- Items are disassembled and thoroughly cleaned with detergent and water to remove soil, blood, body fats, and other substances.

- Lumens are brushed and flushed under water with a cleaning solution and rinsed thoroughly.
- Items are placed in a closed sterilization container or tray, validated for flash sterilization, in a manner that allows steam to contact all instrument surfaces.
- Measures are taken to prevent contamination during transfer to the sterile field.

Flash-sterilized items are to be used immediately and not stored for later use.[3]

Table 5 provides examples of typical flash sterilization parameters.

IV.b. Packaging and wrapping (eg, textiles, paper/plastic pouches, nonwoven wrappers) should not be used in flash sterilization cycles unless the sterilizer is specifically designed and labeled for this use. (PNDS: I70, I98)

Cycle parameters vary according to sterilizer design.

IV.b.1. Sterilizer manufacturers' written directions should be followed and reconciled with the packaging manufacturer's instructions for sterilization.[3]

IV.c. Process challenge devices (PCDs) should be used with routine process monitoring devices (ie, chemical indicators, biological indicators, physical monitoring devices).[3] (PNDS: I70, I98)

Process challenge and process monitoring devices provide information to demonstrate that conditions for sterilization have been met.

Table 5

EXAMPLES OF TYPICAL FLASH STEAM STERILIZATION PARAMETERS[1]				
Type of sterilizer	**Load configuration**	**Time**	**Exposure Temperature**	**Drying Times**
Gravity displacement	Metal or nonporous items only (ie, no lumens)	3 minutes	270° F to 275° F (132° C to 135° C)	0 to 1 minute
	Metal items with lumens and porous items (eg, rubber, plastic) sterilized together. Complex devices (eg, powered instruments requiring extended exposure times). Manufacturer instructions should be consulted.	10 minutes	270° F to 275° F (132° C to 135° C)	0 to 1 minute
Dynamic air-removal (prevacuum)	Metal or nonporous items only (ie, no lumens)	3 minutes	270° F to 275° F (132° C to 135° C)	N/A
	Metal items with lumens and porous items sterilized together	4 minutes 3 minutes	270° F (132° C) 275° F (135° C)	N/A N/A

- The sterilizer manufacturer's instructions for use of express cycles should be followed. One sterilizer manufacturer provides an express flash cycle that permits flash sterilization with a single-ply wrapper to help contain the device to the point of use. This cycle is not recommended for devices with lumens. Express cycles should only be used if the sterilizer is designed with this feature.
- Steam-flush pressure-pulse: See manufacturers' written instructions for time and temperature.
- This table does not include specific instructions for rigid flash sterilization containers. The container manufacturer's instructions should be followed.

REFERENCE

1. Association for the Advancement of Medical Instrumentation. ANSI/AAMI ST79:2006 and A1:2008 Comprehensive Guide to Steam Sterilization and Sterility Assurance in Health Care Facilities. *Arlington, VA: Association for the Advancement of Medical Instrumentation; 2006:60-72. Adapted with permission.*

IV.c.1. Each sterilization cycle should be monitored to verify that parameters required for sterilization have been met.[3]

IV.c.2. The sterilizer operator should use physical monitoring devices to verify cycle parameters for each load.[3]

Physical monitoring devices (eg, printouts, graphs, gauges) can indicate immediate sterilizer failure. Physical monitors record cycle parameters (ie, time, temperature) for each cycle.

IV.c.3. Biological (BI) and chemical indicators should be used to monitor sterilizer efficacy and assess compliance of monitoring standards established for gravity-displacement and dynamic air-removal sterilizers. Class 5 chemical integrating indicators should be used within each sterilizer container or tray.[3]

IV.d. Users should adhere to aseptic technique for flash-sterilized items during transport to the point of use. It is important that sterilization processing be carried out in a clean environment and that flash-sterilized devices are transferred to the point of use in a manner that prevents contamination.

IV.e. Rigid sterilization containers designed and intended for flash-sterilization cycles should be used. (PNDS: I70, I98)

Rigid flash-sterilization containers
- reduce the risk of contamination during transport to the point of use,
- facilitate ease of presentation to the sterile field, and
- protect sterilized items during transport.[3]

IV.f. Flash-sterilization containers should be used, cleaned, and maintained according to the manufacturer's written instructions.[3]

IV.f.1. Flash-sterilization containers should be opened, used immediately, and not stored for later use.

IV.f.2. Flash-sterilization containers should be differentiated from other types of containers.

IV.g. Flash sterilization should not be used for implantable devices except in cases of emergency when no other option is available.[12] (PNDS: I85, I138)

Implants are foreign bodies and they increase the risk of surgical site infection.[12] Careful planning, appropriate packaging, and inventory management in cooperation with suppliers can minimize the need to flash sterilize implantable medical devices.

IV.h. In an emergency, when flash sterilization of an implant is unavoidable, a rapid-action BI with a Class 5 chemical integrating indicator (or enzyme only indicator) should be run with the load.[3,12] (PNDS: I70, I98)

IV.h.1. The implant should be quarantined on the back table and should not be released until the rapid-action BI provides a negative result.

IV.h.2. If the implant is used before the BI results are known and the BI is later determined to have a positive result, the surgeon and infection prevention and control personnel should be notified as soon as the results are known.

IV.h.3. If the implant is not used, it cannot be saved as sterile for future use. Resterilization of the device is required if the implant is to be used later.[3,12]

IV.i. Documentation of cycle information and monitoring results should be maintained in a log (electronic or manual) to provide tracking of the flashed item(s) to the individual patient.[3,12] (PNDS: I112)

Documentation allows every load of sterilized items used on patients to be traced.

IV.i.1. Sterilization records should include information on each load, including
- the item(s) processed;
- the patient receiving the item(s);
- the cycle parameters used (eg, temperature, duration of cycle);
- the date and time the cycle is run;

- the operator information; and
- the reason for flash sterilization.[3]

Recommendation V

Ethylene oxide (EO) sterilization is a low-temperature process that is appropriate for heat- and moisture-sensitive surgical items when indicated by the device manufacturer.

Ethylene oxide at sterilizing temperatures kills microbes in hard-to-reach areas, and it does so with no damage to devices. Ethylene oxide is an alkylating agent that results in microbial death under controlled parameters. Ethylene oxide substitutes for hydrogen atoms on molecules needed to sustain life and, by attaching to these molecules, EO stops these molecules' normal life-supporting functions. Some of the key molecules that EO disrupts are proteins and DNA. Under low-temperature sterilizing conditions, so much EO is used that this disruption proves lethal to microbial life.[13]

V.a. Ethylene oxide should be used if alternate methods of sterilization are not available compatible with the medical devices being processed.[14]

Health care organizations use 100% concentrations of EO or EO in mixtures with inert diluent gases (eg, carbon dioxide, hydrochlorofluorocarbons [HCFC]) for EO sterilization procedures. Until the 1990s, chlorofluorocarbons (CFCs) were used as diluents for EO. Chlorofluorocarbons cause depletion of the ozone layer and are no longer produced in the United States. Hydrochlorofluorocarbons deplete the ozone layer, but to a lesser degree than CFCs.[14]

V.a.1. Users of HCFCs should be aware of and comply with federal, state, and local regulations regarding HCFC use in EO sterilizers.[15-17]

V.b. The manufacturer's written instructions should be reviewed to determine if a heat- or moisture-sensitive item is compatible with EO sterilization before attempting sterilization by this method. (PNDS: I122)

V.c. Items, including all lumens, should be clean and dry before being packaged for EO sterilization. (PNDS: I75, I98, I122)

Soil inhibits sterilization, and moisture may produce toxic by-products. The combination of water and EO results in the formation of ethylene glycol (ie, antifreeze).

V.d. Sterilizer manufacturers' written instructions should be followed for EO sterilization parameters and placement of items within the sterilizer. (PNDS: I70, I75, I122)

Ethylene oxide sterilizers differ in design and operating characteristics.

V.d.1. Items should be placed in EO sterilizers in baskets or on loading carts in a manner that allows free circulation and penetration of the EO.[15]

V.e. Physical monitors of EO sterilizers should record the essential parameters for sterilization including temperature, exposure time, pressure.[15] (PNDS: I75, I98, I122, I138)

Physical monitors provide real-time assessment and documentation of sterilization cycle parameters. Timely review of graphs, charts, and printouts enhance detection of sterilizer malfunctions and allows for implementation of corrective actions.[3]

V.f. Items sterilized in EO sterilizers should be properly aerated in a mechanical aerator to remove EO. (PNDS: I75, I122)

Ethylene oxide residual absorbed into sterilized items represents a hazard to patients and personnel, if not removed. Ethylene oxide is a known human carcinogen and a chemical that has the potential to cause adverse reproductive effects in humans. The Occupational Safety and Health Administration (OSHA) has established exposure limits for EO in the workplace.[16,18]

Items not sufficiently aerated may cause patient or personnel injury (eg, chemical burns). Aeration is the only safe and effective way to remove EO.[15,16,19]

Adequate aeration times reduce EO vapors and residue to a level safe for exposure of both patients and health care personnel.

Rinsing an inadequately aerated item does not remove EO and can create hazardous by-products.

V.f.1. Sterilized items should be handled as little as possible before aeration to prevent health care personnel from breathing EO gas or coming in contact with EO residues.

- Health care personnel should wear butyl rubber, nitrile, or neoprene gloves that provide protection to the skin when handling unaerated EO-sterilized items.[15]
- Pulling, rather than pushing, sterilizer carts during transfer to aerators directs the flow of EO vapors and residues away from health care personnel.
- When using a separate mechanical aerator, health care personnel should be protected from EO vapors and residue during transfer of sterilized items from the sterilizer to the aerator.
- The transfer of products from a sterilizer to an aerator should be performed in as short a time as possible.

V.f.2. Required aeration times depend on many variables that include, but are not limited to,
- item composition and size,
- item preparation and packaging,
- density of the load,
- type of EO sterilizer used,
- type of aerator used, and
- temperature penetration pattern of the aerator's chamber.[15]

V.f.3. All EO-sterilized items must be completely aerated before they can be used safely.
- Aeration cycles should never be interrupted to remove items for use.
- Items should remain in aerators until the aeration time has been completed.
- Aeration requirements for the most difficult-to-aerate products may require increased time frames. Ethylene oxide vapors and residues diffuse from sterilized items over time. This aeration or degassing process can be expedited by raising the temperature and by increasing the flow of air around the item.
- Whenever possible, EO-sterilized items should be processed in sterilizers that have an integrated aeration cycle.

V.f.4. The device manufacturers' written instructions should be followed for specific aeration requirements.

V.f.5. All aeration cycle parameters should be documented and verified as to the accuracy of the correct aeration time and temperature.

V.f.6. A program for monitoring occupational exposure to EO must be established according to OSHA regulations to accurately determine the permissible airborne concentrations of EO within the health care setting.

Compliance with regulations promotes a safe work environment that is within federal and state mandated limits.[18,20]

V.g. Personnel who have the potential for exposure should wear EO-monitoring badges that meet the National Institute for Occupational Safety and Health standards for accuracy.[15,21,22]

V.g.1. The EO-monitoring program in each organization must comply with OSHA regulations.[16]

General environmental monitoring is not required, although it may provide an indicator of problems with the ventilation or EO system.[15]

Monitoring of short term exposures over a 15-minute period also is required while sterilizer and aeration activities are being performed.

V.h. Health and safety procedures should be developed for health care personnel.

Established procedures help to identify, eliminate, or minimize risk from exposure to hazards as well as facilitate timely response to accidental exposure and emergencies.

V.h.1. Personnel should be informed about the health effects and potential hazards associated with exposure to EO.

V.h.2. Information on the EO health effects and potential hazards should be provided at the time of assignment to an area where EO is used and at least annually thereafter.

V.h.3. Periodic employee and environmental physical assessment and testing should be carried out and documented according to current OSHA regulations.[15,21,23]

V.h.4. Personnel should be familiar with the organization's emergency spill plan.[18]

V.h.5. Personnel should be aware of safety procedures that should be implemented following exposure to EO.

People who have inhaled concentrated EO gas

- should seek fresh air immediately;
- may require the administration of oxygen; and
- may require cardiopulmonary resuscitation, if respiratory or cardiac collapse occurs.[15,19]

The material safety data sheet (MSDS) for the type of ethylene oxide used should be consulted for specific first-aid measures after exposure.

V.i. Documentation of employee breathing zone EO monitoring must be maintained in employees' health records for the duration of employment plus 30 years after termination of employment.[15,23]

Documentation establishes a continuous history of the work environment.

Recommendation VI

Low-temperature hydrogen peroxide gas plasma sterilization methods should be used for moisture-sensitive and heat-sensitive items and when indicated by the device manufacturer.

Low-temperature hydrogen peroxide gas plasma sterilization uses a combination of hydrogen peroxide vapor and low-temperature hydrogen peroxide gas plasma.[74] In this process, microbial life is disrupted when free radicals created from hydrogen peroxide gas plasma interact with microbial cell membranes, enzymes, or nucleic acids.[16]

Items processed using a low-temperature hydrogen peroxide gas plasma sterilization require no aeration because the residuals and by-products are oxygen and water in the form of humidity.[16,25,26] Items are dry at the end of the cycle.

Hydrogen peroxide is a severe irritant, but it is considered nonmutagenic and noncarcinogenic.[16,24,27]

VI.a. The sterilizer manufacturer's written instructions for use, monitoring, and maintenance should be followed when using a low-temperature hydrogen peroxide gas plasma sterilization system. (PNDS: I75, I98, I122)

VI.a.1. Written documentation of the acceptability of low-temperature hydrogen peroxide gas plasma sterilization for specific devices should be obtained from the instrument manufacturer.

VI.a.2.　Devices with lumens should comply with the sterilizer manufacturer's lumen specifications relating to diameter and length of the device.[26,27,28]

VI.b.　Items to be gas-plasma sterilized should clean and dry and packaged in nonwoven polypropylene wraps, high-density polyethylene, or biaxially oriented polyethylene terephthalate polyester film (ie, Mylar®) pouches.

Cellulose-based (eg, paper-based) packaging materials or products and liquids are not suitable for low-temperature hydrogen peroxide gas plasma sterilization.

VI.c.　Trays designed and validated for use with low-temperature hydrogen peroxide gas plasma sterilization should be used.

VI.d.　When loading a low-temperature hydrogen peroxide gas plasma sterilizer, the load configuration and placement of items inside the sterilizers should comply with the sterilizer manufacturer's recommendations. (PNDS: I122)

Proper load configuration allows sterilant contact.[3]

Recommendation VII

Sterilization systems using peracetic acid as a low-temperature liquid sterilant is appropriate for heat-sensitive surgical items that can be immersed and when indicated by the device manufacturer.

Peracetic acid sterilization is a system that uses a chemical formulation of 35% peracetic acid and water. Peracetic acid is an oxidizing agent that is an effective biocide at low temperatures and is effective in the presence of organic matter. It has a chemical formula of acetic acid plus an extra oxygen atom. This extra oxygen atom is highly reactive, reacts with most cellular components, and causes cellular death. The ability of peracetic acid to inactivate many different critical cell systems is responsible for its broad spectrum antimicrobial activity. As peracetic acid returns to acetic acid (ie, vinegar) and the oxygen decomposes, it is rendered nontoxic and environmentally safe.

VII.a.　Items sterilized by liquid peracetic acid sterilization should be used immediately. This sterilization technique should not be used for items to be stored for later use without additional processing. (PNDS: I70, I75, I98: I122)

VII.b.　Sterilization systems using liquid peracetic acid should be used, monitored, and maintained according to the manufacturer's written instructions. (PNDS: I70, I98, I122)

Peracetic acid is an effective sterilizing agent that does not leave toxic residues on sterilized items when items are rinsed properly. Serious injuries (eg, burns) may result if the chemical is not handled, neutralized, and rinsed properly. Peracetic acid is corrosive to the skin at concentrations of 3.4% or higher and corrosive to eyes at concentrations of 0.35% or higher.[26-29]

VII.c.　Health care personnel should clean and process endoscopes and their accessories according to AORN's "Recommended practices for cleaning and processing endoscopes and endoscope accessories,"[30] and the manufacturer's specific instructions when using peracetic acid, as with other sterilization/disinfection processes. (PNDS: I75, I98, I122)

Peracetic acid is an efficient, effective method for cleaning and disinfecting endoscopes and accessories with lumens in order to provide high-quality patient care, ensure equipment integrity, and facilitate rapid turn around on endoscopes and other items that need to be used quickly.[26,29]

VII.d.　When using peracetic acid to sterilize items with lumens, health care personnel should verify proper selection of adapters and connect the device to the appropriate adapters as recommended by the manufacturer of both the device and sterilizer. (PNDS: I70, I75, I98, I122)

Failure to do so may result in failure to sterilize the lumen of the item.

VII.e.　Items sterilized in an automated system using peracetic acid should be transported to the point of use and used immediately. (PNDS: I70, I98, I122)

Items sterilized with peracetic acid are wet and the cassette or container in which they are sterilized is not sealed to prevent contamination, thereby increasing the risk of contamination if not used immediately.

VII.f.　The ability to successfully process devices intended for use with a peracetic acid system should be validated by the device manufacturer and comply with the sterilizer manufacturer's written instructions. (PNDS: I122)

Exposure and cycle times are important factors in assessing the efficiencies of a decontamination or sterilization process.

VII.f.1. Appropriate use of sterilizers should be identified to ensure proper sterilization and prolong the life of instrumentation.

VII.f.2. Documentation of items that can and cannot be processed in peracetic acid should be obtained from the device and sterilizer manufacturers.

Peracetic acid can be corrosive to some items not meant for this type of processing.

Recommendation VIII

Sterilization systems using ozone should be used for moisture and heat-sensitive items when indicated by the device manufacturer.

Ozone is a strong oxidizer, which makes ozone sterilization an effective low-temperature sterilization process. Ozone is generated within the sterilizer using only oxygen and water. On completion of the sterilization cycle, ozone is exhausted through a catalytic converter, where it is converted back into the raw materials of oxygen and water. No aeration of sterilized items is necessary because these by-products are nontoxic.[16,28,29,31]

VIII.a. Manufacturers' written instruction for operating, monitoring, and maintaining ozone sterilizers should be followed. (PNDS: I122)

Ozone has been cleared by the US Food and Drug Administration (FDA) for use in the sterilization of metal and plastic surgical instruments, including some instruments with lumens.

VIII.a.1. All devices should comply with the sterilizer manufacturer's specifications for lumen length and diameter.

VIII.b. Items to be processed in ozone should be packaged in nonwoven pouches or reusable rigid sterilization containers validated by the container manufacturer for use in ozone sterilizers.[28,31] (PNDS: I70, I98, I122)

Cellulose-based packaging materials and products are not suitable for ozone sterilization processes.

Recommendation IX

Dry-heat sterilization should be used to sterilize anhydrous (ie, waterless) items that can withstand high temperatures and when indicated by the device manufacturer.

Sharp instruments that would be damaged by the moisture of steam may be sterilized by dry-heat.[9] Dental instruments, burrs, reusable needles, glassware, and heat-stable powders and oils are examples of items that can withstand the high temperatures generated by dry-heat sterilization. Dry heat is an oxidation or slow burning process that coagulates protein in microbial cells. There is no moisture present in a dry-heat process, so microorganisms are destroyed by a very slow process of heat absorption.

IX.a. Dry-heat sterilizers should be used, monitored, and maintained according to the manufacturer's written instructions. (PNDS: I122)

Dry heat sterilizers may vary in design and performance characteristics.

IX.b. Only packaging and container materials designed to withstand the high temperature of the dry-heat sterilization should be used for this type of processing. (PNDS: I122)

If packaging is not formulated for dry-heat sterilization, pouches may char, compromising the aseptic presentation and storage of sterilized items.

IX.b.1. Closed containers or cassettes may extend the time needed to achieve sterilization; therefore, the use of such containers should be based on manufacturers' instructions and biological indicator monitoring results.

IX.b.2. Manufacturers should be consulted to confirm the compatibility of the packaging material with sterilizer temperatures before packaging materials are selected for dry-heat sterilization.[32]

IX.b.3. When possible, small containers should be used for items to be dry-heat sterilized, and package density should be as low as possible.[32]

Most types of tape are not designed to withstand the high dry-heat sterilization temperatures. Tape adhesive melts when subjected to dry-heat sterilization and may leave a sticky residue on sterilized packages that degrades, leaving baked-on tape residue on the items, or can result in loss of tape adhesion.[32]

IX.c.   The operator should be aware of the hazards associated with dry-heat sterilization and use the appropriate protective equipment (eg, insulated gloves, transfer handles).[32] (PNDS: I122)

Burns are the most common safety hazard associated with dry-heat sterilization.

IX.c.1.   On completion of the sterilization cycle, both the sterilizer chamber and the items in the chamber are very hot and should not be touched.

IX.c.2.   Packages should be cooled before being handled or removed from the dry-heat sterilizer.

IX.d.   Presterilized oils and powders are commercially available and should be considered before purchasing a dry-heat sterilizer.

Dry-heat sterilizers are not commonly available in operating rooms or sterile processing departments.

When used, the main purpose of a dry-heat sterilizer is to sterilize talcum powder for surgical procedures.

Recommendation X

A formalized program between health care organizations and health care industry representatives should be established for the receipt and use of loaner instrumentation.

Implementation of tracking and quality controls and procedures are necessary to manage instrumentation and implants brought in from outside organizations and companies.[33]

X.a.   Interdisciplinary collaboration between the health care organizations' sterile processing, operative services and commercial health care industry representatives should be established.

The systematic management of loaner instrumentation reduces loss and ensures proper decontamination and sterilization through increased communication and accountability.

X.a.1.   The loaner instrumentation process should include, but not be limited to,

- requesting loaner instrumentation or implant; (PNDS: I85)
- receiving loaner items, including a detailed inventory list; (PNDS: I85)
- obtaining manufacturers' written instruction for instrument care, cleaning, assembly, and sterilization; (PNDS: I122)
- cleaning, decontaminating, and sterilizing borrowed instrumentation by the receiving facility, performed in accordance with AORN's "Recommended practices for cleaning and care of surgical instruments and powered equipment;"[2] (PNDS: I70, I98, I138)
- transporting processed loaner instrumentation to the point of use; (PNDS: I98)
- returning items to the sterile processing department following the procedure for decontamination, processing, inventory, and return to the health care industry representative; (PNDS: I98) and
- maintaining historical records of transactions.

X.b.   Personnel should coordinate requests for loaner instrumentation in sufficient time for loaner items to be processed by conventional sterilization methods. (PNDS: I138)

Advance delivery of loaner items to the receiving health care organization ensures sufficient time to permit in-house disassembly, cleaning, packaging, quality assurance testing, and sterilization of the instruments before scheduled procedures.

X.b.1.   Personnel requesting loaner items should specify quantities, estimated time of use and return, and restocking requirements to circumvent the need for flash sterilization.

X.b.2.   Flash sterilization should not be used as a substitute for sufficient instrument inventory resulting from late delivery of loaner instrumentation.

X.c.   Loaner instrumentation sterility assurance should begin on receipt at the point where the health care organization personnel assume responsibility for the items.[3]

Failures in instrument cleaning have resulted in transmission of infectious agents.

X.c.1. All loaner instruments should be considered contaminated and delivered directly to the decontamination area for processing. Instruments should be thoroughly cleaned and dried in a manner consistent with AORN's "Recommended practices for cleaning and care of surgical instruments and powered equipment"[2] and the standards of the Association for the Advancement of Medical Instrumentation before sterilization.[3,15] (PNDS: I70, I98, I122, I138)

X.c.2. Newly manufactured loaner items should be properly decontaminated before sterilization to remove bioburden and substances (eg, oils, greases) remaining on the item during the manufacturing process.[3]

X.c.3. Clean or sterile items transported to sterile processing should be removed from external shipping containers.[3]

External shipping containers may have potentially high microbial contamination due to environmental exposures during transport.

X.c.4. Rigid sterilization containers should be thoroughly inspected on receipt and cleaned and decontaminated according to manufacturers' instructions.

Containers should be inspected for integrity and function.

X.c.5. Loaner items, type, and quantity should be inventoried and documented.

X.c.6. Implants and instruments should be visually inspected for damage.

X.c.7. Manufacturers' instructions on processing and sterilizing loaner items should be followed.

X.c.8. Loaner items should be decontaminated and handled in accordance with organizational policy following the procedure.

X.c.9. Implantable devices should be sterilized with a BI and a Class 5 integrating indicator and documented in accordance with FDA regulations and AORN recommended practices.

Recommendation XI

Sterilized materials should be packaged, labeled, and stored in a manner to ensure sterility, and each item should be marked with the sterilization date.[3,34]

Limiting exposure to moisture, dust, excessive light or handling, and temperature and humidity extremes decreases potential contamination of sterilized items.[3]

XI.a. The shelf life of a packaged sterile item should be considered event-related. (PNDS: I70, I98, I122)

An event must occur to compromise package content sterility. Events that may compromise the sterility of a package include, but are not limited to,
 - multiple handling that leads to seal breakage or loss of package integrity,
 - moisture penetration, and
 - exposure to airborne contaminants.[3,15,32]

XI.b. Sterile packages should be stored under environmentally controlled conditions.[2] (PNDS: I70, I98, I122)

Controlled conditions reduce the risk of contamination.

XI.b.1 The temperature in the sterile storage areas should not exceed 24° C (75° F).

XI.b.2. The storage area should have at least four air exchanges per hour.

XI.b.3. Relative humidity should be controlled, not to exceed 70%.

XI.b.4. Traffic should be controlled to limit access to those trained in handling sterile supplies. (PNDS: I81)

XI.b.5. Supplies should be stored in a manner that allows adequate air circulation, ease of cleaning, and compliance with local fire codes. (PNDS: I98)

XI.b.6. Sterile items should be stored at least eight to 10 inches above the floor, at least 18 inches below sprinkler heads, and at least two inches from outside walls.

XI.b.7. Outside shipping containers should not be allowed in the sterile storage area because they serve as generators of, and reservoirs for, dust. (PNDS: I98)

XI.c.   Storage conditions should be evaluated before policies and procedures on event-related sterility are written for perioperative practice settings. (PNDS: I70, I98, I122, I138)

The shelf life of packaged sterile items is event-related and dependent on packaging material, storage conditions, transport and handling. Adequacy and quality of storage space are factors to be considered when writing policies and procedures.[3]

XI.c.1.   All storage items should be rotated according to the principle of "first in, first out."

Recommendation XII

Transportation of sterile items should be controlled.

Sterility is event-related and depends on the amount of handling, conditions during transportation and storage, and the quality of the packaging material.

XII.a.   Sterile items should be transported in covered or enclosed carts with solid-bottom shelves. (PNDS: I70, I81, I98, I122)

Covered or enclosed carts will protect sterile items from exposure to environmental contaminants during transportation.

XII.a.1.   Carts and reusable covers should be cleaned after each use because contaminants are picked up from the environment during transport.[3]

XII.b.   Written policies and procedures should address prevention of physical damage and maintenance of package sterility during transport.

Procedures for transporting sterile items can help preserve the quality of sterile packages and maintain the integrity of processed items until the time of use.[3,15]

XII.b.1.   Transportation conditions should be evaluated before policies and procedures for the transportation of sterile items are written for perioperative practice settings.[3,15,32] (PNDS: I70, I81, I98, I122, I138)

Recommendation XIII

Competency
An introduction and review of policies and procedures should be included in personnel orientation to sterile processing of surgical instruments in the perioperative setting. Continuing education should be provided for employees when new equipment, instruments, and processes are introduced. (PNDS: I1)

Operator and processing errors are minimized with regularly scheduled education, training, and competency demonstration.[3,15]

XIII.a.   Sterilization-specific education and competency assessment of personnel should encompass all sterilization methodologies in use in the organization, to include
   – operation and maintenance of sterilization equipment;
   – selection and monitoring of sterilization cycles;
   – use of chemical, biological, and physical monitoring measures; and
   – documentation requirements.

XIII.b.   Education should address, but not be limited to,
   – orientation programs to equipment and work area;
   – infection control policy and procedure, including exposure plans;
   – potential hazards in the environment and methods of hazard protection;
   – safe ergonomic practices; and
   – use and location of MSDS.

Recommendation XIV

Documentation
Sterilization records should be maintained for a time specified by the health care organization's policies and in compliance with local, state, and federal regulations.[3,15,32]

Accurate and complete records are required for process verification and used in sterilizer malfunction analyses. Documentation establishes accountability.

XIV.a.   Every sterilization cycle and modality, including steam (eg, wrapped, unwrapped), EO, hydrogen peroxide gas plasma, liquid peracetic acid, ozone, and dry heat should be documented. Documentation should include
   – the assigned lot number;
   – contents of each load; and
   – results of physical, chemical, and biological monitors.

Recommendation XV

Policies and Procedures

Policies and procedures for sterilization processes should be developed, reviewed periodically, and readily available in the practice setting. (PNDS: I1)

Policies and procedures establish authority, responsibility, and accountability and serve as operational guidelines. Policies and procedures also assist in the development of continuous quality improvement activities.

XV.a. Policies and procedures for routine cleaning of sterilizer chambers, carts, and exterior surfaces should be developed and implemented. (PNDS: I122)

XV.b. These recommended practices for sterilization should be used to guide the development of policies and procedures within individual perioperative practice settings.

XV.c. The sterilizer manufacturer's written instructions for cleaning should be reviewed and followed.

XV.d. An introduction and review of policies and procedures should be included in the orientation and ongoing education of health care personnel to assist in the development of knowledge, skills, and attitudes that affect patient outcomes.

XV.e. User manuals for all sterilization equipment should be readily available to the sterilizer operators. (PNDS: I122)

As new technologies are introduced for use in perioperative practice settings, it is imperative that health care personnel strictly follow manufacturers' written instructions for the operation and maintenance of sterilization equipment and are aware of the occupational hazards that different sterilants may pose to patients, health care personnel, and the environment. Compliance with the Safe Medical Device Act of 1990, which was amended in 2000, is required and will contribute to patient safety.[35]

XV.e.1. Equipment manuals should be retained for the life of the sterilizer.

XV.f. When selecting a new sterilization technology, perioperative nurses and nurse managers should follow AORN's "Recommended practices for product selection in perioperative practice settings."[36]

Capital equipment and medical device procurement are collaborative processes requiring clinical, business, financial, and legal acumen. Goals of product standardization and value analysis processes are to select functional and reliable products that are safe, cost-effective, and environmentally conscious and that promote quality care and avoid duplication or rapid obsolescence.

Recommendation XVI

Quality

A quality control program should be established and maintained. (PNDS: I1)

Quality control programs that enhance personnel performance and monitor sterilization efficacy are established to promote patient and employee safety.

XVI.a. The health care organization should establish quality control and improvement programs to monitor the work place environment and practices associated with cleaning, disinfection, and sterilization of surgical instruments.

Monitoring the sterilization process allows results to be compared to a predetermined level of quality. Reviewing the findings provide a method of identifying problems and trends to change and improve practice.

XVI.b. All sterilizer failures and corrective actions should be documented and reported to the infection control professional and/or quality assurance committee, and to administration.

XVI.c. All BI test results, including results from controls, should be interpreted by qualified personnel in the time frame specified by the BI manufacturer and should be included in the sterilization records. (PNDS: I70, I98, I122, I138)

Accurate interpretation and reporting of positive results promotes safe patient care.[3]

XVI.c.1. Positive BI test results should be reported immediately so that appropriate action can be taken.
- The sterilizer printout should first be checked to determine if the cycle parameters were met.

- If retrievable, items processed in the suspect sterilizer (ie, back to the last known negative BI test) should be recalled and reprocessed before use.[3]
- The positive BI vial should be sent to the laboratory for subculturing for bacilli (the recall should not be delayed during this testing).
- All actions taken in response to a positive BI test should be documented.
- A positive control should be placed in each incubator each day a test vial is run and incubated.

XVI.c.2. All control vials should be from the same lot number as the BI test vial for the test to be considered valid.[3]

XVI.d. Processed items should be labeled with lot control numbers to identify the sterilizer used, the cycle or load number, and the date of sterilization. (PNDS: I122)

Lot control numbers allow items to be identified or retrieved in the event of a sterilizer failure or malfunction.[3,15,32]

XVI.d.1. Information should be recorded from each sterilization cycle and should include, but not be limited to,

- identification of sterilizer (eg, "sterilizer #1");
- type of sterilizer and cycle used;
- lot control number; load contents (eg, major set, Kelly clamps);[3]
- critical parameters for the specific sterilization methodology (eg, exposure time, temperature for steam sterilization);
- operator's name; and
- results of sterilization process monitoring (ie, biological, chemical, physical).

XVI.e. Physical monitors should be used to verify time, temperature, and pressure recordings for steam sterilization cycles. (PNDS: I70, I98, I122)

Physical monitoring provides real-time assessment of cycle conditions while providing historical records by means of graphs, printouts, or charts. Reviewing data from physical monitoring can readily identify sterilizer malfunctions to expedite corrective actions.[3]

XVI.e.1. Recordings of physical data should be used, when available, for all sterilization methodologies to ascertain that sterilization systems function within manufacturers' specifications.[3,15]

XVI.e.2. The printout should be reviewed at the end of each cycle and signed by the sterilizer operator verifying that all sterilization parameters were met.

XVI.f. A sterilization chemical indicator should be used inside and outside each package and load sterilized. (PNDS: I122)

The purpose of the external chemical indicator is to differentiate between processed and unprocessed items.

Internal chemical indicators do not establish whether the item is sterile, but they do demonstrate that the contents were exposed to the sterilant.

XVI.f.1. Although external chemical indicators do not verify sterility, they help detect procedural errors and equipment malfunctions; therefore, the color change should be verified before opening.

XVI.f.2. An external chemical indicator should be used on the outside of each package unless the internal chemical indicator is visible.

XVI.f.3. Chemical indicators should be reviewed for a proper endpoint response (eg, color, migration or other change).

XVI.f.4. If the interpretation of the external or internal process monitors suggests inadequate processing, the item should not be used.[3,15,37] (PNDS: I70, I98, I122, I138)

XVI.f.5. The internal chemical indicator should be reviewed for a proper end point response (eg, color, migration, other change) before placing the items or tray on the sterile field.

XVI.g. Quality assurance testing of rigid containers should be performed before initial use, and periodically, according to manufacturers' written instructions.[3] (PNDS: I122, I138)

Rigid sterilization container systems vary widely in design, mechanics, and construction. These variables can affect the performance of characteristics and suitability of containers with sterilization methods.

XVI.g.1. The following measures should be evaluated when conducting periodic product quality assurance testing of sterilization containers for each sterilizer type used:
- sterilization efficacy, and
- drying effectiveness.

Health care organizations are responsible for obtaining and maintaining manufacturers' documentation of methodology and performance testing of the container system.

Health care personnel are responsible for ensuring that container systems are suitable for proposed sterilization uses and are compatible with existing sterilizers.

XVI.g.2. Personnel should perform product testing to verify and collaborate with the sterilizer manufacturer for resolution of technological concerns.

XVI.h. Sterilization conditions such as exposure time should be evaluated with physical, biological, and chemical monitoring by strategically placing monitors alongside each other at locations that present the greatest challenge to air evacuation and sterilant penetration. (PNDS: I70, I122, I138)

Table 6 indicates types and applications of sterilization monitoring devices.

XVI.h.1. Monitors should be used for routine load release, routine sterilizer efficacy monitoring, sterilizer qualification testing (eg, after installation, relocation, malfunctions, major repairs, sterilization process failures) and periodic product quality assurance testing for all sterilization processes. **Table 7** provides recommendations for sterilizer testing process monitoring.[3,15,32,33,38]

XVI.h.2. **Steam sterilizers:** *Geobacillus stearothermophilus* biological indicators should be used for routine load release, routine sterilizer efficacy monitoring, sterilizer qualification testing, and periodic product quality assurance testing.

Routine sterilizer efficacy monitoring should be done weekly, preferably daily, as follows:
- each load containing an implantable device should be monitored with a BI and quarantined until the results of the BI testing are available, and

- one BI PCD should be run in three consecutive empty cycles for sterilizer qualification testing.

If a steam sterilizer is intended to be used for multiple types of cycles (eg, gravity-displacement, dynamic air-removal, flash), each sterilization mode should be tested.[3]

XVI.h.3. **Ethylene oxide sterilizers:** *Bacillus atropheus* (formerly *Bacillus subtilis*) spore testing should be performed with every load.

XVI.h.4. **Low temperature hydrogen peroxide gas plasma sterilizers:** *Geobacillus stearothermophilus* biological indicators are used for routine load release, routine sterilizer efficacy monitoring, sterilizer qualification testing and periodic product quality assurance testing.[28]

Routine sterilizer efficacy monitoring should be done daily, preferably with each load, as follows:
- each load containing an implantable device should be monitored with a BI and quarantined until the results of the BI testing are available,
- one BI PCD should be run in three consecutive empty cycles for sterilizer qualification testing, and
- the sterilizer manufacturer should be consulted for the specific monitoring product(s) to use and the appropriate placement of the product within the sterilizer.

XVI.h.5. **Ozone sterilizers:** *Geobacillus stearothermophilus* biological indicators are used for routine load release, routine sterilizer efficacy monitoring, sterilizer qualification testing and periodic product quality assurance testing.[28]

Routine sterilizer efficacy monitoring should be done daily, preferably with each load, as follows:
- each load containing an implantable device should be monitored with a BI and quarantined until the results of the BI testing are available,
- one BI PCD should be run in three consecutive empty cycles for sterilizer qualification testing, and

Table 6

TYPES AND APPLICATIONS FOR USE OF STERILIZATION MONITORING DEVICES[1,2]		
Monitor	Frequency of Use	Application *(release of sterilizer, package, load)*
Physical Monitors Time, temperature, and pressure recorder displays; digital printouts; and gauges	Should be used for every load of every sterilizer.	Part of load release criteria.
Chemical Indicators (CIs)		
External CIs Class 1 (process indicators)	Should be used on outside of every package.	Part of load and package release criteria.
Bowie-Dick-type indicators Class 2 (Bowie-Dick)	For routine sterilizer testing (dynamic air-removal sterilizers only): Should be run within a test pack each day in an empty sterilizer before the first processed load.	Test of sterilizer efficacy of air removal and steam penetration; part of release criteria for using sterilizer for the day.
	For sterilizer qualification testing (dynamic-air-removal sterilizers only): Should be run within a test pack after sterilizer installation, relocation, malfunction; after major repairs; and after sterilization process failures. Test should be run three times consecutively in an empty chamber after biological indicator (BI) tests.	Part of release criteria for placing sterilizer into service after qualification testing.
Internal CIs	Should be used inside each package.	Part of package release criteria at use site.
	Should be used in periodic product quality assurance testing.	Part of release criteria for changes made to routinely sterilized items, load configuration, and/or packaging. Release criteria should include BI results.
Class 3 (single-variable indicator) Class 4 (multi-variable indicator)[2]	May be used to meet internal CI recommendation.	Part of package release criteria at use site; NOT to be used for release of loads.
Class 5 (integrating indicator) Enzyme-only indicator	• May be used to meet internal CI recommendation. • Within a process challenge device (PCD), may be used to monitor nonimplant sterilizer loads. • Within a PCD, should be used to monitor each sterilizer load containing implants. The PCD should also contain a BI.	• Part of package release criteria at use site. • Part of load release criteria for nonimplant loads. • Part of release criteria for loads containing implants. Except in emergencies, implants should be quarantined until BI results are known.
Biological Indicators	• Within a PCD, may be used to monitor nonimplant loads. • Within a PCD should be used in every load containing implants. The PCD should also contain a Class 5 integrating indicator or an enzyme-only indicator. • Within a PCD, should be used for weekly, preferably daily (ie, each day the sterilizer is used), routine sterilizer efficacy testing. (The PCD may also contain a CI.) Should be run in a full load for wrapped items; for table-top sterilization, should be run in a fully loaded chamber; for flash sterilization, should be run in an empty chamber. • Within a PCD should be used for sterilizer qualification testing (after sterilizer installation, relocation, malfunction, major repairs, sterilization process failures). The PCD may also contain a CI. • Test should be run three times consecutively in an empty chamber except for table-top sterilizers, where the test should be run three times consecutively in a full load. • Should be used for periodic product quality assurance testing.	• Part of load release criteria. • Part of release criteria for loads containing implants. Except in emergencies, implants should be quarantined until BI results are known. • Part of sterilizer/load release and recall criteria. • Part of release criteria for placing sterilizer into service after qualification testing. • Part of release criteria for changes made to routinely sterilized items, load configuration, and/or packaging.

Adapted with permission from Association for the Advancement of Medical Instrumentation.

1. Association for the Advancement of Medical Instrumentation. ANSI/AAMI ST79:2006—Comprehensive Guide to Steam Sterilization and Sterility Assurance in Health Care Facilities. *Arlington, VA: Association for the Advancement of Medical Instrumentation; 2006.*
2. Association for the Advancement of Medical Instrumentation. ANSI/AAMI/ISO 11140-1: Sterilization of health care products—Chemical indicators, Part 1: General requirements. *Arlington, VA: Association for the Advancement of Medical Instrumentation; 2005.*

Table 7

STERILIZATION PROCESS MONITORING RECOMMENDATIONS[1]				
Routine load release		Routine sterilizer efficacy monitoring	Sterilizer qualification testing *(after installation, relocation, malfunctions, major repairs, sterilization process failures)*	Periodic product quality assurance testing
Nonimplants	Implants			
Physical monitoring of cycle. External and internal chemical indicator monitoring of packages. Optional monitoring of the load with a process challenge device (PCD) containing one of the following: • a biological indicator (BI), • a BI and a Class 5 integrating indicator, • a BI and an enzyme-only indicator, • a Class 5 integrating indicator, • an enzyme-only indicator.	Physical monitoring of cycle. External and internal chemical indicator monitoring of packages. Monitoring of every load with a PCD containing a BI and a Class 5 integrating indicator or a PCD containing a BI and an enzyme-only indicator.	Physical monitoring of cycle. External and internal chemical indicator monitoring of packages. Weekly, preferably daily (or each day the sterilizer is used), monitoring of a full load with a PCD containing a BI. (The PCD may also contain a chemical indicator [CI].) In flash sterilization cycles, monitoring is done in an empty chamber. For dynamic air-removal sterilizers, daily Bowie-Dick testing in an empty chamber.	Physical monitoring of cycle. External and internal chemical indicator monitoring of packages. For sterilizers larger than 2 cubic feet and for flash sterilization cycles, monitoring of three consecutive cycles in an empty chamber with a PCD containing a BI. (The PCD may also contain a CI.) For table-top sterilizers, monitoring of three consecutive cycles in a fully loaded chamber with a PCD containing a BI. (The PCD may also contain a CI.) For dynamic air-removal sterilizers, monitoring of three consecutive cycles in a empty chamber with a Bowie-Dick test pack.	Physical monitoring of cycle. Placement of BIs and CIs within product test samples.

REFERENCE

1. Association for the Advancement of Medical Instrumentation. ANSI/AAMI ST79:2006—Comprehensive Guide to Steam Sterilization and Sterility Assurance in Health Care Facilities. Arlington, VA: Association for the Advancement of Medical Instrumentation; 2006. Adapted with permission.

- the sterilizer manufacturer should be consulted for the specific monitoring product(s) to use and the appropriate placement of the product within the sterilizer.

XVI.h.6. **Liquid peracetic acid sterilizers:** *Geobacillus stearothermophilus* biological indicators should be performed daily for routine sterilizer efficacy monitoring.
- The test product used should be designed specifically for use with liquid peracetic acid processes.
- The sterilizer manufacturer's written instructions for use should be followed.

XVI.h.7. **Dry-heat sterilizers:** *Bacillus atropheus* biological indicators should be used for routine load release, routine sterilizer efficacy monitoring, sterilizer qualification testing and periodic product quality assurance testing.

Routine sterilizer efficacy monitoring should be done weekly, preferably daily, as follows:
- each load containing an implantable device should be monitored with a BI and quarantined until the results of the BI testing are available;
- sterilizer qualification testing one BI PCD should be run in three consecutive empty cycles;
- mechanical convection (ie, forced air) dry-heat sterilizers should be monitored according to the manufacturer's recommendations, additional monitoring of three consecutive sterilization cycles should be performed after installation, major repair, redesign, or relocation of sterilizers; and
- this testing is performed in an otherwise empty sterilizer.

XVI.h.8. **Dynamic air-removal steam sterilizers:** A Bowie-Dick air removal test should routinely be performed daily in an empty chamber.
- The air-removal test is designed to detect residual air in the sterilizer chamber.
- The test should be run in accordance with the test manufacturer's instructions before the routine biological indicator testing.

Whenever a dynamic air-removal sterilizer is installed, relocated, malfunctions, undergoes a major repair, or has a sterilization process failure, three consecutive cycles in an empty chamber should be tested with a BI PCD followed by three consecutive cycles in an empty chamber with a Bowie-Dick test.

XVI.i. Preventive maintenance on sterilizers should be performed by qualified personnel on a scheduled basis. (PNDS I122)

Periodic inspections, maintenance, and replacement of components subject to wear (eg, recording devices, steam traps, filters, valves, drain pipes, gaskets) help maintain proper functioning of sterilizers.

XVI.i.1. Inspection and cleaning should be performed as outlined in the manufacturer's written instructions.[3,10,15]

Proper inspection and cleaning minimizes sterilizer downtime and helps prevent sterilizer malfunctions.

XVI.i.2. Preventive maintenance and repairs should be performed by qualified personnel as specified in the manufacturer's written instructions.

XVI.i.3. Maintenance records should be kept for each sterilizer. Accurate and complete records are required for sterilization process verification. Information should include, but not be limited to,
- date of service;
- sterilizer model and serial number;
- sterilizer location;
- description of malfunctions;
- name of person and company performing maintenance;
- description of service and parts replaced;
- results of biological indicator testing, if performed;
- results of Bowie-Dick testing, if performed;
- where appropriate, the name of the person requesting the service; and
- the signature and title of the person acknowledging the completed work.

Glossary

Aeration: Method by which absorbed ethylene oxide (EO) is removed from EO-sterilized items by circulating warm air in an enclosed cabinet specifically designed for this purpose.

Anhydrous: Items that are free of water.

Bioburden: The degree of microbial load; the number of viable organisms contaminating an object.

Biofilm: A thin coating containing biologically active organisms that have the ability to grow in water, water solutions, or in vivo and that coat the surface of structures (eg, teeth, inner surfaces of catheters, tubes, implanted or indwelling devices, instruments, other medical devices). Biofilms contain viable and nonviable microorganisms that adhere to the surface and are trapped within a matrix of organic matter (eg, proteins, glycoproteins, carbohydrates), which prevents antimicrobial agents from reaching the cells.

Biological indicator: A sterilization process-monitoring device commercially prepared with a known population of highly resistant spores that tests the effectiveness of the method of sterilization being used. The indicator is used to demonstrate that conditions necessary to achieve sterilization were met during the sterilizer cycle being monitored.

Chemical indicator: A sterilization-monitoring device used to monitor the attainment of one or more critical parameters required for sterilization. A characteristic color or other visual change indicates a defined level of exposure based on the classification of the chemical indicator used.

Class 5 chemical integrating indicator: A chemical indicator designed to react to all critical parameters over a specified range of sterilization cycles and whose performance has been correlated to the performance of the stated test organism under the labeled conditions of use.

Decontamination: Any physical or chemical process that removes or reduces the number of microorganisms or infectious agents and renders reusable medical products safe for handling or disposal; the process by which contaminants are removed, either by hand cleaning or mechanical means, using specific solutions capable of rendering blood and debris harmless and removing them from the surface of an object or instrument.

Downtime: A period of time when an item or device is not operational.

Dynamic air-removal: Mechanically assisted air removal from the sterilization chamber. Includes prevacuum and steam-flush pressure-pulse steam sterilizers.

Dynamic air-removal test (ie, Bowie-Dick test): A diagnostic test to determine the adequacy of air removal from the chamber of a dynamic-air-removal steam sterilizer. The air-removal test is not a test for sterilization.

Emergency spill plan: A plan of action for any unanticipated release of ethylene oxide or other hazardous chemicals into the workplace.

Flash sterilization: A process designed for the steam sterilization of patient care items for immediate use.

Gravity-displacement sterilizer: Type of sterilization cycle in which incoming air displaces residual air through a port or drain near the bottom of the sterilizer chamber.

Physical monitor: Automated devices (eg, graphs, gauges, printouts) that monitor sterilization parameters for the sterilization method in use.

Process challenge device: A predetermined item/package (ie, test pack) designed to simulate the product to be sterilized and that is used to assess the efficacy of the sterilization process.

Prevacuum steam sterilizer: A steam sterilization cycle in which air is removed from the chamber and load via a series of pressure and vacuum excursions.

Shelf life: The length of time an item is considered sterile and safe to use.

Short-term exposure limits: Durations of exposure to a potentially toxic or harmful substance lasting for less than 15 minutes that cannot be repeated more than four times per day.

Steam-flush pressure-pulse (SPPP): A steam sterilization cycle in which air is removed from the chamber and load via a series of steam flushes and pressure pulses.

Sterilization process monitoring device: A device used to monitor sterilization processes. Sterilization monitoring devices can be biological, chemical, or physical.

REFERENCES

1. Petersen, C, ed. *Perioperative Nursing Data Set.* Rev 2nd ed. Denver, CO: AORN, Inc: 2007.

2. Recommended practices for cleaning and care of surgical instruments and powered equipment. In: *Standards, Recommended Practices, and Guidelines.* Denver, CO: AORN, Inc; 2008:421-446.

3. Association for the Advancement of Medical Instrumentation. *ANSI/AAMI ST79: 2006—Comprehensive Guide to Steam Sterilization and Sterility Assurance in Health Care Facilities.* Arlington, VA: Association for the Advancement of Medical Instrumentation, 2006:4,24-25,36 37,39,54,60,62-74,77-80,83,87,90,110.

4. Alvarado CJ, Reichelderfer M. 1997-1999 APIC Guidelines Committee: APIC guideline for infection prevention and control in flexible endoscopy. *American Journal of Infection Control*. 2000;28:138-155.

5. Recommended practice for traffic patterns in the perioperative practice setting. In: *Standards, Recommended Practices, and Guidelines*. Denver, CO: AORN, Inc; 2007:703-706.

6. Recommended practices for selection and use of packaging systems. In: *Standards, Recommended Practices, and Guidelines*. Denver, CO: AORN, Inc; 2007:607-616.

7. Association for the Advancement of Medical Instrumentation. *ANSI/AAMI/ISO 11607—Packaging for Terminally Sterilized Medical Devices*. Arlington, VA: Association for the Advancement of Medical Instrumentation, 2000.

8. Position statement on ergonomically healthy workplace practices. In: *Standards, Recommended Practices, and Guidelines*. Denver, CO: AORN, Inc; 2007:382.

9. Joslyn LJ. Sterilization by heat. In: *Disinfection, Sterilization, and Preservation*. 5th ed. Block SS, ed. Philadelphia, PA: Lippincott Williams & Wilkins; 2001: 695-728.

10. Association for the Advancement of Medical Instrumentation. *ANSI/AAMI ST8—Hospital steam sterilizers*. Arlington, VA: Association for the Advancement of Medical Instrumentation; 2001.

11. Clement L, Bliley J. Cracking the steam sterilizer door: Dispelling the myth. *Healthcare Purchasing News*. May 2007:40-42.

12. Mangram AJ, Horan TC, Pearson ML, Silver LC, Jarvis WR. Guideline for prevention of surgical site infection, 1999. [Special Report]. *Infection Control and Hospital Epidemiology*. 1999; 20:250-278. Available at *http://www.cdc.gov/ncidod/dhqp/pdf/guidelines/SSI.pdf*. October 26, 2007.

13. Conviser S. The Future of Ethylene Oxide Sterilization. *Infection Control Today*. June 2000. Available at *http://www.infectioncontroltoday.com/articles/061feat4.html*. Accessed October 26, 2007.

14. US Environmental Protection Agency. Code of Federal Regulations Title 40: Protection of Environment, Part 261. Identification and Listing of Hazardous Waste. Available at *http://www.epa.gov/epahome/cfr40.htm*. Accessed October 26, 2007.

15. Association for the Advancement of Medical Instrumentation. *ANSI/AAMI ST41—Ethylene Oxide Sterilization in Health Care Facilities: Safety and Effectiveness*. Arlington, VA: Association for the Advancement of Medical Instrumentation; 2000.

16. Joslyn LJ. Gaseous chemical sterilization. In: *Disinfection, Sterilization, and Preservation*. 5th ed. Block SS, ed. Philadelphia, PA: Lippincott Williams & Wilkins; 2001:337-359.

17. Crane T, Preziotti R. Hospital sterilization after the CFC phase out. [Viewpoint]. *Surgical Services Management*. 1996;2:10-11.

18. US Department of Labor, Occupational Safety and Health Administration. 29 CFR 1910.1047, Ethylene oxide. Available at *http://www.osha.gov/pls/oshaweb/owadisp.show_document?p_table=STANDARDS&p_id=10070*. Accessed October 26, 2007.

19. Material Safety Data Sheet: Ethylene Oxide Sterilant, April 23, 2007. St. Louis, MO: STERIS Corporation: 2007:1-2.

20. US Department of Labor, Occupational Safety and Health Administration. Hazard communication in the 21st century workplace; March 2004. Available at *http://www.osha.gov/dsg/hazcom/finalmsdsreport.html*. Accessed October 26, 2007.

21. Schneider PM. Ethylene oxide sterilization: employee monitoring. In: *Sterilization Technology for the Heath Care Facility*. 2nd ed. Reichert M, Young JH, eds. Gaithersburg, MD: Aspen Publishers; 1997:220-227.

22. National Institute for Occupational Safety and Health. Appendix I Guidelines For Minimizing Worker Exposure To Ethylene Oxide. Current Intelligence Bulletin 35. Available at *http://www.cdc.gov/niosh/81130_35.html#Recommendations*. Accessed October 26, 2007.

23. US Department of Labor, Occupational Safety and Health Administration. 29 CFR 1910.1020, Access to employee exposure and medical records. Available at *http://www.osha.gov/pls/oshaweb/owadisp.show_document?p_table=STANDARDS&p_id=10027*. Accessed October 26, 2007.

24. *Material Safety Data Sheet 09461-0-001: Hydrogen Peroxide Solution, August 7, 2003*. Irvine, CA: Advanced Sterilization Products; 2003:1-8.

25. Rutala WA, Gergen MF, Weber DJ. Comparative evaluation of the sporicidal activity of new low-temperature sterilization technologies: ethylene oxide, 2 plasma sterilization systems, and liquid peracetic acid. *American Journal of Infection Control*. 1998;26:393-398.

26. Jacobs PT, Lin SM. Sterilization processes utilizing low-temperature plasma. In: *Disinfection, Sterilization, and Preservation*. 5th ed. Block SS, ed. Philadelphia, PA: Lippincott Williams & Wilkins; 2001:747-763.

27. Malchesky PS. Medical applications of peracetic acid. In: *Disinfection, Sterilization, and Preservation*. 5th ed. Block SS, ed. Philadelphia, PA: Lippincott Williams & Wilkins; 2001:979-996.

28. Association for the Advancement of Medical Instrumentation. *AAMI ST58 Chemical Sterilization and High Level Disinfection in Health Care Facilities*. Arlington, VA: Association for the Advancement of Medical Instrumentation; 2005.

29. Smith DF. STERRAD 200 Sterilization System. Advanced Sterilization Products: 2000: 1-22. Available at: *http://sterrad.com/SI/Products_&_Services/STERRAD/STERRAD_200_GMP/Literature/200_white_paper.pdf*. Accessed October 26, 2007.

30. Recommended practices for cleaning and processing endoscopes and endoscope accessories. In: *Standards, Recommended Practices, and Guidelines*. Denver, CO: AORN, Inc;2007:531-536.

31. Weavers LK, Wickramanayake GB. Disinfection and sterilization using ozone. In: *Disinfection, Sterilization, and Preservation*. 5th ed. Block SS, ed. Philadelphia, PA: Lippincott Williams, & Wilkins; 2001:205-214.

32. Association for the Advancement of Medical Instrumentation. *ANSI/AAMI ST40—Table-top Dry Heat (Heated Air) Sterilization and Sterility Assurance in Health Care Facilities*. Arlington, VA: Association for the Advancement of Medical Instrumentation; 2004.

33. *ASHCSP/IAHCSMM Position Paper on Loaner Instrumentation.* http://www.iahcsmm.org/current_issues_Joint_paper_loaner_instrumentation.htm. Accessed October 26, 2007.

34. US Department of Health and Human Services; Centers for Medicaid and Medicare Services (CMS) State Operations Manual Appendix L, §416.42 Condition for Coverage: Surgical Services, *http://www.cms.hhs.gov/manuals/downloads/som107ap_l_ambulatory.pdf.* Accessed October 26, 2007.

35. Medical device reporting: manufacturer reporting, importer reporting user facility reporting, distributor reporting; final rule. *Federal Register.* 2000;65 no 17:4112-4121. Also available at *http://www.fda.gov/OHRMS/DOCKETS/98fr/012600c.pdf.* Accessed October 26, 2007.

36. Recommended practices for product selection in perioperative practice settings. In: *Standards, Recommended Practices, and Guidelines.* Denver, CO: AORN, Inc; 2007:637-640.

37. Association for the Advancement of Medical Instrumentation. *ANSI/AAMI/ISO 15882 Sterilization of Health Care Products—Chemical Indicators—Guidance for the Selection, Use, and Interpretation of Results.* Arlington, VA: Association for the Advancement of Medical Instrumentation; 2003.

38. Recommended practices for sterilization in the perioperative setting. In: *Standards, Recommended Practices, and Guidelines.* Denver, CO: AORN, Inc; 2007:673-687.

Resources

Bailey A. Updating sterilization technology. *Infection Control and Sterilization Technology.* 1995;2:31-33.

Bastedo G. Ethylene oxide sterilization. [Viewpoint]. *Surgical Services Management.* 1995;1:14-15.

Bronowicki JP, Venard V, Botte C, et al. Patient-to-patient transmission of hepatitis C virus during colonoscopy. [Brief Report]. *New England Journal of Medicine.* 1997;337:237-240.

Centers for Disease Control and Prevention. Bronchoscopy-related infections and pseudoinfections—New York, 1996 and 1998. *Morbidity and Mortality Weekly Report.* 1999;48:557-576. Available at *http://www.cdc.gov/mmwr/preview/mmwrhtml/mm4826a1.htm.* Accessed August 3, 2007.

Chobin N. Cost analysis of three low-temperature sterilization systems at Saint Barnabas Medical Center. *Journal of Healthcare Materiel Management.* 1994;12:29-32.

DesCoteaux JG, Poulin EC, Julien M, Guidon R. Residual organic debris on processed surgical instruments. *AORN Journal.* 1995;62:23-30.

Gross D. Ethylene oxide sterilization and alternative methods. [Viewpoint]. *Surgical Services Management.* 1995;1:16-18.

Lagergren E. Gas plasma sterilization. [Viewpoint]. *Surgical Services Management.* 1995;1:26-28.

Spry C. Sterilization regulations—who's in charge here? [Focus on Quality]. *Surgical Services Management.* 1995;1:56-59.

Tablan OC, Anderson LJ, Besser R, et al. Guidelines for preventing health care-associated pneumonia, 2003. Recommendations of the Centers for Disease Control and Prevention and the Healthcare Infection Control Practices Advisory Committee. *Morbidity and Mortality Weekly Report.* 2004;53 no RR03:1-36. Available at *http://www.cdc.gov/mmwr/preview/mmwrhtml/rr5303a1.htm.* Accessed August 3, 2007.

Ward SF. Today's new sterilization technology presents new decision variables. [Editorial]. *Surgical Services Management.* 1995;1:4-5.

Publication History

Originally published August 1980, *AORN Journal.* Format revision July 1982.

Revised February 1987, October 1992. Published as proposed recommended practices in July 1994.

Revised; published August 1999, *AORN Journal.* Reformatted July 2000.

Revised November 2005; published March 2006, *AORN Journal.*

Revised 2007; published in *Perioperative Standards and Recommended Practices,* 2008 edition.

Minor editing revisions made in November 2010 for publication in *Perioperative Standards and Recommended Practices,* 2011 edition.

AORN Perioperative Standards and Recommended Practices, 2012 Edition

AORN
Guidelines
and Guidance
Statements

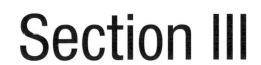

Section III

AORN Perioperative Standards and Recommended Practices, 2012 Edition

AORN Guidance Statement: Environmental Responsibility

Introduction

This document is intended to guide perioperative registered nurses in the development of environmentally responsible practices. This document may be used by health care organizations to provide direction for the creation of environmentally responsible policies and procedures. This guidance document addresses

- infectious and noninfectious waste management;
- recycling practices;
- resource conservation;
- supply conservation and management practices;
- reprocessing, reuse, repair and refurbishing;
- sterilization and disinfection; and
- construction for efficiency and conservation.

It is recognized that not all portions of this document may be usable by all health care organizations because of the varying standards and regulations set forth in various geographic locations. It also is recognized that the perioperative setting is varied and includes hospitals; obstetrical surgical suites; ambulatory facilities; physicians' offices; specialty centers for invasive procedures (eg, cardiac catheterization laboratories, radiology departments, endoscopy suites); and other areas where invasive procedures or interventions are performed.

Background

Nurses comprise a large single group of health care providers and are in a position to influence environmental management practices. Nurses have long played a role in the protection of the environment. In the 1800s, Florence Nightingale was one of the first nurses to advocate for a healthy environment.[1] Nurses have an ethical responsibility to actively promote and participate in resource conservation and to protect the environment.

US health care organizations generate in excess of two million tons of waste annually.[2] Approximately 85% of this waste is noninfectious, with a large amount being generated in the operating room.[3] Inpatient facilities spend more than five billion dollars a year on energy consumption. Health care energy consumption is increasing to support new and existing technology.[4] Sterilizing, heating and cooling processes, and hand sanitization contribute to use of water, a limited natural resource. In addition to waste generation, energy and water consumption has a significant negative impact on the environment.

Guidance Statement

The perioperative registered nurse should serve as a steward of the environment by being knowledgeable about perioperative practices that negatively affect the environment. Perioperative registered nurses should actively promote and participate in resource conservation. Effective resource conservation leads to an improvement of environmental health. The perioperative registered nurse should strive to understand the political, economic, and public health components of environmental responsibility.[5] The following strategies provide a framework on which to build an environmentally responsible practice.

Infectious and Noninfectious Tissue and Waste Management

More than four million tons[2] of general waste are produced annually by US health care facilities.[6] Waste materials can be classified as potentially infectious or noninfectious. Waste management is a major expenditure for health care organizations. Infectious waste management alone can consume as much as 20% of a hospital's annual budget for environmental services.[7]

Waste generated from the operating room includes potentially infectious and noninfectious waste as well as material that requires special disposal (eg, liquid chemicals, hazardous materials). Mercury-based products and dioxin generated by incineration of polyvinylchloride (PVC) are hazardous chemicals. Mercury, a heavy metal and neurotoxin, is a frequent contaminant found in medical waste. Dioxin, a known human carcinogen, has been implicated in cancer of the lung, thyroid, hematopoietic system, and liver as well as soft tissue sarcoma.[8] Polyvinylchloride is found in many medical supplies, packaging, and building materials. The resulting air pollutants from medical waste incineration not only affect the local community, but also can migrate to pollute distant environments and populations.[8] Disposal of mercury and medical waste are subject to regulation by local, state, or federal governmental agencies. Health care organizations must comply with the regulations.[9]

Perioperative nurses can significantly affect waste management practices by encouraging and implementing strategies that promote a safe and healthy environment. These strategies should be cost effective and conserve resources. Strategies

---

that should be considered include, but are not limited to, the following.

- Conduct a survey to assess types of waste generated in perioperative practice settings.
- Conduct a cost analysis of waste management considering
  - the volume of noninfectious waste, and
  - the weight of potentially infectious waste generated and treatment technology available.[7]
- Define potentially infectious waste according to local, state, and federal regulations.
- Provide education to all health care workers, to include, but not be limited to,
  - the definition of potentially infectious waste,
  - the importance of and process for segregation of potentially infectious waste from noninfectious waste,
  - the costs of waste management,
  - the environmental impact of waste disposal,[10] and
  - state and federal guidelines and regulations for disposal of waste.
- Review and update organization-wide waste management policies.
- Limit contents of biohazardous waste containers (eg, red bags) to potentially infectious waste.
- Explore methods of waste segregation, which may include
  - placing noninfectious waste and biohazard containers side by side in a convenient location, and
  - using a bag-in-bag collection system (ie, clear bag inserted inside red bag for collection of waste used to set up for a procedure; clear bag is removed from bag holder but left in room before start of procedure when infectious waste may be generated).[7] Consider risks to health care workers when using this system.
- Eliminate use of mercury-based products—ie, inventory, remove, and replace mercury-containing devices with nonmercury-containing devices (eg, digital thermometers, sphygmomanometers, batteries, bougies, cantor tubes, fluorescent lights).[3]
- Work with waste management services to explore alternatives to incineration, including, but not limited to,
  - microwaving,
  - autoclaving,
  - radiowaving, and
  - electrotechnologies.[11]

- Explore recycling programs for noninfectious waste (eg, paper, irrigation bottles, sterilization wraps and other plastics).
- Evaluate the environmental impact of reusable, reposable, and disposable products.
- Develop an ongoing performance improvement program for waste management.
- Dispose of chemicals in accordance with state and local regulations, including, but not limited to,
  - dilution,
  - inactivation of solution before release, and
  - consideration of a program of controlled release.[12]
- Consider membership in Healthy Hospitals for the Environment (H2E), located online at *http://www.H2E-online.org* (accessed 23 Jan 2006); and Health Care Without Harm (HCWH), located online at *http://www.noharm.org* (accessed 23 Jan 2006).[8]

Recycling Practices

A significant amount of hospital waste is composed of noninfectious material, much of which may be recyclable.[13,14] Recyclable items found in the perioperative environment include, but are not limited to, plastic bottles, sterilization wrap, peel packs, glass, paper, aluminum and metal cans, and corrugated cardboard.[15,16] Only items that are clean and noninfectious, as defined by local, state, and federal regulations, should be recycled.[3] Recycling noninfectious waste materials has environmental and financial benefits that may include[17]

- providing materials for remanufacture,
- preserving resources for future generations,
- decreasing air and water pollution,
- conserving energy, and
- limiting the expansion of landfills and incinerator use.

Health care facilities should modify purchasing and waste disposal practices to favor recycling.[14,16] Perioperative nurses can significantly affect waste management practices by encouraging and implementing recycling strategies that promote a safe and healthy environment. These strategies should be cost effective and conserve resources. Strategies that should be considered include, but are not limited to, the following.

- Perform a waste assessment to identify items appropriate for recycling.
- Investigate available community recycling programs to determine feasibility of participation.

- Obtain recycling containers from local waste management systems.[18]
- Begin with simple items (eg, paper, cardboard, plastics).
- Contact manufacturers regarding recycling programs.
- Identify waste versus recycling receptacles with distinguishing features:
  - use color-coded receptacles (eg, green for paper, silver for metal, blue for plastic); and
  - use a slotted top for paper, a round top for cans.
- Provide receptacles in areas where the waste is generated.
- Provide education to all health care workers regarding recycling practices, including separation procedures.[18]
- Implement a process improvement program to demonstrate changes and to identify additional recycling opportunities.
- Give feedback to health care workers related to the results of the waste management efforts to reinforce this behavior.

Resource Conservation

Health care organizations should conserve finite natural resources such as water, electricity, and natural gas. The average water consumption by US hospitals is 139,214 gallons per day.[19] Health care organizations use 62 billion kilowatt hours of electricity annually, with a higher intensity than other commercial buildings (ie, 26.5 kWh per square foot).[20] The average per square foot consumption of electricity in health care organizations is $1.67, compared to $0.99 per square foot in commercial buildings, and inpatient facilities use more electricity than outpatient facilities.[20] Conserving electricity minimizes air pollution caused by electrical generation and reduces costs.[20]

Heath care organizations also consume large quantities of natural gas (252 billion cubic feet annually) and have a much higher natural gas intensity than the average commercial building (143.0 cubic feet per square foot).[21] The average per square foot consumption of natural gas is $0.48 per square foot compared, to $0.24 per square foot in commercial buildings.[21]

Perioperative registered nurses should actively promote and participate in resource conservation measures for water, electricity, and natural gas. Conservation strategies should be incorporated into daily practice, including, but not limited to, the following:

- Conduct a resource utilization assessment.
- Provide education to health care workers about the importance and benefits of resource conservation.[19,22]
- Create resource conservation suggestion boxes and place in prominent areas.[23,24]
- Install signs encouraging resource conservation.[23,24]
- Develop a team of health care workers (eg, "green team") to evaluate resource conservation opportunities and effectiveness.[16,24]
- To conserve electricity,
  - install occupancy sensors in certain areas of the practice setting to control lighting based on the presence or absence of personnel and patients;[25]
  - turn off lights when rooms are not in use;[26]
  - turn off equipment when not in use;[24]
  - install and use energy-efficient electrical equipment, lights, and appliances;
  - reduce flow to surgical vacuum pumps to minimum acceptable level and maintain proper operation;[23,27] and
  - insulate hot water pipes.[28]
- To conserve natural gas,
  - insulate hot water pipes,[28] and
  - shut off natural gas to equipment and areas that are not in current use.[28]
- To conserve water,
  - ensure the return of sterilizer steam condensate to the boiler tank for reuse;[19,27,28,29]
  - eliminate use of city water for cooling sterilizer condensate, possibly by using holding tanks as an alternative;[23,27,30]
  - establish a preventive maintenance program for the evaluation and replacement of faulty steam traps on sterilizers;[19,23,24,28,31]
  - recirculate noncontact sterilizer cooling water;[30]
  - install flow control fixtures on all faucets;[27,28,31]
  - install scrub sinks with timers and foot or knee controlled turnoff valves;
  - install an on-demand water heater near sinks to avoid running water while waiting for hot water;[31]
  - turn off water while scrubbing until needed for wetting or rinsing hands;
  - evaluate the use of waterless surgical scrub products;
  - evaluate the use of microfiber mops for cleaning;[32]

- install high-pressure, low-volume nozzles on scrub sinks and showers;[29]
- recycle and reduce water use whenever possible;[24]
- operate washers, disinfectors, and steam sterilizers only when full, if possible;[19,23,24,27-29]
- avoid flash sterilization of single items or small loads when possible;[31]
- repair leaks in water lines and faucets;[19,23,31] and
- replace older equipment (eg, sterilizers, ice machines, automated endoscope reprocessors, disinfectors) with water-efficient models.[19,22,29,31]

Supply Conservation and Management Practices

Supply management is essential to ensure that the correct products are available when needed.[33] Cost containment measures that minimize waste production provide economic benefits without compromising quality of care. Effective supply chain management will offer opportunities to minimize process inefficiencies and product waste.

Perioperative nurses can significantly affect supply management practices by encouraging and implementing strategies that promote a safe and healthy environment. The strategies should be cost effective and conserve resources. Strategies that should be considered include, but are not limited to, the following.

- Standardize products, devices, and equipment.[34]
- Collaborate with other health care organizations to purchase partial quantities of infrequently used supplies.
- Preference cards and pick-lists should list the minimum number of items to be routinely opened and specify items to be available but unopened.[33,35]
- Open implantable devices only when the desired specifications are known and confirmed by the surgeon.[35]
- Identify processes or practices that increase efficiency or reduce cost, to include
  - monitoring preference card/pick-list supply utilization and remove items not used;
  - reducing excess supply inventory and returning slow-moving inventory;
  - rotating stock with expiration dates to use oldest inventory first;[36] and
  - evaluating excess supplies from customized packs.

- Evaluate implementation of a value analysis and product standardization program for supply purchase and selection.
- Consider natural resource requirements specific to item (eg, clean water availability).[36,37]
- Consider the impact of the item on the waste stream when purchasing supplies and equipment.[3,16]
- Collaborate with vendors to return unopened, expired items or donate items to charities or nonprofit organizations.[38]
- Purchase items made from recycled products.[39]
- Use double-sided photocopies.[39]
- Use reusable totes and pallets instead of cardboard boxes or wooden pallets for transport of goods.[39]

Reprocessing

Reprocessing single-use devices can potentially reduce the amount of waste entering the waste stream.[39,40,41] A recent estimate shows that facilities with 250 beds or more rely on reprocessing to extend their budgets and reduce waste.[40] In 2004, reprocessing was estimated to have reduced the waste generated by health care organizations by more than 449 tons destined for landfills.[40]

If a health care organization chooses to practice reprocessing of single-use devices as a means of decreasing the amount of waste entering the waste stream, the perioperative registered nurse should investigate and evaluate the environmental impact of reprocessing on the organization's waste stream as well as the total environmental impact. Refer to the AORN guidance statement on the reuse of single-use devices for more tools to use for evaluation of reprocessing[42] and adherence to the US Food and Drug Administration regulations controlling reprocessing of single-use devices.

Reuse, Repair, and Refurbishing

Reuse of medical equipment demonstrates the health care organization's commitment to supply conservation and fiscal responsibility through

- conservation of resources and energy,
- optimization of resources, and
- reduction of the pollution that occurs with waste disposal in the environment.[43] (Pollution is reduced because the final disposal of the item is delayed.[38])

Reuse includes the repair, refurbishing, washing, or recovery of worn or used items.[38] Strategies the perioperative nurse should consider when deciding to purchase reusable items or repair and refurbish an item include, but are not limited to, the following.

- ♦ Identify factors affecting the longevity of instruments and equipment, such as
  - – adequate inventory to reduce frequency of reprocessing and wear;
  - – education of health care workers who use and reprocess instruments;
  - – education of health care workers who operate and maintain equipment; and
  - – adequate storage facilities to protect the instruments and equipment from damage.[44]
- ♦ Implement proactive maintenance, repair, or restoration programs for instruments and equipment to prevent malfunction and maintain integrity.
- ♦ Consider purchasing reusable medical equipment, instruments, and supplies.
- ♦ Educate health care workers regarding their practice accountability for
  - – safe care and handling of instruments and equipment,
  - – environmental and workplace practices supporting care and handling of instruments and equipment, and
  - – repair and refurbishing initiatives of the health care institution.
- ♦ Consider projected life span when purchasing instruments and equipment.
- ♦ Consider reuse of clean items internally (eg, corrugated boxes, packaging materials, interoffice envelopes, furniture).

Sterilization and Disinfection

Various sterilization and disinfection technologies that affect the environment are used in health care settings. Sterilization technologies in current use include steam, dry heat, ethylene oxide gas, hydrogen peroxide gas plasma, and ozone.[45] High-level disinfectants commonly used include liquid chemicals such as peracetic acid, glutaraldehyde, and orthophthalaldehyde. Steam and dry heat are not known to generate by-products harmful to the environment, but these methods of sterilization do consume natural resources (ie, water, electricity, or natural gas).[20] Ethylene oxide gas sterilization and liquid chemical disinfectants can result in harm to the environment if used irresponsibly or contrary to existing local, state, and federal regulations.[46] Ethylene oxide gas, for example, is an air pollutant, a known carcinogen, a potential reproductive hazard, an allergic sensitizer, and a potent neurotoxin.[47] When choosing

a sterilizing or disinfecting method or product, the effect on the environment should be considered.

Perioperative nurses can significantly affect the environment by encouraging and implementing strategies that are cost effective and/or conserve resources. Strategies that should be considered include, but are not limited to, the following.

- ♦ Develop a program for monitoring the environmental effects of sterilization and disinfection products on the environment.
- ♦ Ensure that the necessary equipment and supplies are available to deal with spillage of sterilizing or disinfecting chemicals.
- ♦ Use, maintain, and monitor sterilizers according to the manufacturers' written instructions.[45]
- ♦ Establish, ensure, and maintain proper safety measures for handling hazardous materials (eg, monitoring compliance with emission control regulations for ethylene oxide sterilizers, glutaraldehyde disposal).
- ♦ Provide education for health care workers regarding the environmental impact of the sterilant or disinfectant being used and appropriate safety measures.
- ♦ Use and dispose of liquid chemicals employed in sterilization or disinfection in accordance with manufacturers' written instructions and local, state, and federal governmental agency requirements.
- ♦ When possible, purchase items for which the sterilization or disinfection process has the least potential for harm to the environment.[3]
- ♦ Additional glutaraldehyde precautions include
  - – using fume cabinets,[48]
  - – considering cold sterilization alternatives to glutaraldehyde,[45] and
  - – limiting areas in the facility where glutaraldehyde is used and stored.

Construction for Efficiency and Conservation

Building design, construction, and materials significantly affect the natural environment and health outcomes of patients, staff, and community.[49] Although such a discussion is beyond the scope of this document, perioperative registered nurses involved in the planning, design, and construction of health care facilities should incorporate the principles of "green" building design—ie, designs that are energy efficient and water conserving, among other qualities—wherever possible. Nurses interested in green building codes should refer to Healthy Hospitals for the Environment (H2E), located online at *http://www.H2E-online.org;* Health Care Without Harm (HCWH), located online at *http://www.noharm.org;* or the US Green Building Council, located online at *http://www.usgbc.org* (accessed 23 Jan 2006).[50]

Summary

This document has provided strategies for perioperative registered nurses to use in becoming effective stewards of the environment, addressing

♦ infectious and noninfectious waste management;

♦ recycling practices;

♦ resource conservation;

♦ supply conservation and management practices;

♦ reprocessing, reuse, repair, and refurbishing,

♦ sterilization and disinfection, and

♦ construction for efficiency and conservation.

Glossary

Green building codes: Codes used during building design that require the building to be energy efficient and water conserving, have low environmental impact, and have high indoor air quality, among other requirements.[49,50]

Noninfectious waste: Materials with no inherent hazards or infectious potential (eg, packaging materials, paper).[7]

Potentially infectious waste: The definitions of potentially infectious waste vary from state to state, but for the purposes of this document, potentially infectious waste is waste (eg, blood, body fluids, sharps) that is capable of producing infectious diseases.[7]

Reprocessing of single-use devices: Includes all operations necessary to render a contaminated reusable or single-use device patient-ready. Single-use devices to be reprocessed may be either used or unused. Reprocessing steps include disassembling for cleaning, decontamination, inspecting, packaging, relabeling, sterilization, testing, and tracking.[41]

Reuse: The repeated or multiple use of any medical device, whether marketed as reusable or single use. Repeated/multiple use may be on the same patient or on different patients with applicable reprocessing of the device between uses.[41]

Waste: Waste can be classified as potentially infectious and noninfectious materials. In this document, waste refers to the combination of potentially infectious and noninfectious waste.

REFERENCES

1. "Nurses can make a difference: Environmentally responsive health care," The Nightingale Institute for Health and the Environment, *http://www.nihe.org* (accessed 8 Oct 2005).

2. "Medical waste: The issue," Health Care Without Harm, *http://www.noharm.org/us/medicalWaste/issue* (accessed 8 Oct 2005).

3. A Melamed, "Environmental accountability in perioperative settings," *AORN Journal* 77 (June 2003) 1157-1168.

4. B Scrantom, "Health care: New paths to energy savings," *Building Operating Management* (January 2003), *http://www.facilitiesnet.com/bom/article.asp?id=1522* (accessed 8 Oct 2005).

5. B Sattler, "Pioneering the environmental health frontier," Maryland Nurses Association Newsletter, *http://www.oarm.org/details.cfm?type=news&ID=91* (accessed 14 May 2005).

6. B K Lee, M J Ellenbecker, R Moure-Ersaso, "Alternatives for treatment and disposal cost reduction of regulated medical wastes," *Waste Management* 24 no 2 (2004) 143-151.

7. R Garcia, "Effective cost-reduction strategies in the management of regulated medical waste," *American Journal of Infection Control* 27 (April 1999) 165-175.

8. B Sattler, "The greening of health care: Environmental policy and advocacy in the health care industry," *Policy, Politics & Nursing Practice* 4 (Feb 2003) 6-13.

9. J Andrews, "New diet of products can help hospitals watch their 'waste' lines" *Healthcare Purchasing News* (June 2003) 14-19.

10. C Schierhorn, "Haste makes (infectious) waste: Saving money by segregating hospital refuse," *Health Facilities Management* 15 (Sept 2002) 34-37.

11. M Cox, C Rhett, A Gudmundsen, "Environmental protection through waste management: Implications for staff development," *Journal of Nursing Staff Development* 13 (March–April 1997) 67-72.

12. B Jolibois, M Guerbet, S Vassal, "Glutaraldehyde in hospital wastewater," *Archives of Environmental Contamination and Toxicology* 42 (February 2002) 137-144.

13. F D Daschner, M Dettenkofer, "Protecting the patient and the environment—New aspects and challenges in hospital infection control," *Journal of Hospital Infection* 36 (May 1997) 7-15.

14. Walsh Integrated Environmental Systems, "Environmental impact," *http://www.walshenvironmental.com/products/ben_environmentalimpact.htm* (accessed 9 Oct 2005).

15. "Recycling fact sheet," Health Care Without Harm, *http://www.noharm.org/details.cfm?type=document&id=599* (accessed 9 Oct 2005).

16. "Waste minimization, segregation, and recycling in hospitals," Health Care Without Harm, *http://www.noharm.org/library/docs/Going_Green_4-1_Waste_Minimization_Segregation.pdf* (accessed 9 Oct 2005).

17. "Reduce, reuse, and recycle," US Environmental Protection Agency, *http://www.epa.gov/epaoswer/non-hw/muncpl/reduce.htm* (accessed 9 Oct 2005).

18. "Hospitals and health care institutions," Recycling Works Tipsheet, Pennsylvania Department of Environmental Protection, *http://www.dep.state.pa.us/dep/deputate/airwaste/wm/recycle/tips/hospitals.htm* (accessed 9 Oct 2005).

19. "Water conservation at work,"Southwest Florida Water Management District, *http://www.swfwmd.state.fl.us /conservation/waterwork/checkhospital.htm* (accessed 9 Oct 2005).

20. "A look at health care buildings—How do they use electricity?" Energy Information Administration, *http://www.eia.doe.gov/emeu/consumptionbriefs/cbecs /pbawebsite/health/health_howuseelec.htm* (accessed 9 Oct 2005).

21. "A look at health care buildings—How do they use natural gas?" Energy Information Administration, *http://www.eia.doe.gov/emeu/consumptionbriefs/cbecs /pbawebsite/health/health_howuseng.htm* (accessed 9 Oct 2005).

22. "Green tips," Ontario Ministry of the Environment, *http://www.ene.gov.on.ca/cons/3781-e.htm* (accessed 9 Oct 2005).

23. "Water conservation checklist: Hospitals/medical facilities—Every drop counts!" North Carolina Department of Environment and Natural Resources, Division of Pollution and Environmental Assistance, *http://64.233.161.104/ search?q=cache:7jnhCXPu4uIJ:www.p2pays.org/ref/23 /22006.pdf+water+use* (accessed 9 Oct 2005).

24. "Water conservation @ hospitals," City of Greeley Water Conservation, *http://www.ci.greeley.co.us/cog /PageX.asp?fkOrgId=44&PageURL=Hospitals* (accessed 9 Oct 2005).

25. US Environmental Protection Agency, *Light Brief* (Washington, DC: US Environmental Protection Agency, June 1992) 7000.

26. R Reeves, "Energy conservation important to MHCP," *Entre Nous* (Winter 2004) 8.

27. "Water efficiency and management for hospitals," North Carolina Department of Environment and Natural Resources, Division of Pollution and Environmental Assistance, *http://www.p2pays.org/ref/14/13679.htm* (accessed 9 Oct 2005).

28. "Water conservation ideas for health care facilities," Pennsylvania Department of Environmental Protection, *http://www.dep.state.pa.us/dep/subject/hotopics/drought /facts/health.htm* (accessed 9 Oct 2005).

29. "Water efficiency practices for health care facilities," New Hampshire Department of Environmental Services, *http://www.des.state.nh.us/factsheets/ws/ws-26-14 .htm* (accessed 9 Oct 2005).

30. "Hospital cost reduction case study: Norwood Hospital," Massachusetts Water Resources Authority, *http://www.mwra.state.ma.us/04water/html/bullet1.htm* (accessed 23 Jan 2006).

31. "Water efficiency in hospitals (small to medium), extended care homes, and laundries," Association of Manitoba Municipalities, *http://www.amm.mb.ca/images/re sources/waterefficiency/extcare.pdf* (accessed 26 June 2005).

32. "Using microfiber mops in hospitals," US Environmental Protection Agency, *http://www.epa.gov/region09 /cross_pr/p2/projects/hospital/mops.pdf* (accessed 9 Oct 2005).

33. P Camp, "Controlling costs while maintaining quality care," *Surgical Services Management* 8 (Dec 2002) 24-30.

34. D Karr, "Standardization and cost savings," *Surgical Services Management* 5 (April 1999) 32-38.

35. N Phillips, ed, "Coordinated roles of scrub person and circulator," in *Berry & Kohn's Operating Room Technique,* tenth ed (St Louis: Mosby, 2004).

36. Baker, D; Hale, D. "Potential cost savings opportunities: The supply chain," *SSM* 9 (April 2003) 33-38.

37. "Value analysis helps to tighten surgical products supply chain," *OR Manager* 18 (May 2002) 1, 14-16.

38. *Pollution Prevention Guide for Hospitals,* US Environmental Protection Agency, *http://www.dtsc.ca.gov/Pollution Prevention/p2-hospital-guide.pdf* (accessed 9 Oct 2005).

39. "Green purchasing," Health Care Without Harm, *http://www.noharm.org/greenPurchasing/issue* (accessed 9 Oct 2005).

40. J E Williamson, "Great expectations: Hospitals find FDA regs build stronger case for reprocessing," *Healthcare Purchasing News* (June 2005) 28-32.

41. D Dunn, "Reprocessing single-use devices: The equipment connection," *AORN Journal* 75 (June 2002) 1143.

42. "AORN guidance statement: Reuse of single-use devices," in *Standards, Recommended Practices, and Guidelines* (Denver: AORN, Inc, 2005) 185-191.

43. M Szczepanski, "The nursing process: A tool for healing the environment," *Nursing Management* 24 (Oct 1993) 56-58.

44. "Recommended practices for cleaning and caring for surgical instruments and powered equipment," in *Standards, Recommended Practices, and Guidelines* (Denver: AORN, Inc, 2005) 395-403.

45. "Recommended practices for sterilization in perioperative practice settings," in *Standards, Recommended Practices and Guidelines* (Denver: AORN, Inc, 2005) 459-469.

46. "Ethylene oxide: Hazard summary," US Environmental Protection Agency, *http://www.epa.gov/ttnatw01 /hlthef/ethylene.html* (accessed 9 Oct 2005).

47. A D LaMontagne, K I Kelsey, "Evaluating OSHA's ethylene oxide standard: Exposure determinants in Massachusetts hospitals," *American Journal of Public Health* 91 (March 2001) 412-417.

48. M Jim, "Instrument reprocessing in theatres: Drivers for change," *British Journal of Perioperative Nursing* 12 (January 2002) 34-38.

49. G Vittori, *Green and Healthy Buildings for the Health Care Industry* (Austin, Tex: Center for Maximum Potential Building Systems, 2002).

50. "Is green building budding?" in *The Washington Post* (April 16, 2005), USGBC in the News, *http:// www.usgbc.org/News/usgbcinthenews_details.asp?ID =1485& CMSPageID=159* (accessed 9 Oct 2005).

RESOURCES

Almuneef, M; Memish, Z A. "Effective medical waste management: It can be done," *American Journal of Infection Control* 31 (May 2003) 188-192.

Alt, S. "Think of environment when choosing supplies," *Hospital Materials Management* 26 (Sept 2001) 11.

Association for the Advancement of Medical Instrumentation (AAMI). *AAMI Standards and Recommended Practices: Sterilization, Part 3—Industrial Process Control* (Arlington, Va: AAMI, 1999).

Bultitude, M F, et al. "Prolonging the life of the flexible ureterorenoscope," *International Journal of Clinical Practice* 58 (August 2004) 756-757.

Burdick, J S; Hambrick, D. "Endoscope reprocessing and repair costs," *Gastrointestinal Endoscopy Clinics of North America* 14 (October 2004) 717-724.

"CDC issues new environmental guidelines," *OR Manager* 19 (August 2003) 20, 22.

Cohoon, B D. "Reprocessing single-use medical devices," *AORN Journal* 75 (March 2002) 557-567.

Cys, J. "Speaking of reuse," *Materials Management in Health Care* 12 (June 2003) 26-28.

"FDA wants to know more about reuse of opened-but-unused items," *OR Manager* 18 (September 2002) 1, 7.

"Good manufacturing practices (GMP)/Quality system (QS) regulation," US Food and Drug Administration, *http://www.fda.gov/cdrh/devadvice/32.html* (accessed 9 Oct 2005).

Hensley, S. "More hospitals buy into device recycling," *Modern Healthcare* 29 (February 1999) 88.

"Integrating green purchasing into your environmental management system (EMS), US Environmental Protection Agency, *http://www.epa.gov/epp/ems.htm* (accessed 9 Oct 2005).

International Association of Health Care Central Service Material Management. "IAHCSMM position statement on the reuse of single-use medical devices," presented at the AAMI/FDA Conference on Reuse of Single-Use Devices: Practice, Patient Safety, and Regulation, Washington, DC, May 5, 1999.

Kleinbeck, S V M; English, N L; Hueschen, J H. "Reprocessing and reusing surgical products labeled for single use," *Surgical Services Management* 4 (January 1998) 21-24.

Lewis, C. "Reusing medical devices: Ensuring safety the second time around," *FDA Consumer* 34 (September/October 2000) 8-9.

"New FDA regulations may force hospitals to abandon reprocessing," *Infection Control and Prevention Report* 5 (Sept 2000) 133-136.

Pope, A M; Snyder, M A; Mood, L H. *Nursing, Health, and the Environment: Strengthening the Relationship to Improve the Public's Health* (Washington, DC: National Academy Press, 1995).

"Reuse of single-use devices," (Clinical Issues) *AORN Journal* 73 (May 2001) 957-964.

Schultz, J. *Clinical Study Guide: Minimizing Potential for Endoscope Contamination* (Denver: Healthstream, 2005).

Schultz, J. "Reusing single-use medical devices," *Surgical Services Management* 4 (July 1998) 11-13.

Schroer, P. "Reuse of single-use devices," *Medical Device Technology* 11 (December 2000) 44, 48-53.

Selvey, D. "Medical device reprocessing: Is it good for your organization?" *Infection Control Today*, *http://www.infectioncontroltoday.com/articles/111feat1.html?wts=20051009035349&hc=44&req=Selvey%2c+and+Don* (accessed 9 Oct 2005).

Spry, C; Leiner, D C. "Rigid endoscopes—Ensuring quality before use and after repair," *AORN Journal* 80 (July 2004) 103-109.

"Survey: One-fourth of operating rooms resterilize opened-but-unused medical devices," *OR Manager* 19 (November 2002).

"Survey: ORs are split on reuse of single-use items," *OR Manager* 15 (September 1999) 1, 11, 14 16.

Thomas, L A. "Endoscope precleaning," *Gastroenterology Nursing* 28 (July/Aug 2005) 334-335.

Thomas, L A. "Endoscope staging," *Gastroenterology Nursing* 28 (May/June 2005) 243-245.

Thomas, L A. "Transporting the endoscope," *Gastroenterology Nursing* 29 (March/April 2005) 145-146.

US Food and Drug Administration. "Medical devices; current good manufacturing practice (CGMP) final rule; quality system regulation," *Federal Register* 61 (Oct 7, 1996). Also available at *http://www.fda.gov/OHRMS/DOCKETS/98fr/61FR52654100796.htm* (accessed 9 Oct 2005).

Whelan, C. "Stats: Reprocessing growth," *Materials Management in Health Care* 13 (May 2004) 41-42.

Zafar, A B; Butler, R C. "Effect of a comprehensive program to reduce infectious waste," *American Journal of Infectious Waste* 28 (February 2000) 51-53.

PUBLICATION HISTORY

Approved by the AORN Board of Directors, November 2005. Published in *Standards, Recommended Practices, and Guidelines,* 2006 edition. Reprinted October 2006, *AORN Journal.*

AORN Guidance Statement: The Role of the Health Care Industry Representative in the Perioperative Setting

Introduction

The purpose of this statement is to provide general guidelines to assist the individual facility in developing policies relating to the role of the health care industry representative in the perioperative setting. The term health care industry representative refers to all health care industry employees who provide services in the perioperative setting (eg, clinical consultants, sales representatives, technicians, repair/maintenance personnel). A systematic method of providing education, training, and instruction related to new technology, equipment, techniques, and procedures is essential for perioperative staff to provide safe patient care. The health care industry representative who possesses the requisite education, knowledge, and expertise can play a vital role in providing technical assistance, instruction, and training to perioperative team members.

Background

It may be hazardous to both patients and perioperative team members when clinicians use equipment with which they are unfamiliar. Misuse of complex technology can cause patient injury and even death. Incidents involving new technology and the presence of the health care industry representative in the perioperative setting have been highly publicized, especially when the end result is patient injury or death.[1] Hospitals have been cited and fined for allowing the use of surgical equipment not approved by the hospital; not providing formal training to physicians, nurses, and other perioperative team members on the proper use of the equipment; and permitting an unauthorized person from the medical device company to participate in a procedure.[2]

Tragic incidents have drawn attention to the need for individual facility policies to address formal instruction of physicians, nurses, and other members of the perioperative team on the operation of new medical devices before their use. Policies and procedures should be in place to authorize the introduction of new equipment and the admittance of nonmedical professionals into the room where the surgical or other invasive procedure will be performed. These policies and procedures should delineate acceptable activities and conduct of the health care industry representative in the perioperative setting. The role of the health care industry representative is to provide essential technical training and assistance related to the device for the safe care of the patient. The health care industry representative should not be considered part of the clinical team and should not be requested to perform tasks outside his or her approved role.[1]

All perioperative team members are responsible for acquiring instruction on new procedures, techniques, technology, and equipment with which they are not familiar, before their use in a surgical procedure. The health care industry representative, who has completed specialized training to provide technical instruction and support to the perioperative surgical team expedites the procedure and facilitates desired safe patient outcomes. Health care industry representatives have a valid, but restricted, role in the perioperative setting.[3]

Guidance Statement

A health care industry representative may be present during a surgical procedure under conditions prescribed by the health care organization, in accordance with accreditation requirements, and in compliance with local, state, and federal regulations. In consideration of patient safety and confidentiality, AORN recommends the following precepts to guide policy development.

Perioperative team members are responsible for acquiring instruction on new procedures, techniques, technology, and equipment before their use in a surgical procedure. This instruction may be provided by a health care industry representative and may take place in a formal inservice program or as one-on-one instruction. The facility should maintain evidence of documented competencies for perioperative team members, especially when introducing new procedures, techniques, technology, and equipment.[4]

As the patient's advocate, the RN responsible for the patient's care during the procedure is accountable for maintaining the patient's safety, privacy, dignity, and confidentiality. The RN should monitor the health care industry representative's activities whenever possible and facilitate the representative's service to the perioperative team during the procedure. The RN should monitor and limit the movement and number of people in the operating room during the procedure to prevent increased airborne contamination.[5] The RN should be informed before

2012 Perioperative Standards and Recommended Practices
Last revised: November 2005.

the procedure that a health care industry representative will be present during a specific procedure as well as the purpose for being in attendance.

Policies should be developed in collaboration with the facility's risk manager and/or legal counsel to ensure compliance with applicable local, state, and federal laws.[2]

Conditions should be specified under which the health care industry representative may be present during a surgical or other invasive procedure.

Each facility should develop a system that clearly delineates limits on the health care industry representative's activities in the room where the surgical or other invasive procedure is performed based on community standards, accreditation requirements, and local, state, and federal regulations.

The role of the health care industry representative is to provide technical support, as opposed to direct patient care; the representative should never function as a member of the scrubbed team. The health care industry representative with specialized training and facility approval may perform calibration to adjust devices to the surgeon's specification (eg, pacemakers, lasers).

The health care industry representative with previous perioperative experience (eg, RN, surgical technologist) should be held to the same rules and restrictions as all other health care industry representatives.

Each facility should develop a system that addresses informed patient consent regarding the presence and role of the health care industry representative during an operative or other invasive procedure in both routine and emergency situations. This system should include the name of the representative and documentation of consent in the patient's medical record.[5,6]

Each facility should develop a system which documents that the health care industry representative has completed instruction in the principles of asepsis, fire and safety protocols, infection control practices, bloodborne pathogens, and patients' rights. Based on community standards, this may range from maintaining up-to-date documentation supplied by the representative's employing company to providing facility-specific instruction and training.

The health care industry representative must be aware of and follow the regulations of the federal Health Insurance Portability and Accountability Act[7] and the Bloodborne Pathogens Standard.[8]

The health care industry representative's presence and purpose should be authorized by the designated department administrator and the surgeon in accordance the facility policy.

While in the facility, the health care industry representative should wear identification, preferably a photo identification badge, and be appropriately attired, including personal protective equipment as described in the "Recommended practices for surgical attire" and the "Recommended practices for standard and transmission based precautions in the perioperative practice setting" in the AORN *Standards, Recommended Practices and Guidelines*.

Experienced health care industry representatives who are accompanied by persons in training from their own organization for the purposes of orientation should make prior arrangements with the health care organization and comply with accreditation requirements, and local, state, and federal regulations.

The guidelines of the Association for the Advancement of Medical Instrumentation state: "Medical equipment and other complex devices must be reviewed and approved prior to their use by the facility's service provider."[9] The term *service provider* is defined as an entity with the responsibility to provide inspection and/or other maintenance services on a specific piece of equipment. A service provider may be a department within the health care organization or a contracted provider.[9]

A clearly defined mechanism should exist to address departures from established policy.

REFERENCES

1. E Murphy, "The presence of sales representatives in the OR," *AORN Journal* 73 (April 2001) 822-824.

2. "New York incident underscores need for policy on sales reps in OR," *Operating Room Risk Management* (December 1998).

3. P Lebowitz, M Hart Yeary, "Allowing sales representatives in the OR creates new liability issues," *News & Business* (Nov/Dec 2001).

4. Joint Commission on Accreditation of Healthcare Organizations, *Comprehensive Accreditation Manual for Hospitals: The Official Handbook* (Oakbrook Terrace, Ill: Joint Commission on Accreditation of Healthcare Organizations, 2005).

5. "Recommended practices for traffic patterns in the perioperative practice setting," *Standards, Recommended Practices and Guidelines* (Denver: AORN Inc, 2006) 659-662

6. "Standards for privacy of individually identifiable health information; final rule," 45 CFR Parts 160 and 164, Centers for Medicare and Medicaid Services, *http://www .cms.hhs.gov/hipaa/hipaa2/regulations/privacy/finalrule /PvcFR01.pdf* (accessed 4 Oct 2005).

7. "Administrative simplification in the health care industry," US Department of Health and Human Services,

http://aspe.os.dhhs.gov/admnsimp/index.shtml (accessed 4 Oct 2005).

8. "Bloodborne pathogens and needlestick prevention," Occupational Safety and Health Administration, *http://www.osha.gov/SLTC/bloodbornepathogens/index.html* (accessed 4 Oct 2005).

9. Association for the Advancement of Medical Instrumentation, "Recommended practice for a medical equipment management program," ANSI/AAMI EQ56:1999/(R)2004 (Arlington, Va: Association for the Advancement of Medical Instrumentation, 1999) 4.1.2.1.

RESOURCES

"AORN OR protocol," Healthstream, *http://www.health stream.com/Products/STS/RepDirect/orProtocol.htm* (accessed 4 Oct 2005).

PUBLICATION HISTORY

Approved by the AORN Board of Directors, November 2005. Published in *Standards, Recommended Practices, and Guidelines,* 2006 edition. Reprinted April 2006, *AORN Journal.*

AORN Perioperative Standards and Recommended Practices, 2012 Edition

AORN Guidance Statement: Care of the Perioperative Patient With an Implanted Electronic Device

Introduction

This document is intended to serve as a guide for perioperative nurses involved in the care of surgical patients with implanted electronic devices (IEDs) who are undergoing surgical and other invasive procedures. This document does not address care of patients undergoing surgery for implantation of an electronic device; it covers only issues surrounding the care of patients with existing electronic implants. Because of the rapid advancement of science and medical technology, this document does not presume to address every IED. Manufacturers' written directions for specific devices should be followed. This document is intended to help perioperative nurses provide safe care for patients with IEDs because these patients require extraordinary safety precautions in the surgical environment.

Implanted electronic devices provide a vast number of options in the treatment of many disease processes that cannot be managed with medications alone. Common examples of IEDs include permanent pacemakers, which are used to treat profound bradycardia; implantable cardioverter defibrillators (ICDs), which are used to treat sustained ventricular tachycardia (VT); deep brain stimulators (DBSs), which are used to treat tremors and Parkinson's disease; and spinal cord stimulators (SCSs), which are used to deliver low-voltage stimulation to the spinal cord to block the sensation of pain and to stimulate the sacral nerve for treatment of neurogenic bladder and tremors. Sudden failure of these implanted devices can result in patient injury or sudden cardiac death (SCD).[1] When precautions are implemented, patient risk for injury can be minimized.

The goal of every surgical intervention is to provide optimal patient outcomes while maintaining a safe environment. Some medical equipment devices necessary for performing surgical and other invasive procedures may interfere with the functioning of IEDs. Manufacturers of IEDs recommend precautions for and/or avoiding certain devices that create electromagnetic fields.[2] Because of the potential for interference, patients with IEDs require special safety precautions when undergoing a surgical procedure. The perioperative registered nurse should be knowledgeable about the specific IED and associated precautions that should be implemented to protect the patient from injury.

Implanted electronic devices are widely used in a number of diverse medical applications, ranging from the familiar cardiac pacemaker to the less frequently encountered cochlear implant. The perioperative nurse should be aware that these devices require that special precautions be taken. One predominantly important precaution is managing the sources of inherent electromagnetic interference (EMI) in the perioperative patient care environment. Cardiac patients are particularly at risk because they may be dependent on the proper function of an IED to sustain their lives. Understanding what types of IEDs exist, how they function, and the precautions that must be taken when caring for patients with IEDs is critical for every perioperative nurse because patients with these devices may be encountered in any perioperative environment. The history, application, function, and safety issues of the different types of IEDs will be addressed in this document.

Definitions

For the purposes of this document, the following definitions apply.

Conducted EMI: Occurs when an electromagnetic source comes in direct contact with the body. Can be generated by electrosurgery and defibrillation.[3]

Direct coupling: The contact of an energized metal active electrode tip with another metal instrument or object within the surgical field.

Electromagnetic: Magnetism that is induced by an electric current.[4]

Electromagnetic interference (EMI): Any electromagnetic disturbance that interrupts, obstructs, or otherwise degrades or limits the effective performance of electronics/electrical equipment. *Synonym:* radio frequency interference.[5]

Implanted electronic devices (IEDs): Electronic medical devices that have been implanted in a patient to treat a physiological defect or to replace a sensory function.

Microwave: A short electromagnetic wave between about 1 mm and 1 m in length.

Radiated EMI: Occurs when the body is placed within an electromagnetic field; no contact with the source is necessary. Can be generated by magnetic resonance imaging (MRI), positron emission tomography (PET), and radiation therapy.[3]

Shortwave: A radio wave with a wavelength between 10 m and 100 m.

General Safety Issues and Concerns

Electronic devices implanted in a patient may be affected by other IEDs or medical equipment that a patient may come in contact with in a health care facility. These devices may include

- ◆ cardiac pacemakers or ICDs,
- ◆ electrosurgical devices,
- ◆ ultrasound equipment, or
- ◆ MRI equipment.

All of these devices have the potential to adversely affect an IED.[6] Perioperative registered nurses should be aware of potential patient safety hazards associated with specific IEDs and the appropriate patient care interventions required to protect patients from injury. (See **Exhibit A**, at the end of this document, for a summary of potential patient safety hazards.)

Exposure to shortwave and microwave diathermy should be avoided if an implanted device has metallic leads, even if the implanted device is not turned on. The energy from diathermy can cause tissue heating at the site surrounding the implant and has the potential to cause tissue injury. *Note:* As used here, the term "diathermy" does not include electrocautery and electrosurgical devices or ultrasonic imaging devices.[7] Examples of implants with metallic leads include cardiac pacemakers and defibrillators, cochlear implants, bone growth stimulators, deep brain stimulators, spinal cord stimulators, and other nerve stimulators.[7,8]

General Patient Management

Preoperative

- ■ The perioperative registered nurse should routinely assess patients for the presence of any IEDs.[9] Patient education occurring at the time of the implant surgery should include instructions to the patient to always report the presence of the implant to health care providers, especially when a surgical procedure is necessary.[10] A patient who has an IED should have been given a product identification card at the time of implantation; the patient may have the card with him or her, or the medical record may contain a copy of the card.[10]
- ■ The perioperative registered nurse may contact the patient's implanting surgeon to inform him or her that the patient is scheduled for surgery and ask the implanting physician to send the following IED information to the preoperative assessment nurse, the operating surgeon, and the operative suite:[10,11]

- ■ manufacturer and model of IED,
- ■ location of the device,
- ■ when the device was last evaluated,
- ■ if the device can be turned off before or during surgery,
- ■ what settings should be reprogrammed into the device immediately postprocedure,
- ■ whether the implanting physician wishes to be contacted when the patient enters the postanesthesia care unit (PACU), and
- ■ whether the patient needs to schedule an appointment with the implanting physician.[12]
- ■ The information above should be documented on the medical record before surgery.
- ■ Determine whether electrosurgery and/or defibrillation are necessary for the procedure.
- ■ Contact the appropriate health care industry representative and arrange for his or her presence before, during, and after the surgery, if requested by the physician.[13]
- ■ Notify the anesthesia care provider of the presence of the IED.

Intraoperative

- ■ Notify all perioperative team members that the patient has an IED in place, and review potential safety concerns and equipment conflicts.[11,14]
- ■ The programming device and personnel who are qualified to program the IED should be in the OR before the start of the procedure.[3]
- ■ When electrosurgery is necessary, bipolar electrosurgery should be used.[14]
- ■ If the use of monopolar electrosurgery is required, the current pathway should be perpendicular to the IED's lead system. This can be achieved by manipulating the placement of the patient return electrode; however, a perpendicular pathway is not always a realistic possibility. If monopolar electrosurgery must be used, the active electrode and the dispersive electrode should be located as close together as possible.[3] A reusable, capacitive-coupled return electrode may be used if the perpendicular current pathway does not pass through the IED or the IED lead system.[15]
- ■ Place the active electrode and the dispersive electrode as far from the IED generator and wires as possible.[16]
- ■ The current path from the active electrode to the dispersive electrode should not pass through the area containing the IED or the electrodes.[16]
- ■ Avoid placing the dispersive electrode directly over the site of a metal implant.[15] The dispersive

electrode should be placed in such a way that the current will flow away from the IED. The distance between the dispersive electrode and the active electrode should be as small as possible.[17]

- To prevent EMI, care should be taken not to arc current between the active electrode and another surgical instrument. The instrument and active electrode should be in direct contact before activation.
- If the IED appears to have been inadvertently reprogrammed by the use of electrosurgery, it is advisable to return the device to the appropriate mode before continuing the procedure.[3]
- The humidity and temperature in the OR should be maintained within recommended ranges to reduce the possibility of creating static electricity in the environment. The OR temperature should be between 20° C and 24° C (68° F and 76° F) and humidity should be between 50% and 60%.[18(p147)]
- For patients who have pacemakers and other IEDs in the chest area and who require defibrillation, anterior-posterior-type paddles should be used. The anterior paddle should be placed as far from the pulse generator as possible. This should allow the current to flow away from the IED. The lowest possible defibrillator current setting should be used. Inability to defibrillate at low current settings will necessitate an increase in power, and damage to the IED may be unavoidable.[3]

Postoperative

- If necessary, notify the implanting physician and/or the health care industry representative that electrosurgery or defibrillation was used during surgery. An evaluation of IED function similar to that performed before surgery should be done early in the postoperative period.[3,16]
- Continue to monitor the patient closely during the postoperative period for signs of complications and IED malfunction.

Cardiac IEDs

Implanted electronic devices provide a vast array of treatments for patients with cardiac dysfunctions. The ability to electrically stimulate the chambers of the heart with an implanted device has helped many patients who have cardiac dysfunction and limited options for treating their disease with medications. For this reason, IEDs are popular treatment modalities. Pacemakers, ICDs, and ventricular assist devices (VADs) are three examples of IEDs used today to treat cardiac dysfunction. Specifically, pacemakers are used to treat patients with compromised cardiac output caused by profound bradycardia.[1] Implantable cardioverter defibrillators treat patients with a known risk for SCD caused by ventricular fibrillation (VF).[1] Ventricular assist devices are implantable pumps used for circulatory support in patients with congestive heart failure.[3]

History and Current Application

Pacemakers
Cardiac pacemakers first were introduced in 1954.[19] Pacemakers consist of a power source that delivers an electric impulse that travels along leads that have contact with the heart. Early pacemakers fired at a fixed rate and did not have the ability to sense the patient's heartbeat.[1] As technology improved, pacemakers with the ability to sense the patient's heart rate were introduced, helping to eliminate the hazard of the pacemaker competing with the intrinsic heartbeat and potentially creating a ventricular dysrhythmia.[1] The development of the sensing demand pacemaker in the 1960s brought with it the problem of interference.[3] Specifically, sensing pacemakers were able to sense and react to the changing needs of the heart, but they also could sense and react to electromagnetic signals that were not cardiac in origin.[3] Pacemakers have evolved from the limited capability of stimulating only one chamber of the heart to those capable of stimulating both atrial and ventricular chambers, adjusting rates to physiologic demands, providing telemetric information and autoprogramming and reprogramming functions, and providing antitachycardia functions.[20] The transvenous route performed with fluoroscopy is the most common insertion method.[1]

Implanted cardioverter defibrillators
Implanted cardioverter defibrillators are similar to pacemakers in that they have a power source and leads that attach to the heart and sense the patient's heartbeat. Early ICDs consisted of defibrillating patches placed via thoracotomy on the ventricular epicardium and connected to an internal defibrillator that discharged when it sensed VT or VF.[1] Lowe and Wharton (1955) report that the development of nonthoracotomy lead systems inserted transvenously has made epicardial patch systems rare.[21] The greatest challenge in treating patients with spontaneous VF is that electrical counter shock is the only treatment for

patients at risk for SCD caused by VF;[1] therefore, patients may be totally dependent on the ICD to save their lives. Realizing that patients often died of VT or VF because the necessary equipment and personnel to defibrillate patients were unavailable, Mirowski and his associates (1980) conceived of an implantable device that could sense the dysrythmia and deliver a counter shock to terminate the life-threatening disorder.[22] In 1980, the first device of this kind was implanted at Johns Hopkins Hospital in Baltimore.[1]

Ventricular assist devices

A VAD is a type of mechanical heart that is surgically implanted in the patient's chest during open-heart surgery[20] and that is used to treat patients with end-stage heart failure. Blood fills the device through a cannulation site in the ventricle or atrium. Within the device, a diaphragm is actuated pneumatically, electrically, or magnetically, and it pumps blood into the aorta or pulmonary artery.[18] After the pump is implanted, it needs power to operate. The driveline passes through the skin and attaches to the power base unit, which consists of a system controller and batteries. The power source is worn externally in a holster or waist pack.[19] Government-funded research and development work in cardiac support systems began in 1966. Clinical trials of an air-driven left ventricular assist system started in 1986, and an electric system was tested in 1991. The device has been used in patients aged 11 to 78 years, with an average age of 50 years, and in as many as 4,000 patients in the United States and elsewhere.[19]

Ventricular assist devices initially were used as "bridges to transplantation," helping people survive as they waited for a heart transplant. Today, VADs play another role; they allow disease-weakened hearts to recover. In patients not eligible for heart transplantation, VADs offer permanent support, which is called destination therapy.[19] Clinical trials have demonstrated that destination therapy doubles the one-year survival rate of patients with end-stage heart failure as compared to treatment with medication.[20]

Safety Concerns

Pacemakers, ICDs, and VADs are IEDs that rely on sensing capability for proper function of the device and appropriate treatment being delivered to the patient. Electromagnetic interference is the most common safety issue noted when caring for patients with existing cardiac IEDs, mostly because EMI can alter what the device is sensing. This potentially could change the rhythm or, in some cases, render the device incapable of delivering appropriate treatment.

Electromagnetic interference occurs in two forms: conducted and radiated. Conducted EMI occurs when an electromagnetic source comes in direct contact with the body. This type of EMI can be generated by electrosurgery and defibrillation. Radiated EMI occurs when the body is placed within an electromagnetic field; no contact with the source is necessary. This type of EMI can be generated by MRI, PET, and radiation therapy.[3]

The electrosurgical unit (ESU) is a commonly used device that cuts and coagulates tissue with high-voltage, high-frequency (ie, 10,000 Hz) current.[3(p640)] Practically every surgical intervention requires some form of electrosurgery to help facilitate hemostasis. Some surgical procedures would be nearly impossible to perform without electrosurgery. There are two types of electrosurgical current: monopolar and bipolar. Monopolar current begins at the tip of the instrument, travels through the body, and returns to the generator through a dispersing ground pad. When monopolar electrosurgery is used, surgeons may use the active electrode to pass current through other surgical instruments. If the ESU is activated before the active electrode is in contact with the instrument, the current can arc through the air toward the instrument and demodulate the signal to the IED. If allowed to demodulate, the signal can dip well into the frequency range that pacemakers and ICDs are designed to sense. The result is that the IED might interpret the current as cardiac in origin and respond inappropriately or not respond at all.[3]

Ventricular assist devices also are affected by EMI generated by electrosurgery. Theoretically, the timing circuit of one model can be disrupted, but this rarely is reported. Ventricular assist devices that are run by electricity may exhibit an erratic pattern of current output during electrosurgery use. This results in a significant decrease in device output.[3]

Bipolar electrosurgery does not require a patient-return electrode because the current flows between the two tips of a bipolar forceps that is positioned around tissue to create a surgical effect. Current passes from the active electrode of one tip of the forceps through the patient's tissue to the dispersive electrode of the other forceps tip, thus completing the circuit without entering another part of the patient's body. This means that the current flows only through the area of tissue that is in direct contact with the instrument.[17] Using bipolar electrosurgery rather than monopolar electrosurgery may be advantageous when trying to avoid possible arcing that could demodulate; however, bipolar electrosurgery is much less powerful than monopolar electrosurgery and may be inappropriate for many surgical procedures.

Other dangers inherent to monopolar electrosurgery include burns, triggering ventricular or atrial fibrillation, and loss of battery output. A continuous train of electrical impulses conducted down the lead can induce ventricular or atrial fibrillation, cause thermal burns at the lead-tissue interface, and pass from the leads to the pulse generator and cause irreversible loss of battery output.[3]

Some surgeries and emergency situations employ the use of defibrillation as part of the surgical procedure. Patients with existing pacemakers and ICDs may experience permanent damage to the pulse generator, particularly after repeated attempts at defibrillation. In addition, the current shunted away from the pacemaker or ICD can lead to myocardial burns at the lead-tissue interface.[3]

Patient Management

Preoperative

- If the IED was not evaluated within the previous six months, it should be evaluated for programming, telemetry, thresholds, and battery status.
- If the make and model of the IED is unavailable, a chest x-ray may be helpful in identifying the pacemaker or ICD. Each device has a serial number and a unique silhouette that can be used for device identification.[3] Modern pacemakers employ a variety of different pacing modes, so it is important to be familiar with the North American Society of Pacing and Electrophysiology/British Pacing and Electrophysiology Group (NBG) generic pacemaker codes. The first three letters of the code describe the basic anti bradycardia functions, and the last two letters describe the programmability and antitachycardia functions.[3] Similar coding also is found on ICDs. This code, which is located on the device, also can be identified via chest x-ray.
- For a pacemaker-dependent patient, it is advised that the device be reprogrammed to an asynchronous mode if EMI is likely to cause significant malfunction (eg, monopolar electrosurgery for surgical procedures involving the upper abdomen or chest wall).
- For patients with adaptive-rate devices, including ICDs, this feature should be programmed off

during surgery because exposure to other EMI might cause a device malfunction.[23] Magnet-activated testing should be programmed off.[20]

- For patients with an ICD, tachycardia sensing should be programmed off.[23]
- Patients with a VAD should be evaluated in a similar manner. Most surgical procedures involving patients with VADs take place at institutions that can provide technical and surgical support for these devices.[3]

Intraoperative

- If monopolar electrosurgery must be used, the current pathway should be perpendicular to the pacemaker's lead system when possible. This is done by manipulating the placement of the dispersive electrode; however, a perpendicular pathway is not always a realistic possibility, especially when the IED has a dual lead system.
- If it is impossible to place the pacemaker in a triggered or asynchronous mode and it becomes apparent that the ESU is adversely affecting the pacemaker, the electrosurgery current should be activated for no more than one second at a time, allowing at least 10 seconds for the device to function properly. This will permit the pacemaker enough time to maintain cardiac output. It is widely assumed that placing a magnet over any pacemaker pulse generator will invariably cause asynchronous pacing as long as the magnet remains in place; however, in some pacemakers, the magnet response may have been programmed off. In others, a variety of magnet responses may have been programmed, some of which do not provide immunity to EMI sensing. In still other pacemakers, the device will continue to pace asynchronously or pacing will cease after a programmed number of intervals.[24] If possible, one should determine before EMI exposure what type of pulse generator is present and what must be done to provide protection. If this is not possible, one can observe the magnet response during EMI to ascertain whether there is protection from EMI sensing. During electrosurgery, for example, if the active electrode triggers rapid pacing or inhibits pacing stimuli in a pacemaker-dependent patient despite magnet application, then activation of the ESU should be limited to short bursts.[23]
- The use of electrosurgery also may interfere with the ability of the electrocardiogram (ECG) to monitor the heart, so heart rate and blood pressure should be monitored using an arterial line.

When the ESU is not in use, the ECG should be checked for arrhythmias or alterations in pacemaker function.

■ Patients with VADs that require the use of electrosurgery should have the device placed in the fixed rate mode for the duration of the surgery. Adequate pumping is not possible during electrosurgery, so the ESU should be activated for no more than one second at a time, allowing 10 seconds for the VAD to function properly. Cardiac output should be monitored. It may be necessary for an external hand pump to be available in the OR during surgery.[3]

■ Patients with VADs who require defibrillation may need to have the timing circuit disconnected from the external controller before defibrillation. This may require the use of a fixed rate mode, depending on the type of VAD, during the period of defibrillation, but it will eliminate the possibility of damage to the circuit. During this time, a pneumatic or manually run pump will be needed.[3]

■ In patients with pacemakers and ICDs who require defibrillation, anterior-posterior-type paddles should be used. The anterior paddle should be placed as far from the pulse generator as possible. This should allow the current to flow away from the generator. If the anterior type of paddles must be used, the paddles should be placed along a line perpendicular to the lead(s). This may be difficult if the patient has a dual-lead system. The lowest possible defibrillator current setting should be used. Inability to defibrillate at low current settings will necessitate an increase in power, and damage to the pulse generator may be unavoidable. For these reasons, a temporary pacing system should be available.[3]

Postoperative

■ Inform the cardiologist, cardiothoracic surgeon, and/or the health care industry representative that electrosurgery or defibrillation was used during surgery. An evaluation of pacemaker and ICD function similar to that performed before surgery should be done in the early postoperative period and again 24 to 48 hours later. This is necessary because failure of the device to capture due to damage at the lead-tissue interface may not be apparent until 24 to 48 hours after surgery. If any of the postoperative measurements of the demand or magnet rates vary from those obtained before surgery, one must suspect that the pacemaker has been reprogrammed inadvertently during surgery or has sustained permanent damage.[3]

■ Alteration of the VAD motor current occurs only during exposure to electrosurgery and has no permanent effect on the device. Defibrillation, however, can damage the timing circuit, depending on the model and if the timing circuit is left connected during surgery. The surgeon or cardiologist responsible for the care of the patient should be informed if the circuit is damaged during surgery because repair or replacement should be considered.[3]

Neurostimulators

Deep brain stimulators, SCSs, vagal nerve stimulators (VNSs), and programmable ventricular shunts all are examples of neurological IEDs. Neurological IEDs are devices that help to restore functionality to people who have neurological or sensory impairments. This is accomplished by electrically stimulating the nervous system. Electrodes are placed in specific regions of the nervous system with regard to the patient's pathology. Neurostimulation used to treat movement disorders, such as those caused by Parkinson's disease, involves implanting leads in specific regions of the brain (ie, DBS) that then are connected to a programmable pulse generator. Electrodes may be implanted in the spine (ie, SCS) to control intractable pain, and they also may be used for sacral nerve stimulation to alleviate urinary incontinence and on the left vagus nerve (ie, VNS) to treat intractable seizures.[25]

History and Current Application

In 1964, E. A. Spiegel, MD, and H. T. Wycis, MD, along with their team members at Temple University Hospital, created the first neurological IED.[26] The physicians, however, were reluctant to use a new device, so their first device was never implanted. C. Norman Shealy, MD, is credited with implanting the first neurological IED spinal cord stimulator in 1967.[26] For the past three decades, neurological IEDs have continued to evolve. Thorough patient selection and screening, combined with physician experience, has resulted in a 50% to 60% good long-term results. More than 20,000 DBSs,[27(p76)] 130,000 SCSs,[27(p76)] and 15,000 VNSs have been implanted.[28 (p1,662)]

Deep brain stimulators

The first IED to treat tremors associated with Parkinson's disease was approved by the US Food and Drug Administration (FDA) in August 1997.[29] Deep brain stimulators consist of four electrodes that are placed in the ventricle. These electrodes then are connected to a pulse generator. The pulse generator usually is placed in the subcutaneous tissues in the chest, similar to the cardiac pacemaker.[29] The electrical stimulation blocks the abnormal brain signal that induces tremors. These devices can be turned off and adjusted from high to low frequency settings.

Spinal cord stimulators

The use of electrical stimulation for patients with spinal cord injuries was first attempted in the 1960s.[30] Spinal cord stimulators have been used to stimulate phrenic nerves and the diaphragm to permit a patient freedom from a respirator and to promote easier mobility. Spinal cord stimulators also are used in the treatment of intractable pain. An SCS is used to reduce pain, not eliminate it. Spinal cord stimulator studies have shown a 50% reduction in pain, increased activity levels, and a decreased reliance on narcotic medications.[31(p3)] Spinal cord stimulators have helped patients with chronic pain lead more comfortable and productive lives.

Patients with implanted cardiac pacemakers or defibrillators should not use spinal stimulators. Use of a transcutaneous electrical nerve stimulator unit is acceptable.[32]

Vagal nerve stimulators

In 1985, Zabara[27] developed the concept of vagal stimulation to control seizures; however, it was not until 1997 that the FDA approved the use of VNSs.[27] Vagal nerve stimulators are composed of implantable (eg, generator, leads) and external (eg, computer, software, programming wands) components. The generator or stimulator, which is the main component, is very similar to a cardiac pacemaker. It is a pulse generator that is programmed by a computer, and it runs on battery power. The pulse generator is implanted on the left side of the upper chest just under the skin. The lead is a flexible tube that is attached to the left vagus nerve on the left side of the neck.[33] The pulse generator has a life span of approximately 16 years. The battery life span ranges from six to 10 years.[33(p4)] Vagal nerve stimulators operate by sending electrical signals through the implanted leads via the left vagus nerve to the brain. This signal stimulates the brain to reduce the frequency and duration of seizures.

Programmable ventricular shunts

Ventricular shunts are used to treat patients with hydrocephalus. Shunts are long tubes that draw cerebrospinal fluid (CSF) away from the brain and into a body cavity, such as the chest or abdomen.[34] One of the major setbacks in ventricular shunts is shunt failure. This leads to repeated surgeries to adjust the shunt to drain the CSF. In September 1999, the FDA approved the first programmable shunt.[34] Programmable shunts allow surgeons to adjust the settings on the shunt from outside the body, thereby decreasing the need for repeated surgeries.

Neurostimulators or neurological IEDs are similar to cardiac pacemakers in design. They deliver electrical stimulation to targeted structures in the appropriate area of the nervous system. After it is programmed, a neurological IED can be turned on and off by a patient or clinician using a magnet or a patient-therapy controller. In the OR, because the neurological IED generates electrical impulses, it may be affected by or have an adverse effect on medical equipment (eg, cardiac pacemakers, cardioverters/defibrillators, external defibrillators, ultrasonic equipment, ESU) or procedures (eg, radiation therapy, some MRI procedures).[25]

Safety Concerns

Neurological IEDs, like implantable cardiac devices, generate electrical impulses and have the potential for interference from other medical devices with electromagnetic forces. Electromagnetic interference is the primary concern. In the perioperative setting, many procedures and devices have the potential to cause interference with IEDs, including electrosurgery, defibrillation, MRI, ultrasonic equipment, and other IEDs.[35]

More than 177,000 neurological IEDs have been implanted,[27(p76)] so perioperative team members must be aware of and understand potential complications before patients with IEDs enter the OR. This knowledge can help team members deal with potential complications and possibly prevent patient injury.[3]

Devices and procedures that may cause damage to or interfere with the function of the neurological IED or harm to the patient include defibrillators, cardioverters, electrosurgery, and MRI. If a patient is in ventricular or atrial fibrillation, patient survival always should be the first consideration. Steps should be taken to minimize the electrical circuit flowing through the neurological IED during defibrillation. These steps include

- positioning paddles as far from the neurological IED as possible,
- positioning paddles perpendicular to the neurological IED,

◆ using the lowest clinically appropriate output settings, and

◆ having perioperative team members confirm that the neurological IED is functioning properly after defibrillation.

Use of monopolar electrosurgery may cause the tissue around the leads to be damaged. In addition, the insulation on the leads may be damaged, which could cause device failure or shock the patient.[35] Damage to the neurological IED itself also may occur, and this could cause changes in stimulation settings, changes in parameters, or complete device failure. These are potentially serious risks, so the use of the ultrasonic scalpel is being investigated as an alternative to monopolar electrosurgery. Ultrasonic scalpels do not emit electromagnetic impulses.[3] If electrosurgery is deemed necessary, bipolar electrosurgery is recommended. If bipolar electrosurgery is not a suitable option and monopolar electrosurgery is necessary, the following precautions should be taken.

◆ The neurological IED should be turned off. If this cannot be accomplished by the patient, a staff member, or the physician, the appropriate health care industry representative may need to be notified.

◆ Use only a low voltage mode/setting.

◆ Keep the grounding pad as far from the neurological IED as possible.

◆ After using the ESU, perioperative team members should confirm that the neurological IED is functioning properly.

With the increasing popularity of intraoperative MRI, perioperative team members should be aware of MRI safety issues. Magnetic resonance imaging is not recommended for patients who have a neurological IED. It may cause heating at the lead site, resulting in tissue damage. Magnetic resonance imaging also may cause damage to the neurological IED itself, resulting in patient injury or device failure.[36]

The following devices used in the perioperative setting are unlikely to cause interference with neurological IEDs; however, special precautions should be taken when using them.[36]

◆ Keep the external magnetic coils of neurological IEDs a minimum of 18 inches (45 cm) away from bone growth stimulators.

◆ Turn the neurological IED off when dental drills, ultrasonic probes, diagnostic ultrasound, electrolysis, and lasers are used. Keep the device six inches (15 cm) away from the neurological IED. Keep the laser directed away from the neurological IED.

◆ For questions about precautions when other IEDs are present, contact the manufacturer of the other IED and notify the physicians involved in both therapies.

Patient Management

Preoperative

■ Vagus nerve stimulators can pose a serious risk to a patient's respiratory status. Patients with VNSs may have increased swallowing difficulties, so the risk of aspiration is increased.[33] The perioperative nurse and anesthesia care provider should be aware of the risk of spontaneous airway obstruction.[28]

Intraoperative

■ The patient, physician, a staff member, or the appropriate representative should turn off the IED.

Implantable Hearing Devices

Four types of implantable electronic hearing devices are used today. These devices are cochlear implants, implanted bone conduction stimulators, implantable and semi-implantable hearing aids, and auditory brainstem implants.

History and Current Application

Cochlear implants

Cochlear implants are used for people with sensorineural hearing loss. The first cochlear implant procedures on humans were done in 1961.[37] Graeme Clark and colleagues in Australia began research into cochlear implants in the late 1960s and implanted a multichannel device into the world's first cochlear implant recipient in 1978.[38] Cochlear implants now are the standard treatment for individuals whose ability to hear, even with hearing aids, is so poor that their ability to effectively communicate through speech is affected.[39] Statistics from 2003 indicate that approximately 60,000 people worldwide have received a cochlear implant since 1983.[39(p1)] Cochlear implants are seen more commonly than the other types of implantable hearing devices described here.

Cochlear implants consist of an implant system and an external component. After being implanted, these components work together to allow a patient with sensorineural hearing loss to hear by converting mechanical sound energy into electrical impulses that are transmitted directly to the acoustic nerve.[37]

Cochlear implants consist of internal and external parts. The external parts, which consist of a receiver, speech processor, and transmitting coil, may be removed from the patient at any time. The internal receiver/stimulator is surgically implanted into the patient's inner ear and into the bone behind the ear.[38] The external receiver is worn near the ear and is used to pick up sound.

The external speech processor usually is clipped to the wearer's clothing, or for children, it may be kept in a special backpack. The external transmitting coil is surrounded by the transmitting antenna. This transmitting coil is held in place by two magnets of opposite polarity—one in the transmitting coil and the other implanted within the internal receiver/stimulator. The internal receiver/stimulator is surgically implanted and, in addition to the previously mentioned magnet, contains a multi-channeled electrode. A cochleostomy is made, and the electrode is placed into the cochlea. After all parts are connected, electromagnetic induction will cause stimulation of the cochlear nerve, which allows the patient to perceive sound.[10]

Implantable and semi-implantable hearing aids

Implanted bone conduction stimulators, which also are known as temporal bone stimulators,[40] typically are used for people with a conductive hearing loss.[41] Implantable and semi-implantable hearing aids are implanted in the middle ear[42] or directly stimulate the inner ear.[38] The various designs are categorized by the type of output transducer used. Electromagnetic stimulation of the middle ear was first done in 1957. One of the earliest types used was piezoelectric crystal, which first was used in Japan in about 1978.[40]

The semi-implantable hearing aid allows sound to be produced through direct stimulation of the ossicles.[41] The components of this device include a microphone speech processor, which is connected to a transmitter. This transmitter has an external coil that transcutaneously transmits electrical energy to the internal device. The internal device has an internal receiving coil, which is implanted in the temporal bone. The internal receiving coil is connected to a receiver that provides electrical energy to the mechanical driver. The mechanical driver is attached to the incus. This results in vibration of the ossicles, which allows the patient to hear.[42]

Bone-conduction stimulators

One of the first bone-anchored hearing devices (ie, a temporal bone stimulator) was developed in Sweden in 1977. One brand currently is approved by the FDA.[40] A transcutaneous bone-conduction device was developed in 1986. This device has an external unit and an internal unit. The external unit is composed of a microphone and a sound processor system worn on the user's body and held in place with an implanted magnet assembly behind the user's ear. The internal unit is implanted into the temporal bone.[40] These devices are used in the treatment of severe conductive hearing loss, in patients with mixed hearing loss, and sometimes for patients with sensorineural hearing loss in one ear.[43]

Bone-conduction devices have an external processor, which consists of a microphone, amplifier, and a transducer, a device that connects the bone-anchored implant to the external processor. Both the fixture placed in the mastoid bone and the coupling devices are made of titanium.[42]

Auditory brainstem implants

Auditory brainstem implants are used to restore auditory sensation for patients who are totally deaf. The deafness is due to bilateral eighth cranial nerve lesions or neurofibromatosis Type 2. These patients have undergone surgical removal of a tumor and do not plan to undergo radiation treatment.[44]

One auditory brainstem implant system was approved by the FDA in October 2000.[45] The FDA New Device Approvals notice stated that pre-approval testing involved implantation of this auditory brainstem implant system in 90 patients.[45(p1)] The auditory brainstem implant consists of an implantable receiver/stimulator package, an electrode lead, and an electrode array. The receiver/stimulator comes with a magnet that can be removed via a small incision with local anesthesia if the patient is required to undergo MRI.[43]

Safety Issues and Concerns

Studies have been conducted to determine the compatibility of MRI and cochlear implants.[41] In at least one study, MRI was not an absolute contraindication for these patients. Another study determined that MRI should be done only if there is a strong medical indication for the test.[37] Currently, patients with cochlear implants should avoid undergoing MRI unless it is absolutely necessary because of the possibility that the implant can become inactivated.[46]

Roberts et al studied the effects of EMI on cochlear implants using common dental office equipment. This equipment included a bipolar and monopolar ESU. The ESU was tested using cut

"mild electrical stimulation of the sacral nerve that influences the behavior of the bladder, sphincter, and pelvic floor muscles."[57] This device is used to treat urinary retention and to alleviate urinary urge incontinence and urgency-frequency symptoms of overactive bladder.[55] The second device works by initiating a contraction of the detrusor muscle.

Sacral nerve stimulators as therapy for urinary retention and urinary urge incontinence have been placed in about 10,000 patients. Sacral nerve stimulators that facilitate bladder emptying are less frequently implanted, totaling approximately 2,500 systems.[27(p76)]

These systems basically consist of three components. The first component is the pulse generator, which is battery-powered or controlled by an external portable control unit and programmed by a clinician.[56] The second component consists of electrodes placed intradurally or extradurally. The third component consists of the cables used to connect the pulse generator to the electrodes.[27]

Patient Management

Preoperative

■ The perioperative nurse should follow the instructions of the neurostimulator's manufacturer. To prevent potential injury to the patient, it is important to determine exactly how the device producing the electrical stimulation works and how it may function during a surgical procedure to determine whether the device should be turned off during that time.[17]

Intraoperative

■ Large, reusable, capacitive coupled return electrode systems should not be used.[17]
■ The active electrode should be kept at least six inches from the implanted components of the device. This includes any cables, metallic electrodes, or leads, as well as the electrical components.[17]

Osteogenic Stimulators

Osteogenic (ie, bone-growth) stimulators are used to stimulate bone growth in patients with fresh fractures, to assist in healing postosteotomy, to stimulate grafted bone to vertebrae in spinal fusions, and for treatment of delayed fracture healing or nonunion following a fracture.[57] Implanted osteogenic stimulators deliver electrical impulses directly to the site where bone regrowth needs to occur. Types of bone-growth stimulators currently used include electrical, electromagnetic, and ultrasonic. These devices can be used invasively or noninvasively.

History and Current Application

In 1971, successful healing of a nonunion fracture with electrical stimulation was reported. The female patient had a nonhealing fracture of the medial malleolus for more than two years before it was healed successfully with direct current electrical stimulation.[58] Within the next five years, numerous investigators reported the benefits of various types of electrical energy on bone growth in humans.[58] In 1979, the FDA approved the use of three types of electrical stimulation devices for treatment of long bone nonunion.[58]

The first clinical study on the benefits of electrical stimulation in lumbar spinal fusion was reported in 1974. During the next few years, implantable electrical stimulation devices were used with much success on both anterior and posterior spinal fusions and spinal fractures with nonunion.[58] The FDA approved use of electrical stimulators to be used as an adjunct treatment to spinal fusion in 1987.[59]

Electromagnetic fields typically are used as a noninvasive technique, and direct current electrical stimulation is used when invasive electrical stimulation is indicated.[60] Direct current stimulation involves surgical implantation of electrodes at the desired site for bone growth.[58,61] The negative electrode is placed at the site where bone repair is desired, and the positive electrode is place in nearby soft tissue. A generator is placed in nearby subcutaneous tissue or in an intermuscular plane.

Other techniques of electrical stimulation involve capacitive coupling and inductive coupling pulsed electromagnetic stimulation. These devices either are totally external devices or have a combination of implanted components and external components.[61]

Capacitive coupling for bone growth stimulation is delivered through two charged metal devices attached to a source of voltage that produces an electric field. This form of stimulation is delivered through external electrodes.[58,60]

Inductive coupling involves using single or double coils that deliver an electrical current from an external generator.[60,61] One inductive coupling bone healing system was introduced in 1979, and 300,000 patients have been treated using this system.[62]

Pulsing electromagnetic field therapy involves the use of time-varying current applied to metallic coils. These are applied to the desired treatment area and can be applied externally.[58]

Ultrasonic bone growth stimulators are external devices that apply pulsed ultrasound to the skin over the site of a fracture. This is the newest noninvasive technique and has the advantage that the treatment time may be as short as 20 to 30 minutes per day.

The electrodes and generator of a totally implantable device are made primarily of medical grade titanium containing a lithium battery.[58,63] A portion of one type of a spinal fusion system has a platinum coating.[63] These devices can produce continuous electrical stimulation for about six months.[63] The prevalence of spinal fusion systems is five people per 100,000 in Europe, North America, Australia, and Japan.[64(p904)]

Safety Issues and Concerns

One study measured temperature increases in the area of spinal fusion stimulators when MRI was performed. It was discovered that if a broken lead was present, the temperature was considerably higher than the temperature near an intact lead. This led to the recommendation that before MRI scanning is performed on a patient with a spinal fusion stimulator, it is important to make sure all spinal fusion stimulator leads are intact.[64]

Diathermy used over an area with an implanted bone growth stimulator can cause damage to the tissues surrounding the device or to the electronics of the device itself.[32] The magnetic external coils of a neurological IED should be kept to a minimum of 18 inches (45 cm) from bone growth stimulators.[36]

Patient Management

Preoperative

■ Externally worn spine stimulators should be removed before the surgical procedure.

Intraoperative

■ Electrosurgery should be avoided. Electrosurgical devices can produce radio frequency currents strong enough to cause direct coupling.[32] Direct coupling is the contact of an energized metal active electrode tip with another metal instrument or object within the surgical field.[16] When direct coupling occurs, the active electrode directly touches or comes very close to the implanted device, allowing the implanted device to become energized. This energy will seek a pathway to the return electrode.

This could cause injury to the patient or damage to the implanted device.[32]

■ An ultrasonic scalpel is considered safe to use.[14]

■ Specific instructions on the totally implantable bone growth stimulation system specify when electrosurgery is necessary. Following implantation of this device, the electrode (ie, cathode-negative electrode) should remain connected, and the generator should be removed from the tissues and placed outside of the body until the procedure is completed. The generator should be replaced in the subcutaneous tissue at the end of the procedure.[65]

Gastric Electronic Stimulation

Electronic stimulation applied to appropriate areas in the body is beneficial in treating some disease processes that otherwise are difficult or impossible to treat with medication. Gastroparesis is an example of one such disease. Gastroparesis is characterized by delayed gastric emptying of solids without evidence of mechanical obstruction; it presents with nausea and early satiety in mild cases and chronic vomiting, dehydration, and weight loss in severe cases.[66] Gastric motility is controlled by myoelectric activity of the stomach, so abnormalities in gastric myoelectrical activity may result in gastric motility disorders, such as gastroparesis.[67]

Application of pacing techniques to the gastrointestinal tract is an attractive idea because the stomach, like the heart, has a natural pacemaker, and the myoelectric activity it generates may be entrained by electrical pacing.[67] In 1963, Bilgutay proposed the feasibility of using electrical stimulation in the gastrointestinal tract to treat paralytic ileus.[68] Using transluminal electrical stimulation via a nasogastric tube, researchers observed under fluoroscopy augmented gastric contractions and gastric emptying.[68] By the late 1960s and early 1970s, researchers conducted experiments that studied gastrointestinal myoelectric activity and its relationship with contractile activity. The results of these experiments, coupled with new techniques of recording myoelectric activity, gave rise to further research in gastrointestinal pacing.[68] Scientists today study the effects of varying the parameters of electrical stimulation applied to the wall of the stomach by an implanted device.

One IED derived from the research is the gastric electrical stimulation system. This type of therapy is indicated for the treatment of chronic nausea and vomiting associated with gastroparesis when conventional medication therapies are not providing adequate relief of symptoms for diabetic or idiopathic patients.[69] The components of a gastric electrical stimulation system include

- ♦ an implanted neurostimulator, usually surgically placed in the upper abdominal region;
- ♦ two intramuscular leads with electrodes that are implanted in the muscle wall of the stomach; and
- ♦ a programming device that the physician uses to control and adjust the settings of the neurostimulator.[69]

Patient management

Preoperative
■ The perioperative team should be aware of the manufacturer's written warnings and precautions. The system can affect cardiac pacemakers, cardioverters/defibrillators, external defibrillators, MRI, ultrasonic equipment, electrosurgery, and radiation therapy.[69]

Nursing Process Application

The perioperative nursing vocabulary is a clinically relevant and empirically validated standardized nursing language. It relates to the delivery of care in the perioperative setting. This standardized language consists of a collection of data elements (ie, the Perioperative Nursing Data Set [PNDS]) and includes perioperative nursing diagnoses, interventions, and outcomes.[70] In 1999, the PNDS was recognized by the American Nurses Association committee on nursing practice information infrastructure as a data set useful in the practice of nursing. The perioperative patient focused model provides the conceptual framework for the PNDS and the model for perioperative nursing practice. The patient and his or her family members are at the core of the model. The model depicts perioperative nursing in four domains and illustrates the relationship between the patient, family members, and the care provided by the perioperative professional nurse.

Each data element in the PNDS is represented by a unique identifier. The domains are represented by the letter "D," followed by numbers one to four to indicate the particular domain being addressed. Nursing diagnoses are represented by the letter "X" and a number unique to the diagnosis. Interventions are represented by the letter "I" and a unique number, and outcomes are represented by the letter

"O" and a unique number. These designations are used in this document as appropriate.

Care of the patient must be individualized and appropriate to the specific device involved. Documentation should reflect the unique aspects of each patient's care. The PNDS provides a common language for perioperative nursing documentation. The examples listed below may not apply to all of the various IEDs. Each patient and device must be assessed for appropriate outcomes, nursing diagnoses, and interventions.

Domains
The following is a list of domains that may be associated with the patient undergoing surgical or other invasive procedures with an IED:

- ♦ D1—safety,
- ♦ D2—physiological responses, and
- ♦ D3-B—behavioral responses—patient and family: rights/ethics.[70]

Outcomes
The following is a partial list of nursing outcomes that may be associated with the patient undergoing surgical or other invasive procedures with an IED.

- ♦ O2—The patient is free from signs and symptoms of injury caused by extraneous objects.
- ♦ O4—The patient is free from signs and symptoms of electrical injury.
- ♦ O14—The patient's respiratory status is consistent with or improved from baseline levels established preoperatively.
- ♦ O15—The patient's cardiac status is consistent with or improved from baseline levels established preoperatively.
- ♦ O30—The patient's neurological status is consistent with or improved from baseline levels established preoperatively.
- ♦ O23—The patient participates in decision making affecting the perioperative plan of care.
- ♦ O24—The patient's care is consistent with the perioperative plan of care.[70]

Nursing Diagnoses
The following is a partial list of nursing diagnoses that may be associated with the patient undergoing surgical or other invasive procedures with an IED:

- ♦ X4—Anxiety;
- ♦ X28—Infection, risk for;
- ♦ X29—Injury, risk of;
- ♦ X30—Knowledge, deficient;
- ♦ X47—Sensory perception, disturbed;

◆ X56—Surgical recovery, delayed;

◆ X62—Urinary elimination, impaired;

◆ X64—Verbal communication, impaired;

◆ X72—Intracranial adaptive capacity, decreased; and

◆ X74—Pain, chronic.[70]

Interventions

The following is a partial list of nursing interventions that may be associated with the patient undergoing surgical or other invasive procedures with an IED.

◆ I3—Administers care to invasive device sites.

◆ I11—Applies safety devices.

◆ I30—Develops individualized plan of care.

◆ I37—Evaluates for signs and symptoms of electrical injury.

◆ I38—Evaluates for signs and symptoms of injury as a result of positioning.

◆ I44—Evaluates postoperative cardiac status.

◆ I45—Evaluates postoperative respiratory status.

◆ I46—Evaluates postoperative tissue perfusion.

◆ I47—Evaluates physiological response to plan of care.

◆ I54—Evaluates response to pain management interventions.

◆ I58—Identifies and reports the presence of implantable cardiac devices.

◆ I72—Implements protective measures to prevent injury due to electrical sources.

◆ I92—Obtains consultation from the appropriate health care providers to initiate new treatments or change existing treatments.

◆ I122—Uses supplies and equipment within safe parameters.

◆ I127—Verifies presence of prosthetics or corrective devices.

◆ I138—Implements protective measures prior to operative or invasive procedure.

◆ I145—Implements protective measures during neurosurgical procedures.

◆ I152—Evaluates for signs and symptoms of physical injury to skin and tissue.[70]

Conclusion

This guideline is intended to promote safe care for patients with IEDs who undergo surgical and other invasive procedures. Perioperative registered nurses should be aware of potential patient safety hazards associated with specific IEDs and the appropriate patient care interventions and resources required to protect patients from injury.

Perioperative registered nurses should be knowledgeable about the types of IEDs that may be encountered in the practice setting, how they function, and the precautions that must be taken when caring for patients with these devices. Competency related to specific devices should be measured and documented according to individual facility policy. It is AORN's intent that perioperative registered nurses use this document to assist in the development and implementation of policies and procedures for caring for patients with IEDs who are undergoing surgical and other invasive procedures.

REFERENCES

1. P Seifert, "Surgical interventions," in *Cardiac Surgery: Perioperative Patient Care* (St Louis: Mosby, Inc, 2002) 508-526.

2. "Sources of electromagnetic interference (EMI) for pacemakers, implantable cardioverter defibrillators (ICDs), and heart failure devices," Guidant, Inc, *http://www.guidant.com/patient/living* (accessed 14 Jan 2005).

3. J D Madigan et al, "Surgical management of the patient with an implanted cardiac device: Implications of electromagnetic interference," *Annals of Surgery* 230 (November 1999) 639-647.

4. *Mosby's Medical, Nursing & Allied Health Dictionary*, fifth ed (St Louis: Mosby-Year Book, Inc, 1998) 545.

5. "Electromagnetic interference (EMI)," Institute for Telecommunication Sciences, *http://www.its.bldrdoc.gov/fs-1037/dir-013/_1935.htm* (accessed 12 Nov 2004).

6. "InterStim therapy for urinary control: Product technical manual must be reviewed prior to use for detailed disclosure," Medtronic, Inc, *http://www.medtronic.com/neuro/interstim/interstim_warning.html* (accessed 12 Nov 2004).

7. "Safety alert (May 16, 2001)," Medtronic, Inc, *http://www.medtronic.com/neuro/diathermy_alert/alert_physicians.html* (accessed 12 Nov 2004).

8. D W Fiegal, Jr, "FDA public health notification: Diathermy interactions with implanted leads and implanted systems with leads," US Food and Drug Administration, *http://www.fda.gov/cdrh/safety/121902.pdf* (accessed 14 Jan 2005).

9. "Competency statements in perioperative nursing," in *Standards, Recommended Practices and Guidelines* (Denver: AORN, Inc, 2004) 19-21.

10. C J Linstrom, "Cochlear implantation: Practical information for the generalist," *Primary Care; Clinics in Office Practice* 25 (September 1998) 583-617.

11. "Perioperative management of implanted medical devices—Draft 2" (Williamsport, Pa: Susquehanna Health System, May 2004).

12. "Preadmission testing pacemaker or ICD letter" (Williamsport, Pa: Susquehanna Health System).

13. "AORN statement on the role of the health care industry representative in the operating room," in *Standards, Recommended Practices, and Guidelines* (Denver: AORN, Inc, 2004) 153-154.

14. "Electrosurgical precautions," in *University of Iowa Hospitals and Clinics Policy and Procedure Manual* (Iowa City: University of Iowa HealthCare, February 2004).

15. "MEGA 2000 and patients with pacemakers" (Draper, Utah: Megadyne Medical Products, Inc, 2004).

16. "Recommended practices for electrosurgery," in *Standards, Recommended Practices, and Guidelines* (Denver: AORN, Inc, 2004) 245-259.

17. C Peterson, "Rectifying counts; neurostimulators; double gloving; reprocessing single-use devices; simultaneous counting," (Clinical Issues) *AORN Journal* 76 (September 2002) 510-512.

18. L Rhyne, B C Ulmer, L Revell, "Monitoring and controlling the environment," in *Patient Care During Operative and Other Invasive Procedures*, ed M L Phippen, M P Wells (Philadelphia: W B Saunders Co, 2000) 147.

19. "HeartMate® destination therapy," Hearthope.com, *http://www.hearthope.com/1.html* (accessed 14 Jan 2005).

20. "Ventricular assist device," HeartCenterOnline for Patients, *http://heartcenteronline.com/myheartdr/common/articles.cfm?ARTID-340* (accessed 30 July 2004).

21. J E Lowe, J M Wharton, "Cardiac pacemakers and implantable cardioverter-defibrillators," in *Surgery of the Chest*, sixth ed, D C Sabiston, Jr, F C Spencer, eds (Philadelphia: W B Saunders Co, 1995).

22. M Mirowski et al, "Termination of malignant ventricular arrhythmias with an implanted automatic defibrillator in human beings," *The New England Journal of Medicine* 303 (Aug 7, 1980) 322-324.

23. J L Atlee, A D Bernstein, "Cardiac rhythm management devices (Part II): Perioperative management," *Anesthesiology* 95 (December 2001) 1492-1506.

24. S P Kutalek et al, "Approach to generator change," in *Clinical Cardiac Pacing and Defibrillation*, second ed, K A Ellenbogen, G N Kay, B L Wilkoff, eds (Philadelphia: W B Saunders Co, 2000) 645-668.

25. C M Bernards, "An unusual cause of airway obstruction during general anesthesia with a laryngeal mask airway," *Anesthesiology* 100 (April 2004) 1017-1018.

26. "History of neurostimulation: Part II: Implanted neuroaugmentive devices," The Burton Report, *http://www.burtonreport.com/InfSpine/NSHistNeurostimPartII_ImpNeuroAugmenDevices.htm* (accessed 12 Nov 2004).

27. N J M Rijkhoff, "Neuroprostheses to treat neurogenic bladder dysfunction: Current status and future perspectives," *Childs Nervous System* 20 no 2 (2004) 75-86.

28. H W Roberts, "The effect of electrical dental equipment on a vagus nerve stimulator's function," *Journal of the American Dental Association* 133 (December 2002) 1657-1664.

29. J Weaver, S J Kim, A Torres, "Cutaneous electrosurgery in a patient with a deep brain stimulator," *Dermatologic Surgery* 25 (May 1999) 415-417.

30. "Electrical stimulation in spinal cord injury," International Functional Electrical Stimulation Society, *http://www.ifess.org/Services/Consumer_Ed/SCI.htm* (accessed 14 Jan 2005).

31. "Introduction to neurostimulation," Medtronic, *http://www.medtronic.com/neuro/paintherapies/pain_treatment_ladder/neurostimulation/neuroneurostimulation.html* (accessed 16 Aug 2004).

32. "Bone growth stimulation: Questions and answers," Spine Universe.com, *http://www.spineuniverse.com/displayaritcle.php/article1555.html* (accessed 13 Aug 2004).

33. *Patient's Manual for Vagus Nerve Stimulation with the VNS Therapy™ System* (Houston: Cyberonics, Inc, 2002).

34. C A Liberante, "New relief for constant condition," York Neurosurgical Associates, *http://www.yna.org/new%20pages/YDRhydro.html* (accessed 12 Nov 2004).

35. E Eisenberg, H Waisbrod, "Spinal cord stimulator activation by an antitheft device: Case report," *Journal of Neurosurgery* 87 (December 1997) 961-962.

36. *Deep Brain Stimulation MRI Guidelines* (Minneapolis: Medtronic, April 2002) 1-14.

37. S Roberts et al, "Impact of dental devices on cochlear implants," *Journal of Endodontics* 28 (January 2002) 40.

38. "Cochlear implants: Wiring for sound," Australian Academy of Science, *http://www.science.org.au/nova/029/029key.htm* (accessed 14 Jan 2005).

39. G A Gates, R T Miyamoto, "Cochlear implants," *The New England Journal of Medicine* 349 (July 31, 2003) 421-423.

40. A J Maniglia, "State of the art on the development of the implantable hearing device for partial hearing loss," *Otolaryngologic Clinics of North America* 29 (April 1996) 225-243.

41. J M Black, J Hokanson-Hawks, A Keene, "Assist hearing in profound deafness," in *Medical-Surgical Nursing*, sixth ed (Philadelphia: W B Saunders Co, 2001) 1840-1841.

42. D R McEwen, "Otologic surgery," in *Alexander's Care of the Patient in Surgery*, 12th ed, J C Rothrock, ed (St Louis: Mosby, 2003) 717-749.

43. "Bone-anchored hearing aid," Hear-it, *http://hear-it.org/printpage.dsp?printable=yes&page=2020* (accessed 14 Jan 2005).

44. M Kalamarides et al, "Hearing restoration with auditory brainstem implants after radiosurgery for neurofibromatosis Type 2," *Journal of Neurosurgery* 95 (December 2001) 1028-1033.

45. "New device approvals—Nucleus 24 auditory brainstem implant system," US Food and Drug Administration, Center for Devices and Radiological Health, *http://www.fda.gov/cdrh/pdf/p000015.html* (accessed 22 Aug 2004).

46. S C Smeltzer, B G Bare, "Sensorineural function," in *Brunner and Suddarth's Textbook of Medical Surgical Nursing* (Philadelphia: Lippincott, Williams and Wilkins, 2004) 1744.

47. "Proposed package insert," US Food and Drug Administration, Center for Devices and Radiological Health, *http://www.fda.gov/cdrh/pdf/p000015.html* (accessed 22 Aug 2004).

48. "Is electrosurgery safe for patients with internal or external electronic devices?" *Clinical Information Hotline News* 6 (December 2001) 1-2. Also available at *http://www.valleylab.com/displaynews.cfm?articlepageid=380&menu* (accessed 12 Nov 2004).

49. M Goodman "Chemotherapy: Principles of administration," in *Cancer Nursing*, fifth ed, C H Yarbro et al, ed (Boston: Jones and Bartlett Publishers, 2000) 407-408.

50. N H Fortunato, ed, *Berry & Kohn's Operating Room Technique*, 10th ed (St. Louis: Mosby, Inc, 2004) 114-116.

51. "The Medtronic Mini-Med 2007 implantable insulin pump system," Medtronic, *http://www.minimed.com/patientfam/pf_products_implantpump_no neu.shtml* (accessed 12 Nov 2004).

52. "How pump therapy works," Medtronic, *http://www.minimed.com/patientfam/pf_ipt_ptov_how therapyworks.shtml* (accessed 12 Nov 2004).

53. "Safety information: Medtronic MiniMed," Medtronic, *http://www.minimed.com/common/safety.html* (accessed 12 Nov 2004).

54. P E V van Kerrebroeck, "The role of electrical stimulation in voiding dysfunction," *European Urology* 34 suppl (1998) 27-30.

55. "InterStim therapy for urinary control: Product technical manual must be reviewed prior to use for detailed disclosure," Medtronic, Inc, *http://www.medtronic.com/neuro/interstim/interstim_warning.html* (accessed 12 Nov 2004).

56. J R Vignes et al, "Dorsal rhizotomy with anterior sacral root stimulation for neurogenic bladder," *Stereotactic and Functional Neurosurgery* 76 no 3-4 (2001) 243-245.

57. "The challenge: Treating selected bladder control problems and improving outcomes," Medtronic, *http://www.medtronic.com/neuro/interstim/solution.html* (accessed 12 Nov 2004).

58. M Oishi, S T Onesti, "Electrical bone graft stimulation for spinal fusion: A review," *Neurosurgery* 47 (November 2000) 1041-1055.

59. J Soyhan et al, "Demography, clinical characteristics, psychological and abuse profiles, treatment, and long-term follow-up of patients with gastroparesis," *Digestive Diseases and Sciences* 43 (November 1998) 2398-2404.

60. J T Ryaby, "Clinical effects of electromagnetic and electric fields on fracture healing," *Clinical Orthopedics and Related Research* 355 suppl (October 1998) S205-S215.

61. R K Aaron, D M Ciombor, B J Simon, "Treatment of nonunions with electric and electromagnetic fields," *Clinical Orthopedics* 419 (February 2004) 21-29.

62. "Frequently asked questions," EBI Medical, *http://www.ebimedical.com/patients/faq.cfm* (accessed 12 Nov 2004).

63. "Products: Spine systems—Spine fusion stimulators," EBI Medical, *http://www.ebimedical.com/products/index.cfm?s=0E* (accessed 12 Nov 2004).

64. W Kainz et al, "Electromagnetic compatibility of electronic implants—Review of the literature," *Wiener Klinische Wochenschrift* 113 (Dec 17, 2001) 903-914.

65. "EBI Bone Healing System," EBI Medical, *http://www.ebimedical.com/products/detail.cfm?p=0C* (accessed 12 Nov 2004).

66. K Hornbuckle, J L Barnett, "The diagnosis and work-up of the patient with gastroparesis," *Journal of Clinical Gastroenterology* 30 (March 2000) 117-124.

67. Z Lin et al, "Treatment of gastroparesis with electrical stimulation," *Digestive Diseases and Sciences* 48 (May 2003) 837-848.

68. A M Bilgutay et al, "Gastro-intestinal pacing: A new concept in the treatment of ileus," *Annals of Surgery* 158 (September 1963) 338-348.

69. "Safety information on Enterra therapy," Medtronic, *http://www.medtronic.com/neuro/gastro/indicationsuse.html#enterra* (14 Jan 2005).

70. S Beyea, ed, *Perioperative Nursing Data Set*, second ed (Denver: AORN, Inc, 2002).

PUBLICATION HISTORY
Originally published in *Standards, Recommended Practices, and Guidelines,* 2005 edition. Reprinted July 2005, *AORN Journal.*

Exhibit A: Care of the Patient
With an Implanted Electronic Device

IMPLANTED DEVICE	SAFETY CONCERN	PREOPERATIVE PATIENT MANAGEMENT	INTRAOPERATIVE PATIENT MANAGEMENT	POSTOPERATIVE PATIENT MANAGEMENT
All implanted devices				
	Electrosurgery	Assess patients for the presence of any implanted electronic device (IED). Check for a product identification card if an IED is present. Contact the implanting surgeon to inform him or her that the patient is scheduled for surgery. Obtain and document <ul><li>manufacturer and model of IED,</li><li>location of the device,</li><li>when the device was last evaluated,</li><li>if the device can be turned off before or during surgery,</li><li>settings that should be reprogrammed into the device immediately after the procedure,</li><li>if the implanting physician wants to be contacted when the patient enters the postanesthesia care unit, and</li><li>if the patient needs to schedule an appointment with the implanting physician.</li></ul> Determine if electrosurgery and/or defibrillation is necessary Contact the appropriate health care industry representative and arrange for his or her presence before, during, and after the surgery if requested by the physician. Notify the anesthesia care provider that an IED is present.	Notify all perioperative team members the patient has an IED in place and review safety concerns and equipment conflicts. Be sure the programming device and qualified programming personnel are in the OR before starting the procedure. Suggest the use of a bipolar electrosurgical unit (ESU). Place the dispersive electrode as far from the IED as possible, maintaining a perpendicular pathway for the current to travel and making sure it is not over an implant and the current does not go through the IED. Do not arc current between the active electrode and another surgical instrument. If the IED has been reprogrammed by electrosurgery, stop the procedure and reprogram the device. Maintain the OR temperature between 20° C and 24° C (68° F and 76° F) and humidity between 50% and 60%.	If necessary, notify the implanting physician and/or the health care industry representative that electrosurgery or defibrillation was used during surgery. Early in the postoperative period, do an evaluation of IED function similar to that performed before surgery. Postoperatively, monitor the patient closely for signs of complications and IED malfunction.
	Defibrillation		For patients with IEDs in the chest area who require defibrillation, use anterior-posterior-type paddles. Place the anterior paddle as far from the pulse generator as possible. Use the lowest defibrillator current setting possible.	

IMPLANTED DEVICE	SAFETY CONCERN	PREOPERATIVE PATIENT MANAGEMENT	INTRAOPERATIVE PATIENT MANAGEMENT	POSTOPERATIVE PATIENT MANAGEMENT
Cardiac				
Pacemakers Implantable cardioverter defibrillators (ICDs)	Electrosurgery	1. If the IED has not been evaluated during the previous 6 months, it should be tested for programming, telemetry, thresholds, and battery status. 2. If the make and model of IED is not known, a chest x-ray may be helpful in identifying it. 3. The device should be reprogrammed to an asynchronous mode. 4. Adaptive-rate device features should be programmed off. 5. Magnet-activated testing should be programmed off.	1. The current pathway should be perpendicular to the pacemaker's lead system when possible. 2. The ESU may interfere with electrocardiogram (ECG) monitoring of the heart, so the heart rate and blood pressure (BP) should be monitored through an arterial line. When the ESU is not in use, the ECG should be checked for arrhythmias or alterations in pacemaker function. 3. If it is impossible to place the device in an asynchronous mode, and the ESU is adversely affecting the pacemaker, the ESU current should only be activated for 1 second at a time. Ten seconds should elapse between 1-second activations. 4 Bipolar ESU is recommended. 5. Tachycardia sensing should be programmed off.	1. Inform the patient's cardiologist or cardiothoracic surgeon that ESU or defibrillation was used during surgery. 2. An evaluation of the pacemaker and ICD function should be done in the early postoperative period and again at 24 and 48 hours.
	Defibrillation		1. Position paddles at least 6 inches from the device. 2. Place paddles in the anterior and posterior position. 3. The lowest defibrillator current settings should be used. 4. Have a temporary pacing system available in case of pulse generator damage.	

IMPLANTED DEVICE	SAFETY CONCERN	PREOPERATIVE PATIENT MANAGEMENT	INTRAOPERATIVE PATIENT MANAGEMENT	POSTOPERATIVE PATIENT MANAGEMENT
Cardiac, continued				
Ventricular assist device (VAD)	Electrosurgery	1. If IED has not been evaluated within the previous 6 months, it should be tested for programming, telemetry, thresholds, and battery status. 2. If the make and model of the IED is not known, a chest x-ray may be helpful in identifying it.	1. The ESU may interfere with ECG monitoring of the heart, so the heart rate and BP should be monitored through an arterial line. When the ESU is not in use, the ECG should be checked for arrhythmias or alterations in pacemaker function. 2. The device should be placed in the fixed rate mode for the duration of the surgery. 3. The ESU current should only be activated for 1 second at a time. Ten seconds should elapse between 1-second activations. 4. Cardiac output should be monitored. 5. Have an external hand pump available in the OR.	1. Inform the patient's cardiologist or cardiothoracic surgeon that ESU or defibrillation was used during surgery. 2. The surgeon or cardiologist responsible for the care of the patient should be informed if the circuit is damaged during surgery. Repair or replacement should be considered.
	Defibrillation		1. Disconnect the timing circuit from the external controller before defibrillation. 2. Depending on the type of VAD, a fixed rate mode may be required during defibrillation.	
Neurological				
Deep brain stimulators Programmable ventricular shunts Spinal cord stimulators Vagal nerve stimulators	Electrosurgery	1. Magnetic resonance imaging is not recommended.	1. Bipolar ESU is recommended. 2. The device should be turned off. Notify the appropriate vendor representative. 3. Use only low voltage mode/setting. 4. Keep the grounding pad as far away from the device as possible.	1. Perioperative team members should confirm that the device is functioning properly.
	Defibrillation		1. Position paddles as far away from the IED as possible. 2. Position paddles perpendicular to the IED. 3. Use the lowest output settings.	
	Magnetic resonance imaging (MRI)		1. Magnetic resonance imaging is not recommended.	
	Bone growth stimulator		1. Keep magnetic external coils of a neurological IED a minimum of 18 inches (45 cm) away from bone growth stimulators.	
	Dental drills Ultrasonic probes Diagnostic ultrasound Electrolysis		1. Turn the device off. 2. Keep 6 inches away from device.	

IMPLANTED DEVICE	SAFETY CONCERN	PREOPERATIVE PATIENT MANAGEMENT	INTRAOPERATIVE PATIENT MANAGEMENT	POSTOPERATIVE PATIENT MANAGEMENT
Neurological, continued				
	Lasers		1. Turn the device off. 2. Keep lasers directed away from the device.	
Implantable hearing devices				
Cochlear implants Auditory brainstem implant (ABI) Bone-conduction stimulators	Static electricity	1. Educate patients and staff members that a static electric shock has been known to inactivate cochlear implants.	1. Educate patients and staff members that a static electric shock has been known to inactivate cochlear implants.	1. Perioperative team members should confirm that the device is functioning properly.
	Electrosurgery		1. Bipolar ESU is recommended. 2. Bipolar instruments should be kept more than 10 cm from extracochlear electrodes. 3. Monopolar ESU should not be used in the head and neck area. 4. For patients with ABIs, the bipolar electrode should be kept 1 cm from the ground electrodes of the ABI.	
	MRI	1. Magnetic resonance imaging is not recommended and should only be done if it is a medical necessity.	1. Magnetic resonance imaging is not recommended and should only be done if it is a medical necessity.	
	Miscellaneous		1. Remove external devices after induction of anesthesia. 2. Avoid using ionizing radiation directly over the site of the implant.	
Implantable infusion pumps				
	MRI	1. Magnetic resonance imaging may cause the device to malfunction. 2. Remove the external pump and remote control from the patient's body and the treatment area. 3. Avoid exposure to medical imaging equipment.	1. Remove the external pump and remote control from the patient's body and the treatment area. 2. Avoid exposure to medical imaging equipment.	
	X-ray	1. Remove the external pump and remote control from the patient's body and the treatment area.		

IMPLANTED DEVICE	SAFETY CONCERN	PREOPERATIVE PATIENT MANAGEMENT	INTRAOPERATIVE PATIENT MANAGEMENT	POSTOPERATIVE PATIENT MANAGEMENT
Sacral nerve stimulators				
	Miscellaneous	1. Determine how the device functions and whether it can be turned off.	1. The ESU active electrode should be kept 6 inches from the implanted device.	
Osteogenic (bone-growth) stimulators				
	MRI	1. Before imaging, the stimulator should be tested to make sure all leads are intact.		
	Miscellaneous	1. Externally worn stimulators should be removed before the surgical procedure.		
	Electrocautery		1. Monopolar ESU is not recommended. 2. Ultrasonic scalpel is considered safe. 3. Electrodes should remain connected. 4. The generator should be removed from subcutaneous tissues and placed outside of the body until the procedure is complete.	
Gastric electronic stimulation				
	Miscellaneous	1. Review manufacturers' written warnings and precautions. 2. Devices can affect other IEDs. 3. Device is affected by MRI, ultrasonic equipment, ESU, and radiation therapy.		

I. Overview

A. Introduction

Preamble

Natural rubber latex allergy is a significant medical concern because it affects health care workers, as well as the general population. It crosses racial and ethnic boundaries, and it can affect males or females anytime during their lives.

There is no cure at this time, only prevention. Three types of reactions are associated with latex products. In order of frequency of occurrence they are an irritant reaction, a delayed hypersensitivity reaction (ie, type IV), and an immediate hypersensitivity reaction (ie, type I) (**Table 1**). Any individual who experiences any type of latex-associated reaction should be evaluated by a qualified health care practitioner.

Assumptions

Natural rubber latex allergy can be a serious and potentially life-threatening condition. Health care workers and others who experience repeated exposure to latex allergens can develop a latex sensitivity or allergy. Several hundred cases of severe allergic reactions and anaphylaxis and 17 deaths have been reported to the US Food and Drug Administration (FDA).[1,2]

Sensitivity can be described as development of an immunologic memory to the specific latex proteins; however, the affected individual may be asymptomatic. Allergy is the demonstrated outward expression of the sensitivity (eg, hives, rhinitis, conjunctivitis, anaphylaxis). Sensitivity to natural rubber latex is more common than the actual allergy; however, any individual sensitized to natural rubber latex is at risk of a life-threatening reaction and should be treated in the same way as an allergic individual.

Powdered latex gloves are the most common item contributing to the latex load in health care facilities. Recent estimates have shown a 20-fold increase in medical glove use (in billions of pairs) since the introduction of universal precautions in 1987.[3] During the manufacturing process, powder usually is applied to the glove as cornstarch slurry when the glove still is on the mold or former. When the powder slurry is applied to the glove, the extractable, water-soluble proteins leach from the surface of the glove onto the cornstarch particles. When dry, the glove powder then acts as a vector that carries latex proteins from the glove into the environment.

Health care facilities and providers have an ethical responsibility to prevent latex sensitization in patients and employees by creating an environment in which it is safe to be treated and to work. Many facilities in the United States consciously have moved toward a latex-safe environment by switching from powdered latex gloves (eg, examination, surgical) and other latex products to powder-free products with reduced latex protein content. High-protein, powdered latex gloves and other products that create aerosolization can contaminate a facility's environment with latex allergens.

In 1998, Sussman et al reported a 1% annual incidence of sensitization among powdered latex-glove users, whereas users of powder-free, low-protein, latex gloves reported a 0% sensitization rate.[4] In 1999, Levy et al studied a group of dental students in both France and England, reporting that students who wore protein-rich (ie, high protein), powdered latex gloves had a 15% and a 5% sensitization rate, respectively, while students who wore powder-free, protein-poor (ie, low protein) gloves had a 0% sensitization rate.[5]

It is unsafe to treat latex-allergic individuals in an environment laden with latex allergens. Individuals who have been clinically diagnosed as either sensitive or allergic to natural rubber latex should be treated or work in an environment that is latex-safe, with additional measures taken for the immediate vicinity (ie, room) in which the individual receives or provides care. If the entire care facility is maintained as a latex-safe environment, few additional precautions will be needed for latex-allergic individuals. If the facility is not maintained as latex-safe, comprehensive latex precautions will be required each time a latex-allergic individual presents for care or services.

This revised "AORN latex guideline" is based on research and expert opinion available at the time of its revision. Ongoing and future research likely will enhance and expand current knowledge about this topic.

Review of this document has been solicited from content experts at the American Association of Nurse Anesthetists (AANA), the American College of Surgeons (ACS), the American Society of Anesthesiologists (ASA), the American Academy of Allergy, Asthma, and Immunology (AAAAI), the American

Table 1

TYPES OF REACTIONS TO LATEX[1-4]				
Type of Reaction	**Cause**	**Onset**	**Symptoms**	**Prevention**
Irritant contact dermatitis *(Nonallergic irritation; not a true allergy)*	Frequent hand washing, insufficient rinsing, aggressive scrubbing technique, use of antiseptics, climatic irritation, glove occlusion, glove powder.	Reaction develops gradually over a period of days or weeks.	Scaling, drying, cracking of skin may develop as dermatitis on the backs of the hands. Wearing latex gloves when symptoms are present may increase the risk of developing latex allergy.	Obtain medical diagnosis, dermatology consultation; avoid irritant product; ensure barrier effectiveness of glove material; consider alternative products, cotton glove liners.
Type IV hypersensitivity; T cell-mediated *(Also called delayed cutaneous hypersensitivity; allergic contact dermatitis; chemical allergy)*	Results from exposure to chemicals used in latex harvesting, processing, or manufacturing (eg, thiurams, carbamates, benzothiazoles).	Rash usually begins six to 48 hours after contact and may progress to oozing skin blisters or spread away from the area of skin touched by the latex.	Red, raised, palpable area with bumps, sores, and horizontal cracks may extend up the forearm. May occur after a sensitization period resulting from repeated exposure to latex or irritant chemicals.	Obtain medical diagnosis, dermatology consultation; identify irritant chemical; use alternative glove material without chemical; ensure barrier effectiveness of glove material; consider alternative products, cotton glove liners.
Type I hypersensitivity; immunoglobulin-mediated *(Also called immediate reaction hypersensitivity; latex allergy; protein allergy)*	Results from exposure to proteins in latex on glove surface or bound to powder and suspended in the air, settled on objects, or transferred by touch.	Reactions usually begin within minutes of exposure but can occur as much as two hours later. May fade away rapidly after removing the glove.	Mild reactions involve skin redness, hives, or itching on the skin under the glove. The chronic form may mimic irritant and allergic contact dermatitis. More severe reactions may include facial swelling, rhinitis, eye symptoms, generalized urticaria, scratchy throat, respiratory distress, and asthma. In rare cases, anaphylactic shock may occur.	Obtain medical diagnosis, allergy consultation; substitute nonlatex gloves or other nonlatex products; reduce or eliminate exposure to glove powder; clean powder from environment; consider latex-safe environment.

REFERENCES

1. Latex Allergy: Protect Yourself, Protect Your Patients (Silver Spring, MD: American Nurses Association, 1996).

2. "Preventing allergic reactions to natural rubber latex in the workplace," NIOSH publ no 97-135, National Institute of Occupational Safety and Health, http://www.cdc.gov/niosh/latexalt.html (accessed Sept 4, 2008).

3. Reddy, S, "Latex allergy," American Academy of Family Physicians, http://www.aafp.org/afp/980101ap/reddy.html (accessed Sept 4, 2008).

4. "Potential for sensitization and possible allergic reaction to natural rubber latex gloves and other natural rubber products," Occupational Safety and Health Administration, http://www.osha.gov/dts/shib/shib012808.html (accessed Sept 4, 2008).

College of Allergy, Asthma, and Immunology (ACAAI), the American Nurses Association (ANA), the Association of Practitioners of Infection Control, Inc (APIC), the Spina Bifida Association, and the National Institute of Occupational Safety and Health (NIOSH) division of the Centers for Disease Control and Prevention, as well as the AORN Board of Directors and other recognized experts. This guideline may not apply to every individual and may require modification based on specific needs of a given patient, health care provider, or situation.

Definitions

For purposes of this document the following definitions apply.

- ◆ *Allergen:* A substance that in some individuals can cause an allergic or hypersensitivity reaction but is not normally considered harmful.[6]
- ◆ *Allergenic:* A substance that can elicit a hypersensitivity reaction in certain individuals.[7]
- ◆ *Allergy:* An immune reaction to an environmental agent that results in a symptomatic reaction.[6,7]
- ◆ *Antigen:* Any molecule or substance, more

often a protein, that has the ability to bind to an antibody.[6,7] "The name arises from their ability to generate antibodies."[6]

♦ *Irritant contact dermatitis:* A nonallergic, cutaneous response to an irritant. Normally this reaction is primarily localized to the site of exposure. This is not a latex allergy.

♦ *Allergic contact dermatitis (type IV: T-cell mediated/delayed hypersensitivity):* A delayed, T-cell mediated hypersensitivity response attributed to chemicals (ie, antigens) used in the latex and some synthetic manufacturing processes and absorbed through the skin.[6] This reaction generally is localized to the contact area.

♦ *Latex:* Also known as natural rubber latex, this milky cytosol is acquired by tapping the commercial rubber tree, *Hevea brasiliensis.*

♦ *Latex allergy (type immunoglobulin E [IgE]-mediated/immediate hypersensitivity response):* A localized or systemic allergic response to one or more specific proteins (ie, antigens)[6] found in latex to which the individual has been sensitized and has developed antibodies.

♦ *Latex-free environment:* An environment in which all latex-containing products, not simply gloves, have been removed. This state is considered unattainable due to the ubiquitous nature of latex products.

♦ *Latex-safe environment:* An environment in which every reasonable effort has been made to remove high-allergen and airborne latex sources from coming into direct contact with affected individuals. The airborne latex protein load should be less than 0.6 ng per cubic meter.[8]

♦ *Latex precautions:* Interventions to prevent reactions in people (eg, patients, health care workers) allergic to latex proteins.

♦ *Reactions associated with latex:* Irritant contact dermatitis, allergic type IV cell-mediated contact dermatitis, and type I IgE-mediated latex allergy. Only the type I IgE-mediated response constitutes a true latex allergy.

♦ *Sensitization:* The development of immunological memory in response to exposure to an antigen.

♦ *Sensitivity:* A clinical manifestation of symptoms or response that develops after sensitization.

Prevalence

Numerous studies indicate prevalence rates for IgE-mediated latex allergy from 0.8% to 6.5% of the general population.[1,9-13] Latex allergy is believed to be responsible for 70% of anaphylactic reactions occurring in anesthetized children with myelodysplasia (eg, spina bifida).[12] Further, there is a large population of latex-sensitive individuals. Varying sensitization rates have been reported for both patients with myelodysplasia and health care workers.[14-17] According to Sussman, the prevalence rate of latex sensitization among patients with spina bifida is between 35% and 70%. The sensitization rate for health care workers with significant exposure to latex is reported to be 10% to 17%.[18] Although latex-sensitive individuals do not always present with clinical symptoms, these individuals should be assessed for latex allergy. For those who are latex-sensitive but have yet to manifest frank symptoms, there is no predictor of whether or when they will react; therefore, all individuals presenting with natural rubber latex sensitivity should be treated as if they are allergic.

In 1992, Lagier et al reported a 10.7% latex allergy rate in French perioperative nurses.[19] A study of Canadian perioperative nurses by Mace et al, in 1997, reported a 6.9% latex allergy prevalence.[20] Studies of perioperative personnel demonstrate sensitivity rates between 2.5% and 15.8%. In 1992, Arellano et al reported a 9.9% latex sensitization rate in a study of 101 anesthesiologists, radiologists, and surgeons.[21] In 1996, Grzybowski reported an 8.9% rate for hospital RNs in general, but showed perioperative nurses to be less affected than nurses in other areas. One possible explanation for this disparity was that nurses in the OR who were latex sensitive or allergic may have transferred to other nursing units.[22] In 1997, Konrad et al reported a 15.8% positive skin prick test rate for anesthesiologists.[23] In 1998, Brown et al identified 12.5% of anesthesiologists at a tertiary care hospital as sensitized (ie, IgE antibody positive by skin test or serology) with only 2.5% expressing symptoms.[24]

B. Pathophysiology

The major component of natural rubber latex is the hydrocarbon, cis-1, 4 polyisoprene. Chemicals such as sulfur, ammonia, mercaptobenzothiazole, thiuram, and antioxidants may be added during the manufacturing process. Latex protein content and residual chemical levels differ among producers due to variations in manufacturing processes.

Several natural rubber latex proteins responsible for allergenic reactions have been identified (**Table 2**), and sensitivity appears to differ among risk groups.[25-28] Proteins in natural rubber latex may cause a range of mild to severe or even life-threatening type I allergic

Table 2

KNOWN LATEX ALLERGENS				
Name	*Description*	*MW (kD)*	*Plant family*	*Cross-food*
Hev b 1	Rubber elongation factor	14.6		Papain
Hev b 2	Beta one = third gluconase	34-36	PR2	
Hev b 3	Prenyltransferase	24-27		
Hev b 4	Microhelix	110/50		
Hev b 5	Acidic protein	16-24		Kiwi
Hev b 6.02	Hevein protein	4.7	PR3	Kiwi, avocado, banana
Hev b 7	Patatin homologue	43-46		Potato
Hev b 8	Hevea profilin	14-14.2	Profilin	Pollens, celery
Hev b 9	Hevea enolase	51		Molds
Hev b 10	Mn superoxide dismutase	22-26		Molds
Hev b 11	Class I chitinase	33	PR3	Banana, avocado
Hev b 12	Lipid transfer protein	9.4	PR 14	Peach, stone fruit
Hev b 13	Esterase	42		

Suggested by Robert Hamilton, PhD, Latex Committee, Chairman, American Academy of Asthma, Allergy, and Immunology.

reactions. Dipped products made from liquid natural rubber latex (eg, gloves, balloons, condoms) contain a greater amount of soluble proteins than dry gum rubber or heat molded latex products and, therefore, can release more allergen.[2,9,29]

Several types of synthetic materials also may be referred to as latex (eg, butyl, petroleum-based materials) but these do not contain the proteins that cause allergic reactions. There have been case reports, however, of individuals having a type I natural rubber latex-allergic reaction because synthetic materials may have been mixed with or contaminated with natural rubber latex.[29] Water extractable, residual chemicals found in both latex and synthetic gloves usually are implicated in the development of allergic contact dermatitis in individuals who are presensitized.[30-33]

C. Reactions Associated With Latex and Synthetic Products

Reactions associated with latex and synthetic products include irritant contact dermatitis, allergic contact dermatitis (type IV), and immediate IgE hypersensitivity reactions (type I).[34,35] Only the type I hypersensitivity reaction constitutes a latex allergy. Some individuals may present with a single complaint or a combination of all three reactions listed above. Irritant and allergic contact dermatitis are the most common clinical reactions associated with latex and other additives.[34,35]

Irritant contact dermatitis is the result of damage to the skin, but it is not an allergic reaction. Soaps and cleansers, multiple hand washings, inadequate hand drying, or mechanical irritation (ie, sweating, rubbing inside powdered gloves) may cause skin irritation. It also can be caused by chemicals added during glove manufacture. An acute localized response is evidenced by redness, swelling, burning, and itching. Chronic exposure to the irritant can lead to dry, thickened, and cracked skin. Health care workers experiencing irritant contact dermatitis or skin breakdown should be referred to an occupational health practitioner, allergist, dermatologist, or immunologist for further diagnostic testing. This type of dermatitis is reduced by removing the irritant source after it is identified. Thoroughly washing and drying hands, using only powder-free gloves, changing gloves more frequently, or changing glove types can reduce skin irritation.[11,36,37]

Other palliative measures include using only water- or silicone-based moisturizing creams, lotions, or topical barrier agents. Avoid using oil- or petroleum-based skin agents with latex products. These agents may cause breakdown of the latex product. Some skin care agents may help reduce glove-related problems and have been clinically formulated not to interfere with the glove's barrier integrity. Always check with the manufacturer of the skin care agent to verify that the chosen agent is latex compatible before putting the product into use.[38]

Allergic contact dermatitis (ie, delayed hypersensitivity) is a type IV immune reaction. It is a T-cell mediated allergic reaction and usually is localized

Table 3

ANAPHYLACTIC REACTION ASSESSMENT CRITERIA

Decreased cardiac output

Assess physical status and document changes. Report:

♦ Vital signs, including temperature, pulse rate, blood pressure, cardiac rhythm, respiratory rate.
♦ Lung sounds (eg, rales, wheezing, stridor).
♦ Jugular vein distention, pulmonary pressures.
♦ Skin color, rashes, temperature, moisture.
♦ Changes in level of consciousness or mentation.
♦ Changes in patient's level of anxiety.

Defining characteristics: Hypotension, tachycardia, decreased central venous pressure, decreased pulmonary pressures, decreased cardiac output, oliguria.

Ineffective breathing pattern

♦ Monitor respiratory status and observe for changes.
♦ Monitor arterial blood gases and note changes.
♦ Check breath sounds and report changes.
♦ Monitor chest x-ray reports.

Defining characteristics: Dyspnea, wheezing, tachypnea, cyanosis, stridor, tightness of chest.

Impaired skin integrity

♦ Observe for signs of local or generalized flushing.
♦ Watch for development of rashes; note character.
♦ Assess for swelling/edema.

Defining characteristics: Urticaria, pruritus, edema, angioedema, eczema hypersensitivity, dermatitis erythema, swelling, inflammation, vesiculation, blister formation.

Fluid volume deficit

♦ Assess fluid balance (I & O) every hour.
♦ Assess for edema.

Defining characteristics: Decreased urine output, concentrated urine, decreased venous filling, hypotension, thirst, tachycardia.

Altered renal perfusion

♦ Monitor serum and urine electrolytes and osmolarity and document.
♦ Monitor urine output every hour; document changes.
♦ Monitor laboratory data for elevation in BUN (blood urea nitrogen) and creatinine levels, acid-base imbalances, particularly sodium (Na+) and potassium (K+).

Defining characteristics: Decreased urine output, decreased venous filing, hemoconcentration.

Altered level of consciousness

♦ Obtain neurological checks; report and record any changes.
♦ Observe for seizure activity; report and record changes.
♦ Monitor vital signs.

Defining characteristics: Fainting, changes in alertness, changes in orientation.

Gastrointestinal

Defining characteristics: Abdominal cramping, diarrhea, nausea, and vomiting.

Potential anxiety/fear

♦ Recognize patient's level of anxiety and note signs and symptoms.
♦ Assess patient's coping mechanisms.

Knowledge deficit

♦ Assess patient's knowledge of his or her condition and allergens.

---

to the area of contact. Chemical additives used in the manufacturing processes (eg, accelerators) and not the latex itself causes previously sensitized T-cell lymphocytes to stimulate proliferation of other lymphocytes and mononuclear cells, resulting in tissue inflammation and dermatitis.

The onset of type IV reactions is slow, usually occurring during 18 to 24 hours and peaking at 48 hours after exposure. Reactions may present as pruritis, erythema, swelling, crusty thickened skin, pimples, blisters, and other skin lesions. Symptoms usually resolve within three to four days after exposure.[39,40] Each exposure may lead to increased sensitization and a more severe reaction. Diagnosis is made by a health care provider experienced in chemical allergy testing—patch tests commonly are used. Treatment involves education; thoroughly drying hands; using water- or silicone-based moisturizing creams, lotions, or topical barrier agents; avoiding oil- or petroleum-based products unless they are latex compatible; and avoiding the identified causative agent.[38,41,42] Continued use of latex products when there are breaks in the wearer's skin is believed to contribute to latex protein sensitization. This is due to absorption of solubilized latex proteins associated with the product.[43,44]

Latex allergy (ie, immediate hypersensitivity) is a systemic type I IgE-mediated response to plant proteins in natural rubber latex. In sensitized individuals, an anti-latex IgE antibody stimulates mast cell proliferation and basophil histamine release, leading to local swelling, redness, edema, itching, and systemic reactions, including anaphylaxis.[39,44] Type I reactions are immediate, with the onset of symptoms usually occurring in minutes.[39] Symptoms

Table 4

SAMPLE LATEX ALLERGY QUESTIONNAIRE	Yes	No
1. Have you ever had allergies, asthma, hay fever, eczema, or problems with rashes?	❏	❏
2. Have you ever had respiratory distress, rapid heart rate, or swelling?	❏	❏
3. Have you ever had swelling, itching, hives, or other symptoms after contact with a balloon?	❏	❏
4. Have you ever had swelling, itching, hives, or other symptoms after a dental examination or procedure?	❏	❏
5. Have you ever had swelling, itching, hives, or other symptoms following a vaginal or rectal examination or after contact with a diaphragm or condom?	❏	❏
6. Have you ever had swelling, itching, or hives during or within one hour after wearing rubber gloves?	❏	❏
7. Have you ever had a rash on your hands that lasted longer than one week?	❏	❏
8. Have you ever had swelling, itching, hives, runny nose, eye irritation, wheezing, or asthma after contact with any latex or rubber product?	❏	❏
9. Have you ever had swelling, itching, or hives after being examined by someone wearing rubber or latex gloves?	❏	❏
10. Has a physician ever told you that you had rubber or latex allergy?	❏	❏
11. Are you allergic to bananas, papaya, avocados, kiwifruits, other stone fruits, tomatoes, raw potatoes, or chestnuts?	❏	❏
12. Have you ever had an unexplained anaphylactic episode? If so, please describe.	❏	❏

include rhinitis, conjunctivitis, urticaria, laryngeal edema, bronchospasm, asthma, angioedema, anaphylaxis, and death.[39,45-40] These responses can occur when materials containing latex come into contact with the skin, mucous membranes, or internal tissues. Aerosolization of very small amounts of natural rubber latex proteins may cause some individuals to react after inhaling traces of powder from latex gloves or balloons.[49,50] The severity of repeat reactions is unpredictable; therefore, individuals who have suffered any type I reaction are considered to be at high risk for anaphylaxis.

Latex allergy is diagnosed by a history of type I reactions to latex products, such as gloves, balloons, or condoms, and a skin prick test—no FDA-approved reagent is yet approved in the United States—or serum test to identify IgE antibodies to latex. Individuals may experience irritant, type IV, and type I reactions simultaneously. If a patient or health care worker experiences any form of reaction to a medical device that may contain latex (eg, medical gloves), the individual should be carefully evaluated by a health care provider experienced in latex allergy diagnosis and management. **Table 3** provides anaphylactic reaction assessment criteria with which health care workers should be familiar.

D. Population Affected/Risk Factors

Children with myelodysplasia or a history of multiple surgeries beginning in infancy and any individual with a past history of type I reaction or positive test results to natural rubber latex are at high risk for developing anaphylaxis. People at risk for developing latex sensitization include individuals occupationally exposed to latex (eg, health care workers, food service workers); atopic individuals with a history of asthma, eczema, and rhinitis; people who react to medications; and individuals with multiple environmental allergies. People with a history of type I allergic reactions to certain foods (eg, banana, avocado, chestnut, kiwi) also are at increased risk for latex sensitization. This is because of a cross reactivity that exists between natural rubber latex proteins and certain food allergens.[10,22,24,51] **Table 4** provides a sample

Table 5

LATEX ALLERGY RISK GROUPS

Persons at high risk for systemic reactions
- Children with a history of frequent surgeries or use of instrumentation, particularly if begun in early infancy, as with congenital malformations like myelodysplasia (eg, spina bifida) or genitourinary problems.
- Verifiable history of latex allergic reactions, particularly if intraoperative or asthmatic.
- Positive test results to serum latex antibody test (eg, radioallergosorbent/enzyme-linked immunosorbent assay) or skin prick test.
- History of any immunoglobulin E-mediated symptoms (eg, urticaria, rhinoconjunctivitis, asthma, bronchospasm) when in contact with natural rubber latex products.

Persons at risk for developing latex allergy
- Occupational exposure to latex products, particularly to powdered products such as gloves, or to aerosolized latex proteins.
- History of latex-fruit syndrome or progressive reactions to foods known to cross-react with NRL—including bananas, kiwifruits, avocados, stone fruits, raw potatoes, tomatoes, papayas, or chestnuts—or a history of a latex glove-associated contact dermatitis.

Persons who should be evaluated for latex allergy
- History of any unexplained anaphylaxis—particularly if occurring in a medical or dental setting.
- History of hives or itching after incidental latex exposure, such as dental or gynecological examinations, or on contact with balloons, condoms, or natural rubber latex gloves.
- History of multiple surgical procedures.

Risks suggested by Dr. B. Lauren Charous, Milwaukee Medical Clinic

questionnaire suitable for assessing patients and others for their risk of latex allergy or sensitization.

The ACAAI recommends that individuals with known latex allergy and those at high risk for allergy be treated in a latex-safe environment. Individuals designated as at risk for developing latex sensitization should be assessed carefully, and health care facility protocol should be followed in determining the need for testing for immediate hypersensitivity to natural rubber latex (**Table 5**).[10,12,52,53]

E. Exposure

Systemic exposure to latex can occur through the following routes: mucous membrane, ingestion, inhalation, or intravascular or cutaneous contact. The majority of severe latex reactions result from latex proteins coming in contact with internal tissues during invasive procedures or after contact with mucous membranes of the mouth, vagina, urethra, or rectum.[45,46] Triggering items include latex gloves, latex glove powder, orthodontic elastic, dental dams, nasogastric tubes, balloons, pacifiers, urinary catheters, enema kits, barium enema catheters, condoms, and balloon catheters. Case

reports describe intraoperative anaphylaxis after the peritoneum or other internal tissues are contacted by surgical gloves.[39,45-48]

Inhalation of latex proteins can lead to bronchospasm or laryngeal edema. Aerosolized glove powder is the most common source of latex protein inhalation.[49,50] Latex proteins bind to the glove starch powder during the manufacturing process and are expelled into the air when gloves are opened, donned, or removed.[50] Latex proteins, particularly when bound to starch glove powder and then aerosolized, can and have caused serious health problems for both patients and employees.[3] Use of powdered latex gloves in the same room as a sensitized individual can produce an allergic reaction. Use of powder-free gloves results in only small or negligible amounts of latex in the air.[8,50,54-56]

Cutaneous exposure to latex products can trigger serious systemic reactions in highly sensitized individuals. Examples of products that have triggered reactions include gloves, condoms, anesthesia masks, tourniquets, electrocardiogram electrodes, adhesive tape, elastic bandages, condom catheters, rubber shoes, elastic in clothing, balloons, and racquet handles.

F. Prevention

The goals of prevention are twofold: to prevent reactions in individuals who are latex-sensitized and to prevent initial sensitization of nonsensitized persons. The only effective preventive strategy at this time is latex avoidance. Working in an environment that is free of powdered, high-allergen latex gloves and products will help minimize sensitization of health care workers.[4,5] The NIOSH, AAAAI, ACAAI, and others recommend and encourage the use of low-allergen, powder-free latex gloves as an important factor in developing a latex-safe environment.[8,37,38,41,50,53,55-65] For patients or staff members with a known allergy to natural rubber latex proteins, additional precautions are necessary. The presence of even small amounts of residual aerosolized latex in the air or on surfaces can trigger a life-threatening reaction. Latex-allergic individuals should be treated or work in an environment using strict latex avoidance. Although it is impossible to remove all latex from the environment (eg, wheels on carts), all latex that may potentially contact the individual should be removed.

When establishing a latex-safe environment, pertinent clinical data should be obtained on every latex or latex-containing product used in the facility, with an emphasis placed on the protein and powder content of each product, if powdered gloves or other powdered items are used. Latex products selected for use should be low-allergen and powder-free. The protein content should be less than 50 μg/dm^2 using the American Society for Testing and Materials (ASTM) D5712 total protein test[66] and less than 10 μg per dm^2 by the ASTM D6499 antigen test.[67]

AORN's "Recommended practices for product selection in perioperative practice settings" provides guidance to assist practitioners with product evaluation and selection.[68] A master list or directory of products containing latex and appropriate latex-free substitutes for those products should be maintained by the health care facility and be readily accessible to all health care providers. Since September 30, 1998, the FDA has required that all FDA-cleared medical devices containing natural rubber latex carry a warning statement.[69-71] This statement reads "Caution: This product contains natural rubber latex which may cause allergic reactions." This label warning will facilitate alternative product selection for latex-allergic individuals. This ruling does not include pharmaceuticals or products that are not regulated by the FDA.

A latex-free cart may be helpful for consolidating latex-free items in a single place for ease of location and use. Specialty patient care areas, such as the OR, emergency, and labor and delivery departments, should develop a list of items to meet their special care needs. Emergency carts (ie, code carts) also should contain latex-free items (eg, syringes, latex-free gloves, resuscitation equipment). Manufacturer documentation should be obtained to ensure the latex-free status of contents for all carts (eg, code, latex, other specialty carts). It is important that each cart be latex-free as emergency situations can occur without respect for any individual patient considerations. A sample of items to be included in a latex-free cart can be found in **Table 6**.

Pretreating latex-allergic individuals with certain medication regimens (eg diphenhydramine, ranitidine, corticosteroids) may prevent initial allergy symptoms, but it also may give care providers with a false sense of security.[9,34,39,53] This practice remains controversial. Pretreated latex-allergic individuals may present with anaphylaxis as the first sign observed by the health care team.[72]

The use of medication vials with rubber stoppers also is controversial when caring for latex-sensitive or allergic patients. Protein can be leached from the vial stopper. Even when the single-puncture or the pop-the-top-off method is used, individuals already sensitized to natural rubber latex can react.[73] One study reported that the amount of latex found in a medication vial after 40 punctures was below the level of detection using standardized methods.[74] Another study suggested that medication vials should be changed to synthetic vial tops or be clearly labeled as is required for other medical devices.[75] Coring of the stopper also is a concern. Coring may occur from repetitive puncturing of a multi-use vial stopper. This raises a concern about latex-containing particulate matter potentially contaminating the medication. In two studies, the use of sharp needles reportedly caused coring fragments in 73% of solutions in test vials using multi-dose insulin stoppers.[75,76] Whenever possible, medications should be used from a latex-free vial. When this is not possible, arrangements with the pharmacy should be made in advance so medications can be drawn into a latex-free delivery device under aseptic conditions (eg, inside the pharmacy's hood). If neither of these solutions is possible, the stopper should be removed and the medication withdrawn using a latex-free syringe. AORN does not recommend this practice unless all other options have been exhausted.

Reprocessing instruments previously processed in steam and potentially exposed to latex contamination via sterilization tape, container gaskets, or gloves worn in processing is considered unnecessary by most experts because proteins are denatured by heat and steam.[53,77,78] Health care facilities are cautioned not to heat sterilize a known latex product in an attempt to render it safe for use on a latex-allergic individual.

Sterilization of medical products by means other than heat has not been well studied in relation to latex allergy. Each facility should contact the manufacturer of the sterilizing agent or technology to verify its safe use for individuals with a latex allergy.

G. Managing Latex-Allergic Individuals

Patients

Preparing a health care facility to care for latex-allergic patients is a complex process that can be costly and labor intensive. A multidisciplinary task force to address latex issues should be formed and may include representatives from the following areas:

♦ administration;
♦ risk management;
♦ quality management;
♦ safety management;
♦ surgical services;
♦ sterile processing;
♦ distribution;
♦ anesthesia services;
♦ materiel management;
♦ pharmacy;
♦ laboratory;
♦ infection control;
♦ family medicine;
♦ department of surgery;
♦ department of allergy and immunology; and
♦ various nursing departments (eg, intensive care unit, emergency, medical-surgical, home care, education, occupational health).

The role of the task force is to develop a protocol for creating a latex-safe environment for patients who are latex-allergic. Removing devices and supplies with high latex protein content and discontinuing use of powdered latex products should be an integral part of the protocol. The possible increase in purchase costs for nonlatex items must be weighed against the costs of potential anaphylactic episodes or patient death. The protocol also should include a mechanism for patient education about latex allergy and its management.

Table 6

SUGGESTED CONTENTS FOR A LATEX-SAFE CART
Note: All items must be latex-free.

Safety needles (25 g through 15 g)
Syringes (multiple sizes)
3-way stopcocks
IV tubing
Blood tubing
Tourniquets
Assorted tape (.5″, 1″, 1.5″)
Underpads and small Chux
100% silicone or polyvinyl chloride (PVC) urinary catheters
Silicone or PVC external catheters—pediatric and adult
Urinary drainage system
Feeding tubes (5 Fr to 10 Fr)
Feeding pump bag and tubing
Bulb syringe (60 mL)
Blood pressure cuffs and connecting tubing
Stethoscope
Examination gloves
Sterile gloves
Oxygen delivery supplies (eg, cannula, masks)
Anesthesia breathing bag

Patient safety cannot be compromised. If a facility is maintained as latex-safe, additional preparation for latex-allergic patients may not be necessary. If a facility makes the conscious decision not to continuously maintain a latex-safe environment, special preparation and precautions will be required every time a latex-allergic individual presents for care.[64,79-82]

Employees

Latex-allergic individuals should be counseled about the risk of working in environments with high latex use. They should use only nonlatex gloves and avoid all products containing latex. The ACAAI suggests that these individuals wear an allergic identification bracelet or tag, always carry an epinephrine auto-injector device, and avoid environments where powdered latex gloves are used or balloons are allowed.[52]

For both facility and employee protection, employees new to a facility should be assessed to determine the risk or presence of latex-related problems. This can be done through the employee health service or a similar mechanism during the pre-employment history and physical examination. A simple questionnaire can be used as part of the initial assessment. People at high risk for latex sensitivity should have further evaluation for latex allergy. Individuals considered at high risk

- have existing allergies, particularly to fruits (eg, latex-fruit syndrome)[83];
- have hand dermatitis or eczema; and
- use gloves regularly.

Low-risk employees with a negative clinical history of latex reactions do not need allergy testing, but they should be evaluated if symptoms suggestive of latex sensitivity develop during their employment. For people with contact dermatitis, the causative agent should be identified and avoided if possible. If the dermatitis appears on the hands, the use of glove liners under latex or nonlatex gloves that do not contain the triggering agent has been found to be helpful.[41,52]

All employees should be educated about latex sensitivity and allergy and be able to recognize the symptoms of a latex reaction. Employees should be encouraged to report development of any symptoms to the facility's employee health service or other designated mechanism.

II. Nursing Process Application

A. Perioperative Nursing Vocabulary

The perioperative nursing vocabulary is a clinically relevant and empirically validated standardized nursing language. It relates to the delivery of care in the perioperative setting. This standardized language consists of a collection of data elements (ie, the Perioperative Nursing Data Set [PNDS]) and includes perioperative nursing diagnoses, interventions, and outcomes. In 1999, the PNDS was recognized by the ANA committee on nursing practice information infrastructure as a data set useful in the practice of nursing. The perioperative patient-focused model provides the conceptual framework for the PNDS and the model for perioperative nursing practice.[84] The patient and his or her family members are at the core of the model. The model depicts perioperative nursing in four domains and illustrates the relationship between the patient, family members, and care provided by the perioperative professional nurse. The patient-centered domains are

- D1—safety,
- D2—physiological responses to surgery,
- D3—patient's and family members' behavioral responses to surgery, and

- D4—health system in which perioperative care is provided.

Each data element in the PNDS is represented by a unique identifier. The domains are represented by the letter "D" followed by numbers one to four to indicate the particular domain being addressed. Nursing diagnoses are represented by the letter "X" and a number unique to the diagnosis; interventions are represented by the letter "I" and a unique number; and outcomes are represented by the letter "O" and a unique number. These designations are used in this document as appropriate.

B. Assessment

Perioperative nurses assess, document, and communicate patient status to all members of the health care team. Data collection involves the patient and his or her significant others. Assess for the following risk factors:

- history of multiple surgeries beginning at an early age (eg, spina bifida, urinary malformations);
- food allergies (eg, latex-fruit syndrome);[83]
- exposure to latex; and
- history of allergic reaction to latex.

Assess for inadvertent latex exposure and impending anaphylaxis. **Table 7** provides a summary of symptoms of latex exposure and possible anaphylaxis for both conscious and anesthetized patients.

C. Nursing Diagnosis

The perioperative nurse analyzes the assessment data when determining nursing diagnoses. Following is a partial list of nursing diagnoses that may be associated with latex-allergic individuals ("X" = nursing diagnosis, "D" = domain).

- X 32 (D2)—latex allergy response (risk for);
- X 30 (D3)—knowledge deficient related to latex hypersensitivity (risk for/actual);
- X 50 (D1)—skin integrity, impaired, related to manifestations of allergic reaction (risk for/actual);
- X 7 (D2)—breathing pattern, ineffective, related to facial angioedema, bronchospasm, and laryngeal edema (risk for/actual);
- X 8 (D2)—cardiac output, decreased, related to severe latex-allergic reaction (risk for/actual);
- X 61 (D2)—tissue perfusion, ineffective, renal, related to hypotension and decreased cardiac output (risk for/actual);
- X 18 (D2)—fluid volume, risk for deficient;
- X 11 (D2)—acute confusion related to physiologic condition and decreased circulation;

- X 64 (D3)—verbal communication, impaired, related to hypotension and decreased cardiac output (risk for/actual);
- X 47 (D1)—sensory perception, disturbed, related to hypotension and decreased cardiac output (risk for/actual); and
- X 4 (D1)—anxiety, related to change in physiological status in response to latex.

D. Outcome Identification

The following is a partial list of nursing outcomes that may be associated with the latex-allergic individual ("O" = outcome, "D" = domain).

- O 2 (D1)—The patient is free from signs and symptoms of injury caused by extraneous objects.
- O 3 (D2)—The patient is free from signs and symptoms of chemical injury.
- O 11 (D2)—The patient has wound/tissue perfusion consistent with or improved from baseline levels established preoperatively.
- O 13 (D2)—The patient's fluid, electrolyte, and acid-base balances are consistent with or improved from baseline levels established preoperatively.
- O 14 (D2)—The patient's respiratory status is consistent with or improved from baseline levels established preoperatively.
- O 15 (D2)—The patient's cardiac status is consistent with or improved from baseline levels established preoperatively.
- O 23 (D3)—The patient participates in decision making affecting the perioperative plan of care.

E. Planning

The perioperative nurse develops a plan of care for the latex-allergic patient that prescribes interventions to attain expected outcomes. Interventions and activities are selected according to the procedure to be performed as well as to address the latex allergy. The following is a partial list of interventions that may be associated with the latex-allergic individual ("I" = interventions).

- I 30—Develops individualized plan of care.
- I 139—Implements latex-allergy precautions as needed.
- I 27—Ensures continuity of care.

The natural rubber latex-allergic individual should be identified by the admitting practitioner, and this information should be made available to the entire health care team, thus providing a continuous safe level of care. The latex-allergic individual

Table 7

SYMPTOMS OF LATEX EXPOSURE AND POSSIBLE ANAPHYLAXIS	
Conscious Patient	**Anesthetized Patient**
Itchy eyes	Facial edema
Generalized pruritis	Urticaria
Shortness of breath	Rash
Sneezing	Skin flushing
Wheezing	Bronchospasm
Nausea	Laryngeal edema
Edema	Edema
Vomiting	Hypotension
Abdominal cramping	Tachycardia
Diarrhea	Cardiac arrest
Faintness	
Feeling of impending doom	

should be treated in a latex-safe environment with emphasis placed on the removal of all latex-containing devices and products within the immediate care environment. **Figure 1** provides a simple flow chart to assist with planning for a latex-safe procedure.

F. Implementation

Implementation refers to actually performing the activities comprising the interventions identified in the individualized plan of care. This includes taking latex-allergy precautions as appropriate. If the patient is to be cared for in a facility-wide, latex-safe environment, no additional latex precautions should be needed. If latex or latex-containing products remain in the patient's immediate care environment, those products should be removed.

Nursing interventions are composed of many and varied activities. To care for the latex-allergic individual, some or all the following activities will be appropriate, particularly if the patient is not in a facility-wide latex-safe environment.

Preoperative activities

The following activities should take place before the surgical procedure.

- Notify OR of potential or known latex-allergic patient 24 to 48 hours (or as soon as possible) before scheduled procedure.
- Identify the patient's risk factors for latex allergy and communicate same to health care team.
- Schedule procedure as first case of the day if the facility is not latex-safe.

Figure 1

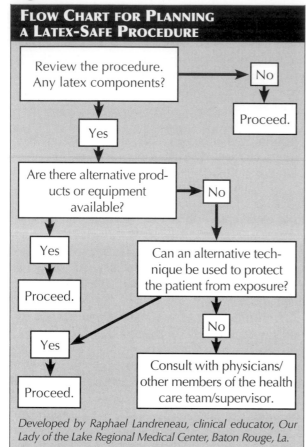

FLOW CHART FOR PLANNING A LATEX-SAFE PROCEDURE

Review the procedure. Any latex components? → No → Proceed.

Yes ↓

Are there alternative products or equipment available? → No → Can an alternative technique be used to protect the patient from exposure?

Yes ↓ Proceed.

Can an alternative technique be used to protect the patient from exposure? → No → Consult with physicians/other members of the health care team/supervisor.

Yes ↓ Proceed.

Developed by Raphael Landreneau, clinical educator, Our Lady of the Lake Regional Medical Center, Baton Rouge, La.

♦ Notify all other care providers of patient's allergy status.

♦ Educate patient about latex-safe plan and ensure involvement of all providers.

♦ Involve patient, family members, and significant others in planning patient's care.

♦ Plan for a latex-safe environment of care.

♦ Secure latex-free products for all latex-containing items on surgeon's preference card and those used by anesthesia care provider.

♦ Notify surgeon if no alternative product is available.

♦ Notify anesthesia care provider if latex-containing product is to be used, and develop plan for emergency care if needed.

♦ Remove all latex items from OR unless no nonlatex alternative exists.
- Remove boxes of latex gloves and replace with nonlatex gloves (eg, sterile, nonsterile).
- Double-check all supplies and equipment for latex and remove any latex-containing items.

Intraoperative activities

The following activities should be performed during the surgical procedure.

♦ Continue implementing the perioperative latex-safe plan of care.

♦ Mark the OR room doors with "Latex precautions" signs.

♦ Mark the patient's admitting bed and transport vehicles.

♦ Provide latex-sensitive patients with a "latex allergy" identification band and ensure that the bed and chart also are clearly labeled.

♦ Remind all health care team members of the necessity for following latex avoidance procedures.

♦ Restrict traffic flow in the room before and during the procedure.

♦ Use latex-free IV tubing or replace injection ports with three-way stopcocks. Tape over any remaining ports to prevent inadvertent use.

♦ Use medication in ampules or latex-free vials when available.

♦ Use latex-free syringes.

♦ Use latex-free blood pressure cuffs and connecting tubing. If they are not available, wrap the patient's arm to prevent blood pressure cuff tubing or tourniquet cuff tubing from coming into contact with the patient's skin.

♦ Do not use latex tourniquets (eg, Penrose drains) to start IV lines or as drains in a wound.

♦ Use a 100% silicone (ie, not silicone coated) or polyvinyl chloride catheter if a urinary catheter is ordered for a procedure.

♦ Verify that additional items requested after the case is in progress are latex-free before delivering them to the sterile field.

♦ Be prepared for the possibility that the procedure may require more than the scheduled equipment (eg, laparoscopy to open).

♦ Monitor for anaphylactic reactions to latex throughout the procedure as reactions may occur immediately after induction (eg, IV exposure) or up to 40 minutes later.

♦ Have IV fluids and medications for treatment of allergic reaction available immediately.

♦ Inform postanesthesia care unit (PACU) staff members in advance of the patient's arrival time.

Postoperative activities

The following activities should be performed after the surgical procedure.

◆ Continue the perioperative latex-safe plan of care.

◆ Ensure that latex-free supplies are available to follow the patient to all future locations within the health care facility.

◆ Provide a latex-free resuscitation bag, oxygen mask, and supplies.

◆ Transport the patient to a latex-safe area.

◆ Provide education for patient and his or her family members or significant others.

If the latex-allergic patient is not cared for in a facility-wide, latex-safe environment, he or she is at risk for reaction upon arrival in the PACU. When the patient re-enters the mainstream care environment, he or she is at risk because of the aerosolized powder-containing latex proteins being transferred through the air or shed from scrub attire of individuals working with or near powdered latex products. In a nonlatex-safe facility, it may be necessary to use a positive pressure isolation room if a latex-safe environment of care has not been previously established in preparation for the patient.

G. Evaluation of Outcomes

The perioperative nurse evaluates the patient's progress toward attainment of outcomes. The perioperative nurse's evaluation should be systematic and ongoing. The patient's progress toward attainment of outcomes should be documented using the recognized, standardized perioperative nursing vocabulary.[84] Outcome indicators will vary according to the specific desired outcome and may include

◆ physiological indicators (eg, neurological status, cardiovascular status);

◆ cognitive indicators (eg, repeats instructions correctly, asks appropriate questions);

◆ affective indicators (eg, verbalizes and demonstrates willingness to comply with treatment regimen); and

◆ supportive resources (eg family members participate in care planning and delivery).

Patient satisfaction
Evaluation of patient progress is based on observations of the patient's responses to nursing interventions and the effectiveness of interventions in moving the patient toward the desired outcome. Desired patient outcomes, nursing interventions, and potentially applicable nursing diagnoses are articulated in the standardized perioperative nursing vocabulary which provides the basis for documentation of perioperative nursing practice. Ongoing assessment should be used to revise diagnoses, outcomes, and the plan of care as needed. Revisions in diagnoses, outcomes, and the plan of care should be documented. The patient, his or her significant others, and other health care providers should be involved in the evaluation process when appropriate.

III. Conclusion

This guideline has been designed to promote a safe health care environment for latex-sensitive and latex-allergic patients and health care workers. The document addresses prevalence, history, pathophysiology, risk factors, prevention, and nursing process applications. This guideline can be used as a resource by facilities developing latex-safe policies, procedures, and protocols. The guideline may not apply to every individual and may require alteration based on specific needs.

REFERENCES
1. P C A Kam, M S M Lee, J F Thompson, "Latex allergy: An emerging clinical and occupational health problem," *Anaesthesia* 52 (June 1997) 570-575.

2. S Reddy, "Latex allergy," *American Family Physician* 57 (Jan 1, 1998) 93-100.

3. M Swanson, D W Olson, "Latex allergen affinity for starch powders applied to natural rubber gloves and released as an aerosol: From dust to don," *Canadian Journal of Allergy and Clinical Immunology* 5 no 8 (2000) 328-336.

4. G L Sussman et al, "Incidence of latex sensitization among latex glove users," *Journal of Allergy and Clinical Immunology* 101 (February 1998) 171-178.

5. D A Levy et al, "Powder-free protein-poor natural rubber latex gloves and latex sensitization," (Research Letters) *JAMA* 281 (March 17, 1999); also available at *http://jama.amaassn.org/issues/v281n11/ffull/jlt0317 -5.html* (accessed 5 July 2003).

6. C A Janeway et al, "The induction, measurement, and manipulation of the immune response," *Immuno Biology: The Immune System in Health and Disease,* fourth ed (New York: Elsevier Science Ltd/Garland Publishing, 1999) 33-75.

7. *Mosby's Medical and Nursing Dictionary* (St Louis: The C V Mosby Co, 1983)

8. X Bauer, Z Chen, H Allmers, "Can a threshold limit value for natural rubber latex airborne allergens be defined?" *Journal of Clinical Allergy and Immunology* 101 (January 1998) 24-27.

9. *Latex Allergy Protocol* (Park Ridge, Ill: American Association of Nurse Anesthetists, 1993) 1-2.

10. G L Sussman, D H Beezhold, "Latex allergy: A clinical perspective," *Surgical Services Management* 3 (February 1997) 25-28.

11. V J Tomazic, "Adverse reactions to natural rubber latex," *FDA User Facility Report* 19 (Spring 1997) 2.

12. F Porri et al, "Prevalence of latex sensitization in subjects attending health screening: Implications for a perioperative screening," *Clinical and Experimental Allergy* 27 (April 1997) 413-417.

13. R Bernardini et al, "Prevalence and risk factors of latex sensitization in an unselected pediatric population," *Journal of Allergy and Clinical Immunology* 101 (May 1998) 621-625.

14. American College of Allergy and Immunology, "Latex allergy: An emerging healthcare problem," *Annals of Allergy, Asthma, and Immunology* 75 (July 1995) 19-21.

15. P Patterson, "Latex allergy: Managers' actions can aid latex-sensitive employees," *OR Manager* 13 (February 1997) 1-10.

16. M Veach, "Latex gloves hand health workers a growing worry," *Latex Allergy News* 4 (December 1997) 1-4.

17. T Kibby, M Akl, "Prevalence of latex sensitization in a hospital employee population," *Annals of Allergy, Asthma, and Immunology* 78 (January 1997) 41-44.

18. G L Sussman, "Latex allergy: An overview," *Canadian Journal of Allergy and Clinical Immunology* 5 (May 2000) 317-322.

19. F Lagier et al "Prevalence of latex allergy in operating room nurses," *Journal of Allergy and Clinical Immunology* 90 (September, 1992) 319-322.

20. S R Mace et al "Latex allergy in operating room nurses," *Annals of Allergy, Asthma, and Immunology* 80 (March 1998) 252-256.

21. R Arellano, J Bradley, G Sussman, "Prevalence of latex sensitization among hospital physicians occupationally exposed to latex gloves," *Anesthesiology* 77 (November 1992) 905-908.

22. M Grzybowski et al "The prevalence of anti-latex IgE antibodies among registered nurses," *Journal of Allergy and Clinical Immunology* 98 (September 1996) 535-544.

23. C Konrad et al, "The prevalence of latex sensitivity among anesthesiology staff," *Anesthesia and Analgesia* 84 (March 1997) 629-633.

24. R H Brown, J A Schauble, R G Hamilton, "Prevalence of latex allergy among anesthesiologists: Identification of sensitized but asymptomatic individuals," *Anesthesiology* 89 (August 1998) 292-299.

25. H Alenius et al, "IgE reactivity to 14-kD and 27-kD natural rubber proteins in latex-allergic children with spina bifida and other congenital anomalies," *International Archives of Allergy & Immunology* 102 no 1 (1993) 61-66.

26. J E Slater, S K Chhabra "Latex antigens," *Journal of Allergy and Clinical Immunology* 89 (March 1992) 673-678.

27. B L Charous, "The puzzle of latex allergy: Some answers, still more questions," *Annals of Allergy* 73 (October 1994) 277-281.

28. H Y Yeang et al, "The 14.6 kd rubber elongation factor (Hev b 1) and 24 kd (Hev b 3) rubber particle proteins are recognized by IgE from patients with spina bifida and latex allergy," *Journal of Allergy and Clinical Immunology* 98 (September 1996) 629-639.

29. J W Yunginger, "Natural rubber latex," *Immunology and Allergy Clinics of North America* 15 (August 1995) 583-595.

30. E M Warshaw, "Continuing medical education: Latex allergy," *Journal of the American Academy of Dermatology* 39 (July 1998) 1-24

31. R M Adams, "Reflecting on developments in occupational dermatitis," *Clinics in Dermatology* 15 (July-August 1997) 473-477

32. S M Wilkinson, M H Beck, "Allergic contact dermatitis from latex rubber," *British Journal of Dermatology* 134 (May 1996) 910-914.

33. M Wyss et al, "Allergic contact dermatitis from natural latex without contact urticaria," *Contact Dermatitis* 28 (March 1993) 154-156.

34. K P Bensky, "Latex allergy: Who, what, when, where, why, and how," *CRNA: The Clinical Forum for Nurse Anesthetists* 6 (November 1995) 177-182.

35. N M Strzyzewski, "Latex allergy: Everyone is at risk," *Plastic Surgical Nursing* 15 (Winter 1995) 204-206.

36. H Zhai, H I Maibach, "Moisturizers in preventing irritant contact dermatitis: An overview," *Contact Dermatitis* 38 (May 1998) 241-244.

37. "Latex allergy: Protect yourself, protect your patients," *Work Place Information Series Brochure*, American Nurses Association, *http://www.nursingworld.org/dlwa/osh/wp7.htm* (accessed 17 Oct 2003).

38. National Institute for Occupational Safety and Health, *NIOSH Alert: Preventing Allergic Reactions to Natural Rubber Latex in the Workplace.* DHHS Publ 97-135 (Cincinnati: National Institute for Occupational Safety and Health, August 1997).

39. D L Hancock, "Latex allergy: Prevention and treatment," *Anesthesiology Review* 21 (September/October 1994) 153-163.

40. A Heese et al, "Allergic and irritant reactions to rubber gloves in medical health services," *Journal of the American Academy of Dermatology* 25 (November 1991) 831-841.

41. ECRI, "Latex sensitivity: Clinical and legal issues," in *Operating Room Risk Management* (Plymouth Meeting, Pa: ECRI, September 1997) 1-9.

42. W Wigger-Alberti, P Elsner, "Preventive measures in contact dermatitis," *Clinics in Dermatology* 15 (July-August 1997) 661-665.

43. M Evangelisto, "Latex allergy: The downside of standard precautions," *Today's Surgical Nurse* (September/October 1997) 28-33.

44. V M Steelman, "Latex allergy precautions: A research-based protocol," *Nursing Clinics of North America* 30 (September 1995) 475-493.

45. G Sussman, S Tarlo, J Dolovich, "The spectrum of IgE-mediated responses to latex," *JAMA* 265 (June 5, 1991) 2844-2847.

46. J G K Axelsson, S G O Johansson, K Wrangsjo, "IgE-mediated anaphylactoid reactions to rubber," *Allergy* 42 (January 1987) 46-50.

47. T Carrillo et al, "Contact urticaria and rhinitis from latex surgical gloves," *Contact Dermatitis* 15 (August 1986) 69-72.

48. A C Gerber et al, "Severe intraoperative anaphylaxis to surgical gloves: Latex Allergy, an unfamiliar condition," *Anesthesiology* 7 (November 1989) 800-802.

49. K J Kelly, G Sussman, J N Fink, "Stop the sensitization," *Journal of Allergy and Clinical Immunology* 98 (November 1996) 857-858.

50. D K Heilman et al, "A prospective, controlled study showing that rubber gloves are the major contributor to latex aeroallergen levels in the operating room," *Journal of Allergy and Clinical Immunology* 98 (August 1996) 325-330.

51. M Ahlroth et al, "Cross-reacting allergens in natural rubber latex and avocado," *Journal of Allergy and Clinical Immunology* 96 (August 1995) 167-173.

52. G Sussman, M Gold, *Guidelines for the Management of Latex Allergies and Safe Latex Use in Health Care Facilities* (Arlington Heights, Ill: American College of Allergy, Asthma, and Immunology, March 1996) 1-25.

53. K T Kim et al, "Implementation recommendations for making health care facilities latex safe," *AORN Journal* 67 (March 1998) 615-632.

54. O Vandenplas et al, "Prevalence of occupational asthma due to latex among hospital personnel," *American Journal of Respiratory Critical Care Medicine* 151 (January 1995) 54-60.

55. O Vandenplas et al, "Latex gloves with a lower protein content reduce bronchial reactions in subjects with occupational asthma caused by latex," *American Journal of Respiratory and Critical Care Medicine* 151 (March 1995) 887-889.

56. B L Charous, P J Scheunemann, M C Swanson, "Dispersion of latex aeroallergen," (Abstract) *Journal of Allergy and Clinical Immunology* suppl (January 1998) S160-S161.

57. American College of Allergy, Asthma and Immunology, American Academy of Allergy, Asthma and Immunology, "AAAAI and ACAAI joint statement concerning the use of powdered and non-powdered natural rubber latex gloves," *Annals of Allergy, Asthma, and Immunology* 79 (December 1997) 487.

58. *Interim Recommendations to Health Professionals and Organizations Regarding Latex Allergy Precautions* (Arlington Heights, Ill: American College of Allergy and Immunology, March 1992) 1-4.

59. D H Beezhold, G L Sussman, "Determining the allergenic potential of latex gloves," *Surgical Services Management* 3 (February 1997) 35-41.

60. C L Romig, "The powdered latex glove war," (Health Policy Issues) *AORN Journal* 66 (July 1997) 152-153.

61. D M Korniewicz, K J Kelly, "Barrier protection and latex allergy associated with surgical gloves," *AORN Journal* 61 (June 1995) 1037-1044.

62. E F O'Boyle, B Brochard, "Latex allergy: Be prepared," *Surgical Services Management* 4 (March 1998) 34-37.

63. M A Young, "Strategies for a latex-safe environment," *Surgical Services Management* 4 (March 1998) 19-24.

64. V M Steelman, "Is it really necessary to go powder-free?" *Infection Control Today* 2 no 4 29-30.

65. R S Holzman, J D Katzk, "Occupational latex allergy: The end of innocence," *Anesthesiology* 89 (August 1998) 287-289.

66. *Standard Test Method for the Analysis of Aqueous Extractable Protein in Natural Rubber and Its Products Using the Modified Lowry Method,* D 5712 (West Conshohocken, Pa: American Society for Testing and Materials, 1999) 1-7.

67. *Standard Test Method for the Immunological Measurement of Antigenic Protein in Natural Rubber and Its Products,* D 6499 (West Conshohocken, Pa: American Society for Testing and Materials, 2003) 1-6.

68. "Recommended practices for product selection in perioperative practice settings," in *Standards, Recommended Practices, and Guidelines* (Denver: AORN, Inc, 2004) 347-350.

69. "Natural rubber-containing medical devices: User labeling, Final rule," *Federal Register* 62 (Sept 30, 1997) 51021-51030.

70. "Guidance on the content and format of premarket notification [510(k)] submissions for testing for skin sensitization to chemicals in latex products, draft document" (Rockville, Md: US Department of Health and Human Services Center for Devices and Radiological Health, Feb 13, 1998) 1-14.

71. "Latex allergy position statements, guidelines, and resources," (Trends) *Surgical Services Management* 4 (March 1998) 56.

72. *Natural Rubber Latex Allergy: Considerations for Anesthesiologists* (Park Ridge, Ill: American Society of Anesthesiologists, 1999).

73. S A Vassallo et al, "Allergic reaction to latex from stopper of a medication vial," *Anesthesia & Analgesia* 80 (May 1995) 1057-1058.

74. J W Yunginger et al, "Latex allergen contents of medical and consumer rubber products," *Journal of Allergy Clinical Immunology* 91 (1993) 241.

75. M N Primeau, N F Adkinson, Jr, R G Hamilton, "Natural rubber pharmaceutical vial closures release latex allergens that produce skin reactions," *Journal of Allergy and Clinical Immunology* 107 (June 2001) 958-962.

76. T Asakura, "Occurrence of coring in insulin vials and possibility of rubber piece contamination by self injection," *Journal of the Pharmaceutical Society of Japan* 121 (June 2001) 459-463.

77. S A Sherman, "Precautions reduce risk of latex reactions," *OR Manager* 9 (August 1993) 17-20.

78. B D Zehr, S Gromelski, D Beezhold, "Reduction of antigenic protein levels in latex gloves after gamma irradiation," *Biomedical Instrumentation and Technology* 28 (November/December 1994) 481-483.

79. G Weinert, "Health care latex allergy costs," *Surgical Services Management* 4 (March 1998) 27-30.

80. K Catalano, "Risk management and latex allergies," *Surgical Services Management* 3 (February 1997) 42-46.

81. C Johns, "A call to action: Latex allergy in the workplace," *Surgical Services Management* 4 (March 1998) 41-44.

82. "Natural rubber latex sensitivity: An AAOHN position statement," American Association of Occupational Health Nurses, Inc, *http://www.aaohn.org/natrubr.htm#latex* (accessed 16 May 1998) 1-3.

83. S Wagner, H Breiteneder, "The latex-fruit syndrome," *Biochemical Society Transactions* 30 (November 2002) 935-940.

84. S Beyea, ed, *Perioperative Nursing Data Set,* second ed (Denver: AORN, Inc, 2002).

RESOURCES

Kim, K, et al. "Implementation recommendations for making health care facilities latex safe," *AORN Journal* 67 (March 1998) 615-632.

Latex Allergy Links, *http://latexallergylinks.tripod.com/* (accessed 19 Oct 2003).

"Natural rubber latex allergy: Considerations for anesthesiologists," American Society of Anesthesiologists, *http://www.asahq.org/publicationsAndServices/latexallergy.html* (accessed 19 Oct 2003).

Phillips, V; Goodrich, M; Sullivan, T. "Health care worker disability due to latex allergy and asthma: A cost analysis," *American Journal of Public Health* 89 (July 1999) 1024-1028.

Steelman, V. "Latex allergy precautions: A research-based protocol," *Nursing Clinics of North America* 30 (September 1995) 475-493.

Sussman, G. "Latex allergy: An overview," *Canadian Journal of Allergy and Clinical Immunology* 5 no 8 (2000) 317-322.

PUBLICATION HISTORY

Originally approved by the AORN Board of Directors in November 1998.

Revised; approved by the AORN Board of Directors in November 2003. Published in *Standards, Recommended Practices, and Guidelines,* 2004 edition; reprinted March 2004, *AORN Journal.*

Part I: Overview

A. Introduction

The "AORN malignant hyperthermia (MH) guideline" was created to provide clarity regarding assessment and treatment of MH and to familiarize perioperative nurses and other health care providers with the resources and tools available for staff development training. This guideline is specific to perioperative care for patients confirmed to have, or who are thought to be susceptible to, MH. This guideline includes the history, pathophysiology, and risk factors of the disease; protocols for treating a patient in MH crisis; considerations for education and counseling for patients and families determined to be at risk for developing MH; evaluation of care after an MH crisis; and a guide for planning staff member education.

This guideline is based on current, available research and incorporates information from the Malignant Hyperthermia Association of the United States (MHAUS) protocol. The MHAUS is a nonprofit organization dedicated to assisting in the diagnosis and treatment of MH. The MHAUS protocol was developed by a panel of experts based on scientific research and is viewed as the national guideline or standard of care for the MH patient.[1] Clinician's may need to tailor this guideline to specific patient needs.

AORN recognizes the numerous types of settings in which perioperative nurses practice. This guideline is intended to be adaptable to various practice settings. These practice settings include traditional ORs, ambulatory surgery units, physicians' offices, cardiac catheterization suites, endoscopy suites, radiology departments, emergency departments, labor and delivery units, and all other areas where operative and other invasive procedures may be performed.

The AORN Board of Directors approved the original guideline in February 1997. This current version of the guideline has been reviewed and updated by the AORN Nursing Practice Committee and approved by the AORN Board of Directors in November 2006. Content experts from various practice disciplines (eg, perioperative nurses, perianesthesia nurses, critical care nurses, nurse anesthetists, anesthesiologists) who have experience in managing MH or specific knowledge about MH were invited to provide feedback for consideration and incorporation into the final guideline.

Definition

Malignant hyperthermia is a rare genetic condition characterized by a severe hypermetabolic state and rigidity of the skeletal muscles. It occurs when affected individuals are exposed to a triggering agent such as inhalation anesthetics and succinylcholine, a depolarizing muscle relaxant.[2,3] The triggering agent causes a series of chain reactions in the body related to an increase in intracellular calcium ion concentration.

"Awake" Malignant Hyperthermia

In 1966 an "awake MH" episode was identified as the Porcine Stress Syndrome when pigs were observed to die rapidly when under stress (eg, fighting). In 1974, studies were done for "human stress syndrome," related to sudden deaths in a MH susceptible family. The deaths were unrelated to surgery and thought to be related to exercise and emotion-induced pyrexia.[1]

Studies have continued since that time focusing on physiological changes resulting from stress-related MH (eg, evidence of pH changes in an MH-susceptible muscle recovering from extreme exercise). In spite of potential correlations between exertional heat stroke and MH, dantrolene sodium is not recommended for routine use when managing heat stroke.[2]

Awake MH triggered by stress is common in MH-susceptible swine, but it is not found to be common in MH-susceptible humans.[3] Humans are not the only species to develop MH crises. Reactions have been described most often in pigs, but there are also reports in horses, dogs, and other animals, which helps facilitate research.

REFERENCES

1. Wingard D W. Malignant hyperthermia: a human stress syndrome? *The Lancet.* [Letter to the Editor].1974; 2: 1450-1451.

2. Rosenberg H, Davis M, James D. Pollock N, Stowell K. Malignant hyperthermia. Orphanet encyclopedia, November 2004. *http://www.orpha .net/data/patho/GB/uk-malignant-hyperthermia.pdf.* Accessed September 7, 2006.

3. Gronert GA, Pessah IN, Muldoon SM, Tautz TJ. Malignant hyperthermia. In: Miller, R D, ed. *Miller's Anesthesia.* 6th ed. Philadelphia, Pa: Elsevier, Churchill Livingstone; 2005: 1169-1190.

Table 1

MALIGNANT HYPERTHERMIA TRIGGERING AND NONTRIGGERING AGENTS[1,2]

Triggering Agents	Nontriggering Agents
Halothane	Barbiturates
Isoflurane	Propofol
Enflurane	Local and regional anesthetics
Sevoflurane	Benzodiazepines
Desflurane	Opiods
Succinylcholine	Ketamine
	Nitrous oxide
	Etomidate
	Nondepolarizing muscle relaxants such as:
	♦ Pancuronium
	♦ Cisatracurium
	♦ Vecuronium
	♦ Rocuronium
	♦ Atracurium
	♦ Mivacurium

REFERENCES

1. McCarthy EJ. Malignant hyperthermia: pathophysiology, clinical presentation, and treatment. *AACN.* [Clinical Issues]. 2004; 15: 232-233.

2. Malignant Hyperthermia Association of the United States (MHAUS). MH susceptible patient FAQs. *http://www.mhaus.org/index.cfm/fuseaction/ Content.Display/PagePK/SusceptFAQ.cfm.* Accessed November 8, 2006.

B. History

The history of MH as a known and described disorder is relatively short. In 1960, a clinician reported the case of a young man with a compound leg fracture who feared general anesthesia because relatives had died while undergoing ether anesthesia. He was given halothane, a new inhalation anesthetic agent. Intraoperatively, he experienced fever, tachycardia, cyanosis, and hypotension, but survived.[4]

Since that time, extensive progress has been made in the diagnosis and treatment of MH. In 1962 an autosomal dominant mode of inheritance was suggested, leading to the thesis that increased skeletal muscle metabolism, not abnormal central temperature regulation, accounted for the hyperthermia seen in MH. In vitro muscle biopsy testing in the early 1970s showed that freshly cut muscle demonstrated contracture responses to caffeine and halothane.[3,5-7] Biopsy testing still is the current method for the diagnosis of MH susceptibility.[3,8-11] Dantrolene sodium was introduced in 1979 as the first effective therapy for MH, and to date it remains the only drug specific to the treatment of MH.[9]

In 1981, MHAUS was formed to provide a central clearinghouse to collect data and to provide education and information to the public on MH. One of the most important features of MHAUS is an emergency hotline, (800) 644-9737 (in US and Canada) or 001-1-315-464-7079 (outside the US), that is available for expert help with the diagnosis and treatment of an ongoing MH episode. The North American Malignant Hyperthermia Registry is a professional subsidiary of MHAUS that collates findings from biopsy centers in the United States and Canada and provides access to specific patient data through their hotline.[1,12,13]

C. Affected Population

All patients undergoing general anesthesia should be screened for a family history of MH. Ethnic groups from all parts of the world are affected. In the United States, Wisconsin, Nebraska, West Virginia, and Michigan have higher reported MH incidences than other states.[14] Males develop reactions more frequently than females. People under 18 years of age have the highest incidence of MH. One study reports that 52% of all reactions occurred in children under the age of 15 years.[15,16] Another study reports patients who are obese or who have muscular physiques have a higher rate of recrudescence.[17]

Incidence and Mortality

Malignant hyperthermia has an autosomal mode of inheritance. Previous uneventful anesthesia does not eliminate the diagnosis of MH, because patients may undergo multiple anesthetics before MH is triggered.[18] Reports vary widely on the incidence of MH. Studies show that in patient populations who have been diagnostically tested there is an incidence of 1:30,000 and 1:37,000.[15] The MHAUS reports that MH occurs as frequently as one in 5,000 patients and may occur as rare as once in 65,000 administrations of general anesthetics with a triggering agent.[14] The MH mortality rate has been reduced from as high as 70% to less than 5%.[19] Four factors are responsible for the significant drop in mortality from MH.

> ♦ There is better screening for MH susceptibility through careful preoperative interviews and caffeine-halothane contracture testing.

- A pharmacologic basis for MH has been established so triggering agents can be avoided when MH is suspected (**Table 1**).
- When an unexpected MH crisis occurs, sophisticated monitoring techniques such as capnography and pulse oximetry give an early warning so diagnosis and treatment can be started immediately.
- The use of dantrolene sodium, a drug specific for the treatment of MH.[11,20]

Socioeconomic Factors in Malignant Hyperthermia

The social and financial ramifications of an MH episode cannot be overstated. Patients who know they are susceptible to this potentially lethal syndrome are likely to have high levels of preoperative anxiety. They need continual reassurance that everyone is aware of the potential for problems and that an anesthesia treatment plan has been developed to avoid an MH occurrence. Beyond the psychological and emotional factors, there are physical sequelae to an episode of MH, and the treatment is expensive.

Making provisions to deal with MH is costly and time-consuming. A comprehensive MH treatment cart should be available, including a supply of dantrolene sodium (see Section III of this guideline for suggested contents to include on a dedicated MH cart). Despite more than 25 years of research, dantrolene sodium is the only clinically available agent for the treatment of MH, and it is expensive.[21,22] The list price of dantrolene sodium in 2006 was $82 per vial, and the shelf life is three years.[23-25]

It is fortunate that an MH occurrence is rare in most settings. Dantrolene sodium may become outdated because it is not used frequently, but the benefit of having an adequate supply of it when a crisis arises will outweigh the cost of not having what is needed during this unexpected emergency.[26] According to the MHAUS, as much as 8 to 10 mg/kg of dantrolene sodium is needed to treat a patient who is having an acute MH crisis.[24,26,27] This means 50 vials must be available to treat a person who weighs 100 to 110 kg (ie, 220 to 250 pounds). (See **Table 2**). Thirty six vials of dantrolene sodium will allow for initial stabilization and treatment while more vials are being acquired to continue treatment. Strategies can be developed and implemented for the cost-effective inventory management of this expensive medication.

Risk Factors

Malignant hyperthermia is a genetic disorder; therefore, during the preoperative interview the perioperative nurse should ask all patients if they have had a family member who experienced an MH episode or died during surgery. Patients also should be asked if they have had an MH episode themselves during surgery. This information should be given to the anesthesia care provider and surgeon.

Other diseases have been associated with MH. There is a definite association with central core disease (CCD), an inherited neuromuscular disorder. Both CCD and MH are caused by a genetic mutation in the skeletal muscle ryanodine receptor type 1 (RYR1), which causes an association between the two disorders. There are also associations between MH and other neuromuscular disorders, such as

- Duchenne muscular dystrophy,
- King-Denborough syndrome,
- Becker muscular dystrophy,
- other myopathies,
- periodic paralysis,
- myotonia congenita,
- Schwartz-Jampel syndrome,
- Fukuyama-type congenital muscular dystrophy,
- mitochondrial myopathy, and
- sarcoplasmic reticulum adenosine triphosphate deficiency.[3,8]

Perioperative nurses also should alert anesthesia care providers about patients who describe a history of nonsurgical related incidences of heat stroke or hyperthermia.[28,29]

Other drugs and physiologic conditions have been known to stimulate a syndrome that closely resembles MH (eg, serotonin syndrome).[30] There remain questions as to whether serotonin has a role in stress-induced episodes of MH.[15] More research is needed to learn if there is a correlation between the relative risk of patients who experienced MH being more susceptible to exertional heat illness, and whether patients who have experienced exertional heat illness may be at risk for MH.[21,28,29] Phenothiazine, haloperidol, and drugs used to treat schizophrenia are some of the medications that may stimulate a condition referred to as neuroleptic malignant syndrome. Physiologic indicators of this MH-like syndrome include muscle rigidity, elevated body temperature, and elevated creatine phosphokinase (CPK). Rhabdomyolysis and myoglobinuria also may occur.[3]

D. Pathophysiology

The primary MH defect resides in the skeletal muscle at the level of calcium release from the sarcoplastic reticulum of the muscle cell. The resultant

Table 2

<table>
<tr><td colspan="4" align="center">**MALIGNANT HYPERTHERMIA MEDICATION CHART**</td></tr>
<tr><td colspan="4" align="center">This chart is intended to provide a guide for calculating patient weight, medication dosage in relation to weight, and the amount of sterile water needed for reconstitution.</td></tr>
</table>

Dantrolene Sodium (Dantrium)

Dosage: 2.5 mg/kg intravenous. **Pediatric dose:** Refer to adult dosing.

Reconstitution: Supplied as a lyophilized powder that contains 20 mg of dantrolene sodium, 3,000 mg of mannitol, and sufficient sodium hydroxide to yield a pH of 9.5 when powder is reconstituted. During an MH crisis, it may take from two to four licensed individuals to reconstitute the required amounts of dantrolene sodium to accomplish rapid administration.

- ♦ Reconstitute each vial by adding 60 mL of preservative-free sterile water. Do not use bacteriostatic water for injection. Warming the mixing solution will help convert the lyophilized powder into solution.
- ♦ Shake vigorously until solution is clear.
- ♦ Do not use glass IV bottles for infusion.
- ♦ Protect from light.
- ♦ Use within six hours after reconstitution.[1,2]

Weight	Initial Dose: 2.5 mg/kg (continuous, rapid IV push)		# of vials to have on hand for four doses**	Sterile water necessary for four doses
10 kg	25 mg	(1.25 vials)	5	300 mL
30 kg	75 mg	(3.75 vials)	15	900 mL
40 kg	100 mg	(5 vials)	20	1,200 mL
50 kg	125 mg	(6.25 vials)	25	1,500 mL
60 kg	150 mg	(7.5 vials)	30	1,800 mL
70 kg	175 mg	(8.75 vials)	35	2,100 mL
80 kg	200 mg	(10 vials)	40	2,400 mL
90 kg	225 mg	(11.25 vials)	45	2,700 mL
100 kg	250 mg	(12.5 vials)	50	3,000 mL

**8-10 mg/kg is needed for an MH crisis; repeat 2.5 mg/kg doses up to four doses.[3,4] Risk of phlebitis is decreased if infused through largest possible vein.[5] Note that dantrolene sodium can be administered for spasticity associated with other clinical conditions. Warnings include caution when a patient has impaired cardiac function or impaired pulmonary function. The liver metabolizes dantrolene sodium, and there is a potential for hepatotoxicity. It is contraindicated when there is active hepatic disease.[3,6]

DO NOT USE CALCIUM CHANNEL BLOCKERS.
May lead to life-threatening hyperkalemia and myocardial depression.[7]

REFERENCES

1. Proctor and Gamble Pharmaceuticals. Dantrium IV®: information for health care professionals. [product information]. Cincinnati, OH: Proctor and Gamble; 2006: 1-6.

2. Rosenberg H. Malignant hyperthermia in the ambulatory setting. *Perioperative Medicine and Pain. [Seminars in Anesthesia]*. 2001; 20: 270-274.

3. Lexi-com. *Drug Information Handbook for Perioperative Nursing*. Adapted from *Anesthesiology and Critical Care Drug Handbook*, 6th ed; and *Drug Information Handbook for Advanced Practice Nursing*, 6th ed. Hudson, Ohio: Lexi-Comp; 2006: 1856, 485-486, 512.

4. Malignant Hyperthermia Association of the United States (MHAUS). Medical professional's FAQs—dantrolene. *http://www.mhaus.org/index.cfm/fuseaction/Content.Display* */PagePK/MedicalFAQs.cfm*. Accessed November 9, 2006.

5. Malignant Hyperthermia Association of the United States (MHAUS). [online brochure]. Drugs, equipment, and dantrolene—managing MH. *http://www.mhaus.org/index .cfm/fuseaction/Content.Display/PagePK/Home.cfm*. Accessed 9 Nov 2006.

6. Krause T, Gerbershagen MU, Fiege M, Weibhorn R, Wappler F. Dantrolene—a review of its pharmacology, therapeutic use and new developments. *Anesthesia*. 2004; 59 (11): 1139-1140.

7. Rosenberg H, Davis M, James D, Pollock N, Stowell K. Malignant hyperthermia: Orphanet Encyclopedia. November 2004. *http://www.orpha.net/data/patho/GB/uk-malignant -hyperthermia.pdf*. Accessed 7 Sept 2006: 8.

Table 2, *continued*

ADDITIONAL MEDICATIONS USED IN THE MANAGEMENT OF AN MH CRISIS					
NOTE: Dosage must be calculated for each patient.					
Weight	Insulin (0.15 units regular insulin/kg)	Glucose (1mL/kg D50W)	Furosemide (Lasix) (0.5–1 mg/kg)	Sodium bicarbonate (NaHCO₃) (1–2 mEq/kg)	Mannitol (Osmitrol) (300 mg/kg IV)
10 kg	1.5 units	10 mL	5–10 mg	10–20 mEq	When mannitol is used for the prevention or treatment of late renal complications of MH, the 3 g of mannitol needed to dissolve each 20 mg vial of IV dantrolene sodium should be taken into consideration.
20 kg	3.0 units	20 mL	10–20 mg	20–40 mEq	
30 kg	4.5 units	30 mL	15–30 mg	30–60 mEq	
40 kg	6.0 units	40 mL	20–40 mg	40–80 mEq	
50 kg	7.5 units	50 mL	25–50 mg	50–100 mEq	
60 kg	9.0 units	50 mL	30–60 mg	60–120 mEq	
70 kg	10 units	50 mL	35–70 mg	70–140 mEq	

Insulin/Glucose Drip: Regular insulin (US brand name: Humulin R) is the only type of insulin that can be administered IV. IV administration requires the use of an infusion pump. Combine 0.15 units/kg of regular insulin in 1mL/kg of 50% glucose for the treatment of hyperkalemia or combine 10 units of regular insulin in 50 mL of 50% glucose. Infusion rate titrated to results of potassium level.[1]

Calcium chloride (CaCl): 2 to 5 mg/kg or calcium gluconate may be used for treatment for life-threatening hyperkalemia. Gluconate may be less potent, but it is less likely to irritate peripheral veins.[2]

Lidocaine or amiodarone may be used to treat arrhythmias.

REFERENCES

1. Lexi-com. *Drug Information Handbook for Perioperative Nursing.* Adapted from *Anesthesiology and Critical Care Drug Handbook,* 6th ed; and *Drug Information Handbook for Advanced Practice Nursing,* 6th ed. Hudson, Ohio: Lexi-Comp; 2006: 1856, 485-486, 512.

2. Malignant Hyperthermia Association of the United States (MHAUS). Medical professional's FAQs—dantrolene. *http://www.mhaus.org/index.cfm/fuseaction/Content.Display/PagePK/MedicalFAQs.cfm.* Accessed November 9, 2006.

intracellular hypercalcemia leads to hypermetabolism, which in turn results in increased sympathetic activity, increased carbon dioxide production, increased oxygen consumption, and disruption of the cell membranes.[7,8,31] Muscle tissue is unable to return to a resting state in the susceptible patient, and because of this the primary signs of MH begin to appear. (See **Figure 1.**)

Malignant hyperthermia may present with a variety of signs and symptoms during an acute phase or present in a more subtle fashion and develop over a course of several hours. These changes in physiological state may not present in any particular sequence. Each of the following signs and symptoms has been associated with an MH crisis.[7,8,15,25,32]

Masseter muscle rigidity that is severe, sustained, and may interfere with intubation should be considered a possible sign of an impending MH episode. The muscle contracture may not be relieved with further doses of succinylcholine or a nondepolarizing muscle relaxant. As many as 50% of pediatric patients and 25% of adults who experience succinylcholine-induced masseter rigidity have tested positive for MH by the in vitro contracture test.[25,33]

Unexplained tachycardia is often the first sign of an acute MH episode. This sign may be mistaken for "light anesthesia" with prompt administration of more anesthetic agents. Progression of the syndrome can lead to dysrhythmias such as ventricular fibrillation and sudden cardiac arrest. Inability to maintain blood pressure may also present at this time.

Hypercarbia may occur due to increase in carbon dioxide (CO_2) production that results in elevated end tidal CO_2 and oxygen consumption. Other respiratory system symptoms may include an

Figure 1

PHYSIOLOGY OF MALIGNANT HYPERTHERMIA		
Physiology of Muscle Contraction/Relaxation in Normal Tissue Versus Malignant Hyperthermia (MH) Crisis[1-4]		
The central regulator of contraction and metabolism in the muscle is calcium. With an MH crisis, biochemical, metabolic, and physiologic conditions are a direct result of sudden and progressive increases in intracellular myoplasmic calcium.		
Normal Muscle Contraction		**Events Triggered by MH** *Note:* Not every symptom will be observed in every patient.
Tubules of sarcoplasmic reticulum (SR) in skeletal muscle contain calcium ions.		Tubules of SR in skeletal muscle contain calcium ions.
Calcium is released into myoplasm from SR through calcium release channels.		Calcium is released into SR through calcium release channels at an abnormally high rate.
The ryanodine receptor is the calcium release channel within the skeletal muscle cell that mediates calcium release.		Abnormalities associated with the function of the ryanodine receptor and the gene encoding for the receptor may account for MH in certain patients.
Calcium ions lead to activation of actin and myosin filaments.		Imbalance in calcium ions within skeletal muscle cells stimulate metabolism. Sustained hypermetabolic state progresses to: ♦ Excess lactate production ♦ High adenosine triphosphate (ATP) consumption ♦ Elevated oxygen (O_2) consumption ♦ Increased carbon dioxide (CO_2) ♦ Elevated heat production
Calcium ions bind to the troponin-tropomyosin complex, shifting it away from actin filaments.		Leads to subsequent loss of cellular integrity due to depletion of ATP.
Myoplasmic calcium is reduced via membrane adenosinetriphosphatase (ATPase) pump which breaks ATP down to adenosine diphosphate + phosphate + heat.		Leads to failure of cellular membrane pumps with subsequent leakage of: ♦ Electrolytes (eg, potassium and calcium) ♦ Enzymes (eg, creatinin-phosphokinase) ♦ Myoglobin from the skeletal cell
Calcium returns to the SR.		Sustained hypermetabolic state progresses to: ♦ Tachycardia due to respiratory acidosis and metabolic acidosis. ♦ End-organ damage.
Muscle relaxation.		Death, if unrecognized and untreated.

REFERENCES

1. McCarthy EJ. Malignant Hyperthermia. *AACN. [Clinical Issue]* 2004; 15: 231-237.

2. Scanlon VC, Sanders T. Essentials of Anatomy and Physiology. 4th ed. Philadelphia, Pa: F A Davis Company; 2003: 135.

3. Thibodeau GA, Patton KT. Anatomy & Physiology. 5th ed. St Louis, Mo: Mosby; 2003: 317-319.

4. Hopkins PM. Malignant hyperthermia: advances in clinical management and diagnosis. British Journal of Anaesthesia. 2000; 85(1): 118-28.

increase in arterial CO_2, and/or respiratory acidosis. Excess CO_2 can cause the CO_2 absorbent canister associated with the anesthesia machine to become discolored and hot to the touch.

Metabolic acidosis has been observed during MH crises. Associated altered laboratory values may include the following:

- Arterial blood gasses (ABGs) may show
  - decreased pH,
  - decreased partial pressure of oxygen in arterial blood (PaO_2),
  - increased partial pressure of carbon dioxide in arterial blood ($PaCO_2$), and
  - increased anion gap.
- Coagulation studies may show
  - prolonged prothrombin time (PT),
  - prolonged partial thromboplastin time (PTT), and
  - decreased platelets.
- Electrolyte imbalances may include
  - increased potassium,
  - increased calcium (but can also be decreased as calcium moves into cells),
  - increased magnesium, and
  - decreased sodium.

Core temperature may increase by as much as $1°$ C ($1.8°$ F) every few minutes. Extreme temperatures of $46°$ C ($114.8°$ F) have been recorded. Skin temperature may read too high or too low. Body temperature increase is often a late sign of MH, because the site of the temperature elevation is skeletal muscle.

Skin changes may include generalized erythmatous flush or mottling of the skin. Cyanosis may present secondary to generalized vasoconstriction and accelerated oxygen consumption by muscles. Diaphoresis may also be present.

Myoglobinuria may become evident as a result of breakdown of muscle tissue.

Renal function may be altered. Due to leakage of muscle contents and filtering by the kidney, myoglobinuria may occur before elevation in creatine kinase (CK) and may cause renal insufficiency. This condition is treated by alkalizing the urine and maintaining a diuresis. The patient's urine may change color to a dark red or brown and will test positive for blood with the use of a urine test strip. If there are no red blood cells in the urine, then the presumptive evidence is myoglobin, and urine and/or blood samples should be sent for quantitative myoglobin. This may take time if the facility has to go off-site for the testing. Laboratory studies may include an increased creatinine.

Rhabdomyolysis occurs when muscle is damaged and intracellular contents begin to leak into the bloodstream. Only laboratory tests reveal rhabdomyolysis. Rigidity may or may not be present. Whole-body rigidity in the presence of profound neuromuscular blockade confirms the MH diagnosis. The absence of muscle rigidity does not rule out MH. In rhabdomyolysis, there may be an increased CK. Creatine kinase may be acutely normal and may not peak until approximately 16 hours after the episode.

Serum studies are late findings and should be used for retrospective diagnosis. These may include the following:

- increased glucose,
- increased lactate,
- increased pyruvate,
- increased lactic dehydrogenase (LDH), and
- increased aldolase.

Part II: Plan of Care

The perioperative nurse develops a plan of care for patients at risk for MH that includes interventions to attain expected outcomes. These outcome statements become a guide for the nursing interventions necessary to achieve the desired results. The individualized plan of care reflects the perioperative assessment and a logical sequence to attain outcomes. Priorities for the provision of nursing care are established by the perioperative nurse in collaboration with other health care providers, the patient, and the patient's significant others. The flow chart in **Figure 2** can be used to assess patients for MH risk in the development of an individualized plan of care for a patient identified as at increased risk for MH.

A. Preoperative Nursing Care

Nursing care begins when the patient is scheduled for any procedure involving general anesthesia. As early as possible in the preoperative phase, the perioperative nurse should ask patients and their families a series of questions to help screen for susceptibility to MH.[25,29,32,34] For example:

- Has anyone ever told you that you had a "bad" reaction to anesthesia?
- Has anyone ever told you that you or a family member had a problem with anesthesia?
- Have you or a family member experienced a high fever while under anesthesia?
- Has anyone ever told you or a family member they had a difficult time opening your jaw during a general anesthetic?

Figure 2

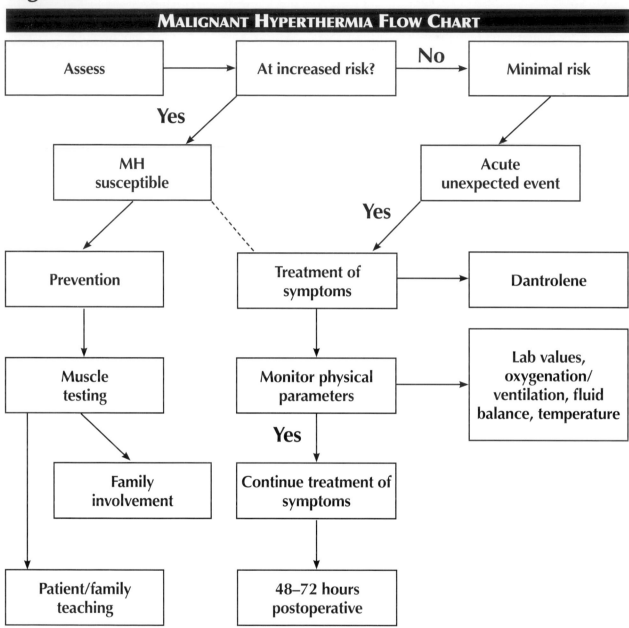

MALIGNANT HYPERTHERMIA FLOW CHART

- Has anyone in your family died unexpectedly in the operating room?
- Have you or anyone in your family experienced sunstroke or heat stroke resulting in hospitalization?
- Have you ever noticed dark "cola-colored" urine after a general anesthetic or after experiencing a heat-related illness?

Opening a discussion using layman's terms may help the patient and family talk about situations that relate to susceptibility for MH. If the perioperative nurse believes a patient is susceptible to MH, the surgeon and anesthesia care provider should be notified. Preoperative education and preparation is crucial for the patient who is identified as susceptible to MH. It is important that the patient and family members understand that answering "yes" to any of the questions above will not mean they will be denied anesthesia during a surgical procedure but that different considerations may be initiated for their anesthesia care. They should participate in decisions about when and where to go for the surgical procedure and understand that counseling is available. Patients who are identified as susceptible to MH can safely undergo surgery in outpatient settings with the use of nontriggering anesthetics and careful monitoring.[24,25,35] More information is provided about this in Section D.

B. Perioperative Nursing Vocabulary

The Perioperative Nursing Data Set (PNDS) is a clinically relevant and empirically validated standardized nursing language. It relates to the delivery of care in perioperative settings. This standardized language consists of a collection of data elements (ie, perioperative nursing diagnoses, interventions, outcomes).[36] In 1999, the PNDS was recognized by the American Nurses Associations' Committee on Nursing Practice Information Infrastructures as a data set useful in the practice of nursing. The perioperative patient focused model provides the conceptual framework for the PNDS and the model for perioperative nursing practice. The patient and his or her family members are at the core of the model. The model depicts perioperative nursing in four domains and illustrates the relationship between the patient, his or her family members, and care provided by the perioperative professional nurse. The patient-centered domains are

- ◆ D1—safety,
- ◆ D2—physiological responses to surgery,
- ◆ D3—patient and family member behavioral responses to surgery, and
- ◆ D4—health system in which perioperative care is provided.

A unique identifier represents each data element in the PNDS. The domains are represented by the letter "D" and are followed by the numbers one to four to indicate the particular domain being addressed. The letter "X" and a number unique to the diagnosis represent nursing diagnoses; the letter "I" and a unique number represent interventions; and the letter "O" and a unique number represent outcomes. These designations are incorporated into this guideline to help perioperative nurses create a flexible plan of care that can be put into action when circumstances change. The plan of care should be a part of the patient's medical record to increase the perioperative nurse's awareness of the patient's needs during an MH crisis, to provide documentation for third-party payers and accreditation agencies, and to meet legal requirements. **Exhibit A**, at the end of this guideline, provides a sample care plan using PNDS terminology and includes the MH protocol.

C. Post-Crisis Patient Care

After the patient has been stabilized in the OR and before transfer to either the postanesthesia care unit (PACU) or a critical care setting, the team should review the protocol checklist to be sure that all recommended testing and treatments have been completed and appropriately documented (**Table 3**).

During the post-acute crisis phase, the patient should be observed in a critical care setting for a minimum of 36 hours after the MH crisis.[31] Arrangements for transfer either directly from the OR to a critical care area or from PACU to a critical care area should be made according to policy. If an MH crisis occurs at an ambulatory surgical setting or facility without critical care services, arrangements should be made for transfer to a facility providing those services via ambulance. A comprehensive status report from the perioperative registered nurse(s) and anesthesia care provider(s) should be given to the accepting critical care area nurse(s) and physician(s). Any time the perioperative team suspects a patient may have experienced an adverse metabolic reaction to anesthesia (AMRA), the attending anesthesia care provider or designated physician should complete an AMRA form and submit it to the North American Malignant Hyperthermia Registry of MHAUS, preferably within 48 hours of the event.[37] The form can be accessed through *https://www.mhreg.org/Downloads.aspx*.

During the post-crisis phase (eg, 24 to 48 hours) dantrolene sodium 1 mg/kg should be administered IV every four to eight hours.[15,31] Each vial of dantrolene sodium contains 3g of mannitol, which is an osmotic diuretic. When additional mannitol is used for the prevention or treatment of late renal complications of MH, the mannitol that exists in dantrolene sodium should be taken into consideration.

Urinary output should be monitored using an indwelling urinary catheter. When rhabdomyolysis is present, vigorous diuresis is necessary.[25] The patient's urine output should be greater than 2mL/kg/hour to prevent renal failure. Furosemide may be used to facilitate sufficient output.[31] Creatine Kinase should be measured every six hours until there is a decrease. If the MH crisis was severe, CK may remain elevated for two weeks. When the patient has improved and is considered stable, CK should be measured on a declining time basis until it is

Table 3

EXAMPLE OF MALIGNANT HYPERTHERMIA (MH) CRISIS CHECKLIST[1]

Note: This checklist is intended to provide a means to quickly summarize what has been done at any point in the MH crisis and what still may need to be done according to the Malignant Hyperthermia Association of the United States (MHAUS) protocol. The actions listed are not necessarily in order, and each action may not be needed for every circumstance. This checklist may be a helpful tool for reporting to personnel in critical care settings.

Check each item when complete

☐ Discontinue volatile agents and succinylcholine.

☐ Hyperventilate patient with 100% oxygen at flows of 10L/min or more.

☐ Dantrolene sodium 2.5mg/kg IV, given rapidly through large bore needle. Administer repeatedly until resolved.

☐ Change breathing circuits.

☐ Change soda lime canister.

☐ Treat hyperkalemia.
▪ Regular insulin; dextrose 50%
▪ For adults, 10mg/kg calcium chloride or 10 to 50mg/kg calcium gluconate

☐ Treat arrhythmias.
▪ Lidocaine or amiodarone
▪ Beta blockers
▪ **DO NOT** use calcium channel blocking agents

☐ Insert arterial line.

☐ Draw arterial blood gasses.
▪ Watch for:
  – decreased pH,
  – decreased partial pressure of oxygen of arterial blood (PaO_2), and
  – increased partial pressure of carbon dioxide of arterial blood ($PaCO_2$).
▪ Administer sodium bicarbonate if metabolic acidosis (1–2mEq/kg) is present.
▪ Venous blood gas (eg, femoral vein) may document hypermetabolism better than arterial values.

☐ Monitor renal function
▪ IV fluids (do not use lactated Ringers because it enhances metabolic acidosis).
▪ Furosemide, if needed.
▪ Urine test strip to check for blood.

Check each item when complete

☐ Insert 3-way indwelling urinary catheter.

☐ Insert central line.

☐ Monitor laboratory studies.
Electrolyte studies, watch for:
▪ increased potassium,
▪ increased calcium,
▪ increased magnesium, and
▪ decreased sodium.

Coagulation studies, watch for:
▪ prolonged prothrombin time,
▪ prolonged partial thromboplastin time, and
▪ decreased platelets.

Serum studies, watch for increased:
▪ creatine phosphokinase,
▪ myoglobin,
▪ creatinine,
▪ glucose,
▪ lactate,
▪ pyruvate,
▪ lactic dehydrogenase, and
▪ aldolase.

☐ Decrease temperature.
▪ Apply cooling blanket.
▪ Infuse cold saline IV.
▪ Monitor with esophageal or rectal temperature probe.
▪ Ice packs to head, axillae, groin, and underneath patient.
▪ Esophageal lavage.
▪ Rectal lavage.
▪ Discontinue cooling measures when body temperature has reached 38° C (100.4° F).

Post Crisis

Complete AMRA form; submit it to the North American Malignant Hyperthermia Registry of MHAUS, preferably within 48 hours of the event. Forms can be accessed at *https://www.mhreg.org/Downloads.aspx* or *https://www.mhreg.org/forms/AMRA_9-1.pdf*.

REFERENCE
1. Malignant Hyperthermia Association of the United States (MHAUS). *Hospital Procedure Manual.* Sherbourne, NY: Malignant Hyperthermia Association of the United States [MHAUS]; 2006.

normal (eg, every four hours during the acute episode to once a week during convalescence).[9]

Cardiac arrhythmias are usually corrected when the anesthesia care provider disrupts the progression of the MH episode and corrects the hyperkalemia. If cardiac arrhythmias caused by the MH crisis continue into the post-acute crisis phase, standard antiarrhythmic agents may be used. Calcium channel blockers should not be used to treat arrhythmias because they can lead to further hyperkalemia and cardiovascular collapse. Sodium bicarbonate, IV glucose, and insulin are used to treat hyperkalemia.[9,19]

The patient should be monitored for signs of recurrence or complications. This includes assessing the patient closely for muscle rigidity. Vital signs, including core body temperature, should be monitored with an esophageal or rectal probe. Cooling methods should be continued until the temperature is 38° C (100.4° F) and falling; then discontinue to prevent temperature from dropping below 36° C (96.8° F).[13,31] End tidal CO_2 is monitored on the intubated patient. Serum and urine studies are performed until the results return to normal. Serum studies include, but are not limited to, ABGs; serum CK, potassium, calcium, and myoglobin; and clotting values. Urine studies include (but are not limited to) urine output and myoglobin levels.[31]

Patients and family members should be informed of symptoms reported by other patients who have received IV dantrolene sodium. Patients may experience a decrease in grip strength and weakness of their leg muscles. This is especially noticeable when going down stairs. Light-headedness may also be noticed for up to 48 hours, and there may be difficulty swallowing or choking when the patient starts taking food.[21,23,27] There is also a risk of phlebitis if the dantrolene sodium was not infused through a large vein.[24,27]

When patients who are MH susceptible have surgery in ambulatory surgery centers (ASCs) and exhibit a mild masseter spasm or severe masseter rigidity, they should not be discharged without further observation. If there were mild symptoms of jaw tension but no increase in CK, and no signs of myoglobinuria, muscle weakness, muscle soreness, hyperthermia, or abnormal electrolytes, patients should be observed for at least 10 hours. Patients may be discharged after 10 to12 hours with instructions to the family to return to an emergency room at the first sign of elevated temperature.[25]

> Expert help is available for diagnosis and treatment of an ongoing MH episode. Call:
>
> **MHAUS Emergency Hotline:**
> **800-644-9737**
> *(US and Canada)*
>
> **001-1-315-464-7079**
> *(outside the US)*

If there are signs of dark or cola-colored urine, increased temperature or pulse rate, or changes in acid-base balance, patients should be admitted and observed overnight. If the jaw rigidity was severe, overnight observation is necessary to observe for progression of symptoms and the potential for an MH crisis. When MH-susceptible patients undergo uneventful general anesthetics in ASCs, they should be monitored for at least one hour in PACU and at least one and a half hours in the phase II PACU or step-down unit before being discharged.[24,35,38]

Malignant hyperthermia occurs most frequently during administration of anesthesia. Initial symptoms are not generally seen in the PACU, especially more than two hours after discontinuing anesthetic agents.[32] When patients present with symptoms of a fever in PACU, it is generally due to sepsis or iatrogenic heating and is not related to MH. Temperature increases after a patient is discharged are not generally related to MH unless there were signs of MH (eg, myoglobinuria, muscle weakness, muscle rigidity) before discharge.[25]

D. Patient/Family Follow-up Education and Counseling

Patients and relatives should understand the importance of informing the entire surgical team (eg, anesthesia care providers, surgeon, perioperative nurses) about a family history of MH before they undergo any future surgical or invasive procedures requiring general anesthesia. It is critical that patients and their relatives receive counseling and education regarding the pathophysiology and management of MH. It is useful for the patient to have a copy of the anesthesia record, laboratory tests, and the PACU/critical care area notes to show to future care providers.

Contact Information for the Malignant Hyperthermia Association of the United States

Mailing address
11 East State St
PO Box 1069
Sherburne, NY 13460

Web page
http://www.mhaus.org

Phone number
607-674-7901 or 800-986-4287

Email address
info@mhaus.org

Patients and their families also should understand that MH is a genetic disease and that it could affect other relatives. An autosomal dominant pattern is inherited when MH is identified in a family member. This translates into the following inheritance patterns:

- Children of the MH-susceptible (MHS) patient have a 50% chance of inheriting the susceptibility.
- Grandchildren of the MH susceptible patient have a 25% chance of testing positive for MH susceptibility.
- The risk to siblings of the MH susceptible patient depends upon the genetic status of the MHS patient's parent. If a parent of the MHS patient has MH susceptibility, the risk to the siblings is 50%.
- More distant relatives have a lesser chance of testing positive for MH susceptability.[3,14,15,39]

Patients are appropriate candidates for muscle biopsy testing if they have a family history of MH or have experienced unexplained hypercarbia and muscle rigidity related to a general anesthetic.[15,40]

The standard diagnostic test for MH is the caffeine-halothane contracture test. This test involves making an incision in the patient's quadriceps muscle, removing a small piece of muscle tissue, and immersing the muscle in a solution of caffeine and/or halothane. Typically, a patient undergoing the diagnostic muscle biopsy will undergo a nerve block or regional anesthetic supplemented with sedation. Occasionally a clinician will supplement the block with a nontriggering general anesthetic. A local anesthetic is contraindicated because it adversely affects the tissue viability when a local anesthetic

agent is directly injected into the muscle that is being biopsied. After the biopsy, there may be a period of two to seven days of relative disability.[15,40] This test cannot be performed on children unless they weigh more than 25 kg and are older than 10 years of age.[41] Testing also cannot be done within 6 months of being treated for an MH crisis.[31]

There are three categories of test results:

- **MH susceptible.** The muscle biopsy has abnormal contractures to both halothane and caffeine.
- **MH negative.** The muscle biopsy has normal contractures, and the patient is not considered susceptible.[3,35]
- **Malignant hyperthermia equivocal.** This is a third category is used in Europe and applies when the biopsied muscle responds abnormally to only one agent.

Patients who are identified as equivocal are considered susceptible, however, until proven otherwise. False negatives can occur with the contracture tests.[3] In this case, if the patient had a suspected family history or personal history of possible MH, the patient should be treated as MH susceptible regardless of a contracture test that showed normal contractures when tested.

The muscle biopsy must be analyzed within five hours of the harvest.[3] This usually means it is necessary for patients and their families to travel to a diagnostic center for the testing. Patients who decide to proceed with this type of diagnostic screening are often responsible for their own costs for the test and the associated travel. There are 22 centers in Europe that do MH diagnostic testing, but there are only eight centers in North America where testing is performed (**Table 4**).

Genetic studies have indicated that a defect in the ryanodine type 1 receptor (RYR1) located on chromosome 19 may be linked with MH. The genetic test is less costly and less invasive than the contracture testing, but it is not a clinical screening test at this time. Ongoing genetic research shows promise for patients and relatives affected by MH.[41-43] Until DNA studies are refined, the caffeine-halothane contracture test for the diagnosis of MH susceptibility continues to be the "gold standard" for testing.[10,40]

The MHAUS goal is to educate the public and offer support to patients and their relatives about MH. Patients and their families should be given information about MHAUS including the website (mhaus.org), phone number (607-674-7901), and the email address (info@mhaus.org).[1] They can receive medical identification bracelets to wear and identification cards to carry in their wallets from MHAUS to use as a communication tool for emergency surgery and documentation for future elective surgeries.

When assessing patients for blood or organ donations, perioperative nurses should know that susceptibility to MH is not "carried" in the blood or organs, so there is no contraindication to blood or organ donation by a person known to be susceptible to MH. Clinicians who identify themselves as MH-susceptible individuals and are working in the OR may want to avoid close proximity to the anesthesia care provider during a mask induction with a triggering agent, but there are no cases reported of a MH crisis related to waste anesthetic gases while working in the OR.[41]

Part III: Evaluation of Caregiver Response to an MH Crisis

When a patient undergoing an invasive procedure is having a MH crisis, decisions need to be made about potentially postponing subsequent invasive procedures throughout the facility. Emergency surgeries should be diverted until the crisis has been resolved. As responders are handling the MH crisis, a designated team (eg, surgical services director or designee, lead pharmacist, lead anesthesia care provider) should assess the availability of crisis management supplies, including dantrolene sodium throughout the facility. If invasive procedures are to be continued, sufficient quantities of dantrolene sodium must be available to treat the patient who is actively in MH crisis for at least 48 hours and as well as enough to treat a potential second patient in MH crisis.

The designated team should develop a communication action plan if invasive procedures will be delayed or cancelled. In small facilities or ambulatory surgery centers, the nursing supervisor or receptionist may be assigned to participate in the communication plan. This decision should not wait for the current crisis to resolve. Facility administrators should establish a policy that clearly identifies who will be responsible for making the decision about other invasive procedures. Consideration should be given regarding whether the full supply of medication needs to be available in-house before proceeding with other invasive procedures or general anesthetics. The policy should also indicate who might need to help with the communication plan if no one from the perioperative team is available due to the MH crisis.

Table 4

TESTING CENTERS AND LABORATORIES

The following medical facilities provide testing in the United States and Canada:

- University of California at Los Angeles, Los Angeles;
- University of Minnesota, Minneapolis;
- University of California Davis, California;
- Thomas Jefferson University, Philadelphia;
- Uniformed Services University of the Health Sciences, Bethesda, Maryland;
- Wake Forest University (Bowman-Gray), Winston-Salem, North Carolina,
- Ottawa Hospital-Civic Campus, Ottawa, Ontario, Canada
- Toronto General Hospital, Toronto, Ontario, Canada.

SOURCE: Malignant Hyperthermia Association of the United States (MHAUS). MH muscle biopsy centers: directory North American malignant hyperthermia muscle contracture testing centers. *http://www .mhaus.org/index.cfm/fuseaction/Content.Display/Pag ePK/BiopsyTestCenters.cfm.* Accessed 12 Sept 2006.

For more information about genetic tests for MH, contact the following laboratories:

- Prevention Genetics LLC, Marshfield, Wisconsin, *http://www.preventiongenetics.com.*
- Center for Medical Genetics, University of Pittsburgh Medical Center, *http://path.upmc .edu/divisions/mdx/diagnostics.html.*

Performance Improvement

After the patient has been transferred out of the OR and a comprehensive report has been provided to the accepting nurses(s) and physician(s), another assessment should be done to consider the availability for crisis management supplies to complete the remainder of scheduled cases. If it is not safe to proceed with scheduled cases, alternate plans may include transferring patients to another facility or rescheduling cases for a later time or date. Immediate steps should be taken to reorder dantrolene sodium and other crisis management supplies necessary to restock the MH cart. **Table 5** shows suggested contents for a dedicated MH cart.[26]

All staff members involved in the MH crisis response should hold a debriefing meeting to evaluate their response as soon as possible. This would include ancillary areas and other departments (eg, critical care, pharmacy, central supply, emergency department). This

Table 5

SUGGESTED CONTENTS FOR A MALIGNANT HYPERTHERMIA (MH) CART				
Medications				
Name	Concentration	Amount	Rationale	Comments
Dantrolene sodium	20 mg vials	36 vials	Skeletal muscle relaxant.	Previously mannitol was included in the list of drugs to be kept on an MH cart. This is no longer necessary because dantrolene sodium has 3 g of mannitol included in each vial.[1]
Preservative-free sterile water (ie, without a bacteriostatic agent)	1,000 mL per bag or bottle	2 bags or bottles	Needed to mix dantrolene sodium.	Contact MHAUS for special supplies for reconstituting dantrolene sodium.
Sodium bicarbonate (NaHCO3) 8.4%	50 mEq	5 syringes	Treats metabolic acidosis.	
Dextrose 50%	50 mL vials	2 vials	Treats hyperkalemia.	
Regular insulin (must be refrigerated)	100 units/mL	1 bottle	Treats hyperkalemia.	Regular insulin is the only type of insulin that can be administered IV.[2] IV administration requires the use of an infusion pump.
Furosemide (eg, Lasix)	40mg/ampule	4 ampoules	Increases urine output.	
Calcium chloride 10%	10 mL vial	2 vials	Treats life-threatening hyperkalemia.	Calcium gluconate or calcium chloride can be used. Calcium gluconate may be less potent, but it is less likely to irritate peripheral veins.[1]
Lidocaine hydrochloride 2% for injection	100 mg/5 mL or 100 mg/10 mL in preloaded syringes	3 syringes	Treats cardiac arrhythmias. Requires the use of an infusion pump to administer accurate dose.	Amiodarone is also acceptable. Previously, procainamide had been a recommended stock drug for MH carts. It is no longer necessary because it has been confirmed that lidocaine does not aggravate MH.[1]
Note: Each facility should decide whether to stock more medications for treating cardiac arrhythmias on the MH cart or whether to use an accompanying code cart for advanced cardiac life support (ACLS) for protocols that may be necessary.				

REFERENCES

1. Malignant Hyperthermia Association of the United States (MHAUS). Medical professional's FAQs—dantrolene. April 2006. Available at *http://www.mhaus.org/index.cfm/fuseaction/Content.Display/PagePK/MedicalFAQs.cfm.* Accessed September 8, 2006.

2. Lexi-Comp. *Drug Information Handbook for Perioperative Nursing.* Adapted from *Anesthesiology and Critical Care Drug Handbook,* 6th ed; and *Drug Information Handbook for Advanced Practice Nursing.* 6th ed. Hudson, Ohio: Lexi-Comp; 2006: 933.

Table 5, *continued*

SUGGESTED CONTENTS FOR A MALIGNANT HYPERTHERMIA (MH) CART		
Supplies		
Description of Item	**Amount**	**Comments**
60 mL Luer-lock syringes	5	Used to dilute dantrolene sodium.
60 mL catheter-tip syringes	6	Used for irrigation (eg, nasogastric tube [NG], indwelling urinary catheter).
10 mL Luer-lock syringes	10	
3 mL syringes	10	For blood gas analysis if arterial blood gas (ABG) kits are not available.
Alcohol prep pads	1 box	
Vial spikes	6	
Elastic tourniquets	4	For drawing blood.
Povidone-iodine paint 4 oz	2 bottles	Prepping arterial line sites.
Sterile gauze 4x4s (boxes of 10)	2	For dressings at IV sites.
Radial artery catheters	2	
Arterial line monitoring kit	1	Sizes appropriate to patient population.
Central venous pressure line kit	1	Sizes appropriate to patient population.
Cassette tubing for IV infusion pumps	4 sets	
Angiocaths: 16 g, 18 g, and 20 g = 2-inch; 22 g = 1-inch; 24 g = 3-inch	6 of each	
Tape (various types)	2 rolls of each	
Small and large adhesive IV dressings	6 of each	
Adult IV drip chambers	4	
IV solution sets with drip chambers	4	These supplies need to be readily available on the anesthesia cart or separately stocked on the MH cart.
IV extension tubing	4	
"T" connectors	4	
Three-way stopcocks	4	
Pediatric arm boards	4	
Adult arm boards	4	
Sharps container	1	

Table 5, *continued*

SUGGESTED CONTENTS FOR A MALIGNANT HYPERTHERMIA (MH) CART		

Anesthesia Equipment

Description of Item	Amount	Comments
Soda lime canister	1	
Adult anesthesia breathing circuits	2	
Pediatric anesthesia breathing circuits	2	
NG tubes (various sizes)	3 each	
Esophageal temperature probes	2	Large size esophageal temp probe can be used as a stethoscope.
General purpose temperature probe	2	General-purpose temperature probe cannot be used as a stethoscope.
Heparinized ABG syringes	6	ABG kits may be used. May also be used to assess lactic acid levels.
Pediatric ambu bags	1	
Adult ambu bag	1	
Extra oxygen tank	1	Readily available if not on MH cart.
Infusion pumps	2	Readily available.

Cooling Supplies

Description of Item	Amount	Comments
Chilled 0.9% Saline for irrigation	6 bottles each, 1 liter and 3 liter	At the time the cart is requested, add these items from the refrigerator.
Clear, large plastic bags	6	Used for ice.
Clear, small or medium plastic bags	6	Used for ice.
Large containers	2	Used for ice.
Ice		Access to ice machine or bags of ice.

Nursing Equipment

Description of Item	Amount	Comments
Large translucent adhesive sterile drape	2	Used for closure of wound.
Closed-system urinary catheter trays	2	
Urinary catheter drainage bags with urimeters	2	
3-way urinary catheters (adult size)	2	
3-way urinary catheters (pediatric sizes)	2	
Rectal tube	1	
Peritoneal lavage trays	2	
Cystoscopy tubing	2	
5-in-1 connectors	2	
Y connectors	2	

Table 5, *continued*

SUGGESTED CONTENTS FOR A MALIGNANT HYPERTHERMIA (MH) CART		

Laboratory Testing Supplies

Description of Item	Amount	Comments
Urine specimen containers	2	Myoglobinuria.
Urine test strips	1 bottle	Test for blood in the urine.
Blood specimen tubes appropriate for the following tests: creatin kinase, myoglobin, chemistry screen, lactic hydrogenase, electrolytes, thyroid studies, prothrombin/partial thromboplastin times, fibrinogen, fibrin split products, complete blood count, platelets.	At least 2 large and 2 small of each tube type	

Forms and Checklists

Blood gas slips	6	
Hematology forms	2	
Chemistry forms	2	
Coagulation forms	2	
Urinalysis forms	2	
Physician order forms	2	
Blood requisition form	2	
MHAUS label on front of cart listing hotline phone number (ie, 800-644-9737)		
MHAUS MH crisis data management sheet		Can be ordered by calling 800-986-4287; or can be printed from *http://www.mhaus.org*.
Anesthesia records	4	This may not be needed if using MHAUS data sheet.
ICU report form or hand-off transfer report form for ambulance (eg, ambulatory surgery center, office-based setting)	1	
Physician consultation form	1	
Medication labels	At least 10	Consider labeling sterile water for "reconstitution only."
Adverse medical reaction to anesthesia report form from North American MH Registry (NAMHR)		Can be printed online: *https://www.mhreg.org*. Contact NAMHR to receive patient packet with ID cards included.
Guides, checklists, worksheets		Training manual (eg, designed by MHAUS or own facility); worksheets and checklists with assignments for responders.
Other supplies are available through MHAUS (eg, hand-held cards, poster, list of duties)		Can be ordered by calling 800-986-4287; or can be printed from *http://www.mhaus.org*.

meeting should address areas that the response team may need to improve for future patients in MH crisis. Points to consider include:

♦ Was the MH cart adequately stocked and immediately available?
♦ Are there additional supplies that should be added to the cart?
♦ Were enough staff members available to manage the crisis effectively?
♦ When staff members responded, were they familiar with tasks expected in an MH crisis?
♦ How long did it take to get the recommended 36 vials of dantrolene sodium supply replaced?
♦ How long did it take to get the MH cart restocked with supplies?
♦ Were scheduled surgeries postponed or cancelled because of inadequate supplies on the cart?
♦ Was an effective communication plan implemented if scheduled surgeries had to be postponed or cancelled?
♦ Was an incident report completed and filed?
♦ Was MHAUS appropriately notified?
♦ Is a process in place to facilitate patient and family MH education and counseling?
♦ Do staff members have other ideas about planning care for a future MH crisis?
♦ Are there plans to have periodic MH crisis drills, including practice sessions to mix dantrolene sodium using outdated vials?
♦ Do policies need to be created or revised?
♦ Has a root-cause analysis been done (MH is considered a sentinel event)?

Every facility should include MH training in the orientation plan for new members of the perioperative team and other teams involved in responding to the crisis. Ongoing periodic reviews should be scheduled. The MHAUS recommendations suggest that the perioperative team initiate mock MH drills at least twice a year to improve staff member efficiency in treating a patient during an MH crisis.[45] Because dantrolene sodium is difficult to mix, some institutions reconstitute the outdated medication in staff member education sessions to give hands-on training during the mock drills. For perioperative nurses, it may also be helpful to include a review of electrolyte imbalances and the shifts in ABGs that occur with respiratory and metabolic acidosis during an MH crisis.

Facilities should identify specific tasks assigned to each member of the response team to effectively manage a MH crisis. Procedure manuals are available through MHAUS to assist in assigning specific tasks and to facilitate staff education.[45] Examples of role delineation are provided in **Table 6**.

Part IV: Summary

This guideline outlines the assessment and treatment of MH and presents resources and tools for staff member development training. Perioperative nurses are committed to providing one standard of care to patients regardless of where an invasive procedure is taking place. Nurses should be prepared to monitor the patient and treat an MH crisis if they are working in any type of facility or department where MH triggering agents are used (eg, OR, labor and delivery, interventional radiology, emergency department).[25]

Perioperative nurses and other health care providers should stay up-to-date with new research and treatment recommendations. For more information about MH, contact the MHAUS at 11 East State St, PO Box 1069, Sherburne, NY, 13460; telephone (607) 674-7901 or 1-800-986-4287; Web site, http://www.mhaus.org.

REFERENCES

1. Malignant Hyperthermia Association of the United States (MHAUS). What is MHAUS? http://www.mhaus.org/index.cfm/fuseaction/Content.Display/PagePK/Home.cfm. Accessed September 10, 2006.

2. Mosby's Dictionary of Medicine, Nursing & Health Professions. 7th ed. St Louis, Mo: Mosby Elsevier; 2006: 1144-1145.

3. Rosenberg H, Dirksen RT. Malignant hyperthermia susceptibility: GeneReviews. http://www.genetests.org. Accessed August 28, 2006.

4. Denborough MA, Forster JFA, Lovell RHR, Maplestone PA, Villiers JD. Anaesthetic deaths in a family. British Journal of Anaesthesia 1962; 34: 395-396.

5. Hopkins PM, Halsall PJ, Ellis FR. Diagnosing malignant hyperthermia susceptibility. [editorial]. Anaesthesia. 1994; 49: 373-375.

6. Kalow W, Britt BA, Richter A. The caffeine test of isolated human muscle in relation to malignant hyperthermia. Journal of the Canadian Anaesthesia Society. 1977; 24: 678-694.

7. Hopkins PM, Malignant hyperthermia: advances in clinical management and diagnosis. British Journal of Anaesthesia. 2000; 85 (1): 118-128.

8. Miller JD, Rosenbaum H, Weiss L. Malignant hyperthermia: UCLA anesthesiology. http://www.anes.ucla.edu/dept/mh.html. Accessed September 22, 2006.

9. Malignant Hyperthermia Association of the United States (MHAUS). Clinical update: managing malignant hyperthermia. http://www.mhaus.org/index.cfm/fuseaction/OnlineBrochures.Display/BrochurePK/3FFCBC12-9479-49. Accessed September 13, 2006.

10. Rosenberg H, Antognini JF, Muldoon S. Testing for malignant hyperthermia [Clinical Concepts and Commentary] Anesthesiology. 2002; 9: 232-237.

Table 6

MANAGEMENT OF A MALIGNANT HYPERTHERMIA (MH) CRISIS

Outline shows examples for delineation of roles.

Anesthesia care provider

- Discontinue volatile agents.
- May hyperventilate patient with 100% oxygen.
- May continue administering nitrous oxide.

Dantrolene sodium
- Administer 2.5mg/kg IV until crisis is resolved.

Treat hyperkalemia (if patient is symptomatic)
- Regular insulin.
- Dextrose 50%.
- 10 mg/kg calcium chloride or 10 to 50 mg/kg calcium gluconate.

Treat arrhythmias
- Administer lidocaine or amiodarone.
- Administer beta blockers.
- Do not use calcium channel blocking agents, which may cause hyperkalemia or cardiac arrest in the presence of dantrolene sodium.

Arterial line placement
Draw arterial blood gasses (ABGs). Based on ABG results, may need to administer sodium bicarbonate to treat metabolic acidosis.

Decrease temperature (if elevated)
- Apply cooling blanket.
- Infuse cold saline IV.
- Apply ice packs to head, axillae, groin, and underneath patient, if possible.
- Discontinue cooling measures when body temperature has reached 38 °C (100.4° F).

Monitor renal function
- Administer IV fluids; avoid lactated Ringer's solution as it may contribute to patient's acidosis.
- Administer furosemide as needed.

Surgical Team

- Complete surgical procedure as soon as possible or stop surgical procedure.
- Communicate closely with anesthesia care provider.
- Cold saline irrigation of body cavity, if needed.
- Prepare for/assist with central line placement.
- Insert urinary catheter (3-way).
- If available, help mix dantrolene sodium or with insertion of additional IV lines.

Circulating RN

- Notify anesthesia team leader.
- Notify OR charge nurse.
- Ask for extra personnel (see "Delegation of Duties").
- Assemble ice packs.
- Obtain basins of ice water (may delegate to clinical assistant [CA] as stated below).
- Apply cold face cloths and towels to exposed body surfaces.
- Ensure appropriate documentation forms are available (eg, laboratory order forms, labels); verify correct patient name, medical record number, and correct test/medication is ordered.
- Nurse-to-nurse report to either postanesthesia care unit (PACU) or intensive care unit (ICU).

Delegation of Duties
Circulating nurse assigns arriving staff members to assist in the following roles:
- Nursing personnel or CA to get MH cart.
- Two to four licensed individuals dedicated to reconstitution of dantrolene sodium.
- Medication nurse to
  - obtain other medicationsused for treatment of MH,
  - contact pharmacy department to obtain more dantrolene sodium as needed, and
  - document medications as they are given.
- Nurse recorder: documentation should include, but not be limited to,
  - vital signs,
  - laboratory reports,
  - fluid intake and output,
  - size of urinary catheter,
  - color of urine (brown-colored urine denotes rhabdomyolysis due to muscle breakdown),
  - type of irrigation used and amounts,
  - placement of central venous line, arterial line, and peripheral IV's.
- Lavage nurse to assist with placement of urinary catheter, nasogastric (NG) tube, rectal tube and/or perform lavage of cold saline to irrigate stomach, rectum, and bladder.
- Assign a person to obtain refrigerated IV fluids for infusion. Avoid lactated Ringer's solution as it may contribute to metabolic acidosis.
- If available, assign someone to set up equipment for invasive monitoring.
- If available, assign someone to obtain blood and urine samples for laboratory analysis.

Table 6, *continued*

MANAGEMENT OF A MALIGNANT HYPERTHERMIA (MH) CRISIS

PACU RN

♦ Responds to OR if available.
♦ Assigns and prepares bed space in PACU:
  – sets up monitors and ensures that cardiac arrest cart is close,
  – prepares containers for ice,
  – fills containers with ice when patient is on the way, and
  – arranges for ventilator according to orders.

Clinical Assistant

♦ Obtains basins of ice water.
♦ Ensures that face cloths and towels are available.
♦ Runner stays available to retrieve supplies and equipment as needed.
♦ Stamps laboratory requisition forms, labels and other documentation forms with patient's name and ID.
♦ Takes worksheet or list of duties to OR front desk to facilitate communication plan.

Anesthesia Technician

♦ Changes soda lime canister and circuit hoses, if requested by anesthesia care provider.
♦ Obtains supplies and equipment for placement of arterial line.
♦ Has two to four infusion pumps available (used to infuse antiarrhythmic medications).
♦ Obtains chilled bags of IV saline and irrigation bottles of saline from refrigerator.
♦ Obtains insulin from refrigerator.
♦ If not already stocked on MH or anesthesia cart, has the following items available:
  – esophageal and rectal temperature probe,
  – various sizes of NG tubes,
  – stopcocks, and
  – phlebotomy supplies and equipment.
♦ Brings defibrillator into room.
♦ Stamps laboratory requisition forms and labels with patient's name.
♦ Changes anesthesia machine, if directed by anesthesia care provider.

OR or Ambulatory Surgery Center Front Desk Personnel

♦ Receives worksheet or list of duties from OR.
♦ Initiates communication plan.

Adapted with permission from Malignant Hyperthermia Association of the United States (MHAUS). Malignant Hyperthermia Event OR Response Protocol Flowchart. In: MHAUS Hospital Procedure Manual. Sherbourne, NY: Malignant Hyperthermia Association of the United States (MHAUS); 2006.

11. Carr, A S, Canaliffe, M, McLeod, E E, Britt, B A. Incidence of malignant hyperthermia reactions in 2,214 patients undergoing muscle biopsy. *Canadian Journal of Anaesthesia*. 1995; 42 (4): 281-286.

12. Malignant Hyperthermia Association of the United States (MHAUS). Hotline information. *https://www.mhaus.org/index.crm/fuseaction/Hotline*.Home.cfm. Accessed August 22, 2006.

13. Malignant Hyperthermia Association of the United States (MHAUS). North American malignant hyperthermia registry. *https://www.mhreg.org/Default.aspx*. Accessed September 6, 2006.

14. Malignant Hyperthermia Association of the United States (MHAUS). What is malignant hyperthermia? *http://www.mhaus.org/index.cfm/fuseaction/OnlineBrochures.Display/BrochurePK*. Accessed August 22, 2006.

15. Rosenberg, H, Davis, M, James, D, Pollock, N, Stowell K. Malignant hyperthermia: Orphanet encyclopedia November 2004. *http://www.orpha.net/data/patho/GB/uk-malignant-hyperthermia.pdf*. Accessed September 7, 2006.

16. Strazis, K P, Fox, A W. Malignant hyperthermia: a review of published cases. *Anesthesia and Analgesia*. 1993; 77: 297-304.

17. Malignant Hyperthermia Association of the United States (MHAUS). Burkman, J M, Posner, K L, Domino, D B. Analysis of the clinical variables associated with recrudescence after malignant hyperthermia reactions. *http://www.mhaus.org/index.cfm/fuseaction/Content.Display/PagePK/AbstractJMBurkman*. Accessed August 28, 2006. This abstract can also be accessed at *http://www.asaabstracts.com/strands/asaabstracts/abstractList.htm;jsessionid=FBA05735125 3B386A3D862B2404C46B4?year=2005&index=12*. Accessed September 20, 2006.

18. Hallsall, P J, Cain, P A, Ellis, F R. Retrospective analysis of anaesthetics received by patients before susceptibility to malignant hyperthermia was recognized. *British Journal of Anaesthesia*. 1979; 51: 949-954.

19. Gronert, G A, Pessah, I N, Muldoon, S M, Tautz T J. Malignant hyperthermia. In: Miller, R D, ed. *Miller's*

Anesthesia. 6th ed, vol 1. Philadelphia, Pa: Elsevier, Churchill Livingstone; 2005: 1169-1190.

20. Sheehan JA. Malignant hyperthermia susceptibility and the trauma patient. Military Medicine. 2005; 170: 510-512.

21. Krause T, Gerbershagen MU, Fiege M, Weibhorn R, Wappler F. Dantrolene—a review of its pharmacology, therapeutic use, and new developments. Anaesthesia. 2004; 59: 364-373, 1139-1140.

22. Podranski T, Bouillon T, Schumacher PM, Taguchi A, Sessler DI, Kurz A. Compartmental pharmacokinetics of dantrolene in adults: do malignant hyperthermia association dosing guidelines work? Anesthesia and Analgesia. 2005; 101: 1695-1699.

23. Proctor & Gamble Pharmaceuticals. Dantrium® information for health care professionals. http://www.pgpharma.com/healthcareprofessional_dantriumiv.shtml. Accessed August 23, 2006.

24. Malignant Hyperthermia Association of the United States (MHAUS). Medical professional's FAQ's—dantrolene. http://www.mhaus.org/index.cfm/fuseaction/Content.Display/PagePK/MedicalFAQs.cfm. Accessed December 5, 2006.

25. Rosenberg H. Malignant hyperthermia in the ambulatory setting. Seminars in Anesthesia, Perioperative Medicine and Pain. 2001; 20: 270-274.

26. Malignant Hyperthermia Association of the United States (MHAUS). Drugs, equipment, and dantrolene—managing malignant hyperthermia: MHAUS online brochure. http://www.mhaus.org/index.cfm/fuseaction/OnlineBrochures.Display/BrochurePK/B5DBDF12-20C3-453. Accessed Sept 8, 2006.

27. Lexi-Comp. Drug Information Handbook for Perioperative Nursing. Adapted from Anesthesiology and Critical Care Drug Handbook, 6th ed; and the Drug Information Handbook for Advanced Practice Nursing, 6th ed. Hudson, Ohio: Lexi-Comp; 2006: 1856, 485-486.

28. Porter AM. Collapse from exertional heat illness: implications and subsequent decisions. Military Medicine. 2003; 168: 76-81.

29. Wappler F, Fiege M, Steinfath M, et al. Evidence for susceptibility to malignant hyperthermia in patients with exercise-induced rhabdomyolysis. Anesthesiology. 2001; 94: 95-100.

30. Rusyniak DE, Sprague JE. Toxin-induced hyperthermic syndromes. The Medical Clinics of North America. 2005; 89: 1277-1296.

31. McCarthy EJ. Malignant hyperthermia. AACN. [Clinical Issues]. 2004; 15: 231-237.

32. Nagelhout JJ, Zaglaniczny KL. Nurse Anesthesia. Second ed. Philadelphia, PA: WB Saunders Company; 2001: 728-732.

33. O'Flynn RP, Shutack JG, Rosenberg H, Fletcher JE. Masseter muscle rigidity and malignant hyperthermia susceptibility in pediatric patients: an update on management and diagnosis. Anesthesiology. 1994; 80:1228-1233.

34. Halaszynski TM, Juda R, Silverman DG. Optimizing postoperative outcomes with efficient preoperative assessment and management. Critical Care Medicine. 2004 April; (Suppl, 32): S76-88.

35. Pollock N, Langton E, McDonnell N, Tiemessen J, Stowell K. Malignant hyperthermia and day stay surgery. Anaesthesia and Intensive Care. 2006; 34: 40-45.

36. Petersen C. Perioperative Nursing Data Set: The Perioperative Nursing Vocabulary. Revised 2nd ed. Denver, CO: AORN, Inc; 2007: 17-18, 29.

37. The North American Malignant Hyperthermia Registry of MHAUS, Report of acute adverse metabolic reaction to anesthesia report (AMRA Report) Version 9.1. https://www.mhreg.org/forms/AMRA_9-1.pdf. Accessed September 6, 2006.

38. Bryson G, Chung F, Cox RG, et al. Patient selection in ambulatory anesthesia—an evidence-based review: Part II. Canadian Journal of Anesthesia. 2004; 51(8):782-794.

39. Malignant Hyperthermia Association of the United States (MHAUS). MHAUS FAQs—molecular genetic testing for MH. http://www.mhaus.org/index.cfm/fuseaction/Content.Display/PagePK/MolecularGeneticsFAQ.cfm. Accessed September 8, 2006.

40. Malignant Hyperthermia Association of the United States (MHAUS). Molecular Genetic Testing for Malignant Hyperthermia Susceptibility. Sherburne, NY: Malignant Hyperthermia Association of the United States [MHAUS]: 2006; also available at Malignant Hyperthermia Association of the United States (MHAUS). Testing for susceptibility to MH; muscle contracture or molecular genetics? http://www.mhaus.org/index.cfm/fuseaction/OnlineBrochures.Display/BrochurePK/71A5AFFC=1BC7-4A. Accessed September 6, 2006.

41. Brandom BW. The genetics of malignant hyperthermia. Anesthesiology Clinics of North America. 2005; 23: 615-619.

42. Sambuughin N, Holley H, Muldoon S, et al. Screening of the entire ryanodine receptor type 1 coding region for sequence variants associated with malignant hyperthermia susceptibility in the North American population. Anesthesiology. 2005; 102: 515-521.

43. Rosenberg, H. Malignant hyperthermia syndrome: from barnyard to molecular genetics laboratory. American Society of Anesthesiologists Newsletter. 2005; 69: also available at http://www.asahq.org/Newsletters/2005/09-05/rosenberg09_05.html. Accessed May 18, 2006.

44. Malignant Hyperthermia Association of the United States (MHAUS). MH susceptible patients FAQs: drugs and MH susceptibility. http://www.mhaus.org/index.cfm/fuseaction/Content.Display/PagePK/SusceptFAQ.cfm. Accessed September 13, 2006.

45. Malignant Hyperthermia Association of the United States (MHAUS). Hospital Procedure Manual. Sherbourne, NY: Malignant Hyperthermia Association of the United States [MHAUS]; 2006.

PUBLICATION HISTORY

Created by AORN Data Elements Coordinating Committee, 1996. Approved by the AORN Board of Directors, February 1997.

Revised by AORN Nursing Practice Committee, 2006. Approved by the AORN Board of Directors, November 2006. Published in Standards, Recommended Practices, and Guidelines, 2007 edition.

EXHIBIT A: Outcome Management of MH Through Application of the PNDS[1]

The Perioperative Nursing Data Set (PNDS) is a clinically relevant and empirically validated standardized nursing language. The tables on the following pages represent a sample care plan for malignant hyperthermia (MH) that uses PNDS terminology to describe the care of patients in the perioperative setting. The diagram below provides more information to assist in reading and understanding the tables.

Nursing assessments for each outcome relate to symptoms covered in the corresponding pathophysiology section incated by the PNDS domain (eg, D2, D3-B). The order of the outcomes is listed in the order the symptoms present as explained in the interpretive statements.

The information in the first column, labeled "Patient who has a personal or familial history of MH," explains the perioperative team's preventive actions to avoid symptoms and crisis.

The second column represents the "Patient who does not have history of MH; unknown risk." This covers basic perioperative competencies and general assessments for all patients. It is included in the care plan as a reminder that any patient could go into an MH crisis, shifting the perioperative nurse's interventions to the third column unexpectedly.

The third column represents the "Patient in crisis; actively having symptoms" and includes the Malignant Hyperthermia Association of the United States (MHAUS) protocol.[2]

Note: Specific clinical interventions are based on the MHAUS protocol, but the protocol may not apply to all patients and should be altered according to specific patient needs.

REFERENCES
1. Beyea SC, ed. *Perioperative Nursing Data Set: The Perioperative Nursing Vocabulary.* Second ed. Denver, CO: AORN, Inc; 2002: 85, 118, 121, 123, 131, 137, 158, 168, 183.
2. Malignant Hyperthermia Association of the United States (MHAUS). Emergency therapy for malignant hyperthermia. *http://www.mhaus.org/index.cfm /fuseaction/OnlineBrochures.Display/BrochurePK.* Accessed September 13, 2006.

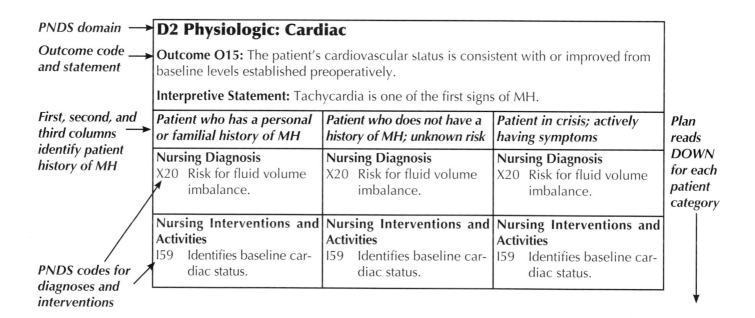

	D2 Physiologic: Cardiac		
PNDS domain →	**Outcome O15:** The patient's cardiovascular status is consistent with or improved from baseline levels established preoperatively.		
Outcome code and statement →	**Interpretive Statement:** Tachycardia is one of the first signs of MH.		
First, second, and third columns identify patient history of MH →	**Patient who has a personal or familial history of MH**	**Patient who does not have a history of MH; unknown risk**	**Patient in crisis; actively having symptoms**
	Nursing Diagnosis X20 Risk for fluid volume imbalance.	**Nursing Diagnosis** X20 Risk for fluid volume imbalance.	**Nursing Diagnosis** X20 Risk for fluid volume imbalance.
PNDS codes for diagnoses and interventions →	**Nursing Interventions and Activities** I59 Identifies baseline cardiac status.	**Nursing Interventions and Activities** I59 Identifies baseline cardiac status.	**Nursing Interventions and Activities** I59 Identifies baseline cardiac status.

Plan reads DOWN for each patient category ↓

D2 Physiologic: Cardiac

Outcome O15: The patient's cardiovascular status is consistent with or improved from baseline levels established preoperatively.

Interpretive Statement: Tachycardia is one of the first signs of MH.

Patient who has a personal or familial history of MH	Patient who does not have a history of MH; unknown risk	Patient in crisis; actively having symptoms
Nursing Diagnosis X20 Risk for fluid volume imbalance.	**Nursing Diagnosis** X20 Risk for fluid volume imbalance.	**Nursing Diagnosis** X20 Risk for fluid volume imbalance. X8 Decreased cardiac output.
Nursing Interventions and Activities I59 Identifies baseline cardiac status.	**Nursing Interventions and Activities** I59 Identifies baseline cardiac status.	**Nursing Interventions and Activities** I59 Identifies baseline cardiac status. ♦ Monitors physiological parameters. ♦ Assists anesthesia provider as appropriate in monitoring – electrocardiogram (ECG); – vital signs (ie, blood pressure, pulse rate, body temperature); – oximetry; – capnometry; – arterial and venous blood gases for unexplained tachycardia; – core temperature, measured via esophageal, tympanic, axillary, rectal, and bladder probes; – serum potassium; – calcium; – clotting studies; – urine color and output; – diaphoresis; – mottling of skin; and – central venous and arterial pressure.
I120 Uses monitoring equipment to assess cardiac status.	I120 Uses monitoring equipment to assess cardiac status.	I120 Uses monitoring equipment to assess cardiac status. Based on cardiac assessment of arrythmias and indicators of cardiac output, follow MH protocol (see *D1 Safety: Medication* section).

D2 Physiologic: Respiratory

Outcome O14: The patient's respiratory function is consistent with or improved from baseline levels established preoperatively.

Interpretive Statement: Irregular breathing, ineffective breathing pattern, and subsequent impaired gas exchange are early stages of an MH crisis.

Patient who has a personal or familial history of MH	Patient who does not have a history of MH; unknown risk	Patient in crisis; actively having symptoms
Nursing Diagnosis X7 Ineffective breathing pattern (risk for).	**Nursing Diagnosis** X7 Ineffective breathing pattern (risk for).	**Nursing Diagnosis** X7 Ineffective breathing pattern. X21 Impaired gas exchange.
Nursing Interventions and Activities I87 Monitors changes in respiratory status.	**Nursing Interventions and Activities** I87 Monitors changes in respiratory status.	**Nursing Interventions and Activities** I87 Monitors changes in respiratory status.
I121 Uses monitoring equipment to assess respiratory status.	I121 Uses monitoring equipment to assess respiratory status.	I121 Uses monitoring equipment to assess respiratory status.
I45 Evaluates postoperative respiratory status.	I45 Evaluates postoperative respiratory status.	I45 Evaluates postoperative respiratory status.
		I110 Recognizes and reports deviations in arterial blood gas (ABG) studies.

D2 Physiologic: Fluid/electrolyte/acid-base balances

Outcome O13: The patient's fluid, electrolyte, and acid-base balances are consistent with or improved from baseline levels established preoperatively.

Interpretive Statement: Due to cardiac arrhythmias and impaired gas exchanges, acid-base imbalance may be the next progression of symptoms when a patient is in MH crisis.

Patient who has a personal or familial history of MH	Patient who does not have a history of MH; unknown risk	Patient in crisis; actively having symptoms
Nursing Diagnosis X18 Risk for fluid volume deficit.	**Nursing Diagnosis** X18 Risk for fluid volume deficit.	**Nursing Diagnosis** X18 Risk for fluid volume deficit. X17 Fluid volume deficit.
Nursing Interventions and Activities I89 Monitors physiologic parameters.	**Nursing Interventions and Activities** I89 Monitors physiologic parameters.	**Nursing Interventions and Activities** I89 Monitors physiologic parameters.

I23 Collaborates in fluid and electrolyte management.	I23 Collaborates in fluid and electrolyte management.	I23 Collaborates in fluid and electrolyte management.
		♦ Measures urine output
		♦ Observes characteristics of any drainage.
		  – Inserts 3-way indwelling urinary catheter.
		  – Monitors urinary output.
		  – Monitors color, amount, and consistency.

D2 Physiologic: Fluid/electrolyte/acid-base balances *(continued)*

Patient who has a personal or familial history of MH	Patient who does not have a history of MH; unknown risk	Patient in crisis; actively having symptoms
		Nursing Interventions and Activities I23 Collaborates in fluid and electrolyte management. (continued) ◆ Administers urinary drainage system care. Maintains aseptic technique during insertion. Secures catheter and places it in view of anesthesia care provider. ◆ Administers drainage tube system care. Maintains clean drainage device site, maintain dressings, and secures device properly.
		I84 Laboratory values (specimen collection) ◆ Manages specimen handling and disposition (eg, blood and urine). ◆ Monitors central venous or pulmonary artery (PA) monitoring as needed; records minute ventilation. ◆ Venous blood gas (eg, femoral vein) values may document hypermetabolism better than arterial values. ◆ Follows coagulation profile. Watches for disseminated intravascular coagulation. ◆ Measure creatinine kinase (CK) every six hours until decreased. If event is severe, CK levels may stay elevated for two weeks.

D2 Physiologic: Fluid/electrolyte/acid-base balances *(continued)*

Patient who has a personal or familial history of MH	*Patient who does not have a history of MH; unknown risk*	*Patient in crisis; actively having symptoms*
		Nursing Interventions and Activities *(continued)* I34 Establishes IV access. ◆ Initiates IV access or helps anesthesia care provider to initiate IV access, if none exists. ◆ Facilitates set-up for central line as needed. ◆ Based on fluid/electrolyte/acid-base assessment, follow MH protocol: – Administers IV fluid therapy. – Administers refrigerated IV normal saline. ***Note:*** Do not use IV lactated Ringer's solution; it may contribute to the patient's acidosis.
		I9 Administers prescribed medications based on ABG results. Based on fluid/electrolyte/acid-base assessment, follow MH protocol (see *D1 Safety: Medication*).
		I153 Evaluates response to administration of fluids and electrolytes. ◆ Creatinine kinase and potassium rise persistently, or urine output falls to less than 0.5 mL/kg/hr; induce diuresis to at least 2 mL/kg/hr to avoid myoglobin-induced renal failure.

D2 Physiologic: Wound/tissue perfusion

Outcome O11: The patient has wound/tissue perfusion consistent with or improved from baseline levels established preoperatively.

Interpretive Statement: When a patient is in an MH crisis, there may not be time to close the wound immediately, acute muscular contraction and changes to tissue profusion may affect the long-term wound healing and the rigorous cooling processes can increase the risk for physical injury to the skin and other tissue being cooled.

Patient who has a personal or familial history of MH	Patient who does not have a history of MH; unknown risk	Patient in crisis; actively having symptoms
Nursing Diagnosis X51 Risk for impaired skin integrity.	**Nursing Diagnosis** X51 Risk for impaired skin integrity.	**Nursing Diagnosis** X50 Impaired skin integrity.
Nursing Interventions and Activities I60 Identifies baseline tissue perfusion.	**Nursing Interventions and Activities** I60 Identifies baseline tissue perfusion.	**Nursing Interventions and Activities** I15 Assesses factors related to risk for ineffective tissue perfusion. ♦ Assesses for muscle rigidity progressing to cyanosis and mottling. ♦ Administers care to incision sites. ♦ Assists with closure of wound as soon as MH is suspected. ♦ If wound closure is not possible, wound should be packed with saline-soaked towels or laparotomy sponges. ♦ May need to irrigate the wound with cool normal saline solution, not lactated Ringer's solution.
Note: Perioperative nurses assume basic assessment of injury to skin and tissue, but I152 is not specifically included in this column to indicate extra levels of assessment are needed for the patient in crisis.	*Note: Perioperative nurses assume basic assessment of injury to skin and tissue, but I152 is not specifically included in this column to indicate extra levels of assessment are needed for the patient in crisis.*	I152 Evaluates for signs and symptoms of physical injury to skin and tissue.
I46 Evaluates postoperative tissue perfusion.	I46 Evaluates postoperative tissue perfusion.	I46 Evaluates postoperative tissue perfusion.

D2 Physiologic: Normothermia

Outcome O12: The patient is at or returning to normothermia at the conclusion of the immediate postoperative period.

Interpretive Statement: When a patient is in an MH crisis there is hyperthermia related to hypermetabolic crisis and muscular contraction, and hypothermia related to rigorous cooling processes used to treat hyperthermia.

Patient who has a personal or familial history of MH	Patient who does not have a history of MH; unknown risk	Patient in crisis; actively having symptoms
Nursing Diagnosis X57　Risk for imbalanced body temperature.	**Nursing Diagnosis** X57　Risk for imbalanced body temperature.	**Nursing Diagnosis** X58　Ineffective thermoregulation. X29　Risk for injury.
Nursing Interventions and Activities I131　Assesses risk for inadvertent hypothermia.	**Nursing Interventions and Activities** I131　Assesses risk for inadvertent hypothermia.	**Nursing Interventions and Activities** I131　Assesses risk for inadvertent hypothermia. ♦ Stop cooling if temperature is 38° C (100.4° F) and falling to prevent it from dropping below 36° C (96.8° F).
I86　Monitors body temperature.	I86　Monitors body temperature.	I86　Monitors body temperature.
	♦ Discontinues cooling measures when patient's temperature reaches 38° C (100.4° F). *Note:* Care should be taken to avoid too rigorous cooling, which can result in inadvertent hypothermia.	I78　Implements thermoregulation measures: ♦ Directly lavage peritoneal and/or thoracic cavity with refrigerated normal saline irrigation fluid (ie, if surgical site is open). ♦ Indirectly lavage stomach (eg, connect nasogastric [NG] tube to refrigerated normal saline irrigation, not lactated Ringer's solution, with cystoscopy tubing). ♦ Lavage rectum (eg, connect a 3-way indwelling urinary catheter with 30-mL balloon to refrigerated normal saline irrigation, not lactated Ringer's solution, with cystoscopy tubing). ♦ Surface-cool patient with ice in plastic bags and a hypothermia blanket to neck, axillae, and groin area. ♦ Discontinues cooling measures when patient's temperature reaches 38° C (100.4° F). *Note:* Care should be taken to avoid too rigorous cooling, which can result in inadvertent hypothermia.

D1 Safety: Medication

Outcome O9: The patient receives appropriate medication(s), safely administered during the perioperative period.

Interpretive Statement: When a patient is in an MH crisis, it is important to have a sufficient number of trained responders. The responders should be familiar with their role in the crisis and be able to access the appropriate supplies and prepare or administer medications efficiently.

Patient who has a personal or familial history of MH	Patient who does not have a history of MH; unknown risk	Patient in crisis; actively having symptoms
Nursing Diagnosis X29 Risk for injury.	**Nursing Diagnosis** X29 Risk for injury.	**Nursing Diagnosis** X29 Risk for injury.
Nursing Interventions and Activities I8 Administers prescribed medications and solutions.	**Nursing Interventions and Activities** I8 Administers prescribed medications and solutions.	**Nursing Interventions and Activities** I8 Administers prescribed medications and solutions. ♦ Anesthesia care provider to discontinue volatile agents and succinylcholine. ♦ Anesthesia care provider hyperventilates patient with 100% oxygen at flows of 10 L/min or more.

		I9 Administers prescribed medications based on ABG results.
		♦ Rapidly administers IV dantrolene sodium 2.5 mg/kg given rapidly through large-bore IV for initial bolus.
		  – Dantrolene sodium should be mixed with sterile water for injection USP (without a bacteriostatic agent; 60 mL per 20-mg vial) and shaken vigorously.
		  – Prewarming (not to exceed 38° C) the sterile water will speed dissolving of dantrolene sodium into solution.
		  – Repeat dosages of dantrolene sodium as necessary; titrate to tachycardia, hyperthermia, hypercarbia, and rigidity.
		  – Although the stated upper dosage of 10 mg/kg is suggested, more may be administered as needed.
		  – For at least 24 hours dantrolene sodium should be administered by infusing 1mg/kg every 4 to 6 hours or 0.25mg/kg/hr.

D1 Safety: Medication *(continued)*

Patient who has a personal or familial history of MH	Patient who does not have a history of MH; unknown risk	Patient in crisis; actively having symptoms

		Nursing Interventions and Activities
		
		I9 Administers prescribed medications based on ABG results. *(continued)*
		
		♦ Administer sodium bicarbonate to correct metabolic acidosis as guided by ABG analysis.
		  – If initial ABG results are not available and there are dysrhythmias or cardiac arrest, consider the most likely cause is due to acidosis and/or hyperkalemia.
		  – Administer initial dose of 1 to 2 mEq/kg of sodium bicarbonate IV and repeat as indicated. Thereafter, dose should be based on ABG results.
		♦ Administer IV glucose and insulin.
		  – To treat hyperkalemia in adults use 10 units regular insulin IV and 50 mL 50% glucose.
		  – To treat hyperkalemia in children, use 0.1 units insulin/kg and 1mL/kg 50% glucose.
		♦ Administer calcium chloride to treat life-threatening hyperkalemia.
		  – For adults, 10mg/kg calcium chloride or 10 to 50 mg/kg calcium gluconate for life-threatening hyperkalemia.
		  – Check glucose levels hourly.
		♦ Administer standard anti-arrhythmic agents if dysrhythmias persist following treatment of acidosis and hyperkalemia.

D1 Safety: Medication *(continued)*

Patient who has a personal or familial history of MH	Patient who does not have a history of MH; unknown risk	Patient in crisis; actively having symptoms
		Nursing Interventions and Activities I9 *Administers prescribed medications based on ABG results. (continued)* ♦ Life-threatening dysrhythmias should not be treated with calcium channel blocking agents because they may cause hyperkalemia or cardiac arrest in the presence of dantrolene sodium. ♦ Avoid using solutions containing potassium.

		I78 Implements thermoregulation measures and applies devices to cool the patient as indicated.
		♦ Recognizes and reports deviation in diagnostic studies.
		♦ Collaborates in maintenance and/or corrective therapy. Requests additional staff members to assist with management of complications.
		♦ Monitors physiological parameters. Assists anesthesia provider as appropriate in monitoring
		  – electrocardiogram (cardiac);
		  – vital signs (ie, blood pressure, pulse rate, body temperature; cardiac);
		  – oximetry (respiratory);
		  – capnometry (respiratory);
		  – arterial and venous blood gases for unexplained tachycardia (fluid and electrolytes);
		  – core temperature (esophageal, tympanic, axillary, rectal, bladder);
		  – serum potassium (electrolytes);
		  – calcium (electrolytes);
		  – clotting studies (electrolytes);
		  – urine color and output (electrolytes);
		  – diaphoresis (fluid electrolytes);
		  – mottling of skin (perfusion); and
		  – central venous pressure and arterial pressure (cardiac).

D1 Safety: Freedom from acquired physical injury.

Outcome O2: The patient is free from signs and symptoms of injury caused by extraneous objects.

Interpretive Statement: When a patient goes into an MH crisis, routine count procedures may be disrupted and additional supplies and equipment are used for thermoregulation. The perioperative nurse should reconcile the surgical count (ie, sponge, sharps, instrument) as soon as possible and anticipate prevention of retained surgical items throughout the MH crisis. The perioperative nurse should identify potential hazards associated with controlling patient temperature and establish safe practices.[3,4,5]

Patient who has a personal or familial history of MH	Patient who does not have a history of MH; unknown risk	Patient in crisis; actively having symptoms
Nursing Diagnosis X29 Risk for injury.	**Nursing Diagnosis** X29 Risk for injury.	**Nursing Diagnosis** X29 Risk for injury.
Nursing Interventions and Activities I76 Implements protective measures to prevent skin or tissue injury due to thermal sources.	**Nursing Interventions and Activities** I76 Implements protective measures to prevent skin or tissue injury due to thermal sources.	**Nursing Interventions and Activities** I76 Implements protective measures to prevent skin or tissue injury due to thermal sources. Inspects skin integrity periodically during, when possible, and after using devices (eg, ice packs, temperature-regulating blankets).
I93 Performs required counts.	I93 Performs required counts.	I93 Performs required counts. ♦ Informs the surgeon and perioperative team as soon as a discrepancy in a surgical count (ie, sponge, sharps, instrument) is identified. ♦ Initiates additional measures for prevention of retained surgical items. ♦ Depending on facility policy and procedure, additional measures may include investigation, reconciliation, and documentation.[4]
I122 Uses supplies and equipment within safe parameters. ♦ Use supplies, equipment, and instruments carefully to avoid compromising patient safety.	I122 Uses supplies and equipment within safe parameters. ♦ Uses supplies, equipment, and instruments carefully to avoid compromising patient safety.	I122 Uses supplies and equipment within safe parameters. ♦ Irrigation/infusion solutions should be warmed or cooled to the temperatures appropriate for the surgical need.[5] ♦ Uses supplies, equipment, and instruments carefully to avoid compromising patient safety.

D2 Physiologic: Pain control

Outcome O29: The patient demonstrates and/or reports adequate pain control throughout the perioperative period.

Interpretive statement: Patients who have experienced an MH crisis have potential for pain not only at the surgical wound site, but also as a result of acute muscle contractions and rigorous cooling processes that may have been implemented.

Patient who has a personal or familial history of MH	Patient who does not have a history of MH; unknown risk	Patient in crisis; actively having symptoms
Nursing Diagnosis X38 (Potential for) Acute pain.	**Nursing Diagnosis** X38 (Potential for) Acute pain.	**Nursing Diagnosis** X38 Acute pain.
Nursing Interventions and Activities I16 Assesses pain control.	**Nursing Interventions and Activities** I16 Assesses pain control.	**Nursing Interventions and Activities** I16 Assesses pain control.
I71 Implements pain guidelines.	I71 Implements pain guidelines.	I71 Implements pain guidelines.
I54 Evaluates response to pain management intervention.	I54 Evaluates response to pain management intervention.	I54 Evaluates response to pain management intervention.
I61 Identifies cultural and value components related to pain.	I61 Identifies cultural and value components related to pain.	I61 Identifies cultural and value components related to pain.
I69 Implements alternative methods of pain control.	I69 Implements alternative methods of pain control.	I69 Implements alternative methods of pain control.
		I118 Transports according to individual needs. ♦ Ensures transfer without tissue injury; altered body temperature; ineffective breathing patterns, altered tissue perfusion; and undue discomfort, pain, or fear. ♦ Gentle handling/movement/positioning.

D3-B Rights/Ethics: Participates in decisions

Outcome O23: The patient participates in decisions affecting his or her perioperative plan of care.

Interpretive Statement: When a patient has a known increased risk for an MH crisis, decisions need to be made about where to have his or her invasive procedure performed, and the patient should be informed about preventive measures.

Patient who has a personal or familial history of MH	*Patient who does not have a history of MH; unknown risk*	*Patient in crisis; actively having symptoms*
Nursing Diagnosis X12 Decisional conflict.	**Nursing Diagnosis** X12 Decisional conflict.	**Nursing Diagnosis** X12 Decisional conflict.
Nursing Interventions and Activities I63 Identifies individual values and wishes concerning care.	**Nursing Interventions and Activities** I63 Identifies individual values and wishes concerning care.	**Nursing Interventions and Activities** I63 Identifies individual values and wishes concerning care.
I79 Includes family members in preoperative teaching.	I79 Includes family members in preoperative teaching.	I79 Includes family members in preoperative teaching.
Discharge planning I80 Includes patient and family members in discharge planning.	**Discharge planning** I80 Includes patient and family members in discharge planning.	**Discharge planning** I80 Includes patient and family members in discharge planning.
I106 Provides instruction based on age and identified needs.	I106 Provides instruction based on age and identified needs.	I106 Provides instruction based on age and identified needs.
I135 Determines knowledge level.	I135 Determines knowledge level.	I135 Determines knowledge level.
I136 Assesses readiness to learn.	I136 Assesses readiness to learn.	I136 Assesses readiness to learn.
I137 Assesses coping mechanisms.	I137 Assesses coping mechanisms.	I137 Assesses coping mechanisms.
I147 Implements measures to provide psychological support.	*Note: Perioperative nurses assume basic role of support, but I147 is not specifically included in this column to indicate that extra levels of support are needed for the patient in crisis or susceptible for MH.*	I147 Implements measures to provide psychological support.
I151 Maintains patient confidentiality.	I151 Maintains patient confidentiality.	I151 Maintains patient confidentiality.

D3-B Rights/Ethics: Consistent care

Outcome O27: The patient receives consistent and comparable care regardless of the setting.

Interpretive Statement: Every patient is at risk for a malignant hyperthermia crisis and deserves to have the same level of care regardless of the setting where the procedure is performed.

Patient who has a personal or familial history of MH	*Patient who does not have a history of MH; unknown risk*	*Patient in crisis; actively having symptoms*
Nursing Diagnosis X44 Protection, ineffective (potential for).	**Nursing Diagnosis** X44 Protection, ineffective (potential for).	**Nursing Diagnosis** X44 Protection, ineffective (potential for).
Nursing Interventions and Activities I1 Acts as a patient advocate by protecting the patient from incompetent, unethical, or illegal practices.	**Nursing Interventions and Activities** I1 Acts as a patient advocate by protecting the patient from incompetent, unethical, or illegal practices.	**Nursing Interventions and Activities** I1 Acts as a patient advocate by protecting the patient from incompetent, unethical, or illegal practices.
I97 Preserves and protects the patient's autonomy, dignity, and human rights.	I97 Preserves and protects the patient's autonomy, dignity, and human rights.	I97 Preserves and protects the patient's autonomy, dignity, and human rights.
I99 Provides care in a nondiscriminatory, nonprejudicial manner regardless of the setting in which care is given. ◆ Adheres to AORN, JCAHO, and other standards of care. ◆ Provides comparable levels of care regardless of the setting in which care is given (eg, inpatient, outpatient, public, private, home, emergency department).	I99 Provides care in a nondiscriminatory, nonprejudicial manner regardless of the setting in which care is given. ◆ Adheres to AORN, JCAHO, and other standards of care. ◆ Provides comparable levels of care regardless of the setting in which care is given (eg, inpatient, outpatient, public, private, home, emergency department).	I99 Provides care in a nondiscriminatory, nonprejudicial manner regardless of the setting in which care is given. ◆ Adheres to AORN, JCAHO, and other standards of care. ◆ Provides comparable levels of care regardless of the setting in which care is given (eg, inpatient, outpatient, public, private, home, emergency department).
I27 Ensures continuity of care. ◆ Hand-off communications include extra focus on patient's susceptibility to MH.	*Note: Perioperative nurses assume basic role of continuity and communications, but I27 is not specifically included in this column to indicate that extra levels of communication are needed for the patient in crisis or susceptible for MH.*	I27 Ensures continuity of care. ◆ Transfers to another facility/department. ◆ Hand-off communications.

D3-B Rights/Ethics: Consistent care (continued)

Patient who has a personal or familial history of MH	Patient who does not have a history of MH; unknown risk	Patient in crisis; actively having symptoms
Nursing Interventions and Activities *(continued)*	**Nursing Interventions and Activities** *(continued)*	**Nursing Interventions and Activities** *(continued)*

I92 Obtains consultation from the appropriate health care provider to initiate new treatments or change existing treatments.
◆ Upon suspicion and/or diagnosis of an MH crisis, notify the following personnel as appropriate:
  – attending anesthesia care provider,
  – attending physician,
  – OR charge nurse,
  – anesthesia technician(s),
  – postanesthesia care unit/intensive care unit,
  – OR cardiopulmonary assistant(s),
  – house supervisor, and
  – pharmacy supervisor.
	I92 Obtains consultation from the appropriate health care provider to initiate new treatments or change existing treatments.
	◆ Upon suspicion and/or diagnosis of an MH crisis, notify the following personnel as appropriate:
	  – attending anesthesia care provider,
	  – attending physician,
	  – OR charge nurse,
	  – anesthesia technician(s),
	  – postanesthesia care unit/intensive care unit,
	  – OR cardiopulmonary assistant(s),
	  – house supervisor, and
	  – pharmacy supervisor.
		I92 Obtains consultation from the appropriate health care provider to initiate new treatments or change existing treatments.
		◆ Upon suspicion and/or diagnosis of an MH crisis, notify the following personnel as appropriate:
		  – attending anesthesia care provider,
		  – attending physician,
		  – OR charge nurse,
		  – anesthesia technician(s),
		  – postanesthesia care unit/intensive care unit,
		  – OR cardiopulmonary assistant(s),
		  – house supervisor, and
		  – pharmacy supervisor.
		◆ Counsel the patient and family regarding MH and further precautions; refer them to MHAUS.
		◆ Fill out and send the Adverse Metabolic Reaction to Anesthesia (AMRA) form and send a letter to the patient and attending physician.
		◆ Refer patient and family to the nearest center for muscle biopsy follow-up.

REFERENCES

1. Peterson C, ed. *Perioperative Nursing Data Set: The Perioperative Nursing Vocabulary*. Rev 2nd ed. Denver, CO: AORN, Inc; 2007: 85, 118, 121, 123, 131, 137, 158, 168, 183.

2. Malignant Hyperthermia Association of the United States (MHAUS). Emergency therapy for malignant hyperthermia. *http://www.mhaus.org/index.cfm/fuseaction/OnlineBrochures.Display/BrochurePK*. Accessed September13, 2006.

3. Malignant Hyperthermia Association of the United States (MHAUS). Clinical update: Managing malignant hyperthermia. *http://medical.mhaus.org/index.cfm/fuseaction/OnlineBrochures.Display/BrochurePK/3FFCBC12-9479-49C3-8A9E0B304EF08746.cfm*. Accessed January 3, 2008.

4. Recommended practice for sponge, sharp, and instrument counts. In: *Standards, Recommended Practices, and Guidelines*. Denver, CO: AORN, Inc; 2006: 459.

5. "Recommended practices for safe care through identification of potential hazards in the surgical environment. In: *Standards, Recommended Practices, and Guidelines*. Denver, CO: AORN, Inc; 2006: 547.

AORN Guidance Statement:
Creating a Patient Safety Culture

Introduction

The purpose of this guidance statement is to assist managers and clinicians in developing policies and procedures related to creating a patient safety culture.

Since the Institute of Medicine (IOM) report released in 1999, the vast majority of patient safety initiatives have focused on micro issues, such as medication errors and wrong-site surgery, with little emphasis on the macro issue of culture. Edgar Schien, professor of management at the Sloan School of Management, Massachusetts Institute of Technology, defines *culture* as the set of shared, implicit assumptions that a group holds and that determines how it perceives, thinks about, and reacts to its various environments.[1] In broader terms, culture is a mindset centering on shared values, attitudes, or beliefs within an organization. As defined in the health care literature, a safety culture is an environment that encourages reporting,[2] ends blame,[3] involves senior leadership,[4] and focuses on systems.[5]

Lucian Leape, adjunct professor of health policy, Harvard School of Public Health, Harvard University, Boston, has stated the single greatest impediment to error prevention is that "we punish people for making mistakes."[6] Medical errors are grossly unreported across the country; only 2% to 3% of major errors are reported,[6] and when reported, they don't create stories or generate action.[7] Analytical methods such as root cause analysis (RCA) and the failure mode and effects analysis (FMEA) will not work in detecting the causes or errors if health care workers are bound by a "code of silence," fear of retribution, or are uncomfortable revealing imperfection in a process for which they are responsible.[8]

To date, most of the work in patient safety has been reactive. As the culture matures with increased information and trust, the emphasis will switch to a more proactive or generative approach.

Background

In review of the literature, few hospitals have assessed their organizations' safety culture, nor have many actually measured the impact of interventions. One study, conducted in April 2001, reported that 15 California hospitals conducted a safety culture survey with two objectives: (1) measure attitudes toward patient safety and organizational culture; and (2) determine how the culture of safety varied among the hospitals and between the various types of health care workers.[9] The majority of the participants in the study responded in ways that indicated a positive safety culture; however, senior leadership gave fewer problematic responses than frontline workers, and clinicians—in particular nurses—were more pessimistic.[10]

Johns Hopkins Hospital conducted a systematic assessment on safety and developed a strategic plan to improve safety.[11] Its study revealed a comparable culture of safety as compared to the airline industry, but identified several areas for improvement. Key messages identified were that senior leaders need to be more visible to frontline caregivers when addressing safety; safety planning must be proactive; physicians are less aware of safety initiatives than nurses; and physicians must actively participate in the education process.[11]

Preamble

The intention of this guidance statement is to provide a framework from which perioperative teams can foster a patient-centric safety culture and assist with the development of policies and procedures that will support that culture. A patient-centric safety culture consists of five major subcultures: reporting, flexible, just, learning,[5] and wary[2] (**Figure 1**).

Reporting Culture

A reporting culture is a culture in which all members of the perioperative team readily report errors and near misses. A reporting culture can be assessed by the types of errors reported by staff. As the safety culture matures, there is increased risk-taking associated with errors reported. In a true reporting culture, individuals report events to allow all staff in the organization to learn from the experience.

Suggested strategies[5-7]

- Focus on both actual events and near misses.
- Use FMEA proactively to anticipate and prevent potential error.
- Discuss close calls, "good catches," and how

Figure 1

PATIENT-CENTRIC SAFETY CULTURE

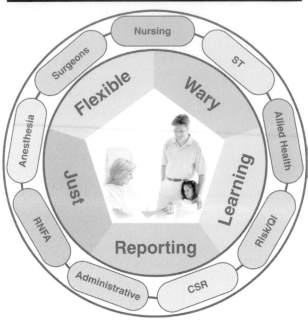

© Kate A. O'Toole. Used with permission.

harm to the patient was avoided or minimized.
- Develop a documentation system that is easy to use.
- Develop a reporting system that focuses on story-telling and knowledge-sharing.
- Focus on individual cases that provide learning opportunities.
- Identify ways to circulate stories and lessons learned throughout the facility.
- Provide feedback to the staff on all issues reported.
- Develop metrics for success (eg, increase number of reports).
- Prioritize improvement initiatives based on themes discovered and potential risks revealed.
- Use a process that emphasizes quality improvement (eg, Plan, Do, Check, Act).

Flexible Culture

A flexible culture is a culture that is nimble enough to keep pace with the rapid changes in health care.

Suggested strategies[7,9-11]
- Identify model for improvement programs that focuses on rapid cycle change.
- Develop processes that ensure shared leadership.

- Shared leadership is a hallmark of the organization.
- An environment of respect, collaboration, and trust exists between all team members and leadership.

Learning Culture

A learning culture is a culture that is capable and ready to gain knowledge from experiences and data, and that is willing to implement major changes as indicated from safety information systems. A learning culture is informed and learns from incidents and near misses.[8]

Suggested strategies
- Foster learning opportunities through open communication.
- Develop the ability to adapt to the changing health care environment and be receptive to change.
- Frontline staff is engaged to use initiative to problem-solve unique situations.
- Individual performance is linked to team performance.

Wary Culture

A wary culture is a culture in which all members of the perioperative team are continually aware of the unexpected. Being vigilant is a healthy state that is a combination of being informed and aware that, at any given moment, an untoward event can occur. Healthy reporting, learning, and flexible cultures will facilitate a wary culture.

Suggested strategies[5,7,12,13]
- Go "looking for trouble"; conduct executive walk-arounds in all perioperative areas.
- Become preoccupied with opportunities for improvement.
- Be willing to challenge assumptions.
- How can we "stop the line" and still stay efficient?
- How can we get better when we know we are the best?

Just Culture

A just culture is a culture that provides an environment of trust where all members of the perioperative team are encouraged to provide safety-related data and are acutely aware of the distinction between acceptable and unacceptable behavior. Errors and mistakes must be evaluated in a manner such that contributing factors are reviewed first, and then accountability is determined in relation to actions. A just culture is not a nonpunitive (ie, blame-free) environment, but rather an environment where actions are analyzed to ensure that individual accountability is established and appropriate actions are taken.[12]

Health care organizations must adopt a disciplinary system theory approach in promoting a just culture that freely reports errors. To understand the interrelationship between discipline and patient safety, four behavioral concepts are examined: human error, negligence, intentional rule violations, and reckless conduct.[7]

When evaluating an adverse event, care must be taken to determine whether human error or misconduct has occurred. Historically, most disciplinary actions are based upon the outcome of the mishap; if a patient is harmed, then that health care worker is considered blameworthy. By assigning blame, the health care organization stands to lose an opportunity to learn from the error and the error may reoccur. Disciplinary policies must balance the benefits of a learning culture with the need to retain personal accountability and discipline.[12] Adverse event investigation tools may be created to augment the use of the suggested strategy identified below.

Suggested strategy

James Reason, professor of psychology, University of Manchester, United Kingdom, created a model to assist managers to determine culpability after an untoward event has occurred.[13] (**Figure 2** is an adaptation of the Reason model applied to the perioperative setting.) Perioperative leadership should apply this model when investigating incidences to determine whether disciplinary action is warranted. Six basic steps are used. It is important to focus on the error and not the outcome.

Step 1. The first line of questioning is to establish intent. Was this action or omission deliberate? If there was deliberate intent, the action or omission is culpable.

Step 2. If no intent is established, then determine whether substance use or abuse was involved. If abuse is determined, culpability is established. If the health care worker is taking a medication for medical reasons and is aware that he or she could be impaired, culpability is present; however, it is not as egregious as abuse.

Step 3. If the health care worker is not under the influence of drugs or alcohol, the next determinant is whether he or she knowingly violated safe operating procedures. This aids in determining reckless behavior. The threshold for reckless behavior is met when procedures are available, correct, and workable, but still are violated by the health care worker. If there are no adequate procedures in place, a systems error has occurred. When evaluating the situation, care must be taken to determine whether "normalization of deviance" is taking place—that is, whether there is a policy or procedure in place, but it not widely followed.

Step 4. If a policy or procedure is violated, a substitution test is conducted. Peers are asked how they would behave in a similar situation. If the peers respond the same as in the error in question, a systems-induced error is established. If they respond differently, possible negligence should be considered.

Step 5. The next question is whether the health care worker has a history of unsafe acts. If the questions in steps 1 through 4 are unsubstantiated, and there is no history of unsafe acts, then it is human error with no culpability. If the health care worker does have a history of unsafe acts, this particular incident may not be culpable; however, the organization should review the record for trends and may consider moving the health care worker to a lower-risk environment.

Step 6. The last question and assessment is where the possibility of mitigating circumstances is examined. Possible factors include stressors (eg, anger, fear, personal issues), distractions, and interruptions (eg, pagers, music, environmental temperature, extraneous conversation, overhead paging). Environmental influences include but are not limited to, physical plant and wrong size room for operative and other invasive procedures (eg, overcrowded, not ergonomic).

It is important to note that the accountability model does not evaluate or determine the proof legally required to prove reckless behavior or criminal negligence. This model should not be used for performance rating of surgical team members. It should be utilized by leadership after all the facts

Figure 2

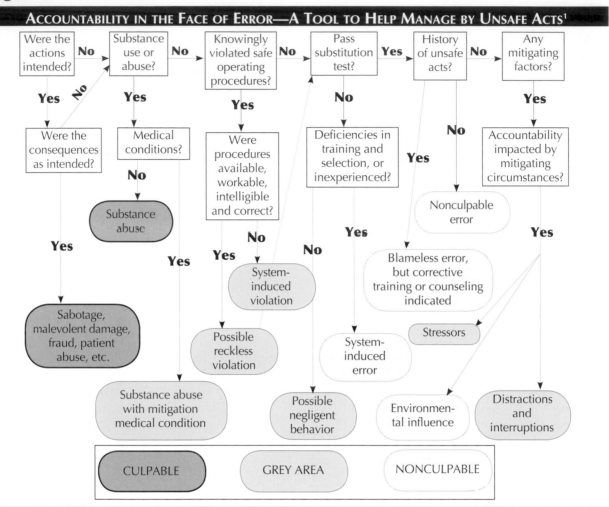

ACCOUNTABILITY IN THE FACE OF ERROR—A TOOL TO HELP MANAGE BY UNSAFE ACTS[1]

Adapted with permission for the perioperative setting . © Managing the Risks of Organizational Accidents, Reason J, 1997, Ashgate Publishing.

have been gathered, but as soon after the event as possible. If more than one person is involved, the model should be applied separately for each person.

Summary

AORN believes all health care organizations must strive to create a culture of safety. Such a culture will provide an atmosphere where all members of the perioperative team can openly discuss errors, process improvements, or system issues without fear of reprisal. A culture of safety places an emphasis on flexibility and learning as a means of improving safety and reducing errors. Characteristics of a culture of safety include the following:

- communication is open and honest;
- the emphasis is on the team rather than the individual;
- standards and practices are developed in a multidisciplinary framework;
- staff members are helpful and supportive of each other;
- staff members trust each other;
- surgical team members have a friendly, open relationship emphasizing credibility and attentiveness;
- the environment is resilient, encourages creativity, and is patient outcomes-driven;
- the focus is on work flow and process; and
- these attributes are supported by an informed culture that learns from incidents and near misses.

A commitment to safety must be articulated at all levels of the organization. Safety must be valued as the top priority, even at the expense of efficiency. Health care organizations must allocate an appropriate amount of resources and provide the necessary incentives or rewards to promote a robust patient safety culture. AORN recognizes that most patient safety initiatives will fail in the absence of a viable safety culture.

Glossary

Accountable: Responsible for one's actions or conduct.

Adverse event: Experiencing harm from error.

Culture: The shared norms, values, and practices associated with a nation, organization, or profession.[14]

Error: Failure of a planned action to be completed as intended, or the use of a wrong plan to achieve an outcome.

Failure mode and effects analysis (FMEA): A proactive tool used to anticipate and prevent the potential for product or process failure.

Just culture: An environment where actions are analyzed to ensure that individual accountability is established and appropriate actions are taken.[15]

Medical error: An adverse event or near miss that is preventable with the current state of medical knowledge.[16]

Near miss: An event or situation that could have resulted in an accident, injury, or illness, but did not, either by chance or timely intervention.[17]

Negligence: Failure to use such care as a reasonable prudent and careful person would use under similar circumstances.[17]

Root cause analysis (RCA): A process for identifying the basic or causal factor(s) that underlie variation in performance, including the occurrence or possible occurrence of a sentinel event.[18]

Safety: Freedom from accidental injury.

Safety culture: An environment that encourages reporting,[5] ends blame,[9] involves senior leadership,[9] and focuses on systems.[5]

REFERENCES

1. E H Schein, *Organizational Culture and Leadership,* second ed (San Francisco: Jossey-Bass, 1992).

2. P Hudson, "Applying the lessons of high-risk industries to health care," *Quality and Safety in Health Care* 12 Suppl 1 (December 2003) i7-i12.

3. L Larson, "Ending the culture of blame: A look at why medical errors happen-and what needs to change," *Trustee* 53 (February 2000) 6-10.

4. H S Ruchlin et al, "The role of leadership in instilling a culture of safety: Lessons from the literature," *Journal of Healthcare Management* 49 (January/February 2004) 47-59.

5. J M Krumberger, "Building a culture of safety," *RN* 64 (January 2001) 32ac2-32ac3.

6. J Reason, *Human Error* (New York: Cambridge University Press, 1990).

7. D Marx, "Patient safety and the 'Just Culture': A primer for health care executives," Medical Event Reporting System for Transfusion Medicine, *http://www.mers-tm .net/support/Marx_Primer.pdf* (accessed 2 Dec 2005).

8. "The IOM medical errors report: 5 years later, the journey continues," *The Quality Letter for Healthcare Leaders* 17 (January 2005) 2-10.

9. V F Nieva, J Sorra, "Safety culture assessment: A tool for improving patient safety in healthcare organizations," *Quality and Safety in Health Care* 12 suppl 2 (December 2003) ii17-23.

10. S J Singer et al, "The culture of safety: Results of an organization-wide survey in 15 California hospitals," *Quality and Safety in Health Care* 12 (April 2003) 112-118.

11. P J Pronovost et al, "Evaluation of the culture of safety: survey of clinicians and managers in an academic medical center," *Quality and Safety in Health Care* 12 (December 2003) 405-410.

12. "Just culture toolkit," The Risk Management and Patient Safety Institute, *http://www.rmpsi.com/education /liveprograms/JustCultureToolkit.pdf* (accessed 2 Dec 2005).

13. J Reason, *Engineering a Safety Culture* (London: Ashgate Publishing, 1997) 209.

14. R L Helmreich, A C Merritt, *Culture at Work in Aviation and Medicine: National, Organizational, and Professional Influences* (Brookfield, Vt: Ashgate, 1998).

15. R H Kilmann, M J Sexton, R A Serpa, eds, "Five key issues in understanding and changing culture," in *Gaining Control of the Corporate Culture* (San Francisco: Jossey-Bass, 1985), 1-17.

16. "Glossary of terms," in *Doing What Counts for Patient Safety: Federal Actions to Reduce Medical Errors and Their Impact,* Quality Interagency Coordination Task Force, *http://www.quic.gov/report%2Dbackup/mederr8 .htm#terms* (accessed 2 Dec 2005).

17. "Sentinel event glossary of terms," Joint Commission on Accreditation of Healthcare Organizations, *http://www.jcaho.org/accredited+organizations/sen tinel+event/glossary.htm* (2 Dec 2005).

18. D E Broadbent, *Third Report: Organising for Safety* (London: Health and Safety Commission, 1993).

RESOURCES

Carroll, J S; Quijada, M A. "Redirecting traditional professional values to support safety: Changing organisational culture in health care," *Quality and Safety in Health Care* 13 suppl 2 (December 2004) ii16-21.

Davies, H T; Nutley, S M; Mannion, R. "Organisational culture and quality of health care," *Quality in Health Care* 9 (June 2000) 111-119.

Hofstede, G H; Hofstede, G J. *Cultures and Organizations: Software of the Mind,* second ed (New York: McGraw Hill, 2005).

Kowalczyk, L. "Hospitals study when to apologize to patients," *Boston Globe,* July 24, 2005. Available at *http://www.boston.com/tools/archives* (fee required).

Barach, P; Small, S D. "Reporting and preventing medical mishaps: Lessons from non-medical near miss reporting systems," *BMJ* 320 (March 18, 2000) 759-763.

"Safety climate survey (IHI tool)," Institute for Healthcare Improvement, *http://www.ihi.org/IHI/Topics/Patient Safety/SafetyGeneral/Tools/Safety+Climate+Survey +%28IHI+Tool%29.htm* (accessed 2 Dec 2005).

Schein, E H. "Culture: The missing concept in organization studies," *Administrative Science Quarterly* 41 no 2 (June 1996) 229-240.

Schein, E H. "Three cultures of management: The key to organizational learning," *MIT Sloan Management Review* 38 (Fall 1996) 9-20. Also available at *http:// sloanreview.mit.edu/smr/issue/1996/fall/1* (accessed 2 Dec 2005).

Wachter, R M; Shojania, K G. *Internal Bleeding: The Truth Behind America's Terrifying Epidemic of Medical Mistakes,* second ed (New York: Rugged Land, 2005).

PUBLICATION HISTORY

Approved by the AORN Board of Directors, November 2005. Published in *Standards, Recommended Practices, and Guidelines,* 2006 edition. Reprinted April 2006, *AORN Journal.*

AORN Guidance Statement: Perioperative Staffing

Introduction

The purpose of this guidance statement is to provide a framework for developing a staffing plan throughout the continuum of perioperative patient care, beginning with scheduling a surgical or invasive procedure through the postoperative phase III/follow-up process. Staffing in the perioperative setting is dynamic in nature and depends on the clinical judgment, critical thinking skills, and administrative skills of nursing management in the perioperative setting. Patients undergoing surgical or invasive procedures require perioperative nursing care provided by a perioperative registered nurse, regardless of the setting. This guidance statement offers suggested staffing strategies to accommodate safe perioperative patient care while promoting a safe work environment.

Background

To provide safe and effective patient care, individual health care organizations should have staffing policies and procedures relevant to individual practice settings. The health care system is affected by increasing demand for health care, continued economic pressures, the looming nursing shortage, and financial ramifications from medico-legal issues. Patient safety is the primary focus of perioperative nurses and other health care providers. Perioperative nursing leaders need to be judicious in meeting the challenge of stretching scarce resources without compromising patient care. Perioperative department nursing leaders have an ethical responsibility to maintain staffing levels that are appropriate for providing safe patient care while they also balance shrinking budgets.

Guidance Statement

Perioperative nurse leaders should identify workforce requirements and the effect of environmental factors on staffing patterns. Surgery is performed in a wide variety of settings with uniquely different needs. Perioperative clinical staffing guidelines should be based on individual patient needs, patient acuity, technological demands, staff member competency, skill mix, practice standards, health care regulations, and accreditation requirements.[1,2] Staffing requirements are relative to department functions and assigned role expectations.

An effective staffing plan is flexible and responsive to short-term and long-term patient and organizational demands. Effective planning involves determining staffing needs, planning for the appropriate staffing mix and number of staff members, budgeting for personnel costs, and scheduling personnel. Perioperative nursing management should determine both direct and indirect patient caregivers for the unit. Additionally, productive and nonproductive time should be considered.[2] The perioperative staffing policy should state the minimum number of nursing personnel that will be provided for various types of surgical procedures. Complexity of the procedure may require more than the minimum number of nursing personnel identified. **Table 1** includes recommended minimum staffing requirements.

Call

The perioperative staffing plan includes provisions for unplanned, urgent, or emergent procedures and how to provide care for patients whose procedures run over scheduled time. Call staffing plans should be based on strategies to minimize long work hours, allow for adequate recuperation, and retain the perioperative RN as circulator. Scheduling requirements for call are subject to facility type, location, nature of services provided, and patient population served. Staffing for call should be provided in accordance with standards of perioperative and perianesthesia nursing practice. Safe call practices should be based on AORN's "Guidance statement: Safe on-call practices in perioperative practice settings."[3-5]

A systematic approach based on the operational needs of the department is required to develop a staffing plan. Identifying the hours of operation defined by the department or facility, in addition to the hours needed to cover off-shift (eg, holidays, nights, weekends) emergent/urgent surgery and the number of operating/procedure rooms is the initial step in determining staffing needs.[6] Review of historical data regarding minutes/hours of service, case volumes, case mix, and technology demands and projections for the coming year are essential for staff scheduling and budgeting. The following formula provides a platform to develop an annual staffing plan and budget. The formula is flexible and can be adapted to meet the specific needs of the perioperative setting. Although the basic formula is based on 100% utilization, it can be modified to coincide with expected volume.

Table 1

MINIMUM STAFFING RECOMMENDATIONS		
Surgical phase	**Minimum requirements**	**Comments**
Scheduling	1 clerical person under the supervision of a perioperative RN	Depending on the size of the facility, this activity may be combined with other business or clerical duties. Additional staff members may be required depending on volume and the hours that the scheduling office is open.
Preplanning	1 RN[1]	Depending on the setting and level of activity, this stage may require additional RNs and ancillary support. This may include preoperative telephone calls/interviews or planning for special supplies and equipment to meet patient needs.
Registration	Clerical person	The number of clerical staff members depends on the setting, level of activity, number of patients scheduled, patient acuity, and types of procedures and may be combined with other tasks.
Day of surgery: Preoperative	1 RN[1]	The number of additional RNs should be based on the number of patients, the number of ORs/procedure rooms, patient acuity, types of procedures, complexity/intensity of patient care requirements, time required to perform tasks, a patient's age-specific needs, and the average time for individual patient preparation. Licensed practical nurses (LPNs) and unlicensed assistive personnel (UAP) may be included in preoperative staffing plans. Unlicensed assistive personnel may be assigned to help with delegated patient care tasks as determined by the RN and according to individual state boards of nursing scope of practice and other local, state, and federal regulations.[2-4]
Intraoperative	1 RN per patient per OR in the role of the circulating nurse.[5] 1 scrub person per patient per room; may be RN, surgical technologist, or LPN. In some circumstances, a scrub person may not be required.	Additional staff members, with appropriate competencies, may be used as appropriate for the following: ♦ moderate sedation—one RN dedicated to monitoring the patient and separate from the dedicated RN circulator; ♦ local anesthesia—depending on patient needs, nursing assessment, and type of procedure, an RN may be needed to monitor the patient in addition to the RN circulator; ♦ complex surgical procedures and patients with compound needs may require an additional RN circulator and scrub person; ♦ technological demands (eg, lasers, robotics, audiovisual equipment, auto transfusion device); ♦ first assist requirements. *Note:* See formula for calculating additional staffing.
Postoperative Phase I level of care[6]	"Two registered nurses, one of whom is a[n] RN competent in Phase I postanesthesia nursing, are in the same unit where the patient is receiving Phase I level of care."[6] Staffing will reflect the American Society of PeriAnesthesia Nurses' (ASPAN's) "Patient classification/ recommended staffing guidelines."	Phase I level of care* Class 1:2—One nurse to two patients who are ♦ One unconscious, stable, without artificial airway, and over the age of 8 years; and one conscious, stable, and free of complications. ♦ Two conscious, stable, and free of complications. ♦ Two conscious, stable, 8 years of age and under, with family or competent support staff member present.[6]

Table 1, *continued*

MINIMUM STAFFING RECOMMENDATIONS		
Surgical phase	**Minimum requirements**	**Comments**
		Class 1:1—One nurse to one patient ♦ At the time of admission, until the critical elements** are met. ♦ Unstable airway.*** ♦ Any unconscious patient 8 years of age and under. ♦ A second nurse must be available to assist as necessary.[6] Class 2:1—Two nurses to one patient ♦ One critically ill, unstable, complicated patient.[6] Additional staff members may include support staff. Unlicensed assistive personnel may be assigned to help with delegated patient care tasks according to local, state, and federal regulations.[4]
Phase II level of care[6]	"Two competent personnel, one of whom is a[n] RN competent in Phase II postanesthesia nursing, are in the same room where the patient is receiving Phase II level of care. A[n] RN must be in the Phase II PACU at all times while a patient is present."[6] Staffing will reflect ASPAN's "Patient classification/recommended staffing guidelines."	Phase II level of care* Class 1:3—One nurse to three patients ♦ Over 8 years of age. ♦ 8 years of age and under with family present.[6] Class 1:2—One nurse to two patients ♦ 8 years of age and under without family or support staff member present. ♦ Initial admission of patient postprocedure.[6] Class 1:1—One nurse to one patient ♦ Unstable patient of any age requiring transfer.[6] Additional staff members may include support staff. Unlicensed assistive personnel may be assigned to help with delegated patient care tasks according to local, state, and federal regulations.[4]

Extended observation level of care (formerly Phase III)[6]	"Two competent personnel, one of whom is a[n] RN possessing competence appropriate to the patient population, are in the same unit where the patient is receiving extended observation level of care. The need for additional RNs and support staff is dependent on the patient acuity, patient census, and the physical facility."[6] Staffing will reflect ASPAN's "Patient classification/recommended staffing guidelines."	Extended observation level of care* (formerly Phase III)
		Class 1:3/5—One nurse to three to five patients
		♦ Examples of patients that may be cared for in this phase include, but are not limited to,
		  – patients awaiting transportation home;
		  – patients with no caregiver;
		  – patients who have had procedures requiring extended observation/intervention (ie, potential risk for bleeding, pain management, postoperative nausea, vomiting); and
		  – patients being held for an inpatient bed.[6]
		
		Additional staff members may include support staff. Unlicensed assistive personnel may be assigned to help with delegated patient care tasks according to local, state, and federal regulations.[4]

* Phases of postanesthesia care were developed by the American Society of PeriAnesthesia Nurses (In. Standards of Perianesthesia Nursing. Cherry Hill, NJ: American Society of PeriAnesthesia Nurses; 2004).

** Critical elements can be defined as:
  – Report has been received from the anesthesia care provider, questions answered, and the transfer of care has taken place.
  – Patient has a secure airway.
  – Initial assessment is complete.
  – Patient is hemodynamically stable.

*** Examples of an unstable airway include, but are not limited to, the following:
  – Requiring active interventions to maintain patency, such as manual jaw lift or chin lift.
  – Evidence of obstruction, active or probable, such as gasping, choking, crowing, wheezing, etc.
  – Symptoms of respiratory distress, including dyspnea, tachypnea, panic, agitation, cyanosis, etc.

Table 1, *continued*

MINIMUM STAFFING RECOMMENDATIONS		
Surgical phase	**Minimum requirements**	**Comments**
Discharge from service	An RN assesses the discharge readiness of the patient and confirms the order from anesthesiologist/surgeon for discharge according to facility protocol.[7]	"The perianesthesia nurse uses sound judgment in determining the appropriate method of communication and mode of transport to transfer care of the perianesthesia patient."[7] 1. "A policy exists to ensure safe transportation of patients. ◆ The professional nurse determines the mode, number, and competency level of accompanying personnel based on patient need. ◆ The professional nurse ensures the availability of appropriate transportation of the patient from the facility. ◆ An appropriate means of transportation from a freestanding facility to a full-service hospital will be used in emergency situations. 2. A professional nurse should accompany patients who ◆ require continuous cardiac monitoring. ◆ require evaluation and/or treatment during transport (ie, vasopressor infusions or pulse oximetry)."[7]
Postoperative follow-up	An RN completes discharge follow-up.[8]	Ambulatory surgery patients are reassessed postoperatively. The time frames for reassessment are based on patient needs and the care, treatment, and services provided. Individual organizations should develop policies and procedures regarding the mechanism chosen (eg, postoperative telephone calls) based on the patients it serves and the services or care it provides.[9,10]

REFERENCES

1. "Standard III: Staffing and personnel management," in Standards of Perianesthesia Nursing (Cherry Hill, NJ: American Society of PeriAnesthesia Nurses, 2004) 14.

2. "AORN official statement on unlicensed assistive personnel" in Standards, Recommended Practices, and Guidelines (Denver: AORN, Inc, 2004) 167-168.

3. "AORN guidance statement: Preoperative patient care in the ambulatory surgery setting," in Standards, Recommended Practices, and Guidelines (Denver: AORN, Inc, 2007) 319-324.

4. "A position statement on registered nurse utilization of unlicensed assistive personnel," in Standards of Perianesthesia Nursing (Cherry Hill, NJ: American Society of PeriAnesthesia Nurses, 2004) 77.

5. "AORN statement on nurse-to-patient ratios," in Standards, Recommended Practices, and Guidelines (Denver: AORN, Inc, 2004) 157-158.

6. "Resource 3: Patient classification/recommended staffing guidelines," in Standards of Perianesthesia Nursing (Cherry Hill, NJ: American Society of PeriAnesthesia Nurses, 2006) 61-62.

7. "Resource 11: Safe transfer of care," in Standards of Perianesthesia Nursing (Cherry Hill, NJ: American Society of PeriAnesthesia Nurses, 2004) 49.

8. "Resource 4: Criteria for initial, ongoing, and discharge assessment and management," in Standards of Perianesthesia Nursing (Cherry Hill, NJ: American Society of PeriAnesthesia Nurses, 2004) 27.

9. "Provision of care, treatment, and services," in Comprehensive Accreditation Manual for Ambulatory Care (Oakbrook Terrace, Ill: Joint Commission on Accreditation of Healthcare Organizations, 2005) PC-1, PC-3.

10. "Follow-up phone calls in outpatient surgery," Joint Commission on Accreditation of Healthcare Organizations, http://www.jcaho.org/accredited+organizations/ambulatory+care/standards/faqs/provision+of+care/anesthesia+care/followup+calls.htm (accessed 14 Dec 2004).

Intraoperative Staffing Formula

Direct staff patient care calculation
- **Step 1**—Number of rooms multiplied by number of hours per day multiplied by number of days per week equals total hours to be staffed per week.
- **Step 2**—Total hours to be staffed per week multiplied by number of people per room equals total working hours per week.
- **Step 3**—Total working hours per week divided by 40 hours equals basic full-time equivalents (FTEs).
- **Step 4**—Calculate benefit relief.
- **Step 5**—Basic FTEs multiplied by benefit hours per FTEs per year divided by 2,080 hours equals relief FTEs.
- **Step 6**—Basic FTEs added to relief FTEs equals total minimum direct care staff members.
- **Step 7**—Calculate indirect care staff members.
- **Step 8**—Calculate call replacement relief.

To determine the number of personnel per room:
- Generally, there are at least two staff members for every surgical or other invasive procedure: one RN in the circulator role and one scrub person.
- The scrub position can be filled by an RN or surgical technologist.
- If half the procedures done in the OR require a third person for part or all of the procedure (eg, to monitor patients receiving sedation, operate complex technology, high patient acuity), use a figure of 2.5 people per room in computing staffing needs.
- If more or less than half of the procedures done in the OR require a third person, or if a percentage of procedures require a fourth person, the number of personnel per room will need to be adjusted accordingly.
- In the following example, a figure of 2.5 people per room is used. The following calculation can be used to determine the RN to technologist ratio of 67%:33% (2:1):

Determine the number of RNs per room by multiplying 2.5 x 67 = 1.7 RNs

Determine the number of technologists per room by multiplying 2.5 x .33 = 0.8 technologists

The above calculation can be applied to any number of total people needed per room. If an institution's FTE is greater or less than 2,080 hours per year, this also must be adjusted in the formula.

Indirect staff calculation
For the purposes of this calculation, indirect staff members include, but are not limited to, the budgeted positions of surgical services director, clinical nurse manager, charge nurse, perioperative educator, schedulers, secretaries, aids, orderlies, and housekeeping personnel as appropriate. The number of indirect care staff members will vary according to function, but a traditional compliment is one indirect caregiver to two direct caregivers.

Call hours replacement calculation
The maximum number of call hours is determined by identifying the number of shifts multiplied by the number of hours multiplied by two FTEs. The actual hours on call personnel are called in to work per year divided by 2,080 equals the replacement FTEs for call-time worked.

Relief replacement
- Benefit hours (ie, nonproductive hours) are hours such as vacation time, holiday time, available sick time (whether paid or unpaid), education days, and any other time that personnel policies determine an employee might take off. The number of benefit hours is proportionate to the amount of vacation time and the number of long-term employees. Some organizations use an established percentage to calculate benefit hours.
- In the OR, benefit hours also include breaks and lunches, unless the OR ceases work during those times.
- When determining relief for lunch, it is necessary to add approximately 15 minutes to the allotted time at either end to allow for nurse-to-nurse report about what has transpired during the procedure in progress. It may take less than seven minutes for the circulating nurse to report to the relief nurse, but relief of the scrub person needs to include time needed to scrub, gown, and glove, so 15 minutes is average.
- When computing relief for breaks and lunches, the number of minutes is multiplied by 260 days (ie, 52 weeks multiplied by five days per week).
- Nonproductive time for orienting new staff members also needs to be included.

Example. *An OR suite has eight rooms, which are to be staffed and available as follows:*
- *8 rooms, 7 AM to 3 PM, Monday through Friday;*
- *2 rooms, 3 to 6 PM, Monday through Friday;*
- *1 room, 6 PM to 7 AM, seven days per week; and*
- *1 room, 7 AM to 6 PM, Saturday and Sunday.*

■ **Step 1**—Number of rooms multiplied by number of hours per day multiplied by number of days per week equals total hours to be staffed per week.

$$8 \times 8 \times 5 = 320$$
$$2 \times 3 \times 5 = 30$$
$$1 \times 13 \times 7 = 91$$
$$1 \times 11 \times 2 = 22$$
463 total hours staffed per week

■ **Step 2**—Total hours staffed per week multiplied by number of people per room equals total working hours per week.

463 hours x 2.5 = 1,157.5 total working hours per week

The following calculation can be used to determine the hours for a 67%:33% RN:technologist ratio.

Determine the number of RNs per room by multiplying 2.5 x .67 = 1.7 RN

Determine the number of technologists per room by multiplying 2.5 x .33 = 0.8 technologists

RNs: 1.7 x 463 hours = 787.1 total RN working hours per week

Surgical technologists: 0.8 x 463 = 370.4 total surgical technologist hours per week

Total working hours per week = 1,157.5

■ **Step 3**—Total working hours per week divided by 40 hours worked per week equals basic FTEs.

1,157.5 ÷ 40 = 28.9 basic FTEs

The following calculation can be used to determine the basic RN FTEs and surgical technologist FTEs for a 67%:33% RN:technologist ratio.

RNs: 787.1 hours ÷ 40 = 19.7 basic RN FTEs
Surgical technologists: 370.4 ÷ 40 = 9 basic surgical technologist FTEs

■ **Step 4**—Calculate benefit relief per employee.

Average vacation hours per year = 100
Holiday hours per year = 56
Available sick hours per year = 96
15 minute break x 260 days ÷ 60 minutes = 65 hours
45 minute lunch x 260 days ÷ 60 minutes = 195 hours
512 hours of benefit relief

Note: Organizations handle benefit hours differently. Benefits hours may include, but are not limited to the following.

■ Vacation hours, holiday hours, and sick hours are grouped together under paid time off (PTO).
■ If sick time is not established and included in the PTO, historical average sick time is used to calculate replacement FTEs.
■ A percentage is used to calculate benefit hours.

■ **Step 5**—Basic FTEs multiplied by benefit hours per FTE per year divided by 2,080 hours equals relief FTEs.

28.9 x 512 hours ÷ 2,080 = 7.1 relief FTEs

The following calculation determines the RN and surgical technologist relief FTEs for a 67%:33% RN:technologist ratio.

RNs: 19.7 x 512 = 10,086.4 ÷ 2,080 = 4.8 RN relief FTEs
Surgical technologists: 9 x 512 = 4,608 ÷ 2,080 = 2.2 surgical technologist FTEs

Calculating the orientation time for new employees depends on several factors, including, but not limited to, the size and type of OR, anticipated turnover time, and increase in the number of staff due to growth of services and volume. For the purposes of the example, if four people with experience were expected to be hired for a year and each receives 12 weeks of orientation, use the following calculation:

4 staff members x 40 hours per week x 12 weeks = 1,920 hours of orientation ÷ 2,080 = 0.9 FTE for orientation

■ **Step 6**—Basic FTEs added to relief FTEs equals total minimum direct care staff members.

28.9 + 7.1 = 36 FTEs

The following calculation is used for a 67%:33% RN:technologist ratio.

RN: 19.7 basic FTEs + 4.8 benefit relief FTEs = 24.5 RN FTEs

Surgical technologist: 9 basic FTEs + 2.2 benefit relief FTEs = 11.2 surgical technologist FTEs

■ **Step 7**—Calculate indirect care staff members.

1 indirect caregiver per 2 direct caregivers =
1.25 x 463 hours per week = 578.8 ÷ 40 =
14.5 FTEs
512 benefit hours x 14.5 = 7,424 ÷ 2,080 =
3.6 relief FTEs
3.6 + 14.5 = 18.1

■ **Step 8**—Calculate call relief (see **Table 2**).
The total number of FTEs calculated in this example is:

Direct caregivers
  RNs: 24.5 FTEs
  surgical technologists: 11.2 FTEs
  call replacements: 1.5 FTEs
  indirect caregivers: 18.1 FTES
  orientation FTEs: 0.9 FTE
Total: 56.3 FTEs

This formula is based on 100% utilization.

Post Anesthesia Care Unit (PACU) Staffing Formula

There are no standardized staffing formulas at this time for calculating perianesthesia staffing in the PACU. Neither the American Society of Perianesthesia Nurses nor AORN have a recommended staffing formula at this time. Refer to **Table 1** for PACU staffing recommendations.

Summary

One of the most important responsibilities of a perioperative nursing leader is the development of an effective staffing plan relative to surgical patients' needs. AORN recognizes there are a variety of settings in which perioperative RNs practice. This guidance statement is intended to serve as a guide for perioperative nursing leaders in developing a staffing plan and is designed to be adaptable to various practice settings.

Glossary

Direct staff members: Personnel directly involved in providing care to patients undergoing surgical or other invasive procedures. These individuals provide direct patient care and include RNs, surgical technologists, nursing assistants, orderlies, RN first assistants, and surgical assistants.[2]

Table 2

CALL RELIEF CALCULATION				
Call coverage	Maximum possible hours			Historical usage in hours
	Hours	Staff	Total	Total
260 night shifts	8 x	2 =	4,160	3,342
52 weekends	48 x	3 =	7,488	5,256
12 holidays	24 x	3 =	864	689
Total			12,512	9,287*

* *The difference between the maximum possible call hours and actual usage of call hours is 3,225 hours worked. The 3,225 call hours worked per year divided by 2,080 hours (ie, one full-time equivalent [FTE]) equals 1.55 FTE replacement for call-time worked.*

Indirect staff members: Personnel who support nonpatient care activities in the perioperative environment. These positions may include the director, manager, charge nurse, educator, secretaries, environmental services personnel, instrument processing personnel, materials management personnel, and clerical/business personnel. The perioperative director, management team members (eg, team leaders, charge nurse), clinical nurse specialists, and educators may be a combination of direct and indirect personnel.[2]

Productive hours: Actual hours worked; includes direct and indirect hours. Worked hours are those needed to staff the unit.[2]

Nonproductive hours: These are paid hours not worked and considered benefit hours (eg, vacation, sick time, funeral leave, holiday).[2]

Editor's note: *This staffing guidance statement was developed by the Nursing Practice Committee in December 2004. AORN would like to thank the American Society of PeriAnesthesia Nurses for their participation in the development of this statement.*

REFERENCES
1. B Fernsebner, "Key factors affecting staffing," *OR Manager* 16 (December 2000) 10-11.
2. K A Halverson Carpenter, "Staffing and scheduling," *Leadership in Action: A Managers Guide to Success* (Denver: AORN, Inc, 2004) 74.
3. "A position statement on on call/work schedule," in *Standards of Perianesthesia Nursing* (Cherry Hill, NJ: American Society of PeriAnesthesia Nurses, 2004) 79.
4. "Proposed AORN position statement for safe on-call practices," pending ratification by the 2005 House of Delegates.

5. "AORN guidance statement: Safe on-call practices in perioperative practice settings," in *Standards, Recommended Practices and Guidelines* (Denver: AORN, Inc, 2005) 193-195.

6. B Fernsebner, "Building a staffing plan based on OR's needs," (Surgical Staffing) *OR Manager* (1996).

RESOURCES

Perioperative Management Resources: Budgeting (Denver: AORN, Inc, 2004).

PUBLICATION HISTORY

Originally published in *Standards, Recommended Practices, and Guidelines,* 2005 edition. Reprinted May 2005, *AORN Journal.*

AORN Guidance Statement: Postoperative Patient Care in the Ambulatory Surgery Setting

Editor's note: Table 1 of this guidance statement was updated in October 2010 to reflect the 2010-2012 American Society of PeriAnesthesia Nurses Standards of Perianesthesia Nursing Practice.

Introduction

This guidance statement provides a framework for health care practitioners to use when developing and implementing policies and procedures for postoperative patient care in the ambulatory surgery setting. AORN defines *postoperative* as "the time [that] begins with admission to the postanesthesia care area and ends with a resolution of surgical sequelae."[1(p31)] This includes the postanesthesia phases I, II, and extended observation (formerly phase III) levels of care. These phases are defined by the American Society of PeriAnesthesia Nurses' (ASPAN's) *Standards of Perianesthesia Nursing Practice* as follows.[2]

Phase I focuses on providing a transition from a totally anesthetized state to one requiring less acute interventions. Recovery occurs in the postanesthesia care unit (PACU). The purpose of this phase is for patients to regain physiological homeostasis and receive appropriate nursing intervention as needed.

Phase II focuses on preparing the patient for self-care, care by family members, or care in an extended care environment. The patient is discharged to phase II recovery when intensive nursing care no longer is needed. In the phase II area, sometimes referred to as the step-down or discharge area, the patient becomes more alert and functional.

Extended observation focuses on providing ongoing care for patients who require extended observation or intervention after transfer from phase I or phase II. Interventions are directed toward preparing the patient for self-care or care by family members. Extended observation is designed for patients who are unable to meet the criteria for discharge from phase II and the ambulatory unit. These patients may need alternative care, such as home health care or a stay in an overnight short-stay hospital unit or recovery center.

This guidance statement is directed specifically to ambulatory surgery centers (ASCs). It also may be used in other ambulatory settings that perform surgery or other invasive procedures. The ambulatory surgery setting is defined as an area where outpatient surgery or other invasive procedures are performed, including, but not limited to, freestanding surgery centers, hospital-based ambulatory surgical units, physicians' offices, cardiac catheterization suites, endoscopy units, and radiology departments.

Perioperative nurses have limited contact with patients before surgery, which may lead to an increased risk for adverse patient outcomes. Ambulatory surgery centers must have consistent approaches to postoperative patient care to ensure patient safety. This guidance statement is intended to promote patient safety in the ambulatory surgery setting.

Guidance Statement

Ambulatory surgery centers should develop written policies and procedures for postoperative patient care. Policies and procedures should include, but not be limited to, the following elements:

- staffing,
- supplies and equipment,
- postanesthesia care,
- fast tracking of patients,
- pain management,
- documentation,
- discharge criteria,
- discharge instructions, and
- monitoring of outcomes.

The criteria in this guidance statement represent the minimum levels of care.

Perioperative Nursing Data Set

The Perioperative Nursing Data Set (PNDS) is a clinically relevant and empirically validated standardized nursing vocabulary describing perioperative nursing. It relates to the delivery of care in all perioperative settings. This standardized language consists of a collection of data elements and includes perioperative nursing diagnoses, interventions, and outcomes. The PNDS should be used to develop ambulatory surgery patient plans of care and to standardize nursing documentation. In addition, PNDS outcomes, as well as outcome indicators, interventions, and nursing diagnoses, can be

- incorporated into competencies, policies and procedures, job descriptions, pathways, guidelines, and care plans;
- linked to the electronic health record;
- used as a tool for teaching new nurses about perioperative nursing; and
- applied in performance improvement projects and benchmarking.

Each data element in the PNDS corresponds to a unique identifier. The domains are represented by the letter "D" followed by numbers 1 to 3 to indicate the particular domain being addressed. Nursing diagnoses are represented by the letter "X" and a number unique to the diagnosis. Interventions are represented by the letter "I" and a unique number, and outcomes are represented by the letter "O" and a unique number. These designations are identified in this document with unique identifiers noted in parentheses. A list of outcomes, interventions, and nursing diagnoses specific to each domain is printed in an appendix of the PNDS reference book.[3]

The PNDS is conceptualized by the perioperative patient focused model. The patient and his or her family members are at the center of the model's framework. The model depicts perioperative nursing in four domains and illustrates the relationship between the patient, family members, and the care provided by the perioperative RN. The patient-centered domains are

♦ D1—patient safety;
♦ D2—physiological responses to surgery; and
♦ D3—patient and family member behavioral responses to surgery, including
  – behavior responses—knowledge, and
  – behavior responses—rights and ethics.[3]

Nursing Care Policies

Perianesthesia nursing care policies and procedures should be available in the PACU and all areas where other postoperative care (phase I, II, or extended observation) is delivered.[4] At a minimum, each nurse should review the policies and procedures periodically, and the review process should be documented. Specific criteria for postanesthesia care policies and procedures should include

♦ assessment of data elements;
♦ supplies and equipment required for each phase of recovery;
♦ postoperative patient care;
♦ emergency medications[5] and equipment;
♦ patient classification;
♦ infection control (O10);
♦ pain management (O20), patient knowledge of pain (O29), and pain control;
♦ documentation of patient care;
♦ patient transfer; and
♦ care of patients receiving moderate sedation.[6]

Staffing

A staffing plan should be developed and used to provide an adequate number and mix of personnel to meet patient care needs.[7,8] The staffing plan should include criteria regarding the number of patients, number of ORs and procedure rooms, average patient length of stay, and intensity of care.[6] An operational patient classification system may help in determining and allocating nursing personnel.[9] The ASPAN "Recommended staffing guidelines" should be used as a guide to calculate requirements for postanesthesia staffing needs (**Table 1**).

Staffing for an ASC PACU should conform to national and state guidelines and regulations for safe postanesthesia nursing care.[4] Additional practice standards that apply to postanesthesia care also should be followed and should include personnel competency requirements that meet state licensure guidelines, organizational guidelines, accreditation and professional standards, procedure-specific training, and professional experience.[10,11] Personnel should be trained in the use of emergency equipment and cardiopulmonary resuscitation for both adult and pediatric patients if pediatric care is provided.[12] Advanced cardiac life support and pediatric advanced life support training, if pediatric care is provided, is recommended for all PACU nurses. All staff members should undergo a comprehensive orientation program, and competencies should be documented.

Supplies and Equipment

A checklist of required supplies and equipment for PACU phase I and PACU phase II should be developed.[13] A method should be in place to ensure all equipment is maintained according to manufacturers' specifications.[14] Equipment must be available to

♦ administer oxygen (I87);
♦ provide suction (I87);
♦ maintain IV access (I34); and
♦ monitor postoperative cardiac status (I44) (I120)
  – blood pressure,
  – heart rhythm and rate, and
  – oxygen saturation.[15]

Emergency equipment, an emergency communication system, and knowledgeable emergency assistive personnel should be readily available.[14,16] Emergency equipment and supplies should include a defibrillator, medications, oxygen, a positive-pressure breathing device, suction equipment, and appropriate nasal and oral airways.[17,18]

Table 1

PRACTICE RECOMMENDATION 1
PATIENT CLASSIFICATION/RECOMMENDED STAFFING GUIDELINES

Staffing is based on patient acuity, census, patient flow processes and physical facility. The perianesthesia registered nurse (RN) uses prudent judgment to determine nurse to patient ratios, patient mix, and staffing mix that reflect patient acuity and nursing intensity.

PREANESTHESIA PHASE

Preadmission

Perianesthesia nursing roles during this phase focus on assessing the patient and developing a plan of care designed to meet the preanesthesia physical, psychological, educational, sociocultural, and spiritual needs of the patient/family/significant other. The nursing roles also focus on preparing the patient/family/significant other for his or her experience throughout the perianesthesia continuum. Interviewing and assessment techniques are used to identify potential or actual problems that may occur.

Staffing for preadmission units (eg, preadmission testing, preanesthesia testing, preoperative assessment clinic, preanesthesia assessment unit, preoperative teaching unit) is dependent on patient volume, patient health status and required support for preanesthesia interventions.

Day of Surgery/Procedure

Perianesthesia nursing roles during this phase focus on validation of existing information and completion of preparation of the patient. The perianesthesia registered nurse continues to assess the patient and develops a plan of care designed to meet the physical, psychological, educational, sociocultural, and spiritual needs of the patient/family/significant other.

Staffing for Day of Surgery/Procedure

Due to the varied complexities of these units, recommended staffing ratios must be determined by individual institutions based on but not limited to the following criteria:

♦ Patient safety
♦ Number and acuity (patient characteristics and requirements of care) of patients
♦ Complexity (management of patient acuity) and intensity of care
♦ Examples include: average time in patient preparation (eg, education, testing, history completion, patient education, preoperative testing, intravenous access, completion of required paperwork/electronic charting, blood product administration)
♦ Medication reconciliation/administration (antibiotics, sedation, anxiolytics, etc.)
♦ Moderate sedation and subsequent monitoring for invasive procedures
♦ Procedures (eg, insertion of invasive lines, regional blocks)
♦ Need for additional monitoring
♦ Additional processes of the specific unit (eg, blending of levels of care, etc.)

POSTANESTHESIA PHASE

Phase I Level of Care

The perianesthesia registered nursing roles during this phase focus on providing postanesthesia nursing care to the patient in the immediate postanesthesia period, and transitioning them to Phase II level of care, the inpatient setting, or to an intensive care setting for continued care (see Blended Levels of Care).

TWO REGISTERED NURSES, ONE OF WHOM IS AN RN COMPETENT IN PHASE I POSTANESTHESIA NURSING, ARE IN THE SAME ROOM/UNIT WHERE THE PATIENT IS RECEIVING PHASE I LEVEL OF CARE.

♦ Staffing should reflect patient acuity. In general a 1:2 nurse-patient ratio in Phase I allows for appropriate assessment, planning, implementing and evaluation for discharge as well as increased efficiency and flow of patients through the Phase I area.
♦ This also allows for flexibility in assignments as patient acuity changes.

Table 1 (continued)

PATIENT CLASSIFICATION/RECOMMENDED STAFFING GUIDELINES

◆ New admissions should be assigned so that the nurse can devote his/her attention to the care of that admission until critical elements* are met.

◆ Staffing patterns should be adjusted as needed based on changing acuity and nursing requirements, and as discharge criteria are met.

Class 1:2 One Nurse to Two Patients

a. One unconscious patient, hemodynamically stable, with a stable airway, over the age of 8 years and one conscious patient, stable and free of complications

b. Two conscious patients, stable, and free of complications

c. Two conscious patients, stable, 8 years of age and under, with family or competent support staff present

Class 1:1 One Nurse to One Patient

a. At the time of admission, until the critical elements* are met

b. Unstable airway

◆ Examples of an unstable airway include, but are not limited to, the following:
  – Requiring active interventions to maintain patency such as manual jaw lift or chin lift or an oral airway
  – Evidence of obstruction, active or probable, such as gasping, choking, crowing, wheezing, etc.
  – Symptoms of respiratory distress including dyspnea, tachypnea, panic, agitation, cyanosis, etc.

c. Any unconscious patient 8 years of age and under

d. A second nurse must be available to assist as necessary

Class 2:1 Two Nurses to One Patient

a. One critically ill, unstable patient

Phase II level of care

Perianesthesia nursing roles during this phase focus on preparing the patient/family/significant other for care in the home or Extended Care level of care.

TWO COMPETENT PERSONNEL, ONE OF WHOM IS AN RN COMPETENT IN PHASE II POSTANESTHESIA NURSING, ARE IN THE SAME ROOM/UNIT WHERE THE PATIENT IS RECEIVING PHASE II LEVEL OF CARE. AN RN MUST BE IN THE PHASE II PACU AT ALL TIMES WHILE A PATIENT IS PRESENT.

Critical elements can be defined as:
- *Report has been received from the anesthesia care provider, questions answered, and the transfer of care has taken place.*
- *Patient has a stable/secure airway.*
- *Initial assessment is complete.*
- *Patient is hemodynamically stable.*
- *Patient is free from agitation, restlessness, combative behaviors.*

Postanesthesia Care

A postanesthesia care policy and procedure should be written for transporting, monitoring, and evaluating patients in the PACU.[19] Patients should have a complete systems assessment during the first few minutes of PACU care.[4] This assessment should include, but not be limited to,

◆ vital signs (I59) (I128) (I16);

◆ respiratory adequacy (I45);
◆ postoperative cardiac status (I59);
◆ peripheral circulation (ie, postoperative tissue perfusion) (I46);
◆ postoperative neurological status (I146);
◆ level of consciousness (I144) (I146);
◆ alertness (I144) (I146);
◆ lucidity (I144) (I146);
◆ orientation (I144) (I146);

Table 1 *(continued)*

PATIENT CLASSIFICATION/RECOMMENDED STAFFING GUIDELINES

♦ Staffing should reflect patient acuity and complexity of care. In general, a 1:3 nurse patient ratio allows for appropriate assessment, planning, implementing care and evaluation for discharge as well as increasing efficiency and flow of patients through the Phase II area. This also allows for flexibility in assignments as patient acuity is subject to change.

♦ New admissions should be assigned so that the nurse can devote his/her attention as needed to appropriate discharge assessment and teaching.

♦ Staffing patterns can be adjusted as needed as acuity/nursing interventions and discharge criteria are met.

Class 1:3 One Nurse to Three Patients

a. Over 8 years of age
b. 8 years of age and under with family present

Class 1:2 One Nurse to Two Patients

a. 8 years of age and under without family or support staff present
b. Initial admission of patient post procedure

Class 1:1 One Nurse to One Patient

a. Unstable patient of any age requiring transfer

Extended Care Level of Care

The nursing roles in this phase focus on providing the ongoing care for those patients requiring extended observation/intervention after transfer/discharge from Phase I and Phase II levels of care.

Two competent personnel, one of whom is an RN possessing competence appropriate to the patient population, are in the same room/unit where the patient is receiving Extended Care level of care. The need for additional RNs and support staff is dependent on the patient acuity, complexity of patient care, patient census and the physical facility.

Class 1:3/5 One Nurse to Three-Five Patients

Examples of patients that may be cared for in this phase include but are not limited to:
1. Patients awaiting transportation home
2. Patients with no care giver
3. Patients who have had procedures requiring extended observation/interventions (eg, potential risk for bleeding, pain management, [postoperative nausea and vomiting], etc.)
4. Patients being held for an inpatient bed

Copyright © 2010. Reprinted with permission from the American Society of PeriAnesthesia Nurses (ASPAN). These guidelines are effective December 27, 2010.

♦ IV patency (I34);
♦ allergies and sensitivities (I123);
♦ pain management (I16);
♦ motor abilities (I146);
♦ return of sensory and motor control in areas affected by local or regional anesthetics (I146);[4]
♦ skin integrity (I38) (I46);[3,4]
♦ temperature regulation (I78);
♦ positioning (I38);

♦ surgical wound site (I4) (I130);
♦ nausea and vomiting (I128) (I153); and
♦ fluid and electrolyte balance (I132).

The postanesthesia nurse should provide ongoing assessments and reevaluations concurrently with nursing interventions.[4,20]

A nursing care plan should be based on the initial patient assessment and documented appropriately. The perioperative nurse analyzes the assessment data to determine nursing diagnoses. Following is a partial list of nursing diagnoses that may be associated with patients undergoing ambulatory surgery:

- X38 (D2)—pain, acute;
- X73 (D2)—nausea;
- X28 (D2)—infection, risk for;
- X26 (D2)—hypothermia; and
- X21 (D2)—gas exchange, impaired.[3]

Postoperative Patient Outcomes

Nursing interventions are initiated to achieve a desired conclusion and/or to reduce the probability of undesired outcomes.[3,21] Following is a partial list of patient outcomes that may be associated with a patient's postoperative experience:

- (O14)—the patient's respiratory status is consistent with or improved from baseline levels established preoperatively;
- (O25)—the patient's right to privacy is maintained;
- (O30)—the patient's neurologic status is consistent with or improved from baseline levels established preoperatively;
- (O19)—the patient demonstrates knowledge of medication management.[3]

Fast Tracking of Patients

Fast tracking is defined as transferring a patient directly from the OR to PACU phase II, bypassing PACU phase I. Policy and procedures should be developed before initiating a patient fast-tracking process.[22-25] Patient education concerning fast tracking begins during the preoperative assessment.

Wherever fast tracking is practiced, a collaborative plan of care should be developed by anesthesia care providers and perianesthesia nurses.[22] The plan should include

- written guidelines addressing patient selection,[26]
- preoperative patient education,
- selection and management of anesthetic agents,
- assessment criteria,
- discharge criteria, and
- monitoring and reporting of patient outcomes.

Pain Management

Policies and procedures for treatment of pain, nausea, and vomiting in the PACU should be written.[27,28] Every patient should receive an initial and ongoing evaluation and assessment of pain. Assessment of pain, the fifth vital sign, includes pain intensity, location, qual-

ity, duration, onset, and treatment effectiveness.[20,27] Each facility should adopt a consistent pain management scale for assessing pain, including scales for special patient populations. Separate documentation should be maintained for each pain site.[27,29]

A policy and procedure that specifies that anesthesia orders take precedence over surgeon's orders for immediate postoperative treatment in the PACU should be developed.[27] Anesthesia orders should be documented and include preferred medications to be used for treating the patient.[27]

Documentation

A comprehensive system for documenting patient events, assessments, and treatments to prevent duplication and provide for a smooth progression of care should be established.[5,30] The PNDS should be incorporated into the nursing documentation.[3] The PACU record should allow for checklist documentation of routine care rather than narrative documentation. Descriptive notes should focus on deviations from expected outcomes and individual patient responses to treatment and interventions.[4]

Postoperative documentation should include the patient's assessment, treatment, and reactions to treatment.[30] Specific documentation should include, but not be limited to,

- respiratory status (I87);
- cardiac status (I44);
- peripheral circulation (I46);
- neurological status (I146);[30]
- pain (I16) (I51), nausea, or vomiting (I128) (I153);
- condition of the surgical site (I130) or bleeding (I132);
- temperature (I86) (I131) (I55);
- chills or shivering (I78) (I89);
- urinary status (I23) (I89) (I153);
- administration of fluids or electrolytes (I5) (I153);
- administration of medication and responses (I8) (I51);[30]
- administration of antibiotics (I7) (I51);
- emotional status (I68) (I137) (I147);[3] and
- unusual events or postoperative complications (I92) (I111).[30]

Discharge Criteria

Discharge policies and procedures should be written and implemented.[31] Discharge criteria should be based on standards or general guidelines for discharging patients established by accrediting organizations and anesthesia and postanesthesia provider associations.[6] The patient's postprocedure status should be assessed before he or she is discharged from the postsedation or postanesthesia recovery room.[20]

The discharge policy should clearly specify who is responsible for discharging the patient from PACU phase I, II, and extended observation.[15] Written criteria should include specific guidelines patients must meet before being discharged to the next level of care or discharged directly home.[28,32] These criteria should include a numeric scoring system to evaluate the patient's condition.[4,31]

Discharge criteria should include an evaluation of the patient for nausea, vomiting, pain, chills, shivering, the surgical site condition, and bleeding. The patient's emotional status, fluid and urinary status, cognitive abilities, peripheral circulation, and temperature also should be evaluated.[4]

Patient Transfer

Whenever a patient is transferred from one level of care to another level of care, the perioperative RN should communicate all pertinent information to the next caregiver. After the perioperative RN completes the final assessment before patient discharge, the perioperative RN will provide a transfer report.[2] Communication between caregivers is essential for patient safety and appropriate and consistent nursing care. Items in the transfer report should include, but are not limited to,

- vital signs (O15) and airway patency (O14);
- level of consciousness (O30);
- muscular strength (O30);[33]
- allergies;
- condition of operative site/dressing (O11);
- location and patency of tubes and/or drains;
- medications given and response to those medications (O9);
- intake and output (eg, IV, estimated blood loss) (O13);[33]
- tests ordered with pertinent results, if available;
- pain level (O29);
- nausea and vomiting (O13);[2]
- psychosocial status (O28) (O31); and
- discharge orders.

An emergency care and transfer plan should be in place, including a formal policy and procedure for hospital admission.[20] Personnel should be familiar with the process for transporting patients according to the

plan. A policy for handling patients who leave the facility against medical advice also should be written.[31]

Discharge Instructions

Written postoperative and follow-up care instructions should be provided to each patient and should reflect the patient's individual informational needs specific to home care, response to unexpected events,[8,15,34] and follow-up by the physician.[16] Discharge instructions should be reviewed with the patient and a responsible adult before discharge.[15,31,35] Discharge information should include medication use, side effects, signs and symptoms to report, and when to contact the health care provider for additional assistance.[27,36]

Monitoring of Outcomes

Policies and procedures for completing discharge follow-up with the patient to assess and evaluate the patient's status should be written.[36-39] Discharge follow-up should include ongoing pain assessment and determination of the efficacy of the prescribed pain medication.[27,40] If a staff member other than a professional nurse conducts the follow-up telephone call, the protocol should include a decision tree with a branch identifying professional nurse interventions for any unexpected outcome. Results of patient follow-up telephone calls should be documented.

The facility should collect data to monitor its performance.[41] Data collected should include patients' perceptions of care, treatment, and provision of services, including specific individual needs and expectations, how well the facility met these needs, surgical site infections, how the facility can improve patient safety, and the effectiveness of pain management, when applicable.[41]

REFERENCES

1. "Competency statements in perioperative nursing," in *Standards, Guidelines, and Recommended Practices* (Denver: AORN, Inc, 2004) 19-31.

2. *Standards of Perianesthesia Nursing Practice* (Cherry Hill, NJ: American Society of PeriAnesthesia Nurses, 2002) 4-5.

3. *Perioperative Nursing Data Set: The Perioperative Nursing Vocabulary*, second ed, S Beyea ed (Denver: AORN, Inc, 2002) 97.

4. R Ferrara-Love, "Immediate postanesthesia care," in *Ambulatory Surgical Nursing*, second ed, N Burden, ed (Philadelphia: WB Saunders Co, 2000) 409-476.

5. S Smith, "Progressive postanesthesia care: Phase II recovery," in *Ambulatory Surgical Nursing*, second ed, N Burden, ed (Philadelphia: WB Saunders Co, 2000) 477-503.

6. D Geuder, "Postoperative patient care," in *Ambulatory Surgery Principles and Practices*, third ed, N J Vinson, ed (Denver: AORN Inc, 2003) 133-144.

7. "Standard III: Staffing and personnel management," in *Standards of Perianesthesia Nursing Practice* (Cherry Hill, NJ: American Society of PeriAnesthesia Nurses, 2002) 14.

8. "Surgical and related services," in *Accreditation Guidebook for Office Based Surgery* (Wilmette, Ill: Accreditation Association for Ambulatory Health Care, 2004) 47-52.

9. J A Kusler-Jensen, "A patient classification system for ambulatory surgery centers," *AORN Journal* 64 (August 1996) 273-277.

10. "Standards for postanesthesia care," in *ASA Standards, Guidelines and Statements* (Park Ridge, Ill: American Society of Anesthesiologists, 2002) 7.

11. "Quality of care provided," in *Accreditation Guidebook for Office Based Surgery* (Wilmette, Ill: Accreditation Association for Ambulatory Health Care, 2004) 19-21.

12. "Management of human resources," in *2004 Comprehensive Accreditation Manual for Ambulatory Care* (Oakbrook Terrace, Ill: Joint Commission on Accreditation of Healthcare Organizations, 2004) HR1-HR12.

13. "Resource 5: Equipment for preanesthesia phase, PACU phase I, phase II, and phase III," in *Standards of Perianesthesia Nursing Practice* (Cherry Hill, NJ: American Society of PeriAnesthesia Nurses, 2002) 32-35.

14. "Facilities and environment," in *Accreditation Guidebook for Office Based Surgery* (Wilmette, Ill: Accreditation Association for Ambulatory Health Care, 2004) 35-38.

15. "Guidelines for ambulatory anesthesia and surgery," American Society of Anesthesiologists, *http://www.asahq.org/publicationsAndServices/standards/04.pdf* (accessed 9 April 2004).

16. D O'Brien, V A Walter, N Burden, "Special procedures in the ambulatory setting," in *Ambulatory Surgical Nursing*, second ed, N Burden, ed (Philadelphia: WB Saunders Co, 2000) 817-842.

17. J Odom, "Conscious sedation/analgesia," in *Ambulatory Surgical Nursing*, second ed, N Burden, ed (Philadelphia: WB Saunders Co, 2000) 309-330.

18. "Resource 6: Emergency drugs and equipment," in *Standards of Perianesthesia Nursing Practice* (Cherry Hill, NJ: American Society of PeriAnesthesia Nurses, 2002) 36-37.

19. "Practice guidelines for postanesthesia care," American Society of Anesthesiologists, *http://www.asahq.org/publicationsAndServices/postanes.pdf* (accessed 29 Sept 2004).

20. "Provision of care, treatment, and services," in *2004 Comprehensive Accreditation Manual for Ambulatory Care* (Oakbrook Terrace, Ill: Joint Commission on Accreditation of Healthcare Organizations, 2004) PC1-PC50.

21. J C Rothrock, *Perioperative Nursing Care Planning* (St Louis: Mosby, Inc, 1990) 497.

22. "A position statement on fast tracking," in *Standards of Perianesthesia Nursing Practice* (Cherry Hill, NJ: American Society of PeriAnesthesia Nurses, 2002) 73.

23. M Mamaril, "Fast-tracking the postanesthesia patient: The pros and cons," *Journal of Perianesthesia Nursing* 15 (April 2000) 89-93.

24. A C Watkins, P F White, "Fast-tracking after ambulatory surgery," *Journal of PeriAnesthesia Nursing* 16 (December 2001) 379-87.

25. P F White et al, "PACU fast-tracking: An alternative to 'bypassing' the PACU for facilitating the recovery process after ambulatory surgery," *Journal of PeriAnesthesia Nursing* 18 (August 2003) 247-253.

26. R I Patel et al, "Fast-tracking children after ambulatory surgery," *Anesthesia and Analgesia* 92 (April 2001) 918-922.

27. K Cunningham, "Pain management," in *Ambulatory Surgery Principles and Practices*, third ed, N J Vinson, ed (Denver: AORN Inc, 2003) 145-149.

28. "Anesthesia services," in *Accreditation Guidebook for Office Based Surgery* (Wilmette, Ill: Accreditation Association for Ambulatory Health Care, 2004) 41-45.

29. D A Krenzischek, L Wilson, "An introduction to the ASPAN pain and comfort clinical guideline," *Journal of PeriAnesthesia Nursing* 18 (August 2003) 232-236.

30. "Management of information," in *2004 Comprehensive Accreditation Manual for Ambulatory Care* (Oakbrook Terrace, Ill: Joint Commission on Accreditation of Healthcare Organizations, 2004) IM1-IM20.

31. R A Marley, B M Moline, "Patient discharge issues," in *Ambulatory Surgical Nursing*, second ed, N Burden, ed (Philadelphia: WB Saunders Co, 2000) 504-526.

32. "Surgical care," in *Guidelines for Optimal Ambulatory Surgical Care and Office-Based Surgery* (Chicago: American College of Surgeons, 2000) 14-20.

33. "Criteria for initial, ongoing, and discharge assessment and management," in *Standards of PeriAnesthesia Nursing Practice* (Cherry Hill, NJ: American Society of PeriAnesthesia Nurses, 2004) 27-31.

34. R A Marley, J Swanson, "Patient care after discharge from the ambulatory surgical center," *Journal of Perianesthesia Nursing* 16 (December 2001) 399-417.

35. R M Tappen, J Muzic, P Kennedy, "Preoperative assessment and discharge planning for older adults undergoing ambulatory surgery," *AORN Journal* 73 (February 2001) 464-474.

36. "Resource 4: Criteria for initial, ongoing, and discharge assessment and management," in *Standards of Perianesthesia Nursing Practice* (Cherry Hill, NJ: American Society for PeriAnesthesia Nurses, 2002) 27-30.

37. "The postop phone call: An effective tool?" *OR Manager* 19 (January 2003) 25-27.

38. K Heseltine, F Edlington, "A day surgery postoperative telephone call line," *Nursing Standard* 13 (November 1998) 39-43.

39. S Barnes, "Not a social event: The follow-up phone call," *Journal of Perianesthesia Nursing* 15 (August 2000) 253-255.

40. M C Redmond, "Extensions of care: Phase III recovery," in *Ambulatory Surgical Nursing*, second ed, N Burden, ed (Philadelphia: WB Saunders Co, 2000) 527-249.

41. "Improving Organizational Performance," in *2004 Comprehensive Accreditation Manual for Ambulatory Care* (Oakbrook Terrace, Ill: Joint Commission on Accreditation of Healthcare Organizations, 2004) P16.

PUBLICATION HISTORY

Originally published in *Standards, Recommended Practices, and Guidelines*, 2005 edition. Reprinted April 2005, *AORN Journal*.

AORN Guidance Statement: Preoperative Patient Care in the Ambulatory Surgery Setting

Introduction

The purpose of this guidance statement is to provide a framework that health care practitioners can use to develop and implement policies and procedures for preoperative patient care in the ambulatory surgery setting. This guidance statement is directed specifically to ambulatory surgery centers (ASCs). It also may be used in other ambulatory settings that perform surgery or other invasive procedures. The ambulatory surgical setting is defined as an area in which outpatient surgery or other invasive procedures are performed, including, but not limited to, freestanding surgery centers, hospital-based ambulatory surgery units, physicians' offices, cardiac catheterization suites, endoscopy units, and radiology departments.

Perioperative nurses have limited contact with patients before surgery, which may lead to an increased risk for adverse patient outcomes. Ambulatory surgery centers must have consistent approaches to preoperative patient care to ensure patient safety. This guidance statement is intended to promote patient safety in the ambulatory surgery setting.

Guidance Statement

Ambulatory surgery centers should develop written policies and procedures for preoperative patient care. Policies and procedures should include, but not be limited to, the following elements:

- staffing,
- preadmission assessment,
- preadmission testing,
- anesthesia evaluation,
- preoperative teaching,
- preoperative nursing assessment,
- documentation of the preoperative nursing assessment,
- fast tracking of patients,
- prevention of postoperative infections, and
- monitoring of outcomes.

The criteria in this guidance statement represent the minimum levels of care.

Perioperative Nursing Data Set

The Perioperative Nursing Data Set (PNDS) is a clinically relevant and empirically validated standardized nursing vocabulary describing perioperative nursing. It relates to the delivery of care in all perioperative settings. This standardized language consists of a collection of data elements and includes perioperative nursing diagnoses, interventions, and outcomes. The PNDS should be used to develop ambulatory surgery patient plans of care and to standardize nursing documentation. In addition, PNDS outcomes, as well as outcome indicators, interventions, and nursing diagnoses, can be

- incorporated into competencies, policies and procedures, job descriptions, pathways, guidelines, and care plans;
- linked to the electronic health record;
- used as a tool for teaching new nurses about perioperative nursing; and
- applied in performance improvement projects and benchmarking.

Each data element in the PNDS corresponds to a unique identifier. The domains are represented by the letter "D," followed by numbers 1 to 3 to indicate the particular domain being addressed. Nursing diagnoses are represented by the letter "X" and a number unique to the diagnosis. Interventions are represented by the letter "I" and a unique number, and outcomes are represented by the letter "O" and a unique number. These designations are identified in this document with unique identifiers noted in parentheses. A list of outcomes, interventions, and nursing diagnoses specific to each domain is printed in an appendix of the PNDS reference book.[1]

The PNDS is conceptualized by the perioperative patient focused model. The patient and his or her family members are at the center of the model's framework. The model depicts perioperative nursing in four domains and illustrates the relationship between the patient, family members, and the care provided by the perioperative RN. The patient-centered domains are

- D1—patient safety;
- D2—physiological responses to surgery; and
- D3—patient and family member behavioral responses to surgery, including
  - behavior responses—knowledge, and
  - behavior responses—rights and ethics.[1]

Nursing Care Policies

Preoperative nursing care policies and procedures should be available in the preoperative care unit.[2] At a minimum, each nurse should review these policies and procedures periodically, and the review process should be documented. Specific criteria for the preoperative care policies and procedures should include

- assessment of data elements;
- preoperative patient care;
- supplies and equipment;
- emergency medications[3] and equipment;
- fast tracking of perioperative patients;
- infection control (O10);
- pain management (O29), patient knowledge of pain, and pain control (O20); and
- documentation of care.

Staffing

A staffing plan should be developed and used to provide an adequate number and mix of personnel to meet patient care needs.[4-6] An adequate number of RNs should be available to provide patient assessments. The staffing plan for the preoperative area should include criteria regarding the number of patients; number of ORs and procedure rooms; types of procedures scheduled; medications to be administered; types of patients (eg, elderly, pediatric); average patient preparation time; preoperative procedures (eg, insertion of invasive lines, radiological studies, regional blocks); patient acuity; and intensity of care.[4,7] Licensed practical nurses (LPNs) and unlicensed assistive personnel (UAP) may be included in preoperative staffing plans. Unlicensed assistive personnel may be assigned to assist with delegated patient care tasks as determined by the RN and according to federal, state, and local regulations.[8] All personnel should be qualified and competent according to state licensure requirements, accreditation and professional standards, procedure-specific training, and experience.[5,9] Personnel should be trained in the use of emergency equipment and cardiopulmonary resuscitation for both adult and pediatric patients if pediatric care is provided.[5] Basic life support training is recommended for all nurses in the preoperative care unit. All staff members should undergo a comprehensive orientation program, and competencies should be documented.

Preadmission Assessment

Specific admission criteria and guidelines should be identified for all perianesthesia care settings, and patients should meet the admission criteria.[10] The perioperative RN should ensure all admissions are

identified as appropriate and evaluated based on written guidelines for preadmission.[10-13]

Preadmission telephone calls or face-to-face interviews should be conducted by a professional RN.[13,14] Pre-established admission criteria should be used to identify patients who need a face-to-face interview versus those who can be interviewed by telephone.

Preadmission nursing assessment criteria should determine preoperative status.[13] The assessment should include, but should not be limited to, the following:

- appropriate baseline physical assessment (I59) (I144);
- allergies and sensitivities (I123);
- signs of abuse or neglect (I113);[15]
- cultural, emotional, and socioeconomic assessment (I57) (I68);
- comprehensive pain assessment (I16) (I17);
- medication history, including nonprescription medications, illicit drugs, and herbal medications and supplements (I30);[16,17]
- anesthetic history;[18]
- results of radiological examinations and other preoperative testing (I30) (I111);
- discharge planning (I30) (I80);
- referrals (I63) (I92);
- identification of physical alterations that require additional equipment or supplies (I64);
- preoperative patient teaching (I135) (eg, medications to be taken or held before surgery, preoperative shower, NPO requirements [I107]);[13,19]
- informed consent and/or knowledge of planned procedure (I32);
- advance directive review (I97) (I103);[20]
- development of a care plan (I30); and
- documentation and communication of all information per facility policy (I27) (I92).[6,12]

Preoperative Testing

Policies and procedures that include criteria for preoperative testing should be developed by each ASC and approved by the appropriate medical staff members. The requested preoperative tests should be based on the patient's clinical conditions.[18,21] The criteria also should identify requirements for medical history and physical examination and documentation of such.[16]

A medical history and physical examination should be conducted before a surgical or invasive procedure and documented on the patient's medical record.[6] The history and physical should be reviewed immediately before surgery, and any changes to the patient's condition should be documented. Facility policy should be congruent with regulation and accreditation agency requirements.

Diagnostic testing to determine the patient's health care needs should be performed in a timely manner as defined by the health care organization.[10] Special screening may be needed for high-risk patients with certain conditions (eg, cardiac disease, obesity, sleep apnea).[22] Specific studies may be conducted for special categories of surgical procedures or type of anesthesia. Findings from the history, physical examination, and designated studies must be documented in the patient's medical record before anesthesia is administered or surgery is performed.[22,23]

Anesthesia Evaluation

An appropriate preanesthesia evaluation and assessment should be conducted by an anesthesia care provider before induction of anesthesia and surgery for patients receiving any type or level of anesthesia.[16,18,24] A preanesthesia assessment must be conducted for each patient to determine whether he or she is an appropriate candidate for moderate or deep sedation or anesthesia. A preanesthesia evaluation may not be required when the patient is only receiving local anesthesia. A patient receiving only local anesthesia may require a preanesthesia evaluation if the patient has significant comorbidities (eg, morbid obesity).

The assessment should include past and present medical and medication history, previous anesthesia experiences, evidence of a patient physical status assessment, American Society of Anesthesiologists physical status classification, results of relevant diagnostic studies, and the planned choice of anesthesia.[16] An anesthesia plan should be developed based on this information.[18]

Preoperative Teaching

A preoperative teaching plan should be developed for each patient. The teaching plan should include preoperative instructions[18] and patient preparation. The plan should address acceptable NPO requirements before surgery; preoperative showers or medications, when ordered; and physical, emotional, social, and procedural issues.[13,19,25,26] The teaching plan should describe perioperative routine care (I56), as well as the preparation phase; length of time in each phase of the perioperative

period; other care providers; use of preoperative medications; management of postoperative pain and nausea; fast tracking, if applicable; discharge criteria; and continuum of care services.[13,27] Preoperative teaching should include the patient's family members or guardian (I79).

Preoperative Nursing Assessment

A perioperative RN should conduct a preoperative nursing assessment on the day of surgery. Perioperative nurses assess, document, and communicate patient status to all members of the health care team. Data collection involves the patient and his or her significant others or guardians. On the day of surgery, the perioperative RN should verify the information obtained during the preadmission assessment. The RN is responsible for ensuring that the preoperative assessment is complete and the patient's emotional needs are met.[13] Assessments for special populations, such as pediatric patients, older adult patients,[27] high-risk patients,[22] and patients with special needs,[13] may require additional preparation.

A preoperative assessment should be completed on admission. Interventions relating to the assessment may include, but are not limited to,

♦ verification of the patient's identity using two identifiers (I26) (eg, patient's name, date of birth, social security number, an assigned identification number)—neither identifier should be the patient's location or diagnosis.[28]
♦ review of preadmission assessment;
♦ appropriate baseline physical assessment (I59) (I144) (I60) (I64) (I66);
♦ review of preoperative status (I27) (I66);
♦ review of medications, including nonprescription medications, illicit drugs, and herbal medications and supplements (I30);
♦ allergies and sensitivities (I123);
♦ NPO status (I107);[22]
♦ hypothermia assessment and management (I131);[29]
♦ pain scale assessment (I16);[30,31]
♦ relevant preoperative needs of the patient and family members (I57) (I63) (I79);
♦ advance directives (I103) (I97);
♦ identification of planned procedure by the patient or his or her significant other or guardian (I32);
♦ verification of surgical site, side, or level, as applicable (I143);[6,17,32]

- prescribed surgical preparation (eg, preoperative shower, enema, medication) (I30);
- prosthetic devices (eg, dentures, hearing aids, contact lenses, glasses) (I90) (I127);
- implantable electronic devices (eg, pacemakers [I58], brain stimulators, pain pumps);
- availability of safe transportation home and aftercare (I35);
- contact information for the patient's support person (I109);
- understanding of preoperative teaching and discharge planning (I135) (I136) (I137) (I62);[16] and
- documentation of information per facility policy (I27) (I92).

A nursing care plan should be based on the patient assessment and documented appropriately. The perioperative RN analyzes the assessment data to determine nursing diagnoses. Following is a partial list of nursing diagnoses that may be associated with patients undergoing ambulatory surgery.

- X30 (D3)—knowledge deficit;
- X34 (D1)—physical mobility, impaired;
- X4 (D3)—anxiety;
- X28 (D2)—infection, risk for;
- X20 (D2)—fluid volume, risk for imbalance—related to altered nutritional state; and
- X26 (D2)—hypothermia.[1]

Preoperative Patient Outcomes

Nursing interventions are initiated to achieve a desired conclusion and/or to reduce the probability of undesired outcomes.[1,33] Following is a partial list of patient outcomes that may be associated with a patient's perioperative experience:

- (O22)—the patient demonstrates knowledge of wound healing;
- (O25)—the patient's right to privacy is maintained;
- (O20)—the patient demonstrates knowledge of pain management.[1]

Communication of the Preoperative Nursing Assessment

Policies and procedures should be written for communicating to the appropriate surgical team members any changes in the patient's status noted during the preadmission interview and assessment. A process should be developed for reporting and acting on abnormal findings (I27) (I30).

Prevention of Postoperative Infections

Prevention of postoperative infection begins in the preoperative period. Outcome O10 states, "the patient is free from signs and symptoms of infection."[1] Policies and procedures for reducing the risk of postoperative infection should be written and followed.[34,35] Prophylactic antibiotics should be considered and used according to the published guidelines, which include, at a minimum, the following elements (I10):[36]

- surgical procedures for which prophylactic antibiotics are recommended;
- the selection of appropriate medications;
- the timing of administering medications;
- the route of administration; and
- the personnel responsible for procuring, preparing, and administering the medication.[37]

Depending on the type of prophylactic medication used, administration should occur between 30 minutes and one hour before incision.[37,38]

Body temperature should be monitored and maintained as close to normothermia as possible during the preoperative period (I86) (I78) (I55).[39] Hypothermia may delay healing and predispose patients to wound infections.[40]

Documentation

Policies and procedures for documenting preoperative patient information should be established. Nursing documentation should incorporate the PNDS.[1] A preadmission checklist should be implemented to ensure all required patient-specific information is documented properly. Documentation requirements include, but are not limited to,

- a preadmission patient survey;
- a preoperative nursing assessment;
- signed consents for surgery and anesthesia (I124);
- written permission to leave postoperative follow-up telephone messages by voice mail or with a designated individual in keeping with the Health Insurance Portability and Accountability Act privacy guidelines (I151);
- history and physical in the patient's medical record;
- test results;
- preanesthesia assessment;
- pain scale assessment (I16);[30,31]
- identified possible risks, such as the potential for malignant hyperthermia or latex allergy (I123);[13]

- surgical procedure and site verification (I26) (I143);[32]
- advance directives (I103); and
- documentation of education and instructions provided (O31) (I27).

Monitoring of Outcomes

The facility should collect data to monitor its performance.[41] Data collected should include patients' perceptions of care, treatment, and provision of services, including specific individual needs and expectations, how well the facility met those needs, surgical site infections, how the facility can improve patient safety, and the effectiveness of pain management, when applicable.[41]

REFERENCES

1. *Perioperative Nursing Data Set: The Perioperative Nursing Vocabulary*, second ed, S Beyea, ed (Denver: AORN, Inc, 2002).

2. R Ferrara-Love, "Immediate postanesthesia care," in *Ambulatory Surgical Nursing*, second ed, N Burden, ed (Philadelphia: WB Saunders Co, 2000) 409-476.

3. S Smith, "Progressive postanesthesia care: Phase II recovery," in *Ambulatory Surgical Nursing*, second ed, N Burden, ed (Philadelphia: WB Saunders Co, 2000) 477-503.

4. "Standard III: Staffing and personnel management," in *Standards of Perianesthesia Nursing Practice* (Cherry Hill, NJ: American Society of PeriAnesthesia Nurses, 2004) 14.

5. "Management of human resources," in *2004 Comprehensive Accreditation Manual for Ambulatory Care* (Oakbrook Terrace, Ill: Joint Commission on Accreditation of Healthcare Organizations, 2004) HR1-HR12.

6. "Surgical and related services," in *Accreditation Guidebook for Office Based Surgery* (Wilmette, Ill: Accreditation Association for Ambulatory Health Care, 2004) 47-52.

7. "Resource 3, patient classification/recommended staffing guidelines," in *Standards of Perianesthesia Nursing Practice* (Cherry Hill, NJ: American Society of PeriAnesthesia Nurses, 2004) 25-26.

8. "AORN official statement on unlicensed assistive personnel," in *Standards, Recommended Practices, and Guidelines* (Denver: AORN, Inc, 2004) 167-168.

9. "Quality of care provided," in *Accreditation Guidebook for Office Based Surgery* (Wilmette, Ill: Accreditation Association for Ambulatory Health Care, 2004) 19-21.

10. "Provision of care, treatment, and services," in *2004 Comprehensive Accreditation Manual for Ambulatory Care* (Oakbrook Terrace, Ill: Joint Commission on Accreditation of Healthcare Organizations, 2004) PC1-PC50.

11. "Standard VI: Assessment," in *Standards of Perianesthesia Nursing Practice* (Cherry Hill, NJ: American Society of PeriAnesthesia Nurses, 2002) 17.

12. "Resource 4: Criteria for initial, ongoing, and discharge assessment and management," in *Standards of Perianesthesia Nursing Practice* (Cherry Hill, NJ: American Society for PeriAnesthesia Nurses, 2002) 27-30.

13. G D Williams, "Preoperative preparation of the ambulatory surgery patient," in *Ambulatory Surgical Nursing*, second ed, N Burden, ed (Philadelphia: WB Saunders Co, 2000) 346-362.

14. D Dunn, "Preoperative assessment criteria and patient teaching for ambulatory surgery patients," *Journal of PeriAnesthesia Nursing* 13 (October 1998) 274-291.

15. "Provision of care, treatment, and services" in *2004 Comprehensive Accreditation Manual for Ambulatory Care* (Oakbrook Terrace, Ill: Joint Commission on Accreditation of Healthcare Organizations, 2004) PC.3.10.

16. R E Grundman, "Preoperative patient care," in *Ambulatory Surgery Principles and Practices*, third ed, N J Vinson, ed (Denver: AORN, Inc, 2003) 109-124.

17. "What's being done to make ambulatory surgery safer?" *OR Manager* 19 (March 2003) 30-35.

18. "Guidelines for ambulatory anesthesia and surgery," American Society of Anesthesiology, http://www.asahq.org/publicationsAndServices/standards/04.pdf (accessed 29 Sept 2004).

19. P Patterson, "NPO status: Have ASCs changed policies?" *OR Manager* 17 (March 2001) 25-27.

20. "Be proactive on advance directives," *OR Manager* 17 (June 2001) 25-26.

21. J M Mathias, "Assess first, test later, centers say," *OR Manager* 17 (May 2001) 26-28.

22. B A Scales, "Screening high-risk patients for the ambulatory setting," *Journal of Perianesthesia Nursing* 18 (October 2003) 307-316.

23. "Clinical records and health information," in *Accreditation Guidebook for Office Based Surgery* (Wilmette, Ill: Accreditation Association for Ambulatory Health Care, 2004) 29-31.

24. "Anesthesia services," in *Accreditation Guidebook for Office Based Surgery* (Wilmette, Ill: Accreditation Association for Ambulatory Health Care, 2004) 41-45.

25. M J Bernier et al, "Preoperative teaching received and valued in a day surgery setting," *AORN Journal* 77 (March 2003) 563-582.

26. "Practice guidelines for preoperative fasting and the use of pharmacologic agents to reduce the risk of pulmonary aspiration: Application to healthy patients undergoing elective procedures," American Society of Anesthesiologists, http://www.asahq.org/publications AndServices/NPO.pdf (accessed 16 April 2004).

27. R M Tappen, J Muzic, P Kennedy, "Preoperative assessment and discharge planning for older adults undergoing ambulatory surgery," (Elder Care) *AORN Journal* 73 (February 2001) 464-474.

28. "2005 National Patient Safety Goals FAQs," Joint Commission on Accreditation of Healthcare Organizations, http://www.jcaho.org/accredited+organizations/patient +safety/05+npsg/05_npsg_faqs.htm (accessed 1 Jan 2005)

29. M C Karlet, "Malignant hyperthermia: Considerations for ambulatory surgery," *Journal of PeriAnesthesia Nursing* 13 (October 1998) 304-312.

30. K Cunningham, "Pain management," in *Ambulatory Surgery Principles and Practices*, third ed, N J Vinson, ed (Denver: AORN, Inc, 2003) 145-149.

31. D A Krenzischek, L Wilson, "An introduction to the ASPAN pain and comfort clinical guideline," *Journal of PeriAnesthesia Nursing* 18 (August 2003) 228-236.

32. "Correct site surgery toolkit" (Denver: AORN, Inc, 2004).

33. J C Rothrock, *Perioperative Nursing Care Planning* (St Louis: Mosby, 1990) 497.

34. "Surveillance, prevention, and control of infection," in *2004 Comprehensive Accreditation Manual for Ambulatory Care* (Oakbrook Terrace, Ill: Joint Commission on Accreditation of Healthcare Organizations, 2004) IC1-IC24.

35. "Facilities and environment," in *Accreditation Guidebook for Office Based Surgery* (Wilmette, Ill: Accreditation Association for Ambulatory Health Care, 2004) 35-38.

36. "Antimicrobial prophylaxis in surgery," *The Medical Letter on Drugs and Therapeutics* 39 (Oct 24, 1997) 97-101.

37. "ASHP therapeutic guidelines on antimicrobial prophylaxis in surgery," American Society of Health-System Pharmacists, *http://www.medqic.org/cms-service/stream/asset/TK8_tagged pdf?asset_id=847853* (accessed 29 Sept 2004).

38. "Suggested recommendations and guidelines for surgical prophylaxis," Medical College of Wisconsin, *http://www.intmed.mcw.edu/drug/SurgProph.html* (accessed 29 Sept 2004).

39. "Recommended practices for safe care through identification of potential hazards in the surgical environment," in *Standards, Recommended Practices, and Guidelines* (Denver: AORN, Inc, 2004) 301-307.

40. A Kurz, D I Sessler, R Lenhardt, "Perioperative normothermia to reduce the incidence of surgical-wound infection and shorten hospitalization," *The New England Journal of Medicine* 334 (May 9, 1996) 1209-1215.

41. "Improving organizational performance," in *2004 Comprehensive Accreditation Manual for Ambulatory Care* (Oakbrook Terrace, Ill: Joint Commission on Accreditation of Healthcare Organizations, 2004) PI6.

PUBLICATION HISTORY

Originally published in *Standards, Recommended Practices, and Guidelines,* 2005 edition. Reprinted April 2005, *AORN Journal.*

AORN Guidance Statement: Safe On-Call Practices in Perioperative Practice Settings

Introduction

The purpose of this guidance statement is to assist managers and clinicians in developing policies and procedures related to safe call practices for perioperative personnel. Providing care for patients requiring urgent or emergent surgery after regular hours of operation is a reality for perioperative nurses. Perioperative personnel are assigned designated times to be available for unplanned, urgent, or emergent procedures or to provide care for patients whose procedures run over the scheduled time. These assignments are referred to as "call."

Many perioperative nurses take call after scheduled hours, on weekends, and on holidays in addition to their daily shift assignments. Call hours vary, but generally are eight to 16 hours on weekdays, 48 to 64 hours on weekends, and 72 hours or more for extended holiday weekends. Actual hours worked during the call period are unpredictable and can range from 30 minutes to the entire length of the call period. Covering call may strain existing resources, create stress for perioperative staff members, affect safe patient care, and increase the potential for occupational injury due to prolonged work hours.

Background

Traditionally, perioperative nurses have worked eight-hour shifts; however, several new trends in perioperative staffing patterns include fewer, but longer, work days in addition to a call schedule. The expansion of work hour flexibility enhances individual nurse satisfaction and accommodates the organization's objectives.[1] Although the call schedule may be assigned on a rotating basis according to patient population, organizational needs, and demographic challenges, perioperative nurses may take extra call to increase compensation (eg, elective overtime). Perioperative nurses also may be mandated to work beyond their scheduled work/call shift to augment staffing requirements, meet unexpected patient needs, or satisfy organizational expectations (eg, mandatory overtime). These new trends in staffing and call hours have converged to create potentially hazardous conditions for patient and employee safety. There is a lack of current research in trending the number of hours worked per day by nurses. Anecdotal reports suggest that perioperative staff nurses are working longer hours with fewer breaks and often have inadequate time for rest between shifts.[2] Twenty-four hour call shifts are becoming more common.[3]

Long hours and prolonged periods of wakefulness are among working conditions that may have a negative effect on human performance.[4-6] It has been reported that 17 hours without sleep can have an adverse affect on performance equivalent to a blood alcohol concentration of 0.05%.[1] At 24 hours without sleep, performance degradation is equivalent to a blood alcohol concentration of 0.10.[7]

Fatigue resulting from working long hours can have a detrimental effect on patient care. Work by Rogers et al demonstrates a link between working long hours and medical errors; the possibility of an error triples after 12.5 hours of work.[3,5] Moreover, this research identified that medication errors, procedural errors, documentation, and transcription errors occur more frequently as work hours increase.[7,8] Studies suggest a correlation between sleep deprivation and negative effects on memory, language/numeric skills, visual attention and concentration.[9-11] In addition to creating a risk to patient safety, research indicates that sleep-deprived and fatigued nurses are at increased risk for personal injury on duty and when driving home after an extended work day.[5,12,13]

The existing nursing shortage is contributing to extended work hours and call shifts for perioperative nurses. It is predicted the number of RNs will fall to 20% below the demand by 2010.[2] More than 126,000 nursing positions currently are estimated to be unfilled.[1] This increases the burden of perioperative nurse fatigue with longer working hours and extended call requirements.

Guidance Statement

Recognizing that long work hours are a growing concern among nursing organizations, regulatory agencies, patient safety organizations, and perioperative nurses, this document offers a framework from which managers and clinicians can develop and implement methodologies to safely establish a call schedule. The call staffing plan retains the perioperative RN as circulator and is consistent with established AORN recommendations for nurse:patient ratios. The call staffing plan should minimize long work hours and allow for adequate recuperation between shifts. This guidance statement may be adapted to any setting in which call schedules are required.

Ultimately, health care organizations are responsible for developing and implementing staffing policies and procedures relevant to individual practice settings. Perioperative nurse leaders should be knowledgeable about emerging research and incorporate new evidence into the development, evaluation, and revision of policies for safe staffing and on-call practices.[6] Health care facilities should develop an organizational culture that promotes and provides safeguards to protect staff members and patients from potential errors and workplace injuries.

Individual facility policy should focus on creating call schedules that consider the effect of working long hours on patient safety as well as on perioperative staff members' well-being.[5,6,14] Safe call practices should be based on the following considerations:

- the type of facility (eg, trauma center, ambulatory surgery center), patient needs, procedure mix, demographics (eg, large metropolitan, rural), and organization structure;
- staff experience, competencies, skill mix; and
- staffing minimums as defined by state regulation, accrediting organization standards, professional organization recommendations, and patient safety requirements.

Suggested Strategies

■ Address staffing limitations in facility-specific policy and procedures based on relevant fatigue-related outcomes studies.

■ Establish a guideline to promote patient and worker safety in relation to the number of hours worked in a 24-hour, seven-day period based on current research. All worked hours should be included. For example, a facility may limit all scheduled and call back hours to 60 hours in a seven-day work week.[6,7]

■ Implement recuperation periods between shifts and establish limits for perioperative call schedules within designated time frames.[5,6]
  ■ Budget enough full-time equivalents (FTEs) to allow for safe staffing levels.
  ■ The budget should include adequate replacement staff members to allow rest periods for personnel who have worked long hours.

■ Establish the number of allowed consecutive hours that may be worked. Identify when the next scheduled work shift may begin. Work hour limitations should be determined in accordance with state regulation, accrediting organization standards, professional organization recommendations, and patient safety requirements.

■ Provide education to increase awareness of perioperative staff members' personal responsibility to arrive at work fully rested.[6,7]

■ Consider call requirements for perioperative staff members based on research indicating a correlation between adverse effects of sleep deprivation and aging.[15]

■ Reduce the amount and frequency of unscheduled overtime or last-minute call assignments.

■ Evaluate economic implications of unsafe call practices in relation to workplace injuries and adverse patient outcomes.

■ Develop performance improvement activities to determine if there is a correlation between workplace injuries, errors, adverse patient outcomes, and the number of hours worked during call.

■ Involve perioperative nurses in developing call schedules and work processes.

■ Develop competency-based orientation programs for new perioperative staff members, including skill acquisition to manage urgent and emergent patient care. The orientation time frame should be determined based on the type of procedures performed and experience of perioperative staff members.

■ Establish a staffing plan to recognize and retain staff members with extended tenure.
  ■ Develop guidelines for self-assignment of call. Management should review the call schedule before posting it to ensure appropriate coverage for patient safety.
  ■ Explore fiscal and operational benefits of establishing a dedicated call team.
  ■ Consider providing sleep rooms to allow perioperative staff members the option to stay at the facility during the call shift to alleviate the potential of sleep deprivation and fatigue. A sleep room also would allow for timely response to urgent and emergent cases.

Summary

Call staffing and the associated long work hours can be challenging for both perioperative staff members and the health care organization. A change in culture is needed to recognize exhaustion as an unacceptable risk to patients and perioperative personnel safety. Perioperative health care providers have a personal responsibility to arrive at work fully rested. Health care organizations have a responsibility to create work and call schedules that consider the effect of long work hours on patient safety as well as perioperative staff members' welfare. The development of standardized safe work hours and call practices should reflect current recommendations emerging from authoritative sources, legislation, and empirical data. Prolonged work periods without adequate rest may contribute to diminished performance by perioperative personnel, placing both patients and workers at risk. This guidance statement may assist managers and clinicians in developing policies and procedures for safe call practices.

REFERENCES

1. "Keeping patients safe: Transforming the work environment of nurses," National Academies Press, *http://www.nap.edu/openbook/0309090679/html/1.html* (accessed 13 Dec 2004).

2. A Page, "Appendix C: Work hour regulation in safety-sensitive industries," in *Keeping Patients Safe: Transforming the Work Environment of Nurses* (Washington, DC: National Academies Press, 2004) 384-435.

3. A E Rogers et al, "The working hours of hospital staff nurses and patient safety," *Health Affairs* 23 (July/August 2004) 202-212.

4. "The effect of health care working conditions on patient safety," *Evidence Report: Technology Assessment* 74 (March 2003) 1-3.

5. M R Rosekind et al, "Managing fatigue in operational settings 1: Physiological considerations and countermeasures," *Hospital Topics* 75 (Summer 1997) 23-30.

6. M Rosekind et al, "Managing fatigue in operational settings 2: An integrated approach," *Hospital Topics* 75 (Summer 1997) 31-35.

7. D M Gaba, S K Howard, "Patient safety: Fatigue among clinicians and the safety of patients," *The New England Journal of Medicine* 347 (Oct 17, 2002) 1249-1255.

8. *Long Working Hours for Nurses Lead to Medical Errors* (news release, Bethesda, Md: Health Affairs, July 7, 2004) 1. Also available at *http://www.rwjf.org/news/newsRelease070604.pdf* (accessed 13 Dec 2004).

9. R P Hart et al, "Effect of sleep deprivation on first-year residents' response times, memory, and mood," *Journal of Medical Education* 62 (November 1987) 940-942.

10. R Rubin et al, "Neurobehavioral effects of the on-call experience in housestaff physicians," *Journal of Occupational Medicine* 33 (January 1991) 13-18.

11. J Robbins, F Gottlieb, "Sleep deprivation and cognitive testing in internal medicine house staff," *Western Journal of Medicine* 152 (January 1990) 82-86.

12. A Gurjala et al "Petition to the Occupational Safety and Health Administration requesting that limits be placed on hours worked by medical residents (HRG publication #1570)," (30 April 2001) Public Citizen, *http://www.citizen.org/publications/release.cfm?ID=6771* (accessed 10 Dec 2004).

13. R G Hughes, A E Rogers, "Are you tired?" *American Journal of Nursing* 104 (March 2004) 36-38.

14. M L Parsons, J Stonestreet, "Staff nurse retention: Laying the groundwork by listening," *Nursing Leadership Forum* 8 (Spring 2004) 107-113.

15. K Reid, D Dawson, "Comparing performance on a simulated 12 hour shift rotation in young and older subjects," *Occupational and Environmental Medicine* 58 (January 2001) 58-62.

RESOURCES

Beck, S M; Wood, D S. "Helping OR staff members cope with the anxiety of being on call," *Surgical Services Management* 3 (November 1997) 39-42.

Dexter, F; O'Neal, L. "Weekend operating room on call staffing requirements," *AORN Journal* 74 (November 2001) 664-671.

Lamberg, L. "Impact of long working hours explored," *JAMA* 292 (July 7, 2004) 25-26.

Lucas, C E, et al. "Mathematical modeling to define optimum operating room staffing needs for trauma centers," *JAMA* 192 (May 2001) 559-565.

Tucker, J B, et al. "Using queuing theory to determine operating room staffing needs," *Trauma Injury, Infection, and Critical Care* 46 (January 1999) 71-79.

Tucker, P. "The impact of rest breaks upon accident risk, fatigue and performance: a review," *Work and Stress* 17 (April 2003) 123-137.

PUBLICATION HISTORY

Originally published in *Standards, Recommended Practices, and Guidelines,* 2005 edition. Reprinted May 2005, *AORN Journal.*

AORN Perioperative Standards and Recommended Practices, 2012 Edition

AORN Guidance Statement: Safe Patient Handling and Movement in the Perioperative Setting

Editor's note: *Ergonomic Tool #3 and related text in this guidance statement were updated in September 2011 to reflect the revised Ergonomic Tool #3 published in the* AORN Journal *(May 2011, Vol 93, No 5, page 591).*

Description of the Problem

Perioperative registered nurses and the perioperative team are routinely faced with a wide array of occupational hazards in the perioperative setting that place them at risk for work-related musculoskeletal disorders.[1-3] Musculoskeletal disorders are injuries or disorders of the muscles, nerves, tendons, joints, cartilage, or spinal discs associated with actions such as overexertion, repetitive motion, and bodily reaction.[4,5] The US Department of Labor does not include injuries caused by slips, trips, falls, motor vehicle accidents, or similar accidents in their definition of musculoskeletal disorders.[4] Musculoskeletal disorders are one of the most frequently occurring and costly types of occupational issues affecting nurses.[2,6,7] More than a third (ie, 36%) of the musculoskeletal injuries that nurses reported requiring time away from work were back injuries.[8] Among the nurses working in the private sector, nearly 9,000 had back injuries.[8,9] One study revealed that 12% of nurses planning to leave the profession indicated that back injuries were either a primary or contributing factor to their decision.[10] While back injuries are one of the most common occupational injuries in the health care industry, injuries of the shoulder and neck were more likely to prevent nurses from performing their work than low back pain.[10-13] The US Department of Health and Human Services report on nursing identified concern for personal safety in the health care environment as the reason given by 18.3% of nurses for leaving the profession.[14]

When the worker's physical ability, task, workplace environment, and workplace culture are not compatible, there is an increased risk of a musculoskeletal disorder.[1,2,15] The connection between physical risk factors and musculoskeletal disorders is greater when exposures are intense and prolonged and when several occupational risk factors are present at the same time.[16] Examples of physical stressors encountered in health care include

- forceful tasks,
- repetitive motion,
- awkward posture,
- static posture,
- moving or lifting patients and equipment,
- carrying heavy instruments and equipment, and
- overexertion.[1-3,11,12,14,17-26]

The perioperative setting poses unique challenges related to the provision of patient care and completion of procedure-related tasks. This highly technical environment is equipment intensive and necessitates the lifting and moving of heavy supplies and equipment during the perioperative team member's work period. Many of the patients having surgical or other invasive procedures are completely or partially dependent on the caregivers due to the effects of general or regional anesthesia or sedation. Patients who are unconscious cannot move, sense discomfort, or feel pain, and they must be protected from injury. This may require the perioperative team to manually lift the patient or the patient's extremities several times during a procedure. The following are among the high-risk tasks specific to perioperative nurses identified that will be addressed in the following discussion of ergonomic tools:

- transferring patients on and off OR beds,[2]
- repositioning patients in the OR bed,[2]
- lifting and holding the patient's extremities,[2]
- standing for long periods of time,[2]
- holding retractors for long periods of time,[2]
- lifting and moving equipment,[2] and
- sustaining awkward positions.

Transferring, lifting, and handling patients has been identified as the most frequent precipitating trigger of back and shoulder problems in nurses.[2,27] Certain patient handling tasks (eg, patient transfers) have been identified as high risk for musculoskeletal injuries to health care workers.[27] Lifting and moving patients is a frequent activity in the perioperative setting; for example, caregivers transfer patients to and from transport carts (eg, stretchers) and the OR bed many times during a typical work shift.

Health care providers often reposition patients once they are on the OR bed to provide appropriate exposure of the surgical site. This high-risk activity requires team members to physically lift and maneuver the patient or a patient's extremity while simultaneously placing a positioning device. The patient's weight may not be evenly distributed; the extremity's mass may be bulky and asymmetric, and it may be difficult to hold the extremity close to the health care provider's body during positioning maneuvers.[28] Additionally, concern for the patient's airway, maintaining his or her body alignment, and supporting the extremities may make it difficult for team members to position themselves in an ergonomically safe position, thus exacerbating physical demands.

Several unique aspects of high-risk patient handling tasks associated with prepping a patient's limb have been identified.[29] Preparing an extremity for surgery generally requires it to be elevated to allow complete circumferential skin preparation. The limb can be suspended by a person holding the limb or by placing the limb in a holding device. In some instances, the limb may be held manually during the entire skin prep while a second person performs the skin prep. The person performing the skin prep may also hold the limb if the limb is small or if only the distal portion needs to be prepped. To maintain asepsis, the person lifting the extremity is forced to hold the limb extended away from his or her body. The size of the limb, length of prep time, posture necessary to hold the extremity, and the physical capability of the person holding the limb all contribute to the ability of the caregiver to safely suspend the limb for the required prep. The following questions should be considered when determining how to safely raise and hold a limb.

- Does the limb need to be raised for the entire surgical skin prep?
- Does the limb need to be lifted by scrubbed or unscrubbed personnel?
- Is the person holding the limb strong enough to perform the task?
- Is there an alternative practice that can be adopted?
- Is there equipment that could be used to support the task?
- Is it possible to hold a heavy limb safely without risk of injury to the nurse or the patient?[29]

Perioperative registered nurses are prone to pain and fatigue from static posture during surgical procedures. The entire perioperative team spends a significant amount of time on their feet during the course of a shift; however, sterile perioperative team members may be required to stand for much longer periods of time. The sterile team members must maintain the integrity of the sterile field, which precludes them from changing levels. They should not alternate between sitting in a chair that is lower than the sterile field and a standing position. Acute and chronic back, leg, and foot pain are frequent complaints resulting from standing in one place for long periods of time. The following factors should be considered during surgical or other invasive procedures. Are the sterile members of the team

- at the appropriate height for the level of the OR bed?
- adopting awkward positions to work effectively?

- positioned in close proximity to the patient to perform required tasks?
- stretching and relaxing muscles regularly?[29]

Perioperative nurses and other perioperative personnel are frequently required to push or pull heavy equipment (eg, OR beds, portable microscopes, video carts). This equipment is very expensive and often must be shared between several individual operating rooms. Unoccupied OR beds are very heavy and difficult to move. Moving an occupied OR bed is not recommended because the risk of injury increases for both the worker and the patient.

Perioperative personnel and central processing personnel are frequently required to carry sets of surgical instruments. Instrument set weights vary and may weigh as much as 40 pounds. Instrument trays are wrapped with impervious nonwoven material or contained in a ridged container system. Both packaging methods can present lifting and carrying problems. Wrapped instrument sets that are too heavy may pose an additional problem because they have no handles and are awkward to carry. Rigid container systems often have handles that make carrying easier, but the weight of the container itself adds to the total weight of a full tray. In an effort to keep costs down and conserve storage space, instrument trays may be inappropriately prepared and too heavy to lift or carry safely. Instrument sets that are flash sterilized require staff members to aseptically remove the hot trays from the sterilizer. The weight of these trays and the height of the person removing them from the sterilizer in relation to the height of the sterilizer chamber contribute to the degree of risk to that individual.

The consequences of musculoskeletal disorders are severe. Employees who experience pain and fatigue are less productive and attentive, more prone to make mistakes, more susceptible to further injury, and may be more likely to affect the health and safety of others. Nurses suffering from disabling back injuries or the fear of getting injured have contributed to the number of nurses leaving the profession, thus increasing the nursing shortage. Workplaces with high incidences of musculoskeletal disorders report increases in lost or modified workdays, higher staff member turnover, increased costs, and adverse patient outcomes.[14,29,30]

Description of the Process

The 2005–2006 Workplace Safety Task Force was charged by AORN President Sharon McNamara, RN, MS, CNOR, to prepare a guidance document for ergonomically healthy workplaces. In addition, the task force was charged with forming a collaborative arrangement with the National Institute for Occupational Safety and Health (NIOSH) and the American Nurses Association (ANA) to work together to discuss, design, and advance the agenda of healthy work sites for perioperative professionals, to include ergonomic safety. This document was developed by AORN with the assistance of a panel of experts from the Patient Safety Center of Inquiry, Tampa, Fla; the James A. Haley Veterans Administration Medical Center (VMAC); the NIOSH Division of Applied Research and Technology Human Factors and Ergonomics Research Team; and ANA.

Members of the task force examined current research, literature, and patient care practices to evaluate and make recommendations to promote patient and caregiver safety when performing activities in a perioperative setting. While there are several high-risk tasks specific to perioperative nurses, the task force identified seven key activities as the starting point for developing recommendations. Some of these recommendations are based upon current technology that can be immediately implemented. Others, such as use of ceiling lifts in operating rooms, are in development or are projected patient handling innovations. This group will continue to examine what is available and encourage manufacturers to develop new and innovative technologies to achieve the optimal safety of the patient and the caregiver. Development of this equipment is critical for successful implementation of these ergonomic tools.

The ergonomic tools developed for this guidance document are based on previous work by Audrey Nelson, PhD, RN, FAAN; experts within the Veterans Administration (VA); and nationally recognized researchers.[28] The ergonomic tools for safe patient handling and movement have been designed with the goal of eradicating job-related musculoskeletal disorders in perioperative nurses. The ergonomic tools and algorithms were developed based on professional consensus and evidence from research. Plans are under way for pilot tests in several facilities.

Ergonomic Tool #1: Lateral Transfer From Stretcher To and From the OR Bed

Transferring a patient to and from the OR bed is one of the first actions of the perioperative team. The AORN "Recommended practices for positioning the patient in the perioperative practice setting" recommends that the perioperative registered nurse perform a preoperative assessment for patient-specific positioning needs.[31] Based on that assessment and using **Ergonomic Tool #1**, the patient will be transferred to and from the OR bed in an ergonomically safe manner.

Task Force Members

Andrea Baptiste, MA (OT), CIE
Ergonomist/Biomechanist
Patient Safety Center of Inquiry
James A. Haley Veterans' Hospital
Tampa, Fla

Edward Hernandez, RN, BSN
OR Nurse Manager
James A. Haley Veterans' Hospital
Tampa, Fla

Nancy Hughes, RN, MHA
Director, Center for Occupational and Environmental Health
American Nurses Association
Silver Spring, Md

Valerie Kelleher
Information Specialist
Patient Safety Center of Inquiry
James A. Haley Veterans' Hospital
Tampa, Fla

John D. Lloyd, PhD, MErgS, CPE
Director, Research Laboratories
Patient Safety Center of Inquiry
James A. Haley Veterans' Hospital
Tampa, Fla

Mary W. Matz, MSPH
VHA Patient Care Ergonomics Consultant and Industrial Hygienist
Patient Safety Center of Inquiry
James A. Haley Veterans' Hospital
Tampa, Fla

Karen Moser, RN, BSN, CNOR
Educator
William S. Middleton VA Hospital
Madison, Wis

Audrey Nelson, PhD, RN, FAAN
Director, Patient Safety Center of Inquiry
James A. Haley Veterans' Hospital
Tampa, Fla

Carol Petersen, RN, BSN, MAOM, CNOR
Perioperative Nursing Specialist
AORN, Inc
Denver, Colo

Lori Plante-Mallon, RN, CNOR
Perioperative RN
Strong Memorial Hospital
University of Rochester Medical Center
Rochester, NY

Kristy Robinson, RN, BSN, CNOR
Perioperative RN
Tampa General Hospital
Tampa, Fla

Manon Short, RPT, CEAS
Injury Prevention Coordinator
Tampa General Hospital
Tampa, Fla

Patrice Spera, RN, MS, CNOR, CRNFA
Director of Clinical Services
Tampa Bay Specialty Surgical Center
Pinellas Park, Fla

Deborah G. Spratt, RN, MPA, CNAA, CNOR
Clinical Specialist
University of Rochester Medical Center
Rochester, NY

Thomas R. Waters, PhD, CPE
Leader of the Human Factors Ergonomics Research Team
National Institute for Occupational Safety and Health
Cincinnati, Ohio

Ergonomic Tool #1

LATERAL TRANSFER FROM STRETCHER TO AND FROM THE OR BED

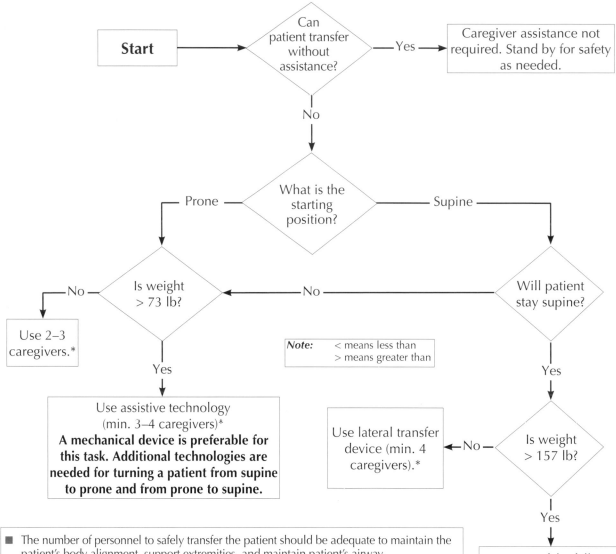

- The number of personnel to safely transfer the patient should be adequate to maintain the patient's body alignment, support extremities, and maintain patient's airway.
- For lateral transfers, it is important to use a lateral transfer device that extends the length of the patient.
- Current technologies for supine-to-prone include the Jackson frame and the spine table.
- Destination surface should be slightly lower for all lateral patient moves.
- A separate algorithm for prone-to-jackknife is not included because this is assumed to be a function of the table.
- If the patient's condition will not tolerate a lateral transfer, consider the use of a mechanical lift with a supine sling.
- During any patient transfer task, if any caregiver is required to lift more than 35 lb of a patient's weight, assistive devices should be used for the transfer.
- While some facilities may attempt to perform a lateral transfer simultaneously with positioning the patient in a lateral position (ie, side-lying), this is not recommended until new technology is available.
- The assumption is that the patient will leave the operating room in the supine position.

* One of the caregivers may be the anesthesia provider.

Supine to Prone Transfer

Assuming that one caregiver or anesthesia care provider supports the patient's head and neck during supine to prone transfers, the patient's remaining body mass equals 91.6% of his or her total body mass.[32] Using the approach for lifting and holding, a maximum two-handed load to achieve 75% US adult female design goal equals 22.2 lb (10.1 kg).* Typically one of the four caregivers moving a patient is the anesthesia care provider who maintains the airway and supports the patient's head. Two caregivers plus the anesthesia care provider can safely transfer a patient weighing up to 48.5 lb (22.0 kg) from supine to prone position. Three caregivers, plus an anesthesia care provider, can safely transfer a patient weighing up to 72.7 lb (33.0 kg). If the patient's weight is greater than 73 lb, it is necessary to use assistive technology and a minimum of three to four caregivers. Although this has been identified as a gap in technology, a mechanical device is preferable for this task and should be developed.

Supine to Supine Transfer

The desirable approach for lateral transfer of a patient involves use of a lateral transfer device (eg, friction-reducing sheets, slider board, and air-assisted transfer device). If only a draw sheet is used without a lateral transfer device, the care provider exerts a pull force up to 72.6% of the patient's weight.[33] Assuming that one caregiver or anesthesia care provider supports the patient's head and neck to maintain the airway during lateral transfers, the remaining mass of the patient's body equals 91.6% of his or her total body mass.[32] Research indicates that for a pulling distance of 6.9 ft (2.1 m) or less, where the pull point (ie, starting point for the hands) is between the caregiver's waist and nipple line, and the task is performed no more frequently than once every 30 minutes, the maximum initial force required equals 57 lb (26 kg) and the maximum sustained force needed equals 35 lb (16 kg).[34] Therefore, each caregiver can safely contribute a pull force required to transfer up to 48 lb (35 lb/0.726 as referenced above). For one caregiver, plus the anesthesia care provider, maximum patient weight equals 52.6 lb (48 lb/0.916 as referenced above). Two caregivers plus the anesthesia care provider can safely transfer a patient up to 104.8 lb (48 x 2)/0.916 as referenced above). Three caregivers plus the anesthesia care provider can safely transfer a patient up to 157.2 lb (48 x 3)/0.916 as referenced above). If the patient is > 157 lb, use an appropriate mechanical lifting device—ie, mechanical lift with supine sling, mechanical lateral transfer device, or air-assisted lateral transfer device—and a minimum of three to four caregivers.

Ergonomic Tool #2: Positioning and Repositioning the Patient on the OR Bed Into and From the Supine Position

The AORN "Recommended practices for positioning the patient in the perioperative practice setting" require that "the perioperative nurse should actively participate in monitoring patient body alignment and tissue integrity based on sound physiologic principles." It further states, "an inadequate number of personnel and equipment can result in patient injury."[31] **Ergonomic Tool #2** provides

---

*Calculation of Design Goal

To accommodate the design goal of 75% of the US adult female working population, **maximum load for a one-handed lift** is calculated to be 11.1 lb (5.0 kg), assuming a worst-case scenario where the patient load may be handled at full arm's length. This is determined by calculating the strength capabilities for the 25th percentile US adult female maximum shoulder flexion moment (25th percentile strength = 31.2 Nm, based on mean of 40 Nm and standard deviation of 13 Nm, therefore 25th percentile = 31.2 Nm)[35] and the 75th percentile US adult female shoulder to grip length (75th percentile length = 630 mm, based on mean of 610 mm and standard deviation of 30 mm).[36] Therefore, maximum one-handed lift is calculated as 31.2 Nm divided by 0.63 m, which equals 49.5 N, or 11.1 lb.

Maximum load (for one person) for a two-handed lift (22.2 lb/10.1 kg) is calculated as twice that of a one handed lift. According to Rohmert, muscle strength capabilities diminish as a function of time.[37] Therefore, maximum loads for two-handed holding of body parts are presented for one-, two-, and three-minute durations. After one minute, muscle endurance has decreased by 48%; by 65% after two minutes; and after three minutes of continuous holding, strength capability is only 29% of initial lifting strength.

Ergonomic Tool #2

POSITIONING/REPOSITIONING THE PATIENT ON THE OR BED INTO AND FROM THE SUPINE POSITION

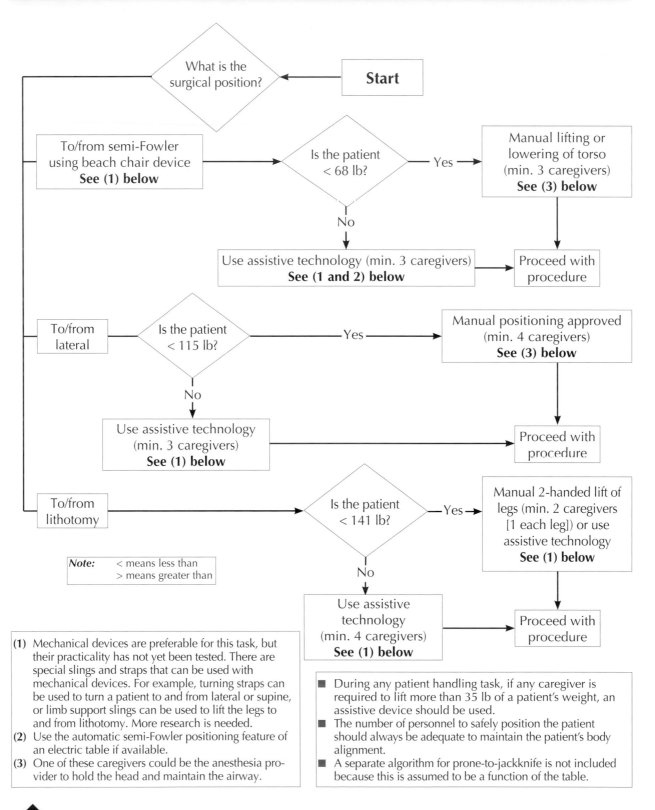

(1) Mechanical devices are preferable for this task, but their practicality has not yet been tested. There are special slings and straps that can be used with mechanical devices. For example, turning straps can be used to turn a patient to and from lateral or supine, or limb support slings can be used to lift the legs to and from lithotomy. More research is needed.

(2) Use the automatic semi-Fowler positioning feature of an electric table if available.

(3) One of these caregivers could be the anesthesia provider to hold the head and maintain the airway.

■ During any patient handling task, if any caregiver is required to lift more than 35 lb of a patient's weight, an assistive device should be used.

■ The number of personnel to safely position the patient should always be adequate to maintain the patient's body alignment.

■ A separate algorithm for prone-to-jackknife is not included because this is assumed to be a function of the table.

evidence-based guidelines to assist the perioperative registered nurse and other team members to position and reposition the patient on the OR bed in a safe manner for the patient and the team.

Moving the Patient Into and Out of a Semi-Fowler Position

The mass of a patient's body from the waist up, including the head, neck, and upper extremities, equals 68.6% of the patient's total body weight.[32] Added to this is the estimated weight of the equipment (20 lb/9.1 kg). To accommodate at least 75% of the US adult female working population, the maximum load for a two-handed lift is 22.2 lb (10.1 kg). This is determined based on 25th percentile US adult female shoulder strength capabilities[35] and 75th percentile US adult female arm length.[36] Therefore, three caregivers together could lift up to 66.6 lb (10.3 kg), which equates to a 68-lb (30.1 kg) patient.* Mechanical devices and a minimum of three caregivers are preferable if the patient weighs more than 68 lb. An example of an appropriate mechanical device is the automatic semi-Fowler positioning feature of an electric OR bed. Further research to address gaps in technology is recommended.

Positioning the Patient Into and From the Lateral Position

Positioning or repositioning a patient into or out of a lateral position involves push/pull forces rather than lifting forces. Assuming that one caregiver or anesthesia care provider supports the patient's head and neck during lateral positioning, the patient's remaining body mass equals 91.6% of total body mass.[32] Based on the Liberty Mutual tables (see **Table 3** under **Ergonomic Tool #7**) for a pulling distance of 6.9 ft (2.1 m) or less, with a pull point (ie, starting position of the hands) between the caregiver's waist height and nipple line, performed no more frequently than once every 30 minutes, maximum initial force equals 57 lb (26 kg), and maximum sustained force equals 35 lb (16 kg).[34] Therefore, two caregivers, plus an anesthesia care provider maintaining the patient's airway, can safely position a patient weighing up to 76 lb (34.5 kg) (35 lb x 2 care providers/0.916 as referenced above). Three caregivers plus an anesthesia care provider can

safely position a patient weighing up to 115 lb (52.2 kg) (35 lb x 3 care providers/0.916 as referenced above). If the patient's weight exceeds 115 lb, lateral positioning devices are needed. Further research is needed to enhance technology to address this task.

Positioning the Patient Into and From the Lithotomy Position

When lifting and holding body parts, the maximum load for a two-handed lift is 22.2 lb (10.1 kg). Each complete lower patient extremity, including thigh, calf, and foot, weighs 15.7% of the patient's total body mass. Therefore, one caregiver can safely perform this task if the patient weighs 141 lb (64.1 kg) or less because each leg is estimated to be less than 22.2 lb.[33]

Caregivers attempting to lift the patient's legs using two hands can each safely lift one leg for patients weighing less than 141 lb. Patients weighing more than 141 lb require assistive technology or four caregivers (ie, two to lift each leg). A mechanical device such as support slings can be used to lift the legs to and from the lithotomy position. Further research is needed to enhance availability of technology to address this task.

Ergonomic Tool #3: Lifting and Holding Legs, Arms, and Head for Prepping in a Perioperative Setting

Introduction

AORN's "Recommended practices for skin preparation of patients" states that "when indicated, the surgical site and surrounding area should be prepared with an antiseptic agent. The prepared area of skin and the drape fenestration should be large enough to accommodate extension of the incision, the need for additional incisions, and all potential drain sites."[38] To accomplish this task, a member of the perioperative team may need to hold the extremity so that the appropriate body part is prepared in the required manner.

Ergonomic Tool #3 shows the calculations for average weight for an adult patient's leg, arm, and head as a function of whole body mass, ranging from slim to morbidly obese body type. Weights are presented both in US (lbs) and metric (kg) units. Maximum lift and hold loads were calculated

---

*__Maximum patient weight__ = (Maximum 2-handed lift (22 lb) x 3 caregivers) − equipment weight (20 lb) = 68 lb
(68 lb) $\qquad$ Percentage of patient weight above the waist (0.686)

Ergonomic Tool #3

LIFTING AND HOLDING LEGS, ARMS, AND HEAD FOR PREPPING

Patient Weight lb (kg)	Body Part	Body Part Weight		Lift 1-hand	Lift 2-hand	Hold 2-hand ≤ 1 min	Hold 2-hand ≤ 2 min	Hold 2-hand ≤ 3 min
≤ 40 lb (≤ 18 kg)	Leg	< 6 lb	< 3 kg					
	Arm	< 2 lb	< 1 kg					
	Head	< 3 lb	< 1 kg					
40-90 lb (18-41 kg)	Leg	< 14 lb	< 6 kg	▓			▓	▓
	Arm	< 5 lb	< 2 kg					
	Head	< 8 lb	< 4 kg				▓	▓
90-140 lb (41-64 kg)	Leg	< 22 lb	< 10 kg	▓		▓	▓	▓
	Arm	< 7 lb	< 3 kg					
	Head	< 12 lb	< 6 kg	▓			▓	▓
140-190 lb (64-86 kg)	Leg	< 30 lb	< 14 kg	▓	▓	▓	▓	▓
	Arm	< 10 lb	< 4 kg					▓
	Head	< 16 lb	< 7 kg	▓		▓	▓	▓
190-240 lb (86-109 kg)	Leg	< 38 lb	< 17 kg	▓	▓	▓	▓	▓
	Arm	< 12 lb	< 6 kg	▓			▓	▓
	Head	< 20 lb	< 9 kg	▓		▓	▓	▓
240-290 lb (109-132 kg)	Leg	< 46 lb	< 21 kg	▓	▓	▓	▓	▓
	Arm	< 15 lb	< 7 kg	▓			▓	▓
	Head	< 24 lb	< 11 kg	▓	▓	▓	▓	▓
290-340 lb (132-155 kg)	Leg	< 53 lb	< 24 kg	▓	▓	▓	▓	▓
	Arm	< 17 lb	< 8 kg	▓		▓	▓	▓
	Head	< 29 lb	< 13 kg	▓	▓	▓	▓	▓
340-390 lb (155-177 kg)	Leg	< 61 lb	< 28 kg	▓	▓	▓	▓	▓
	Arm	< 20 lb	< 9 kg	▓		▓	▓	▓
	Head	< 33 lb	< 15 kg	▓	▓	▓	▓	▓
390-440 lb (177-200 kg)	Leg	< 69 lb	< 31 kg	▓	▓	▓	▓	▓
	Arm	< 22 lb	< 10 kg	▓		▓	▓	▓
	Head	< 37 lb	< 17 kg	▓	▓	▓	▓	▓
> 440 lb (> 200 kg)	Leg	> 69 lb	> 31 kg	▓	▓	▓	▓	▓
	Arm	> 22 lb	> 10 kg	▓	▓	▓	▓	▓
	Head	> 37 lb	> 17 kg	▓	▓	▓	▓	▓

No shading: OK to lift and hold; use clinical judgment and do not hold longer than noted.
Heavy shading (▓): Do not lift alone; use assistive device or more than one caregiver.

based on 75th percentile shoulder flexion strength and endurance capabilities for US adult females, where the maximum weight for a one-handed lift is 11.1 lb and a two-handed lift, 22.2 lb.

The shaded areas of the table indicate whether it would be acceptable for one caregiver to lift the listed body parts or hold the respective body parts for 0, 1, 2, or 3 minutes with one or two hands. Respecting these limits will minimize risk of muscle fatigue and the potential for musculoskeletal disorders. Perioperative registered nurses must use clinical judgment to assess the need for additional staff member assistance or assistive devices to lift and/or hold one of these body parts for a particular period of time.

Rationale and Calculations for Ergonomic Tool #3

NOTE: *These are guidelines for the average weight of the leg, arm, and head based upon the patient's*

weight. Nurses should use their clinical judgment to assess the need for additional staff member assistance or assistive devices to lift and/or hold one of these body parts for a particular period of time. The maximum weight for a one-handed lift is 11.1 lb and for a two-handed lift, 22.2 lb.

Patient weight is divided into 10 categories, ranging from very light (≤ 40 lb) to very heavy (> 440 lb). Normalized weight for each leg, each arm, and the patient's head is calculated as a percentage of total body weight, where each complete lower extremity represents 15.7% of total body mass, each upper extremity (ie, upper arm, forearm, hand) represents 5.1% of total body mass, and the combination of head and neck represents 8.4% of total body mass.[32] All weights are presented in both pounds and kilograms, rounded to the nearest whole unit.

To accommodate 75% of the US adult female working population, maximum load for a one-handed lift is calculated to be 11.1 lb (5.0 kg). This is determined by calculating the strength capabilities for 25th percentile US adult female maximum shoulder flexion moment (the mean equals 40 Newton meters; standard deviation equals 13 Nm)[35] and 75th percentile US adult female shoulder to grip length (the mean equals 610 mm, the standard deviation equals 30 mm).[36] Maximum loads for one person for a two-handed lift (ie, 22.2 lb/10.1 kg) are calculated as twice that of a one-handed lift. Muscle strength capabilities diminish as a function of time; therefore, maximum loads for two-handed holding of body parts are presented for 1, 2, and 3 minute durations.[37] After 1 minute, muscle endurance has decreased by 48%, decreasing by 65% after 2 minutes, and after 3 minutes of continuous holding, strength capability is only 29% of initial lifting strength. If the limits in **Ergonomic Tool #3** are exceeded, additional staff members or assistive limb holders should be used.

Ergonomic Tool #4: Prolonged Standing

Perioperative team members who are scrubbed or first assisting for long periods of time may be susceptible to injuries caused by static load.[39-44] Prolonged standing, trunk flexion, and neck flexion are all components of static load.[45,46] **Ergonomic Tool #4**, which appears on the following page, assists perioperative team members to take protective action to decrease the stress caused by prolonged standing.

Ergonomic Tool #5: Retraction

Sterile perioperative team members or those performing in the role of first assistant may be required to hold retractors or body parts for long periods of time, in addition to standing for long periods of time. Manual retraction used to provide exposure of the operative site for the surgeon often requires first assistants to stand in an awkward posture for long periods of time to grip and pull a retractor or to use their hands to retract or steady organs (eg, heart). The height of the surgical field in relation to the person providing retraction influences the risk for musculoskeletal injury.[47] Prolonged standing, trunk flexion, neck flexion, and arms held higher than the optimal working height place perioperative team members at risk for a musculoskeletal injury.

Ergonomic Tool #6: Lifting and Carrying Supplies and Equipment

Members of the perioperative team may need to lift and carry many different types of unsterile and sterile supplies, instrument trays, and equipment. This tool is intended to assist caregivers in evaluating these tasks and taking measures to protect themselves. Information from Association for the Advancement of Medical Instrumentation, the organization that sets standards for safety and efficacy of medical instrumentation, recommends that instrument trays weigh a maximum of 25 lb.[48]

Manual lifting and carrying of objects is physically demanding and may place the worker at substantial risk of low back pain. The NIOSH has developed an equation for calculating the recommended weight limit and lifting index for assessing the physical demands of manual lifting tasks.[49,50] A description of the NIOSH lifting equation is presented in the section entitled "Other background materials."

Typical lifting tasks performed by perioperative nurses were identified and evaluated for potential risk of low back pain due to manual lifting using the Revised NIOSH Lifting Equation (RNLE). **Ergonomic Tool #6** lists the lifting index values for these tasks. According to NIOSH, tasks with a lifting index value greater than 1.0 place some workers at risk of low back pain and a lifting index value greater than 3.0 places many workers at risk of low back pain. In a subsequent study that examined the effects of the NIOSH lifting index as a predictor, the risk of back pain increases when the lifting index exceeds 2.0.[51] As can be seen in the table, tasks with a lifting index value less than 1.0 can easily be performed

Ergonomic Tool #4

PROLONGED STANDING

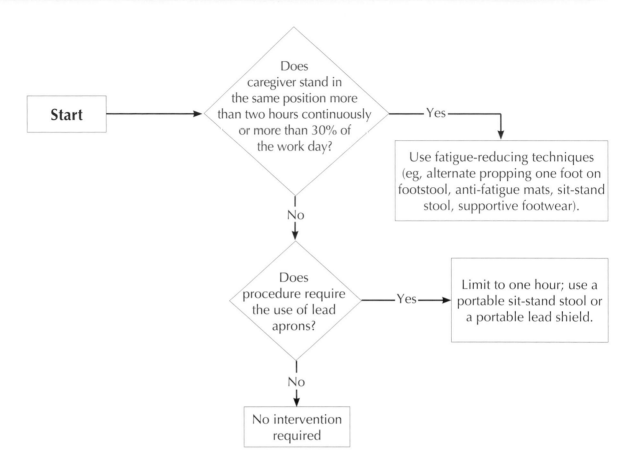

Start → Does caregiver stand in the same position more than two hours continuously or more than 30% of the work day? —Yes→ Use fatigue-reducing techniques (eg, alternate propping one foot on footstool, anti-fatigue mats, sit-stand stool, supportive footwear).

No ↓

Does procedure require the use of lead aprons? —Yes→ Limit to one hour; use a portable sit-stand stool or a portable lead shield.

No ↓

No intervention required

General recommendations

- Caregiver should wear supportive footwear that has the following properties:
  - does not change the shape of the foot;
  - has enough space to move toes;
  - shock-absorbing, cushioned insoles;
  - closed toe; and
  - height of heel in proportion to the shoe.
- Caregivers may benefit from wearing support stockings/socks.
- Anti-fatigue mats should be on the floors.
- Anti-fatigue mats should be placed on standing stools.
- The sit-stand chair should be set to the correct height before setting the sterile field so caregivers will not be changing levels during the procedure.*
- Be aware of infection control issues for nondisposable and anti-fatigue matting.
- Accommodations for pregnancy were considered, but the two-hour limit on prolonged standing covers this condition.
- Scrubbed staff should not work with the neck flexed more than 30 degrees or rotated for more than one minute uninterrupted.
- Two-piece, lightweight lead aprons are recommended.
- During the sit-to-stand break, staff should look straight ahead for a short while.

    * "Recommended practices for maintaining a sterile field," in *Standards, Recommended Practices, and Guidelines* (Denver, Colo: AORN, Inc, 2007) 665-672.

Ergonomic Tool #5

RETRACTION

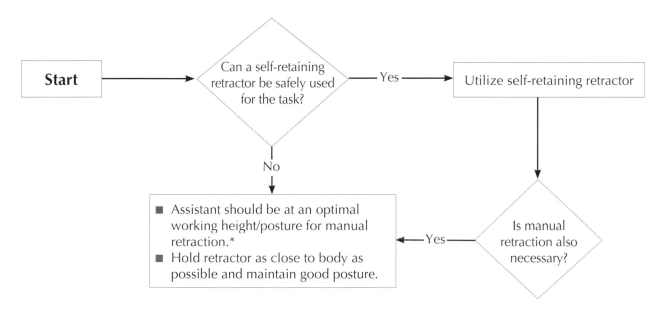

- Arm rests should be utilized as possible and be large enough to allow repositioning of the arms.
- Under optimal working height and posture, an assistive device should be used to lift or hold more than 35 lb.
- Further research is needed to determine time limits for exposure. Since this is a high-risk task, caregivers should take rest breaks or reposition when possible.
- Avoid using the hands as an approach to retraction; it is very high-risk for musculoskeletal or sharps injuries.

  * Optimal working height is defined as area between the chest and the waist height to operative field. Optimal posture is defined as perpendicular/straight-on to the operative field; asymmetrical posture may be acceptable, depending on load and duration; torso twisting should be avoided at all times.

manually. For those tasks with a lifting index value greater than 1.0, however, caution should be used. Alternate handling procedures may help reduce risk of low back pain due to lifting these objects. The list is not all inclusive; the NIOSH equation can be used to calculate a lifting index value for other two-handed manual lifting tasks not on the list.[50]

NOTE: Assistive devices include adjustable-height lift tables, rolling carts, two-wheeled carts, dollies, or mechanical transport devices.

Rationale and Calculations for Ergonomic Tool #6

A series of typical operating room lifting tasks were identified and evaluated with the NIOSH Lifting Equation (NLE) for potential risk of low back pain due to manual lifting of objects in support of patient care (see **Table 1**). The NLE is a tool for assessing

manual lifting of objects that allows the user to calculate the recommended weight limit for a specified two-handed manual lifting task. In addition, the lifting index for the task can be calculated by dividing the actual weight of the load lifted by the recommended weight limit (for details, see "Other background material").

Ergonomic Tool #7: Pushing, Pulling, and Moving Equipment on Wheels

Introduction

Case preparation is a combination of many activities. The movement of patients, supplies, and equipment in and out of the OR contributes to physical stress and should be performed based on scientific evidence. The recommendations in **Ergonomic Tool #7** are a result of research done by

Ergonomic Tool #6

NIOSH LIFTING INDEX VALUE FOR TYPICAL MANUAL LIFTING OF OBJECTS		
Lifting Task	Lifting Index	Level of Risk
3,000 mL irrigation fluid	< 0.2	
Sand bags	0.3	
Linen bags	0.4	
Lead aprons	0.4	
Custom sterile packs (eg, heart or spine)	0.5	
Garbage bags (full)	0.7	
Positioning devices off shelf or rack (eg, stirrups)	0.7	
Positioning devices off shelf or rack (eg, gel pads)	0.9	
Hand table (49" x 28"); largest hand table, used infrequently	1.2	
Fluoroscopy board (49" x 21")	1.2	
Stirrups (two—one in each hand)	1.4	
Wilson frame	1.4	
Irrigation containers for lithotripsy (12,000 mL)	1.5	
Instrument pans	2.0	

No shading   Minimal risk—Safe to lift
Light shading   Potential risk—Use assistive technology as available
Heavy shading   Considerable risk—One person should not perform alone or weight should be reduced

task force members and include some, but not all, of the necessary activities undertaken to prepare for a case.

Pushing forces were measured for equipment listed in the following table. Maximum pushing distances were determined based on Liberty Mutual's psychophysical limits. All results are presented in both US and metric units.

Based on these results, it is clear that pushing an occupied standard hospital bed or standard or specialty OR beds, whether occupied or not, presents a moderate to high risk of injury to the caregiver. For these situations it is strongly recommended that a minimum of two caregivers participate in the transport task, or ideally, that a powered transport device is used.

Recommendations

The recommendations in **Ergonomic Tool #7** are based on Liberty Mutual's psychophysical limits for push forces, where hands are positioned at a middle push point of 3 ft (0.92 m) from the floor or above and task is performed no more frequently than once every 30 minutes.[34]

- ◆ Pushing tasks are ergonomically preferred over pulling tasks.[34]
- ◆ Ensure that handles are at a correct push height of approximately 3 ft (0.92 m) from the floor.[34]
- ◆ For tasks where the push point is lower than 3 ft (0.92 m), maximum and sustained push forces will be decreased by approximately 15%.[34]
- ◆ For tasks performed more frequently than once every 30 minutes, maximum and sustained push forces will be decreased by approximately 6%.[34]
- ◆ If push force limits are exceeded it will be necessary to reduce the weight of the load, use two or more caregivers to complete the task together, or use a powered transport device.
- ◆ Equipment casters need to be properly maintained to assist in moving equipment more easily.
- ◆ For OR equipment not listed above, compare physical effort to that required to push an unoccupied standard hospital bed. If greater effort is required, then additional caregivers and/or use of powered transport device is recommended.

Table 1

		DATA USED TO CALCULATE THE NIOSH LIFTING INDEX VALUES FOR TYPICAL ITEMS LIFTED IN THE OR				
Lifting Task	**Weight**	**Horizontal Distance (inches)**	**Vertical Location-Origin (inches)**	**Vertical Location-Destination (inches)**	**Distance Carried (feet)**	**Lifting Index**
3000 cc IV bags irrigation fluids	2.5 lb	6 in	42 in	30 in	49–118 ft	< 0.2
Sand bags	10.5 lb	12 in	30 in	32 in	20 ft	0.3
Linen bags	15 lb	6 in Set = 10 in	Floor Set = 0 in	42 in	140–251 ft	0.4
Lead aprons	16 lb	13 in	36 in	36 in	N/A on cart	0.4
Custom sterile packs (heart or spine)	12.4 lb	18 in	23 in	32 in		0.5
Garbage bags (full)	23.6 lb	6 in Set = 10 in	Floor Set = 0 in	42 in	140–251 ft	0.7
Positioning devices off shelf or rack (stirrups)	17 lb each (2 stirrups would be 34 lb)	18 in	36 in	36 in		0.7
Positioning devices off shelf or rack (gel pads)	8–25 Set to 25 lb	18 in	36 in	36 in	5–10 ft	0.9
Hand table (49" x 28"); largest hand table, used infrequently	15–27 lb Set to 27 lb	20 in	43 in	32 in	49–118 ft	1.2
Fluoroscopy board (49" x 21")	26 lb	20 in	43 in	32 in	49–118 ft	1.2
Stirrups (2, one in each hand)	34 lb	18 in	36 in	36 in		1.4
Wilson frame	27 lb	32 in	31.5 in	32 in	49–118 ft	1.4
Irrigation containers for lithotripsy (12,000 mL)	0–50 lb Set to 50 lb	6 in Set = 10	63 in (top shelf)	N/A Housekeeping places in bags Set to 33 in	49–118 ft	1.5
Instrument pans	3–38 lb Set to 38 lb	19 in	6–50 in Set to 6 in	Varies Set to 34 in	5–10 ft	2.0

Ergonomic Tool #7

RECOMMENDATIONS FOR PUSHING, PULLING, AND MOVING EQUIPMENT ON WHEELS					
OR Equipment	Pushing		Max Push Distance ft/(m)		Ergonomic Recommendation
Electrosurgery unit	8.4 lbF	(3.8 kgF)	> 200 ft	(60 m)	
Ultrasound	12.4 lbF	(5.6 kgF)	> 200 ft	(60 m)	
X-ray equipment portable	12.9 lbF	(5.9 kgF)	> 200 ft	(60 m)	
Video towers	14.1 lbF	(6.4 kgF)	> 200 ft	(60 m)	
Linen cart	16.3 lbF	(7.4 kgF)	> 200 ft	(60 m)	
X-ray equipment, C-arm	19.6 lbF	(8.9 kgF)	> 200 ft	(60 m)	
Case carts, empty	24.2 lbF	(11.0 kgF)	> 200 ft	(60 m)	
OR stretcher, unoccupied	25.1 lbF	(11.4 kgF)	> 200 ft	(60 m)	
Case carts, full	26.6 lbF	(12.1 kgF)	> 200 ft	(60 m)	
Microscopes	27.5 lbF	(12.5 kgF)	> 200 ft	(60 m)	
Hospital bed, unoccupied	29.8 lbF	(13.5 kgF)	> 200 ft	(60 m)	
Specialty equipment carts	39.3 lbF	(17.9 kgF)	> 200 ft	(60 m)	
OR stretcher, occupied, 300 lb	43.8 lbF	(19.9 kgF)	> 200 ft	(60 m)	
Bed, occupied, 300 lb	50.0 lbF	(22.7 kgF)	< 200 ft	(30 m)	Min two caregivers required
Specialty OR beds, unoccupied	69.7 lbF	(31.7 kgF)	< 100 ft	(30 m)	
OR bed, unoccupied	61.3 lbF	(27.9 kgF)	< 25 ft	(7.5 m)	Recommend powered transport device
OR bed, occupied, 300 lb	112.4 lbF	(51.1 kgF)	< 25 ft	(7.5 m)	
Specialty OR beds, occupied, 300 lb	124.2 lbF	(56.5 kgF)	< 25 ft	(7.5 m)	

No shading   Minimal risk—Safe to lift
Light shading   Potential risk—Use assistive technology as available
Heavy shading   Considerable risk—One person should not perform alone or weight should be reduced

Rationale/Calculations Used for Ergonomic Tool #7

Push forces were measured in Newtons (N) for each item of equipment listed in **Table 2**. Initial forces were measured as the peak force to initially propel the item. Sustained force was measured as the minimum force required to maintain equipment propulsion. Initial-wheels turned were measured as the peak initial force where the wheels on the equipment were turned perpendicular to the desired direction of travel. The average force measured across five repeated trials for each condition and equipment item was computed and converted into US units.

Maximum pushing distances were determined and reported in **Table 2**, based on Liberty Mutual's push force limits.[34] The shortest acceptable push distance, considering both initial and sustained forces, was accepted (see **Table 3**). These values are based on the operator with his or her hands posi-

tioned at a middle push point of 3 ft (0.92 m) from the floor or above and performing a task no more frequently than once every 30 minutes.

Measuring Pushing/Pulling Forces

To measure OR equipment not listed in **Table 2**, a measuring device can be applied to measure applicable pushing/pulling forces. Commercially available measuring instruments can be used to measure push/pull forces (eg, strain gage, force meters, precision springs). A simple low-cost method for measuring the required forces for pushing or pulling objects, such as beds, carts, and transfer equipment, is shown in **Figure 1**. As illustrated, a broom handle or other lightweight cylindrical object can be taped to a bathroom scale and used to measure push forces. Required pull forces would be identical to the required pushing force. The scale is placed against the object to be pushed and a force is then

Table 2

		Trial 1 (N)	Trial 2 (N)	Trial 3 (N)	Trial 4 (N)	Trial 5 (N)	Mean (N)	Mean (lbF)	Max Push Distance (ft)
MEASURED PUSH FORCES FOR OPERATING ROOM EQUIPMENT									
Equipment	**Type of Force**								
Electrosurgical unit	initial force	30	35	35	30	30	32.0	7.2	> 200
	sustained force	10	10	10	10	10	10.0	2.2	> 200
	initial-wheels turned	40	35				37.5	8.4	> 200
OR stretcher, unoccupied	initial force	62	70	65	75		68.0	15.3	> 200
	sustained force	20	20	25	25	25	23.0	5.2	> 200
	initial-wheels turned	113	110				111.5	25.1	> 200
OR stretcher, occupied, 300 lb	initial force	120	120	120	115	120	119.0	26.8	> 200
	sustained force	30	35	30	40	40	35.0	7.9	> 200
	initial-wheels turned	210	180				195.0	43.8	< 50
Bed, unoccupied	initial force	115	120	125	110	105	115.0	25.9	> 200
	sustained force	30	25	30	25		27.5	6.2	> 200
	initial-wheels turned	130	135				132.5	29.8	> 200
Bed, occupied, 300 lb	initial force	170	160	167	135	155	157.4	35.4	> 200
	sustained force	40	50	50	40	60	48.0	10.8	> 200
	initial-wheels turned	230	215				222.5	50.0	< 25
OR bed, unoccupied	initial force	218	275	245	280	270	257.6	57.9	< 25
	sustained force	120	125	120	100	120	117.0	26.3	< 25
	initial-wheels turned	270	275				272.5	61.3	< 25
OR bed, occupied, 300 lb	initial force	425	432	445	405	325	406.4	91.4	< 25
	sustained force	180	180	180			100.0	40.5	< 25
	initial-wheels turned	485	515				500.0	112.4	< 25
Specialty OR beds, unoccupied	initial force	175	182	190	260	200	201.4	45.3	< 25
	sustained force	100	100	100			100.0	22.5	< 100
	initial-wheels turned	305	315				310.0	69.7	< 25

continued on next page

slowly applied to the handle until the object moves. The maximum required pushing force is read off the weight scale. The scale should provide a continuous readout of applied force to obtain the maximum value. To obtain the best estimate of the actual maximum force, the measurement should be repeated several times and the average value should be used for assessment. This force can then be compared to the maximum recommended push force values shown in **Table 3**. For example, assume that the force required to push a cart was measured to be 60 lb. According to **Table 3**, this task would not be acceptable for one caregiver for any distance, but would be acceptable for two caregivers (assuming each pushed 26 lb) for a distance of up to 25 feet. A powered transport device would be recommended if one caregiver is performing the task.

Other Background Materials

The Revised NIOSH Lifting Equation

The Revised NIOSH Lifting Equation (RNLE) provides a mathematical equation for determining the recommended weight limit (RWL) and lifting index (LI) for selected two-handed manual lifting tasks. The RWL is the principal product of the RNLE and is defined for a specific set of task conditions and represents the weight of the load that nearly all healthy workers could perform over a substantial period of time (eg, up to 8 hours) without an

Table 2   continued from previous page

MEASURED PUSH FORCES FOR OPERATING ROOM EQUIPMENT									
Equipment	Type of Force	Trial 1 (N)	Trial 2 (N)	Trial 3 (N)	Trial 4 (N)	Trial 5 (N)	Mean (N)	Mean (lbF)	Max Push Distance (ft)
Specialty OR beds, 300-lb patient	initial force	365	290	320	305	305	317.0	71.3	< 25
	sustained force	140	160	140	115	115	134.0	30.1	< 25
	initial-wheels turned	560	545				552.5	124.2	< 25
Microscopes	initial force	62	75	80	75	75	73.4	16.5	> 200
	sustained force	20	25	20	25	25	23.0	5.2	> 200
	initial-wheels turned	125	120				122.5	27.5	< 50
Case cart, full	initial force	62	108	75	108		88.3	19.8	> 200
	sustained force	30	40	40	40		37.5	8.4	> 200
	initial-wheels turned	122	115				118.5	26.6	> 200
Case cart, empty	initial force	60	65	65	62	65	63.4	14.3	> 200
	sustained force	40	30	35	40	35	36.0	8.1	> 200
	initial-wheels turned	120	95				107.5	24.2	> 200
X-ray equipment, C-arm	initial force	100	75	100	75	85	87.0	19.6	> 200
	sustained force	20	25	25	25	25	24.0	5.4	> 200
	initial-wheels turned	n/a	n/a				n/a	n/a	n/a
X-ray equipment, portable	initial force	60	55	55	60	58	57.6	12.9	> 200
	sustained force	25	30	30	30	30	29.0	6.5	> 200
	initial-wheels turned	n/a	n/a				n/a	n/a	n/a
Video towers	initial force	35	40	40	35	35	37.0	8.3	> 200
	sustained force	15	20	20	15	20	18.0	4.0	> 200
	initial-wheels turned	60	65				62.5	14.1	> 200
Ultrasound	initial force	35	40	45	45	40	41.0	9.2	> 200
	sustained force	20	20	25	20	20	21.0	4.7	> 200
	initial-wheels turned	55	55				55.0	12.4	> 200
Specialty equipment carts	initial force	105	90	120	125	145	117.0	26.3	> 200
	sustained force	25	30	30	25	25	27.0	6.1	> 200
	initial-wheels turned	165	185				175.0	39.3	< 200
Linen cart	initial force	50	70	55	55	65	59.0	13.3	> 200
	sustained force	20	25	20	25	20	22.0	4.9	> 200
	initial-wheels turned	75	70				72.5	16.3	> 200

increased risk of developing lifting-related low back pain. By "healthy workers," NIOSH means workers who are free of adverse health conditions that would increase their risk of musculoskeletal injury.

The concept behind the RNLE is to start with a recommended weight that is considered safe for an "ideal" lift (ie, load constant equal to 51 lb or 23 kg) and then reduce the weight as the task becomes more stressful (ie, as the task-related factors become less favorable). The RWL equation consists of a fixed load constant of 51 lb that is reduced by six factors related to task geometry (ie, location of the load relative to the worker at the initial liftoff and setdown points), task frequency and duration, and type of handhold on the object. Assessment of patient handling tasks was specifically excluded as a restriction for use of the RNLE due to limitations in the data used to derive the equation. For some patient handling tasks, however, where the person being lifted is noncombative or where there is little or no movement of the patient during the lifting task, the RNLE may be applicable, and it should be possible to determine whether the lift exceeds the RWL for those tasks. For example, the RNLE was used to derive the 35-lb weight limit for patient lifting in the VA and AORN ergonomic tools.[52] The precise formulation of the revised lifting equation for calculating the recommended weight limit is based on a multiplicative model that provides a weighting (ie, multiplier) for each of six task variables, which include the

- horizontal distance of the load from the worker (H),
- vertical height of the lift (V),
- vertical displacement during the lift (D),
- angle of asymmetry (A),
- frequency (F) and duration of lifting, and
- quality of the hand-to-object coupling (C).

The weightings are expressed as coefficients that serve to decrease the load constant, which represents the maximum RWL to be lifted under ideal conditions. For example, as the horizontal distance between the load and the worker increases, the recommended weight limit for that task would be reduced from the ideal starting weight (see **Table 4**).

The term *task variables* refers to the measurable task-related measurements that are used as input data for the formula (ie, H, V, D, A, F, C), whereas the term *multipliers* refers to the reduction coefficients in the equation (ie, HM, VM, DM, AM, FM, CM).

The following list briefly describes the measurements required to use the RNLE. Details for each of the variables are presented later in this chapter (see section entitled "Obtaining and using the data").

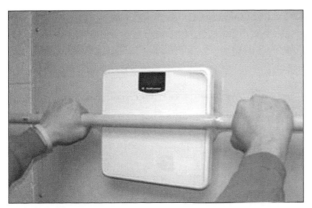

Figure 1. *Simple device for measuring required push force. Photo by Tom Waters, PhD, CPE. Used with permission.*

Table 3

PUSH FORCE LIMITS					
Push/Pull Forces Based on 75% Acceptable for Women Design Goal					
Distance (ft)	25	50	100	150	200
Initial (lb)	51	44	42	42	37
Sustained (lb)	30	25	22	22	15

Adapted from Manual Materials Handling Guidelines, http://libertymmhtables.libertymutual.com/CM_LMTablesWeb/pdf/LibertyMutualTables.pdf. *Reprinted with permission from the Liberty Mutual Research Institute for Safety.*

H = Horizontal location of hands from midpoint between the inner ankle bones. This is measured in centimeters or inches at the origin and the destination of the lift.

V = Vertical location of the hands from the floor. This is measured in centimeters or inches at the origin and destination of the lift.

D = Vertical travel distance in centimeters or inches between the origin and the destination of the lift.

A = Angle of asymmetry; angular displacement of the load from the worker's sagittal plane. This is measured in degrees at the origin and destination of the lift.

F = Average frequency rate of lifting measured in lifts/min. Duration is defined as follows: short-duration (< 1 hour); moderate-duration (> 1 but < 2 hours); or long-duration (> 2 but < 8 hours), assuming appropriate recovery allowances (see **Table 5**).

C = Quality of hand-to-object coupling (quality of interface between the worker and the load being lifted). The quality of the coupling is categorized as good, fair, or poor, depending upon the type and location of the coupling, the physical characteristics of load, and the vertical height of the lift (see **Table 6**).

The LI is a term that provides a relative estimate of the level of physical stress associated with a particular manual lifting task. The estimate of the level of physical stress is defined by the relationship of the weight of the load lifted and the RWL.

Table 4

RECOMMENDED WEIGHT LIMIT			
The recommended weight limit is defined as follows: RWL = LC x HM x VM x DM x AM x FM x CM **Where:**	Variable		Metric	US Customary
	LC =	Load Constant =	23 kg	51 lb
	HM =	Horizontal Multiplier =	(25/H)	(10/H)
	VM =	Vertical Multiplier =	$1-(.003\|V-75\|)$	$1-(.0075\|V-30\|)$
	DM =	Distance Multiplier =	.82 + (4.5/D)	.82 + (1.8/D)
	AM =	Asymmetric Multiplier =	1-(.0032A)	1-(.0032A)
	FM =	Frequency Multiplier =	From Table 5	From Table 5
	CM =	Coupling Multiplier =	From Table 6	From Table 6

The LI is defined by the following equation:

$$LI = \frac{\text{Load weight}}{\text{Recommended Weight Limit}} = \frac{L}{RWL}$$

Where Load weight (L) = Weight of the object lifted (lb or kg).

According to NIOSH, the lifting index may be used to identify potentially hazardous lifting jobs or to compare the relative severity of two jobs for the purpose of evaluating and redesigning them. From the perspective of NIOSH, it is likely that lifting tasks with a lifting index > 1.0 pose an increased risk for lifting-related low back pain for some fraction of the work force.[49] Lifting jobs should be designed to achieve a lifting index of 1.0 or less whenever possible. Some experts believe that worker selection criteria may be used to identify workers who can perform potentially stressful lifting tasks (ie, lifting tasks that would exceed a lifting index of 1.0) without significantly increasing their risk of work-related injury above the baseline level.[49,50] Those who endorse the use of selection criteria believe that the criteria must be based on research studies, empirical observations, or theoretical considerations that include job-related strength testing and/or aerobic capacity testing.

Even these experts agree, however, that many workers will be at a significant risk of a work-related injury when performing highly stressful lifting tasks (ie, lifting tasks that would exceed a lifting index of 3.0). "Informal" or "natural" selection of workers may occur in many jobs that require repet-itive lifting tasks. According to some experts, this may result in a unique workforce that may be able to work above a lifting index of 1.0, at least in theory, without substantially increasing their risk of low back injuries above the baseline rate of injury.

To gain a better understanding of the rationale for the development of the recommended weight limits and lifting index, the *Revised NIOSH Equation for the Design and Evaluation of Manual Lifting Tasks* provides a discussion of the criteria underlying the lifting equation and of the individual multipliers.[49] This article also identifies both the assumptions and uncertainties in the scientific studies that associate manual lifting and low back injuries. For more detailed information about how to use the RNLE, the reader should consult the *Applications Manual for the Revised NIOSH Lifting Equation.*[50]

Glossary

Air-assisted lateral transfer device: A mattress that is inflated with air by a portable air supply, thus facilitating a smoother lateral transfer.

Anti-fatigue mats: A special mat designed with friction-reduction properties, used for workers who stand for long periods of time.

Anti-fatigue technique: Any technique that will reduce fatigue experienced by the worker.

Assistive devices/technology: Equipment that can be used to take all or a portion of a load such as the weight of a body part, off of the person performing a high risk task.

Clinical tools: A standardized process or set of rules by which a provider makes decisions about a complex process (eg, which equipment and techniques to use when performing high-risk patient handling and movement tasks).

Compressive force: Mechanical force directed along the Y (ie, vertical) axis, brought about by the combined effect of internal and external load bearing.

Ergonomics: Applied science of designing and arranging things for people to use efficiently and safely; matching job tasks to workers' capabilities.

Ergonomist: A practitioner in the field of ergonomics.

Friction-reducing devices: Low-friction (slippery) material assistive aids for lateral transfer of patients.

Lateral position: Side-lying.

Lateral transfer: Movement of a patient in a supine position on a horizontal plane, such as transferring a patient from a bed to a stretcher.

Lateral transfer device: A device that is used to move a patient from one surface to another while in a supine position.

lbF: A unit of force equal to the mass of 1 pound with an acceleration equal to 1 gravitational constant (32 ft/s²). Acceleration due to gravity (g) equals 9.8 meters per second squared (9.8 m/s²) or 32 feet per second squared (32 ft/s²).

Lifting index: Relative estimate of physical stress associated with one specific task. It is equal to the load of the object/recommended weight limit.

Table 5

FREQUENCY MULTIPLIERS						
Frequency Lifts/min (F)	Work Duration					
	< 1 Hour		> 1 but < 2 Hours		> 2 but < 8 Hours	
	V < 30	V > 30	V < 30	V > 30	V < 30	V > 30
0.2	1.00	1.00	.95	.95	.85	.85
0.5	.97	.97	.92	.92	.81	.81
1	.94	.94	.88	.88	.75	.75
2	.91	.91	.84	.84	.65	.65
3	.88	.88	.79	.79	.55	.55
4	.84	.84	.72	.72	.45	.45
5	.80	.80	.60	.60	.35	.35
6	.75	.75	.50	.50	.27	.27
7	.70	.70	.42	.42	.22	.22
8	.60	.60	.35	.35	.18	.18
9	.52	.52	.30	.30	.00	.15
10	.45	.45	.26	.26	.00	.13
11	.41	.41	.00	.23	.00	.00
12	.37	.37	.00	.21	.00	.00
13	.00	.34	.00	.00	.00	.00
14	.00	.31	.00	.00	.00	.00
15	.00	.28	.00	.00	.00	.00
> 15	.00	.00	.00	.00	.00	.00

Lithotomy position: Supine position with the hips and knees flexed and the thighs abducted and rotated externally.

Manual retraction: When a member of the perioperative sterile team (ie, scrubbed team) provides exposure of underlying anatomical parts during surgery with his or her hand or by physically holding and/or pulling with a sterile device designed to hold back the edges of tissue and organs.

Maximum sustained force: Force needed to pull or lift for a period of time.

Mechanical lateral transfer device: A powered device that moves a patient horizontally from one surface to another while in a supine position.

Mechanical lift device: Patient transfer device that uses a sling and mechanical lift to transfer patients and/or lift body parts (includes ceiling-mounted and floor-based lifts as well as sit-to-stand lifts).

Musculoskeletal: Relating to or involving the muscles and the skeleton.

Table 6

COUPLING MULTIPLIER		
	Coupling Multiplier	
	V < 30 inches (75 cm)	V > 30 inches (75 cm)
Good	1.00	1.00
Fair	0.95	1.00
Poor	0.90	0.90

Newton (N): A metric unit of measure for forces. (1 Newton = 0.2248 lb)

Newton meter (Nm): A metric unit of measure for moments (ie, force x length). One Newton meter = .738 ft·lb.

Optimal posture: Perpendicular/straight on to the operative field.

Optimal working height: Area between the chest and waist height to the operative field.

Prone: With the front (or ventral) surface of the body positioned face downward.

Recommended weight limit: Recommended weight limit is the principal product of the revised NIOSH lifting equation defined for a specific set of task conditions as the weight of the load that 75% of the population could perform safely.

Revised NIOSH Lifting Equation: Mathematical equation for determining the recommended weight limit and lifting index for selected two-handed manual lifting tasks.

Self-retaining retractor: A sterile device designed to mechanically hold back the edges of tissue and organs to provide exposure to underlying anatomical structures during a surgical procedure.

Semi-Fowler position: The upper half of the body raised to an incline of 30 to 45 degrees; also called the beach-chair position.

Sit-stand stool: A stool that allows the worker to sit or stand while working without changing levels.

Spinal compression: Forces acting along the length of the spine.

Spine loading: Overall mechanical force acting on the spine calculated as root-mean-square value of compressive, lateral, and anterior-posterior components.

Static posture: Postures requiring a sustained position for a long period of time (eg, standing in one position during surgery).

Supine: With the back or dorsal surface of the body positioned downward (ie, lying face up).

REFERENCES

1. B D Owen, A Garg, "Reducing risk for back pain in nursing personnel," *AAOHN Journal* 39 (January 1991) 24-33.

2. B D Owen, "Preventing injuries using an ergonomic approach," *AORN Journal* 72 (December 2000) 1031-1036.

3. J R Garb, C A Dockery, "Reducing employee back injuries in the perioperative setting," *AORN Journal* 61 (June 1995) 1046-1052.

4. "NIOSH facts: Work-related musculoskeletal disorders," National Institute for Occupational Health and Safety, *http://www.cdc.gov/niosh/muskdsfs.html* (accessed 1 Oct 06).

5. A B Hoskins, "Occupational injuries, illnesses, and fatalities among nursing, psychiatric, and home health aides, 1995–2004," Bureau of Labor Statistics, *http://www.bls.gov/opub/cwc/content/sh20060628ar01pl.stm* (accessed 28 Sept 2006).

6. A Converso, C Murphy, "Winning the battle against back injuries," *RN* 67 (February 2004) 52-58.

7. A Nelson, G Fragala, N Menzel, "Myths and facts about back injuries in nursing," *AJN* 103 (February 2003) 32-41.

8. US Department of Labor, "Table R10, Number of nonfatal occupational injuries and illnesses involving-days away from work by occupation and selected parts of body affected by injury or illness, 2001," Bureau of Labor Statistics, *http://www.bls.gov/iif/oshwc/osh/case/ostb1165.pdf* (accessed 1 Oct 2006).

9. "Lost-worktime injuries and illnesses: characteristics and resulting time away from work, 2004," US Department of Labor, Bureau of Labor Statistics, *http://www.bls.gov/news.release/archives/osh2_12132005.pdf* (accessed 28 Nov 2006).

10. D A Stubbs et al, "Backing out: Nurse wastage associated with back pain," *International Journal of Nursing Studies* 23 no 4 (1986) 325-336.

11. B D Owen, "The magnitude of low-back problems in nursing," *Western Journal of Nursing Research* 11 (April 1989) 234-242.

12. A Vasiliadou et al, "Occupational low-back pain in nursing staff in a Greek hospital," *Journal of Advanced Nursing* 21(January 1995) 125-130.

13. M J Lusted et al, "Self-reported symptoms in the neck and upper limbs in nurses," *Applied Ergonomics* 27 no 6 (1996) 381-387.

14. E B Moses, *The Registered Nurse Population: Findings From the National Sample Survey of Registered Nurses, 1992*, (Rockville, Md: US Department of Human Services, 1992) 65; also available at Health Resources and Services Administration, *ftp://ftp.hrsa.gov/bhpr/nursing/samplesurveys/1992sampsur.pdf* (accessed 11 Dec 2006).

15. ECRI, "Workplace hazard reduction through ergonomic evaluation," *Operating Room Risk Management* (September 2005) 1-5.

16. B P Bernard, ed, "Musculoskeletal disorders (MSDs) and workplace factors: A critical review of epidemiological evidence for work-related musculoskeletal disorders of the neck, upper extremity, and low back," US Department of Human Services, National Institute for Occupational Safety and Health, *http://www.cdc.gov/niosh/ergosci1.html* (accessed 16 Feb 2006).

17. C B Stetler et al, "Evidence for prevention of work-related musculoskeletal injuries," *Orthopedic Nursing* 22 (January/February 2003) 32-41.

18. National Occupational Research Agenda for Musculoskeletal Disorders: Research Topics for the Next Decade—A Report by the NORA Musculoskeletal Disorders Team (Washington, DC: US Department of Health and Human Services, 2001) 1-33.

19. P M McGovern, "Toward prevention and control of occupational back injuries," *Occupational Health Nursing* (April 1985) 180-183.

20. G Cust, J C G Pearson, A Mair, "The prevalence of low back pain in nurses," *International Nursing Review* 19 no 2 (1972) 169-179.

21. P Harber et al, "Occupational low-back pain in hospital nurses," *Journal of Occupational Medicine* 27 (July 1985) 518-524.

22. T Videman et al, "Low-back pain in nurses and some loading factors of work," *Spine* 9 no 4 (1984) 400-404.

23. K Williamson et al, "Occupational health hazards for nurses, part 2," Image: *Journal of Nursing Scholarship* 20 (Fall 1988) 162-168.

24. D Stubbs et al, "Back pain research," *Nursing Times* 77 (May 14, 1981) 857-858.

25. F Bell et al, "Hospital ward patient-lifting tasks," *Ergonomics* 22 no 11 (1979) 1257.

26. J Greenwood, "Back injuries can be reduced with worker training, reinforcement," *Occupational Health Safety* (May 1986) 26-29.

27. A L Nelson, G Fragala, "Equipment for safe patient handling and movement," in *Back Injury Among Healthcare Workers*, W Charney, A Hudson, eds (Washington, DC: Lewis Publishers, 2004) 121-135.

28. Patient Safety Center of Inquiry, *Patient Care Ergonomic Resource Guide: Safe Patient Handling and Movement*, A L Nelson, ed (Tampa, Fla: Department of Veterans Affairs, April 2005) 1-71.

29. P Wicker, "Manual handling in the perioperative environment," *British Journal of Perioperative Nursing* 10 (May 2000) 255-259.

30. K Tuohy-Main, "Why manual handling should be eliminated for resident and career safety and how," *Geriaction* 15 no 4 (1997) 10-14.

31. "Recommended practices for positioning the patient in the perioperative practice setting," in *Standards, Recommended Practices, and Guidelines* (Denver: AORN Inc, 2006) 587-592.

32. D B Chaffin, G B J Anderson, B J Martin, *Occupational Biomechanics*, third ed (New York: J Wiley & Sons, 1999) 73.

33. J D Lloyd, A Baptiste, "Friction-reducing devices for lateral patient transfers: A biomechanical evaluation," *American Association of Occupational Health Nurses* 54 (March 2006) 113-119.

34. S H Snook, V M Ciriello, "The design of manual handling tasks: Revised tables of maximum acceptable weights and forces," *Ergonomics* 34 no 9 (1991) 1197-1213.

35. D B Chaffin, G B J Anderson, B J Martin, *Occupational Biomechanics*, third ed (New York: J Wiley & Sons, 1999) 114.

36. S Pheasant, *Bodyspace* (London: Taylor & Francis, Ltd, 1992) 111.

37. D B Chaffin, G B J Anderson, B J Martin, *Occupational Biomechanics*, third ed (New York: J Wiley & Sons, 1999) 49.

38. "Recommended practices for skin preparation of patients," in *Standards, Recommended Practices, and Guidelines* (Denver: AORN, Inc, 2006) 603-606.

39. "Standing problem," *Hazards Magazine*, http://www.hazards.org/standing (accessed 8 May 2006).

40. E Ha et al, "Does standing at work during pregnancy result in reduced infant birth weight?" *Journal of Occupational and Environmental Medicine* 44 (September 2002) 815-821.

41. T B Hendriksen et al, "Standing and walking for > 5 hours per work day increased the risk for preterm delivery," *American College of Physicians* 1 (November/December 1995) 28-30.

42. A P Keomeester, J P J Broesen, P E Treffers, "Physical work load and gestational age at delivery," *Occupational & Environmental Medicine* 52 (May 1995) 313-315.

43. M J Saurel-Cubizolles et al, "Employment working conditions, and preterm birth: Results from the Europop case-control survey," *Journal of Epidemiology and Community Health* 58 (May 2004) 395-401.

44. B Luke et al, "Obstetrics. The association between occupational factors and preterm birth: A United States nurses' study," *American Journal of Obstetrics and Gynecology* 173 (September 1995) 849-862.

45. J Mathias, "New research looks at ergonomic stresses on operating room staff," *OR Manager* 21 (July 2005) 1, 6-7.

46. R Berguer et al, "A comparison of surgeon's posture during laparoscopic and open surgical procedures," *Surgical Endoscopy* 11 (1997) 139-142.

47. R Berquer, W D Smith, D Davis, "An ergonomic study of the optimum operating table height for laparoscopic surgery," *Surgical Endoscopy* 16 (2002) 416-421.

48. Association for the Advancement of Medical Instrumentation, *Comprehensive Guide to Steam Sterilization and Sterility Assurance in Health Care Facilities, ANSI/AAMI ST79:2006* (Arlington, Va: Association for the Advancement of Medical Instrumentation, 2006) 62.

49. T Waters et al, "Revised NIOSH equation for the design and evaluation of manual lifting tasks," *Ergonomics* 36 no 7 (1993) 749-776.

50. T Waters, A Garg, V Putz-Anderson, *Applications Manual for the Revised NIOSH Lifting Equation*, NIOSH publication no 94-110 (Cincinnati, Ohio: Department of Health and Human Services, National Institute for Occupational Safety and Health, Division of Biomedical and Behavioral Science, January 1994) 1-119.

51. T R Waters et al, "Evaluation of the revised NIOSH lifting equation: A cross-sectional epidemiologic study," *Spine* 24 (February 1999) 386-394.

52. T R Waters, "Using the NIOSH Lifting Equation to Determine Maximum Recommended Weight Limits for Manual Patient Lifting Tasks," presentation at the 6th Annual Safe Patient Handling and Movement Conference, Clearwater Beach, Fla, 1 March 2006.

PUBLICATION HISTORY

Approved by the AORN Board of Directors, November 2006.

This document was formerly published as part of *AORN Guidance Statement: Safe Patient Handling and Movement in the Perioperative Setting*. Denver, CO: AORN, Inc; 2007.

AORN gratefully acknowledges the following individuals for reviewing the content of this guidance document:

Darlene Ace, MS
Industrial Hygienist; Environmental Health and Safety Specialist
University of Rochester
Environmental Health & Safety
Industrial Hygiene Unit
Rochester, NY

Kay Ball, RN, BSN, MSA, CNOR, FAAN
Nurse Consultant/Educator
K & D Medical Inc.
Lewis Center, Ohio

Joan Blanchard, RN, MSS, CNOR, CIC
Perioperative Nursing Specialist
AORN Center for Nursing Practice
Denver, Colo

Jay Bowers, RN, BSN, CNOR
Charge Nurse
West Virginia University Hospitals
Morgantown, WVa

Byron Burlingame, RN, MS, CNOR
Perioperative Nursing Specialist
AORN Center for Nursing Practice
Denver, Colo

Camille Collette, RN, MS, CNOR
Patient Safety Coordinator
Risk Management, Health Care
Quality
Beth Israel Deaconess
Medical Center East
Boston, Mass

Alice Comish, RN, BSN, CNOR
Director, Surgical Technology
Program
Our Lady of the Lake College
Baton Rouge, La

Ramona Conner, RN, MSN, CNOR
Perioperative Nursing Specialist
AORN Center for Nursing Practice
Denver, Colo

Bonnie Denholm, RN, MS, CNOR
Perioperative Nursing Specialist
AORN Center for Nursing Practice
Denver, Colo

Guy Fragala, PhD, PE, CSP
Director of Compliance Programs
Environmental Health and
Engineering
Newton, Mass

Sharon Giarrizzo-Wilson, RN, MS, CNOR
Perioperative Nursing Specialist
AORN Center for Nursing Practice
Denver, Colo

Judi Goldberg, RN, BSN, CNOR
Clinical Educator
The William W. Backus Hospital
Norwich, Conn

Linda Groah, RN, MSN, CNOR, CNAA, FAAN
Chief Operating Officer
San Francisco Medical Center
Kaiser Foundation Hospital
San Francisco, Calif

Pamela C. Hagan, MSN, RN
Chief Programs Officer
American Nurses Association
Silver Spring, Md

Katherine Halverson-Carpenter, RN, MBA, CNOR
Director, Perioperative Services
University of Colorado Hospital
Denver, Colo

Stephen D. Hudock, PhD
Ergonomics, Certified Safety
Professional
Team Leader, Human Factors and
Ergonomics Research
National Institute for Occupational
Safety and Health
Robert A. Taft Laboratories
Cincinnati, Ohio

Stephanie Lackey, RN
Clinical Nurse Manager
Fannin Surgicare
Houston, Tex

Nancy Menzel, PhD, RN, COHN-S
Associate Professor
School of Nursing
University of Nevada Las Vegas
Las Vegas, Nev

Donna Pritchard, RN, BSN, MA, CNOR, CAN
Director Perioperative Service
Kingsbrook Jewish Medical Center
Brooklyn, NY

Patricia Seifert, RN, MSN, CNOR, CRNFA, FAAN
Education Coordinator, CVOR
Inova Fairfax Hospital
Falls Church, Va

Victoria Steelman, PhD, RN, CNOR
Advanced Practice Nurse
Perioperative Nursing
University of Iowa Healthcare
Iowa City, Iowa

Dawn L. Tenney, RN, MSN
Associate Chief Nurse
Perioperative Services
Massachusetts General Hospital
Boston, Mass

Dawn M. Yost, RDH, RN, BSN, CNOR
Perioperative Nurse Clinician/
Preceptor
West Virginia University Hospitals
Morgantown, WV

AORN Guidance Statement: Sharps Injury Prevention in the Perioperative Setting

Introduction

The purpose of this guidance document is to assist perioperative registered nurses in the development of sharps injury prevention programs using identified best practices to reduce percutaneous injuries. It also suggests strategies to overcome obstacles to compliance with established sharps safety protocols.

The perioperative setting is a high-risk environment, and perioperative RNs are routinely faced with high risk for exposure to bloodborne pathogens from percutaneous injuries. Although the scope of the problem is not completely known, the National Institute for Occupational Safety and Health (NIOSH) estimates that 600,000 to 800,000 percutaneous injuries occur annually among heath care workers.[1] Percutaneous injuries primarily are associated with occupational transmission of the hepatitis B virus (HBV), hepatitis C virus (HCV), and HIV, but they may be implicated in the transmission of more than 20 other pathogens.[2] Understanding the etiology of percutaneous injuries in the perioperative setting is paramount to developing a safe prevention program.

Background

Percutaneous injuries occur throughout all health care facilities, and many occur in the perioperative setting.[3,4] Exposure to bloodborne pathogens occurs during all phases of the perioperative process. Research indicates that injuries from sharp devices or instruments occur in 7% to 15% of all surgical procedures. Procedures identified as posing the highest risk of injury are thoracic, trauma, burn, emergency orthopedic, major vascular, intra-abdominal, and gynecologic surgeries.[5] Risk of a sharps injury increases during more invasive, longer procedures that result in higher blood loss.[6] Fatigue resulting from working extended hours in combination with the fast pace of the perioperative environment also may contribute to increased risk of percutaneous injuries.[7-9]

Nurses comprise the largest segment of health care workers and are reported to sustain the highest number of percutaneous injuries overall.[2] Observational studies have demonstrated that perioperative personnel experience the highest percutaneous injury rates, but 70% to 96% of exposures were underreported.[5] Surgeons and first assistants have the highest risk of injury and sustain more than half (ie, 59%) of percutaneous injuries in the perioperative setting.[6] Scrub personnel experienced the second highest frequency of percutaneous injury, followed by anesthesia care providers and circulating nurses.[6]

Injuries from hollow bore needles constitute the majority of injuries and pose the highest risk of exposure to bloodborne pathogens.[10] Although the risk of injury from hollow bore needles is prevalent in the perioperative setting, the epidemiology of sharps injuries in the OR is different from that of other locations in health care. Suture needles have been identified as the most frequent mechanism of percutaneous injury in the OR; they are involved in as many as 77% of such injuries.[4,6] Scalpels are the second most frequent mechanism of injury, followed by retractors, skin or bone hooks, and sharp electrosurgical tips.[11,12]

Percutaneous injuries often are self-inflicted. Studies indicate that 6% to 16% of these injuries occur during hand-to-hand passing of sharp instruments, suture needles, and other sharp devices. The most common body part injured is the nondominant hand. Injuries from suture needles occur most often

- ◆ when loading the needle holder or repositioning the needle;
- ◆ during hand-to-hand passing of sharp devices between scrub personnel and the surgeon;
- ◆ during suturing, particularly muscle and fascia (eg, wound closure) when the needle is being manipulated and guided with fingers;
- ◆ when retracting or stretching tissue with hands;
- ◆ when the surgeon sews toward his or her own or an assistant's hand;
- ◆ when tying suture with the needle attached;
- ◆ after the suture has just been used and remains unattended on the operative field—even if suture is unattended on the field for only a short time, the needle holder can fall off the field onto a health care worker's foot, or scrubbed personnel may reach for it in an attempt to prevent it from sliding off the field; and
- ◆ when placing the used needle in an overfilled sharps container.[3]

Injuries from scalpels most often occur
- ◆ when loading or removing a disposable scalpel blade on a reusable knife handle;
- ◆ during hand-to-hand passing of the scalpel;

♦ during dissection when the tissue is being retracted or spread with hands;

♦ when cutting toward the surgeon's or an assistant's fingers;

♦ immediately before or after use when the scalpel is left on the operative field unattended— even if this is for only a short time, the scalpel can fall off the field onto a health care worker's foot, or scrubbed personnel may reach for it in an attempt to prevent it from sliding off the field; and

♦ when the scalpel is placed in an over-filled or poorly located sharps container.[3]

Glove barrier failure is a common occurrence in the perioperative setting. Glove failures can be caused by punctures, tears by sharp devices, or spontaneous failures. These failures expose the wearer to bloodborne pathogens. Studies have demonstrated that glove perforations often occur after an average of 40 minutes of use during surgical procedures. When two pairs of gloves are worn (ie, double gloving), in most instances, only the outer glove is perforated when punctured by a sharp device. In addition, research demonstrates that when two pairs of gloves are worn and a puncture occurs, the volume of blood on a solid sharp device (eg, suture needle) is reduced by as much as 95%. There is evidence that double gloving can reduce the risk of exposure to blood and body fluids, if the outer glove is punctured, by as much as 87%.[6]

The Occupational Safety and Health Administration (OSHA) requires health care organizations to protect their workers and have a written exposure control plan. Protection occurs by using universal precautions, engineering controls, work practice controls, organizational controls, and communication. The standard also requires employers to maintain a log of injuries from contaminated sharps.[13]

Guidance Statement

The perioperative environment poses unique challenges for reducing the risk of injuries from sharp devices. Surgery involves precise, regimented actions that require planning, communication, and team work. These same elements can be employed to mitigate the inherent hazards associated with sharp devices encountered in the perioperative setting. Perioperative RNs should actively participate in the development and implementation of strategies to reduce the risk of sharps injuries to health care team members.

Perioperative nursing management should work with the facility risk manager or safety officer to identify the types of sharp devices and how they are used in the perioperative setting. Both perioperative nursing management and the risk manager or safety officer should have a thorough understanding of OSHA's standards.[3]

By law, an effective sharps injury and bloodborne pathogen exposure control program must be written, communicated to all workers in the perioperative setting, and uniformly supported and enforced by perioperative leadership.[2,13] A multidisciplinary team is key to the success of this process. This team, using steps consistent with the continuous quality improvement process, must conduct a baseline assessment and set priorities for developing an action plan.[2,6]

Perioperative-Specific Risk Reduction Strategies

■ Adopt and incorporate safe habits into daily work activities when preparing and using sharp devices.

■ Focus attention on the intent of the action when working with sharp items, and minimize rushing and distractions while applying safety techniques during critical moments.

■ During preparation for operative or other invasive procedures:
  ▪ inspect the surgical field for adequate lighting and space to perform the procedure;
  ▪ organize the work area so that the sharps are always pointed away from staff members;
  ▪ establish a separate area to place a reusable sharp for safe handling during the procedure;
  ▪ use standardized sterile field set-ups; and
  ▪ include identification of the neutral zone in the preoperative briefing.[14]

■ During the operative or other invasive procedure:
  ▪ wear two pairs of gloves (ie, double gloving);
  ▪ monitor gloves for punctures;
  ▪ encourage the use of blunt suture needles;
  ▪ use neutral or hands-free technique for passing sharp items whenever possible or practical, instead of passing hand-to-hand;
  ▪ give verbal notification when passing a sharp device;
  ▪ keep visual contact with the procedure site and the sharp device;
  ▪ take steps to control the location of the sharp device;

- be aware of other staff members in the area when handling a sharp device;
- keep track of and account for all sharp items throughout the procedure;
- contain used sharps on the sterile field in a designated, disposable, puncture-resistant needle container, and replace it as necessary;
- check to be sure the disposable, puncture-resistant needle container is securely closed before handing it off the field;
- load suture needles using the suture packet to assist in mounting the suture needle in the needle holder, and use the appropriate instrument to adjust and unload the needle;
- remove the needle from the suture before tying, or use "control-release" sutures that allow the needle to be removed with a straight pull on the needle holder;
- activate the safety feature of a safety engineered device immediately after use according to manufacturers' instructions;
- keep hands away from the surgical site when sharp items are in use (eg, suturing, cutting);
- use one-handed or blunt instrument-assisted suturing techniques to avoid finger contact with the suture needle or tissue being sutured;
- provide a barrier between the hands and the needle after use; and
- use gloves and an instrument to pick up sharp items (eg, suture needles, hypodermic needles, scalpel blades) that have fallen on the floor.[2,3,6,13-17]
■ During postprocedure clean up:
- inspect the surgical setup used during the procedure for sharps;
- transport reusable sharps in a closed, secure container to the designated clean-up area;
- inspect the sharps container for overfilling before discarding disposable sharps in it;
- make sure the sharps container is large enough to accommodate the entire device;
- avoid bringing hands close to the opening of a sharps container;
- do not place hands or fingers into a container to dispose of a device; and
- keep hands behind the sharp tip when disposing.[3,14,18]

Health care organizations and their employees are responsible for actively participating in strategies to reduce percutaneous injuries. The employing facility should provide an environment that reduces the risk of percutaneous injuries from contaminated sharp devices. A well-developed safety program and support from management sends a clear message to employees about the organization's commitment to preventing injuries and keeping employees safe. Fewer percutaneous injuries are reported in organizations that have a strong culture of safety. Individual health care workers have a responsibility to be educated about the prevalence and mode of transmission of bloodborne pathogens and to use measures to protect themselves.[19]

Individual Perioperative RN's Responsibilities

■ Observe local, state, and federal regulations (eg, OSHA regulations).
■ Comply with methods to protect yourself from disease transmission (eg, get the hepatitis B vaccination).
■ Use devices with safety features that are provided by your employer.
■ Prevent hollow bore percutaneous injuries during injections or bodily fluid retrieval by using
- needleless systems or sharps with engineered sharp injury protection devices whenever possible;
- retractable, protective sheath or self-resheathing, self-blunting, or hinged re-cap needles to administer local anesthetics and other injectable medications;
- blunt cannulas to withdraw medications and fluids from vials; and
- the one-handed recapping technique, only if no other alternatives exist.
■ Practice using safety devices to establish familiarity and experience with them before using them in practice.
■ Actively participate in the safety conversion process and help others adapt to the change.
■ Use personal protective equipment.
■ Use sharps receptacles that are
- identifiable (ie, orange, orange-red), closable, and labeled with the biohazard symbol;
- appropriately sized with a full line that is readily visible;
- puncture resistant and leak proof;
- located close to the point of use;
- maintained upright when in use; and
- routinely replaced and not allowed to overfill.
■ Participate in education about bloodborne pathogens, and follow recommended infection prevention practices.

■ Support and guide perioperative team members to follow these risk reduction strategies.

■ Encourage perioperative staff members to proactively report hazards that pose a threat of percutaneous injury.

■ Know the location in your department of the exposure control plan.

■ Follow exposure control policy if injured (ie, wash site with soap and water, provide immediate care to the exposure site).[9,13]

Employer Responsibilities

■ Comply with local, state, and federal regulations regarding percutaneous injury prevention.

■ Create a safety-oriented culture.

■ Encourage timely reporting of all percutaneous injuries by all perioperative team members.

■ Analyze needle-stick and other sharps-related injuries in the perioperative setting to identify hazards and injury trends.

■ Establish a communication mechanism to seek input from perioperative team members regarding risks specific to the perioperative setting.

■ Provide training for all perioperative personnel that includes risk reduction strategies designed specifically to address the risks encountered in the perioperative setting.

■ Evaluate and select safety devices that are acceptable to all members of the perioperative team who use them. The safety device should provide features that work effectively, are reliable, do not compromise patient or worker safety, and are ergonomically designed to the acceptable specifications of the users.

■ Provide and have readily available the appropriate sharps safety devices, and provide adequate training on their use.

■ Evaluate the effectiveness of established risk reduction strategies and products, provide feedback, and modify them as necessary to reduce the risk of percutaneous injuries.[7]

■ Establish staffing patterns that minimize extended work hours and allow for adequate recuperation to decrease the risk of fatigue-related injuries.[20]

Overcoming Obstacles to Compliance

Psychosocial and organizational factors may impede change. An employee's risk-taking personality profile, perception that the organization is not committed to worker safety, and a perceived belief that there is a conflict between providing optimal patient care and protecting oneself from exposure contribute to an employee's resistance to changing to safer practices.[2] For example, although percutaneous injuries continue to occur in the perioperative setting, 71% of respondents in a national survey indicated that they have not evaluated blunt-tip suture needles for use in the OR, and only 2% of respondents have fully implemented blunt-tip suture needles. Only 14% of respondents had implemented safety scalpels into their ORs.[4]

Changes in attitudes about risk of exposure must occur before practice can change to comply with sharps safety protocols. It is difficult to change ingrained habits. People are most likely to change behavior when they perceive a significant personal risk. Education about the risk of contracting a bloodborne disease from a percutaneous injury with a contaminated sharp device should be presented in the early stages of a health care worker's career in order to develop safe practice habits.[5]

Surgery involves precise, regimented actions requiring planning, communication, and team work. These same elements can be employed to overcome obstacles to compliance with measures meant to mitigate the inherent hazards of sharp devices encountered in the perioperative setting. Suggested strategies to overcome obstacles to compliance include the following.

■ Use frequent and multiple training methods that include audiovisual aids, articles, hands-on clinical practice, and visual reminders (eg, laminated posters).

■ Develop a multidisciplinary sharps injury prevention education plan.

■ Incorporate sharps injury prevention instruction into initial nursing education to promote well-established, safe habits.

■ Include sharps injury prevention strategies during orientation of new employees.

■ Form a multidisciplinary sharps safety committee that includes, but is not limited to, perioperative RNs, surgeons, anesthesia care providers, surgical technologists, and first assistants. This team could be asked to
  ▪ help with the selection and evaluation of acceptable safety devices (eg, scalpels that employ a one-handed technique or are totally disposable) and
  ▪ work with physicians to explore alternative techniques, such as adhesive skin closures;

alternatives for securing catheters; use of blunt suture needles, rounded scalpels, or stapling devices, when procedurally appropriate; and use of alternative methods for cutting tissue (eg, harmonic scalpel, rounded scissors, laser devices, electrosurgery active electrodes).

■ Network with other facilities to learn about their success stories.

■ Collaborate with personnel who use the device, and facilitate change instead of dictating change.

■ Inform perioperative team members about current research on disease transmission from percutaneous injuries and relate it to the individual's experience.

■ Work with resisters to gain buy-in to the sharps safety program.

■ Remove as many conventional sharp items as possible from stock.

■ Create a culture of safety in which every team member is empowered to call attention to deficiencies in sharps management.[2,9,12,13]

Selecting and Evaluating New Products

As risk reduction strategies are identified, a multidisciplinary team should evaluate and select the best products to meet the facility's needs. An ongoing review process should be developed to assess, evaluate, and modify the plan as needed. Product evaluation and selection should include the following.

■ Assemble a multidisciplinary team to develop, implement, and evaluate a process for selecting products to reduce sharps injury in the OR. Staff members who work with the product are key components of the team. A strong interdisciplinary commitment to best practices and worker safety is the optimal foundation necessary for change to occur.

■ Review the literature for research about the mechanism, frequency, time, and place of injuries, as well as the role and body part of the person sustaining the percutaneous injury to determine priority areas on which to focus.

■ Identify the products to be evaluated. Focus on their intended use in the facility and identify any special technique or design factors that will influence safety, efficiency, and user acceptability. Seek data from all sources on the safety and overall performance of the devices.

■ Ensure that participants in the evaluation represent all of the end users. To ensure a successful evaluation, users must have adequate training.

Use clear, objective, consistent criteria to evaluate safety devices.

■ Continue to monitor a safety device after it has been implemented to assess performance and to identify if there is a need for additional training.[2,10]

Summary

Occupational exposure to bloodborne pathogens via percutaneous injuries is one of the most serious dangers perioperative team members face on a daily basis. The risk of sustaining a percutaneous injury can be decreased through employee education, clear communication, device engineering, and focused work practice controls. Risk reduction strategies should include specific practices aimed at reducing the unique risks of percutaneous injuries encountered in the perioperative environment. AORN recognizes the various settings in which perioperative RNs practice, and the suggested risk reduction strategies in this guidance statement are intended to be adaptable to any setting where surgical or other invasive procedures are performed.

REFERENCES

1. "AORN position statement on workplace safety," in *Standards, Recommended Practices, and Guidelines* (Denver: AORN, Inc, 2004) 169-171.

2. "Workbook for designing, implementing, and evaluating a sharps injury prevention program," Centers for Disease Control and Prevention, *http://www.cdc.gov/sharpssafety* (accessed 5 Jan 2005).

3. ECRI, "Sharps injuries in the operating room—A new focus for OSHA," *Operating Room Risk Management* (December 2004) 1-5.

4. J Perry, G Parker, J Jagger, "EPINet report: 2001 percutaneous injury rates," *Advances in Exposure Prevention* 6 no 3 (2003) 32-36.

5. C L Holodnick, V Barkauskas, "Reducing percutaneous injuries in the OR by educational methods," *AORN Journal* 72 (September 2000) 461-476.

6. R Berguer, P J Heller, "Preventing sharps injuries in the operating room" *Journal of the American College of Surgeons* 199 (September 2004) 462-467.

7. K Hanecke et al, "Accident risk as a function of hour at work and time of day as determined from accident data and exposure models for the German working population," *Scandinavian Journal of Work, Environment, and Health* 24 suppl (1998) 43-48.

8. T Roth, T A Roehrs, "Etiologies and sequelae of excessive daytime sleepiness," *Clinical Therapeutics* 18 (July/August 1996) 562-576.

9. Battelle Memorial Institute, JIL Information Systems, "An overview of the scientific literature concerning fatigue, sleep, and the circadian cycle," Air Line Pilots Association, *http://cf.alpa.org/internet/projects/ftdt/backgr/batelle.htm* (accessed 5 Jan 2005).

10. National Institute for Occupational Safety and Health, "Preventing needlestick injuries in health care settings," publ 2000-108 (Washington, DC: US Department of Health and Human Services, November 1999).

11. J Jagger, M Bentley, P Tereskerz, "A study of patterns and prevention of blood exposures in OR personnel," *AORN Journal* 67 (May 1998) 979-987.

12. S Wasek, "10 practical ways to implement safety devices," *Outpatient Surgery Magazine* 4 (December 2003).

13. "Regulations (Standards–29 CFR) Bloodborne pathogens 1910.1030," Occupational Safety and Health Administration, *http://www.osha.gov/pls/oshaweb /owadisp.show_document?p_table–STANDARDS&p_id =10051* (accessed 5 Jan 2005).

14. "Recommended practices for maintaining a sterile field," in *Standards, Recommended Practices, and Guidelines* (Denver: AORN, Inc, 2004) 367.

15. C Twomey, "Does double gloving double the protection?" *Infection Control Today, http://www.infectioncontrol today.com/articles/051feat3.html* (accessed 5 Jan 2005).

16. "Recommended practices for sponge, sharp, and instrument counts," in *Standards, Recommended Practices, and Guidelines* (Denver: AORN, Inc, 2004) 230-231.

17. "Recommended practices for environmental cleaning in the surgical practice setting," in *Standards, Recommended Practices, and Guidelines* (Denver: AORN, Inc, 2004) 273-279.

18. "Recommended practices for standard and transmission-based precautions in the perioperative practice setting," in *Standards, Recommended Practices, and Guidelines* (Denver: AORN, Inc, 2004) 361.

19. "AORN guidance statement: Safe on-call practices in perioperative practice settings" in *Standards, Recommended Practices, and Guidelines* (Denver: AORN, Inc, 2005) 193-195.

20. K Royer, "Primer on prevention of sharps injuries" (Sharps Safety) *Outpatient Surgery Magazine* 5 (September 2004) 50.

PUBLICATION HISTORY

Originally published in *Standards, Recommended Practices, and Guidelines,* 2005 edition. Reprinted March 2005, *AORN Journal.*

AORN Guidance Statement: Reuse of Single-Use Devices

Introduction

Today's economic environment has compelled health care organizations to explore methods to reduce health care costs. One prospective approach to controlling rising costs is to reprocess single-use medical devices. Reprocessing is rigorously regulated by the US Food and Drug Administration (FDA). AORN, the Association of periOperative Registered Nurses, recognizes the need for each health care facility to provide safe, cost-effective, quality care to patients and realizes that many facilities in today's marketplace are reprocessing and reusing devices labeled for single use. These devices are reprocessed either within the facility or by an external third party contracted to provide the reprocessing service.

Background

As surgery evolved and increased in complexity, the number of single-use devices utilized during surgery increased and continues to rise. In response to this trend, the practice of reprocessing and reusing single-use medical devices began during the 1970s.[1] As technology led to a wide variety of materials used in device manufacture and devices became more complex, concern for patient safety, informed consent, and ethical practice intensified. In the late 1990s, the FDA determined that increased regulation of reprocessing was needed to promote safe practice and protect the public's safety. Although original equipment manufacturers have been regulated for many years, the FDA determined that they, along with third-party reprocessors and hospital reprocessors, should be regulated uniformly according to the Food, Drug, and Cosmetic Act. The FDA sought the expertise of manufacturers, reprocessors, hospitals, users, and other interested parties in developing a regulatory document, and in August 2000, it published its rule governing the reprocessing/reusing of devices labeled for single-use only. The document is applicable to both hospitals and third-party reprocessors.

Reprocessing of single-use devices (SUDs) is additionally addressed in the Medical Device User Fee and Modernization Act of 2002 (MDUFMA), which establishes new statutory requirements for SUDs, including labeling to identify the devices as reprocessed, submission of validation data for many reprocessed SUDs, and submission of pre-market notification (510[k]) with validation data for some SUDs that previously were exempt from 510(k) submission requirements. Firms and hospitals that are reprocessing are considered by the FDA as manufacturers and therefore must comply with statutory and regulatory requirements.[2] In addition, the FDA has published an approved list of single-use devices that are acceptable for reprocessing and a list of items that may not be reprocessed. In essence, the regulations regard reprocessors in the same way as original equipment manufacturers.[3,4]

Guidance Statement

Reprocessing single-use medical devices is chosen by some health care facilities as a cost containment effort and to reduce the amount of waste generated. It is the role and responsibility of each health care facility to determine whether and to what extent it will engage in such practice. As licensed professionals, perioperative nurses must demonstrate accountability to the nursing profession, to other members of the health care team, and to the public they serve.[5] AORN, the professional organization of and for perioperative nurses, believes certain basic tenets must underpin any reprocessing program. The foremost concern is for the patient's safety. Therefore,

- if a device cannot be cleaned, it cannot be reprocessed and reused;
- if sterility of a post-processed device cannot be demonstrated, the device cannot be reprocessed and reused;
- if the integrity and functionality of a reprocessed SUD cannot be demonstrated and documented as safe for patient care and/or equal to the original device specifications, the device cannot be reprocessed and reused; and
- if anything is opened it needs to be decontaminated before reprocessing.

Per requirements of the MDUFMA regulation, the FDA has published a list of reprocessed SUDs that have 510(k) approval/clearance; whose manufacturers have provided supplemental data on functionality, cleaning, and sterility; and which now are on the published list of devices that are acceptable for reprocessing.[2]

2012 Perioperative Standards and Recommended Practices

Although some operational savings may be realized by reusing certain devices, any cost-benefit analysis would necessarily include labor costs; program costs, including quality system requirements such as sterility and post-processing device testing (see section on quality system requirements); documentation costs; and the potential cost of device failure. Using the results of a thorough cost-benefit analysis, each provider facility must make an informed choice as to whether it wishes to invest the necessary resources to develop a safe reprocessing system within the facility. Use of an external reprocessor presents a different, but related, set of factors for consideration. When a decision is made in favor of using an external reprocessing company, it is the user facility's responsibility to assess the quality of services provided under the contractual arrangement.[6] The user facility should review the processes used by the contracted agent and determine whether correct procedures are being followed.[7] Regardless of whether an internal reprocessing program is developed or an external reprocessing company is selected, the user facility should be aware that the FDA views any reprocessor as a manufacturer and, as such, subject to federal regulations.[3,8,9]

Federal Regulatory Requirements

In August 2000, the FDA issued guidance on the practice of reprocessing and reusing medical devices intended to be used only once. The FDA's goal in issuing this regulation was to ensure a reprocessing and reuse regulatory program that is based on good science and protects the public health. At the same time, the FDA intended to ensure equitable regulatory requirements for all parties engaged in reprocessing. In the guidance document,[10] the FDA indicates that hospitals and third parties that reprocess SUDs are subject to the same regulations as the original equipment manufacturers. The MDUFMA also addressed reprocessing of SUDs by amending the federal Food, Drug and Cosmetic Act (the Act) and establishing new statutory requirements applicable to reprocessed SUDs, including requirements for

♦ quality system regulations,
♦ medical device reporting,
♦ registration and listing,
♦ labeling,
♦ premarket approval and premarket notification,
♦ medical device corrections and removals, and
♦ medical device tracking.[2]

Quality System Regulation

All manufacturers, including hospital and third-party reprocessors, are subject to the FDA Good Manufacturing Practices (GMP) requirements. These requirements are presented in the quality system regulation that governs the methods, facilities, and controls used for designing, manufacturing, packaging, labeling, storing, installing, and servicing medical devices.[3] Quality system refers to the organizational structure, responsibilities, procedures, processes, and resources for implementing quality management. For device manufacturers, including reprocessors, this system is required in addition to any quality improvement program that may be in place as required by other regulatory bodies. The quality system regulation addresses the areas shown in **Table 1**.[11]

Medical Device Reporting (MDR)

Under MEDWATCH, the FDA's medical device reporting program resulting from the Safe Medical Devices Act of 1990 (Public Law 101-629),[12] both manufacturers and users are required to report deaths or serious injuries to the FDA if it can be reasonably determined that a medical device may have caused or contributed to the incident. Manufacturers also must report certain device malfunctions.[13] Because the FDA considers reprocessors to be manufacturers when they reprocess an SUD,[9] hospital reprocessors have dual reporting responsibility. They are subject to manufacturer's reporting requirements (21 CFR, Part 803 Subpart E)[14] as well as those for the device user facility (21 CFR, Part 803, Subparts A and C).[15,16] Although user facilities must report only deaths or serious injury, manufacturers' reporting requirements are more extensive and require additional supplemental information. Manufacturers (reprocessors) also must report any event that requires the manufacturer (reprocessor) to take immediate remedial action. The Jan. 26, 2000, issue of the *Federal Register* contains the most recent MDR requirements. Hospitals that reprocess SUDs are subject to both user facility reporting and the more comprehensive manufacturer reporting requirements.[17]

Registration and Listing

All persons or entities owning or operating establishments that manufacture, prepare, or process devices must register with the FDA. The FDA uses this information to identify and locate establishments that it is

Table 1

QUALITY SYSTEM REGULATION[1]	
Area Addressed	**Code of Federal Regulations**
Management responsibility	21 CFR, Part 820.20, 22, 25
Design controls	21 CFR, Part 820.30
Document controls	21 CFR, Part 820.40
Purchasing controls	21 CFR, Part 820.50
Product identification and traceability	21 CFR, Part 820.60, 65
Production and process validation	21 CFR, Part 820.70, 72, 75
Acceptance activities such as inspections, tests, or other verification activities	21 CFR, Part 820.80, 86
Nonconforming product control	21 CFR, Part 820.90
Corrective and preventive action	21 CFR, Part 820.100
Labeling and packaging controls	21 CFR, Part 820.120, 130
Handling, storage, distribution, and installation controls	21 CFR, Part 820.120, 140, 150, 160
Records including device master record, device history record, quality system record, and complaint files controls	21 CFR, Part 820.180, 181, 184, 186, 198
Servicing controls	21 CFR, Part 820.200
Use of statistical techniques to establish, control, and verify the acceptability of process capability and product characteristics	21 CFR, Part 820.250

1. *"Quality system regulation,"* CFR 21 Part 820, US Food and Drug Administration, http://www.accessdata.fda.gov/scripts/cdrh/cfdocs/cfCFR/CFRSearch.cfm?CFRPart=820 *(accessed 3 Oct 2005).*

required to inspect. When registering, the following information must be provided:

- name and address,
- business names used,
- business name of owner or operator, and
- establishment type.

When registering for the first time, a specific FDA form is required. An additional registration form must be submitted annually thereafter. In addition to registering with the FDA, each reprocessing entity must provide a list of the devices it intends to reprocess. A separate listing form must be submitted for each device to be reprocessed. Devices are listed by category. The following information is required:

- FDA classification name,
- FDA product code,
- brand name, and
- common or usual name.

Additional information about registration and listing is available in the *Code of Federal Regulations* (21 CFR, Part 807).[18] The necessary forms can be obtained from the Office of Compliance, Center for Devices and Radiologic Health (HFZ-307), US Food and Drug Administration, 2094 Gaither Road, Rockville, MD 20850. The Center for Devices and Radiologic Health (CDRH) offers an additional document, *CDRH Guidance for Industry: Instructions for Completion of Medical Device Registration and Listing Forms FDA 2891, 2891a, and 2892.* This document can be obtained from the Division of Small Manufacturers Assistance (DSMA) at telephone number 800-638-2041 or 301-638-2041; e-mail *DSMA@CDRH.fda.gov*.

Labeling

The FDA directions for labeling can be found in 21 CFR, Part 801.[19] The term *labeling* includes package inserts as well as the information printed on the actual label of the package. Labeling requirements include the name and location of the manufacturer (reprocessor) and adequate direction for the device's intended use. If the manufacturer (reprocessor) knows of uses other than the intended use of the device, FDA requires the manufacturer (reprocessor) to provide adequate labeling for alternate uses of the device as are known. In addition, MDUFMA added new labeling requirement for reprocessed SUDs (Section 502[v] of the Act). Beginning after January 26, 2004, reprocessed SUDs that are introduced into interstate commerce must prominently and conspicuously bear the statement "Reprocessed device for single use. Reprocessed by [insert the name of the manufacturer that reprocessed the device]."[2] For additional information about labeling requirements, obtain a copy of the FDA guidance document *Labeling Regulatory Requirements for Medical Devices* from *http://www.fda.gov/cdrh/dsma/470. pdf* or contact the Division of Small Manufacturers Assistance (DSMA) by phone at 800-638-2041 or 301-638-2041; e-mail *DSMA@CDRH.fda.gov*.

Premarket Approval and Premarket Notification

After registering with the FDA and submitting a list of devices to be manufactured (reprocessed) and distributed for use, the registered entity must meet premarket submission requirements for each listed device. Certain devices may be exempt from the premarket submission requirement. If exempt, the device need only be listed with the FDA. Additional information about exemptions can be found in 21 CFR, Part 807.75.[20] The FDA has defined a phase-in period for premarket submissions to accommodate entities that are presently engaged in reprocessing. Following the phase-in period, a premarket submission must be submitted for any new device to be manufactured (reprocessed) at least 90 days before beginning distribution of the device.

There are two types of premarket submissions: a premarket notification, or 510(k), and a premarket approval (PMA) application. The type of submission required is based on the device classification, as defined in 21 CFR, Part 814.[21] Unless specifically exempted, a premarket notification (510[k]) is required for all Class I and Class II devices. A premarket notification (510[k]) submission must contain enough information for the FDA to determine whether the particular device is "substantially equivalent" to another device that has been previously judged to be safe and effective and has been cleared for marketing/ reprocessing. The predicate device selected must have the same intended use as the device for which the 510(k) is submitted. The predicate device may be the original SUD of the original equipment manufacturer (OEM) provided that the 510(k) compares the unique characteristics of the submitted device to those of the predicate device so the FDA can determine equivalency with respect to safety and effectiveness. The following information is required for a premarket notification (510[k]) submission:

- device trade name, proprietary name, usual name, or classification name;
- entity registration number;
- device classification;
- action taken to determine device performance standards;
- proposed labels, labeling, and advertisements to describe the device, its intended use, and the directions for its use, including photos and/or engineering drawings if appropriate;
- appropriate data to show that the registered entity has considered the consequences and effects any changes or modifications in the device might have on the safety and effectiveness of the device;
- 510(k) summary or 510(k) statement as defined in 21 CFR, Part 807.92, 93;[22]
- financial disclosure statement;[9]
- statement certifying truth, accuracy, and completeness of material submitted; and
- any other information requested by the FDA.

For specific guidance on preparing 510(k) submissions, consult *Regulatory Requirements for Medical Devices*, available at *http://www.fda.gov/cdrh /manual/510kprt1.html*, or contact the Division of Small Manufacturers Assistance. Locate other relevant guidelines at *http://www.accessdata.fda.gov/ scripts/cdrh/cfdocs/cfGGPSearch.CFM*.

All Class III devices require a PMA. A PMA application must include valid scientific evidence demonstrating the safety and effectiveness of the original and/or reprocessed device. Each PMA application should evaluate the unique characteristics of the submitted device. Clinical data (eg, results of clinical trials) may be required. Some clinical trials require FDA approval of an investigational device exemption (IDE) application for the device(s) to be studied. For additional information, consult the following sources:

- ♦ 21 CFR, Part 814.20;[21]
- ♦ 21 CFR, Part 812;[22]
- ♦ *Device Advice: Premarket Approval (PMA),* available at *http://www.fda.gov/cdrh/devadvice /pma* (accessed 3 Oct 2005);
- ♦ *Guidance for Institutional Review Boards and Clinical Investigators,* "Significant risk and nonsignificant risk medical device studies," available at *http://www.fda.gov/oc/ohrt /irbs/devices.html* (accessed 3 Oct 2005); and
- ♦ *Device Advice: Clinical Trials and Investigational Device Exemption (IDE),* available at *http://www.fda.gov/cdrh/devadvice/ide /application.shtml* (accessed 3 Oct 2005).

The FDA also requires a satisfactory inspection of the manufacturing (reprocessing) facilities before approving a PMA application. The application should include a comprehensive manufacturing (reprocessing) section that clearly identifies all manufacturing (reprocessing) controls. Under MDUFMA, some SUDs that previously were exempt from 510(k) submission requirements under Sections 510(l) or (m) of the Act are no longer exempt and are required under Section 510(o)(2) of the Act to submit 510(k) notifications that include validation data. Validation data also was required for some reprocessed SUDs that already had been cleared under 510(k). Under Section 510(o) of the Act, reprocessors that either did not submit validation data for those reprocessed SUDs within specified time frames or received "not substantially equivalent letters" from the FDA can no longer legally market those reprocessed devices. Finally, under Section 515(c)(2) of the Act, reprocessors of Class III SUDs are required to submit premarket reports instead of premarket approval applications.[2]

Medical Device Corrections and Removals

Device correction and/or removal from the point of use must be promptly reported to the FDA when the correction or removal is initiated by the manufacturer (reprocessor) to reduce a health risk to the user or to correct a violation of the Food, Drug, and Cosmetic Act. For example, if a facility reprocessed an SUD that resulted in a patient's adverse reaction and the hospital chose to remove the remainder of the lot of those reprocessed SUDs from circulation to decrease the possibility of other patients having adverse reactions, that action would be a removal and the facility would be required to report the removal to the FDA. Corrections are defined as

the repair, modification, adjustment, relabeling, destruction, or inspection of a device without its physical removal from its point of use.[23]

Removal is defined as

the physical removal of a device from its point of use to some other location for repair, modification, adjustment, relabeling, destruction, or inspection.[23]

Distributed devices withdrawn from the marketplace due to a minor violation of the Food, Drug, and Cosmetic Act or as a matter of stock rotation need not be reported. Stock recoveries need not be reported, nor should devices removed for routine servicing. The term *stock recoveries* refers to devices that have been prepared for use, but have not left the physical premises and jurisdiction of the manufacturer (reprocessor)—eg, devices that have not left the reprocessing area. However, each correction and/or removal must be documented regardless of whether it is reported to the FDA.

When a report must be filed with the FDA, the report must be filed within 10 days of the correction/removal action. The report should include the following information:

- ♦ registration number of the entity manufacturing/reprocessing the device;
- ♦ date of the report;
- ♦ sequence number of the report from that entity;
- ♦ name, address, and telephone number of the reporting entity;
- ♦ name, title, address, and telephone number of individual responsible for the correction/ removal action;
- ♦ brand name, classification name, and common name of the device and its intended use;
- ♦ marketing status of the device;
- ♦ model, catalog, and code number of the device and the manufacturer's (reprocessor's) lot, serial, or other identification number for the device;
- ♦ description of event leading to correction/ removal action;
- ♦ any injuries resulting from device use;

- total number of devices manufactured (reprocessed) subject to the correction/removal action;
- date of manufacture/distribution/reprocessing and expected shelf life of the device;
- name, address, telephone number of all to whom the device has been distributed and the number of devices distributed to each; and
- copies of all communication regarding the correction/removal action and the names and address of all recipients of the communication.

For additional information about correction and removal requirements, consult 21 CFR, Part 806.

Medical Device Tracking

Medical device tracking is intended to ensure that manufacturers (reprocessors) of certain devices can locate those devices should corrective action and/or notification about such devices become necessary. Original equipment manufacturers are subject to the medical device tracking regulation only when the FDA issues a tracking order for a device manufactured by the OEM. Reprocessors are subject to the medical device tracking regulation only when the FDA issues an order for the specific device(s) being reprocessed. For additional information on device tracking, including the types of devices currently subject to tracking orders, consult *Guidance on Medical Device Tracking,* available at *http://www.fda.gov /cerh/modact/tracking/pdf* or from the Center for Devices and Radiologic Health (CDRH) at 301-827-0111. Request document number 169.

Definitions

Class I medical device: A medical device for which general controls provide reasonable assurance of the safety and effectiveness of the device or, if there is insufficient evidence to reasonably ensure safety and effectiveness, the device is not life-supporting or life-sustaining, its use is not substantially important in preventing impairment of human health, and/or its use "does not present a potential unreasonable risk of illness or injury."[23]

Class II medical device: A medical device for which general controls alone do not provide reasonable assurance of device safety and effectiveness but for which there is sufficient information to establish special controls (eg, performance standards, guidelines, patient registries, postmarket surveillance) to provide that assurance.[23]

Class III medical device: A medical device for which neither general controls nor special controls provide reasonable assurance of device safety and effectiveness and the device is life-supporting or life sustaining or its use "is of substantial importance in preventing impairment of human health" or "presents a potential risk of illness or injury."[23]

Opened-but-unused device: A device whose sterility is compromised before being introduced onto the sterile field and which is not contaminated with blood and/or other potentially infectious materials (OPIM) external to the sterile field.[24]

Reprocessing: Includes all operations to render a contaminated reusable or single-use device patient ready. Single-use devices to be reprocessed may be either used or unused. Reprocessing steps include cleaning, decontamination, and sterilization/ disinfection.[9]

Resterilization: The repeated application of a process intended to remove or destroy all viable forms of microbial life, including bacterial spores.[9] Because sterility is not an absolute, the accepted sterility assurance level (SAL) is usually defined as 10^{-6}.

Reuse: The repeated or multiple uses of any medical device whether marketed as reusable or single-use. Repeated/multiple use may be on the same patient or on different patients with applicable reprocessing of the device between uses.[25]

Single-use device (SUD): A device intended by the manufacturer to be used on one patient during one procedure. The device is not intended for reprocessing and/or use on another patient or on the same patient at another time. Device labeling may or may not identify the device as single-use or disposable, but manufacturer instructions for reprocessing are absent.[9]

Third-party reprocessor: A business establishment, separate from the user facility and the device manufacturer, one of whose primary businesses is to reprocess single-use/disposable medical devices.

REFERENCES

1. "Reuse of single-use devices," *AORN Journal* 73 (May 2001) 957-966.

2. "Medical Device User Fee and Modernization Act (MDUFMA) of 2002," PL 107-250, 107th Congress, *http://www.fda.gov/cdrh/mdufma* (accessed 3 Oct 2005).

3. "Guidance for industry and for FDA staff: Enforcement priorities for single-use devices reprocessed by third parties and hospitals," (Aug 14, 2000) US Food and Drug Administration, *http://www.fda.gov/cdrh/reuse/1168.html* (accessed 3 Oct 2005).

4. "Medical devices; reprocessed single-use devices; termination of exemptions from premarket notification; requirement for submission of validation data," US Food

and Drug Administration, *http://www.fda.gov/OHRMS /DOCKETS/98fr/03-16109.html* (accessed 3 Oct 2005).

5. "AORN explications for perioperative nursing," in *Standards, Recommended Practices, and Guidelines* (Denver: AORN, Inc, 2005) 86-115.

6. Joint Commission on Accreditation of Healthcare Organizations, "Standard LD.3.50: Services provided by consultation, contractual agreements, or other agreements are provided safely and effectively," in *Comprehensive Accreditation Manual for Hospitals* (Oakbrook Terrace, Ill: Joint Commission on Accreditation of Healthcare Organizations, 2005) LD 13.

7. "Letter re: Reusable medical devices rented or leased from third parties," US Food and Drug Administration, *http://www.fda.gov/cdrh/comp/rentleasethird.html* (accessed 23 Aug 2005).

8. "Quality system regulation, Definitions," CFR 21, Part 820.3, US Food and Drug Administration, *http:// www.accessdata.fda.gov/scripts/cdrh/cfdocs/cfCFR /CFRSearch.cfm?fr=820.3* (accessed 3 Oct 2005).

9. "Letter to American College of Healthcare Executives: Reuse of single-use or disposable medical devices," US Food and Drug Administration, *http:// www.fda.gov/cdrh/comp/policymayaply.html* (accessed 3 Oct 2005).

10. Center for Devices and Radiological Health, US Food and Drug Administration, US Department of Health and Human Services, *Enforcement Priorities for Single-Use Devices Reprocessed by Third Parties and Hospitals* (Washington, DC: US Government Printing Office, Aug 14, 2000).

11. "Quality system regulation," CFR 21, Part 820, US Food and Drug Administration, *http://www.accessdata .fda.gov/scripts/cdrh/cfdocs/cfCFR/CFRSearch.cfm?CFR Part=820* (accessed 3 Oct 2005).

12. "Safe Medical Devices Act of 1990," Public Law 101-629, *http://thomas.loc.gov/cgi-bin/query/C?c101:./temp /~c101exIXhd* (accessed 23 Aug 2005).

13. "Medical device reporting: General provisions," CFR 21, Part 803.1, US Food and Drug Administration, *http://www.accessdata.fda.gov/scripts/cdrh/cfdocs/cfcfr /CFRSearch.cfm?fr=803.1* (accessed 3 Oct 2005).

14. "Manufacturer reporting requirements," CFR 21, Part 803, Subpart E, US Food and Drug Administration, *http://www.accessdata.fda.gov/scripts/cdrh/cfdocs/cfcfr /CFRSearch.cfm?CFRPart=803* (accessed 23 Aug 2005).

15. "Medical device reporting: General provisions," CFR 21, Part 803, Subpart A, US Food and Drug Administration, *http://www.accessdata.fda.gov/scripts/cdrh /cfdocs/cfcfr/CFRSearch.cfm?CFRPart=803* (accessed 23 Aug 2005).

16. "User facility reporting requirements," CFR 21, Part 803, Subpart C, US Food and Drug Administration,

http://www.accessdata.fda.gov/scripts/cdrh/cfdocs/cfcfr /CFRSearch.cfm?CFRPart=803 (accessed 23 Aug 2005).

17. US Department of Health and Human Services, "Medical device reporting: Manufacturer reporting, importer reporting, user facility reporting, distributor reporting," *Federal Register* 65 (Jan 26, 2000) 4112-4121.

18. "Establishment regulation and device listing for manufacturers and initial importers of devices," CFR 21, Part 807, US Food and Drug Administration, *http://www .accessdata.fda.gov/scripts/cdrh/cfdocs/cfcfr/CFR Search.cfm?CFRPart=807* (accessed 23 Aug 2005).

19. "Labeling," CFR 21, Part 801, US Food and Drug Administration, *http://www.accessdata.fda.gov/scripts /cdrh/cfdocs/cfcfr/CFRSearch.cfm?CFRPart=801* (accessed 23 Aug 2005).

20. "Exemption from premarket notification," CFR 21, Part 807, US Food and Drug Administration, *http://www .accessdata.fda.gov/scripts/cdrh/cfdocs/cfcfr/CFRSearch. cfm?fr=807.65* (accessed 23 Aug 2005).

21. "Premarket approval of medical devices," CFR 21, Part 814, US Food and Drug Administration, *http://www .accessdata.fda.gov/scripts/cdrh/cfdocs/cfcfr/CFRSearch. cfm?CFRPart=814* (accessed 23 Aug 2005).

22. "Investigational device exemptions," CFR 21, Part 812, US Food and Drug Administration, *http://www. accessdata.fda.gov/scripts/cdrh/cfdocs/cfcfr/CFRSearch. cfm?CFRPart=812* (accessed 3 Oct 2005).

23. "Medical devices: Reports of corrections and removals, definitions," CFR 21, Part 806.2, US Food and Drug Administration, *http://www.accessdata.fda.gov/scripts /cdrh/cfdocs/cfcfr/CFRSearch.cfm* (accessed 3 Oct 2005).

24. "Guidance for industry and for FDA staff: Enforcement priorities for single-use devices reprocessed by third parties and hospitals," US Food and Drug Administration, *http://www.fda.gov/cdrh/reuse/1168.html#_Toc492780057* (accessed 2 Feb 2006).

25. Center for Devices and Radiological Health, US Food and Drug Administration, US Department of Health and Human Services, "FDA's proposed strategy on reuse of single-use devices, docket no 99N-4491," *Federal Register* 64 (Nov 3, 1999) 59782-59783.

Resources

Medical Device Quality Systems Manual: A Small Entity Compliance Guidance, US Food and Drug Administration, *http://www.fda.gov/CDRH/DSMA/GMP MAN.HTML* (accessed 3 Oct 2005).

Publication History

Originally published in *Standards, Recommended Practices, and Guidelines,* 2005 edition. Reprinted November 2006, *AORN Journal.*

AORN Perioperative Standards and Recommended Practices, 2012 Edition

Additional Resources

Section IV

AORN Perioperative Standards and
Recommended Practices, 2012 Edition

Listing of AORN Position Statements

The following is a listing of AORN's official position statements on a variety of topics. These position statements represent the Association's official position on current health care issues affecting perioperative nursing practice and the profession. AORN position statements are approved by the AORN Board of Directors. All current AORN position statements are available online at *http://www.aorn.org/PracticeResources/AORNPositionStatements*.

AORN Position Statements as of November 2011:

Allied Health Care Providers and Support Personnel in the Perioperative Practice Setting
Care of the Older Adult in Perioperative Settings
Creating a Practice Environment of Safety
Criminalization of Human Errors in the Perioperative Setting
Entry into Practice
Environmental Responsibility
Ergonomically Healthy Workplace Practices
Healthy Perioperative Work Environment
Immediate Use Steam Sterilization
Noise in the Perioperative Practice Setting
One Perioperative Registered Nurse Circulator Dedicated to Every Patient Undergoing A Surgical or Other Invasive Procedure
Operating Room Staffing Skill Mix for Direct Caregivers
Orientation of the Registered Nurse and Certified Surgical Technologist to the Perioperative Setting
Patient Safety
Patients and Health Care Workers with Bloodborne Diseases
Perioperative Advanced Practice Nurse
Perioperative Care of Patients With Do-Not-Resuscitate (DNR) Orders
Preventing Wrong-Patient, Wrong-Site, Wrong-Procedure Events
Responsibility for Mentoring
RN First Assistants
Role of the Health Care Industry Representative in the Perioperative/Invasive Procedure Setting
Safe Work On-Call Practices
Surgical Smoke and Bio-Aerosols
Value of Clinical Learning Activities in the Perioperative Setting in Undergraduate Nursing Curricula
Workplace Safety
Policy for Sunset of AORN Position Statements

AORN Perioperative Standards and Recommended Practices, 2012 Edition

Policy and Procedure Template for Use with Recommended Practices

The following template and samples are provided to assist the health care organization in creating policies and procedures for the perioperative practice setting that incorporate AORN recommended practices. The template includes a suggested policy format and an explanation of the intended content of each section. Also included in this appendix are two policy and procedure samples: "Fire safety" and "Correct site, correct procedure, and correct patient for invasive or surgical procedure."

Although the template and these sample documents are copyrighted by AORN, we have designed them to be used without restriction in your workplace. In addition, AORN has developed a CD-ROM that contains a collection of sample policies and procedures based on AORN recommended practices released in the past few years. These 15 policy and procedure documents, formatted in Word®, are fully customizable by the user to suit any perioperative work setting.

Editor's note: *Word is a registered trademark of Microsoft Corp, Redmond, WA.*

AORN's *Policy and Procedure Templates*, 2nd edition

Contents

- Attire
- Correct Site, Correct Procedure, and Correct Patient for Invasive or Surgical Procedure
- Disinfection—High-Level
- Electrosurgery
- Fire Safety
- Flexible Endoscopes and Accessories—Cleaning and Processing
- Hand Hygiene—Perioperative
- Laser Safety
- Minimally Invasive Surgery—Managing the Patient Care and the Risks Related to
- Moderate Sedation—Managing the Adult Patient Receiving
- Positioning
- Product Selection
- Retained Surgical Items—Prevention of
- Surgical Smoke Evacuation Policy
- Transfer of Patient Care Information

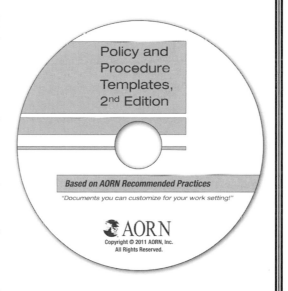

This CD-ROM is available for purchase from the AORN Bookstore at http://www.aornbookstore.org.

Policy Template

INSERT POLICY TITLE AND ANY FACILITY-SPECIFIC INFORMATION HERE

Purpose:

> The purpose statement is the intention of the policy. It is a concise summary with brief highlights. The purpose statement may be based on the Perioperative Nursing Data Set (PNDS) outcome statements or on the purpose statement of the recommended practice related to the policy and procedure.

Insert brief purpose statement here.

Policy:

> The policy is a statement describing activities that must be completed, including requirements from regulatory and accrediting agencies. Recommendations or intervention statements from the recommended practice may be used as policy statements. The recommendations are signified by a Roman numeral (eg, I, II, III) in bold font. The intervention statements are signified by a Roman numeral followed by an alpha character (eg, I.a., I.b., I.c.). The "should" statements in the recommended practice may be changed to *must* or *will*, and several recommendations may be grouped into one policy statement.

It is the policy of *[name of facility]* that:

Procedure Interventions:

> The procedure consists of statements describing the sequence of steps necessary to accomplish the purpose of the policy. Intervention statements or activity statements from the recommended practice may be used as steps in the procedure. The intervention statements are signified by a Roman numeral followed by an alpha character (eg, I.a., I.b., I.c.). The activity statements are signified by a Roman numeral followed by an alpha character followed by an Arabic numeral (eg, I.a.1., I.a.2., I.a.3.). The "should" statements in the recommended practice may be changed to must or will or may be converted into action statements. If the intervention cannot be delegated, the procedure statements may include a reference to the title of the person required to complete the intervention (eg, "The perioperative registered nurse assesses the patient"). If the task may be delegated, the procedure may be described in an action statement (eg, "Remove all contaminated supplies from the operating room").

Insert the specific sequence of steps required to achieve the purpose and the policy.

Documentation:

> The documentation section of the recommended practice may be used to assist in determining the facility's baseline for documentation.

Insert here the information your facility requires to be documented, the area on the chart where this information is to be documented, and who is responsible for the documentation.

Competency:

> The competency section of the recommended practice may be used to assist in determining the facility's baseline competencies.

INSERT HERE a statement of the knowledge, skills, and abilities your facility deems necessary for the person to successfully perform the steps in this policy and procedure.

Definitions:

> The glossary section of the recommended practice may be used as a guideline for determining the definitions used in the policy and procedure.

INSERT HERE the definitions of any words or phrases used that have a new or unfamiliar use in this policy and procedure.

References:

> Suggested references may include the most current edition of the AORN *Perioperative Standards and Recommended Practices*.

INSERT HERE a list of the references used to compile the policy and procedure, using the format chosen by your facility.

Administrative Approval:

> Insert here the publication history of the document and the signatures of the person or persons in a leadership role who are responsible for the policy and procedure (eg, educator, manager, director, vice president of nursing; also may include the responsible physician) in accordance with organizational policy.

Date of original approval, review, or revision.

Created: _____

Reviewed: _____

Revised: _____

Approval signature(s) with position title and date of signature:

_____	_____	_____
Signature	*Title*	*Date*
_____	_____	_____
Signature	*Title*	*Date*
_____	_____	_____
Signature	*Title*	*Date*

Policy & Procedure

VERIFICATION OF CORRECT SITE, CORRECT PROCEDURE, AND CORRECT PATIENT FOR INVASIVE OR SURGICAL PROCEDURES

Purpose:

To provide steps to assist in minimizing avoidable risks during invasive or surgical procedures. The expected outcome is that the patient's procedure is performed on the correct site, side, and level.

Policy:

It is the policy of *[insert name of facility]* that the following steps must be completed before every invasive or surgical procedure, unless noted on the exception list. This policy shall be followed for all invasive or surgical procedures throughout the facility.

> - In the preprocedure/preoperative area, a confirmation of the correct site, procedure, and patient shall occur.
> - In the preprocedure/preoperative area, the patient shall be involved whenever possible. If the patient is unable to participate, a designated caregiver shall participate.
> - All patients who undergo an invasive or surgical procedure involving laterality, multiple structures (eg, fingers and toes), or multiple levels (eg, spinal surgery) must have their surgical sites marked.
> - If a patient refuses site marking, the patient's physician will review the rationale for site marking and the implications for refusing site marking.
> - A licensed independent practitioner or other provider who is privileged or permitted to perform the intended invasive or surgical procedure [determined by facility] will mark the procedure/surgical site before the patient enters the procedure/operating room unless the anatomical site is exempt per policy guidelines.
> - A discrepancy at any point in time must be resolved before continuing the procedure. All team members and the patient, if possible, must agree on resolution of the identified discrepancy.
> - A time out will be performed for all cases, including those not requiring site marking.
> - Two patient identifiers [determined by facility] will be used to verify a patient's identity (eg, full name, date of birth). A patient room number should not be used as a n identifier.
> - If a treatment (eg, anesthesia block) or medication administration (eg, eye drops) must be performed before the site has been marked (in the holding area), the patient verification process as outlined above must be followed.
> - Site marking may be waived in a life-threatening emergency at the discretion of the operating physician, but a time out should be conducted unless there is more risk than benefit for the patient.
> - Bedside procedures (eg, chest tube/central line insertion):
>   - ❖ The person performing the procedure must identify the patient and confirm all data, including consent, history and physical, radiographs, and any other information [determined by facility], and must be in continuous attendance. He or she may perform the procedure without marking the site.
>   - ❖ A time out still must occur before the start of the procedure.

Procedure Interventions:

> - **Scheduling and preadmission testing**
>   - ❖ Obtain the following information when scheduling an invasive or surgical procedure:
>   - • the correct spelling of the patient's full name;

Insert facility name here or use a header or footer

- date of birth;
- procedure to be performed;
- physician's name;
- implants required, if applicable; and
- facility-required booking data.
❖ Write out fully on the procedure/operating room schedule and on all relevant documentation (eg, consents) the words right, left, or bilateral for scheduled procedures that involve anatomical sites that have laterality.

➢ **Preprocedure/preoperative verification**
The registered nurse or other health care provider (eg, radiographer, phlebotomist, respiratory therapist) should
❖ verify the patient's identity using at least two identifiers (eg, full name, date of birth) [*determined by the facility*];
❖ verify the scheduled invasive or surgical procedure as stated by the patient and compare to the posted schedule, consents, radiographic films, site mark (if applicable), and any other information in the medical record [*determined by facility*];
❖ involve the patient in the process, to the fullest extent possible, with verbal and visual responses (eg, stating name, pointing to correct site location);
❖ use a designated caregiver [*determined by facility*] if the patient is a minor, incompetent, sedated, has a language barrier, or is a trauma/emergency victim, to complete the identifiers and verify the site mark; and
❖ clarify any discrepancies in data with the physician.

➢ **Marking the surgical site**
❖ Use a sufficiently permanent marker.
❖ The mark may be placed on the day of the invasive or surgical procedure or before as long as the mark is visible at the time of the invasive or surgical procedure.
❖ Before marking the site, verify the patient's identity, consent, medical record data, and any other information [determined by facility], including radiographs and history and physical, as applicable, to confirm accuracy.
❖ Ask the patient or designated caregiver [*determined by facility*] to state the procedure and site and side of surgery and have the patient provide visual clues, if appropriate, such as pointing.
❖ The designated person will mark the site at or adjacent to the incision site at a location that will be visible after the patient is prepped and draped.
❖ The person marking the site will use his or her initials for the mark.
❖ Spine surgery requires a two-stage marking process.
  - Preoperatively, the person doing the marking does so on the patient's skin at the level of the procedure (eg, cervical, thoracic, lumbar). The skin mark indicates anterior vs. posterior and right vs. left.
  - Intraoperatively, x-rays with immovable markers will be used to determine exact location and level of surgery. The operating physician will review the x-rays for confirmation.
❖ For procedures involving laterality of organs where the incision or approach may be from the mid-line or from a natural orifice, the site is marked and the laterality noted using one of the alternative methods listed below. The person doing the marking should not
  - place the skin mark on an open wound or lesion or

Insert page number in your facility's style

- mark nonoperative sites unless medically indicated (eg, pedal pulse markings, no blood pressure cuff).
- ❖ If the patient refuses site marking, the patient's physician will review with the patient the rationale for site marking and the implications for refusing site marking. If the patient still refuses site marking, the person responsible for marking the site should use an alternative method before the case proceeds.
- ❖ For sites that cannot be easily marked (eg, mucosal surfaces, perineum, premature infants, teeth extractions), alternative methods may include
  - a temporary, unique wrist band on the side of the procedure that contains the patient's name and a second identifier for the intended procedure and site for cases that are impossible or impractical to mark (eg, interventional procedures such as cardiac catheterization, pacemaker insertion);
  - a mark at or near the insertion site that will remain visible after completion of the skin prep and sterile draping (eg, minimal access procedures intended to treat a lateralized internal organ); and
  - documentation, dental radiographs, or dental diagrams that indicate the name and number of the operative tooth.

➤ **Taking a time out**

Time outs will be performed before all surgical or invasive procedures. Time outs will

- ❖ cause all other activities to be suspended (unless there is a threat to patient safety) during the time out;
- ❖ be initiated by a designated team member (eg, RN circulator);
- ❖ involve all members of the surgical team;
- ❖ address the following standard information:
  - correct patient identity,
  - correct side and site are marked,
  - consent form is present and accurate,
  - agreement on the procedure to be done,
  - correct patient position,
  - confirm that relevant images and results are properly labeled and appropriately displayed,
  - confirm that antibiotics have been administered,
  - confirm that the skin prep has dried, and
  - prosthesis is present, if applicable;
- ❖ be performed in the location of the procedure and after the patient is prepped and draped;
- ❖ be performed before each procedure if two procedures are being performed on the same patient; and
- ❖ reconcile problems if the responses among team members differ. The reconciliation process [*determined by facility*].

Documentation:

➤ A variance report should be completed if the time out does not occur and the site is not marked (if required).

➤ The nurse will document the patient's inability and/or refusal to allow documentation and the alternative method used to mark the site.

➤ Record, at a minimum, the following items:

Insert facility name here or use a header or footer

- ❖ who marked the site, date, and time;
- ❖ the time of pause (names are not required because it is assumed that all people listed on the operative record at the start of the procedure were present); and
- ❖ any other items required by the facility.

Competency:

The perioperative registered nurse should be clinically competent and possess the skills necessary to verify the correct site, correct procedure, and correct patient for invasive or surgical procedures. The competencies include the ability to

- ➢ assess the patient;
- ➢ verify the correct site, correct patient, and correct procedure;
- ➢ mark the surgical site (if applicable);
- ➢ initiate the time-out; and
- ➢ document the process.

Definitions:

Time out: The pause in patient care activity conducted by the surgical team immediately before starting the procedure to conduct a final assessment that the correct patient, site, positioning, and procedure are identified and that, as applicable, all relevant documents, related information, and necessary equipment are available.

References:

Petersen C, ed. *Perioperative Nursing Data Set*. 3rd ed. Denver, CO: AORN, Inc; 2010. In press.

National Patient Safety Goals 2009. Joint Commission. *http://www.jointcommission.org/Patient Safety/NationalPatientSafetyGoals*. Accessed December 22, 2009.

Administrative Approval:

Date of original approval, review, or revision:

Created: _____

Last Revised: _____

Last Reviewed: _____

Next Review: _____

Approval signature(s) with position title and date of signature:

Signature	_Title_	_Date_
Signature	_Title_	_Date_
Signature	_Title_	_Date_

Insert page number in your facility's style

Policy & Procedure

FIRE SAFETY IN PERIOPERATIVE SETTINGS

Purpose:

To provide guidance to perioperative personnel in preventing fires during surgical and other invasive procedures and responding appropriately if a fire should occur. Fires are considered a preventable occurrence. The expected outcome is that the patient will be free from signs and symptoms of injury related to thermal sources.

Policy:

It is the policy of [*insert name of facility*] that:

> - All perioperative team members are responsible for preventing fires.
> - All perioperative team members are responsible for participating in departmental fire safety training.
> - Department-specific fire drills will occur quarterly during each shift during which the perioperative department is operational.
> - A mock evacuation scenario will occur as one of the fire drills on an annual basis.
> - On an annual basis each member of the perioperative team shall be able to:
>   - ❖ demonstrate fire extinguishing techniques, including the use of fire-fighting equipment;
>   - ❖ identify department evacuation routes for each room;
>   - ❖ identify fire extinguisher locations;
>   - ❖ locate medical gas panel and demonstrate its operation including turning off medical gases in case of an emergency situation; and
>   - ❖ identify electrical panel locations and procedure for turning off the system.
> - A fire risk assessment will be performed before each surgical or other invasive procedure in which all three of the parts of the fire triangle (ie, fuel, ignition source, oxidizer) come together.
> - Personnel not directly involved in patient care should report to the staff lounge or other location as dictated by organization-wide fire policy when the fire alarm sounds.
> - The decision to evacuate the surgical suite will be made by the RN in charge at the time of the situation, in collaboration with the surgeon, anesthesia care provider, and the fire department personnel, if available.

Procedure Interventions:

The following interventions should be followed to prevent fire on or in a patient.

> - **Scope of a fire risk assessment:**
>   - ❖ Assess the flammability of all materials used on or around the patient, including but not limited to the following:
>   - • liquids (eg, alcohol-based skin prep solutions);
>   - • ointments (eg, petroleum- or oil-based lubricants);
>   - • gases (eg, oxygen, methane, anesthetic agents, alcohol vapor);
>   - • plastics;
>   - • paper or gauze materials;

Insert facility name here or use a header or footer

- surgical drapes;
- foam positioning devices;
- adhesive or plastic tapes; and
- endotracheal tubes.

➤ **Performing a fire risk assessment:**
 ❖ The RN circulator will report fire risk assessment as A, B, C, D, or E or any combinations of the letters before the procedure begins. The designation A, B, C, D, E is determined by the code assigned to each of the critical questions **in bold** below having an affirmative response. The procedure may be any one letter or any combination of the letters.

 A. Is an alcohol-based prep agent or other volatile chemical being used preoperatively?
  ○ **Actions:**
   ▪ Prevent pooling of skin prep solutions on or around the patient.
   ▪ Remove prep-soaked linen and disposable prepping drapes before placing surgical drapes.
   ▪ Allow skin prep agents to dry and fumes to dissipate before draping the patient and using an ignition source.
   ▪ Conduct a skin prep "time out" to validate that the prepping agent is dry before draping the patient.
   ▪ Allow chemicals (eg, alcohol, collodion, tinctures) to dry thoroughly and vapors to dissipate before using an ignition source (eg, electrosurgical unit [ESU], laser).

 B. Is the surgical procedure being performed above the xiphoid process?
  ○ **Actions:**
   ▪ Coat the head and facial hair near the surgical site with water-soluble surgical lubricant to decrease flammability.
   ▪ Use an adhesive incise drape.

 C. Is open oxygen or nitrous oxide being administered?
  ○ **Actions:**
   ▪ Use the same strategies as described below to manage the risks of oxygen and nitrous oxide.
   ▪ Configure surgical drapes to allow sufficient venting of oxygen delivered to the patient via mask or nasal prongs.
   ▪ Deliver 5 L to 10 L/min of air under the surgical drapes to flush out excess oxygen via a separate administration system, if oxygen is being administered via mask or nasal prongs.
   ▪ Titrate oxygen to the lowest percentage necessary to support the patient's physiological needs.
   ▪ Stop supplemental oxygen or nitrous oxide for one minute before using electrosurgery, electrocautery, or laser for head, neck, or upper chest procedures.
   ▪ When possible, use cuffed endotracheal tubes.
   ▪ Inflate endotracheal tube cuff with tinted saline (eg, methylene blue).
   ▪ Evacuate surgical smoke to prevent accumulation in small or enclosed spaces (eg, back of throat).
   ▪ Pack wet sponges around the back of the throat to help retard oxygen leaks.
   ▪ Suction oropharynx deeply before using ignition source if oxygen is used.
   ▪ Check anesthesia circuits for possible leaks.
   ▪ Turn off the flow of oxygen at the end of each procedure.

Insert page number in your facility's style

Insert facility name here or use a header or footer

D. Is an ESU, laser, or fiber-optic light cord being used?
- Actions—ESU use:
  - Place the patient return electrode on a large muscle mass close to the surgical site.
  - Keep active electrode cords from coiling.
  - Store the ESU pencil in a safety holster when it is not in use.
  - Keep surgical drapes or linens away from the activated ESU.
  - Moisten drapes if absorbent, towels, and sponges that will be in close proximity to the ESU active electrode.
  - Do not use an ignition source to enter the bowel when it is distended with gas.
  - Keep ESU active electrode away from oxygen or nitrous oxide if possible.
  - Keep the active electrode tip clean.
  - Use only active electrodes or return electrodes that are manufacturer approved for the type and model of ESU being used.
  - Use only approved protective covers as insulators on the active electrode tip (ie, NOT red rubber catheter or packing materials).
  - Activate the active electrode only when it is in close proximity to the target tissue and away from other metal objects that could conduct heat or cause arcing.
  - Inspect minimally invasive electrosurgical electrodes for impaired insulation and remove the electrode from service if insulation is not intact.
  - Use cut or blend settings instead of coagulation when possible.
  - Use the lowest possible power setting for the ESU.
  - Only the person controlling the active electrode activates the ESU.
  - Remove the active electrode tip from the electrosurgical or electrocautery unit before discarding.
- Actions—laser use:
  - Use a laser-resistant endotracheal tube during upper airway procedures.
  - Place wet sponges around the tube cuff if laser is being operated in close proximity to the endotracheal tube (ET).
  - Use wet sponges or towels around the surgical site for all laser procedures.
  - Only the person controlling the laser beam activates the laser.
  - Verify that water and the appropriate type of fire extinguisher are available before using the laser.
- Actions—fiber-optic light cord use:
  - Place the light source in standby mode or turn it off when the cable is not in active use (eg, used within 5 to 10 seconds).
  - Inspect light cables before use and remove from service if broken light bundles are visible.
  - Secure the working end (ie, the end that is inserted into the body) of the telescope or cord on a moist towel or away from any drapes, sponges, or other flammable materials.

E. Are there other possible contributors?
- Actions:
  - Select defibrillator paddles that are the correct size for the patient.
  - Use only manufacturer recommended product for defibrillator paddle lubrication.
  - Use appropriate defibrillator paddle placement allowing optimal skin contact.
  - Slowly drip saline on a moving drill, burr, or saw blade.
  - Place drills or saws on the Mayo stand or back table when they are not in use.

Insert page number in your facility's style

Insert facility name here or use a header or footer

➤ **Procedure interventions for prevention of fire on or in equipment**
- ❖ Inspect electrical cords and plugs for integrity and remove them from service if they are broken.
- ❖ Check biomedical inspection stickers on equipment for currency and remove the equipment from service if they are not current.
- ❖ Keep fluids off electrical equipment (eg, ESU, laser).
- ❖ Do not bypass or disable ESU or laser safety features (eg, turning audible alarms down).
- ❖ Use medical devices according to manufacturers' recommendations.

➤ **Procedure interventions for handling a fire on a patient**
- ❖ Small flames or a small area:
  - Communicate the presence of the fire to team members.
  - Pour saline or water on the fire slowly to prevent spreading.
  - Place your arm between the patient's head and the fire, then lay a wet towel or sponge over the flame and sweep it toward the patient's feet.
  - Lift the material used to smother the flame to vent heat.
  - Remove burning material from the patient.
  - Assess the surgical field for a secondary fire on the underlying drapes or towels.
  - Assess the patient for injuries and report to a physician.
  - Activate alarms, if necessary.
  - Notify the appropriate chain of command.
- ❖ Large flames or a large area:
  - Communicate the presence of the fire to team members.
  - Communicate with the anesthesia care provider to stop the flow of breathing gases to the patient.
  - If drapes are involved remove the drape to the ground, rolling it on itself to smother the fire.
  - Avoid moving the drape into what may need to be the team members' route to evacuate the room.
  - Assess the surgical field for a secondary fire on the underlying drapes or towels.
  - Assess the patient for injury and report injuries to a physician.
  - Verify the flames are extinguished and use a fire extinguisher, if necessary.
  - Employ the PASS technique when using a fire extinguisher.
    - P = pull
    - A = aim
    - S = squeeze
    - S – sweep
  - Activate alarms, if necessary.
  - Notify the appropriate chain of command.

➤ **Procedure interventions for handling a fire in a patient**
- ❖ Communicate the presence of the fire to all team members.
- ❖ Consult with the anesthesia care provider to determine the necessary actions to take to extinguish an airway fire.
- ❖ Assist the anesthesia care provider with:
  - disconnecting and removing the breathing circuit,
  - turning off the flow of oxygen,
  - removing the ET tube and any segments of the burned tube that remain in the airway,
  - pouring saline or water into the airway if instructed,

Insert page number in your facility's style

Insert facility name here or use a header or footer

- • re-establishing the airway, and
- • examining the airway.
- ❖ Assess the surgical field for a secondary fire on the underlying drapes or towels.
- ❖ Assess the patient for injury and report injuries to a physician.
- ❖ Activate alarms, if necessary.
- ❖ Notify the appropriate chain of command.

➢ **Procedure interventions for handling a fire on a piece of equipment**
- ❖ Communicate the presence of the fire to all team members.
- ❖ Disconnect equipment from its electrical source.
- ❖ Shut off the electricity to the piece of equipment at the electrical panel, if it is not possible to remove the plug from the outlet.
- ❖ Shut off gases to equipment, if applicable.
- ❖ Assess the size of the fire and determine whether equipment can be removed from the room safely or if the room needs to be evacuated.
- ❖ Extinguish the fire using a fire extinguisher, if appropriate.
- ❖ Activate alarms, if necessary.
- ❖ Notify the appropriate chain of command.

➢ **Procedure interventions for handling a fire in another area of the building**
- ❖ All operating and procedure rooms will be notified of the presence of a fire in another area of the building by the person in charge.
- ❖ No elective cases will be started.
- ❖ Prepare to evacuate.

➢ **Procedure interventions for evacuation**
- ❖ **Use RACE**
  - • **RESCUE:**
    - ○ Determine the best method to remove the patient (eg, procedure bed, gurney, carry) from the area.
    - ○ Determine the safest location to receive the patient.
    - ○ Get adequate assistance.
    - ○ Remove the patient and staff members from the room containing the fire or smoke.
  - • **ALARM:**
    - ○ Communicate to the entire perioperative suite, especially the adjoining rooms.
    - ○ Follow the hospital-wide procedure for activating the organizational alarm system.
    - ○ Call the local fire department, if necessary.
  - • **CONTAIN:**
    - ○ Close the doors to the involved room.
    - ○ Shut off medical gases to the involved room.
    - ○ Turn off electricity to the involved room.
  - • **EVACUATE:**
    1. When: When a danger is posed to patients in adjoining areas from fire or smoke.
    2. Where:
       a. Transfer the patients to an area that is beyond the first set of smoke barriers.
       b. Determine the best area in which surgery may be finished safely.
    3. How: Transfer patients by carrying them, using a gurney or moving the procedure bed with the patient remaining on the bed.

Insert page number in your facility's style

Insert facility name here or use a header or footer

Other Procedure Interventions:

> ➤ Save all involved materials and devices for later investigation.
> ➤ Provide all involved materials and devices to quality/risk management personnel.

Documentation:

> ➤ Fire risk assessment score.
> ➤ Time fire risk assessment was performed.

Competency:

All personnel will receive education, training, and competency validation on fire prevention, including but not limited to the following:
> ➤ identifying the elements of the fire triangle;
> ➤ performing and documenting the perioperative fire risk assessment;
> ➤ using fire extinguishers and other fire-fighting equipment;
> ➤ identifying department evacuation routes for each room;
> ➤ locating available fire extinguishers;
> ➤ identifying medical gas panel locations and explaining gas panel operation including turning them off in an emergency situation;
> ➤ locating ventilation and electrical systems and explaining the procedure for turning off the system;
> ➤ determining whether to evacuate the environment or not;
> ➤ performing appropriate rescuer methods;
> ➤ describing how and when to activate the fire safety/evacuation plan;
> ➤ discussing how and when to contact the local fire department; and
> describing the roles and responsibilities of each team member in various fire scenarios.

References:

Petersen C, ed. *Perioperative Nursing Data Set.* 3rd ed. Denver, CO: AORN, Inc; 2010.

Recommended practices for electrosurgery. In: *Perioperative Standards and Recommended Practices.* Denver, CO: AORN, Inc; 2010:105-125.

Recommended practices for laser safety in practice settings. In: *Perioperative Standards and Recommended Practices.* Denver, CO: AORN, Inc; 2010:133-138.

Recommended practices for minimally invasive surgery. In: *Perioperative Standards and Recommended Practices.* Denver, CO: AORN, Inc; 2010:139-174.

Recommended practices for a safe environment of care. In: *Perioperative Standards and Recommended Practices.* Denver, CO: AORN, Inc; 2010:217-240.

National Fire Protection Association, NFPA 101—Life Safety Code, 2009 Edition. Quincy, MA: National Fire Protection Association; 2009.

Guidance article: new clinical guide to surgical fire prevention. *Health Devices.* 2009;38(10):314-332.

Insert page number in your facility's style

Insert facility name here or use a header or footer

Administrative Approval:

Date of original approval, review, or revision:

Created: _____

Last Revised: _____

Last Reviewed: _____

Next Review: _____

Approval signature(s) with position title and date of signature:

Signature	*Title*	*Date*
Signature	*Title*	*Date*
Signature	*Title*	*Date*

AACD Glossary of Times Used for Scheduling and Monitoring of Diagnostic and Therapeutic Procedures

The following glossary was developed by the Association of Anesthesia Clinical Directors (AACD) and was approved by their board of directors in October 1995. It has been endorsed by AORN, Inc, and the Society for Technology in Anesthesia and has been accepted without revision by the American Society of Anesthesiologists Committee on Quality Improvement and Practice Management. It is reprinted here with permission of the AACD.

Background

Elevated concerns regarding the economics of health care are dramatically intensifying the pressure for health care providers to establish critical pathways and/or total quality management programs. In addition, negotiating fiscally sound managed care contracts with health maintenance organizations and health insurance carriers, as well as meeting state and federal government documentation requirements, requires justification for each aspect of patient care as well as improved techniques in cost factor analysis and accounting. Few hospital administrators would deny that operating rooms/procedure rooms (OR/PR) are expensive to run, and all would concur that economic analyses of running OR/PRs are not readily available.

During the planning for multicenter studies of OR/PR scheduling, utilization, and efficiency, members of the Association of Anesthesia Clinical Directors (AACD) felt semantics were introducing a major impediment to data comparison and economic analysis. To provide a universal lexicon for the acquisition of data, the AACD has developed a glossary which inclusively, yet restrictively, defines the procedural times that permit comprehensive analyses of OR/PR scheduling, utilization, and efficiency. The AACD proposes adopting this lexicon as a standardized "Glossary of Times Used for Scheduling and Monitoring of Diagnostic and Therapeutic Procedures."

The glossary is divided into four sections: 1) Procedural Times, 2) Procedural and Scheduling Definitions and Time Periods, 3) Utilization and Efficiency Indices, and 4) Patient Categories. The terms defined under Procedural Times are listed in what is the usual chronological order, while terms defined in the other sections are presented in alphabetical order.

1. Procedural Times

(For purposes of analyzing efficiency, each of the times defined below may be further classified by the subscripts S and A, for "Scheduled" and "Actual," respectively.)

1.1 Patient in Facility (PIF) = Time patient arrives at health care facility (applicable to outpatient or same day admission patients).

1.2 Patient Ready for Transport (PRT) = Time when all preparations required prior to transport (eg, labs, consent, gowning) have been completed.

1.3 Patient Sent-for (PS) = Time when transporting service is notified to deliver patient to the OR/PR.

1.4 Patient Available (PA) = Time the patient arrives in the OR/PR preprocedure area.

1.5 Room Set-up Start (RSS) = Time when personnel begin setting up, in the OR/PR, the supplies and equipment for the next case.

1.6 Anesthesia Start (AS) = Time when a member of the anesthesia team begins preparing the patient for an anesthetic.

1.7 Room Ready (RR) = Time when room is cleaned and supplies and equipment necessary for beginning of next case are present (see Discussion).

1.8 Patient In Room (PIR) = Time when patient enters the OR/PR.

1.9 Anesthesiologist, First Available (AFA) = Time of arrival in OR/PR of first anesthesiologist who is qualified to induce anesthesia in patient (see Discussion).

1.10 Procedure Physician, First Available (PPFA) = Time of arrival in OR/PR of first physician/surgeon qualified to position and prep the patient (see Discussion).

1.11 Anesthesiologist of Record In (ARI) = Time of arrival in OR/PR of anesthesiologist of record (see Discussion).

1.12 Anesthesia Induction (AI) = Time when the anesthesiologist begins the administration of agents intended to provide the level of anesthesia required for the scheduled procedure.

1.13 Anesthesia Ready (AR) = Time at which the patient has a sufficient level of anesthesia established to begin surgical preparation of the patient, and remaining anesthetic chores do not preclude positioning and prepping the patient (see Discussion).

1.14 Position/Prep Start (PS) = Time at which the nursing or surgical team begins positioning or prepping the patient for the procedure.

1.15 Prep-Completed (PC) = Time at which prepping and draping have been completed and patient is ready for the procedure or surgery to start.

1.16 Procedure Physician of Record In (PPRI) = Arrival time of physician/surgeon of record (see Discussion).

1.17 Procedure/Surgery Start Time (PST) = Time the procedure is begun (eg, incision for a surgical procedure, insertion of scope for a diagnostic procedure, beginning of exam under anesthesia [EUA], shooting of x-ray for radiological procedure).

1.18 Procedure/Surgery Conclusion Begun (PCB) = Time when diagnostic or therapeutic maneuvers are completed and attempts are made by the physician or surgical team to end any noxious stimuli (eg, beginning of wound closure, removal of bronchoscope).

1.19 Procedure Physician of Record Out (PPRO) = Time when physician/surgeon of record leaves the OR/PR (see Discussion).

1.20 Procedure/Surgery Finish (PF) = Time when all instrument and sponge counts are completed and verified as correct; all postoperative radiological studies to be done in the OR/PR are completed; all dressings and drains are secured; and the physician/surgeons have completed all procedure-related activities on the patient.

1.21 Patient Out of Room (POR) = Time at which patient leaves OR/PR.

1.22 Room Clean-up Start (RCS) = Time housekeeping or room personnel begin clean-up of OR/PR.

1.23 Arrival in PACU/ICU (APACU) = Time of patient arrival in PACU or ICU.

1.24 Anesthesia Finish (AF) = Time at which anesthesiologist turns over care of the patient to a postanesthesia care team (either PACU or ICU).

1.25 Room Clean-up Finish (RCF) = Time OR/PR is clean and ready for set-up of supplies and equipment for the next case.

1.26 Ready-for-Discharge from Postanesthesia Care Unit (RDPACU) = Time that patient is assessed to be ready for discharge from the PACU.

1.27 Discharge from Postanesthesia Care Unit (DPACU) = Time patient is transported out of PACU.

1.28 Arrival in Same Day Surgery Recovery Unit = Time of patient arrival in same day surgery recovery unit.

1.29 Ready-for-Discharge from Same Day Surgery Recovery Unit (RDSDSR) = Time that patient is assessed to be ready for discharge from the same day surgery recovery unit.

1.30 Discharge from Same Day Surgery Recovery Unit (DSDSR) = Time patient leaves SDSR unit (either to home or other facility).

2. Procedural and Scheduling Definitions and Time Periods

(For purposes of analyzing efficiency, each of the time periods defined below may be further classified by the subscripts E and A for "Estimated" and "Actual," respectively.)

2.1 Anesthesia Preparation Time (APT) = Time from Anesthesia Start to Anesthesia Ready Time.

2.2 Average Case Length (ACL) = Total hours divided by total number of cases performed within those hours.

2.3 Block Time (BT) = Hours of OR/PR time reserved for a given service or physician/surgeon. Within a defined cutoff period (eg, 72 hours prior to day of surgery), this is time into which only the given service may schedule. (NB: In some institutions, this is known as available or allocated time.)

2.4 Case Time (CT) = Time from Room Set-up Start to Room Clean-up Finished (see Discussion).

2.5 Early Start Hours (ESH) = Hours of Case Time performed prior to the normal day's start time when it is not expected that the Patient Out of Room Time will be before the normal start time for that day.

2.6 Evening/Weekend/Holiday Hours (EWHH) = Hours of Case Time performed outside of Resource Hours.

2.7 In-own Block Hours (IBH) = Hours of Case Time performed during a service's own Block Time. (NB: For a case to be counted in IBH, it must begin during that given service's Block Time.)

2.8 Open Time (OT) = Hours of OR/PR time not reserved for any particular service, into which any service or physician/surgeon may schedule according to the rules established by the given institution. (NB: In some institutions, this is known as discretionary time).

2.9 Outside-own Block Hours (OBH) = Hours of Case Time performed during Resource Hours but outside of the service's Block Time.

2.10 Overrun Hours (OVRH) = Hours of Case Time completed after the scheduled closure time of the OR/PR (ie, after the end of that day's Resource Hours).

2.11 Released Time (RT) = Hours of OR/PR time that are released from a service's Block Time and converted to Open Time (typically done when a service anticipates that it will be unable to use the Block Time due to meetings or vacation).

2.12 Resource Hours (RH) = Total number of hours scheduled to be available for performance of procedures (ie, the sum of all available Block Time and Open Time). This is typically provided for on a weekly recurring basis, but may be analyzed on a daily, weekly, monthly, or annual basis (see Discussion).

2.13 Room Clean-up Time (RCT) = Time from Patient Out of Room to Room Clean-up Finished.

2.14 Room Close (RC) = Time at which the room should be empty and the assigned personnel free to be discharged.

2.15 Room Open (RO) = Time when appropriate staff are scheduled to be present and are expected to have the OR/PR available for patient occupancy.

2.16 Room Set-up Time (RST) = Time from Room Set-up Start to Room Ready.

2.17 Service = A group of physicians or surgeons that together perform a circumscribed set of operative or diagnostic procedures (eg, cardiothoracic surgery, interventional radiology). Generally, any member of a service may schedule into that service's block time. Similarly, OR/PR time used by a given physician or surgeon is credited to his/her service's Total Hours.

2.18 Surgical Preparation Time (SPT) = Time from Position/Prep Start to Procedure/Surgery Start Time.

2.19 Start Time (ST) = Patient In Room Time (see Discussion).

2.20 Total Cases (TC) = Cumulative total of all cases done in a given time period. May be subdivided by service or physician/surgeon.

2.21 Total Hours (TH) = Sum of all Case Times for a given period of time. TH = IBH + OBH + EWHH. May be subdivided by service or individual physician/surgeon.

2.22 Turnover Time (TOT) = Time from prior Patient Out of Room to succeeding Patient In Room Time for sequentially scheduled cases (see Discussion).

3. Utilization and Efficiency Indices

3.1 Adjusted-Percent Service Utilization (ASU) = (IBH + OBH) x 100 ÷ BT. This measures the percentage of time a service utilizes their Block Time during Resource Hours. It is adjusted, compared to Raw Utilization, in that it gives a service "credit" for the time necessary to set up and clean up a room, during which time a patient cannot be in the room. It may exceed 100% because of the inclusion of cases performed during Resource Hours that are Outside-own Block Hours (see Discussion).

3.2 Adjusted-Percent Utilized Resource Hours (AURH) = (Total Hours-Evening/Weekend/Holiday Hours) ÷ Resource Hours x 100. This calculation provides the percentage of time that the OR/PRs are being prepared for a patient, are occupied by a patient, or are being cleaned after taking care of a patient during Resource Hours. It is adjusted, compared to Raw Utilization, in that it includes the time necessary to set up and clean up a room, during which time a patient cannot be in the room (see Discussion).

3.3 Delays may be due to:

3.3.1 Patient issues
  Insurance problems
  Patient arrived late
  Patient ate/drank
  Abnormal lab values
  Surgery issues
  Complications arose

3.3.2 System issues
  Test results unavailable
  Blood unavailable
  Patient not ready on floor
  Transport delay
  Elevator delay
  Previous case ran late
  Case bumped for emergency case
  Equipment unavailable
  Equipment malfunction
  X-rays unavailable
  X-ray technician unavailable
  Delay in receiving floor bed
  Insufficient post procedure care beds
  ICU delay
  Instrument problem

3.3.3 Practitioner issues
  Needs more workup (eg, labs, consults)
  No consent
  Physician/surgeon arrived late
  Anesthesiologist arrived late
  Physician/surgeon unavailable
  Anesthesiologist unavailable
  Inaccurate posting
  Prolonged set-up time

3.4 Early Start = When Patient In Room, Actual, is prior to Patient In Room, Scheduled.

3.4.1 With overlap—When a case starts early but prior to the Room Clean-up Finished, Actual, of the case originally scheduled to precede it (this occurs when either the preceding or following case is moved to a different OR/PR than originally scheduled).

3.4.2 Without overlap—When a case starts early but after the Room Clean-up Finished, Actual, of the case originally scheduled to precede it (this may occur because there is no preceding case or because the preceding case finishes earlier than scheduled).

3.5 Late Start = When Patient In Room, Actual, is after Patient In Room, Scheduled.

3.5.1 With no interference—when the Room Clean-up Finished, Actual, of the preceding case occurs before the Room Set-up Start, Scheduled, of the following case (ie, the OR/PR is available prior to or at the time that preparation for the next case is supposed to begin).

3.5.2 With interference—When Room Clean-up Finished, Actual, of the preceding case occurs after the Room Set-up Start, Scheduled, of the following case (ie, the OR/PR is not available at the time that preparation for the next case is supposed to begin, either because it is still occupied or because it has not been cleaned).

3.6 Overrun = When Room Clean-up Finished, Actual, for the last scheduled case of the day is later than Room Close. This may be caused by a late start; a Case Time, Actual, greater than Case Time, Scheduled; or a combination of late start and longer than scheduled Case Time.

3.7 Productivity Index (PI) = Percent of time per hour that a patient is in the OR/PR during the prime shift time (eg, first 8 hours).

3.8 Raw Utilization (RU) = For the system as a whole, this is the percent of time that patients are in the room during Resource Hours (see Adjusted-Percent Utilized Resource Hours). For an individual service, this is the percent of its Block Time during which a service has a patient in the OR/PR (see Adjusted-Percent Service Utilization).

3.9 Room Gap = Time OR/PRs are vacant during Resource Hours.

3.9.1 Empty Room (or Late Start) Gap (LSG)
Planned—When Patient In Room, Scheduled, is later than Room Open.
Unplanned—When Patient In Room, Actual, is later than Room Open.

3.9.2 Between Case Gaps (BCG)
Planned—When Patient In Room, Scheduled, is later than the Room Clean-up Finished, Actual, of the preceding case.
Unplanned—When Patient In Room, Actual, is later than the Room Clean-up Finished, Actual, of the preceding case.

3.9.3 End of Schedule Gaps (ESG)
Planned—When Room Clean-up Finished, Scheduled, occurs before Room Close.
Unplanned—When Room Clean-up Finished, Actual, occurs before Room Close.

3.9.4 Total Gap Hours (TGH) = LSG + BCG + ESG.

4. Patient Categories

4.1 In-house (IH) = Patient admitted to and residing in the hospital prior to scheduled surgery/procedure.

4.2 Outpatient (OP) = Patient who is coming in on the day of surgery/procedure and is expected to return home following the procedure.

4.3 Same Day Admit (SDA) = Patient who is coming in on the day of surgery/procedure and will be admitted to the hospital following the procedure.

4.4 Overnight-Recovery (ONR) = Patient who comes in on the day of surgery/procedure but requires overnight recovery prior to returning home. These patients are never admitted to the hospital as inpatients, but may remain in the recovery facility for 12 to 23 hours post surgery/procedure.

Discussion

The foregoing list of the procedural times was intentionally made exhaustive in order to be all inclusive. This by no means suggests that all of the data points defined need to be collected by all institutions. Where problems with OR/PR efficiency exist, whether they are real or perceptual, collecting the appropriate times listed above, and calculating the pertinent time periods, will permit objective evaluation of where the real problems lie. Use of common definitions across the country will also permit inter-institutional comparisons that have been previously impossible.

Several terms listed in the "Procedural Times Glossary" have not had heretofore universally accepted definitions. For several of these, the authors, the board of directors of the Association of Anesthesia Clinical Directors, and the Society for Technology in Anesthesia National Database Committee felt that there existed significant controversy over which definition should be chosen. Although for each of these a consensus was generated which led to the definition chosen, general acceptance of these choices may be improved if the logic behind the decision is known. For those terms which created serious debate, the following discussion of terms is provided.

Adjusted-Percent Service Utilization (ASU) = (IBH + OBH) x 100 ÷ BT. This measures the percentage of time a service utilizes its Block Time during Resource Hours. It is adjusted, compared to raw utilization, in that it gives a service "credit" for the time necessary to set up and clean up a room, during which time a patient cannot be in the room. It may exceed 100% because of the inclusion of cases performed during Resource Hours that are Outside-own Block Hours.

Adjusted-Percent Utilized Resource Hours (AURH) = (Total Hours-Evening/Weekend/Holiday Hours) ÷ Resource Hours x 100. This calculation provides the percentage of time that the OR/PRs are being prepared for a patient, are occupied by a patient, or are being cleaned after taking care of a patient during Resource Hours. It is adjusted, compared to raw utilization, in that it includes the time necessary to set up and clean up a room, during which time a patient cannot be in the room.

Raw Utilization (RU) = For the system as a whole, this is the percent of time that patients are in the room during Resource Hours (see Adjusted Percent Utilization Resource Hours). For an individual service, this is the percent of its Block Time during which a service has a patient in the OR/PR (see Adjusted-Percent Utilization).

Frequently, institutions attempt to assess the extent to which a service uses its allotted Block Time by calculating a utilization percentage. Such a calculation should be performed for the system as a whole to measure the extent to which the "normal" hours of operation are actually used for patient care. If one considers only the time that a patient is in the OR/PR (raw utilization), then the percent of time that a service uses its Block Time is artificially lowered because the time necessary to set up and clean up a room, during which time a patient cannot be in the room, is not accounted for. Similarly, the calculation of percentage utilization of Resource Hours is artificially reduced if only Patient In Room time is used. The larger the number of procedures done in a given room during Resource Hours, the greater the error.

Cost-effective utilization requires highly effective scheduling and optimum utilization of the Resource Hours, with minimal overtime and/or uses of more highly paid on-call personnel. For proper assessment of the extent to which a service

or system utilizes its Block or Resource Hours, respectively, the utilization calculations should be adjusted as defined above. For the individual service, this provides a fairer determination of how much of its Block Time is truly used. For the system as a whole, it provides the actual percentage of time that the OR/PRs are being used for patient care. Perhaps as important, it provides an accurate percentage of time that is not used and therefore available for efficiency improvements.

Anesthesiologist, First Available (AFA) = Time of arrival in OR/PR of first anesthesiologist who is qualified to induce anesthesia in patient.

Procedure Physician, First Available (PPFA) = Time of arrival in OR/PR of first physician/surgeon qualified to position and prep the patient.

If delays in starting cases are thought to be due to the late arrival of either a qualified anesthesiologist or surgeon, recording of these times will allow documentation of the extent of that cause of delay.

Anesthesia Ready (AR) = Time at which the patient has a sufficient level of anesthesia established to begin surgical preparation of the patient, and remaining anesthetic chores do not preclude positioning and prepping the patient.

To maximize efficiency, surgical preparation of the patient should begin as soon as an adequate level of anesthesia has been obtained. In some instances however, the anesthesiologist may need to continue anesthetic preparation of the patient (eg, insertion of Swan-Ganz catheter) that precludes moving or prepping the patient. Anesthesia Ready is thus defined as that time when the anesthesiologist may allow surgical preparation to begin.

Anesthesiologist of Record In (ARI) = Time of arrival in OR/PR of anesthesiologist of record.

Procedure Physician of Record In (PPRI) = Arrival time of physician/surgeon of record.

In academic settings, delays may be due to the late arrival of either the attending anesthesiologist or surgeon. Recording of these times will allow one to determine if tardiness of either attending contributes to delays. Further, in the future, accrediting bodies and insurance carriers may require documentation of the time of presence of the physicians of record.

Case Time (CT) = Time from Room Set-up Start to Room Clean-up Finished.

This definition includes all of the time for which a given procedure requires an OR/PR. It allows for the different duration of Room Set-up and Room Clean-up Times that occur because of the varying supply and equipment needs for a particular procedure. For purposes of scheduling and efficiency analysis, this definition is ideal because it includes all of the time that an OR/PR must be reserved for a given procedure.

Procedure Physician of Record Out (PPRO) = Time when physician/surgeon of record leaves the OR/PR.

Because perceptual differences of turnover times abound, it is important to note when the physician of record leaves the OR/PR, as this may be significantly earlier than when the patient leaves the OR/PR. In those situations when an anesthesiologist is supervising another anesthesia care provider (resident or CRNA), the anesthesiologist of record may be in and out of the OR/PR multiple times, and thus no analogous definition has been provided for.

Resource Hours = Total number of hours scheduled to be available for performance of procedures (ie, the sum of all available Block Time and Open Time). This is typically provided for on a weekly recurring basis, but may be analyzed on a daily, weekly, monthly, or annual basis.

For a given institution, this is the time during which an optimum number of appropriate personnel are available to do cases. This may include more than one shift of personnel, or personnel working extended shifts (ie, greater than 8 hours), in order to gain vertical expansion of OR/PR hours. It may also include electively scheduled time on weekends to gain horizontal expansion of OR/PR hours. Resource hours do not include time gained through overtime or use of on-call personnel, even though this time may be routinely accrued at a given institution.

Room Ready (RR) = Time when room is cleaned and supplies and equipment necessary for beginning of next case are present. To maximize efficiency, the patient should be brought into the OR/PR as early as possible. Although some wish to have all the supplies and equipment necessary for the entire case present and open before the patient is brought in, institutions that have minimized turnover times move patients into the OR/PR as soon as it is clean and only the minimum supplies and equipment (ie, those needed to start the case) are present, but not necessarily open. In those institutions, room preparation continues as anesthesia in induced, allowing an overlap of processes (anesthesia induction and room preparation) that saves time.

Start Time (ST) = Patient in Room Time. Significant debate, indeed, even argument, exists over the proper definition of Start Time. Operating and procedural room nurses generally feel that they have properly accomplished their preparatory tasks if the room is ready at the scheduled start time (Room Ready = Start Time, Estimated), regardless of where the patient is at that time. Anesthesiologists often feel that they are "on time" if anesthesia induction has been completed by the scheduled start time (Anesthesia Ready = Start Time, Estimated). Surgeons generally believe start time should be the time at which the procedure is begun (Procedure/Surgery Start Time = Start Time, Estimated). Since Room Set-up Time is procedure specific and therefore generally known at the time of scheduling, one can reasonably predict Room Ready Time. Anesthesia Preparation Time, however, depends on both the procedure and patient needs. It is thus more variable and not known at the time a procedure is scheduled, making accurate prediction of Anesthesia Ready Time impossible.

This variability in Anesthesia Preparation Time also makes prediction of Procedure/Surgery Start Time inaccurate. Variability in Case Times, due to varying length of surgery, makes prediction of Start Times after the first scheduled case of the day even more inaccurate.

Much of the concern over Start Time is for the first case of the day, particularly when a service or surgeon follows herself/himself in the same OR/PR throughout the day. Prediction, then, of accurate Start Times for the first case of the day appears to be most critical. Once the procedure is known, it is almost always possible to have the Room Ready at any time that is desired for the start of the day. It should also be possible, and desirable for maximizing efficiency, to have the patient in the room for the first case of the day as soon as the room is ready. For maximizing scheduling accuracy and attempting to encourage the most efficient patient flow, the authors have elected to define Start Time as Patient In Room Time.

Turnover Time (TOT) = Time from prior Patient Out of Room to succeeding Patient In Room Time. Strong perceptual differences exist over the definition of Turnover Time. Anesthesiologists and OR/PR nurses usually consider turnover time to be the time between cases when the room is not occupied by a patient. Surgeons consider any time when they are unable to operate as "down time," and thus more often consider turnover time to be the time between the end of surgery on one case and the beginning of surgery on the next case. The latter may appear to be particularly long to an academic surgeon who leaves an OR before the wound is closed (allowing the residents to close and dress the incision) and does not re-enter the OR until the next patient is ready for incision.

As with Start Time, the variability of Anesthesia Preparation Time (APT) makes prediction of turnover times inaccurate if APT were to be included. Thus, to maximize scheduling accuracy and to encourage distinction of time spent preparing the OR/PR from time spent preparing the patient, the authors have elected to define Turnover Time as time from prior Patient Out of Room to succeeding Patient In Room Time for sequentially scheduled cases. As this definition attempts to include the time spent cleaning and preparing the OR/PR for the next case, it should only be calculated if a subsequent case is scheduled to immediately follow. With nonsequential cases, idle time between Room Clean-up Finished for the prior case to Room Set-up Start for the subsequent case should be identified and recorded under the appropriate room-gap category.

Editor's note: The Association of Anesthesia Clinical Directors changed its name to the American Association of Clinical Directors in 2004. The purpose of the society is to provide a forum for anesthesiologists whose primary responsibility is operating room management. *("About us," American Association of Clinical Directors,* http://aacdhq.org *[accessed 28 Dec 2006].)*

AORN Perioperative Standards and Recommended Practices, 2012 Edition

Registered nurse first assistant (RNFA) education programs are designed to provide RNs with the educational preparation necessary to assume the role of the first assistant during operative and other invasive procedures.

The "AORN Standards for RN first assistant education programs" serve as the foundation upon which RNFA programs are developed and implemented. These standards are intended to guide program administrators and faculty members in designing and evaluating curricula. These standards are broad in scope, definitive, relevant, and attainable, and they provide the framework for RNFA education.

Standard I

Requirements for RNFA education programs shall include the following:

Programs shall
A. be equivalent to one academic year of formal, post-basic nursing study.
B. award college credits and degrees or certificates of RNFA status upon satisfactory completion of all requirements.
C. be associated with schools of nursing at universities or colleges that are accredited for higher education by an accrediting agency that is nationally recognized by the Secretary of the US Department of Education.

The schools of nursing shall be approved by a state licensing jurisdiction for nursing programs at the university, college, or community college level or by another agency that is nationally recognized by the Secretary of the US Department of Education as a specialized accrediting agency for nursing programs.
D. recognize the "AORN position statement on RN first assistants."[1]
E. address all of the content in the *Core Curriculum for the RN First Assistant*.[2]

Standard II

Preadmission requirements for RNFA education programs shall include the following:

A. General admission requirements as determined by each educational institution.
B. Proof of licensure to practice as an RN in the state in which the clinical internship will be undertaken.

C. Verification of certification as one of the following:
1. CNOR® or CNOR eligible. If the student is not certified at time of admission, certification must be submitted before program completion.
2. Board certified or board eligible as an advanced practice registered nurse (APRN). APRNs without experience in intraoperative patient care must undergo an assessment regarding clinical skills and knowledge. Assessment should be completed by the program instructor or perioperative educator at the facility where the clinical experience will be completed. Assessment should include aseptic technique, scrubbing, gowning, gloving, creating and maintaining a sterile field, and positioning the patient. If it is determined that skills or knowledge are deficient, faculty members in the educational institution shall develop a plan to remediate identified deficiencies.
D. Cardiopulmonary resuscitation (CPR) or basic cardiac life support certification (BCLS) is required; advanced cardiac life support (ACLS) is preferred.
E. Letters of recommendation attesting to the years of experience as an RN and knowledge, judgment, and skills specific to surgical patient care.

Standard III

The didactic component of the curriculum for RNFA education programs shall be designed and evaluated based on a course description that identifies course content, course length, faculty composition, instruction and evaluation methodologies, and instructional resources.

A. Course content shall emphasize the expanded functions unique to the RNFA during operative and other invasive procedures, including, but not limited to,
1. preoperative patient management in collaboration with other health care providers, such as
   - performing focused preoperative nursing assessments and
   - communicating and collaborating with other health care providers regarding the patient's plan of care;

2. intraoperative performance of surgical first-assisting techniques such as
   - using instruments and medical devices,
   - providing surgical site exposure,
   - handling and/or cutting tissue,
   - providing hemostasis, and
   - suturing; and
3. postoperative patient management in collaboration with other health care providers in the immediate postoperative period and beyond, such as,
   - participating in postoperative rounds, and
   - assisting with discharge planning and identifying appropriate community resources as needed.[1]

B. The following topics provide content for remediation for the APRN, who as an RNFA student candidate, may not have perioperative experience and whose perioperative skills and knowledge are found to be deficient (as described in Standard II.C.2).
   1. anesthesia;
   2. aseptic technique;
   3. documentation;
   4. electrosurgery;
   5. endoscopic surgery;
   6. environmental sanitation and terminal cleaning;
   7. hemostasis, sponges, and drains;
   8. introduction to perioperative nursing;
   9. laser safety;
   10. latex allergy;
   11. medications and solutions;
   12. patient and family member education;
   13. perianesthesia nursing;
   14. perioperative assessment;
   15. positioning the patient;
   16. professionalism;
   17. safety in the surgical suite;
   18. scrubbing, gowning, and gloving;
   19. skin preps;
   20. specimens;
   21. sterilization and disinfection;
   22. surgical draping;
   23. surgical instruments;
   24. the surgical environment; and
   25. wound closure and healing.
      The APRN also may gain these skills and knowledge by completing a basic perioperative orientation program (eg, Periop 101: A Core Curriculum™).

C. The course shall be a minimum of one academic semester of study, including student assignments, classroom instruction, and laboratory practicums.

D. A multidisciplinary faculty shall include a minimum of
   1. a perioperative nurse with a master of science in nursing degree;
   2. an RNFA or, preferably, a certified registered nurse first assistant (CRNFA®); and
   3. a board-certified surgeon.

E. Instructional methodologies shall include, but not be limited to, lecture, interactive discussion, independent study, instructional media, demonstration/return demonstration, and laboratory practicums.

F. Evaluation methodologies shall include, but not be limited to, written examinations, laboratory practicums, and independent critical thinking assignments.

G. Instructional resources shall include
   1. the *Core Curriculum for the RN First Assistant*[2] and
   2. texts or other instructional media that include anatomy and physiology, operative and other invasive procedures, and preoperative and postoperative patient assessment and management.

Standard IV

Successful completion of all requirements of the didactic component shall be required for matriculation into the clinical component.

Standard V

The clinical component of the curriculum for RNFA education programs shall be designed and evaluated based on a course description that identifies course content, course length, faculty composition, instructional and evaluation methodologies, and instructional resources.

A. Course content shall emphasize the expanded functions unique to the RNFA intern during operative and other invasive procedures, including, but not limited to,
   1. preoperative patient management in collaboration with other health care providers, such as
      - performing focused preoperative nursing assessments,
      - communicating and collaborating with other health care providers regarding the patient plan of care;

2. validated documentation of the intraoperative surgical first-assisting clinical experience, including, but not limited to,
   – using instruments and medical devices,
   – providing surgical site exposure,
   – handling and/or cutting tissue,
   – providing hemostasis, and
   – suturing; and

3. postoperative patient management in collaboration with other health care providers in the immediate postoperative period and beyond, such as
   – participating in postoperative rounds and
   – assisting with discharge planning and identifying appropriate community resources as needed.[1]

B. The clinical course shall be a minimum of one academic semester and shall include, but not be limited to,
   1. a minimum of 120 clock hours of intraoperative first assisting hours and
   2. additional hours of other patient care management as described in section A.

C. A multidisciplinary faculty shall include
   1. a board-certified surgeon in the RNFA intern's primary area of practice,
   2. an RNFA program faculty member, and
   3. an RNFA/CRNFA mentor if available and/or desired by the student.

D. Instructional methodologies shall include, but not be limited to, physician-supervised clinical activities, assigned independent learning activities, a self-evaluative learning diary, a clinical case study project, and a surgical intervention participation log.

E. Evaluation methodologies shall include, but not be limited to, completion of assigned independent learning activities, a self-evaluative learning diary, a clinical case study project, preceptor evaluations, a surgical intervention participation log, and mentor evaluations when applicable. Students must satisfactorily complete all requirements. The RNFA program faculty members shall review all documentation. The surgeon preceptor shall provide a summative evaluation of achievement of competence and a letter of recommendation based on all required learning activities, as shall the RNFA/CRNFA mentor when applicable.

F. Instructional resources shall include
   1. *Core Curriculum for the RN First Assistant*,[2]
   2. texts or other instructional media, and
   3. consultation and collaboration with other health care providers.

Editor's note: CNOR and CRNFA are registered trademarks of the Competency and Credentialing Institute, Denver, CO. *Periop 101: A Core Curriculum* is a trademark of AORN, Inc, Denver, CO.

Glossary

CNOR: The documented validation of the professional achievement of identified standards of practice by an individual registered nurse providing care for patients before, during, and after surgery.

CRNFA: The documented validation of the professional achievement of identified standards of practice by an individual registered nurse first assistant providing care for patients before, during, and after surgery.

Faculty: A person who is appointed by the educational institution to design, teach, or evaluate a course of instruction.

Intraoperative first assisting hours: Calculated from the time of the incision until the dressing has been applied.

Mentor: One who provides encouragement and acts as a guide and facilitator while modeling professional nursing behaviors.

Preceptor: One who teaches, counsels, inspires, serves as a role model, and supports the growth and development of the novice for a fixed and limited period.

REFERENCES
1. AORN position statement on RN first assistants. AORN, Inc. *http://www.aorn.org/PracticeResources /AORNPositionStatements/Position_RNFA*. Accessed March 3, 2011.
2. Vaiden RE. *Core Curriculum for the RN First Assistant*. 4th ed. Denver, CO: AORN, Inc; 2005.

PUBLICATION HISTORY
Originally published March 1995, *AORN Journal*, as "AORN recommended education standards for RN first assistant programs."

Revised December 2004; approved by the AORN Board of Directors in February 2005.

Revised June 2007; approved by the AORN Board of Directors July 2007. Published in: Burlingame BL. *RN First Assistant Guide to Practice*. 3rd ed. Denver, CO: AORN, Inc; 2007.

Revised January, 2011; approved by the AORN Board of Directors in February 2011 for publication online at aorn.org and subsequent publication in the *AORN Journal* and online in the *Perioperative Standards and Recommended Practices*.

AORN Perioperative Standards and Recommended Practices, 2012 Edition

Quality and Performance Improvement Standards for Perioperative Nursing

The 2002 AORN Nursing Practices Committee (NPC) was charged with the review and revision of the "Quality improvement standards for perioperative nursing" developed by the 1990 NPC.

Over time, health care has used many different terms to denote the processes used to improve patient care, such as quality assurance (QA), continuous improvement (CI), and continuous quality improvement (CQI). Quality cannot be assured, but it can be measured, assessed, and improved. Perioperative nurses should strive continuously to improve the care provided to patients in the perioperative setting.

Quality improvement (QI) and performance improvement (PI) are the newest terms used in the quest for excellence. They are two different methodologies that are linked together and continuously developing. "QI examines processes in order to improve them. PI addresses human performance within organizations at the individual, process, and organizational levels."[1] The origin of QI is based in industry and has more of a management and process focus; PI focuses more on the people, their motivation, and the tools (eg, work design, technical support, supervision, safety) they use to achieve the goals of the organization.

Government-funded peer review organizations (PROs), Medicare/Medicaid reimbursement regulations, laws generated at the federal and state levels, and private health insurers' standards have refocused the efforts required to assess patient care systematically. The recent focus of regulatory bodies and the Joint Commission on Accreditation of Healthcare Organizations (JCAHO) has placed greater emphasis on patient safety and reducing the errors that have resulted, at times, in patient deaths. The Institute of Medicine's 1999 report, *To Err Is Human: Building a Safer Health System*," states, "Although there are many kinds of standards in health care, especially those promulgated by licensing agencies and accrediting organizations, few standards focus explicitly on issues of patient safety."[2]

The Joint Commission states, "The goal of the improving organization performance function is to ensure that the organization designs processes well and systematically monitors, analyzes, and improves its performance to improve patient outcomes. Value in health care is the appropriate balance between good outcomes, excellent care and services, and costs. To add value to the care and services provided, organizations need to understand the relationship between perception of care, outcomes, and costs, and how the three issues are affected by processes carried out by the organization. An organization's performance of important functions significantly affects the quality and value of its services."[3] JCAHO bases its evaluation of an institution's QI/PI activities on

♦ designing processes,
♦ monitoring performance through data collection,
♦ analyzing current performance, and
♦ improving and sustaining improved performance.

An effective quality/performance improvement plan should be consistent with the philosophy, mission, and strategic goals of the organization. Departmental initiatives should be systematic, written, and communicated to leaders, practitioners, and staff. The plan should provide reliable data that is integrated into an organization-wide plan. Implementation of QI/PI standards may provide the basis for selecting mechanisms that measure outcomes and maintain systems to analyze and trend data and corrective actions that result in improved, safer patient care.

Staff participation and a multidisciplinary approach to the program enhance the awareness of personnel providing direct and indirect care and enable challenges to be funneled into opportunities for improvement. Documentation should show that all aspects of care in the department conform to contemporary standards of clinical practice and that data are used to study and improve the quality of care.

AORN's *Standards, Recommended Practices, and Guidelines* should be used as a resource when establishing a QI/PI program. Organizations, depending on their size, resources, and commitment to QI/PI, may have a central department, task force, or steering committee to oversee, expedite, and guide departments in achieving the goals of their QI/PI plan.

Standard I

Assign responsibility for monitoring and evaluation activities.

Interpretive statement 1:
The director and/or the designee (eg, manager or other individual[s] responsible for the department) assume overall responsibility for the monitoring

and evaluation processes within the department and in the department's participation in the organization-wide performance improvement plan.

Criteria:

1. The director actively participates in and supports the program.
2. The director may select an individual (ie, designee) to be responsible for the department's overall participation in the QI/PI plan.
3. The director/designee selects the individual/team responsible for each QI/PI project. The team may include, but is not limited to,
   - staff nurses,
   - ancillary staff members,
   - educators,
   - medical director/chief of services,
   - members of the medical staff,
   - OR director/supervisor,
   - QI/PI coordinator, and
   - representatives from any departments involved in the process.
4. The director collaborates with other disciplines and departments that share responsibility for QI/PI activities.

Interpretive statement 2:

The director/designee or other responsible individual(s) develops a mechanism for ensuring that departmental initiatives are congruent with the organization-wide QI/PI plan. The departmental initiatives are integrated and communicated throughout the organization.

Criteria:

1. The plan reflects a departmental and organization-wide commitment to patient care excellence.
2. The plan is communicated through organization-wide and unit-based staff development programs.
3. The plan is evaluated and revised at least annually to determine program appropriateness and effectiveness.
4. The plan describes the roles and responsibilities of those involved in quality improvement/performance improvement. This plan may be in the form of a narrative statement, outline, flow chart, or team charter.
5. The plan describes the monitoring and evaluation activities. These may include, but are not limited to,
   - delineating scope of care,
   - identifying important functions and processes,
   - prioritizing areas for improvement,
   - collecting and analyzing data,
   - evaluating patient care,
   - resolving problem areas and/or improving processes that affect patient care,
   - documenting results,
   - communicating findings, and
   - maintaining improvements.
6. The plan identifies collaborating disciplines/departments that share responsibilities and are interdependent in QI/PI. These activities may include, but are not limited to,
   - contracted services,
   - engineering,
   - environmental services,
   - infection control,
   - laboratory,
   - materials management,
   - medical staff,
   - nursing units,
   - pharmacy,
   - radiology,
   - risk management/safety, and
   - special care units.
7. The plan describes the schedule of the quality QI/PI plan. This may include, but is not limited to, schedule of meetings, schedule of times, and locations of monitoring and evaluation activities.
8. The plan reflects the uniqueness of nursing activities performed in the perioperative setting and the outcomes of perioperative patient care.

Standard II

Delineate the scope of patient care activities or services.

Interpretive statement:

The scope of patient care activities or services describes who is served, what services are provided, who provides the services, physical sites, and times that services are provided.

Criteria:

1. The patient population assessment/description may include, but is not limited to,
   - patient acuity,
   - patient socioeconomic status,
   - demographics,
   - support systems, and
   - clinical conditions/diagnoses.

2. Customers are identified, and they are relevant to the type of service provided. Customers may include, but are not limited to,
   - employees,
   - patients,
   - families,
   - practitioners,
   - purchasers, and
   - suppliers.

3. Clinical care activities and nursing services are determined. These may include, but are not limited to,
   - circulating;
   - scrubbing;
   - first assisting;
   - patient education;
   - resource nurses/advanced practitioners (eg, clinical nurse specialists, nurse practitioners); and
   - others identified in AORN's *Standards, Recommended Practices, and Guidelines.*

4. Services provided in the department are inventoried. Services may include, but are not limited to,
   - cardiovascular/thoracic,
   - endoscopy,
   - general surgery,
   - ophthalmology,
   - orthopedics,
   - otolaryngology,
   - obstetrics and gynecology,
   - neurosurgery,
   - pediatrics, and
   - pain management.

5. Departmental practitioners are listed by job title and level of expertise. Individuals who contribute to departmental care and activities may include, but are not limited to,
   - advanced practice nurses,
   - registered nurses,
   - licensed practical/vocational nurses, and
   - unlicensed assistive personnel.

6. Other practitioners/personnel who share patient care responsibilities are listed. These may include, but are not limited to,
   - ancillary departments,
   - contracting agencies,
   - employed caregivers, and
   - physicians.

7. The physical site is described. The description may include, but is not limited to,
   - number and type of suites/rooms,
   - their proximity to each other, and
   - support areas.

8. Dates, days, and hours of operation are described.

9. Suites/rooms are identified by type of service provided.

10. Staffing plans/patterns that support services are identified.[4] A rationale is given for the chosen staffing, and a mechanism is in place to evaluate the effectiveness.

Standard III

Identify processes impacting the quality and safety of patient care.

Interpretive statement:
High-volume, high-risk, and/or problem-prone processes are identified.

Criteria:

1. High-volume types of patient care activities are those performed on a frequent or daily basis to a large volume of patients. High-volume types include, but are not limited to,
   - procedures that occur frequently (eg, cholecystectomy, laparoscopy, cataract extraction);
   - nursing activities frequently performed for patients (eg, placement of electrosurgical dispersive pad, administration of medication, aseptic technique); and
   - nursing care that affects a large number of patients (eg, patient assessments, patient education, discharge planning, intravenous therapy, pain management).

2. High-risk processes are those that carry a greater potential for liability and/or patient injury. High-risk areas may include, but are not limited to,
   - patients at risk of serious consequences (eg, patients with a history of difficult airway management or a high risk assessment for DVT/PE, physiologically compromised patients, elderly patients, children, neonatal patients);
   - complex or high-risk procedures that are performed infrequently;
   - care delivered that was inconsistent with nursing standards or guidelines (eg, incorrect counts, wrong site/side surgery or failure to verify procedure[s] or patient identity, medication errors, improper positioning, breaks in aseptic technique, lack of appropriate patient education);

- acts of omission/commission;
- patients receiving moderate or deep sedation (refer to JCAHO Standards [TX2]); and
- patients undergoing multiple procedures or recurrent surgeries.

3. Problem-prone processes identify departmental problem areas. Problem-prone areas may include, but are not limited to,
   - procedures and/or care that cause patient and/or staff anxiety;
   - activities known to generate a number of incident reports;
   - activities needing increased efficiency (eg, surgery schedule management, instrument processing); and
   - equipment known to have a high risk or incidence of user error (eg, new equipment, infrequently used equipment, equipment that has been modified).

Standard IV

Systematic performance measures (ie, indicators) and/or priority areas are identified as opportunities for improvement based on the functions and processes of the perioperative episode.

Interpretive statement:
Performance measures (ie, indicators) should relate to the structure, process, or outcome of care and/or service.

Criteria:
1. Structure measures based on the AORN "Standards of perioperative administrative practice" relate to physical, fiscal, and organizational elements that require
   - establishing, controlling, and monitoring a safe perioperative environment (eg, technical and aseptic practice, electrical safety, physical facilities, occupational safety);
   - assessing, managing, and monitoring fiscal resources (eg, equipment, supplies, personnel, time); and
   - communicating and implementing organizational elements (eg, standards of nursing practice, such as care and professional performance, policies and procedures, staffing patterns, orientation, staff development activities, quality assessment plans).
2. Process measures based on the AORN "Standards of perioperative clinical practice" and

"Standards of perioperative professional practice" focus on activities of the nurse or process of nursing that require
   - implementation of the nursing process;
   - management of complications; and
   - adherence to policies and procedures (eg, correct site/side and identity verification, safe medication administration, specimen labeling, counting, positioning).
3. Outcome measures based on the AORN "Perioperative patient outcomes" relate to patient status following delivery of care that requires
   - emphasis on adverse events and complications; and
   - evaluation of measurable changes in patient health status (eg, free from injury, infection, nerve damage, altered skin integrity).
4. When selecting performance measures (ie, indicators), consideration should be given to the following issues:
   - departmental and organizational quality and safety goals;
   - accreditation standards and regulatory requirements;
   - perioperative clinical and service topics of national or local interest;
   - topics of greatest concern to patients and the community; and
   - trends of near misses for the purposes of improving processes.

Standard V

Establish performance expectations.

Interpretive statement 1:
The baselines for each of the measures are determined based on the measurement of the current process.

Criteria:
1. Baseline data should be gathered to establish the current level of performance.
2. Baseline data is used as a starting point for measurement.

Interpretive statement 2:
The baseline is evaluated and a determination is made whether there is an opportunity for improvement.

Criteria:
1. Evaluation of the baseline may be accomplished through analysis of collected data, peer review, literature review, etc.

2. A plan for improvement is thoughtfully designed. Tools such as flowcharts and process diagrams may be used to assist in identifying areas of the process with potential for failure.

Standard VI

Collect and organize data for evaluation.

Interpretive statement 1:
Data sources and methods of data collection/organization for each indicator are identified to establish a baseline of performance.

Criteria:
1. Existing sources of data are used. These may include, but are not limited to,
   ♦ surgery schedule log,
   ♦ staffing schedule,
   ♦ incident reports,
   ♦ perioperative documentation,
   ♦ occurrence screens,
   ♦ patient questionnaires,
   ♦ patient records,
   ♦ personnel credentialing/inservice records, and
   ♦ postoperative visit/call log.
2. Other sources for data collection are used. These may include, but are not limited to,
   ♦ direct observation of and inquiries regarding staff and patient care activities, and
   ♦ physical site inspections.
3. Individuals collecting data have appropriate skill levels for the task being monitored and have the information system—or access to an individual who does—for inputting data and formulating meaningful reports.
4. Methods of data collection are concurrent and retrospective. These methods may include, but are not limited to,
   ♦ chart review,
   ♦ departmental reporting forms,
   ♦ focused review,
   ♦ occurrence screening,
   ♦ peer review,
   ♦ interviews, and
   ♦ questionnaires/surveys.
5. Personnel are provided adequate time to participate in data collection and entry.
6. Personnel are encouraged to report incidents, adverse events, and hazardous conditions without fear of punitive action or retribution.

Interpretive statement 2:
The frequency of data collection and the sample size are sufficient to accumulate the necessary data.

Criteria:
1. The frequency of data collection is determined by the type of care or activity being monitored. This may include, but is not limited to,
   ♦ the number of patients affected,
   ♦ the degree of risk involved,
   ♦ the frequency of the event,
   ♦ the significance of the event or activity being monitored, and
   ♦ the extent to which the important aspect of care has been demonstrated to be problem free.
2. Data collection includes all sentinel events (eg, deaths, serious perioperative complications, near misses).
3. Data collection for performance measures is ongoing. A calendar of events is established to determine frequency of data collection for each indicator.
4. Sampling can be used to gather measurement data. Criteria such as volume, risk, and new procedure or provider can be used to determine an adequate sample size.[5]

Interpretive statement 3:
Data are organized, synthesized, and reported to allow for an accurate analysis of performance.

Criteria:
1. The quality of the data is evaluated to determine accuracy. This may be evaluated by answering questions such as the following.
   ♦ Have all cases that were to be included in the study population been identified and reviewed?
   ♦ Have all required data fields on the data collection instrument been completed?
   ♦ Did the data gatherer(s) follow their explicit data collection instructions?
   ♦ If the data were entered into a computerized database, did the edit/validation checks confirm the accuracy of the data?
   ♦ If the data were obtained through electronic data transfer, did the edit/validation checks confirm the accuracy of the data?
2. Data collected over a period of time for each measure are aggregated for analysis purposes.
3. Aggregated measurement data are used to identify trends or patterns of performance that

might not otherwise be evident in case-by-case review.

4. Statistical analysis techniques and comparative measurement data from outside sources are used to evaluate aggregated measurement data to identify significant undesirable variation from expected performance.

Standard VII

Evaluate care based on data collected.

Interpretive statement 1:
Analysis and evaluation of ongoing, collected data determines the need for action to improve the process(es).

Criteria:
1. Action is taken on adverse trends and patterns. The goal is for the care given to be congruent with perioperative nursing standards.
2. Analysis and evaluation of data collection is timely and provides efficacious opportunities for modifying actions/processes.

Interpretive statement 2:
Measurement data are compared with performance expectations.

Criteria:
1. Performance expectations are compared with actual performance to evaluate compliance with perioperative nursing standards of care and other important aspects of patient care and service.
2. Analysis of measurement data determines the need for more in-depth evaluation and/or initiation of an improvement project.
3. When performance consistently meets or exceeds expectations, the need for continued monitoring of that aspect of care/service is evaluated.
4. Evaluation of performance measurement data is timely.

Interpretive statement 3:
Initiate evaluation of important single events.

Criteria:
1. When an important single event occurs, a root cause analysis will be initiated in accordance with the organization's patient safety policies.
2. People knowledgeable about the systems and processes that affected the occurrence of the event are involved in the evaluation.

3. Evaluation of important single events are coordinated with other involved disciplines or departments.

Standard VIII

Take actions to improve care and services.

Interpretive statement 1:
Action plans/solutions are developed, supported, and approved at the appropriate levels and enacted to solve problems or improve care.

Criteria:
1. Identify the cause(s) of undesirable performance.
2. Corrective action plans are developed based on a thorough understanding of the process problems that are contributing to undesirable performance.
3. Actions are taken to correct defects in systems and/or processes. Actions may include revision of policies and procedures, staffing modifications, judicious use of equipment and supplies, and/or correction of communication or teamwork problems.
4. Relevant knowledge-based information is considered when developing action plans.
5. The plan of corrective action includes who or what is expected to change, individual(s) responsible for implementing the change, what action is needed to bring about the change, and when the change is expected to occur.
6. The action plan/solutions are forwarded to the body that has the authority to act, if the needed action exceeds the authority of the department. This may include, but is not limited to, the
   ♦ administration,
   ♦ board of trustees,
   ♦ chief of service,
   ♦ nursing/medical staff peer review committees,
   ♦ ethics committee, and
   ♦ OR committee.

Interpretive statement 2:
Actions for improvement are appropriate to the cause, scope, and severity of the problem.

Criteria:
1. Active reporting of errors and breaches in patient safety should be embraced without punitive action.
2. Whenever possible, corrective actions should be of a nonpunitive nature. They should be viewed

as an opportunity for education and process improvement of the individual(s) involved, the department, and even the institution.

3. Punitive measures can be counterproductive to the goals of QI/PI and should only be used when appropriate (eg, blatant failure to follow policy resulting in injury and/or liability).
4. Actions are taken to correct knowledge deficits. Actions related to insufficient knowledge may require staff development, referral to other resources, and/or recommendations for continuing education.
5. Actions are taken to correct defects in the system. Actions related to systems may require revision of policies and procedures, staffing modifications, judicious use of equipment and supplies, a change in process, and/or correction of communication problems.
6. Actions are taken to correct deficient behavioral performances. Actions related to behavior or performance may require, but are not limited to,
   ♦ education and training;
   ♦ mentoring;
   ♦ counseling;
   ♦ increased supervision;
   ♦ peer review; and
   ♦ transfer, suspension, termination, or other disciplinary action.

Standard IX

Assess the effectiveness of action(s) and document outcomes.

Interpretive statement 1:
Actions are evaluated based on outcomes.

Criteria:
1. Actions delegated to individuals or disciplines for problem solving are monitored.
2. Effectiveness of actions is assessed through continuous monitoring of care. If an opportunity to improve care is identified and improvement does not occur, the action needs to be reevaluated.
3. A time line is established for reevaluation.
4. Further investigation of the cause of the problem and evaluation to identify the less obvious elements that contributed to the failure of the action plan must take place.

Interpretive statement 2:
Document the action plan and the method of communication.

Criteria:
1. A system is established to document the problem-solving process and the effectiveness in improving care or resolving the problem.
2. A system is established to document the results of the action plan, including trends and patterns that affect action.

Standard X

Communicate relevant information to the appropriate individuals, organization-wide, while maintaining confidentiality.

Interpretive statement 1:
The written organization-wide QI/PI plan identifies appropriate channels of communication.

Criteria:
1. Intradepartmental communication channels include, but are not limited to,
   ♦ minutes of departmental meetings,
   ♦ staff meetings, and
   ♦ summary reports.
2. Conclusions, recommendations, actions, and findings are communicated to
   ♦ departmental staff,
   ♦ appropriate medical staff committees,
   ♦ administration,
   ♦ interdisciplinary committees,
   ♦ organization-wide QI/PI committee,
   ♦ governing body, and
   ♦ accreditation and/or regulatory agencies as appropriate.
3. Confidentiality of QI/PI data is maintained. Maintenance of QI/PI data and all related communications shall comply with
   ♦ federal Health Insurance Portability and Accountability Act (HIPAA) privacy and confidentiality regulations,
   ♦ pertinent state regulations governing privacy and confidentiality of peer review and quality/performance data, and
   ♦ organizational privacy and confidentiality policies and procedures.

Interpretive statement 2:
Personnel are informed of the conclusions, recommendations, actions, and findings.

Criteria:
1. Regularly scheduled staff and/or departmental meetings include quality improvement/performance improvement reports and activities.

2. Identified opportunities to improve care are addressed through staff development offerings, deploying changes in process and practice to staff.

Interpretive statement 3:

Results of the organization-wide quality improvement/performance improvement monitoring activities provide the opportunity to improve care and may have applicability in other areas in the organization.

Criteria:

1. Medical staff, administration, and the governing body use outcomes to determine clinical privileges and credentialing decisions.
2. Departmental managers use outcomes to objectively monitor staff performance, develop short- and long-range plans, measure performance, and contain costs.
3. Clinical practitioners use the outcomes of the QI/PI activities for self-assessment and peer review activities.

Models and Improvement Processes

The models and processes for performing QI/PI are numerous. More than one model can be used in an effective QI/PI program. No matter which method or model is used, the goal is to "Do the right thing, and do the right thing well."[3] AORN and the NPC are not endorsing any one model or any accrediting body. **Note:** More information is available in the *Notes* and *Resources* listed, or by using the Internet and searching under the terms *quality improvement* and *performance improvement*.

Glossary

Assessment: For purposes of performance improvement, the systematic collection and review of patient-specific data.

"For purposes of patient assessment, the process established by an organization for obtaining appropriate and necessary information about each individual seeking entry into a health care setting or service. The information is used to match an individual's need with the appropriate setting, care level, and intervention."[6]

Baseline: "A set of critical observations or data used for comparison or a control."[7]

Clinical practice guidelines: Systematically developed statements to assist practitioner and patient decisions about appropriate health care for specific clinical circumstances.

Concurrent: An activity that takes place in real time; care in progress.

Failure Mode and Effects Analysis (FMEA): A proactive approach to prevent or lessen the chances of a sentinel event from occurring, or reducing the risk/liability when an event occurs. This differs from root cause analysis, which is done after a sentinel event occurs and is a retrospective review of a process or processes. As with other QI/PI models, FMEA is an analysis technique drawn from non-medical industry. FMEA is an exercise that allows identification of the probabilities for "failure" at any point in the implementation of a process. In utilizing this technique, three questions must be answered:

♦ What are the steps of the process?
♦ Where is the process most likely to fail?
♦ How can we minimize the effects of these failures?

FMEA incorporates many of the same tools that are used in other QI/PI models. In determining the possible effects of potential failures, it is possible to quantify the likelihood, severity, and probability of detecting and preventing each failure. This allows providers to determine how critical each failure will be and give it a priority ranking. It allows one to avoid errors or failures before putting new processes in place.

JCAHO, in its leadership standards, addresses the requirements for the use of FMEA and root cause analysis by organizations seeking accreditation. These requirements are specific to the level of care provided by the organization.

Focused review: A formal review of one particular indicator, procedure, or practitioner over a specified time frame. It can be retrospective or concurrent.

Goal: The result that a department, service, or organization aims to accomplish. Also, a statement of attainment/achievement that is proposed to be accomplished or attained.[8]

Hazard analysis: The process of collecting and evaluating information on the circumstances leading to a higher risk for adverse outcomes. These circumstances or conditions are not related to the disease process or the condition for which the patient is being treated.

High risk: Patients at risk if the aspect of care is not provided correctly and in a timely manner. It may be that the patients themselves are at risk due to physical status, or it may be that the complexity and/or risk of complications related to the procedure puts the patients at risk.

High volume: The procedures or treatments that occur frequently, on a regular basis, or affect a large patient population.

Important aspects of care: Clinical or service-related activities that involve a high volume of patients, entail a high degree of risk for patients, or tend to produce problems for staff or patients. Such activities are deemed most important for purposes of monitoring and evaluation.[8]

Indicator: Well-defined, measurable, objective statement related to the structure, process, or outcomes of care; direct attention to problems or opportunities to improve care.[8]

Methodology: The strategies, models, or steps for gathering and analyzing the data in the quality improvement/performance improvement process.

Near miss: "Any process variation that did not affect the outcome, but for which a recurrence carries a significant chance of a serious adverse outcome. Such a near miss falls within the scope of the definition of a sentinel event, but outside the scope of those sentinel events that are subject to review by the Joint Commission under its Sentinel Event Policy."[6]

Nursing process: A systematic approach to nursing practice utilizing problem-solving techniques, including the components of assessment, planning, implementation, and evaluation.

Occurrence screens: Data that are used to identify individual variations in care, which are reviewed and confirmed by peer review and entered into a database to identify trends and/or patterns.[8]

Outcome identification: The intended, or realistically expected, correction of the patient's problem by a certain point in time.

Peer review: The examination and evaluation by associates of a practitioner's clinical practice. Individuals are evaluated by recognized, established standards. Physicians review physicians, registered nurses review registered nurse, etc.

Performance expectation: The desired condition or target level for each performance measure.

Performance measure: A quantitative tool (eg, rate, ratio, index, percentage) that provides an indication of an organization's performance in relation to a specified process or outcome. (See also *process measure* and *outcome measure*.)[6]

Population: The entire set of individuals sharing some common characteristics (eg, all patients with a particular disease, undergoing the same procedure, or of the same demographics).

Problem-prone: Those processes or steps that commonly generate incidents or barriers for patients and/or staff.

Process: A goal-directed, interrelated series of actions, events, mechanisms, or steps. An interrelated series of events, activities, actions, mechanisms, or steps that transform inputs into outputs.[6]

Retrospective: A review that begins with a current manifestation and links this effect to some occurrence in the past; post-discharge or post-procedure; not concurrent.

Root cause analysis: "A process for identifying the basic or causal factors that underlie variation in performance, including the occurrence or possible occurrence of a sentinel event. A root cause analysis focuses primarily on systems and processes, not individual performance. It progresses from special causes in clinical processes to common causes in organizational processes and identifies potential improvements in processes or systems that would tend to decrease the likelihood of such events in the future, or determines, after analysis that no such improvement opportunities exist."[9]

Sentinel event: "An unexpected occurrence involving death or serious physical or psychological injury, or the risk thereof. Serious injury specifically includes loss of limb or function. The phrase 'or the risk thereof' includes any process variation for which a recurrence would carry a significant chance of a serious adverse outcome. Such events are called 'sentinel' because they signal the need for immediate investigation and response."[9]

Standard: "A statement that defines the performance expectations, structures, or processes that must be substantially in place in an organization to enhance the quality of care."[6]

Structure: Organizational characteristics, fiscal resources, and management qualifications of health professionals; physical facilities and equipment; environment where care takes place.[10]

REFERENCES

1. T Bornstein, "Quality improvement and performance improvement. Different means to the same end?" *QA Brief* 9 (Spring 2001) http://www.qaproject.org/pdf/engv9n1.pdf (accessed 5 March 2003).

2. Institute of Medicine, *To Err is Human: Building a Safer Health System* (Washington, DC: National Academy Press, 2000) 114.

3. Joint Commission on Accreditation of Healthcare Organizations, "Improving organization performance," in *Hospital Accreditation Standards* (Oakbrook Terrace, Ill: Joint Commission on Accreditation of Healthcare Organizations, 2002) 161, 163.

4. Joint Commission on Accreditation of Healthcare Organizations, "Management of human resources," in *Hospital Accreditation Standards* (Oakbrook Terrace, Ill: Joint Commission on Accreditation of Healthcare Organizations, 2002) 234.

5. Joint Commission on Accreditation of Healthcare Organizations, "Management of information," in *Hospital Accreditation Standards* (Oakbrook Terrace, Ill: Joint Commission on Accreditation of Healthcare Organizations, 2002) 254.

6. Joint Commission on Accreditation of Healthcare Organizations, "Glossary," in *Hospital Accreditation Standards* (Oakbrook Terrace, Ill: Joint Commission on Accreditation of Healthcare Organizations, 2002) 331, 346, 351, 354, 360.

7. *Merriam-Webster's Collegiate Dictionary,* 10th ed (Springfield, Mass: Merriam-Webster, Inc., 1993) 95.

8. L A Kepler, E A Stuart, J Kiefel, "Ten-step template," *QRC Advisor* 6 (April 1990) 1-3.

9. Joint Commission on Accreditation of Healthcare Organizations, "Sentinel events," in *Hospital Accreditation Standards* (Oakbrook Terrace, Ill: Joint Commission on Accreditation of Healthcare Organizations, 2002) 51, 52.

10. Joint Commission on Accreditation of Healthcare Organizations, "Official accreditation policies and procedures," in *Hospital Accreditation Standards* (Oakbrook Terrace, Ill: Joint Commission on Accreditation of Healthcare Organizations, 2002) 48-49.

RESOURCES

AORN, Inc. *Standards, Recommended Practices, and Guidelines.* Denver: AORN, Inc. Annual edition.

Joint Commission Resources. *Failure Mode and Effects Analysis in Health Care: Proactive Risk Reduction.* Oakbrook Terrace, Ill: Joint Commission on Accreditation of Healthcare Organizations, 2002.

Joint Commission Resources. *A Guide to Performance Measurement for Hospitals.* Oakbrook Terrace, Ill: Joint Commission on Accreditation of Healthcare Organization, 2000.

Joint Commission Resources. *A Pocket Guide to Using Performance Improvement Tools.* Oakbrook Terrace, Ill: Joint Commission on Accreditation of Healthcare Organization, 1996.

Joint Commission Resources. *Tools for Performance Measurement in Health Care: A Quick Reference Guide.* Oakbrook Terrace, Ill: Joint Commission on Accreditation of Healthcare Organization, 2002.

Organizational Dynamics. *Quality Action Teams: Team Members' Workbook.* Burlington, Mass: Organizational Dynamics, 1987.

Schroeder, P, ed. *Journal of Nursing Care Quality* Published quarterly by Lippincott Williams & Wilkins, Philadelphia.

Shewhart, W A; Deming, W E. *Statistical Method from the Viewpoint of Quality Control.* New York: Dover Publications, 1986.

Spath, P L. *Fundamentals of Health Care Quality Management.* Forest Grove, Ore: Brown-Spath & Associates, 2000.

PUBLICATION HISTORY

Originally published as "Quality improvement standards for perioperative nursing" in the 1992 *Standards and Recommended Practices for Perioperative Nursing.*

Revised; approved by the AORN Board of Directors in June 2003.

This document was previously published as part of the "Standards of perioperative nursing" as Exhibit D in the 2009 edition of *Perioperative Standards and Recommended Practices.*

H

N

AORN Perioperative Standards and
Recommended Practices, 2012 Edition